Women's Sexual Function and Dysfunction

Study, Diagnosis and Treatment

Women's Sexual Function and Dysfunction

Study, Diagnosis and Treatment

Edited by

Irwin Goldstein MD
Editor-in-Chief, *The Journal of Sexual Medicine*
Milton, MA, USA

Cindy M Meston PhD
Department of Psychology
University of Texas at Austin
Austin, TX, USA

Susan R Davis MBBS, FRACP, PhD
Women's Health Program
Department of Medicine
Central and Eastern Clinical School
Monash Medical School, Alfred Hospital
Prahran VIC
Australia

Abdulmaged M Traish PhD
Laboratory for Sexual Medicine Research
Boston University School of Medicine
Boston, MA, USA

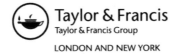

Taylor & Francis
Taylor & Francis Group

LONDON AND NEW YORK

© 2006 Taylor & Francis, an imprint of the Taylor & Francis Group

First published in the United Kingdom in 2006 by Taylor & Francis, an
imprint of the Taylor & Francis Group, 2 Park Square, Milton Park,
Abingdon, Oxon OX14 4RN

Tel.: +44 (0)20 7017 6000
Fax.: +44 (0)20 7017 6699
E-mail: info.medicine@tandf.co.uk
Website: http://www.tandf.co.uk/medicine

Although every effort has been made to ensure that all owners of copyright
material have been acknowledged in this publication, we would be glad to
acknowledge in subsequent reprints or editions any omissions brought to
our attention.

A CIP record for this book is available from the British Library

Library of Congress Cataloging-in-Publication Data

Data available on application

ISBN 1 84214 263 1
ISBN 978 1 84214 263 9

Distributed in North and South America by

Taylor & Francis
2000 NW Corporate Blvd
Boca Raton, FL 33431, USA

Within Continental USA
Tel: 800 272 7737; Fax: 800 374 3401
Outside Continental USA
Tel: 561 994 0555; Fax: 561 361 6018
E-mail: orders@crcpress.com

Distributed in the rest of the world by
Thomson Publishing Services
Cheriton House
North Way
Andover, Hampshire SP10 5BE, UK
Tel.: +44 (0)1264 332424
E-mail: salesorder.tandf@thomsonpublishingservices.co.uk

Composition by Phoenix Photosetting, Chatham, Kent

Printed and bound in Spain by Grafos SA, Arte Sobre Papal

Dedication

Women's Sexual Function and Dysfunction: Study, Diagnosis, and Treatment is dedicated to all women who, in pain or dissatisfaction, were, and continue to be, unable to have or endure sexual relations. It is dedicated to those patients who have been victims of the taboos, fears, uncertainties, and forbidden context of women's sexual dysfunction, and have been either dismissed or informed that this was "all in their heads", that "nothing could be done", that "they already had their children", or that they should "become a good actress". This book is dedicated to those women, yet to present for evaluation, who may now seek and find successful, evidence-based treatment in a new era of integrated biologic and psychologic management. It is for all of them that this multidisciplinary book was written.

We also dedicate this book to those basic science researchers and health-care professionals, past, present, and future, many of whom are strong advocates of the International Society for the Study of Women's Sexual Health (ISSWSH). Despite limited funding and often prejudiced colleagues, you continue to focus on women's sexual health issues and advance our scientific understanding of function and dysfunction.

It is for all of you that this multidisciplinary book has been written.

Finally, we dedicate this book to our colleagues who submitted chapters, to our associate editors, who diligently edited the chapters, and to our spouses, children, parents, families, and significant others who endured the many long hours required to realize this final magnificent, amazing, and awesome contribution to the field of women's sexual health – *thank you!*

Contents

Contributors

Craig J Alexander PhD
Department of Physical Medicine and Rehabilitation
University of Alabama School of Medicine
Birmingham, Alabama
USA

Stanley E Althof PhD
Professor of Psychology
Case Medical School
Executive Director, Center for Marital and Sexual Health of
South Florida
West Palm Beach, Florida
USA

Alan M Altman MD
Assistant Clinical Professor of Obstetrics, Gynecology and
Reproductive Biology
Harvard Medical School
Boston, Massachusetts
USA

Alison Amsterdam MD
Fellow, Gynecology Service
Department of Surgery
Memorial Sloan-Kettering Cancer Center
New York, New York
USA

Lillian Arleque EdD
Educational Consultant
Executive Leadership Coach to Educational Consultant
Andover, Massachusetts
USA

Gloria Bachmann MD
Professor of Obstetrics and Gynecology and Medicine
Robert Wood Johnson Medical School
University of Medicine and Dentistry of New Jersey
New Brunswick, New Jersey
USA

John Bancroft MD
Senior Research Fellow
The Kinsey Institute for Research in Sex, Gender and
Reproduction
Indiana University
Bloomington, Indiana
USA

Linda Banner PhD
Health Psychologist and Certified Sex Therapist
Research Consultant
Stanford Medical School
San Jose, California
USA

David H Barlow PhD, ABPP
Professor of Psychology and Psychiatry
Director, Center for Anxiety and Related Disorders
Boston University
Boston, Massachusetts
USA

Jennifer L Barsky MS
Graduate Trainee in Clinical Psychiatry
Department of Psychology
Rutgers, The State University of New Jersey
New Brunswick, New Jersey
USA

Edgardo F Becher MD, PhD
Professor of Urology
University of Buenos Aires School of Medicine
Buenos Aires
Argentina

Sophie Bergeron PhD
Associate Professor of Sexology
Department of Sexology
University of Québec at Montreal
Montréal, Québec
Canada

Yitzchak M Binik PhD
Professor of Psychology
Director, Sex and Couple Therapy Service
McGill University Health Center (Victoria Hospital)
Montréal, Québec
Canada

Andrea Bradford MS
Department of Psychology
University of Texas at Austin
Austin, Texas
USA

Ulrike Brandenburg MD
Division of Gynaecology, Breast-Centre
Department for Psychooncology/Sexual Science
University Hospital Aachen
Aachen
Germany

Alberto Briganti MD
Department of Urology
Università Vita - Salute
San Raffaele Hospital
Milan
Italy

Lori A Brotto PhD
Assistant Professor in Obstetrics and Gynecology
University of British Columbia
Vancouver, British Columbia
Canada

Candace S Brown PharmD
Professor, Departments of Pharmacy, Obstetrics and
Gynecology, and Psychiatry
University of Tennessee Health Science Center
Memphis, Tennessee
USA

Jeanne Carter PhD
Assistant Attending Psychologist
Department of Psychiatry/Gynecology Service
Memorial Sloan-Kettering Cancer Center
New York, New York
USA

Salvatore Caruso MD
Professor of Gynecology
Research Group for Sexology
Department of Microbiological and Gynecological Science
University of Catania
Catania
Italy

Paula M Castaño MD, MPH
Assistant Clinical Professor of Obstetrics and Gynecology
Columbia Presbyterian Medical Center
Department of Obstetrics and Gynecology
New York, New York
USA

Anita H Clayton MD
Professor of Psychiatric Medicine
University of Virginia
Charlottesville, Virginia
USA

Giulia d'Amati MD, PhD
Associate Professor of Pathology
Department of Experimental Medicine and Pathology
"La Sapienza" University
Rome
Italy

Anne R Davis MD, MPH
Assistant Professor of Obstetrics and Gynecology
Columbia Presbyterian Medical Center
Department of Obstetrics and Gynecology
New York, New York
USA

Susan R Davis MBBS, FRACP, PhD
Professor of Women's Health
Department of Medicine (CECS)
Monash University
Alfred Hospital
Prahran, Victoria
Australia

Elise JB De MD
Assistant Professor of Urology
Division of Urology
Albany Medical Center
Albany, New York
USA

Dina M Deldon-Saltin DO
Instructor in Obstetrics and Gynecology
University of Massachusetts Medical School
Worcester, Massachusetts
USA

Lorraine Dennerstein MBBS, PhD, DPM, FRANZCP
Professor, Office for Gender and Health
Psychiatry Department
University of Melbourne
Melbourne, Victoria
Australia

Stanley H Ducharme PhD
Professor of Rehabilitation Medicine
Assistant Professor of Urology
Boston University School of Medicine
Boston, Massachusetts
USA

Amy Easton PhD
Laboratory of Neurobiology and Behavior
The Rockefeller University
New York, New York
USA

Francesca Ferdeghini MD
Resident in Obstetrics and Gynecology
Research Center for Reproductive Medicine
Department of Obstetrics and Gynecology
IRCCS Policlinico San Matteo
University of Pavia
Italy

David M Ferguson PhD, MD, FACCP
Consultant
Clinical Research Services Consulting
Grand Marais, Minnesota
USA

William A Fisher PhD
Professor, Department of Psychology
Professor, Department of Obstetrics and Gynaecology
University of Western Ontario
London, Ontario
Canada

Jean L Fourcroy MD, PhD, MPH
Assistant Professor of Surgery
Uniformed Services University of Health Sciences
Walter Reed Army Hospital, Urology
Bethesda, Maryland
USA

Richard C Friedman MD
Clinical Professor of Psychiatry
Weill Medical Center, Cornell University
Payne Whitney Clinic
New York, New York
USA

Axel R Fugl-Meyer MD, PhD
Professor of Neuroscience, Rehabilitation Medicine
Department of Neuroscience
Uppsala University
Uppsala
Sweden

Kerstin S Fugl-Meyer PhD
Associate Professor
Andrology Center
Karolinska University Hospital
Stockholm
Sweden

Amy L Gamez MS, APRN, BC
Clinical Research Director
South Florida Medical Research
Co-Director, The Miami Center for Sexual Health
Miami, Florida
USA

Uri Gedalia MD
Neuro-Urology Unit
Rambam Health Care Campus and
The Rappaport Faculty of Medicine
Technion Israel Institute of Technology
Haifa
Israel

Michaela Georgescu MA
Doctoral Candidate in Clinical Psychology
Center for Studies in Behavioral Neurobiology
Department of Psychology
Concordia University
Montréal, Québec
Canada

Annamaria Giraldi MD, PhD
Specialist Registrar and Lecturer in Sexology
Division of Sexological Research, Sexological Clinic
Rigshospitalet
University of Copenhagen
Copenhagen
Denmark

François Giuliano MD, PhD
Urologist, Associate Professor of Therapeutics
Neuro-Urology Unit
Department of Neurological Rehabilitation
Raymond Poincare Hospital, Garches
Pelvipharm Laboratories
Gif-sur-Yvette
France

Dale B Glasser PhD
Medical Director, Urology
Pfizer Inc.
New York, New York
USA

Andrew T Goldstein MD
Instructor, Division of Gynecologic Specialties
Department of Gynecology and Obstetrics
The Johns Hopkins Medical Institutes
Center for Vulvovaginal Disorders
Washington, DC
USA

Irwin Goldstein MD
Editor-in-Chief
The Journal of Sexual Medicine
Milton, Massachusetts
USA

Sue W Goldstein AB
Editorial Assistant
The Journal of Sexual Medicine
Milton, Massachusetts
USA

Cynthia A Graham PhD, M App Sci, BA
Research Tutor; Associate Research Fellow
Oxford Doctoral Course in Clinical Psychology
Oxford, UK
The Kinsey Institute for Research in Sex, Gender and
Reproduction
Indiana University
Bloomington, Indiana
USA

Alessandra Graziottin MD
Director, Center of Gynecology and Medical Sexology
Hospital San Raffaele
Resnati, Milan
Italy

Ilan Gruenwald MD
Neuro-Urology Unit
Rambam Health Care Campus and
The Rappaport Faculty of Medicine
Technion Israel Institute of Technology
Haifa
Israel

André T Guay MD, FACP, FACE
Clinical Assistant Professor of Medicine (Endocrinology)
Harvard Medical School
Boston, Massachusetts
Director, Center for Sexual Function
Lahey Clinic Northshore
Peabody, Massachusetts
USA

Elaine Hatfield PhD
Professor of Psychology
Department of Psychology
University of Hawaii
Honolulu, Hawaii
USA

Richard D Hayes BSc(Hons)
Office for Gender and Health, Department of Psychiatry
School of Population Health, Department of Public Health
University of Melbourne
Melbourne, Victoria
Australia

Kimberly D Hearn PhD
Assistant Professor
Health Education Department
Borough of Manhattan Community College
New York, New York
USA

Julia R Heiman PhD
Professor of Psychology and Clinical Psychiatry
Director, The Kinsey Institute for Research in Sex, Gender
and Reproduction
Indiana University
Bloomington, Indiana
USA

Paula L Hensley MD
Associate Professor of Psychiatry
Department of Psychiatry
University of New Mexico
Albuquerque, New Mexico
USA

Hollis Herman MS, PT, OCS, BCIA-PMDB
Physical Therapist
Private Practice
Healthy Women
Cambridge, Massachusetts
USA

Richard F Hoyt PhD Jnr
Associate Professor of Anatomy and Neurobiology
Department of Anatomy and Neurobiology
Boston University School of Medicine
Boston, Massachusetts
USA

Emmanuele A Jannini MD
Associate Professor of Endocrinology and Medical Sexology
Department of Experimental Medicine
University of L'Aquila
L'Aquila
Italy

Erick Janssen PhD
Associate Scientist
The Kinsey Institute for Research in Sex, Gender and
Reproduction
Indiana University
Bloomington, Indiana
USA

Julie A Johnson PsyD
Sex Therapist
Department of Urology
Boston University
Boston, Massachusetts
USA

Véronique Julia-Guilloteau PhD
Research Scientist
Pelvipharm Laboratories
Gif-sur-Yvette
France

Dongwoo Kang MD
Director, Korean Institute for Sexual and Couple's Health
(KISCH)
Shinsa-dong, Kangnam-gu
Seoul
Korea

Jeong-han Kang MA
Department of Sociology
University of Chicago
Chicago, Illinois
USA

Susan Kellogg-Spadt PhD, CRNP
Assistant Professor of Obstetrics and Gynecology
Robert Wood Johnson Medical School
University of Medicine and Dentistry of New Jersey
Piscataway, New Jersey
Pelvic and Sexual Health Institute
Drexel University
Philadelphia, Pennsylvania
USA

Samir Khalifé MD, FRCS(C), FACOG
Jewish General Hospital
Montréal, Québec
Canada

Noel N Kim PhD
Research Assistant Professor of Urology
Department of Urology
Boston University School of Medicine
Boston, Massachusetts
USA

Michael L Krychman MD
Co-Director of Sexual Medicine
Assistant Clinical Attending, Gynecology Service
Department of Surgery
Memorial Sloan-Kettering Cancer Center
New York, New York
USA

Marie-Andrée Lahaie BA
Doctoral Candidate in Clinical Psychology
Department of Psychology
McGill University
Montréal, Québec
Canada

Edward O Laumann PhD
George Herbert Mead Distinguished Service Professor of
Sociology
Department of Sociology
University of Chicago
Chicago, Illinois
USA

Anna W Lee PhD
Laboratory of Neurobiology and Behavior
The Rockefeller University
New York, New York
USA

Sandra R Leiblum PhD
Professor of Psychiatry
Director of the Center for Sexual and Relationship Health
Department of Psychiatry
Robert Wood Johnson Medical School
University of Medicine and Dentistry of New Jersey
Piscataway, New Jersey
USA

Andrea Lenzi MD
Professor of Endocrinology
Department of Medival Physiopathology
Unit of Andrology, Reproductive Physiopathology and
Endocrine Diagnosis
"La Sapienza" University
Rome
Italy

Roy J Levin MSc, PhD
Reader in Physiology (Retired)
Department of Biomedical Science
University of Sheffield
Honorary Research Associate
Sexual Physiology Laboratory
Porterbrook Clinic
Sheffield
UK

Harold I Lief MD
Emeritus Professor of Psychiatry
University of Pennsylvania
Philadelphia, Pennsylvania
USA

P O Lundberg MD, PhD
Professor of Neurology
Department of Neuroscience and Neurology
University Hospital
Uppsala
Sweden

Peter J Lynch MD
Frederick G Novy, Jr Professor of Dermatology
University of California, Davis and University of California,
Davis Health System
Sacramento, California
USA

Scott R Maitland BA, ARDMS
Sonographer
Center for Sexual Medicine
Boston Medical Center
Boston, Massachusetts
USA

Kenneth R Maravilla MD
Professor, Departments of Radiology and Neurological Surgery
University of Washington School of Medicine
Director, MR Research Laboratory
Director, Neuroscience Core for the Center on Human
Development and Disability
Seattle, Washington
USA

Lynette J Margesson MD, FRCPC
Adjunct Assitant Professor of Medicine (Dermatology) and
Obstetrics and Gynecology
Dartmouth Medical School
Hanover, New Hampshire
USA

Cindy M Meston PhD
Associate Professor of Psychology
University of Texas at Austin
Austin, Texas
USA

Jessica A Mong PhD
Assistant Professor
Department of Pharmacology and Experimental Therapeutics
University of Maryland
Baltimore School of Medicine
Baltimore, Maryland
USA

Francesco Montorsi MD
Associate Professor of Urology
Department Of Urology
Universita' Vita Salute San Raffaele
Milan
Italy

David R Moore PhD
Assistant Professor of Psychology
Department of Psychology
University of Puget Sound
Tacoma, Washington
USA

Ricardo Munarriz MD
Assistant Professor of Urology
Center for Sexual Medicine
Department of Urology
Boston University School of Medicine
Boston, Massachusetts
USA

Sandra Garcia Nader MD
Fellow, Department of Urology
Unidad de Urología y Sexología del Country
Sanitas International
Bogotá
Colombia

Rossella E Nappi MD, PhD
Assistant Professor of Obstetrics and Gynecology
Research Center for Reproductive Medicine
Department of Obstetrics and Gynecology
IRCCS Policlinico San Matteo
University of Pavia
Pavia
Italy

Margaret Nichols PhD
Executive Director
Institute for Personal Growth, P. C.
Highland Park, New Jersey
USA

H George Nurnberg MD
University of New Mexico Health Sciences Center School of
Medicine
Department of Psychiatry
University of New Mexico
Albuquerque, New Mexico
USA

Helen E O'Connell MD, MMed, MBBS, FRACS (Urol)
Chief, Neurourology and Continence Unit
Department of Urology
Royal Melbourne Hospital
Department of Surgery
University of Melbourne
Melbourne
Australia

Lucia F O'Sullivan PhD
Assistant Professor
Department of Family and Social Medicine
Albert Einstein College of Medicine
New York, New York
USA

Anthony Paik PhD
Assistant Professor
Department of Sociology
University of Iowa
Iowa City, Iowa
USA

Sharon J Parish MD
Assistant Professor of Medicine
Albert Einstein College of Medicine
Departmemt of Internal Medicine
Montefiore Medical Center
Bronx, New York
USA

Kwangsung Park MD, PhD
Professor and Chairman
Department of Urology
Chonnam National University Medical School
Gwangiu
Republic of Korea

Manjari Patel MD
Physician
Robert Wood Johnson Medical School
University of Medicine and Dentistry (UMDNJ)
New Brunswick, New Jersey
USA

Kimberley A Payne BA
Doctoral Candidate
Department of Psychology
McGill University
Montréal, Québec
Canada

Michael A Perelman PhD
Clinical Associate Professor of Psychiatry, Reproductive Medicine and Urology
Co-Director, Human Sexuality Program
The New York Presbyterian Hospital
Weill Medical College of Cornell University
New York, New York
USA

Donald W Pfaff PhD
Professor and Head of Laboratory
Neurobiology and Behavior
The Rockefeller University
New York, New York
USA

James G Pfaus PhD
Professor
Center for Studies in Behavioral Neurobiology
Department of Psychology
Concordia University
Montréal, Québec
Canada

Franco Polatti MD
Professor of Obstetrics and Gynecology
Research Center for Reproductive Medicine
Department of Obstetrics and Gynecology
IRCCS Policlinico San Matteo
University of Pavia
Pavia
Italy

Nicole Prause BA
Clinical Science Graduate
Department of Psychology
Indiana University
The Kinsey Institute for Research in Sex, Gender and Reproduction
Bloomington, Indiana
USA

Caroline F Pukall PhD
Assistant Professor of Psychology
Department of Psychology
Queen's University
Kingston, Ontario
Canada

Richard L Rapson PhD
Professor of History
Department of History
University of Hawaii
Honolulu, Hawaii
USA

Alessandra H Rellini MA
University of Texas at Austin
Austin, Texas
USA

Patrizio Rigatti MD
Professor and Chairman
Department of Urology
Universita' Vita Salute San Raffaele
Milan
Italy

Linda J Rosen PhD
Consultant
Belle Mead, New Jersey
USA

Raymond C Rosen PhD
Professor of Psychiatry and Medicine
Department of Psychiatry
Robert Wood Johnson Medical School
University of Medicine and Dentistry of New Jersey
Piscataway, New Jersey
USA

Andrea Salonia MD
Department of Urology
Scientific Institute
Hospital San Raffaele
University Via-Salute San Raffaele
Milan
Italy

Michael Sand RN, MPH
Deputy Director, Scientific Affairs
Bayer HealthCare
Wuppertal
Germany

Kalavampara V Sanjeevan MBBS, MS, MCh (Urol)
Fellow and Senior Specialist in Urology
Amrita Institute of Medical Sciences
Kochi, Kerala
India

Lisa A Scepkowski MA
Doctoral Candidate in Clinical Psychology
Center for Anxiety and Related Disorders
Boston University
Boston, Massachusetts
USA

Anneliese Schwenkhagen MD
Gynaekologicum Hamburg
Cooperating Partner of the Department of Obstetrics and
Gynecology
Unviversity of Lübeck
Hamburg
Germany

Robert Taylor Segraves MD, PhD
Professor of Psychiatry
Case School of Medicine
Cleveland, Ohio
USA

Marca L Sipski MD
Department of Physical Medicine and Rehabilitation
University of Alabama School of Medicine
Birmingham, Alabama
USA

Richard Spark MD, FACE
Director, Steroid Research Laboratory
Beth Isreal Deaconess Medical Center
Boston, Massachusetts
Clinical Associate Professor of Medicine (Endocrinology)
Harvard Medical School
Boston, Massachusetts
USA

Frank Z Stanczyk PhD
Professor of Research
Obstetrics and Gynecology and Preventive Medicine
University of Southern California Keck School of Medicine
Los Angeles, California
USA

Elizabeth Gunther Stewart MD, FACOG
Assistant Professor of Obstetrics and Gynecology
Harvard Medical School
Boston, Massachusetts
USA

Bronwyn G A Stuckey MBBS, FRACP
Clinical Associate Professor
Keogh Institute for Medical Research
Department of Endocrinology and Diabetes
Sir Charles Gairdner Hospital
School of Medicine and Pharmacology
University of Western Australia
Australia

Abdulmaged M Traish PhD
Professor of Biochemistry and Urology
Departments of Biochemistry and Urology
Boston University School of Medicine
Boston, Massachusetts
USA

Trudy Van Houten PhD
Lecturer in Anatomy, Program in Medical Education
Harvard Medical School
Clinical Instructor in Radiology
Radiology Department, Brigham and Women's Hospital
Boston, Masachusetts
USA

Kalli Varaklis MD FACOG
Assistant Clinical Professor of Obstetrics and Gynecology
Maine Medical Center
Portland, Maine
USA

Yoram Vardi MD
Professor of Urology
Neuro-Urology Unit
Rambam Health Care Campus and
The Rappaport Faculty of Medicine
Technion Israel Institute of Technology
Haifa
Israel

Ezio Vincenti MD, PhD
Professor of Anesthesiology and Intensive Care
Division of Anesthesiology and Intensive Care
Dolo, Venice
Padua University
Italy

Kirsten von Sydow PhD
Clinical Psychologist and Psychotherapist
University of Hamburg
Psychological Institute
Hamburg
Germany

Kristene E Whitmore MD
Professor of Urology and Obstetrics and Gynecology
Director, Pelvic and Sexual Health Institute
Drexel University
Philadelphia, Pennsylvania
USA

Markus Wiegel MA
Doctoral Candidate in Clinical Psychology
Center for Anxiety and Related Disorders
Boston University
Boston, Massachusetts
Abel Screening Inc.
Atlanta, Georgia
USA

Claire C Yang MD
Associate Professor of Urology
University of Washington
Seattle, Washington
USA

Ugur Yilmaz MD
Department of Urology
University of Washington
Seattle, Washington
USA

Aline P Zoldbrod PhD
Licensed Psychologist and Certified Sex Therapist
Private Practice
Lexington, Massachusetts
Consulting Sex Therapist
Center for Sexual Function
Lahey Clinic Northshore
Peabody, Massachusetts
USA

Preface

Women's Sexual Function and Dysfunction: Study, Diagnosis, and Treatment is the first comprehensive, multidisciplinary textbook to integrate both psychologic and biologic aspects of women's sexual health. The goal of this textbook is to disseminate, for the first time, state-of-the-art, scientific, evidence-based information on the study, diagnosis, and treatment of women's sexual health concerns. It is the long-range intention that this textbook be revised regularly to continue to make available to the reader the inevitable advances in the field.

The target audience for this textbook is broad, including: (1) all health-care professionals who treat women for general health issues and specifically for sexual health concerns; (2) all health-care professionals who treat men for sexual health issues and who may wish to expand their horizons and engage in treatment of the couple; (3) all basic science investigators who research the epidemiology, physiology, and pathophysiology of women's sexual function and dysfunction; (4) women's health educators, specifically women's sexual health educators and those interested in the history of women's sexual health research and the International Society for the Study of Women's Sexual Health (ISSWSH); and (5) affected women and their families and friends, although this textbook is not tailored for the lay audience.

All women have the right to optimize their health, including sexual health. Health-care providers for woman's health issues need access to evidence-based knowledge concerning women's sexual health issues. To this end, the ISSWSH was established (see Chapter 1.2) by researchers and practitioners in various disciplines in a common cause. As the first multidisciplinary organization devoted solely to women's sexual function and dysfunction from a biopsychosocial model, the ISSWSH provides the opportunity for researchers and clinicians from around the world to bring their various perspectives and share experience and knowledge in the field of women's sexual health. The society mirrors the goals and intention of the textbook; therefore, the editors decided to donate 100% of the profits from this and future textbooks directly to ISSWSH. The editors concluded that what was of benefit for the textbook, was of benefit for the field and for the ISSWSH. Not surprisingly, all contributors agreed to participate under these circumstances. This textbook is the magnanimous expression of an idyllic spirit that permeates researchers and health-care professionals in the field of women's sexual health.

The process of planning the textbook required development of a table of contents fluid enough to incorporate new chapters as editors realized there were areas not originally included. The editors engaged and motivated numerous experts from multiple disciplines to contribute to this textbook. These contributors are specialists of both genders and provide psychologic and biologic input from broad, international and multicultural backgrounds. We have thus drawn on the intellectual resources for this textbook from many members of the ISSWSH. Consequently, this textbook has 128 contributors from five continents. Most of the editors, associate editors, and authors are members of ISSWSH, including many of the past and present officers of the society.

Women's Sexual Function and Dysfunction: Study, Diagnosis, and Treatment is divided into four sections. Each section presents the overall theme of the essential integration of psychologic and biologic components of women's sexual health. The first section covers the history of sexual dysfunction research from Kinsey to the present and the history of the ISSWSH. The second section engages the multitude of psychologic and biologic etiologic factors involved in women's sexual function and dysfunction, including many special issues concerning female sexual dysfunction syndromes as well as psychologic and biologic factors affecting the couple. The third section addresses the myriad of issues and factors involved in psychologic and biologic diagnosis and treatment of women with sexual health concerns, including management of special issues, difficult cases, and strategies to integrate medical and psychologic management. The fourth and final section relates to education and outreach for female sexual dysfunction, including educational strategies to expand women's sexual health awareness in medical school and in the lay audience.

A critical goal was to provide basic and practical information to health-care practitioners to enable them to provide sensible and realistic care for affected women.

While the mental health community has long recognized women's sexual dysfunction, the medical and scientific communities only recently acknowledged the biologic contributions. Building on the early physiologic studies of scientists such as Roy J Levin and Gorm Wagner, contemporary basic science researchers in women's sexual health are continuing and broadening the investigation of the physiologic contribution to women's sexual function. *Women's Sexual Function and Dysfunction: Study, Diagnosis, and Treatment* repeatedly cultivates and promotes the concept that correct management of a woman with sexual health concerns includes both psychologic and biologic components.

We are aware that there are several areas of repetition in this book. For example, material on how to perform a sexual history and genital physical examination in a woman with sexual dysfunction is replicated several times throughout the text. This reflects the multidisciplinary nature of this book and the varying perspectives in the study, diagnosis, and treatment of women's sexual health disorders. In addition, not all chapter requests were fulfilled. Specifically, chapters on psychologic etiology, cultural factors, and feminist approaches to sexuality education were not completed and therefore have not been included in this first printing. As we are made aware of the shortcomings of this textbook, we intend that revisions will address inadvertently deficient areas.

Because the intended readers of this book are from many different disciplines sharing the common purpose of studying, diagnosing, and treating women with sexual health concerns, it became apparent to us that there was a need for a common language. As experts in their unique niche areas of sexual medicine, authors often were highly specialized and used abbreviations known within their area of expertise. We have tried to eliminate such abbreviations whenever possible so that all readers can understand all chapters. It is our hope that this textbook successfully enables the dissemination of scientific and practical information concerning state-of-the-art management of women's sexual health. The information contained within these covers is state of the art at the time of publication. For timely updates on new research, we recommend that readers join the ISSWSH.

We, the editors, sincerely hope you will find reading *Women's Sexual Function and Dysfunction: Study, Diagnosis, and Treatment* to be as rewarding as we have found writing and editing this first textbook.

Acknowledgments

The editors wish to acknowledge the dedication and commitment of many colleagues without whom this project would not have been completed. We are indebted to the associate editors of the book: Lori A Brotto, PhD; Annamaria Giraldi, MD, Sue W Goldstein, AB; André Guay, MD; Emmanuele A Jannini, MD; Noel N Kim, PhD; Rossella E Nappi, MD, PhD; Sharon Parish, MD; Kwangsung Park, MD, PhD; and Alessandra H Rellini, MA. We take this opportunity to thank all the authors who took valuable time from their already busy lives to write chapters for this book. In particular, we would like to thank those who authored more than one chapter, as this demonstrated dedication and commitment to the field that will be appreciated by all who read this work.

In addition, we would like to thank Nick Dunton and Oliver Walter of Taylor and Francis; Nick for having the insight to want this book to be published, and Oliver for having the patience to work with us constantly. We especially would like to thank Sue W Goldstein, who, in addition to acting as an associate editor, took responsibility for keeping everyone informed and on time; without her efforts, this project would not have come to fruition.

We also wish to acknowledge those authors who lost loved ones during this time, yet persevered through their personal pain to help bring you, the reader, this timely body of knowledge.

Section 1

HISTORY

Fifty years of female sexual dysfunction research and concepts: from Kinsey to the present

Linda J Rosen, Raymond C Rosen

Introduction

Research and theory in female sexual dysfunction are evolving rapidly. New theories and conceptualizations of the field are being developed in the urgent attempt to keep up with the rapid flow of new knowledge and theory, but many questions and controversies remain unresolved. Despite advances in and increasing attention to the topic of female sexual dysfunction, there are still fundamental disagreements concerning the definition and classification of female sexual dysfunction and the proper perspective on treatment. This introductory chapter addresses these issues primarily from an historical perspective, detailing the specific contributions of pioneering sex researchers and therapists, including Alfred Kinsey, William Masters and Virginia Johnson, Helen Singer Kaplan, John Bancroft, and others. In reviewing their broader and individual contributions, we will consider also the emergence of key themes and topics in the field.

In recent decades there have been major advances in our understanding of sexual psychophysiology and pharmacology, and the role of sex steroid hormones, and a growing awareness of cultural factors affecting sexuality. Looking back 50 years, we are aware of rapid and steady growth of knowledge about normative sexual behavior in women (and men), and the evolution of current definitions of normal and "problematic" sexual function in women. However, certain core issues, such as the role of

relationship and interpersonal factors in determining sexual dysfunction, remain relatively unexplored. Biologic factors have undoubtedly received greater attention in the overall field of sexual dysfunction research in the past two decades. This has not been true historically, however, as this chapter will illustrate.

The overall purpose of this chapter is to identify and comment on evolving concepts of female sexual dysfunction. While the chapter proceeds chronologically, several themes and concepts will interweave and inform the discussion:

- Important historical changes have influenced medical and scientific conceptions of female sexuality. The past 50 years has witnessed the sexual revolution of the 1960s and 1970s (paralleled by the widespread use of the birth control pill and other effective forms of contraception), the growth of the pharmaceutic industry, and the development of both prescription and nonprescription products that affect sexual function.
- There is greater understanding of variations in female sexuality between and within different cultural groups. This context-dependent view of female sexuality predates Kinsey, although his work contributed greatly to recognition of the importance of social factors in sexual behavior. The debate on the relative influences of culture and society on female sexuality, compared with biologic and intrapsychic factors, continues unabated to this day.

- In the past decade there have been significant developments in medical, biologic, and pharmacologic approaches to sexuality. This has been described as the "medicalization" of sexuality by those who take issue with the emphasis on pharmaceutic or medical solutions to sexual problems, while some view these new and potentially effective medical treatments to age-old problems in women as presenting new and significant professional challenges. This is a highly controversial and complex area with significant implications for our understanding of female sexual function and dysfunction.

- Changing views of female sexuality have been paralleled, and perhaps influenced by, changes in research methodologies. From Kinsey's original interview techniques and Masters and Johnson's direct observation of human sexual response, research has expanded greatly in recent years to incorporate new methods for investigating brain physiology, hormonal changes, and genital blood flow during sexual response. New quantitative and qualitative research methods and survey approaches have also been developed.[1,2]

- Beginning with Masters and Johnson's four-phase conceptualization of sexual response, models of normative sexual function have undergone several significant transformations. Recent advances include the emergence of nonlinear models of sexual response in women (e.g., Basson[3]). These models have served as the basis of proposed diagnostic classifications and management recommendations for female sexual dysfunction.

- The terminology and diagnostic classification of sexual difficulties in women have evolved markedly from earlier value-laden and pejorative terms in the 1950s, such as "frigidity" and "nymphomania", to more descriptive and scientifically objective terms, such as "female sexual arousal disorder" and "hypoactive sexual desire disorder". This terminological and conceptual shift began with Kinsey, and continues to the present day.

Alfred Kinsey

Today, more than five decades since the publication of *Sexual Behavior in the Human Male*[4] and *Sexual Behavior in the Human Female*,[5] Alfred Kinsey's research remains among the most reliable sources of information about sexual behavior in America. It is not uncommon for present-day researchers to use Kinsey's data as a yardstick for measuring change. Kinsey was the researcher who brought sex research, and views of female sexuality in particular, from the last vestiges of the Victorian era into the modern age. In addition to its effects on the scientific community, Kinsey's groundbreaking studies brought human sexuality fully into the public consciousness.

Alfred Charles Kinsey was born in Hoboken, New Jersey, in 1894; he was a sickly child brought up in a strongly religious household who developed a passion for the outdoors and nature, and rejected religion. He studied biology at Bowdoin College,

and pursued doctoral studies at Harvard, where he was an instructor in biology and zoology. His interest in the collection and taxonomy of gall wasps began at this time, and there are noted parallels between this early interest in taxonomy and his later collection of thousands of individual sex histories and categorization of sexual behavior. In 1920, Kinsey became an assistant professor at Indiana University, where he pursued his interest in gall wasp taxonomy for nearly 20 years. It was in the summer of 1938 that Kinsey began to teach a marriage course, which grew in popularity and brought students to Kinsey with questions about their sexuality. The Institute for Sex Research (still functioning at Indiana University in Bloomington) grew out of Kinsey's efforts to answer students' questions by accumulating information about sexual behavior.

Kinsey's taxonomic approach is well known: he is thought to have studied human sexuality in much the same way that a biologist might study the sex lives of any other animal – categorizing sexual behavior in an objective fashion and making no value judgments about this behavior. Indeed, Kinsey may have cultivated the impression that his work was purely empirical because he assumed that this would be more acceptable to the public. However, a closer reading of his books shows that Kinsey often had strong opinions about human sexuality. Kinsey's sexual "ideology" might be said to include an insistence on tolerance of the enormous variability of sexual activity, and his emphasis on naturalism.[6] Kinsey believed that many sexual problems resulted from social training that went against the natural sexual tendencies of other mammals.

Sexual Behavior in the Human Female was published in 1953 amidst a storm of public and scientific controversy. Kinsey removed female sexuality from the realm of moralism and examined it scientifically. While his work on male sexuality was greeted with some shock, the female volume produced outrage. Instead of the Victorian view that masturbation in females was unhealthy and dangerous, Kinsey reported a consistent relationship between premarital masturbation and orgasm during marital intercourse. Among the volume's most significant conclusions, however, was the great similarity between sexual behavior in males and females. Kinsey emphasized the essential similarity in anatomic structures essential to sexual response and orgasm, and wrote that "males would be better prepared to understand females, and females to understand males, if they realized that they were alike in their basic anatomy and physiology." While he emphasized the similarity in anatomy and physiology, Kinsey did recognize the influence of hormonal factors on levels of sexual response, although he rejected the idea that hormones affect the types of sexual activity engaged in. Kinsey also rejected the prevailing wisdom, based on psychoanalytic concepts, that masturbation interfered with the development of "vaginal orgasms", which were a sign of sexual maturity in women. Instead, he observed that the vagina had few nerve endings in most women, and that the clitoris and labia were the major sources of female sexual sensation. In a chapter on the physiology of sexual response and orgasm, Kinsey concluded that orgasm was essentially the same in males and females, and rejected the common notion that females are slower in their capacity to reach orgasm.

Kinsey's influence on our current understanding of female sexual dysfunction can be illustrated by his discussion of "female frigidity". On the basis of the nearly 5000 "sex histories" contributed by women to the Kinsey project, he concluded that frigidity – defined as the absence of orgasm – was relatively rare, with 9 of 10 women reporting having experienced orgasm by age 35. An additional 8% reported experiencing arousal without orgasm. Kinsey concluded that essentially all women were physiologically capable of arousal and orgasm. However, he did discover wide variations in female sexual behavior; the age of first orgasm ranged from 9% by 11 years of age to 50% by age 20. More than two out of three women experienced their first orgasm before marriage. There were also great variations in the nature of stimulation leading to the first orgasm, with masturbation the stimulus for 40%, and heterosexual petting the stimulus for about one in four women. Only 17% of women reported having their first orgasm during marital intercourse.

Women also varied in the frequency of orgasm, in the methods used most often to reach orgasm, and in the proportion of sexual encounters that culminate in orgasm. In Kinsey's statistical portrait of sexual behavior, the average husband starts marriage having already experienced 1523 orgasms, compared with the average wife's 223 premarital orgasms. Women are also less likely to achieve orgasm during marital sex, and have more variability in their sexual response than men do. Women reported that they were less likely to make use of sexual outlets such as masturbation and nocturnal sex dreams, had fewer sexual fantasies, and experienced less arousal from visual stimulation than men. From this evidence, Kinsey concluded that females were not as sensitive to psychologic influences. This point of view is not accepted today, when sex differences in arousal are more likely to be attributed to social learning.

Kinsey examined the question of why some women were much more likely than others to experience orgasm regularly. He found that education was not a very significant factor, neither was social status (as measured by the father's occupation). Women born in the 1920s were more likely to experience orgasm regularly than women born in the 1890s, but this effect was also small. The best predictor of marital orgasm for women was their premarital experience – orgasm through masturbation, "petting", or intercourse before marriage was correlated with greater orgasmic responsiveness during marital intercourse. The problem of "frigidity", then, was not really a sexual dysfunction so much as a result of the fact that women more easily reach orgasm during masturbation than during intercourse. According to Kinsey, "frigidity" results from the repression of female sexual responsiveness, especially the occurrence of masturbation among girls and young women.

In his conclusion to *Sexual Behavior in the Human Female*, Kinsey considered the reasons for the male/female differences in psychosexual response that he had reported. In this discussion, Kinsey discredited the notion that hormonal factors produced these gender differences. He distrusted endocrinologic explanations of sexual differences, and cautioned against "over-enthusiastic advertising by some of the drug companies" and journalistic accounts of scientific research that lead people to believe that sexual behavior could be controlled though hormonal manipulation. These are controversial and timely comments today.

Kinsey was the first great modernizer in the field of human sexuality, recognizing the potential of women to be sexual creatures, and documenting the multiple variations in female sexual activity. His contributions to our understanding of female sexuality are monumental and lasting.

Masters and Johnson

The publication of *Human Sexual Response*[7] and *Human Sexual Inadequacy*[8] was the next milestone in the history of sex research. The two authors of these volumes, William Masters and Virginia Johnson, advanced the work begun by Kinsey in several ways. The first volume provided an extensive and detailed portrait of how the male and female body responds to sexual stimulation. The information upon which it was based was collected in a little more than a decade, and was derived from direct laboratory observation of more than 10 000 male and female orgasms. The second volume was a similarly extensive description of the causes of sexual "inadequacy", as well as a presentation of therapeutic techniques to be used to overcome sexual dysfunction in both sexes.

William Masters was born in Cleveland, Ohio, in 1915 and studied medicine at the University of Rochester with a view to establishing a career in research. Masters trained in obstetrics and gynecology, and in addition to his medical practice, he published research on a variety of related topics, including a series of papers on hormone replacement. Like Kinsey, he felt hampered by a lack of reliable information to provide to his patients. Although Masters was certainly not the first scientist to study human sexual response directly, his research on this topic was the most extensive and detailed at this time. Virginia Johnson, born in Missouri in 1925 and with a background in psychology and sociology, joined Masters' project initially as a research assistant and interviewer. Beginning with a population of prostitutes in the St Louis area, Masters conducted interviews in which he learned a great deal about sexual response patterns and techniques. He concluded that the prostitute population was not appropriate for physiologic study, but did learn how to approach more respectable volunteers who would be willing to participate in direct laboratory observations of sexual response.

A total of 694 individuals, including 276 married couples, ranging in age from 18 to 89, participated in the research program over a 10-year period. More than 14 000 sexual acts were observed and measured. Most subjects were paid volunteers who readily agreed to masturbate or to have intercourse with their partners while being filmed or recorded by physiologic measurement devices. Among the most noteworthy findings of this research were the remarkable similarities in male and female sexual physiology, the role of vaginal lubrication in female sexual arousal, and the physiology of multiple orgasms. Out of this work came the widely influential "four-stage model" of the sexual response cycle. The Masters and Johnson sexual response cycle served as the basis for their classification and subsequent treatment approach; deviations from the "normal" sexual response cycle constituted sexual inadequacies or dysfunction. Notable in this model is the absence of a "desire" phase, since desire is basically a subjective experience difficult to measure within a physiologically based model.

The result of their research program was an extremely detailed description of the major physiologic changes associated with sexual arousal and orgasm in males and females: changes in blood flow, vaginal lubrication, nipple enlargement, and other physiologic changes were described. Further, these physiologic changes were described over the course of the "sexual response cycle," so that the changes take place progressively over time and in specific sequence. The four-stage model of Masters and Johnson serves as the central organizing schema for their observations of male and female sexual physiology, as well as the basis for their subsequent classification of sexual dysfunction.

The model includes the well-known phases of excitement, plateau, orgasm and resolution. Each phase is associated with specific genital and extragenital changes, and focuses almost exclusively on bodily responses to sexual stimulation, with minimal attention to cognitive or subjective aspects of sexual response. Within this model, Masters and Johnson emphasize the essential similarities in the male and female physiologic responses to sexual stimulation, drawing parallels at different phases of the cycle. For example, during the excitement phase, female vaginal lubrication is compared directly to penile engorgement and erection in the male, particularly in respect to parameters such as "reactive intensity", response timing, and age-related changes. In their discussion of the vaginal–clitoral orgasm distinction, they again emphasize the relative uniformity of male and female orgasmic processes.

The overall contribution of this research to the understanding of sexual response is undisputed, but there have also been frequent criticisms of their work. Masters and Johnson acknowledged that their sample was unrepresentative in regard to age, race and educational status. Further, it seems plausible that individuals willing to perform sexual activities in the laboratory are not representative of the general population, and that the laboratory setting may have influenced the character of the sexual responses observed. Robinson[6] has drawn attention to the largely contrived separation of sexual response into four discrete stages, especially the distinction between excitement and plateau, and suggests that the process of arousal is better conceptualized as a continuous progression of events. Another criticism of the Masters and Johnson model is the relative lack of synthesis of cognitive-affective states with the physiologic processes of sexual arousal.[9] Subjective factors are generally overlooked in their model. Moreover, even when discussing changes in physiologic activity, they fail to provide an explanation for the observed patterning of autonomic, somatic, and central concomitants of sexual response. While Masters and Johnson have enumerated the specifics of physiologic response in great detail, there is a lack of explanatory concepts for integrating these separate response dimensions. Overall, one is left with an impressive but essentially disjointed description of physiologic events.

Human Sexual Inadequacy was based on Masters and Johnson's therapeutic experiences with 790 patients, whose complaints fell into six major categories: for males, primary impotence (32 cases), secondary impotence (213 cases), premature ejaculation (186 cases), and ejaculatory incompetence (17 cases); for females, primary orgasmic dysfunction (193 cases) and situational orgasmic dysfunction (149 cases). The absence of sexual desire disorders in their case series is noteworthy. Although Masters and Johnson's research focused on the specific physiologic changes taking place during sexual activity, their therapeutic model emphasized psychologic and social factors. Their women patients frequently described what they called "psychosocial repression", in which "normal" and "natural" sexual responsiveness is inhibited by negative sexual messages, with religious orthodoxy identified as a significant source of sexual misconceptions.

Prior to 1970, most forms of female sexual dysfunction were referred to by the pejorative term "frigidity". With the publication of *Human Sexual Inadequacy*, female sexual dysfunction began to be classified according to which specific phase of the four-stage arousal sequence was most affected. Masters and Johnson highlighted the importance of differential diagnosis based on the patient's sexual history. They distinguished between primary and secondary, or situational, forms of orgasmic dysfunction, thus refining the treatment mechanisms to be used. However, the conceptualization and definition of sexual desire problems did not take place for almost a decade, until the separate contributions of Harold Lief and Helen Singer Kaplan. These were followed by the "psychosomatic circle of sex" concept, developed by John Bancroft.

Sexual response and psychiatry: contributions of Lief, Kaplan, and Bancroft

Harold Lief

The first of three influential psychiatrists and sex therapists, Harold Lief addressed the need to include a desire or libido phase of sexual response, and a clinical approach for evaluating and treating disorders of this phase. Lief deserves credit for being among the first authorities to comment on the need for a greater focus on problems of sexual desire.[10] Lief noted in an early paper that a substantial proportion of patients presenting at sex therapy clinics could not be diagnosed according to the classification proposed by Masters and Johnson. He proposed that the new diagnostic term "inhibited sexual desire" (formerly "low libido") be added to the classification of sexual dysfunction in women and men, and he suggested specifically that the diagnosis be applied to women who chronically fail to respond to sexual initiation. This proposal had immediate and lasting effects on the American Psychiatric Association's *Diagnostic and Statistical Manual of Mental Disorders* (DSM) classification. Lief observed that a large number of referrals for sex therapy (almost 50% in one early study) were due to a loss of sexual interest, in addition to problems of arousal or orgasm.

Another of Lief's key contributions to the field was to focus attention on the role of sex hormones, and testosterone in particular, in the conceptualization of sexual desire phase disorders ("inhibited sexual desire"). Lief noted that testosterone is important for maintaining normal sexual desire or drive in both males and females; he considered studies of hypogonadal men and oophorectomized women in his model, and menstrual cycle effects on sex steroid hormones.[11] In short, Lief drew attention to both the importance of sexual desire as a core issue in our understanding of sexual function and the significance of endocrinologic factors in understanding hypoactive sexual desire disorder. Studies in recent years, and many chapters in this book, illustrate the relevance and clinical importance of these observations.

Helen Singer Kaplan

Helen Singer Kaplan's model of sexual function and dysfunction is grounded in her experiences as a sex therapist.[12,13] Noting the relative neglect of motivational factors in the Masters and Johnson model, Kaplan criticized the field of sex therapy for failing to address the importance of sexual desire deficits in clinical disorders of sexual function. Accordingly, she recommended reconceptualizing the sexual response cycle to include three stages – desire, excitement, and orgasm; she observed that sexual dysfunction fell into these three categories, and that it is possible to be "inhibited" in one of these areas and still function normally in the other two.

The inclusion of "desire" as a separate stage of the sexual response cycle may have been Kaplan's most significant contribution. Unlike excitement or orgasm, sexual desire does not necessarily involve the genital organs; rather, it involves sensations that motivate a person to seek out or become available to sexual experience. The desire stage is comparable to the traditional concept of "libido", and Kaplan identifies the source of libido as activation of certain centers in the limbic system. The second stage, excitement, is identified with reflex genital vasocongestion in both sexes. The third stage, orgasm, consists of reflex pelvic muscle contractions. A key postulate of this model is that the three phases of sexual response are mediated by separate but interrelated neurophysiologic mechanisms. While desire is believed to be mediated by central (i.e., brain) mechanisms, excitement and orgasm are associated with the stimulation of peripheral reflex pathways in the lower spinal cord. Although this distinction is appealing in some respects, Kaplan provided little direct evidence to support the differentiation of drive as centrally mediated in contrast to excitement and orgasm as peripherally based processes.

Kaplan argued that a disturbance in one of the three stages of sexual response does not necessarily imply that there are difficulties with the other stages. For example, a woman with low desire may be reluctant to initiate sex, but may still have pleasurable arousal and orgasm responses if she is induced or pressured into sexual activity. Problems with sexual desire are among the most difficult to modify, according to Kaplan, and accounted for a significant number of failures in her sex therapy program. Similarly, Kaplan cautioned that anorgasmia (lack of orgasm) should not be confused with uninterest in sex or with difficulty in becoming sexually aroused. In fact, she believed that failure to reach orgasm during intercourse was not necessarily a dysfunction at all, but perhaps a normal variation of female sexuality. For some women, the stimulation provided by intercourse is insufficient to trigger orgasm.

Criticisms of Kaplan's three-phase model include the discontinuity between the centrally mediated desire phase and the peripherally mediated excitement and orgasm phases, and the lack of elaboration of the excitement and orgasm phases. Kaplan describes these phases in purely reflexive terms, and focuses exclusively on peripheral physiologic changes in defining excitement and orgasm. She strongly emphasizes the similarities between male and female physiologic responses during excitement and orgasm, but overlooks the role of extragenital or subjective changes during the latter phases of the response cycle.

John Bancroft

Bancroft[14] described four essential features of sexual arousal: (1) sexual appetite or drive, (2) central arousal, (3) genital responses, and (4) peripheral arousal. Included in the category of sexual appetite or drive, according to Bancroft, are both motivational factors and sexual arousability. Other authors, such as Basson,[3] have viewed sexual arousability as a dimension separate from desire. Bancroft's second component, central arousal, refers to central nervous system activation and attentional factors that underlie psychologic processing of sexual stimuli. In recent years, Bancroft and Janssen[15] expanded this component of the model to include the processes of activation or excitation, and inhibition of central nervous systems. These processes are conceptualized to determine the degree and type of psychologic mechanisms in sexual dysfunction, which Bancroft and Janssen further speculate is related to neurochemical processes in the brain and spinal cord, such as alpha-adrenergic tone. Some pharmacologic studies provide support for this hypothesis.[16] The third and fourth components, genital responses and peripheral arousal, have received the most extensive discussion to date, and have been the focus of much research in the past two decades.[9]

Bancroft postulates a "psychosomatic circle of sex". In this model, thoughts and feelings about sex are integrated into several layers of processing of sexual stimuli in the brain, spinal cord, and peripheral genital reflexes of men or women. Bancroft described a "central arousability system" consisting of connections or circuits in the medial preoptic areas of the hypothalamus, prefrontal cortex, and other brain and spinal centers of coordination. At this time, there is evidence of the role of spinal integrating neurons in control of rhythmic contractions during orgasm in males and females. Brain centers involved in arousal and orgasm have been similarly investigated by radioimaging methods such as positron emission tomography (PET) and magnetic resonance imaging (MRI). Other investigators have used peripheral measuring devices (e.g., vaginal photoplethysmography, Doppler ultrasound, genital MRI) for physiologic assessment of sexual response in women. These latter techniques are also described in later chapters.

Leonore Tiefer and the feminist perspective of women's sexuality

Leonore Tiefer and others present a "social constructionist" model or perspective on female sexuality; in this view, definitions and categories of sexuality are the product of a specific social and historical environment.[17] Deconstruction is the process of analyzing existing categories to assess their current validity and usefulness. Tiefer applies this analysis to the sexual response cycle model of human sexual function that originated with Masters and Johnson, and continues to play a prominent role in discussions of female sexual function and dysfunction.

Tiefer argues that the Masters and Johnson model was assumed before the collection of the research data, and in fact actually guided the selection of subjects and research methods. For example, Masters and Johnson selected only women able to be sexually responsive in the laboratory setting, although their responsiveness is not likely to be generalizable to all women. Similarly, the sample was not representative in terms of socioeconomic status, or in what is described as "sexual enthusiasm". Tiefer also points out the potential problems associated with experimenter bias – Masters and Johnson acted as both researchers and "therapists" with many of their subjects – and the bias introduced by the definition of "effective sexual stimulation" as that which advances the subject through the sexual response cycle.

These limitations and biases are important in the study of female sexual dysfunction generally, since Masters and Johnson's model has so long been the reference standard against which "normal" sexual function is measured. Deviations from the model are, by definition, outside the "norm" and therefore a sign of dysfunction. Among the limitations of this model, according to Tiefer, are a focus on sexuality as the performance of a "fragmented series of body parts" rather than a whole, that sexual dysfunction occurs when a body part does not function according to norms, and that dysfunction can be diagnosed adequately by medical tests and technology.

Masters and Johnson emphasized the similarities in male and female sexual response, and constructed the sexual response cycle to show the parallels between men and women. In presenting a feminist critique of the sexual response cycle, Tiefer suggests that insisting on the essential similarities between male and female sexual response may actually obscure some important differences. Men and women are raised with different sexual values and expectations, and the social and emotional meaning of sex is unlikely to be gender neutral. By reducing sexual response to a series of physiologic changes, Tiefer argues, the sexual response cycle ignores the context and meaning of sexuality, factors that are critical in the understanding and treatment of female sexual dysfunction.

In *A New View of Women's Sexual Problems*,[18] Tiefer and others criticize the DSM, the classification scheme used to categorize women's sexual problems, as excessively medical, genitally focused, and mechanistic. In this "new view", the pharmaceutic industry has coerced sex research in the direction of developing physical treatments for sexual problems, to the exclusion of sociocultural, psychologic, or social approaches. The medicalization of sexuality began in earnest with the US Federal Drug Administration (FDA)'s approval of sildenafil, and the growth of a new medical area of "male sexual dysfunction". The development of female sexual dysfunction has followed. In Tiefer's view, female sexual dysfunction is the pharmaceutic industry's concept, which supports the development of pharmaceutic/medical treatment, and is at odds with the complexity of women's sexual problems.

The working group that produced the "new view" argues for a change in the nomenclature and classification of women's sexual problems that is based on recognition of the differences between men and women, the relational context of sexuality, and the differences among women. This new classification scheme defines women's sexual problems as "discontent with any emotional, physical or relationship aspect of sexual experience, including problems due to socio-cultural, political or economic factors, relationship factors, psychological factors, or medical factors".

Rosemary Basson and the reconceptualization of female sexual dysfunction

Advances in the understanding of female sexuality are based in part on new research on changes related to aging, reproductive events, and relationship duration, as well as the importance of mental well-being and other psychologic and biologic factors. Recently, Basson has used these data to reconceptualize women's sexual response and to expand and revise current definitions of female sexual dysfunction.[19]

Basson's model contrasts with the more traditional models formulated by Masters and Johnson and Helen Singer Kaplan, in which sexual activity is a "linear progression of discrete phases plus a focus on genital arousal/congestion, rather than the subjective experience". There are many facets of a woman's sexual function and dysfunction that do not fit the more traditional views of the past 50 years. For example, research indicates that the awareness of sexual desire is not the most frequent reason women engage in sexual activity, that sexual fantasies may be a technique for focusing sexual thoughts rather than an indication of desire, and that a woman's experience of sexual arousal has relatively little to do with her perception of genital changes. In contrast to Kaplan's notion that sexual dysfunction could occur in one part of the sexual response cycle without affecting other parts, new evidence demonstrates that correlation or comorbidity of dysfunction is common.

Basson emphasizes that women have many reasons for engaging in sex, and that these reasons – the desire for emotional intimacy, for example – may have little or nothing to do with feelings of sexual desire. Further, she describes a potential "disconnect" between a woman's feelings of sexual arousal and the physiologic changes, such as genital vasocongestion, that typically accompany sexual arousal. Basson's model of the sexual response cycle is circular, and includes the multiple sexual and nonsexual reasons for engaging in sex, the psychologic and biologic influences on arousability, and subjective feelings of arousal and desire. Within this model, there are many factors that may instigate sex, and a variety of potential positive outcomes, with a range of sexual response cycles in different women. Factors that may interfere with a satisfactory cycle include: minimal emotional intimacy; lack of appropriate sexual stimuli; negative psychologic factors such as distraction and fear; and fatigue, depression or medication effects that reduce arousability. According to Basson, even when a dysfunction is logical and adaptive, it can still cause a woman to feel considerable personal distress and require treatment.

Subjective arousal plays a central role in this model. Feelings of subjective arousal do not correlate well with psychophysiologic measures of genital congestion. Indeed, emotions and thoughts have a stronger influence on the subjective experience of arousal than feedback from genital congestion. It is also possible for a woman to experience healthy sexual vasocongestion without having any feelings of sexual arousal or excitement.

Basson et al.[20] presented revised and expanded definitions of women's sexual dysfunction developed by an international committee organized by the American Foundation for Urological Disease. These new definitions include sexual desire disorder (the absence of not only sexual thoughts and desire but also responsive desire), sexual arousal disorder (subdivided into subjective arousal disorder, genital arousal disorder, and combined arousal disorder), orgasmic disorder (lack of orgasm despite high sexual arousal), dyspareunia and vaginismus, and persistent sexual arousal disorder (the presence of persistent genital congestion that is inappropriate and intrusive).

The pharmaceutic era: will there be a "drug" for women?

The development of selective phosphodiesterase type 5 inhibitor drugs (sildenafil, tadalfil, and vardenafil) has irrevocably altered medical and societal concepts of sexual dysfunction, and how we view sexual problems in the "sildenafil age". These drugs have been widely used in men (about 30 million current users worldwide), and tested in more than 100 prospective, randomized, controlled trials. Although initially questioned for their cardiac safety, these drugs (selective phosphodiesterase type 5 inhibitors) have been shown to be generally safe and effective in men, with additional beneficial effects on mood in men for whom the drugs are effective.[21] Despite their success in the treatment of erectile dysfunction problems in men, selective phosphodiesterase type 5 inhibitors have not had consistent success in studies in women.[22] The paucity of well-controlled studies may be due, in part, to methodological problems in conducting clinical trials in women.[23] While sildenafil has been shown in some studies to increase vaginal blood flow and genital vasocongestion in response to sexual stimulation in women,[24,25] results from clinical trials in outpatient settings have been difficult to interpret.

Based on the inconsistent results obtained, Pfizer announced in early 2004 that it was discontinuing its clinical development program of selective phosphodiesterase type 5 inhibitors for sexual arousal disorder in women. The company indicated that it would continue to investigate female sexual dysfunction generally and to consider development of other treatments. The androgen patch for women, which was developed by Procter & Gamble for women with hypoactive sexual desire disorder, has similarly been withdrawn recently from FDA review. Despite these apparent setbacks, basic and clinical research in female sexual dysfunction has expanded with the entry of the pharmaceutic industry into this area and has made significant advances in recent years. Later chapters in this volume provide strong evidence of this trend. However, a comprehensive and holistic approach to management of sexual dysfunction in women, which takes medical and psychosocial factors into account, is now needed. We hope this volume will support this overall direction of change and provide specific signposts.

References

1. Tiefer L, Rosen R, Giami A et al. Qualitative health research and sexual dysfunction. In TF Lue, R Basson, R Rosen et al., eds. *Sexual Medicine: Sexual Dysfunction in Men and Women*. Paris: Editions 21, 2004.
2. Rosen R, Hatzichristou D, Broderick G et al. Clinical evaluation and symptom scales. In TF Lue, R Basson, R Rosen, et al., eds. *Sexual Medicine: Sexual Dysfunction in Men and Women*. Paris: Editions 21, 2004.

3. Basson R. The female sexual response: a different model. *J Sex Marital Ther* 2000; 26: 51–65.

4. Kinsey AC, Pomeroy WB, Martin CE. *Sexual Behavior in the Human Male*. Philadelphia: WB Saunders, 1948.

5. Kinsey AC, Pomeroy WB, Martin CE et al. *Sexual Behavior in the Human Female*. Philadelphia: WB Saunders, 1953.

6. Robinson P. *The Modernization of Sex*. New York: Harper & Row, 1976.

7. Masters WH, Johnson VE. *Human Sexual Response*. Boston: Little, Brown, 1966.

8. Masters WH, Johnson VE. *Human Sexual Inadequacy*. Boston: Little, Brown, 1970.

9. Rosen RC, Beck JG. *Patterns of Sexual Arousal*. New York: Guilford Press, 1988.

10. Lief HI. Inhibited sexual desire. *Med Aspects Hum Sex* 1977; 7: 94–5.

11. Lief HI. Foreword. In S Leiblum, R Rosen, eds. *Sexual Desire Disorders*. New York: Guilford Press, 1988: vii–xii.

12. Kaplan HS. *The New Sex Therapy*. New York: Brunner/Mazel, 1974.

13. Kaplan HS. *Disorders of Sexual Desire*. New York: Brunner/Mazel, 1979.

14. Bancroft JH. *Human Sexuality and Its Problems*. New York: Churchill Livingstone, 1983.

15. Bancroft J, Janssen E. The dual control model of sexual response: a theoretical approach to centrally mediated erectile dysfunction. *Neurosci Biobehav Rev* 2000; 24: 571–9

16. Rosen RC, Phillips NA, Gendrano NC et al. Oral phentolamine and female sexual arousal disorder. *J Sex Marital Ther* 1999; 25: 137–44.

17. Tiefer L. Historical, scientific, clinical and feminist criticism of "the human sexual response cycle" model. *Annu Rev Sex Res* 1991; 2: 1–23.

18. Kaschak E, Tiefer L, eds. *A New View of Women's Sexual Problems*. New York: Haworth Press, 2001.

19. Basson R. Pharmacotherapy for sexual dysfunction in women *Expert Opin Pharmacother* 2004; 5: 1045–59.

20. Basson R, Berman J, Burnett A et al. Report of the international consensus development conference on female sexual dysfunction: definitions and classifications. *J Urol* 2000; 163: 888–93.

21. Rosen RC, Seidman SN, Menza MA et al. Quality of life, mood, and sexual function: a path analytic model of treatment effects in men with erectile dysfunction and depressive symptoms. *Int J Impot Res* 2004; 16: 334–40.

22. Rosen R, McKenna K. PDE-5 inhibition and sexual response: pharmacological mechanisms and clinical outcomes. *Annu Rev Sex Res* 2002; 13: 36–88.

23. Islam A, Mitchel J, Hays J et al. Challenges in conducting multi-center clinical trials in female sexual dysfunction: baseline differences between study populations. *J Sex Marital Ther* 2001; 27: 525–30.

24. Berman J, Berman L, Linh H et al. Effect of sildenafil on subjective and physiologic parameters of the female sexual response in women with sexual arousal disorder. *J Sex Marital Ther* 2001; 27: 411–20.

25. Laan E, Van Lunsen R, Everaerd W et al. The enhancement of vaginal vasocongestion by sildenafil in healthy premenopausal women. *J Womens Health Gend Based Med* 2002; 11: 357–65.

1.2 History of the International Society for the Study of Women's Sexual Health (ISSWSH)

Sue W Goldstein

Psychologic care for women with sexual dysfunction has been available from mental health practitioners for many years. The medical community, on the other hand, has generally ignored women's sexual health. The advent of sildenafil as a safe and effective, government-approved therapy for men with erectile dysfunction in the late 1990s triggered and empowered women distressed by their own sexual dysfunctions to demand safe and effective therapies for themselves, especially from sexual medicine, biologically-focused health-care professionals. Sexual dysfunctions are well recognized to be byproducts of mind, body, and relationship issues. It is critical for maximal clinical success in sexual medicine to offer both psychologically and medically oriented interventions. When sildenafil was released to the public, there were essentially no groups of health-care professionals that equally concentrated on both psychologically and biologically based investigations in women's sexual health. The demand for such multidisciplinary resources is central to the recent development of the International Society for the Study of Women's Sexual Health (ISSWSH).

The purpose of this chapter is to trace the inception and early years of ISSWSH, believed to be the first organization of its kind. ISSWSH is devoted exclusively to women's sexual health, and membership is uniquely multidisciplinary, more or less equally divided into psychologically and biologically motivated health-care professionals. The membership of organizations such as the American Association of Sex Educators,

Counselors, and Therapists (AASECT) is primarily the mental health community, and the International Society for Sexual Medicine (ISSM) was originally designed as an organization for urologists. In contradistinction, ISSWSH was meant from the outset to be multidisciplinary, to engage clinicians and researchers encompassing basic science and clinical research in psychologic and biologic aspects of women's sexual health. This chapter will also highlight some of the pioneers in this field, who had the passion and commitment and foresight to work together for a common cause.

The organization's original name was the Female Sexual Function Forum (FSFF). ISSWSH was officially born in Boston on 28 October 2001 after the membership of the FSFF approved the society's name change and initials and agreed upon the first ISSWSH board of directors. Sandra Leiblum, of the USA, was the organization's first president, under the original name FSFF. Her successor was Alessandra Graziottin, of Italy, who was, therefore, technically the first ISSWSH president.

The original assembly of experts that would be remembered as the antecedent to ISSWSH was held in the spring of 1997 in Hyannis, Cape Cod, Massachusetts, and chaired by Raymond Rosen, PhD, and Michael O'Leary, MD. This meeting was conceived for the purpose of discussing clinical research outcome data in sexual dysfunction in both men and women. Attendance was by invitation only and consisted of experts from Australia, Canada, Europe, and the USA (Fig. 1.2.1).

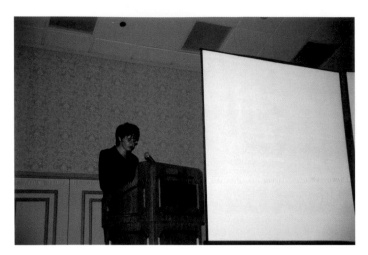

Figure 1.2.1. Ellen Laan presenting her data on women's sexual health at the first Cape Cod conference.

While the bulk of the data were available for men only, the excitement of the attendees grew from the innovative and thought-provoking discussions on women's sexual health. This was one of the first international, multidisciplinary meetings to include speakers on endocrinology, gynecology, internal medicine, neurology, psychiatry, psychology, urology, etc., for scientific discussion of physiology, pathophysiology, diagnosis, and treatment outcome on an equal footing regarding both men's and women's sexual health.

The first multidisciplinary meeting dedicated exclusively to evidence-based outcome data in female sexual dysfunction (FSD) was held again by the same meeting organizers in the same location the following year in June 1998. The aim of this second meeting was to bring international, multifaceted experts together to discuss basic science and clinical management in various physiologic and psychologic aspects of FSD (Fig. 1.2.2). Several meeting highlights were memorable and noteworthy. In the middle of the meeting, the power failed, leaving the

meeting room in complete darkness. A psychologist with her own sexual dysfunction discussed her positive anecdotal experiences with enhanced orgasmic function on sildenafil when the lights went out. The lively spirit and discussion persisted and ultimately when the light returned, she continued with her interesting story. The timing of the darkness with the discussion of woman's selective phosphodiesterase type 5 treatment was ironic and resulted in smiles on many of the attendees' faces. A second highlight was of more academic significance. Attending the meeting alongside the experts was Tom Bruckman, at that time director of the American Foundation for Urologic Disease (AFUD). Prior to the Saturday lunch break, there had been an energetic discussion on the lack of an up-to-date consensus on nomenclature and classification in the field of FSD, in particular, that engaged biologic aspects of sexual dysfunction, hindering contemporary usage of a common scientific language. During lunch, Tom Bruckman and others were optimistically discussing plans to organize an international consensus development conference on FSD to discuss definitions and classifications (Fig. 1.2.3). In the months following the second Cape Cod meeting, Bruckman and the American Foundation for Urologic Disease would sponsor a multiphase process, including an initial planning committee meeting with Irwin Goldstein and Ray Rosen as cochairs, in August 1998 in Amsterdam, and a consensus panel meeting involving use of the Rand methodology for consensus development. A total of 19 panelists from five countries with a wide background of disciplines convened outside Boston on 22 October 1998 (Fig. 1.2.4). A subsequent focus group discussion ensued in Boston on 5 December 1998, and the communications from the expert panel led to the publication of a paper on the subject in the *Journal of Urology* in 2000.[1]

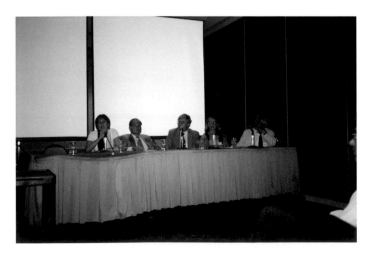

Figure 1.2.2. Discussion panel at the second Cape Cod conference.

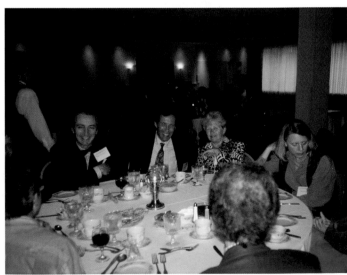

Figure 1.2.3. Lunch at the second Cape Cod conference, including conference cochairs Michael O'Leary and Raymond Rosen talking with Jean Fourcroy and Julia Heiman.

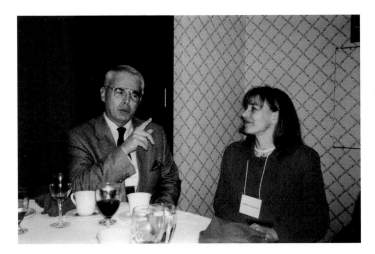

Figure 1.2.4. Leonard Derogatis and Alessandra Graziottin in discussion at the International Consensus Development Conference on Female Sexual Dysfunction: definitions and classifications sponsored by AFUD.

As a result of the Cape Cod conference and the planning of a consensus panel meeting in the Boston area in October, the Boston University School of Medicine departments of Continuing Medical Education (CME) and Urology teamed to host the first of several annual CME courses on FSD entitled "New Perspectives in FSD". The 2-day meeting was held immediately after the consensus panel meeting in October 1998 in a suburb of Boston, and was chaired by Irwin Goldstein, MD.[1,2] Approximately 200 people from diverse disciplines and various regions of the world attended. The format of this meeting was limited to invited speakers, with no peer-reviewed abstract submission process. Whenever possible, however, basic science and clinical researchers who brought slides concerning individual investigations were given limited time at the podium. The enthusiasm for learning and sharing ideas and thoughts among the multidisciplinary attendees in women's sexual health was infectious. Additional meeting highlights included a presentation of Gorm Wagner's movie on the physiologic changes in women during sexual stimulation. A Halloween visit to a local castle, a traditional New England clambake, and dancing to a live band fostered the needed bonding of this multidisciplinary group.

The response to the initial "new perspectives" meeting in Boston was overwhelming. There was a definite interest in and a crucial need for in-depth knowledge of women's sexual function and dysfunction, but there was a paucity of evidence-based information. Planning began immediately for a second new perspectives meeting. The meeting was lengthened to 2½ days to accommodate the expanded format that included podium and poster presentations based on submitted abstracts, in addition to 13 grand master lectures and invited speakers. Essay submissions were solicited for prizes offered in four basic areas: basic science in psychology, basic science in biology, clinical psychology, and clinical biology. This second new perspectives conference in October 1999 was held in a business hotel in downtown Boston.

Outside the doors of the hotel, a group of proponents of Leonore Tiefer's "*New View*"[3] picketed, hoping for some positive attention from the media and support from meeting registrants. Their demonstration was peaceful and reminded attendees that there was a need to be sensitive to the issue of "medicalizing" FSD. Approximately 450 people attended the new perspectives conference. In anticipation of interest in forming a society devoted to better understanding of the physiology, pathophysiology, and management of female sexual function and dysfunction, a business meeting was scheduled as part of the program. Attendees voted to develop a list-serve and name the FSFF. The only criterion for joining the list-serve was being a health-care professional with an interest in the field. The list-serve facilitated communication among people of various geographic locations, disciplines, and perspectives, and started participants thinking about the need for a more formal organization.

The following year's conference in Boston was thus named the FSFF. In anticipation of the growing attendance, the meeting was moved into a larger conference hotel in Boston, Goldstein acting as chair once again. The format was similar to the year before, with more abstracts submitted and accepted. By the time on-site registrations were counted, there were nearly 700 people at the FSFF meeting. The hot topic was the use of androgens in women, with standing room only on Sunday morning to hear numerous questions and answers on the topic. A formal business meeting with elections took place, and the seeds of ISSWSH were sown. The passion, hard work, and dedication of a few had brought this original continuing medical education meeting to the annual meeting of an international organization. This last Boston University-sponsored meeting would set the tone for future ISSWSH meetings, with state-of-the-art lectures, controversial symposia, and abstracts judged on scientific merit.

Sandra Leiblum was elected inaugural president of the FSFF, with a full board of directors consisting of Alessandra Graziottin as vice president, Irwin Goldstein as secretary, André

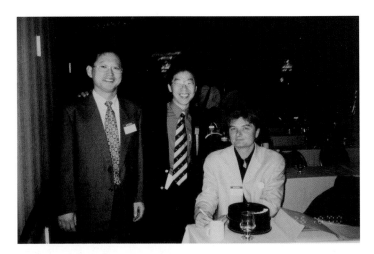

Figure 1.2.5. Colleagues from Korea and France preparing for their presentations at the 2000 meeting of the Female Sexual Function Forum.

Guay as treasurer, and directors-at-large Anne Davis, Moustafa Eyada, François Giuliano, Roy Levin, Rosella Nappi, Kwangsung Park and Leonore Tiefer. Irwin Goldstein acted as meeting chair one last time, Abdul Traish as scientific program chair, and Mitch Tepper as online services chair. Other chair positions would be determined by a set of bylaws, which were necessary for the organization to become a legal entity. Ira Sharlip, who had written bylaws for the Sexual Medicine Society of North America, was asked to chair this committee. The bylaws designated that half the board positions would terminate each year, providing continuity in the organization, and that the board and each committee would be balanced in terms of gender, geography, and discipline.

To enable the dissemination of information presented at this meeting, podium and poster presenters were invited to submit manuscripts for publication in a FSFF-sponsored journal supplement. A total of 27 published papers were dedicated to a multidisciplinary collection of manuscripts on sexual function and dysfunction in women. State-of-the-art lecturers were invited to submit manuscripts to a peer-reviewed journal where the papers would be published as a group.

Although it was held just weeks after the 9/11 tragedy, approximately 400 people came to Boston from around the world for the FSFF meeting, a tribute to the interest in and desire to learn about this field (Fig. 1.2.6). The W J Weiser Company had been hired to manage FSFF. Irwin Goldstein, as both meeting chair and secretary, and his colleague Abdul Traish, scientific program chair, worked together to ensure the success of this meeting. The format continued to include state-of-the-art lectures, symposia, podium presentations, and moderated posters. Topics included cancer, childbirth, cultural aspects of FSD, diagnostic studies, sexually transmitted diseases, vulvar pain, and androgen insufficiency, as interest in the controversial area of androgens continued (Fig. 1.2.7). Again, all presenters were offered the opportunity to submit

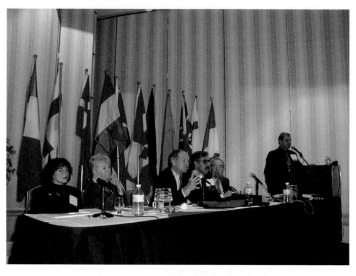

Figure 1.2.7. Androgen panel in 2001 with Aline Zoldbrod, Jean Fourcroy, Fernand Labrie, Abdul Traish, Richard Spark, and André Guay at the podium.

manuscripts to be considered for an ISSWSH-sponsored journal supplement.

At the 2001 business meeting, the bylaws that had been written during the course of the year were approved by the membership (Fig. 1.2.8). After much heated discussion, the organization was renamed the ISSWSH. This name reflected the international nature of the organization. The annual meeting and the list-serve (see below) with instant communication to members around the world would allow communication on a daily basis as well as in-depth annually.

ISSWSH is "a multidisciplinary, academic clinical and scientific organization whose purposes are: (1) to provide opportunities for communication among scholars, researchers, and

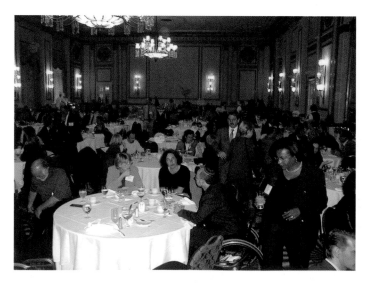

Figure 1.2.6. Lunch during the 2001 meeting.

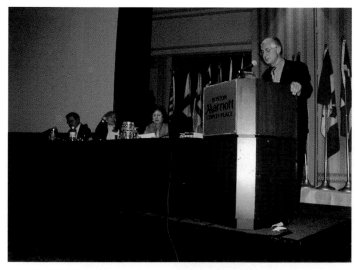

Figure 1.2.8. Irwin Goldstein delivering the secretary's report with André Guay, treasurer; Alessandra Graziottin, vice president; and Sandra Leiblum, president, on the dais.

practitioners about women's sexual health; (2) to support the highest standards of ethics and professionalism in research, education, and clinical practice of women's sexual health; and (3) to provide the public with accurate information about women's sexual health".

The elected board met for the first time in Boston (Fig. 1.2.9). Membership fees were levied, and applications were required for current and future members. Membership became limited to those who could demonstrate an involvement with female sexual function and/or dysfunction. Affiliate membership was granted to those working in industry, while honorary membership could be awarded by the board to individuals who demonstrated a serious interest in female sexuality or had made an important contribution to the field but did not qualify for active membership. While the cost of membership was the same for active and affiliate members, the ability to hold office or serve as a committee chair was restricted to active and honorary members. Privileges afforded to all members included discounted registration fees and access to the list-serve. Started by Irwin Goldstein for members of the Female Sexual Function Forum, the list-serve was made a resource for difficult case questions among the ISSWSH membership under online services chair Mitch Tepper. The final important decision by the board that first year was that the directors-at-large would add a year to their original terms of service, rather than half rotating off in 2001, to aid in the development of the new society.

The board "met" throughout the year by teleconference and e-mail, voting on issues that did not require face-to-face discussions. Then, in October 2002, the Vancouver meeting became truly international, leaving Boston for the first time (Fig. 1.2.10). Approximately 400 members and future members came to Vancouver for the ISSWSH meeting. The number of abstracts had increased and quality of submissions had improved. Deemed necessary during the previous year, the bylaws were amended at the business meeting; and the contract

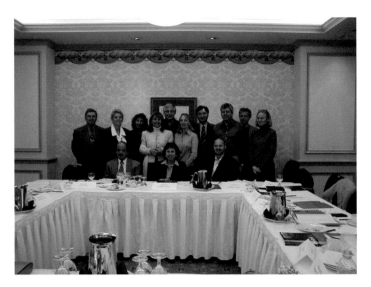

Figure 1.2.10. The board of ISSWSH in 2002 in Vancouver.

with the management company was renewed for 3 years. The organization was truly established.

This ISSWSH meeting was held shortly after the publication of the Women's Health Initiative. In response to the growing interest in this area, a lunchtime seminar was added to the program to include the latest information. Although it was still difficult to understand the integration between the biology and psychology of women's sexual function and dysfunction, members were becoming more open to the concept. Discussion and questions were the heart of the meeting, as the organization encompassed people of various disciplines with diverse areas of knowledge and expertise as well as varied opinions. The scientific program committee had each symposium span both the biologic and psychologic realms, in the basic science and the clinical arenas. Topics included further discussion on the role of androgens, vulvar vestibulitis syndrome, and sexual arousal, as well as a symposium on diabetes, multiple sclerosis, spinal cord injury, and female sexuality. A wide range of topics was discussed in the state-of-the-art lectures, symposia, podium, and moderated poster presentations. Both the membership and the board of directors were feeling their way with a new society in a new field, but there was a strong impetus to continue broadening knowledge with diversity of thought and research. ISSWSH was more than a name and a logo – it was a vibrant organization paving a path in a new direction (Figs 1.2.11 and 1.2.12).

In 2003, the organization finally left North America. ISSWSH met in Amsterdam under the leadership of Cindy Meston. The board discussion focused on the decrease in meeting attendance by Americans when the location moved to Europe. Irwin Goldstein was asked to chair a development committee to work with industry on long-term goals to help ISSWSH become financially stable, modeled on similar committees in sexual medicine societies. Sandra Leiblum, the chair of the affiliations committee, recommended that ISSWSH establish collaborative relationships when the benefit(s) to

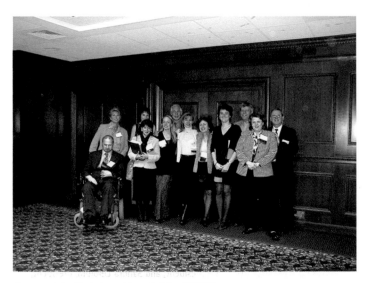

Figure 1.2.9. First elected board of the ISSWSH.

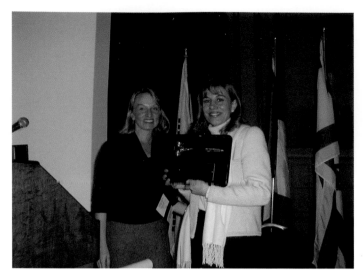

Figure 1.2.11. Incoming president Cindy Meston presenting outgoing president Alessandra Graziottin with a plaque commemorating her year as president of ISSWSH.

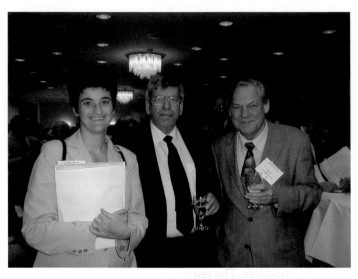

Figure 1.2.13. Annamaria Giraldi, Roy Levin, and Per Lundberg socializing in Amsterdam.

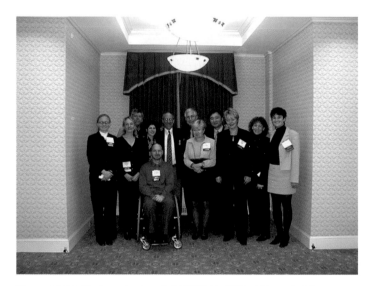

Figure 1.2.12. The incoming board of ISSWSH in 2002 at the end of the Vancouver meeting.

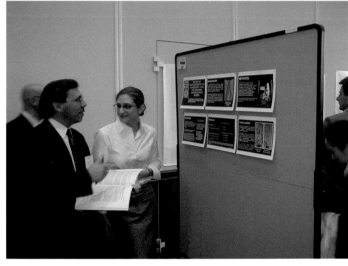

Figure 1.2.14. Lisa Scepkowski explaining her poster to Marc Gittelman in Amsterdam.

ISSWSH would be equal to or greater than the benefit(s) to the other organization. The board voted to become a member society of the World Association of Sexual Health (WAS).

At the 2003 meeting, symposia topics included desire, epidemiologic studies, neurologic aspects of FSD, and new ways of defining and researching FSD. Members heard fascinating state-of-the-art lectures on the necessity of estrogens as well as androgens for modulation of sexual function in women and on neuronal progestin receptors. In an effort to get significant numbers of registrants and appropriate industry support for future meetings, locations were discussed for meetings several years into the future (Figs 1.2.13 and 1.2.14).

Incoming president Lorraine Dennerstein initiated many new developments at the second board meeting in Amsterdam, including recruitment of young researchers to ISSWSH to grow the membership, a newsletter to be edited by Lori Brotto, and more focus on financial stability supported by the new development committee. The board heard a presentation from Wolf Utian regarding the inception and growth of the North American Menopause Society (NAMS), a possible model for ISSWSH. The board had the energy to strive for a stronger, more exciting year to come.

The 2004 annual meeting returned to North America, taking place in Atlanta, Georgia. ISSWSH collaborated with the National Institutes of Health (NIH), cosponsoring the meeting on "Vulvodynia and Sexual Pain Disorders in Women" held the day before. Many people attended both meetings, as their content was complementary rather than repetitive. In addition, several pharmaceutical companies chose to hold their advisory board meetings before and after the meeting, thus supporting ISSWSH and giving both increased visibility and credibility to the young society.

Prior to the opening of the meeting and concomitant with the meeting of the board of directors, a half-day precourse on the "Practical Management of Women's Sexual Dysfunction" from the psychologic and biologic points of view was offered for the first time, taught by the first and second presidents and first secretary of ISSWSH. This course was designed in response to the increasing demand for instruction in the "how to's" of diagnosis and treatment. The enrollment exceeded expectations, with 160 attendees. The response triggered the board's decision to develop a program of educational courses, with Irwin Goldstein as chair of the committee, including the precourse, practical courses running concurrently with the scientific sessions of the annual meeting, and free-standing courses at other locations and times of year (Fig. 1.2.15).

Symposia topics at the 2004 annual meeting included the old favorite, sex steroid hormones, the effect of illness and its treatment on FSD, reproductive concerns, and sexually transmitted diseases. The theme of the conference was sexuality in context, with broadened topics to increase attendance and interest in the society. There were approximately 350 people registered for the year's meeting – a significant increase from 2003. In addition to the traditional prize essays, a new award was named for a member of the board of directors who had passed away unexpectedly in August. The Björn Lundquist New Investigator Award was given for the first time, including a monetary prize, as part of an outreach initiative to encourage students and new researchers (Fig. 1.2.16). Posters were judged

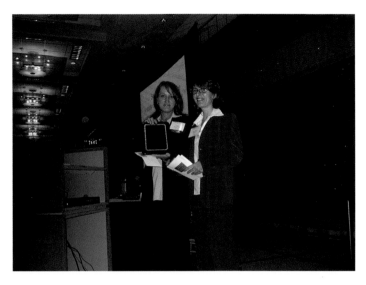

Figure 1.2.16. Board member Lori Brotto presenting the first Björn Lundquist New Investigator Award to Alessandra Rellini.

and authors awarded certificates in the areas of basic science in psychology, basic science in biology, clinical psychology, and clinical biology. The scientific quality of abstracts was significantly better than in the past, leading to an increased number of podium presentations.

The organization continues to grow as more and more investigators and practitioners become interested in the field of FSD. The list-serve, now under the watchful eye of Alan Altman, has become a much-needed and much-used resource by members around the world whose intellectual curiosity or practical needs require answers to questions at any given time. Members support members by offering opinions and advice. Members know that if they read one of the many entries by André Guay, for example, they will be given insight into androgen therapy by a respected source without having to leave their own offices. ISSWSH serves in this way not only as a force for unification of this multidisciplinary field, but also as a resource for dissemination of the material which we are discovering every day.

Conclusion

To offer optimum opportunities for members and nonmembers to question and learn about women's sexual health, ISSWSH will continue to make changes to the meeting format. The 2005 annual meeting will be held in Las Vegas, Nevada, under the leadership of ISSWSH's first male president, Stan Althof, and the 2006 meeting, moved from October to March, is scheduled for Lisbon, Portugal. In 2007, to commemorate the original Cape Cod conference 10 years ago, ISSWSH will return to the area. The annual meeting will continue to rotate from the North American East Coast, to the West Coast, to Europe until such time as the membership numbers can support its going to

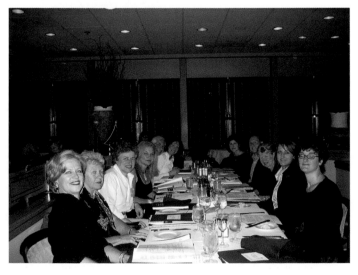

Figure 1.2.15. The board of ISSWSH in 2004 in Atlanta.

other continents. Fortunately for everyone, electronic communication brings the international membership together and shall remain a vital part of the organization.

The increased strength of abstract submission for each year's annual meeting is a result of increased knowledge in the field of women's sexual function and dysfunction. This directly reflects the increased interest, increased research, and increased sharing of information on sexual function and dysfunction in women that is the ultimate purpose of the ISSWSH. The organization may be young, but its membership is vibrant and focused on learning more about women's sexual health

References

1. Basson R, Berman J, Burnett A et al. Report of the International Consensus Development Conference on female sexual dysfunction: definitions and classifications. *J Urol* 2000; 163: 888–93.

2. Tiefer L. The "consensus" conference on female sexual dysfunction: conflicts of interest and hidden agendas. *J Sex Marital Ther* 2001; 27: 227–36.

3. Kaschak E, Tiefer L, eds. *A New View of Women's Sexual Problems*. New York: Haworth Press, 2001

Section 2

PSYCHOLOGIC & BIOLOGIC ETIOLOGIC FACTORS

EPIDEMIOLOGY OF FEMALE SEXUAL DYSFUNCTION

2.1 Prevalence of women's sexual problems in the USA

Anthony Paik, Edward O Laumann

Introduction

Since Kinsey's study of female sexuality,[1,2] the epidemiology of women's sexual problems, generally, and female sexual dysfunction, specifically, have attracted substantial professional interest and controversy. While the underlying reasoning for early epidemiologic studies rested on the paucity of prevalence estimates, the burgeoning literature of today is generating heated debate. Some promote prevalence estimates of women's sexual problems as identifying an underrecognized, public-health concern;[3] others critically assess these estimates as being flawed[4] or, more conspiratorially, intended for manufacturing new markets for pharmaceutic companies and clinicians.[5,6] Amid the din of scholarly recriminations, both factions share a fundamental assumption: they attach great significance to prevalence estimates, suggesting a need for reviewing how surveys have been used to define, measure, and report the prevalence of both female sexual dysfunction and female sexual problems. Understanding how surveys have been used to develop prevalence estimates can shed light not only on the methodological validity of prevalence estimates vis-à-vis one another, but also on the significance of these estimates for the wider culture.[7]

The purpose of this chapter is to provide an overview of epidemiologic studies reporting prevalence estimates of female sexual problems in the USA. This chapter is organized as follows. We first review epidemiologic concepts, focusing on issues of definition and classification, measurement, and study validity. Next, we report prevalence data of female sexual problems in the USA. We limit our discussion to prevalence estimates for general populations, which include representative samples or broadly representative clinical samples, such as those drawn from gynecologic or family-practice settings. Lastly, we conclude with a discussion of the methodological limitations of these epidemiologic studies and suggest future directions in this area.

The epidemiology of women's sexual problems

We draw on a number of concepts from psychiatric epidemiology in this review of the literature. One of the basic epidemiologic measures of outcome occurrence is *prevalence*, defined as the proportion of a population exhibiting a health condition during a specified time interval.[8] While prevalence can refer to any time period, researchers typically distinguish among point (current), period, and lifetime prevalence. However, given the importance of epidemiologic estimates of women's sexual problems, it is important to recognize that many factors of study design can affect estimated prevalence, making validity an important methodological concern.

An important, related conceptual issue is the definition of the health condition. Despite widespread usage of the term *sexual dysfunction* among epidemiologic studies, most of these studies rely not on clinical diagnosis of dysfunction, but on self-reports of symptoms of sexual problems. Thus, we use the term *sexual dysfunction* only when clinically diagnosed, regardless of the terminology used by the epidemiologic study. We use the term *sexual problem* to refer to reported symptoms, which reflects the latent population in which a subset exhibit manifest sexual dysfunction, but also recognize that many reported symptoms are not necessarily perceived subjectively as problematic or consistent with a dysfunction. Nevertheless, we apply the term *sexual problem* to reported symptoms, since it is not currently clear whether sexual problems should be exclusively defined by respondents.

The validity of prevalence estimates of women's sexual problems rests on two fundamental issues. The first deals with a general issue in epidemiology: a study's overall methodological quality, which can be assessed by various criteria indexing internal and external validity. According to Prins et al.,[9] *internal validity* refers to the quality of a study's design, which includes assessing data collection procedures, measurement instruments, definition of the health condition, and informativity of reported prevalence; *external validity* refers to the generalizability of a study, which is affected by the characteristics of the source population, sampling, eligibility criteria, and response rates.

The second issue focuses more specifically on the measurement of women's sexual problems, which includes topics of definition, classification, and the psychometric properties of measurement instruments. That is, researchers' decisions about theoretic concepts and the collection of this information via indicators are quite important for the validity of prevalence estimates. The first deals with the theoretic and conceptual models used. Prevalence studies typically adopt one of the prevailing definitional and classification systems for sexual dysfunctions, such as the American Psychiatric Association's *Diagnostic and Statistical Manual for Mental Disorders*, 4th edition (DSM-IV) or the World Health Organization's *International Classification of Diseases* (ICD-10). However, we note that there is considerable debate about the appropriateness of these definitions, as well as recent attempts to create international consensus about female sexual dysfunction.[10–12] Clearly, the type of definitions used will affect prevalence estimates of women's sexual problems.

Related to issues of definition and classification is the problem of measurement. Measurement instruments consist of questions, or items, which prompt respondents about symptoms. Sexual problems are assessed in surveys by various questions, in the form of *scales* or *schedules*.[13] Scales refer to a question or a set of questions (i.e., single vs multiple indicators), with response categories that can be dichotomous, ordered, or continuous, and that are designed to measure a dimension of a trait or domain. In general, the reliability of scales increases with more items. Other researchers use schedules that are designed to assess the presence or absence of a syndrome, such as a sexual dysfunction. Schedules are used to classify individuals as presenting a diagnostic category of a health condition such as a specific sexual dysfunction. The psychometric properties of scales and schedules – their *reliability* and *validity* – are an important concern. Reliability of measures refers to the reproducibility of results, while validity refers to the extent to which measurements reflect the theoretic concept of interest.[14]

An important measurement issue for prevalence estimates is the problem of *caseness*, which refers to the operationalized criteria, or case criteria, through which researchers designate the existence of a case that meets their theoretic definition of a sexual problem.[15] In general, highly restrictive criteria yield lower prevalence estimates and identify more severe cases; however, they may also exclude many individuals who are still being negatively affected by sexual problems.

Below, we apply these epidemiologic concepts in our review of prevalence studies of women's sexual problems in the USA. We focus on epidemiologic studies of sexual problems, sexual dysfunctions, sexual disorders, or sexual distress. We include studies, published from 1970 to June 2004, which estimated prevalence of one or more sexual problems for general populations in the USA. Thus, we exclude studies utilizing samples comprising only patients with specific health conditions, such as studies focusing on sexual problems among patients with diabetes, cancer, or surgical procedures, for example, or those studying patients at clinics for sexual problems. To increase our coverage, we did include studies relying on samples of women at gynecologic or family-practice clinics, but we focus most of our attention on those employing probability samples. We also exclude studies that lacked systematic sampling criteria, such as recruitment methods based on self-selected volunteers (e.g., responses to magazine advertisements).

We identified prevalence studies of women's sexual problems by two strategies. We first identified studies in reference lists from existing reviews of the literature.[16–20] We then searched MEDLINE (1966–Jun 2004) and PSYCHINFO (1974–Jun 2004), using the search terms *epidemiologic* or *prevalence* plus one of the following terms: *sexual dysfunction, sexual function disturbances, sex, disorder, psychosexual disorder, dyspareunia, vaginismus, anorgasm, vaginal dry, frigidity, sexual arousal, inhibited sexual desire, hypoactive sexual desire, sexual distress, sexual aversion, orgasmic disorder, inhibited female orgasm, or inhibited sexual desire.*

Prevalence studies of sexual problems among US women

Table 2.1.1 lists 15 studies, published in 1970–2004 that produced prevalence estimates of one or more sexual problems among US women in general populations. One paper is listed three times because it presents prevalence estimates from three separate data sets: two community studies and one national study.[22] There are currently four national data sets with some information about women's sexual problems. Two studies, which have representative samples of noninstitutionalized adults, data collected through in-person interviews, and high response rates, are the most generalizable.[23–25] The remaining two national studies are less able to be generalized because one[22] suffers from sample attrition in a longitudinal cohort, while the other[21] has a low response rate (53%) and includes only individuals who meet the following criteria: (1) English is the first language of the respondent, (2) the respondent has been in a heterosexual relationship for 6 months or more, and (3) the respondent is non-Hispanic white or non-Hispanic black.

Seven data sets are used to estimate prevalence for specific communities or regions in the USA. Four of these derive from communities included in the Epidemiologic Catchment Area Study, 1980–5.[22,29,30] The external validity of these studies also appears to be superior, with high response rates and the added

Table 2.1.1. Epidemiologic studies reporting the prevalence of women's sexual problems in the USA

Study	Mode of Sampling	Response Data	Sample administration	Age rate	Size	Range	Restrictions
National							
[21]Bancroft et al., 2003	Probability	Kinsey Institute Study, 1999–2000	Telephone	53%	987	20–65	English as first language; >= 6 months in a heterosexual relationship; white and black respondents only.
[22]Golding et al., 1998	Longitudinal cohort	National Study of Health and Life Experiences for Women, 1991	In-person interview	NA	963	21+	None reported.
[23]Klassen and Wilsnack, 1986	Probability	Drinking and problem drinking among women, 1981	In-person interview, SAQ	87%	917	21+	None reported.
[24, 25]Laumann et al., 1999	Probability	National Health and Social Life Survey, 1992	In-person interview	79%	1,511	18–59	Sexually active in last year.
Community							
[26]Diokno et al., 1990	Probability	Washtenaw County, MI	Clinical interview	65%	1,956	60+	None reported. Size includes men and women.
[27]Gold et al., 2000	Random plus snowball	Study of Women's Health across the Nation, 1995–7	Telephone and in-person	NA	16,065	40–55	None reported.
[22]Golding et al., 1998	Probability	Los Angeles ECA Study, 1980–5	In-person interview	68%	1,428	18+	None reported.
[22]Golding et al., 1998	Probability	North Carolina ECA Study, 1980–5	In-person interview	79%	1,703	18+	None reported.
[28]Johannes and Avis, 1997	Longitudinal cohort	Massachusetts Women's Health Study, 1988–89	In-person interview, SAQ	NA	360	51–62	Initial cohort (1982) was pre-menopause only.
[29]Johnson et al., 2004	Probability	St Louis ECA Study, 1981–2	In-person interview	87%	1,801	18–96	None reported.
[30]Samuels et al., 1994	Probability	Eastern Baltimore Mental Health Survey, 1981	Clinical interview	75%	810	18–64	Excluded persons with dementia or delirium.
Clinical							
[31]Bachmann et al., 1989	Consecutive intercept	Gynecologic clinic	Clinical interview	100%	887	12–78	None reported.
[32]Jamieson and Steege, 1996	Consecutive intercept	Five primary care practices, 1993	Self-completed	83%	581	18–45	Sexually active and menstruating.
[33]Levine and Yost, 1976	Random	Gynecology clinic at a medical center	In-person interview	79%	59	30–39	None reported.
[34]Nusbaum et al., 2000	Complete population	Routine gynecologic care at a medical center, 1992–3	Mail	65%	964	18–87	Excluded persons with cognitive dysfunction, poor English, and those unavailable for follow-up.
[35]Rosen et al., 1993	Unspecified	Outpatient gynecologic service at a medical center	Self-completed	NA	329	18–73	Respondents were in relationships or sexually active.
[36]Schein et al., 1988	Consecutive intercept	Primary care clinic	Self-completed	64%	148	18–78	Excludes acutely ill and new patients.

advantage of being explicitly designed for estimating prevalence of sexual dysfunctions and sexual problems based on *Diagnostic and Statistical Manual for Mental Disorders*, 3rd edition (DSM-III), criteria. In addition, there are three studies of middle-aged or older women, but all of these appear to have lower external validity for various reasons, including sample attrition in a longitudinal cohort,[28] nonrepresentative sampling procedures,[27] and high proportion of missing data.[26]

Finally, there are six studies based on clinical samples drawn from women attending gynecologic or family-practice clinics.[31-36] While these samples are not representative of a general population in a technical sense, they may reflect the prevalence of sexual problems among women seeking routine medical checkups, particularly gynecologic care. Nevertheless, we believe that these studies have the lowest external validity and tend to recruit women who are, on average, less healthy.

Below we review prevalence estimates, presented in Table 2.1.2, for the following sexual problems identified in the literature: problems with sexual desire and interest; problems with sexual arousal, which includes lubrication difficulties; problems with orgasm; problems with painful sex; and combined measures of sexual dysfunctions. Several studies also assessed several other sexual problems, typically associated with assessments about one's partnership, but we did not include this information in this review.

Problems with sexual desire/interest

We identified eight studies published since 1970 that reported estimates, ranging from 7% current to 31% lifetime prevalence, for problems with sexual desire or sexual interest. Population-based estimates of lifetime prevalence for problems with sexual desire/interest among adult women are 11% in a study using the Diagnostic Interview Schedule for DSM-III (DIS-III)[29] and 31% in a study using simple dichotomous measures to measure the proportion of women who have never been interested in or never enjoyed sex (5%) and those who experienced this problem after an initial period of enjoyable sex (26%).[23] The one clinic-based study reported a lifetime prevalence of concern about low sexual desire at 29%.[34] In contrast, a national survey of adult women, which also used a simple dichotomous measure, reported a 1-year prevalence for lack of interest in sex for several months to be 31%;[24] however, a latent structure model presented in the appendices of this paper, which was reported in detail elsewhere because of space limitations,[25] categorized 22% of women nationally as having low desire. In terms of current prevalence, a national study reported that 7% of women nationally had never thought about sex in the last month,[21] while clinic-based estimates were 10–21%.[31,32,36]

Variation in estimated period-specific prevalence appears to reflect differences in measurement and operational criteria.

Table 2.1.2. Prevalence of Women's Sexual Problems by Type and Prevalence Period

Study	Definition of Problem or Question	Response category	Criteria for problem designation	Overall Prevalence	Comments
Problems with Sexual Desire/Interest					
Prevalence - current-last 2 months					
[31]Bachmann et al., 1989	Problem/difficulty with desire	Open-ended	Positive response	21%	
[4]Bancroft et al., 2003	Frequency of thinking about sex in the last month	3-point scale	Never	7%	
[32]Jamieson and Steege, 1996	Currently experiencing less interest in sex	NA	NA	10%	
[36]Schein et al., 1988	Multiple items for sexual desire or libido	NA	NA	18%	14% of sample lack sexual desire with partner
Prevalence - last 3-12 months					
[24]Laumann et al., 1999	Lacked interest for several months last year	Dichotomous	Positive response	31%	
[25]Laumann et al., 2001	Low desire	Probabilistic	Latent structure modeling	22%	
Prevalence - ever					
[29]Johnson et al., 2004	Lack of pleasure with sex for several months and importance of sex	Dichotomous w/ probes	DIS for DSM-III criteria	11%	Excludes problems due to medical conditions or medication
[23]Klassen and Wilsnack, 1986	No interest or enjoyment ever	Dichotomous	Positive response	5%	Designated as a "primary" sexual dysfunction

Table 2.1.2. (Continued)

Study	Definition of Problem or Question	Response category	Criteria for problem designation	Overall Prevalence	Comments
[23]Klassen and Wilsnack, 1986	Initially enjoyable sex; no interest or enjoyment for two months or more ever	Dichotomous	Positive response	26%	Designated as a "secondary" sexual dysfunction
[34]Nusbaum et al., 2000	Sexual concerns about lack of interest	5-point scale	High frequency (unspecified)	29%	

Problems with Arousal/Lubrication

Prevalence – current-last 2 months

[31]Bachmann et al., 1989	Problem/difficulty with arousal, lubrication, or anxiety	Open-ended	Positive response	13%	
[4]Bancroft et al., 2003	Sum of three items measuring arousal in the last month	4-point scale	NA	12%	
[4]Bancroft et al., 2003	No lubrication or reported vaginal dryness during intercourse	Dichotomous	Positive response	31%	
[27]Gold et al., 2000	Vaginal dryness in the last 2 weeks	Dichotomous	Positive response	13%	
[32]Jamieson and Steege, 1996	Currently experiencing less pleasure with sex	NA	NA	2%	
[36]Schein et al., 1988	Multiple items for arousal problems with partner	NA	NA	50%	22% of sample have arousal problems during masturbation

Prevalence – last 3-12 months

[24]Laumann et al., 1999	Sex not pleasurable for several months last year	Dichotomous	Positive response	23%	
[24]Laumann et al., 1999	Trouble lubricating for several months last year	Dichotomous	Positive response	20%	
[25]Laumann et al., 2001	Arousal problems	Probabilistic	Latent structure modeling	14%	

Prevalence – ever

[29]Johnson et al., 2004	Trouble becoming aroused for 2 months or more	Dichotomous w/ probes	DIS for DSM-III criteria	4%	Excludes problems due to medical conditions or medication
[33]Levine and Yost, 1976	Problems with arousal	NA	NA	12%	
[34]Nusbaum et al., 2000	Sexual concerns about lubrication	5-point scale	High frequency (unspecified)	19%	
[35]Rosen et al., 1993	Lack of pleasure with sexual activity	5-point scale	50% of the time or more	20%	
[35]Rosen et al., 1993	Lack of lubrication	5-point scale	50% of the time or more	23%	

Orgasm Problems

Prevalence – current-last 2 months

[31]Bachmann et al., 1989	Problem/difficulty with anorgasmia	Open-ended	Positive response	4%	

Table 2.1.2. (Continued)

Study	Definition of Problem or Question	Response category	Criteria for problem designation	Overall Prevalence	Comments
[4]Bancroft et al., 2003	Frequency of orgasm in the last month	Count	NA	9%	
[32]Jamieson and Steege, 1996	Decreased frequency of orgasm	NA	NA	8%	
[36]Schein et al., 1988	Multiple items for orgasm problems with partner	NA	NA	18%	15% of sample have orgasm problems during masturbation
Prevalence - last 3-12 months					
[28]Johannes and Avis, 1997	Difficulty reaching orgasm during the last 6 months	5-point scale	More than 25% of the time	41%	
[24]Laumann et al., 1999	Inability to orgasm for several months last year	Dichotomous	Positive response	25%	
Prevalence - ever					
[29]Johnson et al., 2004	Bothered by inability to experience orgasm for several months	Dichotomous w/ probes	DIS for DSM-III criteria	16%	Excludes problems due to medical conditions or medication
[23]Klassen and Wilsnack, 1986	No orgasms ever with partner	Dichotomous	Positive response	5%	Designated as a "primary" sexual dysfunction
[23]Klassen and Wilsnack, 1986	Initially able to orgasm; inability to orgasm for two months or more ever	Dichotomous	Positive response	18%	Designated as a "secondary" sexual dysfunction
[23]Klassen and Wilsnack, 1986	Reaching orgasm	6-point scale	25% of the time or less	25%	
[33]Levine and Yost, 1976	Inability to achieve orgasms	NA	NA	5%	
[34]Nusbaum et al., 2000	Sexual concerns about orgasm difficulties	5-point scale	High frequency (unspecified)	26%	
[35]Rosen et al., 1993	Difficulty reaching orgasm	5-point scale	50% of the time or more	30%	
Problems with Pain during/after Sex					
Prevalence - current-last 2 months					
[31]Bachmann et al., 1989	Problem/difficulty with pain during sex	Open-ended	Positive response	48%	
[4]Bancroft et al., 2003	Pain during sex 50% of the time or more in the last month	Dichotomous	Positive response	3%	
[26]Diokno et al., 1990	Pain with intercourse	Dichotomous	Positive response	13%	Only $n = 164$
[32]Jamieson and Steege, 1996	Currently experiencing pain during/after sex	4-point scale	NA	45%	
[36]Schein et al., 1988	Multiple items for dyspareunia	NA	NA	21%	
Prevalence - last 3-12 months					
[28]Johannes and Avis, 1997	Pain during the last 6 months	5-point scale	More than 25% of the time	13%	
[24]Laumann et al., 1999	Pain during sex for several months last year	Dichotomous	Positive response	15%	

Table 2.1.2. (Continued)

Study	Definition of Problem or Question	Response category	Criteria for problem designation	Overall Prevalence	Comments
[25]Laumann et al., 2001	Pain	Probabilistic	Latent structure modeling	7%	
Prevalence - ever					
[32]Jamieson and Steege, 1996	Pain for more than 1 year duration	NA	NA	20%	
[29]Johnson et al., 2004	Sexual relations ever physically painful	Dichotomous w/ probes	DIS for DSM-III criteria	19%	Excludes problems due to medical conditions or medication
[23]Klassen and Wilsnack, 1986	Sexual relations have been sometimes so painful to prevent intercourse	Dichotomous	Positive response	17%	Designated as a "primary" sexual dysfunction
[23]Klassen and Wilsnack, 1986	Sexual relations sometimes physically painful	Dichotomous	Positive response	36%	Designated as a "secondary" sexual dysfunction
[34]Nusbaum et al., 2000	Sexual concerns about dyspareunia	5-point scale	High frequency (unspecified)	10%	
[35]Rosen et al., 1993	Painful intercourse	5-point scale	50% of the time or more	11%	

Other problems

Prevalence - current-last 2 months

Study	Definition of Problem or Question	Response category	Criteria for problem designation	Overall Prevalence	Comments
[31]Bachmann et al., 1989	Problem/difficulty with vaginismus	Open-ended	Positive response	6%	
[4]Bancroft et al., 2003	Distress about sexuality in the last 4 weeks	4-point scale	Moderate and a great deal	15%	
[36]Schein et al., 1988	Multiple items for being frightened about sex	NA	NA	4%	

Prevalence - last 3-12 months

Study	Definition of Problem or Question	Response category	Criteria for problem designation	Overall Prevalence	Comments
[24]Laumann et al., 1999	Anxiety about performance for several months last year	Dichotomous	Positive response	12%	

Prevalence - ever

Study	Definition of Problem or Question	Response category	Criteria for problem designation	Overall Prevalence	Comments
[35]Rosen et al., 1993	Anxiety or inhibition with sexual activity	5-point scale	50% of the time or more	23%	
[35]Rosen et al., 1993	Vaginismus	5-point scale	50% of the time or more	12%	

Combined measures of sexual problems

Prevalence - current-last 2 months

Study	Definition of Problem or Question	Response category	Criteria for problem designation	Overall Prevalence	Comments
[4]Bancroft et al., 2003	Interest, arousal, lubrication, orgasm, or pain	Dichotomous	One or more	45%	
[32]Jamieson and Steege, 1996	Decreased orgasm, pleasure, interest, or frequency	NA	One or more	22%	
[30]Samuels et al., 1981	Any sexual dysfunction - DSM-III	Psychiatric examination	Clinical diagnosis	3%	No gender-specific prevalence

Table 2.1.1. (Continued)

Study	Definition of Problem or Question	Response category	Criteria for problem designation	Overall Prevalence	Comments
Prevalence - ever					
[29]Johnson et al., 2004	Desire, arousal, orgasm or pain ever	Dichotomous w/ probes	One or more	33%	Excludes problems due to medical conditions or medication
[23]Klassen and Wilsnack, 1986	Desire, orgasm, or vaginismus	Cumulative score (0-3)	One or more	35%	Designated as "primary" sexual dysfunctions
[22]Golding et al., 1998	Pain or sex not pleasurable for several months ever	Dichotomous	One or more	28%	LA-ECA
[22]Golding et al., 1998	Pain or sex not pleasurable for several months ever	Dichotomous	One or more	18%	NC-ECA
[22]Golding et al., 1998	Pain or no interest in sex ever	Dichotomous	One or more	56%	NSHLEW

NA = not available; LA-ECA = Los Angeles Epidemiological Catchment Area; NC-ECA = North Caroline Epidemiological Catchment Area; NSHLEW = National Study of Health and Life Experiences in Women

Studies employing single items with dichotomous response categories,[23,24] as opposed to gradated scales or multiple measures, tended to generate the largest prevalence estimates. Similarly, clinic-based estimates were generally higher than those reported in population-based studies. In terms of operational criteria, most of these studies use researcher-defined criteria for designating sexual problems and did not report asking whether respondents perceived these symptoms or conditions as problems. Only two studies used multiple questions to designate caseness: one study used the Diagnostic Interview Schedule III algorithms, which were specifically designed to estimate prevalence of inhibited sexual desire as defined by DSM-III,[29] while the other used a latent structure model fitted to actual response patterns.[25] These two studies are not only highly generalizable, but also offer superior measures for psychometric properties, suggesting that 11–22% of adult women nationally experienced difficulties or problems with sexual desire for several months. Overall, 5% of women nationally have never been interested in sex, and 11–22% have had low desire for several months. Nevertheless, there appears to be a need for scales or schedules that include fine-grained response options, multiple items, and assessment of whether respondents' view a reported symptom of low desire as problematic.

Problems with sexual arousal, including lubrication difficulties

Ten studies reported prevalence estimates for problems with excitement, lubrication difficulties, or arousal in general. Prevalence estimates for problems with excitement or pleasure are 2% currently,[32] a 1-year prevalence of 23%,[24] and a lifetime prevalence of 20%.[35] For lubrication difficulties or vaginal dryness, prevalence estimates are 13–31% currently,[21,27] a 1-year prevalence of 20%,[24] and a lifetime prevalence of 19–23%.[34,35] Unfortunately, there are no population-based estimates of life-

time prevalence for either problems with excitement/pleasure or lubrication difficulties/vaginal dryness.

Several studies reported prevalence estimates for arousal problems in general, which were all tapped with multiple items. In terms of lifetime prevalence, a community study, which used the DIS-III, estimated 4% prevalence of difficulty in becoming aroused for 2 months or more.[29] In contrast, a national study reported a 1-year prevalence of 14% for arousal problems among women.[25] Another national study reported that 12% of women were currently experiencing arousal problems,[21] while clinic-based estimates were 12–50%.[31,33,36]

Prevalence estimates for arousal problems are also limited in several ways. Most researchers use varying definitions to tap arousal problems. Moreover, single-item measures of specific symptoms, such as lubrication difficulties or vaginal dryness, tend to be more liberal than multiple-indicator assessments of arousal problems. Among the three population-based studies assessing arousal problems, measurement strategies vary: one study employed a simple count procedure with no reported psychometric properties;[21] not surprisingly, the constructed arousal measure had no concurrent validity. Alternatively, the other two studies used the DIS-III[29] and a concurrently validated, latent-structure modeling approach,[25] respectively, suggesting that the prevalence of arousal problems among US women runs from 4%, based on DSM-III criteria, to 14% more generally.

Problems with infrequent orgasms

Eleven studies reported prevalence figures for infrequent orgasm or difficulty in reaching orgasm in the range 4–41%. In terms of lifetime prevalence, one population-based study, using DSM-III criteria, estimated that 16% of women were bothered by inability to experience orgasm for several months,[29] while another reported that 5% of women nationally have never had an orgasm; another 18% had this problem for 2 months or more, and 25% had trouble reaching orgasm more than 50% of the time.[23] Three clinical studies reported estimates of 5% for inability to reach orgasm,[33] 26% for concern about orgasm difficulty,[34] and 30% for difficulty in reaching orgasm more than 50% of the time.[35] Similarly, another national study estimated a 1-year prevalence of 25% for reported inability to orgasm for several months.[24] In contrast, a community study reported a 1-year prevalence of 41% for orgasm problems,[28] but this high estimate appears to reflect the narrow age range of older women (ages 51–62) included in this study. For current prevalence, a national study estimated orgasm problems among 9% of women,[21] while clinic-based studies ranged from 4% to 18%.[31,32,36]

In general, definition, measurement, and operational criteria of orgasm problems across these studies were quite heterogeneous. Some researchers assessed orgasm problems by asking about the frequency of orgasm and used ordered scales for response categories; others assessed the presence of orgasm problems with dichotomous measures. However, none of these studies appear to have investigated whether respondents viewed reported inability to orgasm as problematic. Only one population-based study used multiple items from the DIS-III to designate the presence of orgasm problems;[29] thus, its estimate of 16% appears to be the best available. Another study also generated an important baseline estimate: 5% of women nationally have never had an orgasm.[23]

Problems with pain during/after sex

Eleven studies reported prevalence estimates of 3–48% for pain during or after sex. Lifetime estimates from population-based studies were 17% and 19%,[9,23] while clinic-based studies reported prevalence of 10–20%.[32,34,35] Six-month prevalence was reported as 13%,[28] while another study reporting 1-year prevalence found that 15% of women reported pain during sex for several months,[24] but classified only 7% by the study's latent structure model.[25] In terms of current prevalence, two population-based studies reported estimates of 3% and 13%,[21,26] while estimates from clinic-based studies were much higher at 21–48%.[31,32,36]

Variation in reported estimates appears to reflect methodological differences. Studies using single-item indicators generated higher prevalence estimates; moreover, dichotomous indicators appear to yield higher estimates than ordered scales. In terms of operational criteria, most of these studies again used researcher-defined criteria. Two population-based studies with high external validity did use multiple measures to designate caseness: one study used the DIS-III and produced an estimated prevalence of 19%,[29] while the other used a latent structure model that classified 7% of women as having pain with sex.[25] Thus, these two estimates suggest a range of 7–19% for pain with sex.

Overall prevalence of sexual problems

Several studies reported prevalence estimates for other sexual problems, such as anxiety about sex or vaginismus, and for combined measures of female sexual problems; we focus on the latter in this section. One study analyzed three different probability samples[22] and reported lifetime prevalence estimates of 18% and 28% for pain during sex or nonpleasurable sex, and 56% for pain during sex or lack of interest in sex. Two population-based surveys, using similar instruments, estimated that 33%[29] and 35%[23] of women have experienced a problem with desire, arousal, orgasm, or pain. One national study estimated a 1-month prevalence of 45% for experiencing a current sexual problem;[29] however, this study reported no concurrent validity in their measures of sexual problems. Nevertheless, it is important to remember that these proportions reflect the percentage of women reporting symptoms. It is not clear whether women view these symptoms as problematic, or, more importantly, whether a trained clinician would view these symptoms as dysfunctional. Indeed, one population-based study that incorporated a psychiatric examination in its study design found that only 3% of men and women had a clinically diagnosed sexual dysfunction,[30] by DSM-III criteria, suggesting that roughly 1 in 10 cases of reported sexual problems actually exhibits female sexual dysfunction. However, it would be misleading to assume that those cases of sexual problems that do not meet the criteria for female sexual dysfunction are not problematic.

Finally, these combined measures raise the issue of copresence of symptoms. An important epidemiologic question centers on the extent to which reported symptoms are copresent. Only one study reports the extent to which symptoms are copresent.[25] This study reported an oft-cited prevalence of 43% for sexual problems among adult women; however, this statistic actually represents the size of three classes, low desire (22%), arousal problems (14%), and pain (7%), which are constituted by patterns of copresent symptoms. Future research should be devoted to investigating these patterns by more fine-grained measures than simple dichotomous indicators.

Conclusion

We reviewed 15 studies of general populations reporting prevalence estimates of sexual problems among adult women in the USA. Studies with high internal and external validity presented estimates of 5–22% for problems with sexual desire, 4–14% for problems with arousal, 5–16% for orgasm problems, and 7–19% for problems with painful sex. In general, these estimates are approximately the same or slightly higher than prevalence estimates reported in several population-based studies of northern European women, which were 5–16% for low desire, 6–8% for arousal problems, 4–10% for orgasm problems, and 3–18% for sexual pain.[18] Our review also identified four studies, which have not been listed in prior reviews, reporting prevalence estimates based on epidemiologic catchment area data, which was collected with the DIS-III as well as through clinical examination.

However, we strongly emphasize that reported sexual problems in almost all epidemiologic studies do not connote clinical diagnosis of female sexual dysfunction. As we mentioned above, one population-based study, which did not report gender-specific prevalence but did use clinical diagnosis, found an overall prevalence of 3% for any sexual dysfunction in the general population as defined by DSM-III criteria. Thus, most epidemiologic results should be viewed as the latent population of women with sexual problems in which a subset exhibits manifest female sexual dysfunction. Nevertheless, there is still an association between certain sexual problems and negative health outcomes when the former are specified carefully.

Continuing methodological heterogeneity appears to be producing wide variation in estimates. First, there appears to be a strong need for consistent definitions of sexual problems, an issue that continues to produce disagreement despite attempts to produce an international consensus.[10–12] Important omissions in many studies' definitions of sexual problems are assessments of whether the respondent views a particular symptom as a problem and whether a symptoms is recurrent or frequent. Second, there is a widespread use of measures with unknown psychometric properties. Standardization in schedules and scales as well as use of multiple items would certainly increase the validity of these measures. Researchers also need to demonstrate that their measures of sexual problems have concurrent validity.

Finally, several issues require increased attention. Further investigation needs to be done on the copresence of symptoms. Moreover, researchers should devote more attention to relational contexts when assessing sexual problems. Many studies assessed the prevalence of problems with desire, arousal, orgasm, and pain without investigating the nature of the corresponding sexual relationships. Thus, overall, as demand for epidemiologic analyses has increased in recent years, our review has shown that many prevalence studies of women's sexual problems are limited by methodological and substantive issues.

References

1. Kinsey AC, Pomeroy WB, Martin C et al. *Sexual Behavior in the Human Female*. Philadelphia: WB Saunders, 1953.
2. Gebhard PH, Johnson AB. *The Kinsey Data: Marginal Tabulations of the 1938–1963 Interviews Conducted by the Institute for Sex Research*. Philadelphia: WB Saunders, 1979.
3. Rosen RC. Female sexual dysfunction: industry creation or under-recognized problem? *BJU Int* 2003; 93: 3–4.
4. Bancroft J, Loftus, J, Long JS. Distress about sex: a national survey of women in heterosexual relationships. *Arch Sex Behav* 2003; 32: 193–208.
5. Moynihan R. The making of a disease: female sexual dysfunction. *BMJ* 2003; 326: 45–47.
6. Tiefer L. The selling of "female sexual dysfunction". *J Sex Marital Ther* 2001; 27: 625–8.
7. Ericksen JA. *Kiss and Tell: Surveying Sex in the Twentieth Century*. Cambridge, MA: Harvard University Press, 1999.
8. Kramer M. A discussion of the concepts of incidence and prevalence as related to epidemiological studies of mental disorders. *Am J Public Health* 1957; 47: 826–40.
9. Prins J, Blanker MH, Bohnen AM et al. Prevalence of erectile dysfunction: a systematic review of population based studies. *Int J Impot Res* 2002; 14: 422–32.
10. Basson R, Berman J, Burnett A et al. Report of the International Consensus Development Conference on Female Sexual Dysfunction: definitions and classification. *J Sex Marital Ther* 2001; 27: 83–94.
11. Tiefer L. The "consensus" conference on female sexual dysfunction: conflicts of interest and hidden agendas. *J Sex Marital Ther* 2001; 27: 227–36.
12. Bancroft J, Graham CA, McCord C. Conceptualizing women's sexual problems. *J Sex Marital Ther* 2001; 27: 95–103.
13. Murphy JM. Symptom scales and diagnostic schedules in adult psychiatry. In MT Tsuang, M Tohen, eds. *Textbook in Psychiatric Epidemiology*, 2nd edn. New York: Wiley, 2002: 273–332.
14. Goldstein JM, Simpson JC. Validity: Definitions and Applications to Psychiatric Research. In MT Tsuang, M Tohen, eds. *Textbook in Psychiatric Epidemiology*, 2nd edn. New York: Wiley, 2002: 149–63.
15. Prince M. Measurement in psychiatry. In M Prince, R Stewart, F Tasmin et al., eds. *Practical Psychiatric Epidemiology*. Oxford: Oxford University Press, 2003: 13–41.
16. Nathan SG. The epidemiology of the DSM-III psychosexual dysfunctions. *J Sex Marital Ther* 1986; 12: 267–81.
17. Spector IP, Carey MP. Incidence and prevalence of the sexual dysfunctions: a critical review of the empirical literature. *Arch Sex Behav* 1990; 19: 389–408.
18. Simons JS, Carey MP. Prevalence of sexual dysfunctions: results from a decade of research. *Arch Sex Behav* 2001; 30: 177–219.
19. Dunn KM, Jordan K, Croft PR et al. Systematic review of sexual problems: epidemiology and methodology. *J Sex Marital Ther* 2002; 28: 399–422.
20. Lewis RW, Fugl-Meyer KS, Bosch R et al. Definitions, classification, and epidemiology of sexual dysfunction. In RC Rosen et al., eds. *Sexual Dysfunctions: Second International Consultation on Sexual Dysfunction*. London: Health Productions, 2004: 3–37.
21. Bancroft J, Loftus, J, Long JS. Distress about sex: a national survey of women in heterosexual relationships. *Arch Sex Behav* 2003; 32: 193–208.
22. Golding JM, Wilsnack SC, Learman LA. Prevalence of sexual assault history among women with common gynecologic symptoms. *Am J Obstet Gynecol* 1998; 179: 1013–19.
23. Klassen AD, Wilsnack SC. Sexual experience and drinking among women in a US national survey. *Arch Sex Behav* 1986; 15: 363–92.
24. Laumann EO, Paik A, Rosen RC. Sexual dysfunction in the United States: prevalence and predictors. *JAMA* 1999; 281: 537–44.
25. Laumann EO, Paik A, Rosen RC. Sexual dysfunction in the United States: prevalence and predictors. In EO Laumann, RT Michael, eds. *Sex, Love, and Health in America: Private Choices and Public Policies*. Chicago: University of Chicago Press, 2001.
26. Diokno AC, Brown MB, Herzog AR. Sexual function in the elderly. *Arch Intern Med* 1990; 150: 197–200.

27. Gold EB, Sternfeld B, Kelsey JL et al. Relation of demographic and lifestyle factors to symptoms in a multi-racial/ethnic population of women 40–55 years of age. *Am J Epidemiol* 2000; 152: 463–73.

28. Johannes Cb, Avis NE. Gender differences in sexual activity among mid-aged adults in Massachusetts. *Maturitas* 1997; 26: 175–84.

29. Johnson SD, Phelps DL, Cottler LB. The association of sexual dysfunction and substance use among a community epidemiological sample. *Arch Sex Behav* 2004; 33: 55–63.

30. Samuels JF, Nestadt G, Romanoski AJ et al. DSM-III personality disorders in the community. *Am J Psychiatry* 1994; 151: 1055–62.

31. Bachmann GA, Leiblum SR, Grill J. Brief sexual inquiry in gynecologic practice. *Obstet Gynecol* 1989; 73: 425–7.

32. Jamieson DJ, Steege JF. The prevalence of dysmenorrhea, dyspareunia, pelvic pain, and irritable bowel syndrome in primary care practices. *Obstet Gynecol* 1996; 87: 55–8.

33. Levine SB, Yost MA. Frequency of sexual dysfunction in a general gynecological clinic: an epidemiological approach. *Arch Sex Behav* 1976; 5: 229–38.

34. Nusbaum MRH, Gamble G, Skinner B et al. The high prevalence of sexual concerns among women seeking routine gynecological care. *J Fam Pract* 2000; 49: 229–32.

35. Rosen RC, Taylor JF, Leiblum SR et al. Prevalence of sexual dysfunction in women: results of a survey study of 329 women in an outpatient gynecological clinic. *J Sex Marital Ther* 1993; 19: 171–88.

36. Schein M, Zyzanski SJ, Levine S et al. The frequency of sexual problems among family practice patients. *Fam Pract Res J* 1988, 7: 122–34.

2.2 Prevalence data in Europe

Axel R Fugl-Meyer, Kerstin S Fugl-Meyer

This chapter is intended to provide an up-to-date, evidence-based overview of the European epidemiology of female sexual dysfunction since the mid-1980s. Descriptive and analytic female sexual dysfunction literature was identified through searching conventional databases, books, literature surveys[1-3] and references. The literature was evaluated for validity with the 15-item (scores: yes – 1; no – 0; maximum 15) checklist suggested by Prins et al.[4] Our criterion for inclusion in this chapter was a score of at least 8. In the text, Prins (P) scores are given in parentheses. Table 2.2.1 should give the reader pertinent characteristics of the majority of the selected descriptive epidemiologic studies. Four are from the UK,[5-11] four from the Nordic countries,[12-18] one from France,[19,20] one from Germany,[21] and one a recent multicountry investigation.[22]

One must first ask an ontologic question: are there female sexual dysfunctions? In Europe, it has been suggested that female sexual dysfunction is an invention which, through medicalization, paves the road for drug companies.[23,24] We think that this suggestion is a caricature. However, several indices for

classifying female and male sexual dysfunctions appear rather tailor-made for certain clinical trials. Quite clearly, adherence solely to a biologic model of women's sexual response imposes physiologic restrictions on definitions. It has been suggested that female sexual dysfunction may best be conceptualized as a global inhibition of sexual response due to intrapersonal factors,[25] because many cases of female sexual dysfunction can be regarded as adaptations to sexual relationship problems.[26] In other words, female sexual dysfunction must be seen in a multifaceted socio-psycho-biologic context.

Widely different definitions, mostly following the very medicalized International Classification of Impairments, Disabilities, and Handicaps (ICIDH)[27] or the *Diagnostic and Statistical Manual of Mental Disorders*, third and fourth editions (DSM-III or -IV),[28] make valid comparisons of different investigations difficult. In fact, Dunn et al.[3] found that meta-analyses are currently meaningless to perform. Another problem is the scaling of the severity of sexual dysfunctions. While some investigators use the dichotomy of dysfunction versus no dysfunction,

Table 2.2.1. Some methodological details of reasonably valid European descriptive epidemiologic investigations of female sexual dysfunction

Country and ref	Method I/T/Q R/N Scale steps	Performed/ published	Time frame	Age (years)	Respondent (response rate)	Validity (Prins score)
UK[5]	I, R, 5	NG/1988	1 year	35-59	436 (72%)	12
UK[6]	I, R, 2	1993/1997	2 years	>55	2011 (61%)	10
UK[7-9]	Q, NG, 2	1996/1998-2000	Current	18-75	657 (33%)	10
UK[10,11]	T, N, 2	1999-2001/2003	1 or 6 months last year	16-44	NG (65%)	12
France[19,20]	T, N, 4	1991-2/1998	Lifelong	18-69	1137 (70%)	11
Germany[21]	I, R, 2	2002/2004	1 year	30, 45, 60	278/(?)	9
Iceland[13]	I, N, 2	1987-8/1993	Lifelong	55, 57	417 (75%)	14
Denmark[14]	Q, N	NG/1998	Current	18-88	686 (55%)	8
Sweden[12,15-17]	I, N, 6	1996/9-2004	1 year	18-74	1335 (59%)	14
Finland[18]	I, N, 6	1992/1995	1 year	18-74	1146 (78%)	13
Northern Europe[22]	T, N, 4	NG/2004	At least 2 months last year	40-80	1741 (?)	9
Southern Europe[22]	T, N, 4	NG/2004	At least 2 months last year	40-80	1753 (?)	9

I: person-to-person interview; N: nationally representative; NG: representativity not given; Q: mailed questionnaire; R: regionally representative; T: telephone interview.

others use scales with 3–6 gradations, which then may be reduced to 2–4 classes of function/dysfunction. A further problem is the different age strata studied, and even the time-frames for the dysfunctions vary from lifetime, through parts or periods of 1 year to the current situation. It is hardly surprising, therefore, that an international committee[29] recently recommended international consensus on definitions and classification of sexual dysfunction.

Prevalence

The prevalence of female sexual dysfunction in Europe, as reported in reasonably valid descriptive investigations, can be seen in Table 2.2.2, where, as far as possible, the definitions of Basson et al.[30] are followed. For some (total) populations, it has been possible to classify different female sexual dysfunctions as manifest (occurring at least quite often) or mild (occurring sporadically) as suggested elsewhere.[17,29] The authors are, however, aware of the three-grade (mild, moderate, or severe) classification developed in the USA.

Sexual interest/desire

It must first be emphasized that sexual desire cannot readily be distinguished as an entity, as desire and the psychologic aspects of sexual arousal are confluent. Table 2.2.2 shows that a manifestly low level of sexual interest prevails in 10–51% of subjects. The use of different age strata is problematic in comparing the data on low sexual interest. In several countries, there is a clear decline in sexual interest at or above the age of 60. One example of the impact of different time frames was found by Mercer et al.,[11] who, when studying relatively younger women, found that a 6-month prevalence of 10% increased to 41% when the question covered a 1-month period during the past year.

The German[21] prevalence of low sexual interest appears exceedingly high, increasing from about 40–50% in 30- and 45-year-old women to 86% by the age of 60. On the other hand, in Sweden[17] (1-year time frame), 54% reported mild dysfunction in sexual interest in addition to the 33% with manifest dysfunction.

The reader can also find large variation in dysfunction of sexual desire, sometimes, unfortunately, labeled "libido", ranging from a maximum, age-dependent 35% (1 year) prevalence in Finland to 8% (lifetime) in France, where 55% reported mild desire dysfunction. In a Nordic country, the ratio desire/interest (Table 2.2.2) was about 0.3–0.4 for the age span 18–49, increasing to 0.8–0.9 for those age 50 and above. This indicates that at least up to a relatively advanced age, the dysfunctions of sexual interest and desire are, to some extent, separate entities.

Arousal/lubrication

We have found no study that distinctly separates genital from psychologic arousal or explicitly combines these. In Icelandic women in their mid-50s, low level of (lifetime) sexual excitation was reported by as little as 6%, as defined by DSM-III, while Dunn et al.[7] found that 17% of their 18–75-year-old British women currently had arousal dysfunction.

Insufficient lubrication generally appears to occur in about 10–15% of adult European women, peaking around levels of 25–35% after the age of 50. Additionally, nearly half of Swedish women aged 18–74 years have mild lubrication dysfunction. In a regional Nordic questionnaire study, however, investigating the prevalence of genitourinary and other climacteric symptoms in 61-year-old women (P:10), Stenberg et al.[31] found that 43% had "trouble with" vaginal dryness.

Orgasm

Even the prevalence of manifest orgasmic dysfunction varies quite considerably within and between different geographic areas, and may or may not be age dependent. While the overall prevalence of orgasmic dysfunction occurring frequently or periodically in an area labeled "northern Europe" (i.e., Austria, Belgium, Germany, Sweden, and the UK) has been found to be 10%, it has been reported in "southern Europe" (i.e., France, Italy, and Spain as well as Israel) to be 17%.[22] In one regional British investigation,[5] 16% of 35–59-year-old women had orgasmic dysfunction, ranging from 5% in those aged 35–39 to 35% in 55–59-year-olds. In another report from that investigation[32] covering the same 3-month period, however, clearly higher age-dependent results emerged, the overall prevalence being 38% (range 19–68%). In addition, 45% of the total sample achieved orgasm in half or less of their sexual intercourse encounters, classified here as mild dysfunction. The percentages of mild dysfunction in France (lifetime) and Sweden (12 months) were 44% and 60%, respectively, yielding totals of orgasmic dysfunction of 82% in the Swedish and 55% in the French women. The prevalence of manifest orgasmic dysfunction reported by Hawton et al.[32] is overshadowed only by that in the German[21] regional investigation.

While the (lifetime) prevalence of manifest dysfunction in France and the UK is approximately the same rate as that found in the pan-European investigation,[22] higher 1-year prevalence has been ascertained (age independent) in 17–29% of Swedish and British women.[7] Anorgasmia, one category of orgasmic dysfunction, was found to have a prevalence of less than 10% in Iceland and Denmark. Hence, the prevalence of orgasmic dysfunction appears to vary so widely that at the moment there is no conclusive evidence. In a small but extremely well-defined (P:14), regionally representative investigation of women in Denmark, Eplov[33] found that 33% of women at the age of 40 had a relatively low level of desire. Twenty years later at age 60, this was the case for 37%. At this time, 50% reported no change in desire, while more frequent or less frequent desire was reported by 25%, respectively. At age 40 and again 20 years later, 16% rarely or never experienced orgasm. Even mild orgasmic dysfunction was similar at ages 40 and 60 (65% and 69%, respectively).

Table 2.2.2. Prevalence of manifest female sexual dysfunction as reported in valid descriptive epidemiologic European investigations. When possible, prevalence of mild (sporadically occurring) dysfunctions for total samples are given (in parentheses)

Country	Age cohorts	Interest (I) Desire (D) MaD (MiD)	Lubrication MaD (MiD)	Orgasm MaD (MiD)	Dysparuenia MaD (MiD)	Sexually satisfied
UK[5]	35–59	I. 17%	17%	16%	8%	–
	35–39	4%	8%	5%	0%	–
	40–44	8%	12%	8%	1%	–
	45–49	16%	16%	14%	9%	–
	50–54	29%	26%	22%	17%	–
	55–59	28%	22%	35%	17%	–
UK[6]	55–84	–	8%	–	2%	–
	55–64	–	11%	–	3%	–
	65–74	–	7%	–	1%	–
	75–84	–	7%	–	< 0.5%	–
UK[7–9]	18–75	–	28%	27%	18%	75%
UK[10,11]	16–44	I: 10%[a]	3%	4%*	–	–
		41%[b]	9%	14%*		
France[19,20]	18–69	D: 8% (55%)	–	11% (44%)	5% (43%)	48%
Germany[21]	30, 45, 60	I: 51%	–	38%	14%	32%
	30	50%	–	38%	16%	–
	45	42%	–	33%	8%	–
	60	86%	–	61%	26%	–
Iceland[13]	55, 57	D: 16%	–	4%*	3%	–
Denmark[14]	18–88	D: 11%	–	7%*	3%	67%
	18, 23	6%	–	11%	3%	65%
	28, 33	13%	–	9%	4%	55%
	38, 43	17%	–	7%	4%	68%
	48, 53	14%	–	6%	5%	67%
	58–88	10%	–	3%	1%	63%
Sweden[12,15–17]	18–74	I: 33% (54%) D: 14%	13% (49%)	22% (60%)	6% (33%)	56%
	18–24	I: 21% D: 8%	11%	27%	6%	59%
	25–34	I: 37% D: 11%	10%	24%	6%	60%
	35–49	I: 29% D: 8%	6%	17%	4%	57%
	50–65	I: 41% D: 32%	24%	22%	8%	52%
	66–74	I: 47% D: 44%	26%	19%	12%	47%
Finland[18]	18–74	D: 35%	15%	–	7%	83%
	18–24	15%	8%	–	9%	–
	25–34	26%	10%	–	5%	–
	35–44	21%	9%	–	1%	–
	45–54	29%	16%	–	4%	–
	55–64	51%	35%	–	19%	–
	65–74	55%	34%	–	27%	–
Northern Europe[22]	40–80	I: 17%	13%	10%	6%	–
Southern Europe[22]	40–80	I: 21%	12%	17%	9%	

MaD: manifest dysfunction; MiD: mild dysfunction. (a) denotes 6-month and (b) 1-month prevalence; * denotes anorgasmia

Dyspareunia

Manifest genital pain at intercourse is also reported by a large range of women. In the UK (Table 2.2.2), two investigations have found the overall prevalence to be less than 10%. This is reasonably consistent with most European epidemiologic studies. In a well-defined, subarctic sample (P:12) of 3024 women aged 20–60, Danielsson et al.[34] found the prevalence of manifest dyspareunia to be 13% in those aged 20–29, with a nearly linear decrease over age cohorts down to 7% of those aged 50–60 years. In contrast, the Finnish study showed an increase in prevalence of dyspareunia at about the age of 55.

Overall, high prevalence of about 14–18% has been found in Germany,[21] in the UK,[7] and in yet another Swedish investigation.[31] Again, methods and definitions may play a role here, as mild dyspareunia has been found to prevail in 43% of French (lifetime) and in 33% of Swedish (1-year) nationally representative women.

Vaginismus is a rare condition. According to the only European epidemiologic study of which we are aware,[17] the prevalences of mild (occurring sporadically) and manifest (occurring at least quite often) vaginismus are 5% and 1%, respectively. This seems to agree with the only other truly epidemiologically anchored investigation of vaginismus, in which Kadri et al.[35] found the prevalence in Morocco to be 6%.

In conclusion, it appears that there is a clear lack of investigation on female sexual dysfunction by common methods of sampling, definition, classification of severity, and time-frame. Moreover, while there are a series of reports from western and northern European countries, there is a paucity from the southern and eastern parts.

Different sexual dysfunctions quite often occur together. For example, manifest orgasmic dysfunction in 18–74-year-old women is accompanied by manifestly low levels of sexual interest in 53% of Swedish women and 28% have insufficient lubrication. Indeed, in univariate analyses, all female sexual dysfunctions are significantly ($p < 0.001$) associated.[16] In addition, at least in Sweden, all female sexual dysfunctions are significantly associated with partner's erectile and ejaculatory dysfunctions.

The *incidence* of female sexual dysfunction in Europe is very sparsely studied. In the Finnish[18] and Swedish[16] studies, women aged 18–74 reported a 5-year incidence rate of decreased desire in the order of 40–45%. In both countries, as might be expected from the increasing prevalence of low level of desire, this incidence increased with age. The incidence rate of prolonged and severe dyspareunia in Sweden in 1998[34] (P:12) was inversely related to age, being 4.3 per 100 women-years for 20–29-year-olds and then successively decreasing to 2.3 and about 1.0 for age cohorts 30–39 and 40–49, respectively, down to 0.5 for those aged 50–60 years.

How distressed?

There are only a few valid epidemiologic studies on the prevalence of distress accompanying female sexual dysfunction. In the mid-1990s, a pan-European (Denmark, France, Germany, Italy, the Netherlands, and the UK) investigation[36] (P:10) found that 3.4% of women aged 55–64, compared with 0.9% of those aged 65–75, felt that dyspareunia was "an irritating problem". It appears that only one other epidemiologic investigation[17] has discussed the prevalence of distress caused by female sexual dysfunctions *per se*. Manifest dyspareunia was, as shown in Table 2.2.3, accompanied by manifest personal distress for the vast majority of sexually active 18–65-year-old women. Much the same was the case for lubrication insufficiency. Manifest dys-

Table 2.2.3. Prevalence of manifest and mild sexual dysfunctions (*per se*) and distress caused by them

	Dysfunction (*per se*)		Dysfunction is distressful Manifestly/mildly
Sexual interest	Manifest (29%)	→	47%/40%
	Mild (60%)	→	2%/54%
Lubrication	Manifest (12%)	→	61%/28%
	Mild (50%)	→	1%/57%
Orgasm	Manifest (22%)	→	44%/40%
	Mild (60%)	→	1%/60%
Dyspareunia	Manifest (5%)	→	72%/20%
	Mild (34%)	→	2%/60%

functions of sexual interest and orgasm were clearly less frequently (about 45%) followed by manifest distress. Moreover, Table 2.2.3 shows that about 90% of all manifest female sexual dysfunctions lead to some degree of distress. Slightly more than half of those with mild female sexual dysfunction experienced distress, although this was nearly exclusively mild.

How satisfied?

The level of sexual satisfaction varies widely across and within European countries. Thus, in the UK, one study found that, independent of age, 75% of women aged 18–75 years were satisfied with their current sex life. In clear contrast, an investigation of 16–44-year-old British women found that less than half were satisfied (Table 2.2.2). Two Scandinavian studies have revealed that about half (Sweden) and up to two-thirds (Denmark) of sexually active women are satisfied or very satisfied with their sex life. Although some female sexual dysfunctions increase at age 50 and higher, the proportion of sexually satisfied women apparently does not decrease appreciably as a function of (higher) age.

As previously pointed out, all female sexual dysfunctions *per se* are closely associated with each other and with the women's perception of the partner's sexual dysfunctions. Relating overall sexual satisfaction univariately to any particular dysfunction therefore appears to be quite a strongly contaminated measure. Logistic regression[17] found that the likelihood (odds ratio: OR) of distressful lubrication insufficiency being associated with overall sexual dissatisfaction (as opposed to satisfaction) was 1.3. Distressing orgasmic dysfunction and dyspareunia lead to four- and fivefold greater likelihood of being sexually dissatisfied. In Sweden,[16] the (adjusted) risk of not being overall sexually satisfied is about five- to sixfold greater if the woman has distressingly low levels of sexual interest or orgasmic dysfunction and threefold greater with lubrication insufficiency, while distressful dyspareunia and vaginismus (i.e., pain syndromes) did not contribute significantly to this logistic regression model.

And the risks?

We shall address first the somatic risks of female sexual dysfunction, then partner relationship factors, and finally other psycho-socio-demographic risk factors. Generally speaking, *less than good health* – as experienced by the woman – has been shown by some, although not all, authors to have a negative significant effect on different parameters of female sexual function.

Urogenital conditions

In an Austrian investigation (P:11) of 159 gynecologic or urogynecologic patients,[37] the prevalence of female sexual dysfunction was about 50%, and no age dependency was found. The only remarkable discrepancy from most descriptive epidemiologic investigations was a quite high prevalence of dyspareunia (24% in the gynecologic and 18% in the urogynecologic groups). In women treated for early cervical carcinoma (stages IB–IIA), Bergmark et al.,[38] covering the total Swedish population (P:13), reported that after treatment (different modalities), 25% had manifestly increased level of distress with low sexual interest, while 20% became distressfully dyspareunic and about 30% reported distress due to lubrication insufficiency and orgasmic dysfunction, respectively. In this context, it appears relevant to mention that Mannaerts et al.,[39] in a small Dutch series (P:10) of patients treated with high-dose, external radiotherapy plus surgery with intraoperative radiotherapy found that in 50% of the women treated the preoperative ability to reach orgasm had disappeared at follow-up.

We have not been able to locate any conclusive European evidence on the effect of hysterectomy on sexual life. Other than a beneficial effect on dyspareunia (from 50% preoperatively to 10% at follow-up), it appears that the quality of postoperative sexual life is primarily determined by preoperative sexual factors.[40]

Recently, an (P:14) Italian investigation[41] of women with lower urinary tract symptoms (LUTS) and/or incontinence found that they had significantly more dysfunctions of desire and lubrication and more dyspareunia than controls. In Denmark[42] (P:12), lower urinary tract symptoms have been found to be an independent risk factor for "sexual dysfunction" in 40–65-year-old women. The impact of urinary incontinence on the prevalence of female sexual dysfunction has been surveyed internationally by Shaw,[43] who found impairment in sexual function to range from as low as under 1% to 64%. However, in the UK,[5] stress urinary incontinence has been identified as a risk factor for sexual interest, desire, "arousal", lubrication, orgasm, dyspareunia, and even vaginismus. In a small-scale, retrospective Swedish study of 44 women aged 34–62 years,[44] stress incontinence appeared to lead to reduction in lubrication (55%), orgasmic dysfunction (39%), and dyspareunia (33%), while 64% of women were sexually satisfied. One year after surgery, hardly any changes were detectable.

Cardiovascular conditions

In France, in a prospective study of 142 women treated with antihypertensive drugs (response rate: 74%; P:9), Hanon et al.[45] found that 41% had a decreased level of interest. Compared with male peers, however, women had less sexual dysfunction. In the UK,[7] use of antihypertensive medication was likely to be accompanied to a significant degree (OR: 0.3) by orgasmic dysfunction.

In Belgian women with type I diabetes mellitus, Enzlin et al.[46] (P:10) concluded that insufficient lubrication, orgasmic dysfunction, and dyspareunia were almost twice as prevalent in women with diabetic complications than in those without.

Neurologic conditions

Although there is a group of publications on the impact of neurologic conditions on the sexual function of European women, none seem to be adequately epidemiologically anchored for citation under evidence-based circumstances.

Partner relationship

Single women are more likely to have female sexual dysfunction (manifest low level of sexual interest, insufficient lubrication, orgasmic dysfunction, and dyspareunia) than women who have a steady partner. On the other hand, in 18–24-year-old women, the relationship duration has been demonstrated to influence sexual interest negatively.[12] In a heterosexual student population of German women aged 19–32, Klussmann[47] (P:11) found a significant decline in sexual interest if the duration was over 3 years.

The quality of the relationship is a major predictor of several sexual dysfunctions. A poor quality is more likely (logistic regression) to occur with women who have manifestly distressing dysfunctions of sexual interest (OR: 5.6), lubrication (OR: 4.0), and orgasm (OR: 4.5), and twice as likely to prevail in women with mildly distressing dysfunction of sexual interest (OR: 2.2).[48] In the UK, marital difficulties are very likely to be accompanied by arousal problems (OR: 6.8) and orgasmic dysfunction (OR: 5.1).[8] Moreover, "northern European" women who worry about the future of their partner relationship are nearly three times more likely than those who are optimistic to have lubrication dysfunction, while "southern European" women have a higher likelihood of having dyspareunia.[22]

Probably the greatest risk factors for distressful female sexual dysfunction within a stable heterosexual relationship are the male partner's sexual dysfunctions. Thus, if the partner has erectile dysfunction, there is a more than a 30-fold greater risk of the women having a mildly or manifestly distressing low level of sexual interest. If the partner has delayed ejaculation, the risk of the woman's having manifest or mild lubrication dysfunction is high (OR: 18.2 and 7.7, respectively). Erectile dysfunction and early ejaculation are also very sizeable predictors for women's capacity to reach orgasm. ORs for erectile dysfunction and early ejaculation being associated with manifestly distressing orgasmic dysfunctions are about 14 and 4, respectively; while ORs for these two male dysfunctions as predictors of mildly distressing orgasmic dysfunctions are about 3.5.[48] In the Czech Republic, Raboch and Raboch[49] (P:8) found in 21–40-year-old women significant (univariate) associations between distressful orgasmic dysfunction (as opposed to nondistressful) and husbands' "weak sexual desire" or "weak sexual potency".

Psychiatric/psychologic conditions

There is clear evidence that mood disorders influence sexual functions negatively. In the UK,[8] significant ORs (1.8–4.5) linked depression and anxiety to dysfunctions of arousal, lubrication, orgasm, and dyspareunia. In both northern (OR: 2.2) and southern Europe (OR: 1.7), depression was significantly linked to lack of sexual interest, and in "southern Europe" to lubrication (OR: 1.8) and orgasm (OR: 1.6) dysfunctions as well.[22] In a prospective investigation of Spanish women and men treated with selective serotonin reuptake inhibitors (SSRI), Arias et al.[50] clearly identified increased risks of "sexual dysfunctions" for both genders, but significantly more so for men than for women.

Lifetime sexual abuse is a sizeable negative predictor for current sexual dysfunctions. Thus, Swedish women[51] who have ever been sexually abused have a significantly higher number of sexual dysfunctions than the nonabused, and sexual abuse is a strong predictor of later manifestly distressing orgasmic dysfunction (OR: 4.3).

It has been reported from the Czech Republic[49] that women who lost a parent early in life, who had three or more siblings, or who had an unhappy childhood to a significant degree ($p < 0.01$) had a high frequency of distressful orgasmic dysfunction. Among a wealth of sociodemographic variables studied in northern and southern Europe[22] and Sweden,[50] relatively few have emerged as significant predictors of female sexual dysfunction. In northern Europe, "belief in religion guiding sex" is positive for orgasmic function (OR: 2.3), while such a belief is negative for southern European women's lubrication function (OR: 0.6).[22] As might be expected, having young offspring living at home is associated with distressful dysfunction of sexual interest.[50] In northern Europe, relatively low educational level appears[22] to constitute a risk factor for lubrication and orgasmic dysfunctions, and to some extent for having dyspareunia. This has not been found in Sweden.[50] In contrast to erectile dysfunction,[29] smoking has not been found to influence women's sexual function negatively.

Treatment seeking

Do women with female sexual dysfunction seek professional help? Across European investigations, the proportion of women who have at least one manifest female sexual dysfunction is 35–55%. It must be remembered, though, that female sexual dysfunctions, in particular, low interest and distress caused by female sexual dysfunctions, are far from congruent categories.

For example, while 47% of all women aged 18–74 in a Nordic country have at least one manifest female sexual dysfunction, 24% feel that this is accompanied by manifest personal distress (the corresponding proportions for men are 23% and 13%) – still impressive numbers at the population level. However, only a small fraction of the manifestly distressed women (16%) had sought professional help during the last year; most frequently from gynecologists/midwives.[52] In the UK,[8] 39% of women from a regionally representative sample aged 18–75 wished to receive help for "sexual problems", but only 8% of these had sought help, most commonly from general practitioners (GPs). In another recent British nationally representative investigation of 16–44-year-old women, 21% with female sexual dysfunction had sought help, usually from their GP.[11] The big question is, to what extent is society prepared to meet the demands for sexual medicine/sexology consultation even if just half of those with manifestly distressing female sexual dysfunction would actually seek any kind of professional help?

The problem of the ontology of female sexual dysfunction may, therefore, simply be a semantic one. As pointed out by Bancroft et al.,[53] the term "dysfunction" is defined by the dictionary as "malfunctioning, as of a structure of the body". Consequently, several years ago, we[12] argued in favor of substituting "dysfunction" for "disability", denoting incapacity to reach (sexual) goals. This definition was discussed by the definitions committee of the World Health Organization,[29] but was discarded, as it might confuse existing concepts.

References

1. Spector IP, Carey MP. Incidence and prevalence of the sexual dysfunctions: a critical review of the empirical literature. *Arch Sex Behav* 1990; 19: 389–407.
2. Simons JS, Carey MP. Prevalence of sexual dysfunctions: results from a decade of research. *Arch Sex Behav* 2001; 30: 177–219.
3. Dunn KM, Jordan K, Croft PR. Systematic review of sexual problems: epidemiology and methodology. *J Sex Marital Ther* 2002; 28: 399–422.
4. Prins J, Blanker MH, Bohnen AM et al. Prevalence of erectile dysfunction: a systematic review of population based studies. *Int J Impot Res* 2002; 14: 422–32.
5. Osborn M, Hawton K, Gath D. Sexual dysfunction among middle-aged women in the community. *BMJ* 1988; 296: 959–62.
6. Barlow DH, Cardozo LD, Francis RM et al. Urogenital ageing and its effect on sexual health in older British women. *Br J Obstet Gynaecol* 1997; 104: 87–91.
7. Dunn KM, Croft PR, Hackett GI. Sexual problems: a study of the prevalence and need for health care in the general population. *Fam Pract* 1998; 15: 519–24.
8. Dunn KM, Croft PR, Hackett GI. Association of sexual problems with social, psychological, and physical problems in men and women: a cross sectional populations survey. *J Epidemiol Community Health* 1999; 53: 144–8.

9. Dunn KM, Croft PR. Satisfaction in the sex life of a general population sample. *J Sex Marital Ther* 2000; 26: 141–51.

10. Johnson AM, Mercer CH, Erens B et al. Sexual behaviour in Britain: partnerships, practices, and HIV risk behaviours. *Lancet* 2001; 358: 1835–42.

11. Mercer CH, Fenton KA, Johnson AM et al. Sexual function problems and help seeking behaviour in Britain: national probability sample survey. *BMJ* 2003; 327: 426–7.

12. Fugl-Meyer AR, Sjögren Fugl-Meyer K. Sexual disabilities, problems and satisfaction. *Scand J Sexol* 1999; 2: 79–105.

13. Lindal E, Stefansson JG. The lifetime prevalence of psychosexual dysfunction among 55 to 57 year olds in Iceland. *Soc Psychiatry Epidemiol* 1993; 28: 91–5.

14. Ventegodt S. Sex and the quality of life in Denmark. *Arch Sex Behav* 1998; 27; 295–307.

15. Fugl-Meyer KS. Sexual disabilities and sexual problems. In *Sex in Sweden*. Stockholm: National Institute of Public Health, 2000: 199–216.

16. Sjögren Fugl-Meyer K, Fugl-Meyer AR. Sexual disabilities are not singularities. *Int J Impot Res* 2002; 14: 487–93.

17. Öberg K, Fugl-Meyer AR, Fugl-Meyer KS. On categorization and classification of women's sexual dysfunction. An epidemiological approach. *Int J Impot Res* 2004; 16: 261–9.

18. Kontula O, Haavio-Mannila E. *Sexual Pleasures. Enhancement of Sex Life in Finland, 1991–1992*. Aldershot: Dartmouth, 1995.

19. Groupe ACSF, Bajos N, Giami A et al., eds. *Comportements sexuels et sida en France*. Paris: Les Éditions INSERM, 1998.

20. Bejin A. Sexual pleasures, dysfunctions, fantasies and satisfaction. In A Spira, N Bajos et le groupe ACSF, eds. *Les comportements sexuels en France*. Paris: La Documentation Française, 1993: 194–202.

21. Matthiesen S, Hauch M. Wenn sexuelle Erfahrungen zum Problem warden. *Familiendynamik* 2004; 29: 139–60.

22. Laumann EO, Nicolosi A, Glasser DB et al. Sexual problems among women and men aged 40–80 y: prevalence and correlates identified in the Global Study of Sexual Attitudes and Behaviors. *Int J Impot Res* 2005; 17: 39–57.

23. Moynihan R. The making of a disease: female sexual dysfunction. *BMJ* 2003; 326: 45–7.

24. Hart G, Wellings K. Sexual behaviour and its medicalisation in sickness and in health. *BMJ* 2002; 324: 896–900.

25. Hartmann U, Heiser K, Ruffer-Hesse C et al. Female sexual desire disorders: subtypes, classification. Personality factors and new directions for treatment. *World J Urol* 2002; 20: 79–88.

26. Bancroft J. The medicalisation of female sexual dysfunction: the need for caution. *Arch Sex Behav* 2002; 31: 451–5.

27. World Health Organization. *ICD-10: International Statistical Classification of Diseases and Related Health Problems*. Geneva: World Health Organization, 1992.

28. American Psychiatric Association: *DSM-IV: Diagnostic and Statistical Manual of Mental Disorders*, 4th edn. Washington, DC: American Psychiatric Press, 1994.

29. Lewis RW, Fugl-Meyer KS, Bosch R et al. Definitions, classification, and epidemiology of sexual dysfunctions. In *Sexual Medicine. Sexual Dysfunctions in Men and Women*. Paris: Health Publications, 2004: 37–72.

30. Basson R, Leiblum S, Brotto L et al. Definitions of women's sexual dysfunction reconsidered: advocating expansion and revision. *J Psychosom Obstet Gynecol* 2003; 24: 221–30.

31. Stenberg Å, Heimer G, Ulmsten U et al. Prevalence of genitourinary and other climacteric symptoms in 61–year-old women. *Maturitas* 1996; 24: 31–6.

32. Hawton K, Gath D, Day A. Sexual function in a community sample of middle-aged women with partners: effects of age, marital, socioeconomic, psychiatric, gynaecological, and menopausal factors. *Arch Sex Behav* 1994; 23: 375–95.

33. Eplov LF. Sexuality: its theory and a prospective population investigation in Copenhagen County with special focus on the impact of aging and personality traits [in Danish]. PhD thesis. Copenhagen: Copenhagen University, 2002.

34. Danielsson I, Sjöberg I, Stenlund H et al. Prevalence and incidence of prolonged and severe dyspareunia in women: results from a population study. *Scand J Public Health* 2003; 31: 113–18.

35. Kadri N, Mchichi Alami KH et al. Sexual dysfunction in women: population based epidemiological study. *Arch Women Ment Health* 2002; 5: 59–63.

36. Barlow DH, Samsioe G, van Geelen JM. A study of European women's experience of the problems of urogenital ageing and its management. *Maturitas* 1997; 27: 239–347.

37. Geiss IM, Umek WH, Dungl A et al. Prevalence of female sexual dysfunction in gynaecological and urogynaecological patients according to the international consensus classification. *Urology* 2003; 62: 514–18.

38. Bergmark K, Åvall-Lundqvist E, Dickman PW et al. Patient-rating of distressful symptoms after treatment for early cervical cancer. *Acta Obstet Gynecol Scand* 2002; 81: 443–54.

39. Mannaerts GH, Schijven MP, Hendrikx A et al. Urologic and sexual morbidity following multimodality treatment for locally advanced primary and locally recurrent rectal cancer. *Eur J Surg Oncol* 2001; 27: 265–72.

40. Helström L, Lundberg PO, Sörbom D et al. Sexuality after hysterectomy: a factor analysis of women's sexual lives before and after subtotal hysterectomy. *Obstet Gynecol* 1993; 81: 357–62.

41. Saloni A, Zanni G, Nappi R et al. Sexual dysfunction is common in women with lower urinary incontinence: results of a cross-sectional study. *Eur Urol* 2004; 45: 642–8.

42. Hansen BL. Lower urinary tract symptoms (LUTS) and sexual function in both sexes. *Eur Urol* 2004; 46: 229–34.

43. Shaw C. A systematic review of the literature on the prevalence of sexual impairment in women with urinary incontinence and the prevalence of urinary leakage during sexual activity. *Eur Urol* 2002; 42: 432–40.

44. Berglund A-L, Fugl-Meyer KS. Some sexological characteristics of stress incontinent women. *Scand J Urol Nephrol* 1996; 30: 207–12.

45. Hanon O, Mounier-Vehier Cl, Fauvel J-P et al. Troubles de la sexualité chez les hypertendus traités. Resultats d'une enquête nationale. *Arch Mal Coeur Vaiss* 2002; 95: 673–7.

46. Enzlin P, Mathieu C, van den Bruel A et al. Sexual dysfunction in women with type I diabetes. *Diabetes Care* 2002; 25: 672–7.

47. Klussmann D. Sexual motivation and the duration of partnership. *Arch Sex Behav* 2002; 31: 275–87.

48. Öberg K, Fugl-Meyer KS. On Swedish women's distressing sexual dysfunctions, some concomitant conditions and life satisfaction. *J Sex Med* 2005; 2: 169–180.

49. Raboch J, Raboch J. Infrequent orgasms in women. *J Sex Marital Ther* 1992; 18: 114–20.

50. Arias F, Padin JJ, Rivas MT et al. Disfunciones sexuales inducidas por los inhibidores de la recaptación de serotonina. *Aten Primaria* 2000; 26: 389–94.

51. Öberg K, Fugl-Meyer KS, Fugl-Meyer AR. On sexual well-being in sexually abused Swedish women: epidemiological aspects. *Sex Relatsh Ther* 2002; 17: 329–41.

52. Fugl-Meyer AR, Fugl-Meyer KS. Treatment seeking for sexual problems among Swedish women and men. Proceedings of 16th World Congress of Sexology (WAS). Havana, Cuba, 2003.

53. Bancroft J, Loftus J, Scott Long J. Reply to Rosen and Laumann. *Arch Sex Behav* 2003; 32: 213–16.

2.3 Worldwide prevalence and correlates

Jeong–han Kang, Edward O Laumann, Dale B Glasser, Anthony Paik

Introduction

The debate continues on the nature of gender differences in sexual problems.[1] One feature of this debate centers on the extent to which biologic, psychosocial, and cultural factors each contribute to these various difficulties. Yet, assessments of their relative influence on the prevalence of sexual problems have been hampered by the lack of systematic, cross-cultural population studies. A recent review of 52 studies on sexual dysfunctions, for example, found that few were based on broadly representative samples, and even fewer included information on multiple sexual problems.[2] With most epidemiologic studies focused on North American and Western European populations, findings from other regions of the world are often based on smaller studies involving clinical series or other samples that are not broadly representative. The Global Study of Sexual Attitudes and Behaviors (GSSAB) was recently conducted to investigate health status, as well as attitudes, beliefs, behaviors, and satisfaction regarding sex and relationships among middle-aged and older adults in 29 countries.

The objectives of the current analysis of the GSSAB include the following: (1) to estimate the prevalence of sexual problems among women for five regional clusters; (2) to identify factors that increase the likelihood of reporting selected, common sexual problems by regional cluster.

Methods

The GSSAB is the first large, multicountry survey to study systematically attitudes, beliefs, and behavior regarding sexual relationships among middle-aged and older adults. The survey involved 13 882 women and 13 618 men, aged 40–80 years, in 29 countries, representing many world regions. We selected women of 18 countries for the current analysis (n = 7361) that

will represent regions of the world, excluding Europe and the USA. European countries and the USA have been analyzed in Chapters 2.2 and 2.1, respectively, of this volume. For the purposes of this chapter only, "Western" shall refer to the Western regions, excluding Europe and the USA. In Canada, Australia, New Zealand, and Brazil, samples were based on random-digit-dialing, and respondents were selected randomly within households by asking for the person between 40 and 80 years of age with the most recent birthday. Sampling in Middle Eastern countries (Algeria, Egypt, Morocco, and Turkey) employed a door-to-door protocol, where households were selected by random starting points, and study staff contacted every third house in several major cities. In Asian countries (China, Hong Kong [although Hong Kong is part of China, it is listed separately because of its distinct socioeconomic and cultural characteristics], Korea, Indonesia, Malaysia, the Philippines, Singapore, Taiwan, and Thailand), an intercept protocol was employed in major cities. Both the door-to-door and intercept protocols represent accepted survey methods for each country, but are likely to be more reflective of their urban populations. A female sample size of 750 was used in Australia, Turkey, and Japan. A female sample size of 250 was used in New Zealand, Algeria, China, Hong Kong, Taiwan, Indonesia, Malaysia, the Philippines, Singapore, and Thailand. In the remaining countries, the female sample sizes were as follows: Canada, 500; Brazil, 471; Mexico, 252; Egypt, 318; Morocco, 253; and Korea, 600.

In Canada, Australia, New Zealand, and Brazil, telephone interviews were conducted via computer-assisted telephone interview (CATI). Due to the sensitive nature of the topic, refusals were not called back. The door-to-door and intercept protocols employed in Algeria, Egypt, Morocco, Turkey, China, Korea, Taiwan, Indonesia, Malaysia, the Philippines, Singapore, and Thailand used self-completed questionnaires. There were two exceptions to this data collection strategy. In Japan, a mailed, self-completed questionnaire was used, and in Mexico, a mixed-mode method of in-person and telephone interviews was employed. The mean overall response rate was 19%, the mean rate for the telephone interviews being 15%, 30% for the self-completed questionnaires, and 33% for the mailed, self-completed questionnaires used in Japan. Response rate ranged from 8% to 55% in the various countries.

Verbal consent was obtained from all study participants. They were also informed about the following issues: (1) all information obtained would be used in aggregate only, (2) responses were voluntary, (3) the confidentiality and the privacy of their responses were protected because no personal identifiers were coded into the interview instruments, (4) no list of respondents was retained, and (5) 'refusers' were not called back in an effort to convert them to participating respondents.

The questionnaire asked for information about demographics, health, relationships, and general satisfaction with life as a whole, as well as individual behavior, practices, attitudes, and beliefs regarding sexuality. The presence of sexual problems was assessed by the following question: "During the last 12 months have you ever experienced any of the following for a period of 2 months or more when you: (1) lacked interest in having sex; (2) were unable to reach climax (experience orgasm); (3) reached climax (experienced orgasm) too quickly; (4) experienced physical pain during sex; (5) did not find sex pleasurable; and (6) had trouble becoming adequately lubricated?" Respondents were permitted to answer yes to all that applied. For those indicating the presence of a specific sexual problem, the relative severity was assessed in a follow-up question: "For each of these experiences, how often would you say this has occurred during the last 12 months? Would you say that this has occurred occasionally, sometimes, or frequently?"

We restricted our analyses to only those respondents who had had intercourse at least once in the year prior to being interviewed. This procedure reduced our sample size to 4705 women and tended to drop older respondents, who were sexually inactive more frequently. Thus, the prevalence of sexual problems was calculated by dividing the total number of self-reports for each problem by the total number of respondents who were sexually active in the year prior to being interviewed. Country-specific data were grouped into clusters, according to geographic proximity, shared cultural backgrounds, and similar modes of data collection. Using the age distribution of the entire sample in the GSSAB for women, we age-standardized the prevalence estimates for each regional cluster.

A number of possible correlates of sexual problems were investigated. These included age, self-reported measures of general health status, current level of physical activity, self-report of a diagnosed vascular condition (including hypertension, diabetes, heart disease, high cholesterol, and having had a stroke), self-report of a diagnosis of depression, having had a hysterectomy, and whether respondents currently or formerly smoked. Respondents also reported how often they thought about sex – a proxy for their current level of sexual libido – and whether they agreed with the belief that aging reduced sexual desire and/or behavior. Other self-reported measures included

educational attainment, whether respondents believed that their religion guided their sexual behavior, experience with divorce and financial problems in the 3-year period prior to being interviewed, the expected time horizon of their current relationships, the frequency of engaging in sex, whether they usually engaged in foreplay, and whether they were sexually exclusive.

We utilized logistic regression in this study. This approach produced adjusted odds ratios (ORs), which indicate the odds of reporting the particular sexual problem among those with a given characteristic (such as poor health) relative to people in a reference category (such as good health), controlling for all other factors in the regression analysis. In these analyses, the presence of a sexual problem included only those respondents who reported "*sometimes*" or "*frequently*" having the problem (that is, those who indicated "*occasionally*" were recoded to indicate no sexual problem). In order to evaluate the validity of pooling a specific country with the others in a regional cluster, we employed a series of interaction models between covariates and country dummy variables to test whether a specific country could be pooled in an analysis. Countries with covariate patterns that were significantly different from the pooled sample were dropped from the analysis (results are available upon request). Thus, we dropped the following countries: (1) Algeria, Taiwan, Indonesia, the Philippines, and Singapore in logistic regressions of orgasm problems; and (2) Mexico, Egypt, Taiwan, and the Philippines in logistic regressions of lubrication difficulties.

Results

Table 2.3.1 presents the prevalence of sexual problems of 2 months' or more duration, subdivided by frequency of occurrence. In most cases, the reported prevalence of sexual problems was higher in East Asia and Southeast Asia than in the other regions of the world. Lack of interest in sex and inability to reach orgasm were the most common sexual problems across the five regions, ranging from 28% to 43% and 22% to 41%, respectively. Lubrication difficulties were relatively common and showed similar prevalence across most regions, with the notable exceptions of East Asia and Southeast Asia, where the prevalence was approximately 10 percentage points higher than that reported in other regions. We analyzed factors associated with the likelihood of reporting sexual problems among women. We focused on more severe problems: only those respondents indicating a periodic (sometimes) or frequent sexual problem in the 12 months prior to being interviewed were coded as having that particular problem (that is, those who indicated "occasionally" were recoded to indicate no sexual problem). Here we present detailed analyses of two selected problems: the inability to reach orgasm and lubrication difficulties.

Table 2.3.2 presents logistic-regression results for factors associated with the likelihood of reporting an inability to reach orgasm. Age does not appear to be systematically associated with this problem, although several regions show some positive

Table 2.3.1. Prevalence (%) of women's sexual problems by region and severity

	Lack of sexual interest	Inability to reach orgasm	Orgasm too quickly	Pain during sex	Sex not pleasurable	Lubrication difficulties
"West"[a]	33.6 (30.3, 36.9)	25.0 (22.0, 27.9)	9.2 (7.4, 11.0)	12.1 (10.0, 14.2)	19.8 (17.0, 22.6)	27.8 (24.7, 30.8)
Occasionally	12.1 (9.8, 14.4)	8.6 (6.6, 10.5)	4.5 (3.3, 5.7)	4.0 (2.8, 5.1)	6.9 (5.1, 8.7)	7.0 (5.3, 8.8)
Periodically	13.9 (11.5, 16.3)	11.2 (9.0, 13.4)	3.8 (2.5, 5.0)	5.5 (3.9, 7.1)	9.0 (7.0, 11.0)	11.6 (9.4, 13.9)
Frequently	7.3 (5.5, 9.1)	4.6 (3.3, 5.9)	0.8 (0.3, 1.3)	2.5 (1.6, 3.5)	3.6 (2.5, 4.8)	9.1 (7.1, 11.0)
Central/South America[b]	28.1 (24.1, 32.2)	22.4 (18.7, 26.1)	18.3 (14.9, 21.8)	16.6 (13.4, 19.8)	19.5 (16.1, 22.9)	22.5 (18.8, 26.3)
Occasionally	7.8 (5.4, 10.5)	6.7 (4.5, 8.9)	5.0 (3.1, 6.8)	2.6 (1.4, 3.9)	5.6 (3.5, 7.7)	4.3 (2.4, 6.2)
Periodically	12.8 (9.8, 15.8)	12.1 (9.2, 14.9)	9.6 (6.8, 12.3)	8.4 (6.1, 10.6)	8.8 (6.5, 11.1)	11.7 (8.9, 14.5)
Frequently	7.4 (5.0, 9.8)	3.7 (2.0, 5.3)	3.8 (2.3, 5.4)	5.6 (3.4, 7.9)	5.2 (3.3, 7.0)	6.5 (4.3, 8.7)
Middle East[c]	43.4 (38.6, 48.3)	23.0 (18.4, 27.7)	10.0 (6.9, 13.1)	21.0 (16.2, 25.8)	31.0 (26.1, 36.0)	23.0 (18.1, 27.8)
Occasionally	14.3 (11.0, 17.6)	6.1 (4.7, 7.6)	3.8 (2.7, 5.0)	6.6 (5.1, 8.1)	9.2 (6.1, 12.3)	10.7 (6.8, 14.6)
Periodically	18.3 (13.7, 22.8)	10.9 (7.7, 14.0)	5.2 (2.3, 8.0)	9.0 (5.2, 12.8)	13.6 (10.4, 16.9)	7.0 (5.4, 8.5)
Frequently	10.9 (6.6, 15.2)	6.0 (2.4, 9.7)	1.0 (0.5, 1.6)	5.4 (1.7, 9.0)	8.2 (4.4, 12.0)	5.3 (1.7, 9.0)
East Asia[d]	34.8 (32.0, 37.7)	32.3 (29.5, 35.1)	17.6 (15.2, 20.0)	31.6 (28.8, 34.4)	29.7 (26.9, 32.4)	37.9 (35.0, 40.7)
Occasionally	7.4 (5.8, 9.0)	9.0 (7.4, 10.7)	6.2 (4.7, 7.7)	11.2 (9.3, 13.0)	8.6 (6.9, 10.2)	10.1 (8.4, 11.8)
Periodically	13.8 (11.8, 15.9)	11.9 (10.0, 13.9)	7.0 (5.4, 8.6)	11.8 (9.8, 13.9)	10.4 (8.6, 12.1)	15.6 (13.4, 17.9)
Frequently	13.6 (11.4, 15.9)	11.3 (9.3, 13.3)	4.3 (3.0, 5.6)	8.6 (6.7, 10.5)	10.7 (8.7, 12.8)	12.1 (9.9, 14.3)
Southeast Asia[e]	43.3 (38.1, 48.6)	41.2 (36.0, 46.4)	26.3 (21.4, 31.2)	29.2 (24.1, 34.3)	35.9 (31.0, 40.7)	34.2 (28.9, 39.5)
Occasionally	9.5 (5.6, 13.4)	7.3 (4.4, 10.3)	6.6 (3.0, 10.3)	6.7 (3.3, 10.1)	8.2 (4.7, 11.7)	6.5 (3.6, 9.4)
Periodically	23.7 (19.1, 28.4)	26.8 (21.7, 31.9)	17.7 (13.3, 22.1)	19.8 (14.9, 24.6)	22.9 (18.2, 27.7)	20.7 (16.1, 25.2)
Frequently	10.1 (6.3, 13.9)	7.1 (4.1, 10.2)	2.0 (0.0, 4.3)	2.7 (1.3, 4.1)	4.7 (2.8, 6.7)	7.1 (3.6, 10.6)

Note: based on reports from sexually active respondents. 95% confidence intervals in parentheses. Percentage in the first row of each region panel indicates the regional average of sexual dysfunction, defined as an experience of dysfunction for a period of 2 months or more. The difference between the regional average and the sum of the three levels of severity of sexual dysfunction indicates the proportion who failed to specify the level of severity. All prevalences are adjusted according to the age distribution of the total of sexually active women in the GSSAB survey.

[a] Includes Australia, Canada, and New Zealand ($n = 1044$).
[b] Includes Brazil and Mexico ($n = 588$).
[c] Includes Algeria, Egypt, Morocco, and Turkey ($n = 967$).
[d] Includes China, Hong Kong, Japan, Korea, and Taiwan ($n = 1417$).
[e] Includes Indonesia, Malaysia, Philippines, Singapore, and Thailand ($n = 689$).

associations. Poor health tends to increase the likelihood of orgasm difficulties, most prominently in the "Western" regions (OR = 1.7) and Asian (OR = 1.5 for East Asia and OR = 2.0 for Southeast Asia) populations. In contrast, thinking about sex is associated with a decreased likelihood of this problem. Most other factors, including physical inactivity, vascular diseases, having had a hysterectomy, smoking, and belief that aging reduces sexual interest or activity, show inconsistent associations. Financial problems and depression consistently show positive associations; however, few of the odds ratios reach statistical significance. Relationship characteristics, such as partnership status, the frequency of sex, and foreplay, are generally nonsignificant, although women who have low expectations about the future viability of their relationship(s) are consistently more likely to report this problem.

Table 2.3.3 presents logistic-regression results for factors associated with the likelihood of reporting lubrication difficulties. Increasing age shows a curvilinear association with the likelihood of reporting this problem in all the world regions

except for Southeast Asia and South America. Women aged 50-59 years in comparison with those aged 40–49 years are roughly twice as likely to report lubrication difficulties across several regions, including the "West" (Western regions excluding the USA or European countries) (OR = 1.9), East Asia (OR = 2.2), and the Middle East (OR = 2.6). However, their counterparts, who are 70–80 years old, are no more likely to report this problem than the youngest cohort in the "West" or Central/South America. Most physical status factors are not associated with lubrication difficulties. With the exception of southern Europe, belief in religion guiding sex is associated with consistently raised odds ratios, although statistical significance at 5% is seen only in East Asia. Women with lower educational attainment are less likely to report problems with lubrication in several world regions. Moreover, women who have been diagnosed with depression in the past are greater than one and one-half times more likely to report this problem in "Western" (OR = 1.6), Central/South American (OR = 1.8), Middle Eastern (OR = 1.6), and Southeast Asian (OR = 1.6) country clusters.

Table 2.3.2. Factors associated with women's inability to reach orgasm by region

	"West"	C/S America	Middle East	East Asia	SE Asia
Age (years)					
40–49	Referent	Referent	Referent	Referent	Referent
50–59	1.6* (1.0, 2.6)	0.7 (0.4, 1.3)	2.7* (1.5, 5.0)	1.1 (0.8, 1.7)	1.4 (0.5, 3.4)
60–69	1.2 (0.6, 2.2)	1.3 (0.6, 2.9)	2.8* (1.4, 5.7)	1.1 (0.7, 1.8)	3.1† (0.9, 10.7)
70–80	0.6 (0.2, 2.1)	0.3† (0.1, 1.2)	3.9 (0.8, 20.3)	0.8 (0.4, 1.7)	n.a.
Education					
at least some college	Referent	Referent	Referent	Referent	Referent
secondary/high school	0.8 (0.5, 1.2)	1.6 (0.7, 3.6)	1.1 (0.5, 2.2)	1.3 (0.9, 2.0)	0.7 (0.3, 1.8)
primary school or less	1.6 (0.4, 6.5)	1.8 (0.8, 3.9)	1.7 (0.6, 2.7)	1.2 (0.7, 2.2)	0.3* (0.1, 0.9)
Divorce in past 3 years	0.7 (0.3, 2.0)	1.4 (0.2, 13.0)	1.7 (0.6, 5.2)	0.7 (0.1, 3.7)	1.2 (0.3, 4.9)
Financial problems in last 3 years	1.5 (0.9, 2.6)	1.1 (0.6, 1.9)	1.1 (0.6, 2.0)	0.7 (0.4, 1.2)	2.8* (1.2, 6.2)
Fair/Poor overall health (vs good)	1.7† (1.0, 2.9)	0.9 (0.5, 1.6)	1.4 (0.7, 2.6)	1.5* (1.1, 2.1)	2.0† (0.9, 4.3)
Level of physical activity					
average and above	Referent	Referent	Referent	Referent	Referent
lower than average	1.1 (0.7, 1.9)	0.4* (0.1, 1.0)	1.8 (0.8, 3.8)	0.9 (0.6, 1.4)	2.2* (1.0, 4.6)
Vascular diseases	1.1 (0.7, 1.7)	1.7† (1.0, 3.0)	0.8 (0.4, 1.3)	1.1 (0.8, 1.6)	1.0 (0.3, 2.9)
Hysterectomy	0.7 (0.5, 1.2)	0.8 (0.4, 1.5)	1.1 (0.5, 2.6)	1.0 (0.6, 1.9)	0.4* (0.2, 1.0)
Depression diagnosed	1.4 (0.8, 2.2)	1.7† (1.0, 3.1)	1.3 (0.7, 2.3)	1.2 (0.6, 2.5)	2.7† (0.8, 8.7)
Smoking					
never	Referent	Referent	Referent	Referent	Referent
smoked before	1.4 (0.9, 2.2)	1.1 (0.6, 2.1)	1.7 (0.8, 3.5)	0.6 (0.3, 1.2)	1.7 (0.3, 9.4)
currently smoking	2.0* (1.2, 3.5)	1.1 (0.5, 2.0)	2.0* (1.1, 3.6)	1.0 (0.6, 1.8)	0.6 (0.2, 2.1)
Belief that aging reduces sex interest/activity	1.3 (0.8, 2.2)	0.9 (0.5, 1.5)	0.8 (0.5, 1.4)	1.3† (1.0, 1.8)	0.6 (0.3, 1.5)
Belief in religion guiding sex	1.3 (0.9, 2.0)	1.6 (0.9, 2.7)	1.0 (0.6, 1.8)	1.2 (0.7, 2.1)	1.9 (0.8, 4.4)
Partnership status					
exclusive and committed	Referent	Referent	Referent	Referent	Referent
exclusive but not committed	1.3 (0.7, 2.4)	0.3† (0.1, 1.1)	0.2 (0.0, 1.8)	0.4 (0.1, 1.6)	0.1* (0.0, 0.7)
nonexclusive	1.5 (0.3, 7.6)	0.4 (0.1, 1.8)	0.3† (0.1, 1.2)	1.3 (0.6, 3.0)	0.6 (0.1, 2.7)
Future of the relationship					
high hope	Referent	Referent	Referent	Referent	Referent
worried	4.5* (2.2, 9.1)	2.2† (1.0, 5.0)	1.3 (0.5, 3.8)	1.7† (1.0, 2.8)	1.1 (0.3, 3.3)
no future	1.8 (0.7, 5.0)	2.4* (1.0, 5.4)	2.9† (0.8, 8.7)	2.9* (1.5, 5.5)	0.3 (0.1, 2.1)
Frequency of sexual relationship					
several times per week	Referent	Referent	Referent	Referent	Referent
two to three times per month	1.3 (0.8, 2.0)	1.0 (0.5, 1.7)	1.1 (0.6, 1.9)	1.4 (0.8, 2.2)	0.8 (0.3, 2.1)
less than monthly	1.0 (0.5, 1.8)	1.1 (0.4, 2.8)	1.2 (0.4, 3.1)	1.3 (0.7, 2.3)	0.8 (0.2, 3.0)
Usually doesn't engage in foreplay	1.5 (0.7, 2.9)	2.1* (1.2, 3.8)	0.8 (0.4, 1.5)	1.6* (1.1, 2.3)	1.3 (0.5, 3.8)
Thinking of sex					
never or < 1/month	Referent	Referent	Referent	Referent	Referent
a few times/month	0.6 (0.3, 1.2)	0.8 (0.4, 1.6)	0.6 (0.3, 1.1)	0.6* (0.4, 0.9)	0.6 (0.2, 1.5)
a few times/week	0.4* (0.2, 0.9)	0.5 (0.1, 1.8)	0.6 (0.2, 2.4)	n.a.	0.2 (0.0, 4.1)
Chi-square	95.6	46.2	78.0	96.4	42.7
d.f.	27	26	27	27	25
Observations	928	531	749	1159	235

Note: odds ratios from logistic regression and their 95% confidence intervals in parenthesis. Based on reports from sexually active women. Country differences in each region controlled.
"West" includes Australia, Canada, and New Zealand.
Central/South America includes Brazil and Mexico.
Middle East includes Egypt, Morocco, and Turkey.
East Asia includes China, Hong Kong, Korea, and Japan.
Southeast Asia includes Malaysia and Thailand.
*$p \leq 0.05$; †$p \leq 0.10$.

Table 2.3.3. Factors associated with women's lubrication difficulties by region

	"West"	C/S America	Middle East	East Asia	SE Asia
Age (years)					
40–49	Referent	Referent	Referent	Referent	Referent
50–59	1.9* (1.2, 2.8)	1.0 (0.5, 1.9)	2.6* (1.3, 5.0)	2.2* (1.5, 3.3)	0.7 (0.4, 1.3)
60–69	1.7† (0.9, 2.9)	1.6 (0.7, 4.0)	3.2* (1.4, 6.9)	3.3* (2.0, 5.3)	0.9 (0.4, 2.1)
70–80	1.0 (0.4, 2.5)	0.6 (0.1, 2.8)	4.6† (0.9, 23.4)	3.0* (1.4, 6.5)	n.a.
Education					
at least some college	Referent	Referent	Referent	Referent	Referent
secondary/high school	0.7† (0.5, 1.1)	1.1 (0.5, 2.3)	0.6 (0.2, 1.5)	1.0 (0.7, 1.6)	0.7 (0.4, 1.1)
primary school or less	1.4 (0.4, 4.6)	0.8 (0.4, 1.7)	0.5† (0.3, 1.1)	1.0 (0.6, 1.8)	0.5* (0.2, 1.0)
Divorce in past 3 years	0.4 (0.1, 1.4)	n.a.	n.a.	1.2 (0.2, 6.8)	2.1 (0.7, 6.2)
Financial problems in last 3 years	0.8 (0.5, 1.3)	1.1 (0.6, 2.0)	1.4 (0.6, 3.0)	1.2 (0.8, 2.0)	2.0* (1.2, 3.5)
Fair/poor overall health (vs good)	1.3 (0.8, 2.2)	0.7 (0.3, 1.2)	1.7† (0.9, 3.2)	1.5* (1.1, 2.0)	1.4 (0.8, 2.5)
Level of physical activity					
average and above	Referent	Referent	Referent	Referent	Referent
lower than average	1.0 (0.6, 1.7)	0.9 (0.4, 2.1)	1.7 (0.9, 3.6)	1.1 (0.7, 1.7)	2.0* (1.2, 3.3)
Vascular diseases	1.2 (0.8, 1.7)	1.0 (0.6, 1.8)	0.5* (0.3, 0.9)	0.9 (0.6, 1.3)	0.9 (0.5, 1.7)
Hysterectomy	0.8 (0.5, 1.2)	1.1 (0.5, 2.1)	0.8 (0.3, 2.1)	1.2 (0.6, 2.2)	0.8 (0.3, 1.9)
Depression diagnosed	1.6* (1.0, 2.6)	1.8† (1.0, 3.4)	1.6 (0.8, 3.3)	1.2 (0.5, 2.7)	1.6 (0.7, 3.6)
Smoking					
never	Referent	Referent	Referent	Referent	Referent
smoked before	0.9 (0.6, 1.3)	1.0 (0.5, 1.9)	2.5* (1.1, 5.5)	0.6 (0.3, 1.2)	1.2 (0.4, 3.8)
currently smoking	1.5† (0.9, 2.5)	0.6 (0.3, 1.4)	1.5 (0.7, 3.1)	1.3 (0.7, 2.4)	1.3 (0.6, 3.0)
Belief that aging reduces sex interest/activity	1.2 (0.7, 1.8)	1.1 (0.6, 1.9)	1.0 (0.6, 1.8)	1.4* (1.0, 2.0)	1.3 (0.8, 2.1)
Belief in religion guiding sex	1.4† (1.0, 2.0)	1.6 (0.9, 2.9)	1.4 (0.8, 2.7)	1.7* (1.0, 2.9)	1.7† (0.9, 2.9)
Partnership status					
exclusive and committed	Referent	Referent	Referent	Referent	Referent
exclusive but not committed	0.8 (0.4, 1.6)	0.3† (0.1, 1.0)	0.7 (0.1, 4.0)	0.3 (0.1, 1.4)	0.9 (0.2, 4.0)
nonexclusive	0.5 (0.1, 3.7)	0.4 (0.1, 1.8)	2.0 (0.5, 8.6)	1.0 (0.4, 2.5)	1.1 (0.4, 3.1)
Future of the relationship					
high hope	Referent	Referent	Referent	Referent	Referent
worried	3.5* (1.8, 6.9)	1.9 (0.8, 4.4)	1.2 (0.4, 3.5)	1.0 (0.5, 1.8)	1.0 (0.4, 2.7)
no future	1.0 (0.3, 3.9)	1.7 (0.6, 4.8)	1.0 (0.2, 4.9)	1.6 (0.8, 3.1)	0.4 (0.1, 3.1)
Frequency of sexual relationship					
several times per week	Referent	Referent	Referent	Referent	Referent
two to three times per month	1.4† (1.0, 2.2)	1.6 (0.9, 2.9)	1.0 (0.5, 1.9)	1.0 (0.6, 1.6)	0.9 (0.5, 1.6)
less than monthly	1.6† (0.9, 2.8)	1.3 (0.4, 4.1)	1.6 (0.7, 3.8)	1.2 (0.7, 2.1)	0.7 (0.3, 1.5)
Usually doesn't engage in foreplay	1.1 (0.6, 1.9)	1.1 (0.5, 2.1)	1.1 (0.6, 2.0)	1.4* (1.0, 2.1)	0.9 (0.5, 1.7)
Thinking of sex					
never or < 1/month	Referent	Referent	Referent	Referent	Referent
a few times/month	0.5* (0.3, 1.0)	1.2 (0.5, 2.9)	0.7 (0.4, 1.4)	0.9 (0.6, 1.3)	0.8 (0.4, 1.4)
a few times/week	0.5† (0.2, 1.0)	0.5 (0.1, 1.9)	0.7 (0.2, 2.8)	0.7 (0.1, 4.7)	0.5 (0.1, 2.2)
Chi-square	90.4	26.7	53.9	116.2	39.9
d.f.	27	24	26	28	27
Observations	928	374	694	1167	548

Note: odds ratios from logistic regression and their 95% confidence intervals in parenthesis. Based on reports from sexually active women. Country differences in each region controlled.
"West" includes Australia, Canada, and New Zealand.
Central/South America includes Brazil.
Middle East includes Algeria, Morocco and Turkey.
East Asia includes China, Hong Kong, Korea, and Japan.
Southeast Asia includes Indonesia, Malaysia, Singapore, and Thailand.
*$p \leq 0.05$; †$p \leq 0.10$.

We also examined several additional sexual problems by logistic regression, including a lack of interest in sex (Table 2.3.4), pain during sex (Table 2.3.5), and nonpleasurable sex (Table 2.3.6). Lack of interest in sex is associated with the belief that aging reduces sexual desire and activity (OR 1.2–1.8), thinking about sex infrequently (thinking about sex more frequently is associated with OR 0.3–1.0), depression (OR 1.3–1.6), low expectations about the future of the relationship (lower expectations are associated with OR of 1.3–3.6 in all regions except Southeast Asia [OR = 0.5]), and infrequent sex (less frequent sex is associated with OR of 1.0–3.1 within all regions except East Asia [OR = 0.9]) (Table 2.3.4). Factors associated with pain during sex include younger age (the effect shows considerable variability between regions), poor health (OR 1.0–1.7), infrequent sex (OR 1.1–2.4), and low expectations about the future of the relationship (there was some variability between regions; however, lower expectations were usually associated with increasing likelihood of the problem [Table 2.3.5]). With respect to nonpleasurable sex among women, thinking about sex infrequently (with thinking of sex never or less than once a month as the referent, sexually active women who thought about sex at least a few times a month had OR of 0.1–0.7), the belief that aging reduces sexual interest or activity (OR 1.3–1.8 in all regions except Central South America [OR = 0.9]), depression (OR 1.0–3.9), and low expectations about the future of their relationship (OR from 1.0 to 4.7 in all regions except Southeast Asia [OR = 0.9]) all elevate the likelihood of reporting this problem (Table 2.3.6).

Discussion

In this research, we have examined a number of factors that may be contributory in the etiology of sexual problems in women. The unique strength of this study is its cross-cultural emphasis. With a sample drawn from 18 countries, we identified several factors that increased the likelihood of a sexual problem in multiple regions of the world. So, for example, the significant effects of age and depression across world regions support both physiologic and psychologic arguments about the etiology of sexual problems. The GSSAB also provides extensive variation with respect to sexual attitudes, beliefs, and behaviors, and we observed many effects that were significant only in certain regions of the world. Future research should investigate the significance of these contingent effects.

While the prevalence of most sexual problems tends to increase with age,[3–7] we found that older age, net of other factors, consistently increased the likelihood of most sexual problems among men, but not women (results for men are not presented here).[8] Only lubrication difficulties were positively associated with older age. Studies in elderly individuals have indicated that the effects of aging may be of less importance if the effects of the relationship are taken into account.[9] Since the more physiologic sexual problems clearly have a significant biologic component, it is not surprising that lubrication difficulties are associated with increased age.[9] However, this study does demonstrate that aging effects are more relevant to men then women.

Mental health and stress are also thought to influence sexual function. In the GSSAB, depression was associated with the likelihood of lubrication difficulties in some regions of the world, while stress from financial problems was positively associated with the inability to reach orgasm among women. We also found some evidence that education was positively associated with the likelihood of lubrication problems. Thus, the findings of the current analyses demonstrated some effects of psychosocial context in terms of the significance of stressful events, education level, and the occurrence of depression. Previous studies have reported that depression, stress, and emotional problems can be related to a reduced interest in sex as well as other sexual problems.[3,5] Socioeconomic factors have also been shown to have an effect on sexual function in both women and men.[3]

Relationship issues also play a role in the etiology of sexual problems.[10–13] In relationships in which partners show that they care for one another in everyday matters and communicate effectively about their sexual needs, one would anticipate a relatively low risk of sexual problems. In contrast, where there are difficulties in the overall relationship, one would expect this to have a negative impact on sexual function. In the current analysis, low expectations about the future of the relationship increased the likelihood of an inability to reach orgasm among women. Finally, having infrequent sex also increased the likelihood of lubrication difficulties.

The GSSAB has a number of limitations. Methodological issues regarding the study include potentially systematic biases arising from several causes: (1) differences in recruitment of samples and administration of surveys across countries, (2) challenges associated with achieving accurate, valid translations of the survey instrument in multiple languages to ensure the comparability of questions and responses, (3) the adequacy of pooling diverse population samples into regional clusters that are sufficiently homogeneous for comparative statistical analysis, (4) variation in the quality of the country-specific survey organizations across countries, and (5) the attainment of modest response rates.

Thus, while these data are broadly inclusive, they may not be truly representative of each country's entire adult and older populations because of the relatively modest response rates attained in the countries with the random-digit-dialing protocol and because the door-to-door and intercept protocols drew heavily on urban populations. In general, low completion rates can be of concern because they may be indicative of possible selection bias in the way subjects are recruited, and these issues raise some questions about the accuracy of our prevalence estimates. Prior research has concluded that different modes of administration (telephone and personal survey) resulted in few differences in reports of sexual behaviour.[14] We have also tested the effects of the different modes of interview used in the GSSAB and found no effect.[15]

Table 2.3.4. Factors associated with the lack of interest in having sex among women by region

	"West"		C/S America		Middle East		East Asia		SE Asia	
Age (years)										
40–49	Referent		Referent		Referent		Referent		Referent	
50–59	1.2	(0.8, 1.8)	0.8	(0.4, 1.3)	1.1	(0.7, 1.8)	1.6**	(1.1, 2.4)	1.5	(0.8, 3.0)
60–69	1.0	(0.6, 1.7)	1.7	(0.9, 3.3)	1.5	(0.8, 2.7)	1.8*	(1.1, 2.8)	1.1	(0.4, 2.9)
70–80	0.5	(0.2, 1.2)	0.8	(0.3, 2.0)	2.7+	(1.0, 7.5)	1.3	(0.7, 2.3)	1.8	(0.4, 7.3)
Education										
at least some college	Referent		Referent		Referent		Referent		Referent	
secondary/high school	0.8	(0.5, 1.1)	1.5	(0.7, 3.2)	1.2	(0.7, 2.3)	1.2	(0.8, 1.8)	0.6+	(0.3, 1.1)
primary school or less	0.5	(0.2, 1.6)	1.4	(0.7, 3.0)	0.8	(0.5, 1.4)	1.2	(0.8, 2.0)	0.4*	(0.2, 0.9)
Divorce in past 3 years	0.6	(0.2, 1.6)	1.2	(0.2, 8.1)	0.9	(0.3, 3.0)	0.9	(0.1, 6.0)	n.a.	
Financial problems in last 3 years	1.2	(0.7, 1.9)	1.2	(0.8, 2.0)	1.7*	(1.0, 2.8)	1.1	(0.7, 1.8)	2.0*	(1.0, 4.0)
Fair/poor overall health (vs good)	1.3	(0.8, 2.1)	0.9	(0.5, 1.5)	1.0	(0.6, 1.6)	1.6**	(1.2, 2.1)	2.3**	(1.3, 4.3)
Level of physical activity										
average and above	Referent		Referent		Referent		Referent		Referent	
lower than average	1.2	(0.7, 1.9)	1.3	(0.7, 2.4)	1.7*	(1.0, 3.0)	1.1	(0.8, 1.6)	0.9	(0.5, 1.8)
Vascular diseases	1.2	(0.8, 1.7)	1.2	(0.7, 2.0)	1.0	(0.6, 1.5)	1.0	(0.7, 1.4)	2.1*	(1.1, 4.0)
Hysterectomy	1.3	(0.8, 2.0)	0.8	(0.5, 1.5)	1.1	(0.6, 2.1)	0.9	(0.5, 1.7)	0.3*	(0.1, 0.9)
Depression diagnosed	1.5+	(1.0, 2.4)	1.6+	(1.0, 2.7)	1.5+	(1.0, 2.4)	1.3	(0.5, 3.2)	1.3	(0.5, 3.8)
Smoking										
never	Referent		Referent		Referent		Referent		Referent	
smoked before	1.0	(0.7, 1.6)	1.1	(0.7, 1.9)	1.2	(0.6, 2.5)	1.3	(0.8, 2.2)	1.4	(0.3, 7.7)
currently smoking	1.6+	(1.0, 2.4)	0.8	(0.5, 1.4)	1.3	(0.8, 2.1)	0.8	(0.4, 1.3)	0.4+	(0.2, 1.1)
Belief that aging reduces sex interest/activity	1.7*	(1.1, 2.5)	1.5+	(0.9, 2.4)	1.2	(0.8, 1.8)	1.7**	(1.3, 2.4)	1.3	(0.7, 2.4)
Belief in religion guiding sex	1.2	(0.8, 1.7)	1.1	(0.7, 1.8)	1.1	(0.7, 1.7)	1.6	(0.9, 2.9)	3.2*	(1.3, 8.0)
Partnership status										
exclusive and committed	Referent		Referent		Referent		Referent		Referent	
exclusive but not committed	0.6	(0.3, 1.3)	0.8	(0.3, 1.8)	0.9	(0.3, 3.0)	0.5	(0.2, 1.5)	n.a.	
non-exclusive	0.4	(0.0, 3.4)	0.5	(0.1, 2.2)	0.9	(0.2, 4.1)	0.6	(0.3, 1.5)	1.3	(0.3, 5.0)
Future of the relationship										
high hope	Referent		Referent		Referent		Referent		Referent	
worried	3.6**	(1.7, 7.6)	2.2*	(1.1, 4.3)	1.6	(0.6, 4.2)	1.3	(0.7, 2.4)	0.5	(0.1, 2.5)
no future	3.6**	(1.8, 7.4)	2.4*	(1.2, 4.9)	1.9	(0.7, 4.7)	3.1**	(1.6, 6.0)	1.3	(0.1, 25.2)
Frequency of sexual relationship										
several times per week	Referent		Referent		Referent		Referent		Referent	
two to three times per month	2.3**	(1.6, 3.4)	1.1	(0.7, 1.9)	1.8**	(1.2, 2.8)	0.8	(0.5, 1.2)	1.6	(0.8, 2.9)
less than monthly	2.7**	(1.6, 4.4)	1.5	(0.7, 3.2)	3.1**	(1.5, 6.5)	0.9	(0.6, 1.4)	1.0	(0.4, 2.5)
Usually doesn't engage in foreplay	1.7+	(0.9, 3.1)	1.4	(0.8, 2.4)	0.9	(0.6, 1.5)	1.1	(0.7, 1.6)	1.3	(0.7, 2.8)
Thinking of sex										
never or < 1/month	Referent		Referent		Referent		Referent		Referent	
a few times/month	0.4**	(0.3, 0.7)	0.6	(0.4, 1.1)	0.6*	(0.4, 0.9)	0.3**	(0.2, 0.5)	1.0	(0.5, 2.0)
a few times/week	0.3**	(0.1, 0.5)	0.3+	(0.1, 1.2)	0.4+	(0.1, 1.1)	0.7	(0.3, 1.6)	0.2+	(0.0, 1.3)
Chi-square	124.56		49.56		68.77		173.36		78.94	
d.f.	27		26		26		28		24	
Observations	1011		599		668		1144		356	

Note: Odds ratios from logistic regression and their 95% confidence intervals in parenthesis. Based on reports from sexually active women. Country differences in each region controlled.

"West" includes Australia, Canada, and New Zealand;

East Asia includes China, Hong Kong, Taiwan, and Japan;

Southeast Asia includes Indonesia and Malaysia;

South America includes Brazil and Mexico;

Mid-east includes Algeria and Turkey.

$\dagger p \leq 0.10$; * $p \leq 0.05$; ** $p \leq 0.01$.

Table 2.3.5. Factors associated with pain during sex among women by region

	"West"		C/S America		Middle East		East Asia		SE Asia	
Age (years)										
40–49	Referent		Referent		Referent		Referent		Referent	
50–59	0.5+	(0.3, 1.0)	0.8	(0.4, 1.6)	1.0	(0.5, 1.9)	1.1	(0.7, 1.6)	2.1*	(1.1, 4.0)
60–69	0.8	(0.3, 1.9)	1.2	(0.5, 2.9)	0.9	(0.4, 2.0)	1.3	(0.8, 2.1)	1.5	(0.7, 3.5)
70–80		n.a.	0.6	(0.1, 2.4)	1.9	(0.5, 7.9)	1.1	(0.5, 2.1)	1.1	(0.4, 3.0)
Education										
at least some college	Referent		Referent		Referent		Referent		Referent	
secondary/high school	1.0	(0.5, 1.9)	1.2	(0.5, 2.5)	0.9	(0.4, 2.1)	1.0	(0.7, 1.5)	0.7	(0.4, 1.3)
primary school or less	0.5	(0.0, 6.2)	0.7	(0.3, 1.6)	1.1	(0.5, 2.1)	1.2	(0.7, 2.1)	0.5	(0.2, 1.2)
Divorce in past 3 years	0.2	(0.0, 2.0)	0.7	(0.1, 7.4)	1.1	(0.3, 4.4)	1.7	(0.4, 7.2)	0.3	(0.0, 3.4)
Financial problems in last 3 years	1.7	(0.8, 3.5)	2.2*	(1.2, 4.0)	1.0	(0.5, 1.9)	1.6*	(1.0, 2.5)	1.1	(0.6, 2.1)
Fair/poor overall health (vs good)	1.7	(0.8, 3.4)	1.1	(0.6, 2.2)	0.9	(0.5, 1.9)	1.6**	(1.2, 2.3)	1.6	(0.9, 2.7)
Level of physical activity										
average and above	Referent		Referent		Referent		Referent		Referent	
lower than average	0.8	(0.4, 1.8)	0.5	(0.2, 1.3)	2.0*	(1.1, 3.7)	0.8	(0.5, 1.2)	2.2*	(1.1, 4.4)
Vascular diseases	1.0	(0.5, 1.7)	1.3	(0.7, 2.5)	1.4	(0.7, 2.7)	1.1	(0.8, 1.5)	1.4	(0.8, 2.4)
Hysterectomy	0.4**	(0.2, 0.8)	1.5	(0.7, 3.0)	0.4*	(0.2, 0.9)	1.2	(0.7, 2.2)	0.1**	(0.0, 0.3)
Depression diagnosed	1.5	(0.7, 3.1)	1.5	(0.7, 2.9)	1.6	(0.8, 3.1)	1.3	(0.6, 2.9)	1.8	(0.8, 3.9)
Smoking										
never	Referent		Referent		Referent		Referent		Referent	
smoked before	1.6	(0.8, 3.1)	1.1	(0.6, 2.2)	1.1	(0.5, 2.7)	0.4*	(0.2, 0.8)	0.6	(0.2, 2.1)
currently smoking	1.1	(0.5, 2.6)	1.2	(0.5, 2.5)	1.0	(0.5, 1.9)	1.0	(0.6, 1.7)	0.3*	(0.1, 0.9)
Belief that aging reduces sex interest/activity	1.9+	(0.9, 3.8)	0.5*	(0.3, 1.0)	0.6+	(0.4, 1.1)	1.1	(0.8, 1.6)	0.8	(0.5, 1.5)
Belief in religion guiding sex	1.6	(0.8, 2.9)	1.7	(0.9, 3.2)	1.5	(0.8, 2.8)	0.9	(0.5, 1.7)	3.5**	(1.5, 8.1)
Partnership status										
exclusive and committed	Referent		Referent		Referent		Referent		Referent	
exclusive but not committed	1.3	(0.5, 3.4)	0.3*	(0.1, 1.0)	1.6	(0.5, 5.5)	0.7	(0.2, 1.9)	0.7	(0.1, 4.6)
nonexclusive	3.1	(0.3, 29.1)	1.9	(0.5, 6.9)	1.4	(0.3, 6.3)	0.4	(0.1, 1.7)	1.5	(0.4, 6.5)
Future of the relationship										
high hope	Referent		Referent		Referent		Referent		Referent	
worried	3.4*	(1.2, 9.3)	1.5	(0.6, 3.6)	2.4+	(0.9, 6.3)	0.8	(0.4, 1.4)	1.3	(0.4, 4.4)
no future	2.9+	(0.8, 9.8)	0.7	(0.2, 2.0)	0.5	(0.1, 2.4)	1.3	(0.7, 2.5)	1.7	(0.4, 6.5)
Frequency of sexual relationship										
several times per week	Referent		Referent		Referent		Referent		Referent	
two to three times per month	1.4	(0.7, 2.6)	2.4*	(1.2, 4.5)	1.1	(0.6, 2.0)	1.2	(0.8, 1.9)	1.2	(0.6, 2.2)
less than monthly	1.4	(0.6, 3.4)	1.7	(0.5, 5.4)	1.3	(0.5, 3.3)	1.6*	(1.0, 2.4)	1.2	(0.6, 2.4)
Usually doesn't engage in foreplay	1.8	(0.8, 4.2)	1.1	(0.5, 2.5)	0.8	(0.5, 1.6)	1.3	(0.9, 1.9)	0.8	(0.4, 1.6)
Thinking of sex										
never or < 1/month	Referent		Referent		Referent		Referent		Referent	
a few times/month	0.7	(0.3, 1.6)	0.6	(0.3, 1.3)	1.0	(0.5, 1.8)	0.8	(0.5, 1.2)	1.5	(0.8, 2.9)
a few times/week	0.5	(0.2, 1.4)	0.4	(0.1, 1.5)	0.2	(0.0, 2.0)		n.a.	5.7**	(1.7, 19.5)
Chi-square	50.7		44.0		49.1		99.2		80.2	
d.f.	25		25		27		27		27	
Observations	815		430		840		1366		531	

Note: Odds ratios from logistic regression and their 95% confidence intervals in parenthesis. Based on reports from sexually active women. Country differences in each region controlled.
"West" includes Australia and Canada;
East Asia includes China, Hong Kong, Korea, and Japan;
Southeast Asia includes Indonesia, Philippine, and Malaysia;
South America includes Brazil;
Mid-east includes Algeria, Morocco, and Turkey.
+ $p \le 0.10$; * $p \le 0.05$; ** $p \le 0.01$.

Table 2.3.6. Factors associated with finding sex nonpleasurable among women by region

	"West"		C/S America		Mideast		East Asia		SE Asia	
Age (years)										
40–49		Referent		Referent		Referent		Referent		Referent
50–59	1.2	(0.7, 2.0)	0.8	(0.4, 1.7)	1.1	(0.7, 1.8)	1.3	(0.9, 1.9)	1.0	(0.6, 1.9)
60–69	1.6	(0.8, 3.1)	1.0	(0.4, 2.6)	1.5	(0.8, 2.7)	1.4	(0.9, 2.3)	0.5	(0.2, 1.2)
70–80	0.7	(0.2, 2.5)			0.9	(0.2, 4.5)	0.9	(0.4, 2.0)	1.3	(0.1, 18.7)
Education										
at least some college		Referent		Referent		Referent		Referent		Referent
secondary/high school	0.8	(0.5, 1.2)	1.7	(0.7, 3.8)	1.1	(0.5, 2.0)	1.1	(0.7, 1.6)	0.5*	(0.3, 0.9)
primary school or less	0.8	(0.2, 3.7)	0.6	(0.2, 1.5)	1.0	(0.6, 1.6)	1.4	(0.8, 2.4)	0.4*	(0.2, 0.9)
Divorce in past 3 years	0.9	(0.3, 3.0)			0.6	(0.1, 2.1)	1.0	(0.2, 3.9)	0.6	(0.2, 2.4)
Financial problems in last 3 years	2.2**	(1.3, 3.8)	1.1	(0.6, 2.0)	1.4	(0.9, 2.4)	1.0	(0.6, 1.6)	1.6+	(0.9, 3.0)
Fair/poor overall health (vs good)	1.9*	(1.0, 3.7)	1.3	(0.6, 2.7)	0.9	(0.6, 1.5)	1.3+	(1.0, 1.8)	1.4	(0.8, 2.3)
Level of physical activity										
average and above		Referent		Referent		Referent		Referent		Referent
lower than average	1.0	(0.5, 2.0)	1.9	(0.8, 4.6)	2.9**	(1.7, 5.1)	1.3	(0.9, 2.0)	2.5**	(1.5, 4.2)
Vascular diseases	0.7	(0.5, 1.2)	0.9	(0.5, 1.8)	1.4	(0.9, 2.2)	1.1	(0.8, 1.5)	1.2	(0.7, 2.2)
Hysterectomy	1.3	(0.7, 2.2)	1.1	(0.5, 2.4)	1.7	(0.8, 3.7)	1.0	(0.6, 1.7)	0.8	(0.4, 1.9)
Depression diagnosed	1.1	(0.6, 2.0)	1.0	(0.5, 1.9)	1.9**	(1.2, 3.2)	1.6	(0.8, 3.2)	3.9**	(1.5, 10.2)
Smoking										
never		Referent		Referent		Referent		Referent		Referent
smoked before	1.4	(0.9, 2.3)	0.8	(0.4, 1.7)	1.0	(0.5, 2.0)	0.6	(0.3, 1.2)	2.7	(0.8, 9.2)
currently smoking	1.4	(0.8, 2.5)	0.9	(0.4, 2.1)	1.0	(0.6, 1.7)	1.1	(0.6, 2.0)	1.4	(0.6, 3.0)
Belief that aging reduces sex interest/activity	1.8*	(1.1, 3.1)	0.9	(0.5, 1.9)	1.3	(0.8, 2.1)	1.4*	(1.0, 1.9)	1.3	(0.7, 2.2)
Belief in religion guiding sex	1.4	(0.9, 2.2)	0.8	(0.4, 1.6)	0.9	(0.6, 1.5)	1.6+	(1.0, 2.5)	1.0	(0.6, 1.9)
Partnership status										
exclusive and committed		Referent		Referent		Referent		Referent		Referent
exclusive but not committed	0.7	(0.4, 1.4)	0.1*	(0.0, 0.7)	2.1	(0.8, 5.9)	0.7	(0.2, 2.4)	0.8	(0.3, 2.5)
non-exclusive	2.4	(0.4, 14.1)	1.2	(0.4, 3.4)	1.1	(0.3, 4.1)	1.8	(0.8, 3.8)	0.7	(0.2, 2.1)
Future of the relationship										
high hope		Referent		Referent		Referent		Referent		Referent
worried	4.7**	(2.3, 9.9)	2.1	(0.8, 5.6)	1.0	(0.4, 2.6)	2.4**	(1.4, 4.0)	0.8	(0.3, 2.5)
no future	1.4	(0.4, 5.3)	1.4	(0.5, 4.3)	1.2	(0.4, 3.8)	3.3**	(1.7, 6.3)	3.4+	(0.9, 12.5)
Frequency of sexual relationship										
several times per week		Referent		Referent		Referent		Referent		Referent
two to three times per month	1.6+	(0.9, 2.6)	1.2	(0.6, 2.6)	1.9**	(1.2, 3.1)	1.1	(0.7, 1.6)	0.6+	(0.3, 1.1)
less than monthly	2.0*	(1.0, 3.9)	1.6	(0.5, 5.3)	1.9+	(0.9, 4.0)	0.8	(0.4, 1.4)	1.0	(0.4, 2.1)
Usually doesn't engage in foreplay	1.0	(0.4, 2.1)	3.4**	(1.6, 7.2)	0.9	(0.6, 1.5)	1.8**	(1.3, 2.5)	1.6+	(0.9, 2.9)
Thinking of sex										
never or < 1/month		Referent		Referent		Referent		Referent		Referent
a few times/month	0.3**	(0.2, 0.7)	0.5	(0.2, 1.2)	0.7+	(0.4, 1.1)	0.5**	(0.4, 0.8)	0.7	(0.3, 1.3)
a few times/week	0.2**	(0.1, 0.6)	0.1*	(0.0, 0.8)	0.2*	(0.0, 0.8)	0.6	(0.2, 2.3)	0.4	(0.1, 1.4)
Chi-square		104.5		43.6		80.8		107.0		65.0
d.f.		27		23		27		29		28
Observations		928		351		719		1357		550

Note: Odds ratios from logistic regression and their 95% confidence intervals in parenthesis. Based on reports from sexually active women. Country differences in each region controlled.
"West" includes Australia, Canada, and New Zealand;
East Asia includes China, Hong Kong, Taiwan, Korea, and Japan;
Southeast Asia includes Indonesia, Malaysia, Thailand, and Singapore;
South America includes Brazil;
Mideast includes Algeria, Morocco, and Turkey.
† $p \leq 0.10$; * $p \leq 0.05$; ** $p \leq 0.01$.

As in all cross-sectional surveys, the causal direction of many covariates is not clear. For example, when we observe an association between overall health or depression and a sexual problem, we cannot discern the causal direction in these cross-sectional data. All of our measures are self-reported, and many are based on responses to single items; however, in a multicountry survey of this size, it would not be feasible to include physical examinations. Hence, there is likely to be considerable classification error, which is most likely reflected in the relatively modest sizes of many ORs. Self-reports of sexual conditions and other health conditions are likely to underestimate the true prevalence because the subject may not be aware, may not recall, or may choose not to disclose that she has the problem/condition in question. A subject is unlikely to report a problem/condition that she does not have.

A number of sexual problems were found to be frequent in this large sample of women aged 40–80 years. Among those problems, lack of interest in sex and inability to reach orgasm were the most common across the world regions we investigated. In comparing those regions, Asian regions show the highest prevalence rates across various sexual problems. In terms of risk factors, physical, social/emotional, and relationship factors were all found to have a significant impact on the prevalence of one or more sexual problems. In addition, we observed an important gender difference: increasing age was less consistently associated with sexual problems among women.

Acknowledgments

The GSSAB was funded by Pfizer Inc. We acknowledge the contribution of our colleagues in this study, namely, Alfredo Nicolosi (Italy), Clive Gingell (UK), Edson Moreira (Brazil), and Tianfu Wang (China) for the GSSAB Investigators' Group, and the international advisory board for this study, namely, Jacques Buvat (France), Gerald Brock (Canada), Uwe Hartmann (Germany), Sae-Chul Kim (Korea), Rosie King (Australia), Bernard Levinson (South Africa), Ken Marumo (Japan), and Ferruh Simsek (Turkey).

References

1. Tiefer L. A new view of women's sexual problems: why new? why now? *J Sex Res* 2001; 38: 89–96.
2. Simons JS, Carey MP. Prevalence of sexual dysfunctions: results from a decade of research. *Arch Sex Behav* 2001; 30: 177–219.
3. Laumann EO, Paik A, Rosen RD. Sexual dysfunction in the United States: prevalence and predictors. *JAMA* 1999; 281: 537–44.
4. Parish W, Obhuhova E, Laumann EO et al. Sexual dysfunctions in urban China. *J Sex Marital Ther* [undergoing review].
5. Dunn KM, Croft PR, Hackett GI. Association of sexual problems with social, psychological, and physical problems in men and women: a cross sectional population survey. *J Epidemiol Community Health* 1999; 53: 144–8.
6. Fugl-Meyer AR, Fugl-Meyer KS. Sexual disabilities, problems and satisfaction in 18–74 year old Swedes. *Scand J Sexol* 1999; 2: 79–105.
7. Bacon CG, Mittleman MA, Kawachi I et al. Sexual function in men older than 50 years of age: results from the Health Professionals Follow-up Study. *Ann Intern Med* 2003; 139: 161–8.
8. Laumann EO, Nicolosi A, Glasser DB et al. Sexual problems among women and men aged 40–80 y: prevalence and correlates identified in the Global Study of Sexual Attitudes and Behaviors. *Int J Impot Res* 2005; 17: 39–57.
9. Trudel G, Turgeon L, Piche L. Marital and sexual aspects of old age. *Sex Relatsh Ther* 2000; 154: 381–406.
10. Clement U. Sex in long-term relationships: a systematic approach to sexual desire problems. *Arch Sex Behav* 2002; 31: 241–6.
11. Kaplan HS. *The New Sex Therapy: Active Treatment of Sexual Dysfunctions*. New York: Brunner/Mazel, 1974.
12. Masters WH, Johnson VE. *Human Sexual Inadequacy*. Boston: Little, Brown, 1970.
13. Southern S. Facilitating sexual health: intimacy enhancement techniques for sexual dysfunction. *J Mental Health Counsel* 1999; 21: 15–32.
14. Nebot M, Celentano DD, Burwell et al. AISA and behavioural risk factors in women in inner city Baltimore: a comparison of telephone and face to face surveys. *J Epidemiol Community Health* 1994; 48: 412–18.
15. Nicolosi A, Laumann EO, Glasser DB et al. Sexual behavior and sexual problems after age 40: the Global Study of Sexual Attitudes and Behaviors. *Urology* 2004; 64: 991–7.

Assessing the prevalence of female sexual dysfunction with surveys: what is feasible?

Cynthia A Graham, John Bancroft

There is current widespread interest in the prevalence of "female sexual dysfunction", driven, in part, by industrial hopes that drugs such as sildenafil will have beneficial effects, generating a large market for women as well as men. At the same time, there has also been growing dissatisfaction with the current classification of sexual dysfunction, particularly for women.[1,2]

The purpose of this chapter is to review and evaluate the use of community-based surveys to assess the frequency of sexual dysfunction in women. As a first step, we consider the meaning of the term "female sexual dysfunction". We conclude that, whereas sexual dysfunction is a useful clinical concept, only some of the criteria required to make such diagnoses can be established in large, population-based surveys. However, there are a number of important aspects relevant to prevalence and etiology that can be addressed, and suggestions will be made for improving survey design for such purposes.

In 1999, a paper in the *Journal of the American Medical Association*[3] reported that 43% of American women have a sexual dysfunction. This figure, which will be examined more closely in this chapter, has been extensively cited in the scientific literature, in the media, and in self-help books for women*[4,5] We argue that the very limited questions asked in

this survey fell far short of what is needed to identify a "sexual dysfunction" (see fuller discussion in refs 6 and 7).

What is "sexual dysfunction"?

So what does "sexual dysfunction" mean, and how does it differ from a more general term such as "sexual problem" or "sexual difficulty"? It was probably Masters and Johnson, in 1970, who initiated the current use of the term "sexual dysfunction". It did appear in the medical literature prior to 1970, but always in reference to sexual side effects caused by medication or surgery.[8–10] Although in their first book Masters and Johnson[11] put forward their idea of a sexual response cycle that is basically the same in men and women, in their second book[12] they categorized sexual dysfunction for men and for women quite differently. With the male they focused on "impotence" (primary and secondary), with premature ejaculation and "ejaculatory incompetence" as additional categories. With the female, they focused on "orgasmic dysfunction", with "vaginismus" as an additional, specifically female dysfunction. "Dyspareunia" was considered relevant to both men and women. Kaplan[13] used the concept of "general female sexual dysfunction", noting that this was "usually called frigidity". In addition, she described "orgastic dysfunction", drawing the distinction between "inhibition" of the "vasocongestive" and "orgasm" components of sexual response. Both

*As of 1 March 2004, over 300 citations in the medical and psychological literature were identified by the Institute for Scientific Information's "Web of Science".

Kaplan and Masters and Johnson therefore continued to use the conventional but pejorative terms for the principal types of male and female dysfunction, i.e., "impotence" and "frigidity".

The first two editions of the *Diagnostic and Statistical Manual of Mental Disorders* (DSM-I and -II)[14,15] did not use the concept "sexual dysfunction". DSM-I,[14] under the general heading "psychophysiological autonomic and visceral disorders", included the terms "frigidity", "impotence", "premature ejaculation of semen", and "vaginismus" in a list of supplementary terms for the urogenital system. In the second edition, DSM-II,[15] only dyspareunia and impotence were listed as examples of "psychophysiological genito-urinary disorders".

In 1980, the concept of "psychosexual dysfunction" appeared in the third edition of the DSM (DSM-III).[16] The DSM approach to sexual dysfunction was clearly based on Masters and Johnson's ideas, although, interestingly, not their ideas about sexual dysfunction but rather their concept of the sexual response cycle,[11] modified by Kaplan's[13] addition of "sexual desire" as a separate component. This resulted in male and female diagnostic categories that were conceptually similar: "inhibited sexual desire" (neither "inhibited" nor "sexual desire" were defined), "inhibited sexual excitement", "inhibited orgasm", and "functional dyspareunia", each with a male and female version. "Functional vaginismus" was included as a specifically female dysfunction and premature ejaculation as a male dysfunction.

The current (fourth) edition of the DSM (DSM-IV)[17] defines sexual dysfunction as characterized by disturbance in sexual desire and in the psychophysiologic changes that characterize the sexual response cycle, and as causing marked distress and interpersonal difficulty. The concept of "inhibition" no longer features. Thus, there is hypoactive sexual desire disorder and sexual aversion disorder, defined in the same way for men and women. Female sexual arousal disorder is defined as "a persistent or recurrent inability to attain, or to maintain until completion of the sexual activity, an adequate lubrication-swelling response of sexual excitement", and for the male version, erection is the relevant response. Orgasmic disorder (i.e., delayed or absent orgasm) and dyspareunia are defined in basically the same way for men and women. Vaginismus is a specifically female disorder.

The *International Statistical Classification of Diseases and Related Health Problems* (ICD-10)[18] covers sexual dysfunctions in one and a half pages, compared with nearly 30 pages in the current DSM. The basic categories of dysfunction are similar to those of the DSM, but there are few, if any, actual diagnostic criteria given for any of the dysfunctions. The ICD-10 also does not require that personal distress or interpersonal problems be present for a diagnosis to be made. Instead, it states, "sexual dysfunction covers the various ways in which an individual is unable to participate in a sexual relationship as he or she would wish".

be used by some sections of the medical profession. Both terms can be regarded as male-centered; impotence, from erectile failure, rendering the man powerless; frigid indicating absence of warmth, with a consequent chilling effect on the male partner. The use by the DSM of the "sexual response cycle" as a predictable sequence of basically physiologic events, essentially the same in women and men, can be seen as an attempt to redress the societal view, which has prevailed in the past, that women's sexuality is something fundamentally different from that of men. Since such a distinction was central to the long-standing societal repression of female sexuality, challenging this distinction had obvious sociopolitical significance, and may have been regarded by some as "politically correct" for that reason.

However, although Masters and Johnson proposed a "sexual response cycle" that in physiologic terms was basically the same for women and men (and we accept Tiefer's[19] criticisms of that concept), they also emphasized the impact of sociocultural factors on women's sexuality. "Negation of female sexuality, which discourages the development of an effectively useful sexual value system, has been an exercise of the so-called double standard and its socio-cultural precursors".[12] They add, "Socio-cultural influence more often than not places woman in a position in which she must adapt, sublimate, inhibit or even distort her natural capacity to function sexually in order to fulfill her genetically assigned role. *Herein lies a major source of woman's sexual dysfunction*". Masters and Johnson did not appear to equate the sexual dysfunctions of men and women, either in their diagnostic categories, or in the above, telling statement. But if their other ideas on the sexual response cycle were used by clinicians to achieve "political correctness" through the DSM process, "political correctness" can be regarded as no longer the same on this issue. There is now growing recognition of, and emphasis on, gender differences in sexuality. Alternative models of sexual response[20] and new, women-centered definitions of sexual problems in women[21] have been proposed. In a recent national survey of heterosexual American women,[6] the main predictors of distress about sex were not the more physiologic factors that are the basis of the DSM-IV (e.g., lubrication, frequency of orgasm) but were factors related to a woman's mood and the subjective quality of the sexual interaction with the partner. And, as early studies evaluating the effects of sildenafil in women have proven disappointing,[22] even the pharmaceutical industry is moving toward a "politically correct" view that there are fundamental differences between men and women's sexuality. Pfizer recently publicly announced that, after 8 years of work, they had terminated their research program evaluating the effects of sildenafil on women, citing greater complexity of women's sexual response and a "disconnect between genital changes and mental changes" in women as reasons.[23]

"Political correctness"

The term "frigidity" has more or less disappeared from clinical and research use, although the term "impotence" continues to

The issue of distress

Although an essential criterion for the DSM-IV[17] diagnosis of any sexual dysfunction is that the problem causes "marked distress or interpersonal difficulty", this is a relatively recent development. In the revised third edition of the DSM (DSM-III-R),[24] distress or interpersonal difficulty was not required. Why this requirement that a sexual problem cause "marked distress" before being considered a "dysfunction" was added to the DSM-IV is not clear. The recent International Consensus Development Conference Report, written by a multidisciplinary group of experts who reappraised the DSM categories and proposed a slightly modified classification system for female sexual dysfunction,[25] recommended that the presence of "personal distress" be a requirement for any diagnosis, as distinct from the "marked distress or interpersonal difficulty" required in the DSM. The rationale for this emphasis on specifically "personal" distress, while excluding interpersonal distress, was not given. The issue of "distress" is particularly relevant to low sexual desire, which is often not a cause of concern for the individual but may cause problems in the relationship; in such cases, using the new consensus classification system, a diagnosis of sexual dysfunction would not be given. The whole issue of "distress" as an essential diagnostic criterion is complex. Distress, it could be argued, is a reaction to the dysfunction and thus has no explanatory value. It is of clinical relevance, but mainly because it determines whether the individual is motivated to change or wants help; the person who is not distressed by the dysfunction, or whose sexual relationship is not affected by it, is unlikely to seek treatment. It does not help in deciding which treatment is most likely to be effective. On the other hand, if our goal is to conceptualize "sexual dysfunction" in women's terms, capturing the problems and difficulties which are the principal concern for women, then we need to understand what worries or distresses them. But it may well turn out not to be the DSM diagnostic criteria.

Previous community-based surveys

In a review article on the prevalence of sexual dysfunctions, Simons and Carey[26] pointed to a lack of methodological rigor in many of the studies. Of the 52 studies reviewed, more than one-third did not provide *any* operational definition of the dysfunction being assessed. Moreover, of studies that purportedly used the DSM criteria to establish sexual dysfunction, few assessed the presence of "marked distress or interpersonal difficulty" or the absence of an Axis I disorder (both essential criteria for a DSM diagnosis).

Recently, Bancroft and colleagues[6] compared their survey of women with four earlier studies involving substantial community based samples of women.[3,27–30] Three relevant conclusions were drawn from this comparison: (1) arbitrary definitions of what constituted a "sexual problem" were used, resulting in considerable variability across studies in the prevalence of specific sexual problems; (2) there was limited overlap between women who defined themselves as having a sexual problem and those assigned to one of the researcher-defined problem categories; (3) a strong association was found between the presence of "sexual problems" and other problems in the women's lives, most notably mood problems and relationship difficulties.[3,6,28,30]

In 2003, two new British studies using community-based samples were reported. Mercer and colleagues[31] used secondary data from a national probability sample survey of sexual attitudes and lifestyles carried out in 2000.[32,33] In this survey, which obtained a response rate of 65.4%, and included 5530 women aged 16–44 years who reported at least one heterosexual partner in the previous year, 53.8% of the women indicated at least one sexual problem lasting *at least 1 month* during the previous year, the most common problem being "lacked interest in sex" (40.6% of women vs 17.1% of men). "Persistent problems" were defined as those lasting at least 6 months; 15.6% of women reported at least one persistent problem, with 10.2% citing lack of interest in sex as a persistent problem (compared with 1.8% of the men). Overall, 21.0% of women and 10.5% of men had sought help for a sexual problem in the previous year. The striking contrast between the prevalence of "short duration" (53.8%) and "persistent" problems (15.6%), particularly relating to sexual interest, confronts us with the possibility that transient impairment may result from situational factors, and may not indicate "dysfunction" *per se*. On the other hand, recurrence of short-term adaptive impairments of this kind may indicate vulnerability to sexual problems.[34] We will consider this further later in the chapter.

Nazareth and colleagues[35] assessed prevalence of sexual dysfunction in a sample of 1065 women and 447 men attending general practitioners in England. This paper, published in the *British Medical Journal*, is brief. We also find it perplexing. Much is made in the paper of the use of ICD-10 diagnostic criteria, "stringently applied", yet, as stated earlier, ICD-10 gives little more than headings and brief descriptions, and certainly no diagnostic criteria. In this study, the "diagnostic criteria" are based on the past 4 weeks. While this time period may be preferable to obtain reliable estimates of frequencies (see below), no clinician is going to make a diagnosis of sexual dysfunction based only on the past 4 weeks.

In an early but still highly relevant review of the survey literature, Nathan[36] suggested five ways in which epidemiologic data on rates of sexual dysfunction could prove useful: service planning, prevention efforts (e.g. by highlighting high-risk groups), providing normative data, generating hypotheses about causal factors, and, lastly, by providing data that might challenge existing definitions of "dysfunction". Recent survey efforts have focused on the first of these applications, but much less attention has been paid to the other four possibilities. For example, in reporting their conclusion that 43% of women have a sexual dysfunction, Laumann and colleagues[3] stated that "with the affected population rarely receiving medical therapy for sexual dysfunction, service delivery efforts should be augmented to target high-risk populations", what has been described as a clear example of "medicalization".[37]

How do we conceptualize women's sexual problems? The need for a theoretical approach

Simons and Carey[25] concluded that use of "a common classification system", such as the DSM, will lead to better surveys. We would argue that any such classificatory system should be based on good, clinically relevant research that identifies what women see as important sexual problems. This does not appear to be the case with the DSM. Research has shown that sexual satisfaction for many women is closely linked to relationship factors, such as feeling "connected" with a sexual partner.[6,38] As Tiefer[21] has argued, the DSM "bypasses" these relational aspects of women's sexuality and assumes an exclusively individual approach to sexuality. Other researchers have highlighted the importance of partner-related factors to women's sexual satisfaction.[38,39] In a survey, Ellison[38] asked over 2000 women to distinguish between experiences that they considered "problems" and those that they thought of as "just the way life is". Experiences such as feeling "too tired" or "too busy" for sex were less likely to be reported as problems and were most likely to be considered as "just the way life is". At a minimum, studies should assess whether women perceive situations such as inability to reach orgasm as a "problem" or not. It is also important to establish whether a woman is receiving what is for her appropriate stimulation during sexual activity with her partner. In some cases, a woman's failure to experience an orgasm may have more to do with her partner's behavior than whether she is "dysfunctional". But we also need a much better understanding of how women *experience* sexual problems, in their own terms. To do this requires research, with both nonclinical and clinical samples, into basic questions such as how women experience sexual desire and arousal.

Notably absent from this literature is a theoretical approach which might enable us to conceptualize sexual dysfunctions in ways that are relevant and appropriate to each gender, and which can be empirically tested. Recently, the dual control model has been presented as one way to fill this gap.[40,41] This postulates that, for the majority of individuals, inhibition of sexual response is an adaptive mechanism that reduces the likelihood of sexual responses in circumstances where they would be inappropriate or disadvantageous, a mechanism of relevance across species. This reintroduces the concept of inhibition, but with the important difference that it is not necessarily dysfunctional. If we accept this basic premise, we are then faced with the fundamental challenge of distinguishing between a reduction in sexual responsiveness that is appropriate or adaptive given the current circumstances, and one that is a manifestation of some malfunctioning of the sexual response system that might appropriately be called a dysfunction. This may result from increased inhibition or reduced excitation. The focus of any intervention, for the first pattern, would then be the circumstances that elicited the adaptive response (e.g., improving a relationship problem, or dealing with stressful life circumstances). The focus for the second pattern would involve, in some way, treating the sexual dysfunction.

Keeping this fundamental distinction in mind, we can then look at each individual's case through three conceptual "windows".[6]

(1) Through the first window, we look at the woman's current situation. To what extent are problems in her relationship with her sexual partner, or in her life more generally, resulting in adaptive inhibition of sexual responsiveness?

(2) Through the second window, we consider the individual's sexual history. To what extent has the current pattern of nonresponsiveness been evident earlier in her life? Here we can use a second basic premise from the dual control model: that individuals vary in their propensity for sexual inhibition. Our attempts to measure such propensities in men[42] and, more recently, in women (Graham, Sanders, and Milhausen, unpublished data) have supported this premise; the majority of individuals score somewhere in the middle, what we can call "adaptive", range for inhibition proneness. But some individuals score high in this respect, and we have found a strong association between such scores and clinically established erectile dysfunction in men (Bancroft, Herbenick, Barnes et al., unpublished data). We have also found that men scoring low on inhibition are more likely to take sexual risks.[43,44] Comparable research with women is still at an early stage, but we anticipate similar associations, with the possibility that inhibition proneness may play a greater role in the sexuality of women, with a wider range of inhibition-inducing circumstances, and hence with a greater likelihood of inhibition being "adaptive" rather than dysfunctional. The origins or determinants of such individual differences, whether they be genetic factors or early learning, or the effects of early traumatic sexual experiences, remain to be established.

(3) Through the third window, we can look for evidence of aging, medical problems, hormonal changes or the side effects of drugs, which might directly impair sexual functioning.

We can meaningfully consider problems explained through the second and third windows as "sexual dysfunctions". To make these distinctions requires careful clinical assessment, and a not inconsiderable amount of clinical judgment, taking into account a woman's ethnic, cultural, religious, and social background as well as age and experience, current health status, frequency and duration of the sexual problems, and distress.

The importance of establishing norms from community surveys is particularly pertinent to studying the prevalence of "sexual desire problems". Prevalence rates for low sexual desire vary greatly across different studies, more so than for other dysfunctions[6] but are consistently higher for women than for men.[3,31] Surveys reporting prevalence rates for sexual desire disorders have typically asked women about whether they have experienced "problems" such as "lacking desire for sex"[3] or "decreased interest in sex".[29] Yet, rarely have researchers looked at how women interpret "lacking desire for sex". This is particularly important given the comorbidity between arousal and desire disorders[25] and the observation that women often do not differentiate "arousal" from "desire".[38,45] Although there are no established norms, there is an extensive literature on gender differences in the frequency of thoughts and fantasies about sex, the desired frequency of sexual activity and of initiating sex.[46] Research has consistently found that men report more frequent sexual thoughts and fantasies. In one study of 40-year-old Danish women, 33% reported that they never experienced "spontaneous libido", yet most of those women enjoyed sexual activity once their partners had initiated it.[47] With our theoretical model, there is also the question of whether inhibition of sexual interest, as an "adaptive" reaction to current circumstances, and hence transitory, is more common in women than in men. This is highly relevant to deciding whether in a particular case "low sexual desire" should be regarded as a dysfunction. And we are still left with the question of how appropriate it is to assess the frequency of sexual thoughts as an indicator of "sexual interest" in women. As Heiman[48] has argued, we need to consider what we specifically want to capture in our assessment of sexual desire in women; "desire" is an elusive concept.

Designing better community–based studies – methodological issues

Survey design

Most community-based surveys have been and will continue to be cross-sectional. Longitudinal studies have obvious and considerable advantages, although because of their long-term nature, they are exceptionally difficult to implement. Dennerstein and colleagues[39] have reported on a prospective, population-based study of Australian-born women, assessed annually for 8 years, as they progressed through the menopausal transition. The purpose of this study was not to establish prevalence of sexual dysfunction, but to assess factors that affect women's sexual functioning and how these change over time. Another longitudinal study that, while principally focused on issues on mental health, assessed sexual problems is the Zurich cohort study.[34] A sample of men and women were interviewed on four occasions over a 10-year period, between the ages of 20 and 30. Women were more likely than men to report chronic or recurrent sexual difficulties, problems that were also more strongly associated with minor psychiatric or personality problems.

Longitudinal studies involving repeated assessment over a relatively short period (e.g., 2 years) are becoming increasingly feasible with the development of established survey panels (see below).

Obtaining a sample

Surveys that aim to establish prevalence of sexual problems and associated factors clearly need to be representative, if any generalization to the general population is to be made. This presents a challenge. Currently, the only feasible way to generate a representative national sample is to employ one of the survey organizations that have the mechanisms for sampling in place.[3,31] This is extremely costly. Whereas a few years ago, random digit dialing was the usual method for generating a sample, this is no longer considered acceptable as a result of problems with telephone surveys in general (discussed further below). Obtaining a sample of a known but limited population, such as general practitioner's lists,[35] is more feasible, but problems of generalizability and participation biases remain.

When selecting a representative sample, the specific aims of the project should be taken into consideration. Thus, if age is an important factor, the use of probability-based oversampling of otherwise underrepresented age groups will allow sufficient power to test the age-related hypotheses. Other examples of groups that, if a focus of the study, may require oversampling are gay men and lesbian women, celibate individuals, and various ethnic groups.

For studies that focus on relationships between factors of possible causal relevance, rather than prevalence rates, less representative samples can be useful, provided that the limitations of the sample and the need for replication are kept in mind.

Methods of data collection

Surveys conventionally have used self-report questionnaires, interview methods, or a combination of the two. There are advantages and disadvantages with each of these methods. In face-to-face interviews, the interviewer can clarify the meaning of questions and probe for more detailed responses if necessary,[3,32] but this also can result in greater variance in how questions are asked and meanings conveyed. The training of the interviewer is of crucial importance here, as are possible biases related to the gender, age, and ethnic background of the interviewer.[49] A disadvantage of interviews, particularly for large-scale surveys, is that they are expensive and labor-intensive. Problems of underreporting of sexual problems due to concerns about stigmatization may also be more likely if interviews are used, particularly when conditions of privacy cannot be assured. In Laumann et al.'s survey,[3] 21% of the face-to-face interviews were conducted with a third person present (most often children or stepchildren, but in some cases spouses or sexual partners). Although this may not be a problem for many survey topics, asking questions about sensitive issues such as sex requires confidentiality if not anonymity.

Telephone surveys have been used in several of the large-scale acquired immune deficiency syndrome (AIDS) behavioral surveys, such as the survey carried out in France.[50] In a direct comparison of telephone survey and face-to-face interviewing, although questions were more easily answered on the telephone, they were more likely to be influenced by social desirability than with the interview method.[51] Although telephone surveys are less expensive than interviews, it has become increasingly difficult to recruit participants by telephone.

The use of various kinds of computer-assisted interviews in surveys has increased. There are a number of advantage of these methods: use of "branching" and "skip" questions, checks for inconsistencies, and automatic data entry and "time stamping", as well as the increased confidentiality and anonymity that they provide respondents. Studies have found that computerized methods elicit more accurate reports of "sensitive" behaviors such as same-sex sexual activity.[52] If a method such as audio-computer-assisted self-interview (A-CASI) is used in a respondent's home, an interviewer might be present to answer questions about the survey, although this adds to the expense. Such methods have been incorporated into recent telephone surveys, either with the interviewer entering the participant's responses directly into a computer (computer-assisted telephone interview [CATI]), or with respondents entering responses directly into the computer with touch-tone telephones (telephone-audio-computer-assisted self-interview (T-ACASI).[6] Such methods do not, however, solve the participation problems with telephone surveys.

A newly emerging method, which has not as yet been used to collect sexuality-related information, but is being increasingly used for health-related surveys, and which, in our view, has considerable potential, is the use of Internet panels. An example of this is the Knowledge Networks Panel,[53] which involves approximately 40 000 individuals aged over 18. In return for receiving cable connections and computer facilities, an individual agrees to complete a short survey every few weeks. This is a fairly representative sample demographically, although the representation is limited by the original use of random digit dialing for establishing the panel. There are a number of distinct advantages to this approach. First, all of the advantages of computerized interviewing are present. A substantial amount of information about the panelists is already available, which not only can be used to augment the data collected in a specific survey, but also allows better description of those who decline to participate. A large number of individuals can be screened before selecting probability-based subsamples, and a substantial number of questions can be asked by using a series of short surveys. Second, repeated surveying allows assessment of stability of responses and change over time. In a recent comparative study of this Internet approach and telephone interviewing, Chang and Krosnik (unpublished data) found the Internet method to have some advantages in terms of data quality. It remains to be seen whether this approach is effective in collecting sexuality-related data.

Survey questions

Surveys assessing the prevalence of factors relevant to sexual dysfunction need careful consideration of issues such as question wording and comprehension. Items should be as clear and specific as possible.[54] Pretesting of items, either with individuals or focus groups, should be utilized,[55] and checked in pilot surveys where subjects can be asked, after completing the survey, how they interpreted the questions.

Assessing the frequency of sexual activity or sexual problems raises important methodological issues, mainly because of recall error; accuracy of retrospective recall of sexual behavior declines significantly with longer recall periods.[56,57] At the same time, assessing the duration of a problem is clearly important, and often requires reporting over relatively long time periods. This is where the "windows" concept, described earlier, can be useful. Assessment of a short and recent time period[6,27,35] allows reasonably accurate assessment of the current situation (i.e., through the first "window"). Care should be taken, however, with how such frequency is recorded. With a short time interval, such as a month, the number of occasions of sexual activity can be realistically recorded, followed by the proportion of those occasions in which a particular response (e.g., orgasm, vaginal lubrication) did not occur.[6]

In addition to the recent time period, it is clearly important to establish how long a particular pattern has been evident, partly to enable a more comprehensive assessment through the "first window" (e.g., did this altered pattern precede or follow some other factor of potential causal relevance?), but also to address the questions through the "second window" (e.g., Is this a lifelong pattern? Have their been periods of "normality"?). A combination of a relatively precise frequency for a recent time period, and a more realistic estimate of duration or intermittence is therefore appropriate.

Relatively little systematic attention has been paid to assessing duration of a problem or pattern of behavior. In the study by Mercer and colleagues,[31] participants were asked: "In the last year … have you experienced any of the following for one month or longer?" This was followed by the same list of seven "problems" used in Laumann et al.'s study.[3] For any item that was answered "yes", respondents were asked: "For how long did that period last when you …?" (this sequence of questioning was facilitated by computer-assisted self-interview). There were four response options: at least 1 month, but less than 3 months; at least 3 months, but less than 6 months; at least 6 months, but less than 1 year; and 1 year or longer. In contrast, Laumann et al.[3] simply asked whether the participant had experienced each of the seven difficulties "for several months or longer" during the previous year, with the response options "yes" or "no".

Ernst and colleagues[34] showed the benefits of a longitudinal study, with their finding that women, more often than men, reported relatively transient "disturbances" of sexual function that were nevertheless recurring. This pointed not only to circumstantial factors inducing the disturbance (i.e., "first window'), but also a vulnerability to such factors (i.e., "second window").

The use of standardized or psychometrically validated measures in community-based surveys has been infrequent. A small number of studies have used structured interviews, such as the Diagnostic Interview Schedule (DIS), to estimate the prevalence of psychosexual dysfunction.[26] In some cases, it has been stated that such measures permitted clinically accurate identification of the DSM or ICD diagnostic categories,[35,58] although such claims do not bear close examination.

Recently, there has been much emphasis on the need for "validated" measures of sexual problems, particularly for use in clinical trials of female sexual dysfunction.[25] A number of brief, self-report measures have been developed, such as the Female Sexual Function Index (FSFI)[59] and the Sexual Function Questionnaire (SFQ).[60] However, most of these measures were developed for use with clinical populations and to assess outcome after therapy, that is, change in sexual functioning, rather than the presence or absence of sexual dysfunction.[61] Few measures have been validated by comparison with other questionnaires; most have established "construct validity" only by differentiating between clinical and nonclinical populations. Development of questionnaires explicitly designed to assess sexual dysfunction in community-based surveys is required.

Exploring causal relationships

Which associated factors should be assessed will vary with the hypotheses being tested. Increasingly, surveys are showing an important relation between mood and sexual functioning, particularly in women, and some appropriate measure of mood and well-being, such as the Short-Form Health Survey (SF12),[62] should be considered. The more subjective features of the woman's sexual relationship with her partner are also emerging as important, and warrant direct and well-considered inquiry. Issues relevant to the "third window", such as current physical health or use of medication, together with duration, also require attention.

In evaluating the relevance of the woman's previous history to her current sexual functioning, earlier traumatic sexual experiences, including child sexual abuse, should be considered. The age of onset of sexual activity, including masturbation, may be informative. Evidence suggests considerable individual variability in women for when they first become interested and responsive sexually.[63,64] It remains to be determined whether women with later (or earlier) onset of sexual responsiveness are more vulnerable to later sexual problems.

Conclusions

Previous reviews in this area have stressed the need for standard definitions of sexual dysfunction[65] and the use of a common classification system.[26] At this stage, we would recommend something different. Firstly, before adopting standard definitions, it seems that considerable progress needs to be made in understanding the nature of women's sexual problems. Qualitative approaches could be particularly valuable in providing insights into factors that influence distress about a sexual problem.[66] While a common classification system would be extremely useful, and enable comparison across studies, if the typology of sexual problems does not reflect the reality of women's experiences, "standardization" across studies does not, in our view, equal improvement. To date, the rationale for revising the DSM

diagnostic categories of sexual dysfunction has not been made clear, resulting in changes that appear to be arbitrary. It has even been suggested that we should preserve the current DSM diagnostic categories of sexual dysfunction to maintain "continuity in research and clinical practice",[25] but this could effectively turn our attention away from important research questions.

In this chapter we have argued that much of the information required to arrive at a clinical diagnosis of sexual dysfunction is difficult if not impossible to obtain in large, community-based surveys. However, establishing the prevalence of problematic patterns of sexual response in women and their association with factors of potential causal relevance is clearly needed. Of crucial importance is the distinction between inhibition of sexual interest or response that is "adaptive" given the current circumstances, and inhibition or lack of responsiveness, which is "dysfunctional", a distinction which is probably more crucial for women than for men.

References

1. Segraves RT. Editor's comments. *J Sex Marital Ther* 2001; 27: 81.
2. Tiefer L. Critique of the DMS-III-R nosology of sexual dysfunctions. *Psychiatr Med* 1992; 10: 227–45.
3. Laumann EO, Paik A, Rosen RC. Sexual dysfunctions in the United States: prevalence and predictors. *JAMA* 1999; 281: 537–44.
4. Foley S, Kope SA, Sugrue DP. *Sex Matters for Women: A Complete Guide to Taking Care of Your Sexual Self*. New York: Guilford Press, 2002.
5. Leiblum S, Sachs J. *Getting the Sex You Want: A Woman's Guide to Becoming Proud, Passionate, and Pleased in Bed*. New York: Crown Publishers, 2002.
6. Bancroft J, Loftus J, Long JS. Distress about sex: a national survey of women in heterosexual relationships. *Arch Sex Behav* 2003; 32: 193–208.
7. Bancroft J, Loftus J, Long JS. Reply to Rosen and Laumann (2003). *Arch Sex Behav* 2003; 32: 213–16.
8. Shader RI. Sexual dysfunction associated with thioridazine hydrochloride. *JAMA* 1964; 188: 1007–9.
9. May RE. Sexual dysfunction following rectal excision for ulcerative colitis. *Br J Surg* 1966; 53: 29–30.
10. Bernstein WC, Bernstein EF. Sexual dysfunction following radical surgery for cancer of the rectum. *Dis Colon Rectum* 1966; 9: 328–32.
11. Masters WH, Johnson VE. *Human Sexual Response*. Boston: Little, Brown, 1966.
12. Masters WH, Johnson VE. *Human Sexual Inadequacy*. Boston: Little, Brown, 1970.
13. Kaplan HS. *The New Sex Therapy*. New York: Brunner/Mazel, 1974.
14. American Psychiatric Association. *Diagnostic and Statistical Manual of Mental Disorders* (DSM-I). Washington, DC: 1952.
15. American Psychiatric Association. *Diagnostic and Statistical*

Manual of Mental Disorders, 2nd edn (DSM-II). Washington, DC: 1968.

16. American Psychiatric Association. *Diagnostic and Statistical Manual of Mental Disorders*, 3rd edn (DSM-III). Washington, DC: 1980.

17. American Psychiatric Association. *Diagnostic and Statistical Manual of Mental Disorders*, 4th edn (DSM-IV). Washington, DC: 2000.

18. World Health Organization. *ICD-10: International Statistical Classification of Diseases and Related Health Problems*, 10th edn. Geneva: 1992.

19. Tiefer L. Historical, scientific, clinical and feminist criticisms of "The human sexual response cycle". *Annu Rev Sex Res* 1999; 2: 1–23.

20. Basson R. The female sexual response: a different model. *J Sex Marital Ther* 2000; 26: 51–64.

21. Tiefer L. Arriving at a "new view" of women's sexual problems: background, theory, and activism. In E Kaschak, E Tiefer, eds. *A New View of Women's Sexual Problems*. Binghamton: Haworth Press, 2001: 63–98.

22. Basson R, McInnes R, Smith MD et al. Efficacy and safety of sildenafil citrate in women with sexual dysfunction associated with female sexual arousal disorder. *J Womens Health* 2002; 11: 367–77.

23. Harris G. Pfizer gives up testing Viagra on women. *New York Times* 2004; Feb 28.

24. American Psychiatric Association. *Diagnostic and Statistical Manual of Mental Disorders*, 3rd edn rev. (DSM-III-R). Washington, DC: 1987.

25. Basson R, Berman J, Burnett A *et al*. Report of the International Consensus Development Conference on Female Sexual Dysfunction: definitions and classification. *J Urol* 2000; 163: 888–93.

26. Simons JS, Carey MP. Prevalence of sexual dysfunctions: results from a decade of research. *Arch Sex Behav* 2001; 30: 177–219.

27. Dunn KM, Croft PR, Hackett GI. Sexual problems: a study of the prevalence and need for health care in the general population. *Fam Pract* 1998; 15: 519–24.

28. Dunn KM, Croft PR, Hackett GI. Association of sexual problems with social, psychological, and physical problems in men and women: a cross sectional population survey. *J Epidemiol Community Health* 1999; 53: 144–8.

29. Fugl-Meyer AR, Fugl-Meyer K. Sexual disabilities, problems and satisfaction in 18–74 year old Swedes. *Scand J Sexol* 1999; 2: 79–105.

30. Osborn M, Hawton K, Gath D. Sexual dysfunction among middle-aged women in the community. *BMJ* 1988; 296: 959–62.

31. Mercer CH, Fenton KA, Johnson AM et al. Sexual function problems and help seeking behaviour in Britain: national probability sample survey. *BMJ* 2003; 327: 426–7.

32. Johnson AM, Mercer CH, Erens B et al. Sexual behaviour in Britain: partnerships, practices, and HIV risk behaviours. *Lancet* 2001; 358: 1835–42.

33. Erens B, McManus S, Field J et al. *National survey of sexual attitudes and lifestyles II: technical report*. London: National Centre for Social Research, 2001.

34. Ernst C, Földényi M, Angst J. The Zurich study: XXI. Sexual dys-

functions and disturbances in young adults. *Eur Arch Psychiatry Clin Neurosci* 1993; 243: 179–88.

35. Nazareth I, Boynton P, King M. Problems with sexual function in people attending London general practitioners: cross sectional study. *BMJ* 2003; 327: 423–9.

36. Nathan SG. The epidemiology of the DSM-III psychosexual dysfunctions. *J Sex Marital Ther* 1986; 12: 267–81.

37. Moynihan R. The making of a disease: female sexual dysfunction. *BMJ* 2003; 326: 45–7.

38. Ellison C. *Women's Sexualities*. Oakland: New Harbinger, 2000.

39. Dennerstein L, Lehert P, Burger H et al. Factors affecting sexual functioning of women in the midlife years. *Climacteric* 1999; 2: 254–62.

40. Bancroft J. Central inhibition of sexual response in the male: a theoretical perspective. *Neurosci Biobehav Rev* 1999; 23: 763–84.

41. Bancroft J, Janssen E. The dual control model of male sexual response: a theoretical approach to centrally mediated erectile dysfunction. *Neurosci Biobehav Rev* 2000; 24: 571–9.

42. Janssen E, Vorst H, Finn P et al. The Sexual Inhibition (SIS) and Sexual Excitation (SES) Scales. I. Measuring sexual inhibition and excitation proneness in men. *J Sex Res* 2002; 39: 114–26.

43. Bancroft J, Janssen E, Strong D et al. Sexual risk taking in young heterosexual men. The relevance of personality factors. *J Sex Res* 2004; 41: 181–92.

44. Bancroft J, Janssen E, Strong D et al. Sexual risk taking in gay men: the relevance of sexual arousability, mood and sensation seeking. *Arch Sex Behav* 2003; 32: 555–73.

45. Graham CA, Sanders SA, Milhausen RR et al. Turning on and turning off: a focus group study of the factors that affect women's sexual arousal. *Arch Sex Behav* 2004; 33: 527–38.

46. Baumeister RF, Catanese KR, Vohs KD. Is there a gender difference in strength of sex drive? Theoretical views, conceptual distinctions, and a review of relevant evidence. *Pers Soc Psychol Rev* 2001; 5: 242–73.

47. Garde K, Lunde I. Female sexual behaviour. A study in a random sample of 40-year-old women. *Maturitas* 1989; 2: 225–40.

48. Heiman JR. Sexual desire in human relationships. In W Everaerd, E Laan, S Both, eds. *Sexual Appetite, Desire and Motivation: Energetics of the Sexual System*. Amsterdam: Royal Netherlands Academy, 2001: 117–34.

49. Catania JA, Binson D, Canchola J et al. Effects of interviewer gender, interviewer choice, and item wording on responses to questions concerning sexual behavior. *Public Opin Q* 1996; 30: 345–75.

50. Spira A, Bajos N, the ACSF Group. *Sexual Behaviour and AIDS*. Aldershot: Avebury, 1994.

51. ACSF principal investigators and their associates. Analysis of sexual behaviour in France (ACSF). A comparison between two modes of investigation: telephone survey and face-to-face survey. *AIDS* 1992; 6: 315–23.

52. Turner CF, Miller HG, Rogers SM. Survey measurement of sexual behavior: problems and progress. In J Bancroft, ed. *Researching Sexual Behavior: Methodological Issues*. Bloomington, IN: Indiana University Press, 1997: 37–60.

53. Knowledge Networks, Inc. 1350 Willow Rd., Menlo Park, CA 94025 [www.knowledgenetworks.com\ganp].

54. Fenton KA, Johnson AM, McManus S et al. Measuring sexual behaviour: methodological challenges in survey research. *Sex Transm Infect* 2001; 77: 84–92.

55. Catania JA, Turner H, Pierce RC et al. Response bias in surveys of AIDS-related sexual behavior. In DG Ostrow, RC Kessler, eds. *Methodological Issues in AIDS Behavioral Research*. New York: Plenum Press, 1993: 133–62.

56. Catania JA, Gibson DR, Chitwood DD et al. Methodological problems in AIDS behavioral research: influences on measurement error and participation bias in studies of sexual behavior. *Psychol Bull* 1990, 108: 339 62

57. Graham, CA. Catania JA, Brand R et al. Recalling sexual behavior: a methodological analysis of memory recall bias via interview using the diary as the gold standard. *J Sex Res* 2003; 40: 325–32.

58. Lindal E, Stefansson JG. The lifetime prevalence of psychosexual dysfunction among 55- to 57-year-olds in Iceland. *Soc Psychiatry Psychiatr Epidemiol* 1993; 28: 91–5.

59. Rosen R, Brown C, Heiman J et al. The female sexual function index (FSFI): a multidimensional self-report instrument for the assessment of female sexual function. *J Sex Marital Ther* 2000; 26: 191–208.

60. Quirk FH, Heiman JR, Rosen RC et al. Development of a sexual function questionnaire for clinical trials of female sexual dysfunction. *J Womens Health* 2002; 11: 277–89.

61. Daker-White G. Reliable and valid self-report outcome measures in sexual (dys)function: a systematic review. *Arch Sex Behav* 2002; 31: 197–209.

62. Ware JE, Kosinski M, Keller S. A 12–item Short-Form Health Survey (SF-12): construction of scales and preliminary tests of reliability and validity. *Med Care* 1996; 34: 220–33.

63. Reynolds MA, Herbenick DL, Bancroft J. The nature of childhood sexual experiences: two studies 50 years apart. In J Bancroft, ed. *Sexual Development in Childhood*. Bloomington: Indiana University Press, 2003.

64. Bancroft J, Herbenick D, Reynolds M. Masturbation as a marker of sexual development. In J Bancroft, ed. *Sexual Development in Childhood*. Bloomington: Indiana University Press, 2003.

65. Dunn KM, Jordan K, Croft PR et al. Systematic review of sexual problems: epidemiology and methodology. *J Sex Marital Ther* 2002; 28: 399–422.

66. Tiefer, L, Rosen R, Giami A et al. Qualitative health research and sexual dysfunction. In TF Lue, R Basson, R Rosen et al., eds. *International Consultation in Sexual Medicine*. Paris: 2004: 161–70.

PSYCHOLOGY

Women's sexuality in context: relationship factors and female sexual function

David R Moore, Julia R Heiman

The great majority of sexual behaviors occur in the context of a relationship between two individuals who feel emotionally connected. Studying sexuality within a relationship is fundamental to the understanding of diagnosis and treatment of female sexual problems.[1,2]

The primary goal of this chapter is to summarize the research literature on relationship factors and sexual function in women, with a focus on heterosexual relationships, since same-sex relationships are reviewed in Chapter 8.1 of this volume. We have reviewed empirical literature dating back to 1970, using both the PsycInfo and Medline databases, with attention to predictor and outcome relationship measures. This research is primarily correlational rather than experimental, but is valuable for the themes it reveals.

Several studies prior to 1970 deserve brief mention. Terman and colleagues explored correlations between women's sexual adjustment and marital happiness in a volunteer sample of 792 US couples in intact marriages.[3] Marital satisfaction was negatively correlated with number of sexual complaints and discrepancies in sex drive, and positively correlated with satisfaction ratings of intercourse with spouse, wife's satisfaction with first intercourse, agreeable reactions of spouse to sexual refusals, and wife's orgasmic frequency. Dickinson and Beam studied a volunteer sample of 1000 British women in intact marriages.[4] One of the key findings, shocking at the time, was that nearly 50% of the sample reported being dissatisfied with their sexual relationship. Kinsey and colleagues did not look at relationship factors, except as marker variables (e.g., marital status) to categorize sex behavior.[5] Masters and Johnson studied sexual response in couples and individuals,[6] but did not consider relationship factors until their

treatment study.[7] They considered the "relationship" as important, but focused mostly on individual intrapsychic issues. Their main treatment technique, sensate focus, was a couple's exercise, though they only indirectly measured its efficacy.

Relationship factors and female sexual function

Sex research since 1970 has focused more on the individual with an increasingly physiological perspective. Consequently, few studies have attended to the couple,[8] despite the repeated call from researchers and clinicians for the need to consider sexual dysfunction from a relational perspective.[1,2,9–11] A variety of relationship factors have been shown to be influential in women's sexual function and overall satisfaction with their sexual relationships, as summarized in Tables 3.1.1a and 3.1.1b (general empirical literature) and Table 3.1.2 (therapeutic intervention studies).

Relationship quality and sexual function

Frequency of sex

The association between different measures of relationship quality and coital frequency is not a consistent one. Coital frequency has been positively associated with perceptions of overall relationship quality or marital happiness,[12–14] while sexual inactivity has been found to be more prevalent among unhappily married individuals.[15] Terman et al.'s study[3] found no

Table 3.1.1a.   Summary of empirical research on relationship factors and female sexuality: larger-scale studies ($n > 400$)

Study	n	Sample characteristics	Independent variables	Dependent variables	Methodology	Measurement	Results	Comments
Blumstein & Schwartz 1983[23]	6,038	3656 married couples, 653 heterosex cohab couples; 772 lesbian; 957 gay male couples.	Couple type; rel duration; sex freq; sex satisfxn; several other variables.	Rel satisfxn; sex satisfxn.	Corr design; non-rep sample but inclusive of heterosex and homosex couples.	Self-report: survey; pers interview w/ subsample of 300 couples.	Sex freq: gays > cohab heterosex > married > lesbs. Sex freq neg assoc w/ age and rel duration; sex freq and rel satisfxn (+) assoc w/ sex satisfxn.	Approx 2/3 of all couples satisfied w/ sex life.
Coleman et al., 1983[95]	777	407 F in same-sex rels (18–62 yrs old); 370 heterosex F (17–59 yrs old).	Sex orientn (lesb vs heterosex).	Sex arousal; sex behav (freq of sex); satisfxn w/ curr sex response).	Comp group. Stat controlled for bet-group diffs in age and ed.	Self-report: SAI; single-item ratings.	Lesbs > heteros in: (1) sex freq, (2) org freq and consistency, and (3) sex satisfxn. Lesbs > heteros in arousal to: (1) sex scenarios depicting init (vs rec) of sex stim and (2) sex w/ direct genital stim.	SAI had est R and V.
Cupach & Comstock, 1990[25]	402	Married (avg 10.4 yr) univ students (66% women); RS of 1000; M age 33.	Satisfxn w/ sex comm.	Sex satisfxn; marital qual.	Corr design; RS (40% response rate).	Self-report: DAS; ISS; sex comm satisfxn.	Sex comm satisfxn, sex satisfxn, and marital qual all (+) corr. Sex satisfxn mediated satisfxn w/ sex comm and marital qual.	Measures had est R and V.
Donnelly, 1993[15]	6,029	3,292 F; 2,737 M. NSFH. Natl RS of US pop.	Mar interactn (several variables).	Sex activity/ inact in past month.	Nationwide RS; no control strategies used.	Self-report: pers interview and q-aire (mostly single-items).	Sex inact pred by: low lev of mar happiness, fewer shared activities, higher likelihood of sepn, and fewer arguments over sex.	Sex inact may indicate other mar probs.
Ernst et al., 1993[40]	591	292 M, 299 F; Swiss commun sample (age 20/21 to 29/30) interviewed 4 × over 10 yr.	SD (presence vs absence, severity, chronicity); gender.	Rel stress and conflict); sev other non-rel factors.	Longitud'l; desc study; nat existing comp group (ppts who did not report SD).	Self-report: series of pers interviews.	25% F reported sex difficulties. at each asst, inhib desire 2–3 × more freq among F. SD and distress assoc w/ rel stress and conflict (for both M and F).	
Edwards & Booth, 1994[26]	2,033	RS married persons; longitud'l study (1980–1992); 65% completion rate.	Happiness w/ sex rel; loss of interest in sex; presence of X-marital sex.	Marital happiness, stab, and interaxns; confl freq and severity.	Lg scale RS; longitud'l; corr design.	Self-report: interviews; brief q-aires (sev single-item measures).	Sex satisfxn mod corr w/ mar happiness, (+) interaxns, and well-being. Lost interest in sex corr w/ mar unhappiness and neg interaxns. ↓ happiness w/ sex rel pred ↓ mar happiness and divorce.	

[text continues on page 78]

Table 3.1.1a. (Continued)

Study	n	Sample characteristics	Independent variables	Dependent variables	Methodology	Measurement	Results	Comments
Rao & DeMaris, 1995[18]	13,017	Data from NSFH.Wtd rep US sample. M ages = 28.8 (F), 31.4 (M). 84% married.	Rel status (married vs cohab); rel duration; rel qual; no. child; other vars.	Coital freq (in past mo).	Lg rep sample; corr design.	Self-report: interview (mostly single-item global ratings).	Rel duration pred lower coital freq. Sex freq of cohab > married couples. F rel qual mod pred > sex freq. Ppts w/ 1 child reported < coital freq than non-parents; parents of 2+ children had = coital freq w/ childless ppts.	
Call et al., 1995[12]	7,463	6,785 married individuals, 678 cohab; rep nat'l sample from NSFH.	Marital duration, marital happiness.	Sex freq in past mo.	Lg rep sample; corr design.	Self-report: pers interviews; q-aires.	Besides age, mar happiness strongest pred of sex freq over time. Mar duration neg assoc w/ sex freq.	R and V of q-aires not reported.
Haavio-Manila & Kontula, 1997[24]	2,250	Rep Finnish sample (1,104 F, 1,146 M). 76% response rate. Ages 18–74 yr. M ages = 43.1 (F), 41.3 (M).	Gender; sex comm w/ partner; rel satisfxn; sex assert; freq, variety; org consist.	Sex satisfxn/ enjoyment.	Corr design.	Self-report: interview (mostly global, single-item Qs) and q-aires.	F < M in sex satisfxn. Sex satisfxn and rel happiness corr (esp for F). Sex satisfxn pred by younger age (F), sex assert, sex variety, and org consist. Ease of sex comm w/ partner mod ccrr w/ sex satisfxn.	Specific q-aires used not specified (unclear psychometric properties).
Dunn et al., 1999[38]	1,768	979 F, 789 M (18–75 yr). Anon SRS from UK.	Mar probs.	Sex probs (arousal, org dysfx, inhib enjoyment, dyspareunia).	SRS; commun sample; corr design.	Self-report: q-aire dev for this survey.	For F (but not for M), mar difficulties strongly assoc w/ SD (esp arousal probs, org dysfx, and inhib enjoyment).	
Laumann et al., 1999[80] [See also Laumann et al., 1994[78]]	3,159	NHSLS Natl prob sample; 1,410 M, 1,749 F, ages 18–59. > 79% response rate.	Mar status; health/lifestyle factors; soc status; sev indexes of sex exp and behav.	Sex dysfx (low desire, arousal or org dysfx, perform anx, painful sex, no pleasure).	Rep sample of men and women in US households; corr design.	Self-report: pers survey.	SD fairly prevalent in gen pop, esp for F (43% F vs 31% M). Pre- and post-mar status assoc w/ greater risk for SD. Being married assoc w/ lower risk for SD.	For F esp, SD also strongly and (–) assoc w/ pers happiness.
Klusmann, 2002[76]	1,865	967 F, 898 M in L-T rels. From lg rep German student sample. M ages = 24.8 (F), 25.7 (M).	Rel duration; gender.	Sex freq; sex satisfxn; sex desire; desire for rel closeness.	Rep sampling; corr design.	Self-report: global single-item Qs in survey q-aire.	Sex freq neg corr w/ rel duration (Mdn 10×/mo in 1st yr; 5×/mo in 5th yr of rel). As rel duration increased: F sex desire decreased and desire for closeness increased.	Results interpreted in terms of evolutionary psychology.

Table 3.1.1a. (Continued)

Study	n	Sample characteristics	Independent variables	Dependent variables	Methodology	Measurement	Results	Comments
Trudel, 2002[96]	996	496 F, 500 M; all cohab or married. 54% resp rate. M ages = 42 (F), 47.6 (M). M rel duration = 18.4 yr (M), 16.8 yr (F).	Sex satisfxn; sex attitudes, and behav; gender; age group (> 60, < 60).	Rel satisfxn/adj; sex satisfxn.	RS strategy; corr design.	Self-report: telephone survey; rel satisfxn assessed by 10 items from DAS; add'l single-item, global Qs.	Rel satisfxn pred by: (1) sex satisfxn (except F > 60), 2) good sex comm (for M and F < 60), (3) satisfxn w/ sex partner (F only), and (4) sex variety (for M < 60). Sig pred of sex satisfxn: (1) qual of sex comm (except for M > 60), (2) satisfxn w/ sex partner (M and F < 60), and (3) sat sfxn w/ orgasm (M and F < 60).	Role of sex comm, variety, and pres of org in L-T rels may vary as fx of age and gender.
Bancroft et al, 2003[97]	987	SRS of White and Black F 20–65 yr (M = 40.4). All ppts in rel at least 6 mos.	Emot'l well-being; subj sex resp; sex behav; physiologic sex fx (lubr probs, pain).	Distress re: (1) sex rel w/ partner, and (2) one's sexuality.	Corr design.	Self-report: mostly single-item ratings in phone survey; 2 multi-item q-aire scales from SF12 (qual of life measure).	Strong pred of sex distress: neg emot'l well-being, followed by neg feelings re sex contact w/ partner and lack of closeness w/ partner. Physiologic indicators weak pred of sex distress (phys response and subj SA) or nonsig pred (probs w/ lubr, org, pain).	
Liu, 2003[79]	1,550	Married ppts from NHSLS data set. M age = 38.3. 82% White, 10% Black. M rel duration = 13.8 yr.	Duration of marriage; gender.	Qual of mar sex: phys pleasure and emot'l satisfxn from spousal sex.	Corr design. Stat controlled for sev demo vars and sex freq.	Self-report: pers interview (vars measured w/ single-item, global indexes from NHSLS interview).	Mar duration and cohab before marriage had small neg effect on qual of sex w/ spouse. Freq of sex (+) assoc w/ sex qual F < M in satisfxn w/ spousal sex.	Small prop of variance in marital sex qual accounted for (5%).

Abbreviations: adj = adjustment; anon = anonymous; asst = assessment; comm = communication; commun = community; comp = compariso'n; confl = conflict; corr = correlational, correlated; consist = consistency; desc = descriptive; DAS = Dyadic Adjustment Scale; demo = demographic; diff(s) = difference(s); est = established; F = female; fx = function; ISS = Index of Sexual Satisfaction; inact = inactivity; init = initiating, initiated; interaxn(s) = interaction(s); lg = large; lev = level; L-T = long-term; M = male; mar = marital; Mdn = median; mod = moderately; NHSLS = National Health and Social Life Survey; NSFH = National Survey of Families and Households; org = orgasm; ppts = participants; pers = personal; phys = physical; pred = predicted, predictor; pres = present; RS = random sample; R and V = reliability and validity; rec = receiving; rel = relationship; rep = representative; resp = response, responded; satisfxn = satisfaction; sepn = separation; SA = sexual arousal; SAI = Sexual Arousability Inventory; SD = sexual dysfunction(al); stab = stability; stat = statistically; SRS = stratified random sample; vars = variables; wtd = weighted X-marital = extramarital.

Table 3.1.1b. Summary of empirical research on relationship factors and female sexuality

Study	n	Sample characteristics	Independent variables	Dependent variables	Methodology	Measurement	Results	Comments
Frank et al., 1976[46]	54	29 mar therapy couples; 25 sex therapy couples. Modal age 31.5.	Group status (mar therapy vs sex therapy).	Multiple measures of sex and mar adj/satisfxn.	Comp group; no other control strategies.	Self-report (marital q-aire; KDS-15).	No diffs bet groups in no. and type of sex difficulties. Sex therapy couples > mar therapy couples in mar satisfxn/adjust and confl res.	
Howard & Dawes, 1976[16]	27	Married couples; demo characs of sample not reported.	Freq of sex w/ spouse; freq of arguments.	Mar happiness.	Corr design.	Self-report: global rating of mar happiness; diary reports of sex and arg freq.	Sex freq did not pred marital happiness. Sex freq relative to no. arguments did sig pred marital happiness.	
Birchler & Webb, 1977[13]	100	50 happily married and 50 unhappily married couples.	Marital happiness (happy vs unhappy).	Sex freq; confl res (no. unresolved probs); rec activities.	Comp group. Specific sample characteristics not reported.	Self-report: mar activities inv; areas of change q-aire.	Happily (vs unhappily) married couples: > sex freq < unresolved probs; and > participation in rec activities together vs alone.	
Frank et al., 1978[37]	100	Married couples, vol sample; mostly White, middle-class; M age = 36.	SD; sex difficulties.	Mar and sex satisfxn.	Corr design.	Self-report: mar q-aire (KDS-15).	>80% of couples satisfied w/ marriage and sex rel, despite high prev of SD (63% F, 40% M). Sex difficulties (e.g., insuff 4play, uninterest in sex) stronger pred of F sex satisfxn than SD.	Mar satisfxn measure R and V not reported.
Peplau et al., 1978[88]	127	Self-id lesbians, ages 18–59 (Mdn = 26). 61% in current same-sex rels.	Prim rel values: dyad attachment vs pers autonomy.	Sex satisfxn (sex and org freq); rel satisfxn/ intimacy.	Corr design.	Self-report (anon q-aire incl several single-item global ratings).	Most ppts reported high sex and rel satisfxn, closeness, and equality. Freq of sex and org (+) assoc w/ sex satisfxn. Dyad attachment (+) assoc with sex satisfxn.	Unreported psychometric properties of measures.
Swieczkowski & Walker, 1978[19]	48	F students, ages 20–35, married at least 2 yr; mostly White, middle-class, childless.	Sex behav and attitudes (incl spec prefs, positions, and variety).	Mar happiness (adj, satisfxn); infidelity; org exp w/ mar sex.	Desc, corr study.	Self-report: Locke–Wallace MAT, multi-item scales designed by researchers.	Org lower dur times of confl & hostility w/ spouse. Happy (vs. unhappy) married: > satisfxn w/ 4play and oth noncoital sex contacts, > prop org w/ spouse, > sex variety, < sex refusal, < infidelity.	MAT had est R and V; other measures unreported R and V.
Hartman, 1980[34]	20	20 fam therapy couples. M age 40 (M), 38 (F). M length of marriage 14 yr.	4 groups: SD, mar confl, SD + mar confl, controls.	Observed couple interaxns.	Incl of comp groups (but small no.). Coders blind to group status.	Self-report (to assign groups); observ'l data.	SD couples: > (+) interaxns. SD and marital adj possibly indep.	Exact group sizes not spec, but low given no. of groups.

Table 3.1.1b. (Continued)

Study	n	Sample characteristics	Independent variables	Dependent variables	Methodology	Measurement	Results	Comments
Heiman, 1980[99]	55	F ages 21–58. 51% unmarried (M age = 32); 49% married (M age = 28).	Mar status; SA in resp to erotic audio, film and sex fantasies.	Physiologic SA to erotic materials; Subj SA at lab & home.	2 exptl sessions (4 mos apart). Exptl stim pres to assess subj and physiologic SA.	Vag resp (VPA); subj SA assessed by global ratings).	Subj SA and vag resp (+) corr, unmarried F, 1 of 2 sessions. At home SA neg corr w/ vag lab resp.	F sex resp is complex, depends on context. F vag resp and subj SA don't nec coincide.
Berg & Snyder, 1981[45]	90	45 sex therapy couples; 45 mar therapy couples. M = 36 yr of age, married 11 yr.	Group status (seeking sex therapy vs mar therapy); gender.	Rel and sex distress.	Comp group; mar therapy couples matched on key demo characs.	Self-report: q-aire w/ est R and V (Marital Satisfaction Inventory).	Both groups had poor mar adj. Sex therapy > mar therapy couples in sex dissatisfxn. Sex therapy < mar therapy couples in global rel distress.	Multidimensional measure w/ est R and V.
Chesney et al., 1981[43]	73	36 sex therapy couples; 37 univ student couples.	Group status (sex therapy vs student comp group).	Rel adj (comm, perceptn of rel).	Comp group (univ sample); no other control strategies.	Self-report: MCI SII; Sex Attitude and Behav Q-aire.	Sex therapy couples vs normals: > comm probs (gen and spec to sex contacts), > disagreements, > neg percepts of re, and < rel satisfxn.	2 measures used had est R and V (MCI, SII).
Persky et al., 1982[14]	30	Couples from yg cohort (n = 11, M age = 24 yr); and older cohort (n = 19, M age = 54 yr).	Mar adj.	Sex adj.	Small but carefully screened sample (for phys and mental health).	Multimethod asst. Self-report (MAT and SII) and obs ratings of dyad interaxn from interv data.	Mar adj (based on self and obs ratings) corr w/ sex adjustmt. Mut supportive/warm couples had greater: sex desire, F sex resp, sex freq, and F sex gratification.	MAT, SII had est R and V; high R for obs ratings.
Greenblat, 1983[77]	80	50 F, 30 M married for < 5 yrs. RS using random digit dialing.	Sex freq in 1st yr of marriage; dur of marriage; pres of children; demo vars.	Sex freq after 1st yr of marriage; subj imp of sex; subj reasons for ↓ sex freq.	RS; exploratory study; no formal hyp testing.	Self-report: pers interview.	↓ in sex freq afte¯ 1st yr of marriage (due to work, parent'g and partner familiarity. Sex freq in 1st yr strongest pred of later sex freq. Most ppts rep that sex was imp, despite sex freq declines.	Unreported R and V of measures. Findings sugg that sex freq doesn't nec reflect stated importance.
Snyder & Berg, 1983[83]	90	45 sex therapy couples (wives and husbands analyzed separately).	Gender (husbands and wives).	SD; sex satisfxn.	No comp group; corr design.	Self-report: 15-item CL for SD; Sex Dissatisfxn Scale (from MSI).	For F, SA and org dysfx most prev complaints. Partner's lack of resp to sex requests and lack of partner affectn pred sex distress stronger than SD.	Sex dissatisfxn Scale validated.

Table 3.1.1b. (Continued)

Study	n	Sample characteristics	Independent variables	Dependent variables	Methodology	Measurement	Results	Comments
Zimmer, 1983[100] Study 1:	59	20 happy couples, 19 mar distressed, 20 SD couples. M age = 33.4 (M), 30.2 (F).	Group status (happy vs mar distress vs SD).	Self-reported comm skills.	Comp groups; no other control strategies.	Self-report: KIP q-aire.	Mar and sex distressed couples vs normals: > comm probs (e.g., more hostile expressions). Few diffs bet mar and sex distressed couples in reported comm.	Reported adeq R; unclear validity of q-aire.
Zimmer, 1983[100] (Cont.) Study 2:	37	10 happy, 6 mar distressed, 10 dep+sex distressed, 11 sex distressed.	Group status (happy vs mar distress vs. sex dist+dep).	Observed interaxns (rated on sev dimensions of comm).	Comp groups.	Observ'l data (videotaped and coded couple interaxns).	Sex distressed couples (esp if dep) vs marital distressed: > neg comm happy couples showed more (+) interaxns.	Adequate interrater R of coding procedure.
Hawton & Catalan, 1986[58]	154	Couples rec CB tx for mult SDs (99 F w/ chief c/o impaired desire and vagin.	Pred of tx outcome: rel qual, sex qual; and tx motivation.	Tx outcome.	No comp/cont group.	Self-report: q-aires assessing rel qual and feelings tow sex.	(+) tx outcome assoc w/ rel qual, sex rel qual, and partner's motivation for tx.	96 couples completed tx.
Heiman et al., 1986[35]	204	94 clin couples (WL for sex therapy); 110 nonclin couples.	Couple type: clin vs nonclin couples.	Sex and mar satisfxn; sev other sex, soc, and mar vars.	Cont group; screened for med and psych probs; no demo diffs bet groups.	Self-report: MAS; SAS; pers history q-aire.	Sex and mar satisfxn indep; clin couples sex distressed in context of (+) mar satisfxn; sex vs mar factors disting clin from nonclin couples.	Standardized measures used to assess sex and mar satisfxn (and soc desirability).
Whitehead & Matthews, 1986[57]	48	Couples w/ chief c/o lack of F sex interest or enjoyment who rec 3-mo tx based on M and J.	Resp to tx: improved (n = 26) and nonimproved (n = 22).	Rel qual; sex rel qual; enjoyment of sex; percept of self and part attractn and love; rel dur; dur of SD.	Comp group (+ vs neg resp to tx); init tx study based on random assign; clearly def groups w/ incl and excl crit.	Self-report: q-aires w/ unrep psychometric prop; blind rater asst of qual of sex and gen rel qual.	Rel qual (+) assoc w/ successful tx outcomes. Improved (vs nonimproved) couples: > self and part ratings of attractn and love, < arguments, < compat interests, < affection and acceptance. Non-sig pred of tx: rel dur, severity of SD, F sex resp.	Sugg import of qual of couples' rel when making tx decisions, also per attractn and love w/in dyads.
Stuart et al., 1987[47]	90	Married F (59 w/ ISD; 31 non-ISD) seeking tx for mar sex prob; M age = 33.5 yr; married avg of 10.2 yr.	Group status (ISD vs non-ISD).	Mar adj; global rel satisfxn and dyad interaxns; sev aspects of sex rel.	Comp/cont group; screened for med illness; excl ambig diag. No demo diffs bet groups.	Self-report: DAS; global measure of rel satisfxn.	ISD (vs non-ISD) group: poorer mar adj, > dissatisfxn w/ confl res, < attractn to spouse, < emot'l closeness, and < romantic feelings. No diffs bet groups in sex freq. ISD > non-ISD in sex refusals.	DAS is standardized measure; other measures unreported psychometric properties.

Table 3.1.1b. (Continued)

Study	n	Sample characteristics	Independent variables	Dependent variables	Methodology	Measurement	Results	Comments
Rust et al., 1988[101]	28	28 sex and mar therapy couples from UK; M = 33.6 yr of age, 10.6 yr rel dur.	Overall mar satisfxn (assessed by GRIMS).	Sex satisfxn and sex fx (assessed by GRISS).	Corr design.	Standardized Self-report q-aires (est R and V).	Sex satisfxn (+) assoc w/ mar qual. Sex dissatisfxn assoc w/ lower perc mar qual for M and F. Stronger assoc found for M vs F.	Prop of couples seeking tx for M vs F SD not stated.
Byers & Heinlein, 1989[21]	77	55 F, 22 M; 65% married, 35% cohab w/ opp-sex partner. Mdn age = 29.6 yr (18–63). M rel dur = 8.7 yr. 52% w/ child.	Mar status; dyad adj; sex pleasure; rel dur; erotophilia; satisfxn w/ sex confl res; gender.	Sex initiatn; accept vs refusal of sex initiatns; freq of considering init sex desp sex interest.	Corr design.	Self-report: global indexes, sev q-aires, including DAS, SOS, and sex activity q-aire (based on diary of sex behav).	Cohab > married in freq sex initiatns. ↑ sex and rel satisfxn assoc w/ ↑ freq initiatns. ↓ sex satisfxn assoc w/ ↑ F sex refusals. ↓ F pleasure assoc w/ dec to not init sex despite interest. M > F in initiatns.	All multi-item q-aires had est R and V.
Kelly et al., 1990[75]	34	24 org F, 10 anorg F; 21–40 yr old, all in rels w/ sex fx'l M; screened for med probs and med use.	Org vs anorg; resp to sex explic vid segments depicting dir and indirect clit stim.	Sex arousal; deg comfort in comm w/ partner re: sex acts; sex attitudes, guilt, knowl.	Controlled, selective incl criteria; comp group. Assessed resp to exptl stim; counterbal order of videos.	Self-report: moment by moment subj SA; q-aire data (unrep R and V).	Anorg > orgasmic F in: discomfort talking w/ partners re sex acts involving direct clit stim (cunnil and partner man'l stim). Anorg > org F in sex myths, guilt. Anorg < org F in sex knowl.	Strongest pred of anorg was comm probs re sex acts likely to result in orgasm.
Hawton et al., 1991[88]	60	Couples rec modif M and J tx for low F sex desire. M ages = 30 (F), 32.9 (M). M rel dur = 9.4 yr. M dur of SD = 6.1 yr.	Pred of tx outcome: ther and pt ratings; sex and gen rel qual; tx motivatn; SD probs and dur.	Completion of tx and tx outcome (change in presenting probs and couples' sex fx post-tx).	No comp/ cont group; tx not std (varied in dur from 2 to 25 sess).	Self-report: rel q-aire (unrep psychometric prop) and ther global ratings of tx outcome.	M partner's motivatn pred tx completion (vs dropout). h/o mar sepn assoc w/ poor tx outcome. Yg age of male partner and shorter dur of presenting prob also pred poorer tx outcomes.	Lack of pred power of rel factors may be due to fact that couples w/ ser mar probs were excl in study.
Kurdek, 1991[29]	220	Couples (49 married, 36 hetero cohab, 58 lesb, 77 gay). M age 31.	Couple type (married, hetero cohab, lesb, gay); sex satisfxn.	Sex satisfxn; rel satisfxn; Sex perfectionism.	Comp groups. Groups equiv on age and ed; diffs in income and rel dur stat contr.	Self-report: anon q-aire. Global ratings and mult items from rel/sex q-aires.	No bet-group dif's in sex and rel satisfxn. Sex satisfxn sig assoc w/ rel satisfxn. Sex perfectionism neg assoc w/ rel satisfxn among hetero cohab and gays.	One of few studies specifically examining homosex and hetero rels.

Table 3.1.1b. (Continued)

Study	n	Sample characteristics	Independent variables	Dependent variables	Methodology	Measurement	Results	Comments
Hurlbert et al., 1993[31]	98	Nondistressed married F, M age 26.7. 68.4% White, 18.4% Black, 9.1% Hisp, 4.1% Asn.	rel closeness; sex assert; response to sex cues; sex freq, desire; org freq.	Sex satisfxn.	Corr design; Select screening proc (excluded mar distress, ETOH abuse, and anorgasmia).	Self-report: Sex diary; RCI; Hurlbert Indices of Assert and Excitability; SOS; ISS.	Rel closeness, erotophilia, and sex assert pred sex satisfxn more strongly than no. orgasms, sex freq, or sex excitability.	All measures had est R and V.
Oggins et al., 1993[102]	373	199 Black, 174 White couples; rep sample of couples obt 1st marriage lic. All F ≤ 31 yr.	Race; gender.	Mar rel qual; sex rel qual.	Rep ethnically diverse sample. Comp group by race; corr design.	Self-report: Individual pers interviews.	Caring and affirmation strongly assoc w/ sex enjoy, esp for F. Neg mar rel (esp irritation w/ spouse) assoc w/ sex upset (but gender and racial diffs seen).	Adeq R and V of measures; findings sugg imp of race and gender diffs.
Trudel et al., 1993[48]	40	20 couples w/ HSD; 20 non-HSD couples; 20-50 yr old; in 1+ yr stable rel.	Group: HSD vs no HSD.	Dyad adj; rel satisfxn, con sensus, aff expression, cohesion.	Comp group; no other control strategies.	Self-report: DAS.	HSD < non-HSD couples in global dyad adj. HSD F < non-HSD F in cohesion, rel satisfxn, consensus, and aff expression.	DAS has est R and V.
Henderson-King & Veroff, 1994[32]	373	199 B, 174 W couples; 4-yr longit'l study RS from marr lic bureau; 65% response rate.	Race, gender; feelings of affirmation vs tension in rel w/ partner.	Sex satisfxn/ dissatisfxn; mar equity, happiness, competence, control.	Nat-existing groups (by race and gender). RS, racially diverse; longit'l, yrs 1 and 3 of marriage.	Self-report; Q-aire data based prim on 2-6 item Likert scales.	Feeling affirmed by partner pred sex satisfxn; tension w/ partner pred sex dissatisfxn (for B and W couples). Sex satisfxn pred mar well-being (but varied by gender and race).	R and V of measures not reported.
Hulbert & Apt, 1994[103]	78	Married couples @ military fam support ctr. M ages = 31 (M), 28 (F). Married avg of 5 yr.	Mar and sex satisfxn (created 4 groups based on cut scores).	Sex desire, freq, interest; arousal and satisfxn w/ sex acts; org freq.	Single sample; groups created using cut scores; no cont strat.	Self-report. Pers Interviews and Q-aires: Index of Marital Satisfxn; ISS; HISD.	For F, mar dissatisfxn assoc w/ < desire, indep of sex satisfxn. Mar and sex satisfxn nct assoc w/ sex freq. Mar satisfied F had > interest, SA, and sex satisfxn. Org freq highest for Sex+mar satisfxn.	All measures had est R and V.
Aron & Henkemeyer, 1995[17]	100	60 F, 38 M (2 did not indicate gender); all married.	Passionate love.	Rel satisfxn; freq of sex (minus arg).	Corr design; stat controlled for soc desirability.	Self-report:DAS; PLS; Add'l q-aires.	For F (but not M), rel satisfxn mod corr w/ passionate love. For M (but not F), passionate love pred sex freq relative to no. arg.	DAS and PLS have est R and V.

Table 3.1.1b. (Continued)

Study	n	Sample characteristics	Independent variables	Dependent variables	Methodology	Measurement	Results	Comments
Beck & Bozman, 1995[22]	48	24 M and 24 F univ students. M age = 23.8, all sex active in heterosex rels.	Gender; 3 exptl conditn (erotic audio: anger, anx, neut sex sitn).	Subj SA; dec to terminate encounter.	Exptl; control condition, counterbal w/in-subj design; manip checks.	Self-report: Subj SA; reported dec to terminate interaction.	Sex encounters marked by anx and anger lowered sex desire, esp for F. Sig more F vs M reported they would end encounter in anger condition.	F arousal may be esp influenced by neg interaxns and emotions.
Lawrance & Byers, 1995[33]	143	90 F, 53 M in heterosex rels (avg 12 yr). 85% married, 12% cohab. M age = 37.4; gen sex satisfied.	Sex rewards/costs; equity of sex costs and rewards w/in dyad; rel satisfxn; gender.	Sex satisfxn.	Repeated assts (over 3 mos); Avoided item overlap in measures bet IVs and DV. No comp group.	Self-report: Exchange Q-aire; GMREL; GMSEX.	High rewards/costs ratio and equity of rewards/costs pred sex satisfxn. Rel satisfxn added to pred of sex satisfxn (and vice versa) beyond vars above. Rewarding sex contacts for F vs M more depend on rel factors.	Measures had est R and V.
Regan & Berscheid, 1995[104]	108	56 F, 52 M (all univ students). M age = 20.2 yrs. 87% white, 98% heterosex.	Gender.	Reported det of sex desire for M vs F.	Corr design; nat occurring groups (M and F).	Self-report: 5 essay Qs, coded for attributions about causes of M and F sex desire.	F sex desire seen as more depend on rel factors and romance. M sex desire viewed more internally driven and depend on erotic factors.	Adeq interrater R of coding proc.
Apt et al., 1996[36]	235	F nurses. M age 36.4; M rel dur = 10.8 yr. ≈ 73% W, 19% Hisp, 9% Black.	5 groups, based on clust analysis of mar and sex satisfxn.	Sex adj, desire, stress, compatibility and sex assert.	Corr design; groups est using clust analysis.	Self-report: Mar satisfxn scale; ISS; HISD; HISC; HISA; Apt Index of Sexual Stress.	Sex and mar satisfxn partly indep. Subgroups of F exp mod satisfxn w/ marriage desp low sex satisfxn (or vice versa). F w/ highest mar and sex satisfxn had > desire/assert and < sex stress.	All measures had est R and V.
Long et al., 1996[70]	250	Univ students (51% F). M age = 22.2 yr. 19% engaged/cohab, 81% dating	Premar sex conflict; Gender.	Sex satisfxn; rel satisfxn; generic conflict; rel qual.	Brief longitud'l (4 mo duration). Corr study.	Self-report: global indexes and q-aires (incl PMSCS).	Higher sex conflict (e.g., conflicts over sex freq or behav) assoc w/ lower sex and rel satisfxn, after controlling for generic conflict.	All but 1 depend measure had est R and V. Init evid of R and V for PMSCS.
Van Lankveld et al., 1996[52]	43	F w/ VVS (avg dur 3.2 yr) and 38 partners. From Dutch OB-GYN clinic. M age 27.5 yr.	Group (F compared to Dutch std group scores for each measure used).	Mar satisfxn; Sex fx; psychologic distress and probs.	Single sample design, w/ sep std samples used as comp groups. Excluded pts w/ vulvovaginitis.	Self-report: sub scale from Maudsley Mar q-aire; q-aire for SD screen; SCL; MMPI.	VVS F (and partners) = "normal" std pops in mar satisfxn, psych distress, and psych probs. VVS pts > distress spec in context of sex contacts w/ partners (same pattern not seen for masturbation).	Standardized q-aires used.

Table 3.1.1b (Continued)

Study	n	Sample characteristics	Independent variables	Dependent variables	Methodology	Measurement	Results	Comments
Hirst & Watson, 1997[87]	189	56 F and 133 M seeking sex tx, either w/o curr partner (58), w/ non-particip partner in tx (92), or w/ particip partner in tx (39).	Group: involvement of partner in tx; motivatn for tx.	Tx outcome (global ther ratings of successful, sufficient, or poor).	Corr design (w/ nat existing groups and no cont strategies); retrospective study.	Self-report: Q-aires (IIP, BDI, SCL-90); ther assts of their outcome (based on case notes; inter-rater R assessed w/ blind raters).	Strongest pred of (+) outcome was partner involvement in tx. Among pts w/ curr partner, 84% whose part attended their had (+) outcome, vs 51% of pts w/ nonparticip partners. Poor outcomes or prem terminatn assoc w/ > interpers probs.	Bet-group diffs in tx, presnt probs and demo vars not contr. Some meas used had est R and V (IIP, BDI, SCL-90).
MacNeil & Byers, 1997[60]	87	53 F, 34 M in hetero L-T rels; M age = 39 yrs; M rel dur=13 yr 85.5% married, 9.2% cohab.	Sex and non sex comm; sex probs and concerns; gender.	Sex satisfxn.	Corr design.	Self-report: PCI; Sex Self-Discl Q-aire; CLs for sex probs and concerns; GMSEX.	Gen comm and discl to partner of sex likes/dislikes sig pred sex satisfxn. Sex comm contrib sig variance in satisfxn beyond nonsex comm alone.	GMSEX has evidence of R and V; PCI has reported evidence of V.
McCabe, 1997[105]	343	145 fx'l (102 F); 198 SD (84 F). Mostly White, middle-class.	Sex fx (sex clinic vs community group).	Reported intimacy; qual of life.	Comp group (vol community sample).	Self-report PAIR; qual of life assessed by ComQual.	SD < fx'l F in intimacy w/ partner and qual of qual of life. F w/ lack of sex desire had less emot'l closeness w/ partner.	PAIR has est R and V.
Purnine & Carey, 1997[84]	76	63 married, 13 cohab couples; 91% W; avg of 2 children and 9.6 yr rel duration.	Understnd of part sex prefs; agreement re sex prefs; dyad adj.	Sex satisfxn; sex adj (no. sex probs).	Corr study; controlled for soc desirability.	Self-report: ISS; Inventory of Dyad Heterosex Prefs; DAS.	M part understnd of F sex prefs and couple compat in sex prefs contrib to F sex satisfxn and sex adj. Dyad adj sig pred F sex satisfxn.	DAS and ISS have est R and V.
Byers et al., 1998[27]	99	52 F, 47 M (all univ students). M age = 19.3 yr. 85% exclusive dating rel.	Sex rewards/ costs; equity re rew/costs; rel satisfxn; self-discl.	Sex satisfxn.	Corr design.	Self-report: Exchange Q-aire; GMSEX; GMREL.	Sex satisfxn sig pred by: rel satisfxn, perceived rewards/costs in sex contacts (after contr for gender and sex-discl).	
McCabe & Cobain, 1998[39]	343	145 fx'l (43 M, 102 F); 198 SD (114 M, 84 F); ages 25-68 yr.	Group: sex fx'l vs SD.	Rel qual; comm; conflict; sex satisfxn.	Comp group: no diffs bet groups on age or SES; ppts screened for med probs.	Self-report: Sex Fx Scale (SFS); Sex Dysfx Scale (SDS).	SD F (esp w/ arousal and desire probs) < fx'l F on rel qual. Rel probs strongly assoc w/ F (but not M) SD.	Adeq psychometric properties for all measures.

Table 3.1.1b. (Continued)

Study	n	Sample characteristics	Independent variables	Dependent variables	Methodology	Measurement	Results	Comments
Byers & Demmons, 1999[69]	99	52 F & 47 M univ students; M age = 19.3 yrs.; M rel duration = 13 mo.	Sex comm; Nonsex discl; Perc costs/ rewards of sex rel.	Sex satisfxn; Rel satisfxn.	Corr design.	Self-report; comm Q-aire; GMSEX; GMREL.	(+) comm to partner about sex prefs contrib to ↑ sex satisfx thru ↑ overall rel satisfxn & more (+) sex exchanges.	All measures had reported R and V except for comm Q-aire.
Davies et al., 1999[30]	72	Heterosex undergrad couples w/ sex rels of 6+ mos. M age = 20 yr; 88% W. M rel dur = 26.9 mos.	Sex desire discrepancies.	Sex satisfxn; rel satisfxn.	Corr design.	Self-report: SDI; ISS; Hendrick's	When F sex desire < M partner's, assoc w/ lower F rel and sex satisfxn. Discrep in desire contrib to F sex satisfxn, after contr for partner's sex satisfxn. Sex satisfxn med'd assoc bet sex desire discrep and rel satisfxn.	All measures had est R and V.
Hurlbert et al., 2000[20]	54	F w/ diag of HSDD; M age = 31 yr; 76% W; 80% mothers; avg marriage 6.3 yr.	Sex compat; Sex satisfxn; Mar satisfxn; Sex stress.	Sex desire; Sex motivatn.	Corr design; Screened for sex abuse, ETOH/ drug abuse, med use, dyspar, and phys illness.	Self-report: sex diaries; HISC; ISS; Index of Mar Satisfxn; Apt Index of Sex Stress.	Higher sex compat assoc w/ > sex motivatn and desire and < sex stress). F mar satisfxn and (+) attitudes tow sex fantasy assoc w/ > sex desire. Sex compat assoc w/ mar satisfxn and sex satisfxn.	Measures had sound psychometric properties.
Birnbaum et al., 2001[49]	98	36 clin anorg F seeking tx for org probs; 26 subclin anorg F; 36 sex fx'l controls. Israeli sample. M ages 28.6 to 32.4.	Group (clin anorg, subclin anorg, org controls).	Sev characs of self-rep intercourse exp.	Comp/cont groups; Clearly spec incl crit. Subclin and clin anorg group matched on org probs. No demo diffs bet groups.	Self-report: WEHI	Anorg > org in aversive feelings and thoughts dur intercourse, isolatn, anx, distracting thoughts, sense of sex inadeq. Anorg < org pleasure, closeness w/ partner in during sex, love, connectn w/ partner). Clin > subclin anorg in disappt w/ partner, sex burnout.	WEHI had prelim evid of R and V. Anorg F had < emot'l connectn w/ partner dur intercourse vs > overall dyad probs.
Hallam-Jones et al., 2001[50]	172	F presenting at dermatol clin in UK; 85 w/ vulvodyn, 87 controls w/ nonvulv dermatol probs. Ages 18-70 yr.	Group (vulvodyn vs control).	Rel satisfxn; sex satisfxn; sex freq; pain freq and severity w/ sex activity; also assessed dep and anx.	Cont group of pts presenting at same clinic.	Self-report: Pers interviews and q-aires (GRIMS, GRISS); HAD (measure of dep and anx).	Vulvodyn F < control F on sex freq, rel and sex satisfxn. Vulvodyn > controls in reporting rel and sex probs caused by their condition, sex pain, dep, anx.	Standardized measures used for all q-aires.

Table 3.1.1b. (Continued)

Study	n	Sample characteristics	Independent variables	Dependent variables	Methodology	Measurement	Results	Comments
Sprecher, 2002[28]	101	Couples dating for avg of 18.6 mos (at 1st of 5 assts). M age = 20.	Sex satisfxn (and change in satisfxn over time) [In one set of analyses, IVs and DVs reversed].	Rel satisfxn; love; commitment; rel stab (also change in vars over time).	Longitud'l study (5 annual assts, 1988 to 1992). Corr design. Avo'ded item-overlap bet measure of love and sex satisfxn.	Self-report: Hendrick's RASs; Lund's Commitment Scale; Braiker and Kelley Love Scale; Add'l global indexes.	Sex satisfxn corr w/ rel satisfxn, commitment, and love. Increase in sex satisfxn assoc w/ increase in rel satisfxn, commitment, and love. Sex satisfxn pred rel stab for M; poor rel. satisfxn pred dissolutn for F.	Adeq int consist for all q-aires; evid of R and V for RAS.
Reissing et al., 2003[51]	87	F (29 w/ vagin, 29 w/ VVS, and 29 no-pain controls). M age 28 yr (18–43). Can sample.	Group (vagin vs VVS vs no-pain).	Rel adj; sex fx; sex self-schema; psychologic distress; other vars.	Cont groups, matched on age, rel status, and parental status; clearly def incl and excl crit.	Self-report; MAT; Sex Self-Schema; Brief Symptom Inventory.	No diffs bet groups in rel adj (based on small subset of sample in committed rels) or psych distress. Vagin group: less (+) sex self schemas. Both pain groups > controls in SD.	Measures used were all standardized.

Abbreviations adeq = adequate; aff = affective; ambig = ambiguous; anorg = anorgasmic; arg = arguments; Asn = Asian; assert = assertiveness; assign = assignment; BDI = Beck Depression Inventory; B = Black; Can = Canadian; characs = characteristics; CL = checklist; clin = clinical; CB = cognitive behavioral; ComQual = Comprehensive Quality of Life scale; confl res = conflict resolution; contr = controlling; counterbal = counterbalanced; crit = criteria; cunnil = cunnilingus; curr = current; DAS = Dyadic Adjustment Scale (for assessment of marital satisfaction); dec = decision, decided; def = defined; deg = degree; depend = dependent; dep = depressed, depression; det = determinants diag = diagnoses; discl = disclosure; dist = distressed; disappt = disappointment; dissatisfxn = dissatisfaction; dir = direct; dur = duration; dyad = dyadic; dyspar = dyspareunia; ed = education; emot'l = emotional; enjoy = enjoyment; ETOH = alcohol; evid = evidence; excl = exclusion, excluded; exp = experience(d); exptl = experimental; explic = explicit; F = female; fam = family; GMREL/GMSEX = Global Measure of Relationship/Sexual Satisfaction; GRIMS/SS = Golomok-Rust Inventory of Marital/Sexual Satisfaction; HAMA = Hamilton Anxiety Scale; HAMD = Hamilton Depression Scale; Hisp = Hispanic; HISC/A = Hurlbert Index of Sexual Compatibility/Assertiveness; HISD = Hurlbert Index of Sexual Desire; hyp = hypothesis; imp = importance; inadeq = inadequacy; incl = inclusion, included; id = identified; indep = independent; ISS = Index of Sexual Satisfaction; init = initiating; int consist = internal consistency; interv = interview; IIP = Inventory of Interpersonal Problems; inv = inventory; knowl = knowledge; M = male; M and J = Masters and Johnson; manip = manipulation; MAT = Marital Adjustment Test; MAS = Marital Attitudes Scale; MCI = Marital Communication Inventory; MSI = Marital Satisfaction Inventory; man'l = manual; mar = marital; Mdn = median; med'd = mediated; modif = modified; nat = naturally; observ'l = observational; obs = observer; observ'l = observational; obt = obtaining; partic = participating; part = partner; PLS = Passionate Love Scale; perc = perceived; PAIR = Personal Assessment of Intimacy in Relationships; prelim evid = preliminary evidence; PMSCS = Premarital Sexual Conflict Scale; premar = premarital; prem = premature; prss = presenting; prev = prevalent; prsnt = presenting; PCI = Primary Communication Inventory; prim = primarily; proc = procedure; prop = properties; rec = receive(d); RAS = Relationship Assessment Scale; RCI = Relationship Closeness Inventory; R and V = reliability and validity; rew = rewards; ser = serious; sess = sessions; sitn = situation; std = standardized; SA = sexual arousal; SAS = Sexual Attitudes Scale; disting = distinguished; SDI = Sexual Desire Inventory; SII = Sexual Interaction Inventory; SOS = Sexual Opinion Survey; spec = specific; stim = stimuli, stimulation; subj = subjective; sugg = suggest(s); SCL = symptom checklist; SCL-90 = Symptom Checklist 90; ther = therapist, therapy; tow = toward; tx = treatment; understnd = understanding; vag = vaginal; VPA = vaginal pulse amplitude; vagin = vaginismus; vid = video; vol = volunteer; vulvodyn = vulvodynia; VVS = vulvar vestibulitis syndrome; WEHI = Women's Experience of Heterosexual Intercourse Scale; WL = wait list; W = white; yg = young; ↑↓ = higher/increased, lower/decreased

Table 3.1.2. Treatment outcome studies relevant to relationship factors and female sexuality

Study	n	Sample Characteristics	Identified Problem	Treatment(s)	Control	Outcome Post-treatment	Follow-up	Comments
Crowe et al., 1981[56]	48	24 couples w/ chief c/o FSD (anorg or desire dysfx); 24 w/ M SD. M ages = 30 (F), 35.5(M).	Mixed SD in F and M. In couples w/ M presenters, 13 F partners diag w/ SD.	(1) Modif M and J tx w/ co-ther (sens focus; genital focus later in tx); (2) Modif M and J tx w/ single ther; (3) Mar therapy + Relax trng. Txs not std.	Random asst to 1 of the 3 txs. Each ther conducted tx w/ all groups. Txs bal for gender of pt and ther. No WL or plac cont.	All 3 tx groups showed sig imprv from pre-tx in sex and rel satisfxn and sex interest. No diffs bet the 3 txs.	1-yr follow-up (n=36). Gains (from pre-tx levels) maintained for all 3 groups.	Change in target behav assessed by self-rep and blind raters.
Hartman & Daly, 1983[59]	12	Couples diag w/ mult SDs (F, mostly prim org dysfx and HSD). M ages = 33.2 (F), 36.7 (M). M dur = 6.2 yr.	Mixed SD. Screened to R/O organic causes, individ psychpath, relev phys illnesses.	(1) Sex ther: CB tx w/ focus on educ, disinhib, sens focus. (2) Mar ther: comm skills and confl res. 5 wkly sess (90 min) in group format w/ husb/ wife ther team. Txs not blind or manualized.	Bal, crossover design. Random asst to mar ther 1st, then sex therapy (or reverse).	Sex ther > mar ther in sex satisfxn (trend tow sig). Couples w/ > pre-tx dyad adj resp best to sex ther 1st; couples w/ < dyad adj resp better to mar ther 1st.	6-rr o follow-up conducted, but data not reported.	Measures had est R and V. Sex ther alone may be eff w/ SD, in abs of ser rel probs.
Libman et al., 1984[85]	23	Married couples (ages 25–44; 1–20 yr rel dur) w/ F c/o sec org dysfx. M dur of SD=10 yr.	F sec org dysfx.	CB tx in: (1) std couple ther or (2) group ther format. Plac/pseudo-tx (minimum contact and biblio-ther/ self-help)	Random asst to couple ther, group ther, or placebo/ pseudo-tx.	Improvements seen for all 3 txs; couple ther slightly > group ther.		Measures had est R and V.
Kilmann et al., 1986[106]	55	Couples c/o sec coital org dysfx (51 married, 1 engaged, 3 cohab). M ages = 32.6 (F), 34.5 (M). M yr cohab = 9.5; M dur of dysfx = 9.6 yr.	F sec org dysfx w/ partner. Excl: organic etiol, dysp/vagin, severe psych probs, ED in partner.	Comm skills trng: sex comm and generic confl res. Sex skills trng: dir masturb and sens focus. Comb comm+ sex skills. Attn plac: lect, educ, and bibliother. All txs manual and conducted by individ ther in groups of 4-6 couples each (8 wk sess).	Random asst to 1 of 6 conditns: (1) comm skills; (2) sex skills; (3) comm+sex skills; (4) sex skills + comm.; (5) attn plac; (6) WL control.	Tx couples > Plac or WL on sex satisfxn and sex harmony. No single tx superior. F w/ no prev coital org > F w/ prev coital org in dyad adj pre- to post-tx.	6-mo follow-up (WL cont group not incl). Tx gains not maint overall. Poorer pre-tx rel adj pred > gains in org freq at follow-up.	2 of 3 q-aires had est R & V. Clearly spec incl and excl crit. Lack of sig follow-up compar may be due to low stat power.
Zimmer, 1987[54]	28	Couples; F partner diag w/ sec org dysfx. High preval of mar and psych distress (50% of pts w/ severe dep).	Mixed sec FSDs (no. pts w/ spec diag not reported). Pts excl w/ organic etiol, SD assoc w/ psych probs.	(1) 9 sess of mar ther (comm/confl res), followed by 12 sess of CB sex tx based on M and J; (2) 9 sess of Plac tx (relaxation, educ), followed by 12 sess of sex ther. Tx manual used.	Random asst to: (1) mar ther+sex ther; (2) plac+ sex ther; or 3) WL cont. No pre-tx (diffs in demo or symptoms).	Mar ther + sex ther > plac + sex ther. Both txs > WL cont on sex and mar adj. Mar + sex ther vs placebo group: < sex probs, > sex desire, > mar adj post-tx.	3-mo follow-up: tx gains maint for both tx groups.	q-aires w/ est R and V; obs couple interaxns (w/ good inter-rater R. High attrition rate for tx groups.

Table 3.1.2. (Continued)

Study	n	Sample Characteristics	Identified Problem	Treatment(s)	Control	Outcome Post-treatment	Outcome Follow-up	Comments
Hurlbert, 1993[71]	39	F (ages 28–38) with HSD.	F HSD.	Std group ther; Std group ther + org consistency trng.	Random asst to std group tx, or group tx + org consist trng.	Combined tx > std tx in SA and sex assertiveness.	3 and 6 mo fu: Combined tx > std tx in SA and assert (and satisfxn 6 mos).	Increase in assert and SA assoc w/ incr in sex satisfxn.
Hurlbert et al., 1993[86]	57	F c/o HSD, ages 25–37 (M 29.6 yr). 68.4% W, 24.6% B, 7% Hisp. Married avg 7.7 yr. M yr of educ = 12.8.	HSD; excl F w/ mental illness, etoh/drug abuse, dysp, relev phys illness, h/o trauma.	10 wkly sess of Org Consistency Trng (dir masturb, sens focus, tech to improve M climax, coital alignmt). Std tx protocol followed by M/F ther team.	Random asst to F-only group format, couple group format, or WL cont.	Partner involvemt in tx assoc w/ superior outcome. Couple tx > F-only group in sex satisfxn and sex compat. Couple tx > WL.	6-mo follow-up: Couple tx superior on 5 of 6 outcome measures; tx gains maint for both tx groups.	All measures used had est R and V.
MacPhee et al., 1995[55]	64	49 couples cohab for 2+ yr; F diag w/ ISD (M dur 6.7 yr); 15 non-ISD cont couples in ther for other probs.	ISD; excl desire-related illnesses or med use, etoh/drug abuse, dom violence, preg, severe mar probs.	Emotion-focused couple ther (integ of experiential and sys approaches); 10 wkly sess. Not manual. Admin by individ ther w/ wkly supervision.	Pts w/ ISD Randomly assigned to tx (n = 25) or WL cont (n = 24). Pre-tx diffs bet groups ruled out or controlled.	Tx > WL on sex desire, dyad adj. Lower pre-tx mar distress pred higher post-tx sex satisfxn, sex freq, and sex desire. ISD < non-ISD in mar distress and sex satisfxn.	3-mo follow-up: dyad adjust further improved for tx couples; sex desire increase maint, desire tow partner decl slightly from post-tx (still higher than pre-tx levels).	4 of 6 measures used had est R and V; several std instrum used.
Trudel et al., 2001[107]	74	Couples diag w/ F HSD (M = 6 yr). Cohab for avg of 13 yr; 20–55 yr old (M age = 37.4 (F), 39.4 (M).	F HSD. Excl ser psych disord or mar probs.	Multimodal CB tx in group format (4–6 couples). 12 wkly (2 hr) sess. Focus on educ, comm skills, sens focus, sex intimacy exerc, and cog restruct. M/F co-ther.	Random asst to tx (n = 38) or WL control (n = 36). No sig diffs bet groups on key demo or study vars.	Tx > WL on HSD sympt improvemt, sex fx / satisfxn, rel adjust, and decrease in (-) sex thoughts. 74% tx F improved.	3-mo and 1-yr follow-up: 64% of tx F still classified as improved. 38% sympt-free at 1-yr follow-up.	Sev std instrum used. Sec finding of study: HSD F said rel factors maj contrib to SD.

Abbreviations: abs = absence; adj = adjustment; asst = assignment bal = balanced; B = Black; CB = cognitive behavioral; comb = combined; compar = comparison; compat = compatibility; comm = communication; confl res = conflict resolution; crit = criteria; decl = declined; demo = demographic; dur = duration; dyad = dyadic; dysfx = dysfunction; dysp = dyspareunia; educ = education; eff = effective; excl = excluded; exclusion; exerc = exercises; F = female; Hisp = Hispanic; imprv = improvement; instrum = instruments; integ = integration; interaxns = interactions; maint = maintained; maj = major; M = male; manual = manualized; mar = marital; M and J = Masters and Johnson; moaif = modified; obs = observed; org = orgasm(ic); plac cont = placebo control; preg = pregnancy; preval = prevalence; prim = primary; psych = psychological/psychiatric; psychpath = psychopathology; R and V = reliability and validity; relev = relevant; resp = responded; sec = secondary; self-rep = self-report(ed); ser = serious; SA = sexual arousal; sev = several; SD = sexual dysfunction; sig = significant, significance; std = standardized; stat = statistical. sys = systems; ther = therapist, therapy; tow = toward; trng = training; tx = treatment; vagin = vaginismus; WL = waitlist; W = white.

association between marital happiness and intercourse frequency. However, individuals reporting a closer match between actual and desired levels of coitus reported more marital happiness. Other research indicates that sexual frequency does not predict marital happiness, but couples with a higher frequency of sex relative to the number of arguments have been found to report more marital happiness.[16] The ratio of sexual frequency to number of arguments has been associated with the woman's (but not the man's) feelings of passionate love for partner.[17] Women's perceptions of equity/fairness in the relationship have also been found to moderately predict coital frequency.[18]

Sexual response

Better relationship adjustment/satisfaction with one's partner tends to be accompanied by greater sexual response.[14,19,20] For example, Hurlbert et al.[20] found that women (but not male partners) who were dissatisfied with their marriage reported lower sexual desire, regardless of their overall sexual satisfaction. Maritally satisfied women reported greater sexual interest, higher levels of sexual arousal, and higher orgasmic frequency. Marital happiness has been found to predict higher frequency of orgasm during spousal intercourse, greater sexual variety, and fewer refusals of sexual initiations.[19,21] Female orgasmic response has been found to be lower in the context of spousal conflict and hostility,[19] and couples marked by mutual warmth, caring, and affection have been reported to exhibit greater female sexual arousal, desire, and enjoyment of sex.[14] In a rare experimental study, responses to erotic audiotapes depicting sexual interactions containing different emotional contexts (anger, anxiety, and neutral/control) were examined.[22] It was found that sexual encounters containing anxiety and anger lowered sexual desire, and that women were significantly more likely than men to terminate sexual encounters when they felt angry.

Sexual satisfaction

Most research has found general relationship satisfaction and sexual satisfaction to be positively correlated in married, cohabitating, and dating couples.[23–29] The limited longitudinal data available indicates that decreased happiness with one's sexual relationship predicts a subsequent decline in relationship satisfaction.[26] However, the more likely conclusion is that sexual and relationship satisfaction are reciprocal.[26,28,30]

Other relationship factors have been shown to relate to sexual satisfaction. In a community sample of married women, self-reported closeness with one's partner was more predictive of sexual satisfaction than the number of orgasms, frequency of sex, or sexual arousal.[31] In one of the few studies including a large number of African-American couples, tension with partner predicted sexual dissatisfaction, whereas affirmation with one's partner predicted sexual satisfaction.[32] Investigations testing the sexual exchange theory[27,33] found that relationship satisfaction contributed unique variance to sexual satisfaction beyond indices of sexual rewards and costs. Likewise, sexual satisfaction significantly added to the prediction of relationship satisfaction beyond indexes of sexual exchange.[27]

Decreased sexual satisfaction has been found to predict subsequent divorce in married couples[26] and relationship dissolution in dating couples.[28] It has also been found that relationship instability may be more related to sexual dissatisfaction in men, and relationship dissatisfaction in women.[28] This is consistent with evidence that relationship satisfaction in women, but not men, is significantly associated with feelings of passionate love toward one's partner.[17]

Sexual and relationship satisfaction can operate at least partially independently of each other.[34–36] In their comparison of sexually distressed, clinical and nondistressed/nonclinical couples, Heiman and colleagues[35] observed that indicators of sexual adjustment, rather than marital satisfaction, distinguished couples seeking sex therapy from nonclinical couples. Clinical couples reported relatively high marital satisfaction despite their sexual distress, suggesting that sexual distress does not inevitably entail serious relationship problems.[35] Some couples experience sexual dysfunction in the absence of marital problems. Likewise, positive sexual function can occur despite relationship difficulties.[34,35,37]

Mixed sexual dysfunctions and difficulties

A large survey of British men and women found that marital difficulties were strongly associated with reported sexual dysfunction (arousal problems, orgasmic dysfunction, and lack of sexual enjoyment) for women only.[38] Other investigations have found that sexually dysfunctional women have significantly more relationship problems (including lower overall relationship quality, poorer communication, and more conflict)[39,40] and impaired emotional closeness and sexual intimacy than sexually functional controls.[41]

Studies comparing couples seeking sex therapy with either nonclinical couples or those seeking marital therapy have typically found significant differences between these groups in overall relationship adjustment.[42] Compared with nonclinical couples, dyads seeking therapy for sexual dysfunction have been found to report more disagreements and lower relationship satisfaction.[43] Metz and Lutz found that both marital and sex therapy couples were less playful and spontaneous in their interactions than couples not seeking intervention for sexual or marital problems.[44] Sex therapy couples, however, reported higher overall relationship satisfaction than their marital therapy counterparts. Less global relationship distress and fewer nonsexual relationship complaints tend to characterize sex therapy versus marital therapy couples.[45,46]

Sexual dysfunction is assumed to be greater among sex therapy than marital therapy couples. However, Frank and colleagues found no significant differences between sex therapy and marital therapy couples in type or number of sexual difficulties, although sex therapy couples did report experiencing better marital adjustment.[46] Couples may self-select to marital or sex therapy despite experiencing similar problems, perhaps reflecting differences in the interpretations of their problems (i.e., as primarily indicative of "relational" or "sexual" difficulties) rather than differences in level of sexual dysfunction.

Specific sexual dysfunctions

Compared with women without hypoactive sexual desire, women with hypoactive sexual desire have been shown to report poorer dyadic adjustment, greater dissatisfaction with conflict resolution in their relationship, and less attraction to and emotional closeness with their spouses.[47,48] Furthermore, women receiving treatment for hypoactive sexual desire have been found to report that relationship factors were major contributors to their sexual problems.[48]

Findings also suggest that women with orgasmic dysfunction, compared with those orgasmic, report less satisfaction in their overall relationships and have sexual interactions that are characterized by less closeness and intimacy, fewer feelings of connection, less mutual love, and more aversive feelings and thoughts during intercourse.[49]

Results of research on sexual pain disorders are less consistent, perhaps because of the several different types of sexual pain dysfunctions. Women with vulval pain, mostly diagnosed with vulvar vestibulitis, have been shown to have lower relationship and sexual satisfaction than control patients with non-vulval pain.[50] Others have found no difference in women with vaginismus or vulvar vestibulitis syndrome, in regards to relationship satisfaction.[51,52]

Relationship quality and the treatment of sexual dysfunction

Interventions that specifically address relationship issues are usually more successful than treatments focused only on the presenting sexual symptoms.[53] Marital therapy plus sex therapy has been found to be superior to education plus sex therapy on both sexual and relational outcomes for mixed female sexual dysfunctions,[54] and relationship-focused treatments have demonstrated positive effects on sexual adjustment and overall relationship quality.[55,56]

Higher pretreatment relationship quality has been associated with successful treatment outcome.[52,57,58] Whitehead and Matthews found that successful treatment response on both sexual and nonsexual measures was predicted by overall relationship quality, but not by severity of sexual dysfunction and an index of female sexual response.[57]

Severity of relationship problems suggests an initial focus on marital therapy. In one study, sexually dysfunctional couples were randomly assigned to receive sex therapy followed by marital therapy or the reverse (marital therapy followed by sex therapy). Couples with poor dyadic adjustment before treatment responded best to marital therapy first, and couples with good pretreatment relationship adjustment responded best to sex therapy first, with few gains resulting from additional marital therapy.[59]

Communication

General (nonsexual) communication

Both self-reported and observed interactions marked by mutual warmth, affection, and support are associated with higher frequency of coital sex, higher female sexual responsiveness, greater sexual desire, and a higher level of women's reported gratification with partnered sex.[14] Compared with a nonhypoactive sexual desire disorder sample, women with hypoactive sexual desire disorder have been found to report greater dissatisfaction with partners' conflict resolution and ability to listen.[47,48] Frequent and severe disagreements have been found to predict loss of interest in sex with one's partner and involvement in extramarital affairs,[26] and the quality of couples' nonsexual communication has been found to predict sexual satisfaction, both concurrently[60] and longitudinally.[61] Zimmer found that sexually distressed couples exhibited more negative interactions than happily married couples or couples seeking therapy for marital problems.[54] Sexually distressed couples' interactions demonstrated fewer expressions of acceptance, less congruence, and more negative nonverbal behaviors. It has also been found that, compared with sexually functional couples, sexually dysfunctional dyads reported more communication and conflict resolution problems.[40,43,62]

In their review of the literature on the role of communication in sexual dysfunction, Metz and Epstein noted that significant sexual difficulties can be experienced in the absence of communication problems.[34,63,64] Hartman concluded that sexual dysfunction (or at least the process of attributing dyadic problems to sexual dysfunction) may actually enhance relationship satisfaction and buffer against relational distress.[34] Couples who attribute their relationship difficulties to sexual dysfunction may be less likely to experience relationship distress than couples who view their problems as reflective of wide-ranging deficits in their relationships.

Research on specific patterns of interaction implicated in sexual dysfunction is scant. This stands in stark contrast to marital interaction research, which has identified several interactional patterns predictive of overall relationship satisfaction, marital stability, and divorce.[65-68] The association between these patterns and sexual satisfaction or sexual function is unknown, as marital researchers have largely ignored sexual relationships of couples.

Taken together, there are several possible ways in which general communication problems may be associated with sexual dysfunction.[63] First, communication problems may directly lead to sexual dysfunction (or conversely, sexual dysfunction may lead to problems in communication). Second, sexual dysfunction may be compartmentalized and hence not affect general communication or relationship distress, possibly buffering the couple from global relational dissatisfaction/distress. Third, sexual dysfunction may emerge independently of relationship conflict, contributing to communication problems via an indirect impact on the affective tone of the relationship.

Sexual communication

Generic communication skills and positive interactions do not necessarily translate to positive communication about sex. It has been found that sexual communication (particularly disclosure of one's sexual likes and dislikes to one's partner) contributes unique variance to sexual satisfaction beyond general communication alone.[60] Individuals are significantly more likely to make nonsexual than sexual disclosures to their partners. It seems that sexual disclosure is more likely if one's partner takes the initiative to discuss sexual issues; nevertheless, partners are much more willing to disclose their sexual *likes* rather than their *dislikes*.[69]

Based on a sample of 6029 women and men from the National Survey of Families and Households, Donnelly found that sexually inactive respondents (defined as no partner sex during the month prior to interview) reported having *fewer* arguments about sex with their partners than sexually active individuals.[15] This finding was interpreted as reflecting resignation to a lower level of sexual interaction among sexually inactive respondents. Studies investigating more global measures of sexual conflict have generally found that higher levels of sexual conflict are associated with lower sexual and relationship satisfaction.[70]

Couples seeking therapy for sexual dysfunction have been found to report more sexual communication problems than nonclinic control couples.[43] Similar findings have been reported for maritally distressed couples, with quality of sexual communication also predicting overall relationship adjustment and quality of global communication.[62]

Sexual communication contributes significantly to sexual satisfaction.[31,48,60,69,71] It has been found that women's sexual assertiveness (in addition to emotional closeness and erotophilia) predicts sexual satisfaction beyond orgasm frequency, rating of sexual excitability, or frequency of coital sex. For women with hypoactive sexual desire disorder, increases in sexual assertiveness after treatment have been associated with subsequent gains in sexual satisfaction.[71]

The effect of sexual communication on sexual and relationship satisfaction may vary by age and gender. The results of one study of 996 women and men obtained from a community sample (selected randomly from a list of telephone subscribers) found that sexual communication was a significant predictor of sexual satisfaction for women and men under 60 years old as well as for women over 60.[96] Good sexual communication was significantly associated with relationship satisfaction only for younger cohorts of women and men, but not for respondents over 60.

Although sexual communication is often nonverbal, subtle, and complex,[72,73] most empirical research has examined verbal expressions of sexual interest.[74] In one study, men were more likely to initiate sex than women. However, after controlling for initiation frequency, women were just as likely as men to respond positively to sexual advances.[21] Women reporting greater sexual and relationship satisfaction initiated more frequently, and those with less sexual satisfaction refused sex more often.[3,21]

Sexual communication satisfaction has been found to contribute significantly to marital quality indirectly through its positive impact on sexual satisfaction.[25] Anorgasmic (versus orgasmic) women have reported more discomfort with sexual communication, especially in discussing sexual activities, such as direct clitoral stimulation, that are most likely to lead to orgasm.[75]

Relationship status: duration, marital status, and sexual orientation

Relationship duration

Research on relationship duration and sexuality has focused almost exclusively on the frequency of coital sex, with the nearly ubiquitous finding that frequency of sex declines with increasing duration of the relationship.[12,18,23,76–78] Coital frequency is highest in committed relationships during the first 2 years, with a steady and gradual decline thereafter.[12,77] Typical reasons given for this decline include familiarity with one's partner (and accompanying lack of novelty or "routine" nature of sex) as well as child-rearing and job demands.[77]

In the National Survey of Families and Households sample, age and marital happiness were stronger predictors of coital frequency than relationship duration.[12] In contrast, Blumstein and Schwartz found that relationship duration uniquely predicted frequency of sex, after controlling for age.[23]

There is evidence that sexual desire changes in committed relationships may vary by gender. In a representative sample of 1865 German students in committed heterosexual relationships, the duration of the relationship was positively associated with tenderness/closeness and negatively associated with desire in women, but not in men.[76]

Changes in the *quantity* of sex are not necessarily mirrored by changes in sexual satisfaction. Greenblat found that individuals continued to report that sex was both satisfying and personally important despite declines in frequency of partner sex.[77]

Using data from the US nationally representative National Health and Social Life Survey, Liu found that marital duration was moderately and negatively associated with reported *quality* of sex with spouse, with women reporting less satisfaction than men with the quality of marital sex.[79] Marital duration nevertheless accounted for a very small proportion of variance in marital quality.

Marital status

Comparisons of cohabiting and married couples have consistently suggested that cohabiting couples engage in higher sexual activity.[18,21,23] Yet, the National Health and Social Life Survey found that being married (relative to single, divorced, widowed, or separated) decreased the risk of sexual dysfunction[80] and that cohabitation had a weak negative effect on reported quality of sex.[79]

Same-sex relationships

Research on homosexual relationships is rare (see Peplau et al.[81] for a review and elsewhere in this volume). The extant research on women in same-sex relationships is somewhat inconsistent in terms of whether lesbians (and bisexuals) are similar to heterosexuals in sexual function and satisfaction. Kinsey et al.[5]

found orgasm frequency to be higher for lesbians than heterosexual women, with 68% of lesbians reporting that they experienced orgasm 90–100% of the time when having sex, compared with 40% of married women. Similarly, only 7% of lesbians reported never reaching orgasm, compared with 17% of married women. Masters and Johnson found that perceived sexual quality was greater for same-sex couples than heterosexual couples.[82] Others have found lesbian couples to have less frequent sexual activity than heterosexual couples.[23]

Partner variables

Individual partner characteristics

Besides the obvious but critical characteristics of being sexually arousing and providing adequate sexual stimulation, several additional characteristics of the male partner have been shown to influence female sexual function and satisfaction. A woman's age, as well as the age and health of her male partner, have been found to be especially salient for women's reported coital frequency.[18] Important contributors to female sexual satisfaction (versus sexual distress) are the partner's understanding of the woman's sexual preferences, his responsiveness to sexual requests, and his empathy.[32,61,83,84] In 45 couples seeking therapy for sexual dysfunction (predominantly arousal and orgasmic problems), the partner's lack of responsiveness to sexual requests more strongly predicted sexual distress than sexual dysfunction itself.[83] The male partner's empathy prior to marriage predicted the woman's (and man's) sexual satisfaction 1 year after the wedding.[61] Feeling affirmed and generally emotionally supported by one's partner has also been found to predict significantly women's sexual satisfaction.[32]

Partner discrepancies and sexual compatibility

Compatibility in sexual preferences has been found to contribute positively to women's sexual satisfaction, whereas sexual conflict (including discrepancies in the frequency of sex, types of desired sexual behaviors, partners' expectations of sex, and other aspects of sexual interactions) has been associated with sexual dissatisfaction and overall unhappiness with the relationship – even after controlling for the level of generic, nonsexual disagreements.[70,84] In a study of undergraduate cohabiting couples, women with lower sexual desire than their male partners reported lower relationship and sexual satisfaction. Sexual desire discrepancies contributed unique variance to women's sexual satisfaction, even after controlling for partners' level of sexual satisfaction.[30]

Partner's involvement in the treatment of women's sexual dysfunction

Partner involvement in treatment is associated with superior treatment outcomes for women with orgasmic dysfunction[85] or hypoactive sexual desire disorder.[86] Women with hypoactive sexual desire disorder who were randomly assigned to a couple's group treatment, as opposed to a women-only group, fared significantly better (at post-treatment and 6-month follow-up) on measures of sexual satisfaction and sexual compatibility.[86] In a study of mixed sexual dysfunctions, 84% of patients whose partners attended therapy experienced positive outcomes compared with 51% of individuals with nonparticipating partners.[87] The treatment motivation of women's partners has also been found to be important, predicting treatment completion (vs dropout), as well as superior outcomes.[88,89]

Postpregnancy and children

While pregnancy is addressed elsewhere in this volume, we would like to highlight a few points, since pregnancy and children affect many women's lives. The transition to parenthood is important and challenging, and associated with dramatic biologic, psychologic, and interpersonal changes that can have a significant impact on women's (and their partner's) sexual function and satisfaction.

Once intercourse resumes after childbirth, the frequency of sexual activity tends to be lower than prepregnancy levels for several months.[90] Sexual problems during the postpartum period are the norm, rather than the exception,[90] with only 14% reporting an absence of sexual difficulties during this time (Hames, 1980; cited in Bitzer and Alder, 2000).[91]

Fortunately, most women and their partners weather this transition without severe marital distress or clinically diagnosable sexual dysfunction.[91] Research by Gottman and his colleagues[92] has identified several factors that appear to buffer couples against relationship distress during the transition to parenthood. Of particular importance are the male partner's attentiveness and expression of fondness and affection toward his spouse, awareness on the part of both partners of each other and of the relationship, and a positive attitude toward conflict resolution.[92] In contrast, husbands' negativity and disappointment with the marriage predict greater relationship distress and declines in marital satisfaction during this transition.[92]

Research on the impact of children on women's sexual function and satisfaction is limited and tends to focus on coital frequency. Fatigue and responsibilities related to child rearing are frequently given as reasons for declines in sexual activity among couples.[77] It has been found that couples with one child in the home report lower coital frequency than nonparenting couples. However, parents with two or more children report equivalent coital frequency to childless couples.[18] These findings suggest that the impact of having children on sexuality may be greatest after the initial transition to parenthood.

Summary and conclusions

It remains surprising that so little empirical research has included sexuality and relationship variables, particularly since sexual frequency and satisfaction relate to relationship quality, strength, durability, and family stability. While more research is clearly needed, it is important to remember that the above work strongly suggests that relationship factors play an important role in women's sexual function and sexual satisfaction.

Caveats are in order with regard to generalizing too broadly from the studies in this area. Many designs are (1) correlational; (2) based on small, nonrepresentative, or specialized samples and (3) incompletely characterized with regard to social variables (e.g., education, social status, and ethnicity), health, or specification of diagnostic category and severity. They are nevertheless a helpful perspective to direct future research.

There is a danger in the common tendency to view sexual dysfunction as a purely physiologic or psychologic phenomenon. As has been recognized by researchers and clinicians, sexuality is a multidimensional phenomenon that is influenced by a complex web of biologic, psychologic, sociocultural, and interpersonal determinants.[1,2,10,93,94] There is consistent evidence that the interpersonal context of one's relationship is particularly fundamental to women's sexual function and satisfaction.

Research on physiologic factors implicated in women's sexual dysfunction, as well as potential physiologically based treatments for these dysfunctions, is important. However, a purely individualistic and physiologic approach is bound to fall short of a thorough understanding of female sexual dysfunction and its treatment.

References

1. Byers ES. Evidence for the importance of relationship satisfaction for women's sexual functioning. In E Kaschak, L Tiefer, eds. *A New View of Women's Sexual Problems*. New York: Haworth Press, 2001: 23–6.

2. Basson R, Leiblum S, Brotto L et al. Definitions of women's sexual dysfunction reconsidered: advocating expansion and revision. *J Psychosom Obstet Gynaecol* 2003; 24: 221–9.

3. Terman LM, Buttenweiser P, Ferguson LW et al. *Psychological Factors in Marital Happiness*. New York: McGraw-Hill, 1938.

4. Dickinson RL, Beam L. *A Thousand Marriages*. Oxford: Williams & Wilkins, 1931.

5. Kinsey AC, Pomeroy WB, Martin CE et al. *Sexual Behavior in the Human Female*. Oxford: Saunders, 1953.

6. Masters WH, Johnson VE. *Human Sexual Response*. Oxford: Little, Brown, 1966.

7. Masters WH, Johnson VE. *Human Sexual Inadequacy*. Boston: Little, Brown, 1970.

8. Aubin S, Heiman, JR. Sexual dysfunction from a relationship perspective. In JH Harvey, A Wenzel, S Sprecher, eds. *The Handbook of Sexuality in Close Relationships*. Mahwah: Erlbaum, 2004: 477–517.

9. Tiefer L. Historical, scientific, clinical and feminist criticisms of "the human sexual response cycle". *Annu Rev Sex Res* 1991; 2: 1–23.

10. Beck JG. Hypoactive sexual desire disorder: an overview. *J Consult Clin Psychol* 1995; 63: 919–27.

11. Heiman JR, LoPiccolo J. Clinical outcome of sex therapy: effects of daily v. weekly treatment. *Arch Gen Psychiatry* 1983; 30: 443–9.

12. Call V, Sprecher S, Schwartz P. The incidence and frequency of marital sex in a national sample. *J Marriage Fam* 1995; 57: 639–52.

13. Birchler GR, Webb LJ. Discriminating interaction behaviors in happy and unhappy marriages. *J Consult Clin Psychol* 1977; 45: 494–5.

14. Persky H, Charney N, Strauss D et al. The relationship of sexual adjustment and related sexual behaviors and attitudes to marital adjustment. *Am J Fam Ther* 1982; 10: 38–49.

15. Donnelly DA. Sexually inactive marriages. *J Sex Res* 1993; 30: 171–9.

16. Howard JW, Dawes RM. Linear prediction of marital happiness. *Pers Soc Psychol Bull* 1976; 2: 478–80.

17. Aron A, Henkemeyer L. Marital satisfaction and passionate love. *J Soc Pers Relat* 1995; 12: 139–46.

18. Rao KV, DeMaris A. Coital frequency among married and cohabiting couples in the United States. *J Biosoc Sci* 1995; 27: 135–50.

19. Swieczkowski JB, Walker CE. Sexual behavior correlates of female orgasm and marital happiness. *J Nerv Ment Dis* 1978; 166: 335–42.

20. Hurlbert DF, Apt C, Hurlbert MK et al. Sexual compatibility and the sexual desire–motivation relation in females with hypoactive sexual desire disorder. *Behav Modif* 2000; 24: 325–47.

21. Byers ES, Heinlein L. Predicting initiations and refusals of sexual activities in married and cohabiting heterosexual couples. *J Sex Res* 1989; 26: 210–31.

22. Beck JG, Bozman AW. Gender differences in sexual desire: the effects of anger and anxiety. *Arch Sex Behav* 1995; 24: 596–612.

23. Blumstein P, Schwartz P. *American Couples*. New York: William Morrow, 1983.

24. Haavio-Manilla E, Kontula O. Correlates of increased sexual satisfaction. *Arch Sex Behav* 1997; 26: 399–418.

25. Cupach WR, Comstock J. Satisfaction with sexual communication in marriage: links to sexual satisfaction and dyadic adjustment. *J Soc Pers Relat* 1990; 7: 179–86.

26. Edwards JN, Booth A. Sexuality, marriage, and well-being: the middle years. In AS Rossi, ed. *Sexuality Across the Life Course*. Chicago: University of Chicago Press, 1994: 233–59.

27. Byers ES, Demmons S, Lawrance K. Sexual satisfaction within dating relationships: a test of the interpersonal exchange model of sexual satisfaction. *J Soc Pers Relat* 1998; 15: 257–67.

28. Sprecher S. Sexual satisfaction in premarital relationships: associations with satisfaction, love, commitment, and stability. *J Sex Res* 2002; 39: 190–6.

29. Kurdek LA. Sexuality in homosexual and heterosexual couples. In K McKinney, S Sprecher, eds. *Sexuality in Close Relationships*. Hillsdale, NJ: Erlbaum, 1991: 177–91.

30. Davies S, Katz J, Jackson JL. Sexual desire discrepancies: effects on sexual and relationship satisfaction in heterosexual dating couples. *Arch Sex Behav* 1999; 28: 553–67.

31. Hurlbert DF, Apt C, Rabehl SM. Key variables to understanding female sexual satisfaction: an examination of women in nondistressed marriages. *J Sex Marital Ther* 1993; 19: 154–65.

32. Henderson-King DH, Veroff J. Sexual satisfaction and marital well-being in the first years of marriage. *J Soc Pers Relat* 1994; 11: 509–34.

33. Lawrance K, Byers ES. Sexual satisfaction in long-term heterosexual relationships: the interpersonal exchange model of sexual satisfaction. *Pers Relatsh* 1995; 2: 267–85.

34. Hartman LM. The interface between sexual dysfunction and marital conflict. *Am J Psychiatry* 1980; 137: 576–9.

35. Heiman JR, Gladue BA, Roberts CW et al. Historical and current factors discriminating sexually functional from sexually dysfunctional married couples. *J Marital Fam Ther* 1986; 12: 163–74.

36. Apt C, Hurlbert DF, Pierce AP et al. Relationship satisfaction, sexual characteristics, and the psychosocial well-being of women. *Can J Hum Sex* 1996; 5: 195–210.

37. Frank E, Anderson C, Rubenstein D. Frequency of sexual dysfunction in "normal" couples. *N Engl J Med* 1978; 299: 111–15.

38. Dunn KM, Croft PR, Hackett GI. Association of sexual problems with social, psychological, and physical problems in men and women: a cross sectional population survey. *J Epidemiol Community Health* 1999; 53: 144–8.

39. McCabe M, Cobain MJ. The impact of individual and relationship factors on sexual dysfunction among males and females. *Sex Marital Ther* 1998; 13: 131–43.

40. Ernst C, Földenyí M, Angst J. The Zurich study. XXI. Sexual dysfunctions and disturbances in young adults: data of a longitudinal epidemiological study. *J Eur Arch Psychiatry Neurosci* 1993; 243(3–4): 179–88.

41. Moore KA, McCabe MP, Stockdale JE. Factor analysis of the Personal Assessment of Intimacy in Relationships (PAIR): engagement, communication, and shared friendships. *Sex Marital Ther* 1998; 13: 361–8.

42. Metz ME, Dwyer SM. Relationship conflict management patterns among sex dysfunction, sex offender, and satisfied couples. *J Sex Marital Ther* 1993; 19: 104–22.

43. Chesney AP, Blakeney PE, Cole CM et al. A comparison of couples who have sought sex therapy with couples who have not. *J Sex Marital Ther* 1981; 7: 131–40.

44. Metz ME, Lutz G. Dyadic playfulness differences between sexual and marital therapy couples. *J Psychol Hum Sex* 1990; 3: 169–82.

45. Berg P, Snyder, DK. Differential diagnosis of marital and sexual distress: a multidimensional approach. *J Sex Marital Ther* 1981; 7: 290–5.

46. Frank E, Anderson C, Kupfer, DJ. Profiles of couples seeking sex therapy and marital therapy. *Am J Psychiatry* 1976; 133: 559–62.

47. Stuart FM, Hammond DC, Pett MA. Inhibited sexual desire in women. *Arch Sex Behav* 1987; 16: 91–106.

48. Trudel G, Boulos L, Benoit M. Dyadic adjustment in couples with hypoactive sexual desire. *J Sex Educ Ther* 1993; 19: 31–6.

49. Birnbaum G, Glaubman H, Mikulincer, M. Women's experience of heterosexual intercourse – scale construction, factor structure, and relations to orgasmic disorder. *J Sex Res* 2001; 38: 191–204.

50. Hallam-Jones R, Wylie KR, Osborne-Cribb J et al. Sexual difficulties within a group of patients with vulvodynia. *Sex Relat Ther* 2001; 16: 113–26.

51. Reissing ED, Binik YM, Khalifé S et al. Etiological correlates of vaginismus: sexual and physical abuse, sexual knowledge, sexual self-schema, and relationship adjustment. *J Sex Marital Ther* 2003; 29: 47–59.

52. Van Lankveld JJDM, Weijenborg PTM, TerKuile MM. Psychologic profiles of and sexual function in women with vulvar vestibulitis and their partners. *Obstet Gynecol* 1996; 88: 65–70.

53. Althof SE, Leiblum SR. Psychological and interpersonal dimensions of male and female sexual function. In T Lue, R Basson, R Rosen et al., eds. *Sexual Medicine: Sexual Dysfunctions in Men and Women*. Paris: Health Publications, 2004.

54. Zimmer D. Does marital therapy enhance the effectiveness of treatment for sexual dysfunction? *J Sex Marital Ther* 1987; 13: 193–209.

55. MacPhee DC, Johnson SM, Van Der Veer MMC. Low sexual desire in women: the effects of marital therapy. *J Sex Marital Ther* 1995; 21: 159–82.

56. Crowe MJ, Gillan P, Golombok, S. Form and content in the conjoint treatment of sexual dysfunction: a controlled study. *Behav Res Ther* 1981; 19: 47–54.

57. Whitehead A, Matthews A. Factors related to successful outcome in the treatment of sexually unresponsive women. *Psychol Med* 1986; 16: 373–8.

58. Hawton K, Catalan J. Prognostic factors in sex therapy. *Behav Res Ther* 1986; 24: 377–85.

59. Hartman LM, Daly EM. Relationship factors in the treatment of sexual dysfunction. *Behav Res Ther* 1983; 21: 153–60.

60. MacNeil S, Byers E. The relationships between sexual problems, communication, and sexual satisfaction. *Can J Hum Sex* 1997; 6: 277–83.

61. Larson JH, Anderson SM, Holman TB et al. A longitudinal study of the effects of premarital communication, relationship stability, and self-esteem on sexual satisfaction in the first year of marriage. *J Sex Marital Ther* 1998; 24: 193–206.

62. Banmen J, Vogel NA. The relationship between marital quality and interpersonal sexual communication. *Fam Ther* 1985; 12: 45–58.

63. Metz ME, Epstein N. Assessing the role of relationship conflict in sexual dysfunction. *J Sex Marital Ther* 2002; 28: 139–64.

64. Roffe MW, Britt BC. A typology of marital interaction for sexually dysfunctional couples. *J Sex Marital Ther* 1981; 7: 207–22.

65. Gottman JM. *What Predicts Divorce? The Relationship Between Marital Processes and Marital Outcomes*. Hillsdale: Erlbaum, 1994.

66. Baucom DH, Epstein N. *Cognitive-Behavioral Marital Therapy*. New York: Brunner/Mazel, 1990.

67. Christensen A, Heavey, CL. Gender differences in marital conflict: the demand/withdraw interaction pattern. In S Oskamp, M Constanzo, eds. *Gender Issues in Contemporary Society*. Newbury Park: Sage, 1993: 113–41.

68. Karney BR, Bradbury TN. The longitudinal course of marital quality and stability: a review of theory, methods, and research. *Psychol Bull* 1995; 118: 3–34.

69. Byers ES, Demmons S. Sexual satisfaction and sexual self-disclosure within dating relationships. *J Sex Res* 1999; 36: 180–9.

70. Long ECJ, Cate RM, Fehensfeld DA et al. A longitudinal assessment of a measure of premarital sexual conflict. *Fam Relat* 1996; 45: 302–8.

71. Hurlbert DF. A comparative study using orgasm consistency training in the treatment of women reporting hypoactive sexual desire. *J Sex Marital Ther* 1993; 19: 41–55.

72. Hickman SE, Muehlenhard CL. "By the semi-mystical appearance of a condom": how young women and men communicate sexual consent in heterosexual situations. *J Sex Res* 1999; 36: 258–72.

73. Cupach WR, Metts S. Sexuality and communication in close relationships. In K McKinnery, S Sprecher, eds. *Sexuality in Close Relationships*. Hillsdale: Erlbaum, 1991: 93–110.

74. Sprecher S, Cate RM. Sexual satisfaction and sexual expression as predictors of relationship satisfaction and stability. In JH Harvey, A Wenzel, S Sprecher, eds. *The Handbook of Sexuality in Close Relationships*. Mahwah, NJ: Erlbaum, 2004: 235–56.

75. Kelly MP, Strassberg DS, Kircher JR. Attitudinal and experiential correlates of anorgasmia. *Arch Sex Behav* 1990; 19: 165–77.

76. Klussmann D. Sexual motivation and the duration of partnership. *Arch Sex Behav* 2002; 32: 193–208.

77. Greenblat CS. The salience of sexuality in the early years of marriage. *J Marriage Fam* 1983; 45: 289–99.

78. Laumann EO, Gagnon JH, Michael RT et al. *The Social Organization of Sexuality: Sexual Practices in the United States*. Chicago: University of Chicago Press, 1994.

79. Liu C. Does quality of marital sex decline with duration? *Arch Sex Behav* 2003; 32: 55–60.

80. Laumann EO, Paik A, Rosen RC. Sexual dysfunction in the United States: prevalence and predictors. *JAMA* 1999; 281: 537–44.

81. Peplau LA, Fingerhut A, Beals KP. Sexuality in the relationships of lesbians and gay men. In JH Harvey, A Wenzel, S Sprecher, eds. *The Handbook of Sexuality in Close Relationships*. Mahwah: Erlbaum, 2004: 49–69.

82. Masters WH, Johnson VE. *Homosexuality in Perspective*. Boston: Little, Brown, 1979.

83. Snyder DK, Berg P. Determinants of sexual dissatisfaction in sexually distressed couples. *Arch Sex Behav* 1983; 12: 237–45.

84. Purnine DM, Carey MP. Interpersonal communication and sexual adjustment: the roles of understanding and agreement. *J Consult Clin Psychol* 1997; 65: 1017–25.

85. Libman E, Fichten CS, Brender W et al. A comparison of three therapeutic formats in the treatment of secondary orgasmic dysfunction. *J Sex Marital Ther* 1984; 10: 147–59.

86. Hurlbert DF, White LC, Powell RD. Orgasm consistency training in the treatment of women reporting hypoactive sexual desire: an outcome comparison of women-only groups and couples-only groups. *J Behav Ther Exp Psychiatry* 1993; 24: 3–13.

87. Hirst JF, Watson JP. Therapy for sexual and relationship problems: the effects on outcome of attending as an individual or as a couple. *J Sex Marital Ther* 1997; 12 : 321–37.

88. Hawton K, Catalan J, Fagg J. Low sexual desire: sex therapy results and prognostic factors. *Behav Res Ther* 1991; 29: 217–24.

89. Hawton K, Catalan J. Prognostic factors in sex therapy. *Behav Res Ther* 1986; 24: 377–85.

90. von Sydow K. Sexuality during pregnancy and after childbirth: a metacontent analysis of 59 studies. *J Psychosom Res* 1999; 47: 27–49.

91. Bitzer J, Alder J. Sexuality during pregnancy and the postpartum period. *J Sex Educ Ther* 2000; 25: 49–58.

92. Shapiro AF, Gottman JM, Carrere S. The baby and the marriage: identifying factors that buffer against decline in marital satisfaction after the first baby arrives. *J Fam Psychol* 2000; 14: 59–70.

93. Heiman JR. Psychologic treatments for female sexual dysfunction: are they effective and do we need them? *Arch Sex Behav* 2002; 31: 445–50.

94. Leiblum SR, Wiegel M. Psychotherapeutic interventions for treating female sexual dysfunction. *World J Urol* 2002; 20: 127–3.

95. Coleman EM, Hoon PW, Hoon EF. Arousability and sexual satisfaction in lesbian and heterosexual women. *J Sex Res* 1983; 19: 58–73.

96. Trudel G. Sexuality and marital life: results of a survey. *J Sex Marital Ther* 2002; 28: 229–49.

97. Bancroft J, Loftus J, Long SJ. Distress about sex: a national survey of women in heterosexual relationships. *Arch Sex Behav* 2003; 32: 193–208.

98. Peplau LA, Cochran S, Rook K et al. Loving women: attachment and autonomy in lesbian relationships. *J Soc Issues* 1978; 34: 7–27.

99. Heiman J. Female sexual response patterns: interactions of physiological, affective, and contextual cues. *Arch Gen Psychiatry* 1980; 37: 1311–16.

100. Zimmer D. Interaction patterns and communication skills in sexually distressed, maritally distressed, and normal couples: two experimental studies. *J Sex Marital Ther* 1983; 9: 251–65.

101. Rust J, Golombok S, Collier J. Marital problems and sexual dysfunction: how are they related? *Br J Psychiatry* 1988; 152: 629–31.

102. Oggins J, Leber D, Veroff J. Race and gender differences in Black and White newlyweds' perceptions of sexual and marital relations. *J Sex Res* 1993; 30: 152–60.

103. Hulbert DF, Apt C. Female sexual desire, response, and behavior. *Behav Modif* 1994; 18: 488–504.

104. Regan PC, Berscheid E. Gender differences in beliefs about the causes of male and female desire. *Pers Relat* 1995; 2: 345–58.

105. McCabe MP. Intimacy and quality of life among sexually dysfunctional men and women. *J Sex Marital Ther* 1997; 23: 276–90.

106. Kilmann PR, Mills KH, Caid C et al. Treatment of secondary orgasmic dysfunction: an outcome study. *Arch Sex Behav* 1986;15: 211–29.

107. Trudel G, Marchand A, Ravart M et al. The effect of a cognitive-behavioral group treatment program on hypoactive sexual desire in women. *Sex Relat Ther* 2001; 16: 145–64.

3.2 Cognitive and affective processes in female sexual dysfunctions

Markus Wiegel, Lisa A Scepkowski, David H Barlow

There is an increasing recognition that important differences exist between male and female sexual response and function. The relational and cultural factors prominent in the development and maintenance of sexual complaints and dysfunction in women have been discussed in previous sections. In addition to these external factors, cognitive and affective processes at the level of the individual influence sexual responding, and include attention and distraction, expectancies, and negative mood states such as anxiety and depression. Differences between men and women in cognitive and affective processes, as they relate to sexual response and function, occur primarily in the context of sexual performance concerns, while the related mechanisms of action are similar in men and women.

Barlow's cognitive-affective model of sexual (dys)function

Over the last two decades, Barlow and colleagues have developed and empirically supported a model of sexual function and dysfunction that focuses on cognitive and affective processes (Fig. 3.2.1).[1,2] This model has recently been updated (Fig. 3.2.2) to incorporate new empirical findings from the fields of sexual and anxiety research.[3–5] In this model, dysfunctional sexual response results from a negative feedback loop (Fig. 3.2.3). Individuals with sexual dysfunction exhibit a "sexually dysfunctional mentality" that includes perceived lack of control over sexual arousal, sexual failure

expectancies, maladaptive causal attributions, and cognitive bias (hypervigilance).

For women with sexual dysfunctions, sexual situations and their associated implied and expressed demands for sexual performance/response result in a state of anxious apprehension that is characterized by heightened autonomic arousal, negative affect, failure expectancies, and shifts in attentional focus to interoceptive cues and negative self-evaluative cognitions. Sexual failure expectancies, concerns regarding negative evaluation by her partner, and sexual (non)response worries can evoke anxious apprehensive states in women. A narrowing of attentional focus, which accompanies heightened levels of sympathetic arousal, increases the salience of nonerotic thoughts and decreases the woman's ability to focus on the erotic and romantic aspects of the sexual situation. Furthermore, her attention shifts to an internal, self-evaluative focus. This shift to an internal attentional focus forms an additional feedback loop within the overall negative feedback cycle and results in a heightened subjective experience of negative affect (Fig. 3.2.3). Increased negative affect and distraction from erotic cues lead to problems in sexual responding. Repeated experiences with sexual response difficulties result in further failure expectancies and can lead to avoidance of potentially sexual situations. In contrast, sexually functional women associate positive affect and sexual success expectancies with sexual stimuli. They are focused on the erotic and romantic cues necessary for sexual response. With increased autonomic arousal (due to sexual stimulation), their attention narrows, focusing more efficiently on the sexual and romantic aspects, resulting in further increases in their sexual arousal.

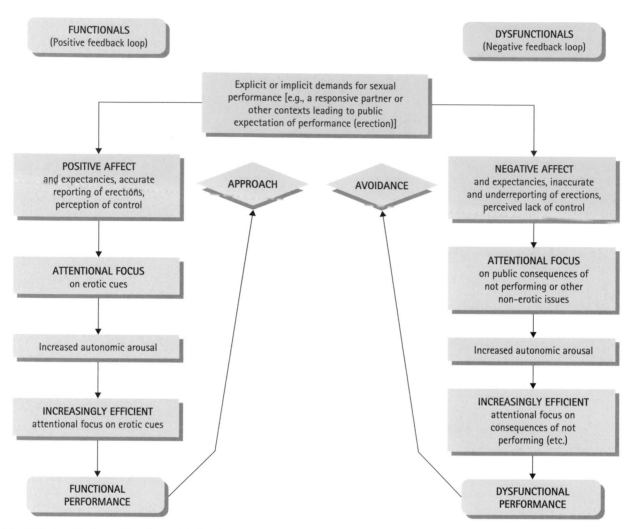

Figure 3.2.1. Original model of sexual function and dysfunction. Reproduced with permission from Barlow[2]. Copyright 1986 by the American Psychological Association.

Sexual performance concerns

Early empirical support for Barlow's model of sexual dysfunction focused primarily on the concepts of performance anxiety and spectatoring and was largely derived from laboratory studies of men with and without erectile dysfunction.[1] A man's ability to attain and maintain adequately a rigid erection is intimately tied to his self-esteem and self-evaluation.[6,7] For women, sexual performance concerns have a different focus because the signs of sexual arousal are less publicly evident. Women experience a wide array of sexual concerns, including worries about pleasing her partner, fears of pregnancy and sexually transmitted infections, fear of partner rejection, and unease related to the ability to reach orgasm.[8,9] One common source of nonerotic cognitive distraction for women that has been empirically studied is the concept of body image self-consciousness.

In Western cultures particularly, women's bodies are evaluated and sexualized with greater frequency than men's bodies.[10,11] Some women may view their sexual attractiveness to their partners as an aspect of sexual performance. To the extent that a woman internalizes the view equating her sexual desirability with her bodily attractiveness (such as thinness), she is prone to heightened awareness of how her body appears to her sexual partners. Such a view is not entirely unrealistic, as demonstrated by the finding that weight gain by women was associated with decreased sexual interest and sexual satisfaction among their husbands, while men's weight gain did not detrimentally affect their wives' sexual interest.[12] Nevertheless, body image self-consciousness has negative effects on female sexual function, above and beyond actual body size or general body image dissatisfaction. Wiederman[13] found that body image self-consciousness was related to lower sexual esteem, less sexual assertiveness, greater sexual avoidance, less sexual experience, and a lower probability of being in a relationship, while statistically controlling for body size, general body dissatisfaction, sexual anxiety, and social avoidance due to negative body image. Importantly, while only 9.6% of the college women studied met criteria for obesity, 35.1% of the sample reported experiencing body image self-consciousness during physical intimacy with a partner at least some of the time.

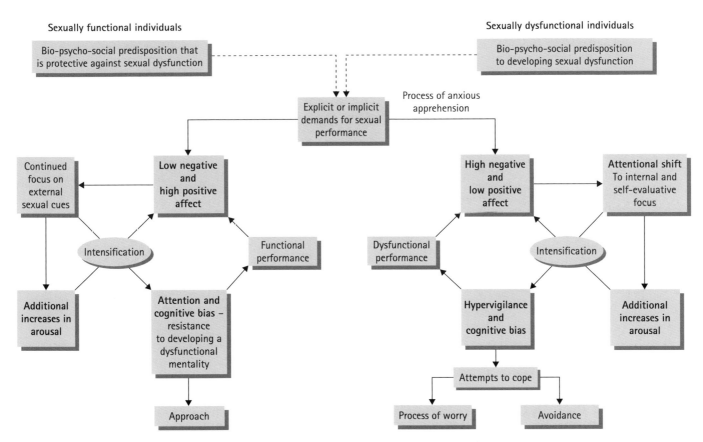

Figure 3.2.2. Updated model of sexual function and dysfunction. Reproduced with permission from Wiegel et al.[4].

Anxious apprehension, anxiety, and cognitive distraction

In women, as in men, sexual performance concerns result in a state of anxious apprehension. The state of anxious apprehension incorporates a sense of uncontrollability focused largely on future negative events, a strong physiologic component [sympathetic nervous system (SNS)], a vigilance (or hypervigilance) for threat-related cues, and a shift in attention to a self-focus (self-preoccupation) in which the evaluation of one's (inadequate) capabilities to cope with the threat is prominent.[5] Sexual arousal is likewise composed of physiologic, cognitive, affective, and behavioral components. Different components of "anxious apprehension" influence the various components of sexual response differentially, and not always in the same direction (i.e., facilitate or decrease). For example, Meston and colleagues[14–18] have attempted to separate the effects of increased SNS arousal from the effects of cognitive and affective components of anxiety on sexual response. In general, these studies found that in women without sexual dysfunction and women with hypoactive sexual desire disorder, heightened SNS activation prior to watching an erotic film increases genital sexual response, as measured by vaginal photoplethysmography. Subjective reports of sexual arousal, on the other hand, do not

seem to be influenced by SNS activation. The implication of this line of research is that the somatic component of anxious apprehension may facilitate genital response, while the negative affective component may concurrently decrease subjective sexual arousal. The cognitive component (selective attentional focus) may either facilitate or interfere with physiologic sexual arousal, depending on whether or not the individual has a sexual dysfunction.

The above-described complex interaction should inform interpretation of empirical research examining the effects of anxiety on sexual response. Studies on the effects of anxiety have yielded numerous conflicting results in both men and women, with some showing detracting effects[8], and others showing enhancement of sexual responding.[19,20] A few key studies with women will be discussed to illustrate the effects of anxiety and distraction on sexual arousal in the framework of a cognitive-affective model.

Palace and Gorzalka[19] found that for both sexually functional and dysfunctional women, exposure to an anxiety-provoking stimulus prior to visual sexual stimulation enhanced physical sexual arousal, compared to a neutral preexposure stimulus. In contrast, anxiety during a sexual encounter was shown by Beggs et al.[8] to reduce significantly physiologic arousal compared with a pleasurable encounter without anxiety. Methodological differences in the timing and type of the

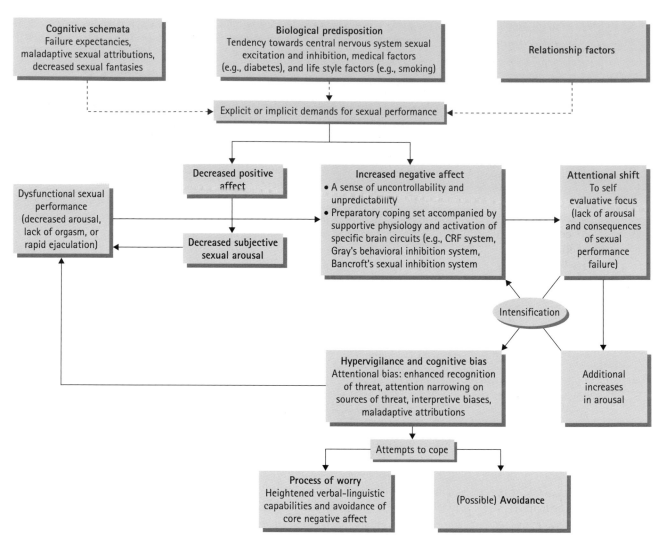

Figure 3.2.3. Detail of updated model of sexual function and dysfunction: sexually dysfunctional individuals. CRF = Corticotropin Releasing Factor. Reproduced with permission from Wiegel et al.[4].

anxiety stimulus (sexually relevant or nonrelevant) account for the opposite valenced effects of anxiety (facilitation vs reduction) on sexual arousal in these two studies.

Palace and Gorzalka[19] presented a nonsexually relevant anxiety stimulus just prior to the erotic stimulus. The anxiety stimulus consisted of a film depicting threatened amputation, which resulted in increased anxiety along with the associated SNS activation. In addition to the facilitative impact of SNS activation on female genital arousal, sympathetic activation also increases the efficiency of attentional focus. Since the anxiety stimulus was not personally relevant to the participants (it was a sexual arousal study, not an amputation study), as the erotic film began, the increasingly efficient attentional focus probably resulted in greater salience of the positive sexual cues. Thus, vaginal vasocongestion was enhanced in both the women with and without sexual dysfunction.

In contrast, Beggs et al. compared the effect of self-generated descriptions of sexual anxiety and sexual pleasure experiences that were then played back to participants as narratives while they underwent physiologic assessment. The anxiety-provoking stimuli were personally relevant to participants and were presented concurrent with the sexual stimuli. Sympathetic activation in the presence of both erotic cues and *sexual anxiety*-provoking cues presumably enhanced attention to the latter since they were a source of threat. Negative sexual cues may have deterred sexual response by eliciting negative affect as well as distracting nonerotic cognitions.

Several studies have documented the detrimental effects of distraction on female sexual response.[21-24] For example, using questionnaires to assess the amount of cognitive distraction recalled during sexual activity with a partner, Dove and Wiederman[23] found that women who reported greater levels of cognitive distraction also reported lower sexual self-esteem, less sexual satisfaction, and experiencing orgasms less consistently than women who reported lower levels of cognitive distractions. These differences remained significant when general life satisfaction, general body dissatisfaction, sexual attitudes, level of sexual desire, and trait self-focus propensity were controlled.

Elliot and O'Donohue[24] attempted to tease apart the differential effects of anxiety and distraction on sexual arousal. The distraction conditions involved dichotic listening tasks in which women either had to listen to (no distraction), repeat forward (low distraction), or repeat backward (high distraction) distracting target sentences while listening to an erotic narrative. Women in the anxiety condition listened to target distracters designed to induce sexually relevant anxiety (e.g., fears of sexually transmitted disease, self-consciousness) and were also told they were being videotaped and evaluated during this task. The comparison group listened to neutral distracters and were not told that they were being taped. Results indicated no significant differences in subjective sexual arousal or physical sexual arousal between the anxiety and comparison groups under the no-distraction condition. However, a manipulation check indicated that the video-related manipulation failed to induce significant anxiety. With the distraction task, levels of anxiety increased as the difficulty of the distraction task increased, as expected. In addition, the group listening to sexually relevant anxiety-producing distracters experienced higher levels of anxiety than the other group at both low and high levels of distraction. Though the data revealed a trend in the predicted direction, there were no significant differences in subjective or physiologic sexual arousal between the two groups at each distraction level. The findings provide preliminary evidence that at low levels of autonomic arousal, a woman is able to attend to sex-related worries as well as the sexual and romantic cues; however, as autonomic arousal increases, whether from sexual or anxious arousal, the focus of attention narrows, increasing the salience of the threatening stimuli and blocking the erotic cues. Unfortunately, with only 48 subjects in this study, it did not have enough power (0.38) to detect significant group differences. The interaction between distraction and anxiety is an important topic for future research.

Mood and affect

Barlow's model[2,4] theorizes that individuals with sexual dysfunctions react to erotic stimuli with greater negative affect, including anxiety and depression. The link between depression and reductions in sexual function has been well established and studied in women.[25] Frohlich and Meston[25] found that women reporting greater depressive symptoms also reported greater difficulties with becoming aroused and reaching orgasm, more experience of pain, as well as reduced sexual satisfaction and pleasure. Surprisingly, the women with greater depressive symptoms reported higher levels of sexual desire.

Beck and Bozman[26] demonstrated that induced anger and anxiety in women reduced sexual desire compared to the control condition, with anger having a more pronounced effect. In this study (which also included men), women listened to three erotic scripts describing sexual interactions ranging from casual contact to foreplay and intercourse between the female participant and a sexual partner. Participants continuously rated their levels of sexual desire (not arousal) with a subjective lever. The anger script included statements by partners regarding reluctance to engage in the sexual activity and self-statements (referring to the participant) indicating feelings of frustration and anger. The anxiety script included statements by the partner regarding the perception of the participant's nervousness and self-statements acknowledging feelings of tension and anxiety. The control script included statements designed to be arousing. The results indicated that both men and women reported the highest levels of sexual desire during the control condition, significantly lower levels during the anxiety condition, and the lowest levels of desire during the anger condition. Another finding of this study was that while female subjects' sexual desire decreased steadily throughout the narrative in the anger and anxiety conditions, male subjects' desire decreased only until the foreplay portion. For men, the detrimental effects of anxiety and anger decreased as the described degree of sexual activity increased, despite many male subjects reporting intent to terminate the narrative because of extreme unpleasantness. Thus, for men, but not for women, increasingly erotic cues and sexual stimulation reduced the impact of negative affect on sexual desire.

Several studies have experimentally manipulated affect during laboratory studies of sexual arousal. Laan et al.[27] used musical selections to induce a positive affect in 51 women and examined its effects on subjective and genital measures of sexual arousal during both fantasy and in response to erotic films. Results indicated no significant effect of the mood induction on post-film/fantasy measures of subjective or genital sexual arousal. There was a marginally significant reduction in negative emotions in response to the erotic film in the mood-induction group compared with the no-induction group.

Other studies have found associations between positive affect and subjective sexual arousal in women.[28,29] In addition, past studies have found that individuals with sexual dysfunction report significantly less positive affect during erotic exposure.[29,30] However, it is difficult to ascertain from available studies what the impact of affect itself is on sexual responding. One possibility is that, as with anxious apprehension, changes in autonomic arousal and attentional focus, rather than negative affect itself, affect sexual response. Although it is possible that depression influences sexual responding via biochemical mechanisms,[31] Bancroft[32] suggested that mood is likely to influence sexual responding by its effect on cognition. Depressed mood is characterized by negative, self-deprecating, rigid thoughts about self and the world, and biased perception of cues. One cognitive component that interacts with affect is self-focused attention.

Self-focused attention

Concerns over her sexual function and response may lead a woman with sexual dysfunction to be hypervigilant for signs of lack of arousal, thereby shifting her attention away from erotic and romantic cues to her unpleasant cognitions. In response to implied or expressed demands for sexual response, her attention shifts from an external focus (on erotic cues) to an internal, predominantly self-evaluative focus, which is analogous to what occurs in performance-related anxiety conditions such as social phobia and test anxiety.[5] She becomes focused on the discrepancy between her perceived current state of sexual performance (e.g., sexual attractiveness) and her internal, a priori standards of sexual performance. This results in a negative evaluation of herself, increased negative affect, and predictions of not being able to cope with the consequences of failing to meet her a priori standards, which further increase anxious arousal. Additionally, an internal focus has been found to increase the intensity with which affective states are experienced. Individuals with a greater tendency to self-focus were found to experience experimental provocation of various emotions as more intense than individuals with a greater disposition to focus externally.[33,34] Thus, focusing on internal proprioceptive sensations not only distracts attention from erotic cues, but also intensifies the experience of negative affect after the emotion has been elicited. Evidence suggests that this shift to an internal, self-evaluative-focused attentional state further increases both arousal and negative affect, thus forming its own negative feedback loop (Fig. 3.2.3).

A further important consequence of self-focused attention is a failure to habituate to external stimuli. This selective internal attentional focus functions as avoidance of the anxiety-producing stimuli; in female sexual dysfunction, this may be the lack of sexual response or the appearance of her body. Paradoxically, women with sexual dysfunction may be more interoceptively aware of the somatic consequences of negative affect, while at the same time less aware of their degree of sexual arousal. Several studies have found that women with orgasm difficulties (i.e., experience orgasm less consistently than comparison women) also showed less awareness of physiologic changes accompanying sexual arousal and orgasm.[35,36]

Expectancies and attributions

Women with and without sexual dysfunction differ in the expectancies with which they enter sexual situations. For example, women with female orgasmic disorder more strongly endorse fears and anxieties related to intercourse.[9] Such negative associations can result from repeated experiences of not being able to achieve orgasm, and these associations may motivate avoidance of future partner sexual activity. A study by Loos et al.[37] explored causal attributions for orgasm among women who consistently experienced orgasms and women who reported experiencing them infrequently. The study showed that women who tended frequently to experience orgasm attributed their orgasms to internal, stable causes, while lack of orgasm was attributed to external, unstable factors. In contrast, women who infrequently experienced orgasm attributed lack of orgasm to internal causes, blaming themselves rather than the situation or their partners, and tended

not to take credit for instances of orgasm, suggesting self-handicapping attributions.

In addition to orgasm, cognitive expectancies also affect women's level of sexual arousal. As in Barlow's[2,4] model, Palace and Gorzalka[19,38–40] have proposed that negative cognitive expectancies in conjunction with a physiologic tendency toward low autonomic lability produce a negative feedback loop resulting in dysfunctional sexual response. Palace[39] presented women with sexual dysfunction false-positive feedback regarding their level of genital arousal to an erotic film in order to manipulate their expectancies. Results indicated that women who received the false-positive feedback not only expected to become more aroused during subsequent erotic films, but actually showed higher levels of genital and subjective sexual arousal to subsequent films than the women who received no feedback. A follow-up analysis demonstrated that among the women who received false-positive feedback, those that reported significantly increased expectancies demonstrated significantly greater increases in physiologic sexual arousal than the women who did not report increased expectancies regarding their sexual arousal.

Conclusion

In summary, it may be that an affect-laden attentional process focusing on sexual performance (e.g., body image for women) and other self-evaluative concerns, combined with a tendency to exhibit biased observation of one's sexual function, may characterize the cognitive-affective processes in female sexual dysfunctions. The basic cognitive and affective mechanisms of action in men and women appear to be similar, while the content of sexual performance concerns differs substantially between men and women.

Much of the empirical inquiry into sexual performance concerns has focused on men and erectile dysfunction; however, cognitive and affective processes may play an even more important and integral role in female sexual response and (dys)function. The cognitive–affective processes described in this chapter may represent the mechanism of action through which negative interpersonal and cultural factors exact their detrimental effects on female sexual response, including impact on a woman's sense of sexual well-being and overall sexual satisfaction. In addition, preliminary findings from psychophysiologic studies indicate that women's genital sexual arousal is less stimulus specific than men's. Chivers et al. found that female genital arousal (vaginal vasocongestion), but not subjective sexual arousal, occurred regardless of the type of stimulus, as long as it was sexual in nature.[41] Furthermore, because it is more difficult for a woman to notice vaginal lubrication and clitoral engorgement than for a man to notice his erection, women are more dependent on interoceptive and contextual cues for feedback regarding their sexual response. As a result, the contextual features of a sexual interaction, both internal and external, largely determine a woman's overall experience during sexual activity, thereby increasing the potential for negative affect, sexual failure expectancies, maladaptive causal attributions, and cognitive bias (hypervigilance) to impair female sexual response.

While the importance of cognitive and affective factors in female sexual (dys)function may be self-evident, the actual cognitive and affective processes are tremendously complex, with different components of affect (e.g., autonomic vs cognitive) influencing the various components and aspects of sexual response differently, and at times in oppositely valenced directions (facilitate and decrease). A bio-psycho-social perspective on the etiology of sexual dysfunction is crucial for developing a comprehensive understanding of the cognitive processes involved in these disorders. Predisposing factors that can lead one to develop the cognitive schemata seen in individuals with recurrent sexual difficulties can be conceptualized similarly to the triple vulnerability theory of the etiology of anxiety disorders.[5,42] In this model, individuals vary in generalized biologic vulnerability factors (e.g., temperament, androgen levels), generalized psychologic vulnerability factors (e.g., perceived uncontrollability of life-events as a result of experience, depression, and anxiety), and specific psychologic vulnerabilities (e.g. sexual attitudes, sexual inhibition as described in the dual control model,[43] sexual self-concept). Factors in each category of vulnerabilities can influence approaches to sexual situations, cognitive processing of sexual stimuli in terms of bias and affective valence, expectancies for successful or unsuccessful sexual outcomes, and coping styles for dealing with occasions of sexual difficulty.

The importance and complexities of female sexual function will provide fertile ground for cognitive and affective research in the future. For example, women experience worry-related anxiety disorders twice as frequently as men. Worry, with its close relationship to depression, autonomic inflexibility, and prominent intrusive negative thoughts, is likely to have a significant impact on women's sexual function, yet little empirical work has examined the impact of worry on female sexual response. Research aimed at increasing the understanding of bio-psycho-social factors involved in female sexual response and dysfunction fuels the hope that more efficacious treatments for the sexual dysfunctions experienced by women are not far behind. Pharmacologic interventions may provide increased physiologic sexual arousal for women, but better understanding of the cultural, interpersonal, cognitive, and emotional factors in female sexual response is required to help women with sexual dysfunctions and complaints to increase their sexual enjoyment, sexual well-being, and overall sexual satisfaction.

References

1. Cranston-Cuebas MA, Barlow DH. Cognitive and affective contributions to sexual functioning. *Ann Rev Sex Res* 1990; 1: 119–61.
2. Barlow DH. Causes of sexual dysfunction: the role of anxiety and cognitive interference. *J Consult Clin Psychol* 1986; 54: 140–8.
3. van den Hout M, Barlow DH. Attention, arousal and expectancies in anxiety and sexual disorders. *J Affect Disord* 2000; 61: 241–56.
4. Wiegel M, Scepkowski LA, Barlow DH. Cognitive-affective processes in sexual arousal and sexual dysfunction. In Janssen E, ed. *The Psychophysiology of Sex*. Bloomington, IN: Indiana University Press (*in press*).
5. Barlow DH. The nature of anxious apprehension. In *Anxiety and Its Disorders: The Nature and Treatment of Anxiety and Panic*, 2nd edn. New York: Guilford Press, 2002: 64–104.
6. Zilbergeld B. *The New Male Sexuality*, rev edn. New York: Bantam Books, 1999.
7. Zilbergeld B. *The New Male Sexuality*. New York: Bantam Books; 1992.
8. Beggs VE, Calhoun KS, Wolchik SA. Sexual anxiety and female sexual arousal: a comparison of arousal during sexual anxiety and sexual pleasure stimuli. *Arch Sex Behav* 1987; 16: 311–19.
9. Birnbaum GE. The meaning of heterosexual intercourse among women with female orgasmic disorder. *Arch Sex Behav* 2003; 32: 61–71.
10. Wolf N. *The Beauty Myth: How Images of Beauty Are Used Against Women*. New York: Anchor Books, 1991.
11. Fredrickson BL, Roberts T. Objectification theory: toward understanding women's lived experiences and mental health risks. *Psychol Women Q* 1997; 21: 173–206.
12. Margolin L, White L. The continuing role of physical attractiveness in marriage. *J Marriage Fam* 1987; 49: 21–7.
13. Wiederman MW. Women's body image self-consciousness during physical intimacy with a partner. *J Sex Res* 2000; 37: 60–8.
14. Meston CM, Gorzalka BB. The effects of sympathetic activation on physiological and subjective sexual arousal in women. *Behav Res Ther* 1995; 33: 651–64.
15. Meston CM, Gorzalka BB. Differential effects of sympathetic activation on sexual arousal in sexually dysfunctional and functional women. *J Abnorm Psychol* 1996; 105: 582–91.
16. Meston CM, Gorzalka BB. The effects of immediate, delayed, and residual sympathetic activation on sexual arousal in women. *Behav Res Ther* 1996; 34: 143–8.
17. Meston CM, Gorzalka BB, Wright JM. Inhibition of physiological and subjective sexual arousal in women by clonidine. *Psychosom Med* 1997; 59: 399–407.
18. Meston CM, Heiman JR. Ephedrine-activated physiological sexual arousal in women. *Arch Gen Psychiatry* 1998; 55: 652–6.
19. Palace EM, Gorzalka BB. The enhancing effects of anxiety on arousal in sexually dysfunctional and functional women. *J Abnorm Psychol* 1990; 99: 403–11.
20. Hoon PW, Wincze JP, Hoon EF. A test of reciprocal inhibition: are anxiety and sexual arousal in women mutually inhibitory? *J Abnorm Psychol* 1977; 86: 65–74.
21. Przybyla DPJ, Byrne D. The mediating role of cognitive processes in self-reported sexual arousal. *J Res Pers* 1984; 18: 43–54.
22. Adams AE, Haynes SN, Brayer MA. Cognitive distraction in female sexual arousal. *Psychophysiology* 1985; 22: 689–96.
23. Dove NL, Wiederman MW. Cognitive distraction and women's sexual functioning. *J Sex Marital Ther* 2000; 26: 67–78.
24. Elliott AN, O'Donohue WT. The effects of anxiety and distraction on sexual arousal in a nonclinical sample of heterosexual women. *Arch Sex Behav* 1997; 26: 607–24.

25. Frohlich P, Meston CM. Sexual functioning and self-reported depressive symptoms among college women. *J Sex Res* 2002; 39: 321–5.

26. Beck JG, Bozman AW. Gender differences in sexual desire: the effects of anger and anxiety. *Arch Sex Behav* 1987; 24: 595–612.

27. Laan E, Everaerd W, van Berlo R et al. Mood and sexual arousal in women. *Behav Res Ther* 1995; 33: 441–3.

28. Laan E, Everaerd W, van Bellen G et al. Women's sexual and emotional responses to male- and female-produced erotica. *Arch Sex Behav* 1994; 23: 153–69.

29. Heiman JR. Female sexual response patterns: interactions of physiological, affective, and contextual cues. *Arch Gen Psychiatry* 1980; 37: 1311–16.

30. Beck JG, Barlow DH. The effects of anxiety and attentional focus on sexual responding. II. Cognitive and affective patterns in erectile dysfunction. *Behav Res Ther* 1986; 21: 1–8.

31. Basson R. Using a different model for female sexual response to address women's problematic low sexual desire. *J Sex Marital Ther* 2001; 27: 395–403.

32. Bancroft J. *Human Sexuality and Its Problems*. New York: Churchill Livingstone, 1989.

33. Wells A, Matthews G. Self-consciousness and cognitive failures as predictors of coping in stressful episodes. *Cognition and Emotion* 1994; 8: 279–95.

34. Ingram R. Self-focused attention in clinical disorders: review and a conceptual model. *Psychol Bull* 1990; 107: 156–76.

35. Andersen BL, Cyranowski JM. Women's sexuality: behaviors, responses, and individual differences. *J Consult Clin Psychol* 1995; 63: 891–906.

36. Hoon EF, Hoon PW. Styles of sexual expression in women: clinical implications of multivariate analyses. *Arch Sex Behav* 1978; 5: 291–300.

37. Loos VE, Bridges CF, Critelli JW. Weiner's attribution theory and female orgasmic consistency. *J Sex Res* 1987; 23: 348–61.

38. Palace EM, Gorzalka BB. Differential patterns of arousal in sexually functional and dysfunctional women: physiological and subjective components of sexual response. *Arch Sex Behav* 1992; 21: 135–59.

39. Palace EM. Modification of dysfunctional patterns of sexual response through autonomic arousal and false physiological feedback. *J Consult Clin Psychol* 1995; 63: 604–15.

40. Palace EM. A cognitive-physiological process model of sexual arousal and response. *Clin Psychol Sci Pract* 1995; 2: 370–84.

41. Chivers ML, Rieger G, Latty E et al. A sex difference in the specificity of sexual arousal. *Psychol Sci* 2004; 15: 736–44.

42. Barlow DH. Unraveling the mysteries of anxiety and its disorders from the perspective of emotion theory. *Am Psychol* 2000; 55: 1245–63.

43. Bancroft J, Janssen E. The dual control model of male sexual response: a theoretical approach to centrally mediated erectile dysfunction. *Neurosci Biobehav Rev* 2000; 24: 571–9.

3.3 Love and passion

Elaine Hatfield, Richard L Rapson

Introduction

Scholars from a variety of academic disciplines (e.g., cross-cultural studies, history, psychology, sociology, neurophysiology, endocrinology) have started to explore the relationships of passionate love with sexual desire, sexual motivation, and sexual behavior. In this chapter, we will review historical and cultural forces that have shaped women's sexual attitudes, sexual feelings, and sexual behavior. We will then discuss the impact of passionate love and other sexual motives on women's sexual desire and pleasure.

Defining passionate and companionate love

Ahdat Soueif, an Arab novelist, described the multitude of meanings that the word *love* possesses in Arabic:

> "Hubb" is love, "ishq" is love that entwines two people together, "shaghaf" is love that nests in the chambers of the heart, "hayam" is love that wanders the earth, "teeh" is love in which you lose yourself, "walah" is love that carries sorrow within it, "sababah" is love that exudes from your pores, "hawa" is love that shares its name with "air" and with "falling", "gharm" is love that is willing to pay the price.[1]

Scholars and laypersons alike have distinguished between two kinds of love: passionate love (i.e., being in love) and companionate love (i.e., loving).[2] Passionate love is a powerful emotional state. It has been defined as "a state of intense longing for union with another".[3] A union with another (i.e., reciprocated love) is associated with fulfillment and ecstasy, while separation (i.e., unrequited love) is associated with feelings of emptiness, anxiety, and despair.[3] Companionate love is a far less intense emotion. It comprises feelings of deep attachment, commitment, and intimacy, and has been defined as "the affection and tenderness we feel for those with whom our lives are deeply entwined".[3] The Passionate Love Scale has long been used to tap the cognitive, emotional, and behavioral incidents of such longing for union.[4]

Historical and cultural factors influencing women's sexual attitudes and behavior

Historical factors

It has been suggested by several social commentators that today women's personal attitudes can lead to problems with sexual desire, sexual arousal, and sexual pleasure. Yet, the idea that throughout history (and today in many cultures) women have been taught that sex is evil, and have been warned not to allow their own passionate and sexual feelings to get out of control,[3,5] suggests that historical factors are probably connected to sexual problems. Historically, in the West, women's sexual attitudes were influenced by an ideology that viewed sexual pleasure as unimportant at best and as shameful at worst. (See the reviews of the historical factors that have influenced women's sexual attitudes and behaviors in non-Western countries.[6-8]) Such notions have likely had strong negative impacts on sexual attitudes, sexual behaviors, and sexual function, both in the past and today.

Western literature abounds in tragic tales of lovers caught up in a sea of passion and violence (Orpheus and Eurydice, Daphnis and Chloe, Dido and Aeneas, Tristan and Isolde, Paolo and Francesca, Romeo and Juliet). While such stories are popular and widely enjoyed today, in the medieval world, religious, medical, and scientific authorities almost uniformly condemned such passion.[3] The early Catholic Church, for example, decreed that all passionate love and sexual pleasure was sinful, whether or not couples were married. The Church urged Christians to be celibate. As Tannahill observed:

> It was Augustine who epitomized a general feeling among the Church Fathers that the act of intercourse was fundamentally disgusting. Arnobius called it filthy and degrading, Methodius unseemly, Jerome unclean, Tertullian shameful, Ambrose a defilement. In fact there was an unstated consensus that God ought to have invented a better way of dealing with the problem of procreation.[9]

Until the eighteenth century, physicians generally assumed that masturbation and so-called excessive sexual activity are unhealthy. A pamphlet by Daniel Defoe, for example, warned about the pitfalls of sexual excess: "Whence come Palsies and Epilepsies, Falling-Sickness, trembling of the Joints, pale dejected Aspects, Leanness, and at last Rottenness, and other filthy and loathsome Distempers, but from the criminal Excesses of their younger times?"[10]

In addition to being suppressed for the aforementioned reasons, sexuality was probably also contained as there was less temptation to indulge in sexual acts in those days than there is today. Twelfth-century troubadours' tales of courtly love defined love affairs as "pure" and "holy" relationships, never to be "tainted" by "crass" physical consummation.[11] By contrast, the lives of commoners were, as Thomas Hobbes notes, "nasty, brutish, and short". Stone[5] points out that at the beginning of the Early Modern Period (1500–1700), most young men and women rarely encountered potential romantic partners who were very sexually appealing. People rarely washed, and had lice, bad breath, rotting teeth, and skin diseases. Women suffered from gynecologic problems (e.g., vaginal infections, ulcers, tumors, and bleeding), which made sexual intercourse uncomfortable, painful, or impossible. Men and women who engaged in sexual relations were likely to catch any number of venereal diseases. Furthermore, it is unlikely that men and women, plagued with malnutrition and exhaustion, often possessed the energy required to indulge in sexual "excess".

Cultural factors

Cultural factors also make it difficult for many women to celebrate passionate love or to experience satisfying romantic and sexual relationships. Cross-cultural researchers argue that romantic love and women's sexual pleasure are more valued in affluent, modern, egalitarian cultures than in traditional, patriarchal societies with strong, extended family ties.[12–14] In modern, urban, egalitarian societies, it is often assumed that the healthy woman is one who experiences pleasurable sex. In more patriarchal cultures, this is not necessarily so. For the So woman of Uganda, for example, penetration is expected to be nonlubricated and painful; it is not surprising that the So have no word for female orgasm (although they do have a word for male ejaculation).[15] In many African cultures, the customs of dry sex, salt cuts, and female genital mutilation further render the issue of female sexual pleasure irrelevant. In a culture in which women prepare themselves to pleasure their husbands by drying their vaginas with powdered stem and leaf mixed with water, wrapped in a nylon stocking and inserted into the vagina for 15 minutes before intercourse, the concept of "female sexual dysfunction" takes on a very different meaning than it holds in other parts of the world.[15] In some African cultures, such as the Hausa of Nigeria, itching vulva, amenorrhea, dyspareunia (i.e., painful intercourse), infertility, and obstructed labor are all considered to be sexual dysfunctions that can be cured by making a "salt cut" on the anterior vaginal wall.[15]

In any multicultural society, women's sexual attitudes are shaped by a variety of inconsistent cultural messages about

sexuality.[6,16] In recent years, globalization and the "women's revolution" have had a profound impact on women's sexual attitudes, desires, and demands.[6] When passionate love is increasingly cherished, when women are no longer entirely dependent on the power of men, and when the ideal relationship is considered to be a committed, stable, and equitable one, more women come to seek sexual pleasure in their love relationships, to have a voice in how and when sexual relations occur, to admit to sexual dissatisfaction, and to seek solutions.

Social psychological perspectives

Passionate love, sexual desire, and sexual satisfaction

Recent research has shed some light onto the impact of passionate love on women's sexual attraction and desire, sexual arousal, and sexual satisfaction. Social psychologists, neuroscientists, and physiologists have started to explore the links between love, sexual desire, and sexual function in both men and women. The first neuroscientists to study passionate love by functional Magnetic Resonance Imaging (fMRI) were Birbaumer and his colleagues,[17] who, as a result of their research, concluded that passionate love is "mental chaos". The neural bases of passionate love were recently studied by Bartels and Zeki.[18,19] They interviewed young men and women from 11 countries and several ethnic groups who claimed to be "truly, deeply, and madly" in love and who scored high on the Passionate Love Scale.[4] Bartels and Zeki[18] concluded that passionate love leads to a suppression of activity in the areas of the brain controlling critical thought. They argued that once an individual gets close to someone, there is less need to assess their character and personality, and thus there is less need to use the frontal lobe critical thinking. Passion also produced increased activity in the brain areas associated with euphoria and reward, and decreased levels of activity in the areas associated with distress and depression. Activity appeared to be restricted to foci in the medial insula and the anterior cingulated cortex, and, subcortically, to the caudate nucleus and the putamen, all bilaterally. Deactivations were observed in the posterior cingulated gyrus and in the amygdala, and were right-lateralized in the prefrontal, parietal, and middle temporal cortices. The authors concluded that the deactivation of networks used for critical social assessment allows individuals to become closer to their loved ones. They argued that this bonding is reinforced by the deactivation of negative emotions and the activation of the reward circuit. This hypothesis fits the observation that love motivates and exhilarates individuals.

Scientific investigations have also validated the link between passionate love and sexuality. Passionate love was found to be closely associated with sexual arousal,[18] sexual desire,[20,21] and sexual motivation.[20,21]

In parallel with this research, social psychologists,

neurobiologists, and physiologists have started to explore the neural and chemical substrates of passionate love, sexual desire, and sexual mating.[20,22–25] Questions that remain to be conclusively addressed include whether romantic and passionate love are emotions,[26,27] and how passionate love, sexual desire, and sexual motivation are related as constructs.[3,26,28–30]

Companionate love, relationship quality and stability, and sexual satisfaction

There is considerable evidence that companionate love, in combination with a variety of factors traditionally thought to contribute to relationship quality and relationship stability, is an important determinant of dating and marital sexual satisfaction. This includes constructs such as affection, intimacy, commitment, the ability to communicate, and the fairness or equity of the relationship.[3,31–34]

Women are more likely than men to view romantic love, emotional intimacy, and commitment as prerequisites for sexual activity and are less likely to be receptive to casual sex.[35,36] Men and women's perceptions of the fairness and equity of their relationships have been found, for example, to be an important determinant of whom they choose for a sexual encounter, how sexual and satisfying their sexual relationships are, and how likely those relationships are to endure.[37] Specifically, researchers have found that:

(1) The more socially desirable people are (i.e., the more physically attractive, personable, famous, rich, or considerate they are), the more socially desirable they will expect an "appropriate" mate to be.
(2) Dating couples are more likely to fall in love if they perceive their relationships to be equitable – that is, if they feel that they and their partners are receiving approximately what they deserve – neither appreciably more nor less than they deserve. They seem to care about fairness and equity in the personal, emotional, and day-to-day rewards involved in a relationship, as well as about the rewards one reaps from simply being in a relationship.
(3) Couples are likely to be romantically matched on the basis of self-esteem, looks, intelligence, education, and mental and physical health or disability.
(4) Couples who perceive their relationships to be fair and equitable are more likely to get involved sexually. When asked about the sexual intimacy of their relationships (e.g., necking, petting, engaging in genital play, intercourse, cunnilingus, and fellatio), couples in equitable romantic relationships tend to report more sexual involvement. In one study, it was found that couples in equitable relationships were generally having sexual relations; couples in inequitable relationships tended to stop before "going all the way".

Partners have also been asked why they make love. Those in equitable affairs were most likely to say that both partners wanted to have sex. Couples in inequitable relationships were less likely to claim that sex had been a mutual decision; many partners felt pressured into having sexual relations in order to keep the relationship alive.

Perhaps it is not surprising, then, to discover that dating and married couples had more satisfying sexual lives if they were in equitable relationships than if they were not. (See a summary of this research.[37,38] For a critique of this research, see Mills and Clark[39]).

Other motives for sex

Thus far, we have focused on one primary motive for sexuality – love. But love is not the only motive women have for engaging in sexual activities. As Levin[40] observed in discussing men's sexuality:

> Coitus is undertaken not only for pleasure and procreation but also to degrade, control and dominate, to punish and hurt, to overcome loneliness or boredom, to rebel against authority, to establish one's sexuality, or one's achieving sexual competence (adulthood), or to show that sexual access was possible (to "score"), for duty, for adventure, to obtain favours such as a better position or role in life, or even for livelihood.

Recently, scientists have begun to investigate the impact of a variety of possible sexual motives on the sexual desire and behavior of women and men.[3,41,42]

In our own cross-cultural work, for example, we found that throughout the world, women assign a wide variety of meanings to passionate love and sexuality, and engage in sexual activities for a wide variety of reasons.[43,44] The three reasons for having sex that are typically reported by women and studied by researchers are passionate love, procreation, and eroticism (i.e., the attainment of physical pleasure; recreational sex; "sport" sex).[41] However, a multitude of other sexual motivations have also been cited, including the desire for spiritual transcendence, duty, conformity, fostering self-esteem and status, kindness, a desire to conquer/possess power over another, submission to others, vengeance, curiosity, money, fostering jealousy, the attainment of health and long life, stress reduction, a desire to save the world, and political revolt.[43,45] Scientists are only beginning to study the wide variety of motives that may spark sexual desire and behavior. Nonetheless, the sparse research suggests that these rarely studied motivations may add appreciably to our understanding of women's sexuality. For example, a series of studies showed that men's and women's desire for power may strongly affect their sexual behavior in that relationship. The desire to dominate or submit to a partner may motivate some sexual behaviors. These behaviors vary from the typical (e.g., kissing and sexual intercourse) to the more unusual (e.g., cross-dressing, sadomasochism, exhibitionism).[45,46]

Critical review of existing literature

The literature has shown a remarkable increase in studies on passionate love in the past four decades. Researchers from a variety of disciplines, such as social psychology, anthropology, evolutionary psychology, and neuroendrocinology, have directed their attention to questions concerning passionate love, sexual desire, and sexual behavior. Some strengths of recent studies on passionate love include the variety of methodologies employed (e.g., primate behavior and fMRI studies), the focus on the majority of women rather than only a few women from elite social classes, and the inclusion of demographic variables as potential mediators or moderators.

Research has yet to answer a number of questions concerning the origins of love and its relationship to sexuality. The evolutionary basis of passionate love is unclear, and it is still debatable whether passionate love is a culturally universal phenomenon. Passionate love and sexual desire have yet to be clearly defined in cognitive, emotional, or behavioral terms, and the distinction between passionate love and sexual desire is ambiguous. More work is also needed to understand the emotional and cognitive consequences of passionate love. Finally, understanding sex differences in the experience of passionate love and sexual desire may enlighten opinion on sexual relationships.

Conclusion

Throughout the world, globalization, the woman's movement, increasing modernization, urbanization, and affluence have combined to produce more positive views of gender and sexual equality, of passionate love and sexual desire, and of love matches (as opposed to arranged marriages), and an increased acceptance of the notion that both men and women are entitled to satisfying sexual lives (see Hatfield and Rapson[3] for a discussion of these issues). Increasingly, societies worldwide are rejecting the notion that passionate love and sexual desire, especially in women, are evil and ought to be punished.[3] The increasing awareness of women's rights to social power, equality, pleasure, and sexual satisfaction may well lead the women of this century to define female sexual satisfaction and sexual function in new ways. We are likely to see a growing emphasis on the importance of female sexual delight and satisfaction, thus suggesting that sexual problems and dysfunctions are something to be cured, not patiently borne.

References

1. Soueif A. *The Map of Love*. London: Bloomsbury, 1999: 386–7.
2. Fehr B, Russell, JA. Concept of love viewed from a prototype perspective. *J Pers Soc Psychol* 1991; 60: 425–38.
3. Hatfield E, Rapson RL. *Love, Sex, and Intimacy: Their Psychology, Biology, and History*. New York: HarperCollins, 1993: 5–9.
4. Hatfield E, Sprecher S. Measuring passionate love in intimate relations. *J Adolesc* 1986; 9: 383–410.
5. Stone L. *The Family, Sex, and Marriage: In England 1500–1800*. New York: Harper & Row, 1977.
6. Hatfield E, Rapson RL. *Love and Sex: Cross–Cultural Perspectives*. Boston, MA: Allyn & Bacon, 1996.
7. Oliver DL. *Native Cultures of the Pacific Islands*. Honolulu: University of Hawaii Press, 1989.
8. Ruan FF. *Sex in China: Studies in Sexology in Chinese Culture*. New York: Plenum, 1991.
9. Tannahill R. *Sex in History*. New York: Stein & Day, 1980: p 14.
10. Defoe, D. *Conjugal Lewdness: or, Matrimonial Whoredom*. London: T. Warner, 1727: p 91.
11. Capellanus A. *Art of Courtly Love*. New York: Columbia University Press, 1990.
12. Goode, WJ. The theoretical importance of love. *Am Sociol Rev* 1959; 24: 38–47.
13. Rosenblatt PC. Marital residence and the function of romantic love. *Ethnology* 1967; 6: 471–80.
14. Simmons CH, Vom Kolke A, Shimizu H. Attitudes toward romantic love among American, German, and Japanese students. *J Soc Psychol* 1986; 126: 327–37.
15. Francoeur RT. Female orgasm, social repression and religion: what we know about the incidence of female orgasm around the world and why it may not be as common as we think. Presentation at the Society for the Scientific Study of Sexuality Western Region Conference, San Diego, 15–18 April 2004.
16. Hatfield E, Rapson, RL, Martel LD. Passionate Love. In: Kitayama S, Cohen D, (Eds) *Handbook of Cultural Psychology*. New York: Guildford Press (*in press*).
17. Birbaumer N, Lutzenberger W, Elbert T et al. Imagery and brain processes. In N Birbaumer, A Öhman, eds. *The Structure of Emotion*. Göttingen: Hogrefe & Huber, 1993: 132–4.
18. Bartels A, Zeki S. The neural basis of romantic love. *Neuroreport* 2000; 11: 3829–34.
19. Bartels A, Zeki S. The neural correlates of maternal and romantic love. *Neuroimage* 2004; 21: 1155–66.
20. Fisher HE. *Why We Love: The Nature and Chemistry of Romantic Love*. New York: Henry Holt, 2004.
21. Fisher HE. The brain chemistry of romantic attraction and its positive effect on sexual motivation. Paper presented at International Academy of Sex Research, 29th Annual Meeting. Bloomington, Indiana, 2004.
22. Carter CS. Neuroendocrine perspectives on social attachment and love. *Psychoneuroendocrinology* 1998; 23: 779–818.
23. Komisaruk BR, Whipple B. Love as sensory stimulation: physiological consequences of its deprivation and expression. *Psychoneuroendocrinology* 1998; 8: 927–44.
24. Marazziti D, Akiskal HS, Rossi A et al. Alteration of the platelet serotonin transporter in romantic love. *Psychol Med* 1999; 29: 741–5.
25. Marazziti D, Canale D. Hormonal changes when falling in love. *Psychoneuroendocrinology* 2004; 29: 931–6.
26. Fisher H, Aron A, Fisher H et al. Early-stage, intense romantic love uses subcortical reward/motivation and attention systems: an

fMRI study of a dynamic network that varies with relationship length, passion intensity, and gender. Presented at Society for Neuroscience 33rd Annual Meeting, November 2004.

27. Shaver PR, Morgan HJ, Wu S. Is love a "basic" emotion? *Pers Relatsh* 1996; 3: 81–96.

28. Beck JG, Bozman AW, Qualtrough T. The experience of sexual desire: psychological correlates in a college sample. *J Sex Res* 1991; 28: 443–56.

29. Diamond LM. Emerging perspectives on distinctions between romantic love and sexual desire. *Curr Dir Psychol Sci* 2004; 13: 116–9.

30. Hatfield E, Rapson RL. Passionate love/sexual desire: can the same paradigm explain both? *Arch Sex Behav* 1987; 16: 259–77.

31. Harvey JH, Wenzel A, Sprecher S. *The Handbook of Sexuality in Close Relationships*. Mahwah: LEA, 2004.

32. McKinney K, Sprecher S. *Human Sexuality: The Societal and Interpersonal Context*. Norwood, NJ: Ablex, 1990.

33. Sprecher S. Sexual satisfaction in premarital relationships: associations with satisfaction, love, commitment, and stability. *J Sex Res* 2002; 39: 190–6.

34. Sprecher S, McKinney K. *Sexuality* (Sage Series on Close Relationships). Thousand Oaks: Sage, 1993.

35. Clark RD III, Hatfield E. Gender differences in receptivity to sexual offers. *J Psychol Hum Sex* 1989; 2: 39–55.

36. Regan PC. Of lust and love: beliefs about the role of sexual desire in romantic relationships. *Pers Relat* 1998; 5: 139–57.

37. Hatfield E, Walster GW, Berscheid E. *Equity: Theory and Research*. Boston: Allyn and Bacon, 1978.

38. Canary DJ, Stafford L. Equity in the preservation of personal relationships. In J Harvey, A Wenzel, eds. *Close Romantic Relationships: Maintenance and Enhancement*. Mahwah, NJ: LEA, 2001: 133–52.

39. Mills J, Clark MS. Viewing close romantic relationships as communal relationships: implications for maintenance and enhancement. In JH Harvey, A Wenzel, S Sprecher, eds. *The Handbook of Sexuality in Close Relationships*. Mahwah: LEA, 2004: 13–26.

40. Levin R. Human male sexuality: appetite and arousal, desire and drive. In CR Legg, D Booth, eds. *Appetite: Neural and Behavioural Bases*. Oxford: Oxford University Press, 1994: 125.

41. DeLamater J, MacCorquodale P. *Premarital Sexuality: Attitudes, Relationships, Behaviour*. Madison: University of Wisconsin Press, 1979.

42. Hill CA, Preston LK. Individual differences in the experience of sexual motivation: theory and measurement of dispositional sexual motives. *J Sex Res* 1996; 33: 27–45.

43. Browning JR, Hatfield E, Kessler D et al. Sexual motives, gender, and sexual behavior. *Arch Sex Behav* 2000; 29: 135–52.

44. D'Emilio J, Freedman E. *Intimate Matters: A History of Sexuality in America*. New York: Harper & Row, 1988.

45. Browning JR, Kessler D, Hatfield E et al. Power, gender, and sexual behavior. *J Sex Res* 1999; 36: 342–7.

46. Kalof L. Sex, power, and dependency: the politics of adolescent sexuality. *J Youth Adolesc* 1995; 24: 229–49.

3.4 Sexual abuse

Alessandra H Rellini

A review of 38 studies reported that across methodologies, samples, and measures, child sexual abuse is a risk factor for adult sexual function.[1] Comparably, sexual abuse that occurs during adulthood has also been found to affect significantly sexual function.[2] Considering that 90 000 children have been reported as having experienced sexual abuse in 2002,[3] and that 17.6% of women are at risk of adult sexual abuse,[4] an alarmingly large proportion of women is at risk of sexual dysfunctions associated with sexual abuse. This chapter provides a review of the association between sexual dysfunction and sexual abuse, followed by a summary of the direct and indirect effects of sexual abuse on sexual function.

Types of sexual concerns

Although the majority of women show a spontaneous remission within the first 4 years after an assault,[5] a large percentage of women continue to report concerns. The prevalence of the sexual dysfunction is highly influenced by the type of sample recruited. While most studies on college students[6,7] report no differences in sexual function between abused and control women, clinical studies[5,8] are usually at the opposite spectrum and report great differences. Studies conducted on community volunteers[9] and random community samples[10,11] also tend to show a greater incidence of sexual dysfunctions in sexual abuse survivors than in nonabused women.

Low sexual desire is the sexual concern most commonly reported by women survivors of sexual abuse, followed by decreased sexual arousal, decreased orgasm, decreased satisfaction, and sexual avoidance.[8,12–14] Desire is significantly lower in both survivors of adult and child sexual abuse than in women who never experienced sexual abuse.[9] Concerns with sexual arousal may be linked to a negative interpretation of physiologic cues typical of the sexual arousal response (e.g., increased heart rate, lubrication). That is, women with a history of sexual abuse may associate cues of the sexual arousal response (i.e., lubrication) with those automatic physiologic responses experienced during the original abuse. Indeed, women with a history of child sexual abuse have reported greater negative affect during increased physiologic sexual arousal induced by sildenafil than controls.[15] Additionally, women with a history of child sexual abuse have reported a lack of feelings during sexual activities with their partners, even in the presence of orgasm.[16] Orgasm disorders are more common in sexual abuse survivors who experienced both child and adult sexual abuse than in survivors of only child or only adult sexual abuse.[14] Researchers have hypothesized that child sexual abuse survivors may have learned at a very young age how to please their partners, but lack experience on how to please their own bodies.[17] Sexual satisfaction is often lower in women with a history of child or adult sexual abuse than in controls.[18–21] Similarly, the concept of sexual pleasure differs between women with a history of sexual abuse and controls. For example, teenagers with a history of child sexual abuse are more likely to distinguish between physical and mental experiences in their narratives of sexual pleasure than nonabused controls.[22] This finding is supported by clinical observations of a separation between body and mind often reported by women with a history of sexual abuse.

In addition to sexual function, sexual risk-taking behaviors are also more common among survivors of child sexual abuse than in women who never experienced sexual abuse. For example, women with a history of child sexual abuse reported more partners and sexual encounters,[23] lower condom efficacy,[24] and less ability to refuse unwanted sex than controls.[25]

Sexual concerns are generally associated with guilt, fear of losing control, humiliation,[26] sexual self-esteem,[27] and perception of severity.[28] Post-abuse variables associated with sexual dysfunctions include avoidance of sexual behaviors[29,30] and partner's sexual dysfunction.[30] Characteristics of sexual abuse known to affect sexual functioning are penetration or genital fondling during the abuse,[31] number of events,[7,28] parental incest,[28] age,[32] and presence of violence at the time of the abuse.[33] However, a variable not found to affect sexuality negatively is the level of dysfunction within the survivor's original family unit.[27]

Trauma model

The lack of a model specifically developed to explain sexual dysfunction in survivors of sexual abuse can be easily overcome by adapting the trauma model developed by J. Herman.[34] This model is particularly useful because it addresses the relation between the self and others as an extension of the original abuse, paralleling the relational nature of female sexuality. Although developed for survivors of child sexual abuse, this model has been extensively used to explain adult sexual abuse. To briefly summarize, survivors of child sexual abuse have to reconcile the perturbing reality that the caregiver is also the cause of their pain and fear. The child often solves the tension between the need to trust the caregiver and the need for self-protection by assuming responsibility for the pain. The survivor may believe her behavior elicited the sexual abuse. In contrast, she may feel love, attachment, and idealization toward the perpetrator. As previously reviewed, problems with sexual desire have been associated with feeling guilty for provoking the perpetrator's sexual attention.[32] Albeit counterintuitive, this gives the child an apparent sense of control over the situation, but at the expense of low self-worth, reduced trust of others, and inflated feelings of guilt and shame. Although survivors of child and adult sexual abuse are usually able to escape the abusive situation, they often bear a damaged view of the self, as well as a number of psychologic symptoms. Herman emphasizes four key feelings common in survivors of sexual abuse: guilt, lack of safety (difficulty in trusting), disconnection from one's needs, and a view of the self as unworthy. Accordingly, consequences of sexual abuse can be subdivided into consequences related to the self (intrapersonal functioning) and consequences affecting relationships (interpersonal functioning).

Intrapersonal functioning

Intrapersonal functioning is one of the most studied aftermaths of sexual abuse and can be further divided into (1) psychologic and psychiatric health, including alcohol/drug abuse and body image, (2) physical health, and (3) cognitive schemas.

Psychologic consequences of trauma

The most common psychologic consequences of sexual abuse are depression, post-traumatic stress disorder (PTSD), dissociation, eating disorders, alcohol/drug abuse, and body dissatisfaction. A study identified depression as the moderator of the relationship between sexual abuse and sexual dysfunction.[20] In both studies, the difference in sexual arousal, orgasm, and desire between women with and without a history of child sexual abuse disappeared after controlling for depression. The sense of worthlessness and negative view of the world, both characteristic of depression, may affect the woman's view of herself as a sexual being. In particular, feeling responsible for the sexual abuse may strengthen a relationship between sexual pleasure and guilt or shame. In fact, child sexual abuse and a less positive sexual schema were found to be closely connected to sexual pain disorders, suggesting that child sexual abuse affects women's view of their sexual self.[35]

PTSD, characterized by symptoms of unwanted memories, avoidant behavior, and hyperarousability, has a high comorbidity with sexual abuse. Unwanted memories appear in the form of visual memories (flashbacks or intrusive memories), as well as bodily (fight or flight reaction) and emotional memories (strong feelings of fear or anxiety). Survivors of adult sexual abuse frequently report flashbacks during sexual activities in the first 4 months after the abuse.[5] Survivors are often unaware of the triggers that evoke these memories. Empirically validated therapies, such as guided exposure, have been developed to help them assimilate their experiences.[36] The goal of guided exposure is to reduce the association between traumatic memories and the fight-or-flight reaction. This is accomplished by guiding the survivor through a detailed recall of the abuse, during which she is encouraged to focus on the details of the memories and the emotions she experienced.[36]

PTSD has been shown to moderate the relationship between sexual dysfunction and sexual abuse.[37,38] In particular, PTSD predicted variance in sexual functioning in sexual abuse survivors even after accounting for other psychologic dysfunctions, characteristics of the abuse, and time elapsed since the abuse.[37] In addition, biologic changes specific to PTSD (i.e., increased sympathetic nervous system activity) may play a role in the relationship between physiologic sexual arousal and child sexual abuse. Specifically, increased sympathetic nervous system activity induced by exercise was found to enhance physiologic sexual arousal in healthy controls but had no effect on the physiologic sexual response of women with an impaired hypothalamus–pituitary–adrenal axis.[38] Finally, sexual abuse survivors with PTSD reported higher levels of negative affect associated with sexual arousal than controls.[33,39] Sexual response can be interpreted by Herman's model as a sign of the responsibility for having invited the sexual abuse.

Dissociation, a symptom often observed in survivors of severe child sexual abuse, is interpreted in Herman's model as a method originally used by the child to distance herself from the abuse. This form of self-defense can later become a problem if the survivor continues to use it as a primary coping mechanism. Sex therapists who treat dissociative clients emphasize the importance of using "grounding" techniques to prevent dissociation during sexual encounters.[40]

Although bulimia is one of the common behavioral consequences of trauma, little is known of its effect on sexual functioning (see review by Wiederman[41]). Given that women with bulimia are reported to have lower sexual self-esteem than controls,[42] bulimics may focus on pleasing their partners more than themselves during sex and this may have a negative impact on their ability to become aroused.[43] Unfortunately, the lack of studies on the relationship between sexual functioning, sexual abuse, and bulimia does not provide more than a tentative explanation of this complicated triad.

Alcohol/drug abuse or dependence is common among women with a history of sexual abuse. Sexual pain is the sexual concern most commonly reported by women with a history of child sexual abuse with alcohol/drug problems. Drugs are often used by child sexual abuse survivors during the sexual encounter to reduce negative emotions (i.e., anxiety, depression, reduced self-esteem) through increasing dissociation and emotional detachment.[44] However, alcohol also inhibits genital sexual response,[45] and this decreases lubrication and may cause more pain due to friction. An additional problem of alcohol is its tendency to make the survivor more prone to further abuse by decreasing her ability to assert her needs during the sexual encounter.

In addition to the link between psychiatric disorders and sexual functioning, the literature also provides evidence for an association between body esteem and sexual functioning in sexual abuse survivors. A variety of clinical observations of abuse survivors pointed to negative feelings toward their bodies, such as detachment, anger, and betrayal. To my knowledge, only one empirical study examined this relationship, and it supported the moderator role of body image in the relationship between adult sexual functioning and childhood sexual abuse.[46]

Physical health

In addition to psychologic difficulties, sexual abuse survivors also reported more gynecologic and psychosomatic problems than women who never experienced sexual abuse. Gynecologic complaints were usually associated with lesions and scar tissue in the hymen, in the posterior forchette, and inside the vagina.[47] Yeast infections and sexually transmitted diseases were also common among sexual abuse survivors. Despite the higher need for clinical attention, the fear of invasive gynecologic examination often deters the survivor from scheduling an appointment. This avoidant behavior may not only exacerbate anxiety associated with sex, but also have negative repercussions on any untreated health conditions. The psychosomatic complaints most frequently reported were stress related headaches, weight change, and back pain. Particular attention should be given to health profiles of survivors who develop PTSD, since this subgroup tend to experience more severe health problems than the normal population.

Adults with PTSD present with an overactive sympathetic nervous system in combination with a deficiency in cortisol levels,[48] indicating an impairment in the negative feedback of the hypothalamus–pituitary–adrenal axis. In healthy individuals, these two systems are responsible for the reaction to stress and the subsequent return to homeostasis. Thus, for a patient with PTSD, the ability to adapt to stress may be impaired. To date, only one study has investigated the relationship between the overactivity of the sympathetic nervous system and sexual functioning in women with PTSD.[38] Although the results supported the theory that the sexual response may be negatively affected by the overactive sympathetic nervous system, further studies need to replicate and expand upon these results.

Cognitive self-schemas

The impact of sexual abuse is not restricted to the behavior and physical health of survivors, but it also infiltrates their self-schemas.[34] Self-schemas are the blueprints people use to organize information and make sense of the world. Trauma survivors often present an altered schema of the self and the world that keeps them in a state of continuous fear and avoidance. A study using explicit measures of sexual schemas asked women to complete questionnaires on their view of sexuality.[35] Women with a history of sexual abuse reported less positive sexual schemas (romantic/passionate and open/direct) than nonabused controls.[35] A study that employed implicit measures of self-schemas asked participants to divide sexual words and adjectives into categories. Women with no history of sexual abuse showed similar networks among themselves, while women with a history of child sexual abuse showed dissimilar networks.[49] These results point to a disruption in the underlying process of sexual information in child sexual abuse survivors. Interestingly, sexual abuse survivors showed a variety of responses to the disruption caused by the sexual abuse rather than a set pattern. Further studies are needed to delineate the nuances of these networks so that they can be targeted during therapy.

Interpersonal difficulties

Intrapersonal difficulties associated with sexual abuse are accompanied by interpersonal difficulties, or difficulties the survivor experiences within relationships. Relationships are very important in the quality of life and healing of the survivor. In fact, satisfaction with an intimate relationship prior to the sexual abuse has been found to protect against the development of sexual concerns.[10] The main problems that plagued the relationships of sexual abuse survivors were difficulties with emotional communication, power and control imbalances, and issues with trust.[30] Sexual communication appeared to be particularly problematic for couples with a history of child sexual abuse (referenced in Compton and Follette[50]). These problems may arise from relational deficits that often are at the base of survivors' psychologic symptoms. The survivor may have difficulties expressing her sexual needs because she may not feel she has the right to pleasure and sexual attention. Moreover, intimate communication was found to predict sexual satisfaction in heterosexual couples,[51] and therefore it is likely that the survivors' communication problems may also affect sexual satisfaction.

The sexual problems observed in survivors of sexual abuse should be observed within the context of the relationship, as these dysfunctions may serve a specific function for the patient and her partner. For example, hypoactive sexual desire may be a way of controlling the power dynamic in the relationship. Given that sexual abuse survivors may be more sensitive to controls and power imbalances than women who never experienced sexual abuse, sex may become an effective way to limit the partner's power in the relationship. Unfortunately, no published studies have investigated the use of sex as a form of control in couples where one partner is a sexual abuse survivor.

Conclusions

In summary, the literature presents evidence that women survivors of sexual abuse are more likely to develop sexual dysfunction than women who never experienced sexual abuse. Since sexuality is a complex bio-psycho-social phenomenon, it is important to take into consideration all aspects of the survivors' lives when assessing or treating their sexual functioning. An accurate and comprehensive evaluation of the sexual dysfunction of survivors of sexual abuse should include questions addressing potential psychologic, cognitive, and medical functioning consequences of the abuse, as well as questions regarding intimacy and communication with the partner. This chapter points to numerous ways in which sexual abuse can affect sexual function. In particular, it brings to light the need for the development of treatments tailored to address individual differences in the history, meaning, and the impact of the abuse on the survivor's life.

References

1. Neumann DA, Houskamp BM, Pollock VE et al. The long-term sequelae of childhood sexual abuse in women: a meta-analytic review. *Child Maltreat* 1996; 1: 6–16.
2. van Berlo W, Ensink B. Problems with sexuality after sexual assault. *Annu Rev Sex Res* 2000; 11: 235–58.
3. National Child Abuse and Neglect Data System. *Child Maltreatment Report 2000*. http://www.acf.hhs.gov/programs/cb/publications/cmreports.htm.
4. Tjaden P, Thoennes N. Prevalence, incidence, and consequences of violence against women: findings from the National Violence Against Women Survey. *National Institute of Justice Centers for Disease Control and Prevention Research in Brief*, 1998: 1–16.
5. Burgess AW, Holmstrom LL. Rape: sexual disruption and recovery. *Am J Orthopsychiatry* 1979; 49: 648–57.
6. Alexander PC, Lupfer SL. Family characteristics and long-term consequences associated with sexual abuse. *Arch Sex Behav* 1987; 16: 235–45.
7. Meston CM, Heiman JR, Trapnell PD. The relation between early abuse and adult sexuality. *J Sex Res* 1999; 36: 385–95.
8. Jehu D. Sexual dysfunctions among women clients who were sexually abused in childhood. *Behav Psychother* 1989; 17: 53–70.
9. Becker JV, Skinner LJ, Abel GG et al. Incidence and types of sexual dysfunctions in rape and incest victims. *J Sex Marital Ther* 1982; 8: 65–74.
10. Dahl S. *Rape – A Hazard to Health*. Oslo: Scandinavian University Press, 1993.
11. Golding JM. Sexual assault history and women's reproductive and sexual health. *Psychol Women Q* 1996; 20: 101–21.
12. Davis JL, Petretic-Jackson PA. The impact of child sexual abuse on adult interpersonal functioning: a review and synthesis of the empirical literature. *Aggress Violent Behav* 2000; 5: 291–328.
13. Leonard LM, Follette VM. Sexual functioning in women reporting a history of child sexual abuse: review of the empirical literature and clinical implications. *Annu Rev Sex Res* 2002; 13: 346–87.
14. Becker JV. Sexual problems of sexual assault survivors. *Women's Health* 1984; 9: 5–20.
15. Berman LA, Berman JR, Bruck D et al. Pharmacotherapy or psychotherapy? Effective treatment for FSD to unresolved childhood sexual abuse. *J Sex Marital Ther* 2001; 27: 421–5.
16. Herman J, Hirschman L. Father–daughter incest. *Signs* 1977; 2: 735–56.
17. Maltz W, Holma B. *Incest and Sexuality: A Guide to Understanding and Healing*. Lexington: Lexington Books, 1987.
18. Fergusson DM, Mullen PE. *Childhood Sexual Abuse: An Evidence Based Perspective*. Thousand Oaks, CA: Sage, 1999.
19. Jackson JL, Calhoun, KS, Amick AE et al. Young adult women who report childhood intrafamilial sexual abuse: subsequent adjustment. *Arch Sex Behav* 1990; 19: 211–21.
20. Bartoi MG, Kinder BN, Tomianovic D. Interaction effects of emotional status and sexual abuse and adult sexuality. *J Sex Marital Ther* 2000; 26: 1–23.
21. Orlando JA, Koss MP. The effects of sexual victimization on sexual satisfaction: a study of the negative-association hypothesis. *J Abnorm Psychol* 1983; 92: 104–6.
22. Tolman DL, Szalacha LA. Dimensions of desire: bridging qualitative and quantitative methods in a study of female adolescent sexuality. *Psychol Women Q* 1999; 23: 7–39.
23. Loeb TB, Williams JK, Carmona JV et al. Child sexual abuse: associations with the sexual functioning of adolescents and adults. *Annu Rev Sex Res* 2002; 13: 307–45.
24. Browne A, Finkelhor D. Impact of child sexual abuse: a review of the research. *Psychol Bull* 1986; 99: 66–77.
25. Heise L, Moore K, Toubia N. *Sexual Coercion and Reproductive Health: A Focus on Research*. New York: Population Council, 1995.
26. Westerlund E. *Women's Sexuality After Childhood Incest*. New York: WW Norton, 1992.
27. Rind B, Tromovitch P, Bauserman R. A meta-analytic examination of assumed properties of child sexual abuse using college samples. *Psychol Bull* 1998; 124: 22–53.
28. Ellis EM, Calhoun KS, Atkenson BM. Sexual dysfunctions in victims of rape: victims may experience a loss of sexual arousal and frightening flashbacks even one year after the assault. *Women's Health* 1980; 5: 39–47.
29. Merrill LL, Guimond JM, Thomsen CJ. Child sexual abuse and number of sexual partners in young women: the role of abuse severity, coping style, and sexual functioning. *J Consult Clin Psychol* 2003; 71: 987–96.
30. Pistorello J, Follette VM. Childhood sexual abuse and couples' relationships: female survivors' reports in therapy groups. *J Sex Marital Ther* 1998; 24: 473–85.
31. Oeberg K, Fugl-Meyer KS, Fugl-Meyer AR. On sexual well-being in sexually abused Swedish women: epidemiological aspects. *Sex Relat Ther* 2002; 17: 329–42.
32. Becker JV, Skinner LJ, Abel GG. Level of postassault sexual functioning in rape and incest victims. *Arch Sex Behav* 1986; 15: 37–49.
33. Schloredt KA, Heiman JR. Perceptions of sexuality as related to sexual functioning and sexual risk in women with different types of childhood abuse histories. *J Trauma Stress* 2003; 16: 275–84.

34. Herman JL. *Trauma and Recovery*. New York: Basic Books, 1992.

35. Reissing ED, Binik YM, Khalife S et al. Etiological correlates of vaginismus: sexual and physical abuse, sexual knowledge, sexual self-schema and relationship adjustment. *J Sex Marital Ther* 2003; 29: 47–59.

36. Foa EB, Dancu CV, Hembree EA. A comparison of exposure therapy, stress inoculation training, and their combination for reducing posttraumatic stress disorder in female assault victims. *J Consult Clin Psychol* 1999; 67: 194–200.

37. Letourneau EJ, Resnick HS, Kilpatrick DG et al. Comorbidity of sexual problems and post-traumatic stress disorder in female crime victims. *Behav Ther* 1996; 27: 321–36.

38. Rellini AH, Meston CM. Psychophysiological sexual arousal in women with a history of childhood sexual abuse. *J Sex Marital Ther* 2005 (*in press*).

39. Heiman JR, Gladue BA, Roberts CW et al. Historical and current factors discriminating sexually functional from sexually dysfunctional married couples. *J Marital Fam Ther* 1986; 12: 163–74.

40. Ashton AK. Structured sexual therapy with severely dissociative patients. *J Sex Marital Ther* 1995; 21: 276–81.

41. Wiederman MW. Women, sex, and food: a review of research on eating disorders and sexuality. *J Sex Res* 1996; 33: 301–11.

42. Katzman MA, Wolchik SA. Bulimia and binge eating in college women: a comparison of personality and behavioral characteristics. *J Consult Clin Psychol* 1984; 52: 423–8.

43. Barlow DH. Causes of sexual dysfunction: the role of anxiety and cognitive interference. *J Consult Clin Psychol* 1986; 54: 140–8.

44. Wilsnack SC, Vogeltanz ND, Klassen AD et al. Childhood sexual abuse and women's substance abuse: national survey findings. *J Stud Alcohol* 1997; 58: 264–71.

45. George WH, Stoner SA. Understanding acute alcohol effects on sexual behavior. *Annu Rev Sex Res* 2000; 11: 92–124.

46. Wenninger K, Heiman JR. Relating body image to psychological and sexual functioning in child sexual abuse survivors. *J Trauma Stress* 1998; 11: 543–62.

47. Emans SJ, Woods ER, Flagg NT et al. Genital findings in sexually abused, symptomatic and asymptomatic girls. *Pediatrics* 1987; 79: 778–85.

48. Southwick SM, Bremner JD, Rasmusson A et al. Role of norepinephrine in the pathophysiology and treatment of posttraumatic stress disorder. *Bio Psychiatry* 1999; 46: 1192–1204.

49. Meston CM, Heiman JR. Sexual abuse and sexual function: an examination of sexually relevant cognitive processes. *J Consult Clin Psychol* 2000; 68: 399–406.

50. Compton JS, Follette VM. Couple therapy when a partner has a history of child sexual abuse. In AS Gurman, NS Jacobson, eds. *Clinical Handbook of Couple Therapy*, 3rd edn. New York: Guilford Press, 2002: 466–87.

51. Meston CM, Trapnell PD. Development and validation of a five factor sexual satisfaction and distress scale for women: the Sexual Satisfaction Scale for Women (SSS-W). *J Sex Med* 2005; 2: 66–81.

ANATOMY

4.1 Anatomy of female genitalia

Helen E O'Connell, Kalavampara V Sanjeevan

Historical, sociocultural, and religious factors appear to have affected the scientific study of female sexual anatomy and physiology. Throughout history, the clitoris was discovered and rediscovered, previous knowledge presumably having been lost or hidden.[1] Famous anatomists argued passionately against the very existence of the clitoris.[2] Moore and Clarke studied anatomic descriptions and diagrams across the twentieth century.[3] Labeling evident in diagrams early in the twentieth century was absent in subsequent editions of the same textbooks. Until the work of De Graaf in the seventeenth century, there was no comprehensive description of female genital anatomy. There was confusion regarding the distinction between the clitoris and labia because of the effects of translation of ancient texts and imprecision of terminology in relation to female genital structures. De Graaf emphasized the importance of using the term "clitoris".[4] Modern textbooks typically provide a complete account of male anatomy only and then highlight the differences as a means of describing female anatomy.[5–7] In the anatomic textbooks, the dorsal nerve of the clitoris is not described but is noted to be "very small and supplies the clitoris".[5] This is an example of the inaccuracy present even in distinguished anatomic textbooks. The dorsal clitoral nerves were visible to the naked eye in every cadaver we studied (i.e. these are not small structures).[8] Near-complete omission of the anatomy of the clitoris has also occurred.[9] In recent years, there have been some dissection and magnetic resonance imaging (MRI) studies of the female genitalia, facilitating a more accurate understanding of the anatomy.[8,10–12] This clarified the accuracy of the work by Kobelt and De Graaf.[13]

For descriptive purposes, reproductive organs lying within the body cavity such as ovaries, uterus, and fallopian tubes are grouped as *internal genitalia*, and sexual or reproductive and adjacent structures outside the body cavity are grouped as *external genitalia* (Fig. 4.1.1).

The external genitalia in women include the structures surrounding the *urogenital cleft*, referred to as the *vulva*. The vulva is comprised of the mons pubis, clitoris, and labia majora and minora. The *mons pubis* forms the anterosuperior limit of the cleft with the *labia majora* on both sides and ending posteriorly at the anterior margin of the *perineal body* (Fig. 4.1.2). Surface anatomy varies considerably. In some women, only the mons and labia majora may be seen unless the labia are parted, while, in others, the labia minora and clitoral glans and/or the hood of the clitoral prepuce may also been seen. The area between the labia minora is called the *vestibule*, although in the literature at times the term "vestibule" has been used synonymously with "introitus" or "vaginal opening".

The mons pubis is a hair-covered mound overlying the pubic symphysis (Fig. 4.1.2). Deep to the fat of the mons pubis lies a "fan-shaped" fibrofatty layer that converges downward from the mons pubis to gain attachment along the body of the clitoris up to its glans. This large superficial component of the *suspensory ligament* of clitoris also extends into the labia majora, and attaches to the crura and bulbs of the clitoris as well. It appears to provide stability to the clitoris and labia.[14] The body of the clitoris projects into the fat of the mons pubis, as is well seen on MRI studies in the sagittal plane.[15]

The labia majora are the two prominent lateral boundaries of the urogenital cleft. Anteriorly, they meet, together forming the *anterior commissure* in front of the glans of the clitoris; posteriorly, they meet, together forming a low ridge of skin called the *posterior commissure*, which is about an inch in front of the anus. Each labium has external pigmented hairy skin, which may be slightly wrinkled in the nonaroused state, and a smooth internal surface. Multiple large, sebaceous follicles line the shiny internal surface. Dissections reveal the highly vascular content of the labia, with the vessels mostly derived from the external pudendal vasculature (Fig. 4.1.3). The labia minora are composed of supple, elastic skin, without any subcutaneous fat but rich in sebaceous glands, flanking the vaginal opening from the clitoral glans anteriorly to the posterior limit of vaginal opening. The size and appearance of the labia minora vary widely. Anteriorly, the labia minora split into two layers, the anterior or upper layer forming the hood of the *clitoral prepuce* and gaining attachment circumferentially to the base of the glans of clitoris. The posterior or lower layer encircles partially

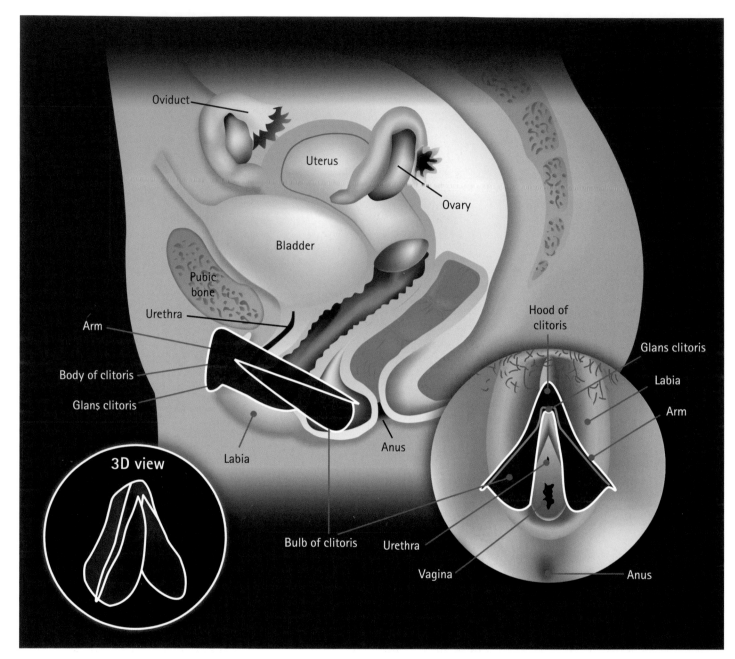

Figure 4.1.1. Composite picture of midsagittal section of female pelvis showing the internal and external genitalia and the clitoro-urethro-vaginal complex. Left inset shows the three-dimensional appearance of clitoris. Right inset shows the vulva and its relation to the clitoris. Reproduced with permission from Williamson S, Nowak R. The truth about women. *New Scientist* 1998; 159: 34–5.

the ventrum of the clitoris to meet the similar layer from the other side to form the *frenulum of clitoris*, which gains attachment to the posteroinferior aspect of glans of the clitoris in the midline.

The clitoris is a complex erectile structure, of which only a tiny portion, the clitoral glans, is appreciable from the surface (Figs 4.1.1 and 4.1.4). The glans projects variably between the anterior bifurcated ends of the labia minora. The *glans clitoris* is the distal extremity of the clitoral body, although the two structures are separate. The body, *corpus clitoris*, is comprised of paired corpora that are joined in the sagittal plane by an incomplete septum. The deep extensions of the corpora diverge under the pubic arch as the *crura*. In postmenopausal cadavers, the body is 0.5–1.0 cm wide, 1–2 cm high, and 2–4 cm long. The body of the clitoris is boomerang-shaped in sagittal section, the bend being maintained by the deep component of the suspensory ligament.[15] In anatomic textbooks, it appears to be flat, but an oblique image reveals the depth of the clitoral body. The body is surrounded by a thick tunica albuginea and has a midline septum between its constituent corpora. Large nerve trunks

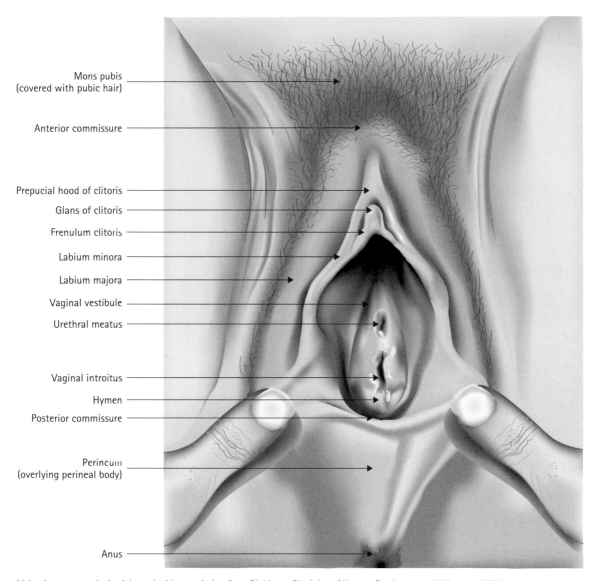

Figure 4.1.2. Vulva in a young virgin. Adapted with permission from Dickinson RL. *Atlas of Human Sex Anatomy.* Williams & Wilkins, 1949.

run along its anterior surface (although they are named the "dorsal" nerves of the clitoris). The nerve trunks run with the corresponding artery and veins on either side of a midline deep dorsal vein of the clitoris.

The *bulbs of the clitoris* lie deep to the thin sheet of *bulbospongiosus muscle*, the fibers of which extend from the perineal body to the body of the clitoris around the vagina and urethra. They are covered by a delicate membrane which is markedly different from the tough capsule, the *tunica albuginea*, which surrounds the corpus clitoris. The bulbs are posteroinferior to the body of the clitoris. They lie lateral to the urethra and superficial to the crura. Their posterior extent varies considerably, but, in younger women, will reach as far posteriorly as the perineal body. In cadaver studies the bulbs are 3–7 cm long, crescentic or triangular in shape, fill the space between the crus and body of the clitoris, and flank the corresponding lateral wall of urethra and distal vagina to a variable extent.[8] Dissection and MRI

studies reveal them very clearly (Figs 4.1.4–4.1.6). The bulbs do not relate consistently to the vestibule, their constant relationship being with the clitoral body, crura, and glans. The bulbs have had a variety of names throughout the literature, most of which do not acknowledge their constant relationship to the rest of the clitoris, urethra, and vagina.

The paired clitoral bulbs appear to be more extensive than the male counterpart. We have progressed very little in the understanding of their physiology from the time of De Graaf, who suggested their role to be "the constriction of the penis" during intercourse. They contain erectile tissue of a different consistency from the body and crura.[16]

The crura, 5–9 cm long and narrower than the body, attach to the deep aspect of the undersurface of the ischiopubic rami on either side and are covered by *ischiocavernosus muscles*. They are composed of typical erectile tissue, like that of the body, and lie adjacent to the dorsal clitoral neurovascular bundle,

The labels in the figure read (top to bottom): Mons pubis (covered with pubic hair), Anterior commissure, Prepucial hood of clitoris, Glans of clitoris, Frenulum clitoris, Labium minora, Labium majora, Vaginal vestibule, Urethral meatus, Vaginal introitus, Hymen, Posterior commissure, Perineum (overlying perineal body), Anus.

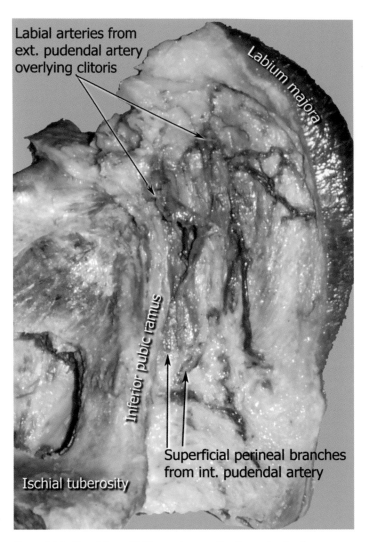

Figure 4.1.3. Vasculature of labium majus revealing the predominant vasculature from the branches of external pudendal artery and some supply from the perineal branches of internal pudendal artery. The highly vascular nature of the labia is not usually observed in anatomy textbooks.

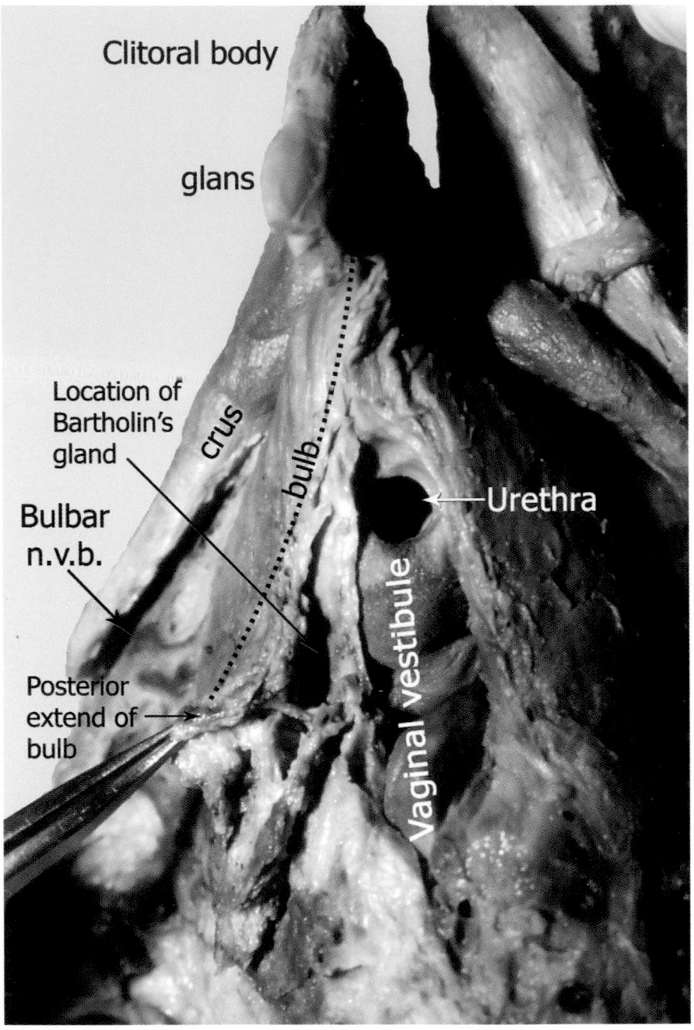

Figure 4.1.4. Anteroposterior view of a dissected specimen of clitoris in a postmenopausal woman. This reveals the relationship between the bulbs, crura, and urethra. The glans is apparent superior to the urethra. The body is best revealed in the sagittal plane, its shape and size not being apparent in the anteroposterior view. n.v.b. = neurovascular bundle.

although no branches appear to surround or perforate the crura of the clitoral body.

The terminal divisions of the pudendal neurovascular bundle are the dorsal clitoral and perineal neurovascular bundles. The dorsal clitoral neurovascular bundle rises along the crus on each side plastered to the periosteum of the ischiopubic ramus (Fig. 4.1.7). This neurovascular bundle supplies the crus, body, and glans of the clitoris, and superficial tissues of the labia. The bulbs and urethra are supplied by the perineal neurovascular bundle. The dorsal nerve of clitoris runs anterosupero-medially from its formation underneath the ischiopubic ramus, and runs along the superior surface of the corpus clitoris, not in the 12 o'clock position, to enter the deep aspect of the glans clitoris. The perineal neurovascular bundle runs medially and more horizontally after its formation, to reach the posterolateral aspect of the bulb. The cavernosal neurovascular bundle runs lateral to the urethra and lies directly on the pelvic aspect of the anterior vaginal wall. The cavernous nerves originate from the vaginal nerve plexus occupying the 2 and 10 o'clock positions on the anterolateral vagina and travel at the 5 and 7 o'clock positions along the urethra.[10] These nerves are microscopic and appear to be a network of fibers rather than discrete nerves.

The clitoris is supported externally by the superficial and deep suspensory ligaments. The deep ligament arises from the undersurface of ischiopubic rami and pubic symphysis. Internally, the clitoris is supported by the urethra and vagina and their attachments to the pelvic floor and bony pelvis.

The urethral orifice (external meatus) is located between the body of the clitoris and the vaginal opening in the midline, about an inch posteroinferior to the glans clitoris. The appearance of the meatus may vary widely from a tiny, inconspicuous, vertical slit, through crescentic or stellate forms to a round aperture, with

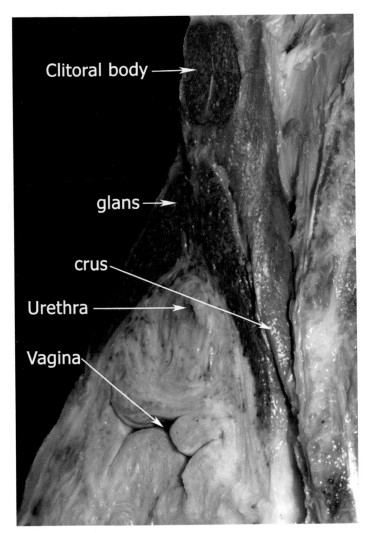

Figure 4.1.5. Coronal cross-section through the midbody of clitoris. Note the bulk of clitoral body, supraurethral portion of the clitoral bulbs and the relationship of clitoral bulb to the lateral walls of the urethra and vagina.

a small bulge or dimple. Surrounding the distal urethra, slightly proximal to the meatus, are several paraurethral glands (Skene's glands), which express prostate-specific antigen (PSA)[17,18] and prostate-specific acid phosphatase (PSAcP).[18] Female ejaculation is reported in some women with orgasmic expulsion of fluid, different from urine, which could be from the periurethral glands, as it contains high levels of PSA.[19] A sexually sensitive area in the anterior vaginal wall is termed the Grafenberg spot, or G-spot.[20] Ultrasound studies have demonstrated that the site of greatest sensitivity corresponds to the location of the external urethral sphincter. There is no consensus, however, regarding "female ejaculation" or presence of the G-spot.[21] It is likely that the increased area of sensitivity reported in some women in relation to the urethra is due to the fact that the urethra is surrounded by erectile tissue. The sexual role of the urethra and the physiology of the clitoris are topics in their infancy.

The vaginal orifice (introitus) is a vertical opening inferior to the urethral meatus. It is irregular at the level of the hymen,

proximal to which the anterior and posterior walls of the vagina meet together, separating the lateral walls, and forming an H- or W-shaped slit.

The vagina extends from the vestibule to the uterine cervix and posterior fornix. This fibromuscular tube is described as having four walls, the anterior, posterior, and right and left lateral walls, the anterior wall measuring 7.5 cm in length and the posterior wall, 9 cm in cadavers. Vaginal to clitoral dimensions are likely to be greater in the live state, but such data are lacking. The uterine cervix projects into the proximal end of the vagina, forming a circular recess, or *fornix*, described as anterior, posterior, or lateral. The anterior wall of the vagina covers the urethral wall. The posterior wall is related to peritoneum lining the rectouterine pouch proximally, connective tissue in the midhalf, and perineal body distally, which separates the vagina from the anal canal. The vagina is attached laterally to the pelvic walls forming a single divider in the middle of the pelvis.[22] The connective tissue supports of the vagina, of extreme importance to pelvic organ support and pelvic organ prolapse, are beyond the scope of this chapter.

The vagina is composed of mucosa (stratified squamous epithelium), a lamina propria, and a muscularis consisting of an inner layer of circular smooth muscle and outer, thicker layer of longitudinal smooth muscle.[23] In the upper third of the vagina, the smooth muscle is clearly separate from the urethra and distinct from the lower two-thirds of the anterior vaginal wall from which the urethra is inseparable. On the lateral aspect of the vaginal muscularis is a venous plexus of variable thickness (Fig. 4.1.8). In younger women, the venous plexus on either side can be over 1 cm in diameter. In older women, and possibly related to hormonal factors, the lateral wall thickness may be less than 0.5 cm. Anterolaterally and distally, the bulbs of the clitoris lie directly deep to the vaginal mucosa.

Branches of the superior and inferior vesical arteries supply the upper and middle thirds of the vagina. These branches anastomose with branches of the uterine artery. In continuity with the urethra, the lower third is supplied by branches of the bulbar artery (branch of the perineal division of the terminal part of the internal pudendal artery). The dorsal clitoral arteries also supply the distal vagina where it is adherent to the urethra and bulbs.

Clarification of vaginal neuroanatomy has been achieved recently.[10] Autonomic nerves form a dense network extending from the rectum to the lateral aspects of the proximal and mid-vagina. On the inner aspect of the pelvis, this vaginal plexus supplies the cavernosal nerves to the clitoris at the level of the proximal urethra. These nerves stain immunohistologically for neuronal nitric oxide synthase (nNOS).

The hymen vaginae is a thin fold of mucous membrane, seen just within the vaginal orifice, that varies greatly in appearance. It may be absent, may or may not rupture with sexual activity, or may rupture in athletics or in certain other physical activities unrelated to sexual activity. Its remnants after its rupture are the small round *carunculae hymenales*. While many misconceptions prevail regarding the anatomy of the

In the figure image the following labels appear: Clitoral body, glans, crus, Urethra, Vagina.

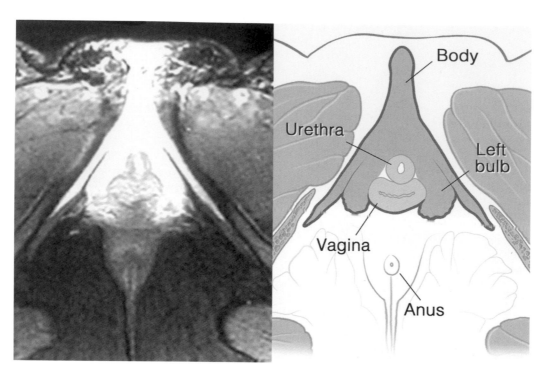

Figure 4.1.6. Magnetic resonance imaging of the clitoris and its components in axial plane: the bulbs, crura, and corpora are well demonstrated. These structures lie ventral and lateral to the urethra and vagina as a cluster or complex. Reproduced with permission from *Journal of Urology*[15].

external genitalia, more has been written about the hymen than any other structure, highlighting the socio-legal implications of female anatomy. Gaping of the hymen can be seen even in sexually nonabused preschool girls.[24]

The *greater vestibular (Bartholin's) glands* are variably depicted throughout anatomic textbooks. Dissections reveal that these glands lie deep to the bulbs; that is, between those structures and the lateral or outer aspect of the distal vaginal

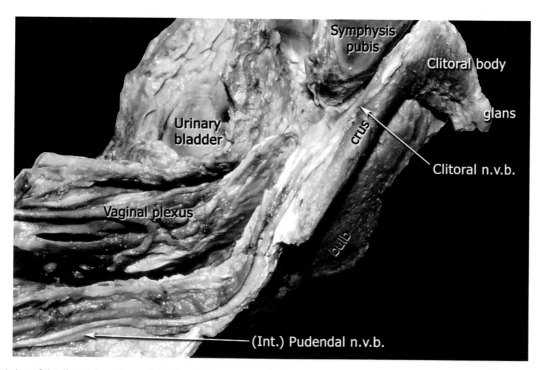

Figure 4.1.7. Lateral view of the dissected specimen of clitoris with its neurovascular bundle. The bundle is clearly seen ascending along the right crus to pass along the superior surface of the clitoral body. n.v.b. = neurovascular bundle.

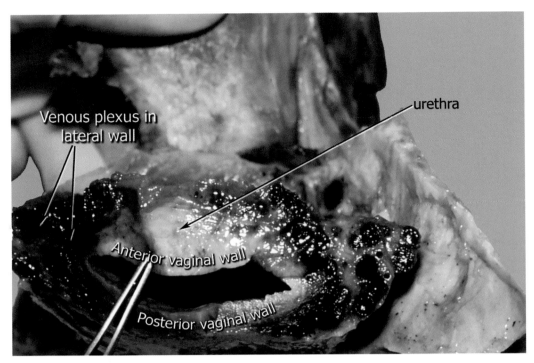

Figure 4.1.8. Axial section through vagina showing the bulk of vaginal muscular wall and paravaginal plexus of veins in a premenopausal cadavar.

wall. A recent MRI study reported the presence of small circular areas of decreased density that presumably represented the greater vestibular glands in all 21 healthy women studied, at the 4 and 8 o'clock positions on the posterolateral aspects of introitus.[11] The greater vestibular glands are tubuloacinar secretory glands that are thought to play a role in lubrication during sexual arousal. Their ducts open on each side into the posterolateral aspect of the vaginal introitus between the labium minora and the hymen.

Conclusions

In recent years, there has been development in the knowledge and review of female genital anatomy. The historical descriptions of Kobelt and De Graaf were comprehensive and, with few exceptions, accurate. Clarification of clitoral anatomy in particular, by dissection and MRI, has led to a new understanding of the relationships between the urethra, distal vagina, and clitoris.

References

1. Park K. The rediscovery of the clitoris. French medicine and the Tribade, 1570–1620. In D Hillman, C Mazzio, eds. *The Body in Parts. Fantasies of Corporeality in Early Modern Europe*. New York: Routledge, 1997: 171–93.
2. Vesalius A. *Observationum anatomicarum Gabrielis Fallopii examen*. Venice: Francesco de' Franceschi da Siena, 1564.
3. Moore LJ, Clarke AE. Clitoral conventions transgressions: graphic representations in anatomy texts, c1900–1991. *Feminist Stud* 1995; 21: 255–301.
4. Jocelyn HD, Setchell BP. Regnier de Graaf on the human reproductive organs. An annotated translation of *Tractatus de Virorum Organis Generationi Inservientibus* (1668) and *De Mulierub Organis Generationi Inservientibus Tractatus Novus* (1962) *J Reprod Fertil Suppl* 1972; 17: 1–222.
5. Williams PL, Bannister LH, Berry MM et al., eds. *Gray's Anatomy*, 38th edn. Edinburgh: Churchill Livingstone, 1995.
6. Sinnatamby CS, ed. *Last's Anatomy: Regional and Applied*, 10th edn. Edinburgh: Churchill Livingstone, 1999.
7. Snell RS. *Clinical Anatomy for Medical Students*, 5th edn. Boston: Little Brown, 1995.
8. O'Connell HE, Hutson JM, Anderson CR, Plenter RJ. Anatomical relationship between urethra and clitoris. *J Urol* 1998; 159: 1892–7.
9. McMinn RMH. *Last's Anatomy: Regional and Applied*, 8th edn. Edinburgh: Churchill Livingstone, 1990.
10. Yucel S, De Souza A Jr, Baskin LS. Neuroanatomy of the human female lower urogenital tract. *J Urol* 2004; 172: 191–5.
11. Suh DD, Yang CC, Cao Y, Garland PA, Maravilla KR. Magnetic resonance imaging anatomy of the female genitalia in premenopausal and postmenopausal women. *J Urol* 2003; 170: 138–44.
12. Baggish MS, Steele AC, Karram M. The relationships of the vestibular bulb and corpora cavernosa to the female urethra: a microanatomic study. II. *J Gynecol Surg* 1999; 15: 171.
13. Lowry TP, ed. *The Classic Clitoris: Historic Contributions to Scientific Sexuality*. Chicago: Nelson-Hall, 1978.

14. Rees MA, O'Connell HE, Plenter RJ, Hutson JM. The suspensory ligament of the clitoris: connective tissue supports of the erectile tissues of the female urogenital region. *Clin Anat* 2000; 13: 397–403.

15. O'Connell HE, DeLancey JOL. Clitoral anatomy in nulliparous healthy premenopausal volunteers using unenhanced magnetic resonance imaging. *J Urol* 2005; 173: 2060–3.

16. O'Connell HE, Hutson HM, Plenter RJ et al. The clitoris: a unified structure. Histology of the clitoral glans, body, crura and bulbs. *Urodinamica* 2004; 14: 127–32.

17. Zaviacic M, Ablin RJ. The female prostate and prostate-specific antigen. Immunohistochemical localization, implications of this prostate marker in women and reasons for using the term "prostate" in the human female. *Histol Histopathol* 2000; 15: 131–42.

18. Tepper SL, Jagirdar J, Heath D, Geller SA. Homology between the female paraurethral (Skene's) glands and the prostate. Immuno-histochemical demonstration. *Arch Pathol Lab Med* 1984; 108: 423–5.

19. Kratochvil S. [Orgasmic expulsions in women]. *Cesk Psychiatr* 1994; 90: 71–7.

20. Lenck LC, Vanneuville G. Sphincter uretral (point G). Corrélations anatomo-cliniques. *Rev Fr Gynecol Obstet* 1992; 87: 65–9.

21. Hines TM. The G-spot: a modern gynecologic myth. *Am J Obstet Gynecol* 2001; 185: 359–62.

22. Wei JT, De Lancey JO. Functional anatomy of the pelvic floor and lower urinary tract. *Clin Obstet Gynecol* 2004; 47: 3–17.

23. Krantz KE. The anatomy of the urethra and anterior vaginal wall. *Am J Obstet Gynecol* 1951; 62: 374–86.

24. Myhre AK, Berntzen K, Bratlid D. Genital anatomy in non-abused preschool girls. *Acta Paediatr* 2003; 92: 1453–62.

4.2 Innervation of the vagina and vulva

Richard F Hoyt Jr

Introduction

The innervation of the female perineum and lower reproductive tract is clinically important in many respects. At one level, appreciation of the gross anatomy of peripheral neural pathways in the pelvis and perineum is the *sine qua non* of nerve-sparing operations designed to minimize disruptions in rectal, bladder, and sexual functions. At another, knowledge of the distribution and function of various nerve fiber types is essential to understanding the physiology and pathophysiology of genital arousal, sexual pleasure, and orgasm. It is therefore surprising that thorough descriptions of the innervation are so difficult to find. In most traditional accounts, the anatomy of the intrapelvic and pudendal nerves in the female is mentioned cursorily as being similar (although smaller in scale) to that in the male, which usually is treated in detail[1-4] (see Chapters 5.3, 5.6, and 16.6 of this volume). More accurate accounts are, however, available in the surgical literature, and a number of recent studies have added significantly to our understanding. The goal of this chapter is to provide a systematic description drawn from a wide variety of sources. With the exception of one or two instances, clearly indicated, attention has been focused throughout on *human female* anatomy.

Basic plan of innervation

Elements of the nervous system

Innervation of the vulva, vagina, and related structures involves motor and sensory aspects of the somatic and visceral nervous systems (see Chapters 4.1 and 4.3 of this volume).

Somatic motor outflow is directed to voluntary, striated, skeletal muscle. At spinal levels, it arises in the ventral gray matter. Multipolar alpha-motor neurons send their axons out of the cord through the ventral roots, to be distributed in the dorsal and ventral primary rami of the spinal nerves.

Somatic sensory nerve cell bodies lie in the dorsal root ganglia of the spinal nerves. There are no synapses in dorsal root ganglia. Each unipolar, primary sensory neuron sends a peripheral process out through a spinal nerve to contact a sensory receptor or end in sensory terminals. It also extends a central process inward via the dorsal root toward the dorsal horn of the spinal gray matter. Somatic sensation can be subdivided into two broad categories: *exteroception* includes thermal, tactile, and pain (nociceptive) sensations from skin and the subcutaneous and deeper somatic tissues; *proprioception* involves the monitoring of stretch, contraction, acceleration, and deceleration in striated muscles, tendons, and joints.

Visceral motor pathways are directed toward cardiac muscle, smooth muscle, vessels, and glands. They require two neurons to convey a signal from the central nervous system to the tissues. These are arranged in series. A preganglionic cell in the brain or spinal cord sends its preganglionic axon into the periphery, where it synapses upon a ganglion cell. The ganglion cell then sends its postganglionic axon on to the target. Visceral motor outflow is subdivided into sympathetic and parasympathetic systems.

- *Sympathetic* motor pathways begin with multipolar preganglionic neurons located in the ventrolateral cell column of the spinal cord, from the first thoracic (T_1) through the second lumbar (L_2) segmental levels. These cells send their preganglionic axons out through the ventral roots and into the ventral rami of the T_1–L_2 spinal nerves. The preganglionic fibers leave each nerve as a "white" communicating ramus by which they enter the sympathetic trunk, an interconnected chain of sympathetic motor ganglia lying alongside the vertebral column from the base of the skull to the coccyx. Many preganglionic fibers end by synapsing in the chain. The ventral ramus of every spinal nerve receives a "gray" communicating ramus, a small bundle of postganglionic axons from ganglion cells in the sympathetic trunk. These fibers run in the spinal nerves and their branches to reach sweat glands, erector pili muscles, and the blood vessels in subcutaneous and deeper musculoskeletal tissues.

A substantial number of preganglionic axons pass through the sympathetic trunk without synapsing. Instead they travel in *splanchnic nerves* to end on prevertebral (preaortic) ganglion cells embedded in an interconnected series of visceral nerve plexuses extending along the aorta and internal iliac arteries. Postganglionic sympathetic fibers are distributed by subsidiary plexuses to reach smooth muscle, blood vessels, and glands in the abdominal and pelvic organs.

● *Parasympathetic* motor pathways begin in brainstem nuclei of certain cranial nerves, including the vagus, and in the ventrolateral cell column of the second, third, and fourth sacral (S_{2-4}) spinal cord segments. Preganglionic axons leave the sacral cord via the ventral roots and emerge from the anterior sacral foramina in the ventral rami of the corresponding spinal nerves. They leave the rami through the *pelvic splanchnic nerves* and enter the pelvic visceral nerve plexus from which they are distributed to ganglion cells in or near the organs. Postganglionic fibers then innervate smooth muscle, certain blood vessels, and glands in the viscera.

Visceral sensory pathways return information from the organs. This input is termed *interoception* and includes pain (nociception), stretch reception, chemoreception, and baroreception. Sensory fibers retrace both sympathetic and parasympathetic outflow pathways. Therefore, visceral afferents enter the T_1–L_2 (sympathetic) and S_{2-4} (parasympathetic) cord segments and the brainstem (parasympathetic). As a rule, pain fibers follow the sympathetic pathway, and most other fibers follow the parasympathetic pathway. In the case of the vulva and the vagina, however, all visceral sensory input passes back along the parasympathetic route through the pelvic plexus and pelvic splanchnic nerves to reach the sacral spinal cord.

Distribution of the neural elements in the vulva and vagina

As summarized in Fig. 4.2.1, skin and subcutaneous tissues of the female perineum are innervated by somatic sensory fibers distributed through branches of the lumbar, sacral, and coccygeal plexuses, all formed by ventral primary rami of spinal nerves. This same distribution includes the lower 2–3 cm of the vagina.

Voluntary striated muscles of the perineum and pelvic floor, including the external urethral and anal sphincters, are innervated by somatic motor and sensory (proprioceptive) fibers of the sacral plexus, either through branches of the pudendal nerve or through branches traveling on the upper surface of the pelvic floor.

Smooth muscle, vessels, and glands in the vagina, cervix, bladder neck, and urethra receive sympathetic and parasympathetic motor innervation through the interconnected pelvic, uterovaginal, and vaginal visceral nerve plexuses (Fig. 4.2.2). This includes the erectile tissues of the clitoris and bulbs of the vestibule.

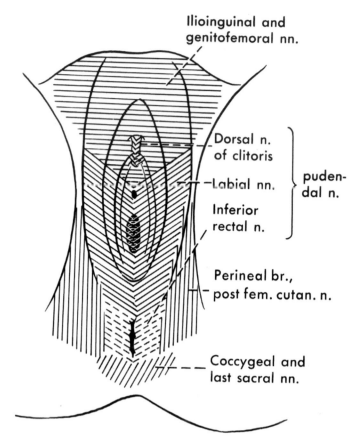

Figure 4.2.1. General distribution of cutaneous nerves to the female perineum. Reproduced with permission from Hollinshead[2] (Fig. 16–2, p 822).

Visceral sensation, including pain, returns from these same organs along the parasympathetic pathway, through the intrapelvic visceral nerve plexuses and pelvic splanchnic nerves, to reach the S_{2-4} segments of the spinal cord.

Pathways of innervation

Somatic pathways

● *Ilioinguinal nerve.* The ilioinguinal is a mixed motor and sensory somatic nerve. It arises from the L_1 ventral primary ramus, passes laterally and downward posterior to the psoas major muscle and behind the parietal fascia on the quadratus lumborum, and iliacus muscles. The nerve then pursues a circumferential course through the anterior abdominal wall, which it supplies. The terminal portion of the nerve emerges through the external inguinal ring below the round ligament of the uterus, accompanies the ligament downward in front of the pubis, and ends by supplying sensory innervation to skin over the mons pubis and portions of the labium majus, labium minus, and vestibule anterior to the urethral orifice.

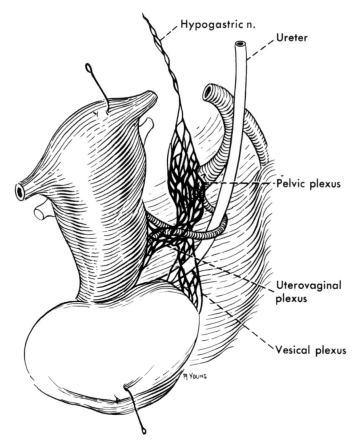

Figure 4.2.2. **The pelvic visceral nerve plexus in the human female. Reproduced with permission from Hollinshead[2] (Fig. 15–36, p 805).

Labels in figure:
Hypogastric n.
Ureter
Pelvic plexus
Uterovaginal plexus
Vesical plexus
R YOUNG

ventral ramus shortly after it emerges through the first anterior sacral foramen. Together, these fibers pass downward and laterally to join the S_{2-4} ventral rami, all of which exit their respective anterior sacral foramina and converge laterally on the greater sciatic foramen. Extrapelvic branches of the sacral plexus exit the pelvic cavity through the greater sciatic foramen and appear in the gluteal region. The superior gluteal nerve leaves above the piriformis muscle; the pudendal, inferior gluteal, and sciatic nerves leave below piriformis, as do the posterior cutaneous nerve of the thigh and the nerves to quadratus femoris and obturator internus muscles.

Deep to the lower part of the gluteus maximus muscle, the posterior cutaneous nerve of the thigh (S_{1-3}) gives rise to its perineal branch, which turns forward below the ischial tuberosity. This nerve runs anteriorly across the hamstring muscles and parallel to the ischiopubic ramus to supply sensory innervation to the lateral aspect of the labium majus.

The S_4 ventral ramus sends a perineal branch through coccygeus or between the coccygeus and levator ani muscles into the ischioanal fossa, where it supplies the posterior part of the external anal sphincter and a small area of skin behind the anal opening. A descending branch from this same ventral ramus joins with the small ventral rami of the 5th sacral and the coccygeal spinal nerves to form a delicate coccygeal plexus on the pelvic surface of the coccygeus muscle. From this plexus, small anococcygeal nerves pass posteriorly through coccygeus and around the lateral margin of the coccyx. They pierce the sacrotuberous ligament and are distributed to skin behind the anal opening and overlying the coccyx.

The sacral plexus also provides branches directly to striated muscles of the pelvic floor. One of these, from the S_4 ventral ramus, enters the pelvic surface of coccygeus. Others, more variable in composition, arise from the S_3 and/or S_4 rami and run forward on the pelvic surface of levator ani. These usually supply the posterior portion of the muscle, principally iliococcygeus, but some fibers may descend through the pelvic floor to end in the external urethral sphincter.

● *Pudendal nerve.* The pudendal nerve is the principal somatic motor and sensory nerve of the perineum. Formed primarily from the 3rd sacral spinal nerve, with lesser contributions from S_2 and S_4, it pursues a short intrapelvic course before passing outward below piriformis with the internal pudendal vessels. The pudendal nerve is the most medial of the neurovascular elements emerging through the greater sciatic foramen. It appears only briefly in the gluteal region, grooving the posterior surface of the ischial spine or the sacrospinous ligament before passing deep to the sacrotuberous ligament and into the perineum. The nerve runs forward against the lateral wall of the ischioanal fossa in the pudendal (Alcock's) canal, a fascial sleeve tethered loosely to the free (medial) surface of the obturator internus muscle. Soon after entering the canal, the pudendal nerve

● *Genitofemoral nerve.* The genitofemoral is a somatic sensory nerve formed behind psoas major by contributions from the L_1 and L_2 ventral primary rami. Descending obliquely, it emerges onto the anterior surface of the muscle. As it continues its downward course, the nerve lies behind the parietal fascia covering psoas and divides at a highly variable point into its femoral and genital branches. The femoral branch passes behind the inguinal ligament lateral to the femoral artery to reach skin of the femoral triangle. The genital branch crosses in front of the external iliac artery, enters the inguinal canal through its deep ring, traverses the canal, and reaches skin over anterior portions of the vulva, overlapping the distribution of the ilioinguinal nerve.

● *Sacral plexus.* Virtually all striated muscles of the perineum and perineal skin behind the urethral orifice are innervated by branches of the sacral plexus, which is formed from lower lumbar and sacral ventral primary rami in front of the sacrum, behind the parietal fascia covering the piriformis and coccygeus muscles.

Fibers from L_4 and L_5 unite to form the lumbosacral trunk, which descends behind the medial portion of psoas major, between the muscle and the sacral promontory. Having crossed the pelvic brim, the trunk joins the S_1

gives off its inferior rectal (inferior hemorrhoidal) branch; shortly thereafter, it ends by dividing into the perineal nerve and the dorsal nerve of the clitoris.

○ *Inferior rectal nerve*. Soon after entering Alcock's canal the pudendal nerve gives off its inferior rectal branch. This leaves the canal through its medial wall and crosses the ischioanal fossa toward the anus. As it does so, it supplies the posterior two-thirds of the external anal sphincter and distributes numerous sensory branches to the lower portion of the anal canal and to skin behind and lateral to the anal opening. Shafik and Doss[5] have described this pattern in some detail. These authors also noted the existence of a discrete labial branch and a motor branch to levator ani; most sources attribute extrapelvic innervation of the levator to perineal branches of the pudendal nerve and 4th sacral ventral ramus and simply mention communications among the three nerves in the ischioanal fossa.

○ *Perineal nerve*. One of two terminal branches of the pudendal nerve, the perineal nerve leaves the distal end of Alcock's canal, directed anteriorly and medially. Again, reports vary, but the general picture is clear. As it approaches the rear edge of the perineal membrane, the nerve gives rise to deep and superficial sets of branches. The medial branches are directed primarily to striated musculature, including the anterior portion of the external anal sphincter, transverse perineal, ischiocavernosus, bulbospongiousus, and levator ani muscles, as well as the external (voluntary) urethral sphincter. The remaining, superficial, branches of the perineal nerve are almost exclusively cutaneous; they form the lateral and medial posterior labial nerves. The lateral set communicates with the perineal branch of the posterior cutaneous nerve of the thigh to supply the lateral margin of the perineum; the medial set runs forward to reach the labia majora and minora, the vestibule, and skin anterior to the anal opening. Somatic sensory innervation to the lower 2–3 cm of the vagina is most likely provided by the medial posterior labial and the inferior rectal nerves.[1]

○ *Dorsal nerve of the clitoris*. This, like the perineal nerve, leaves the distal end of Alcock's canal. It is projected forward and medially through the anterior recess of the ischioanal fossa, running against the margin of the ischiopubic ramus and on the upper surface of the perineal membrane, through which it sends a branch to the corpus cavernosum. Descending through the perineal membrane, it lies between the crus clitoris and the pubic ramus, then crosses medially above the crus, penetrates the suspensory ligament, and gains the dorsum of the clitoral body. Here, at the "hilum" of the clitoris, the dorsal nerve receives an important contribution from the cavernous nerve extending downward along the urethra from the intrapelvic uterovaginal visceral plexus (see below).[6] It then runs distally between the deep fascia and tunica albuginea, separated from the midline by the dorsal artery of the clitoris, giving off branches that spread laterally onto the sides of the corpus. Most are destined for skin of the clitoris and prepuce, but small branches enter the lateral aspect of the tunica albuginea. The dorsal nerve ends in a leash of branches to the glans, especially its dorsal surface.

Visceral pathways

Perineal blood vessels and the sweat glands and erector pili muscles of the skin all receive a postganglionic sympathetic motor innervation. This outflow pathway begins with preganglionic neurons in the L_{1-2} spinal cord segments, whose fibers pass through white communicating rami to synapse on ganglion cells in lumbar and sacral portions of the sympathetic chain. Postganglionic axons traverse gray communicating rami to reach lumbar and sacral spinal nerves and are distributed to the perineum by branches of the ilioinguinal, genitofemoral, posterior femoral cutaneous, and pudendal nerves (Fig. 4.2.1).

The upper vagina, cervix, urethra, greater vestibular glands, and erectile tissues of the clitoris and vestibular bulbs receive sympathetic motor, parasympathetic motor, and visceral sensory innervation. The sympathetic outflow pathway originates in the T_{11}–L_1 spinal cord segments. Preganglionic fibers pass into the sympathetic chain via white communicating rami. Most leave the chain through lumbar splanchnic nerves to enter the interconnected system of visceral nerve plexuses that lie around the abdominal aorta and between the common iliac vessels. Sympathetic fibers continue their descent through the hypogastric nerves on the anterior surface of the sacrum and onto the pelvic floor, where they enter the inferior hypogastric (pelvic) plexus. Here they join preganglionic parasympathetic fibers, which arise in the S_{2-4} cord segments and enter the plexus through pelvic splanchnic nerves from the corresponding ventral primary rami. Intermingled sympathetic and parasympathetic fibers pass through the uterovaginal plexus along the uterine artery to reach the cervix; others turn downward with the vaginal artery, supplying both the vagina and the urethra; and still others continue their descent through the "cavernous nerves" alongside the vagina and urethra to end in the clitoris, bulb of the vestibule, and greater vestibular glands. Sympathetic ganglion cells are scattered along the route. Some lie in the sympathetic chain, but most are located in the pelvic and uterovaginal plexuses. Parasympathetic ganglion cells occur in distal reaches of the uterovaginal plexus and in the vaginal adventitia. Visceral afferent nerves sensing pressure, distention, and pain retrace the paths taken by parasympathetic motor outflow to the region. They enter the 2nd, 3rd, and 4th sacral cord segments, which also receive somatic sensory information from the vulva and perineum through branches of the pudendal nerve. Their cell bodies lie in dorsal root ganglia of the corresponding spinal nerves.

Detailed knowledge of the visceral neural pathways is clinically important not only because elements of the system can be affected by a wide variety of disease processes, but also because they can be damaged by surgical procedures within the female pelvis.

● *Sympathetic trunk.* On each side, the sympathetic trunk enters the abdomen from the thorax by passing behind the medial arcuate ligament on the anterior surface of the psoas major muscle. Lying in the extraperitoneal connective tissue, it descends in front of the origin of psoas from the lumbar vertebral bodies and is overlapped either by the aorta (left side) or by the inferior vena cava (right side). The trunk crosses in front of the lumbar segmental vessels and then behind the common iliac artery and vein to gain the anterior surface of the sacrum. On the sacrum, it courses downward and toward the midline, passing medial to the first three anterior sacral foramina and their emerging S_{1-3} ventral primary rami. After skirting the lateral margin of the fourth anterior sacral foramen and its ventral ramus, the trunk ends independently or joins that of the opposite side in a small *ganglion impar* in front of the coccyx. Ganglionation is highly irregular in the lumbar region, but three or four sacral sympathetic ganglia usually can be identified. Along its course, the sympathetic trunk distributes postganglionic (gray) communicating rami to all lumbar and sacral spinal nerves, and sends four lumbar and two sacral splanchnic nerves into successively lower levels of the continuous abdominopelvic visceral nerve network (see below).

● *Abdominopelvic visceral nerve plexuses.* Organs in the abdominal and pelvic cavities receive their innervation through a longitudinal network of visceral nerve fibers extending from the aortic hiatus in the diaphragm downward onto the pelvic floor. This vertically disposed system lies in the extraperitoneal visceral connective tissue, internal to a plane formed by the aorta and the common and internal iliac arteries. It contains ganglia, microganglia, and isolated ganglion cells (largely if not exclusively sympathetic) embedded in an intermixture of preganglionic and postganglionic sympathetic fibers, preganglionic parasympathetic fibers, and a variety of visceral afferent fibers concerned with pain (nociception), stretch, and other information. Preganglionic sympathetic and accompanying visceral sensory fibers are provided through splanchnic nerves from thoracic, lumbar, and sacral portions of the sympathetic trunk; preganglionic parasympathetic and associated visceral sensory fibers are fed into the network from above, through branches of the vagus nerve, and from below, through pelvic splanchnic nerves from the S_{2-4} ventral rami.

Although the abdominopelvic visceral plexus forms a single continuous network, and should always be thought of as such, the central longitudinal system is usually described as a number of separate units. Beginning above, these are the celiac, intermesenteric (aortic), superior hypogastric, and inferior hypogastric (pelvic) plexuses, the last two being linked across the pelvic brim by the so-called hypogastric nerves. Their extensions pass outward along

visceral branches of the aorta and internal iliac arteries to reach the organs. These subsidiary plexuses generally are named for the vessels they accompany or the organs they supply. For example, the pelvic plexus distributes its fibers to pelvic viscera through its major offshoots, the rectal, uterovaginal, and vesical plexuses.

○ *Celiac plexus.* This is the uppermost – and largest – of the abdominal autonomic plexuses. It lies in front of the aorta just below the aortic hiatus, surrounding the origins of the celiac trunk and superior mesenteric artery. Large, irregular right and left celiac ganglia are embedded in the plexus, along with the superior mesenteric ganglion and smaller aggregates of sympathetic ganglion cells. On each side, a small aorticorenal ganglion lies in the plexus near the origin of the renal arteries. Sympathetic input to the plexus comes through the greater, lesser, and least splanchnic nerves carrying fibers from the T_{5-9} (greater), T_{10-11} (lesser), and T_{12} (least) spinal cord segments. These nerves issue from the thoracic sympathetic trunk and reach the plexus by passing through the crus of the diaphragm or behind the medial arcuate ligament. The plexus also receives fibers from lower thoracic and upper lumbar cord segments through the first lumbar splanchnic nerve. Parasympathetic motor fibers are added to the plexus by branches of the left and right vagus nerves, which have entered the abdomen along with the esophagus. Visceral sensory fibers in the celiac plexus follow both splanchnic and vagal routes.

○ *Intermesenteric plexus.* The intermesenteric, or aortic, plexus extends downward from the celiac plexus as a series of interconnected strands in front of and alongside the aorta between the origins of the superior and inferior mesenteric arteries. Small, discrete sympathetic ganglia and ganglion cells are embedded in the meshwork of nerve fibers, and occasionally a larger, inferior mesenteric ganglion can be identified. The lower part of the intermesenteric plexus receives the second lumbar splanchnic nerve.

○ *Superior hypogastric plexus.* The superior hypogastric plexus is a network of strands continued downward from the aortic plexus in front of the aortic bifurcation and between the right and left common iliac vessels onto the 5th lumbar vertebral body and the sacral promontory. It may contain scattered sympathetic ganglion cells and usually receives the 3rd and 4th lumbar splanchnic nerves. Few, if any, vagal fibers reach the superior hypogastric plexus.

○ *Hypogastric nerve.* Arising from the superior hypogastric plexus in a variety of configurations, ranging from a single strand to a plexiform network, the left and right hypogastric nerves gradually diverge from one another as they descend on the anterior surface of the sacrum. Each nerve passes downward in the visceral pelvic fascia, at first roughly parallel with the ureter but some

2 cm dorsomedial to it. As it does so, it lies between the peritoneum and the lateral wall of the true pelvis, from which it is separated by the internal iliac vessels. In its course, the nerve runs lateral to the rectum and turns forward into the relatively loose connective tissue forming the base (lateral portion) of the crescentic uterosacral fold, whose acute medial margin bounds the rectouterine peritoneal pouch. Here, opposite the rectal ampulla, the hypogastric nerve expands into the pelvic plexus.

○ *Pelvic plexus.* The inferior hypogastric, or pelvic, plexus (Fig. 4.2.2) is a densely woven network of nerve fibers studded with small ganglia and isolated ganglion cells. Most but not all of these are sympathetic in nature. The plexus is roughly 2.5–3.5 cm high and about 5 cm long. It is embedded in a reasonably discrete sheet of extraperitoneal connective tissue (pelvic visceral fascia) medial to the internal iliac vessels and their branches, and it extends anteromedially through the base of the cardinal ligament, directed toward the base of the bladder. Thus, although its origin from the hypogastric nerve is just external to the peritoneum covering the lateral pelvic wall, distal portions of the plexus are situated below the level of the peritoneum and close to the pelvic floor.

Most sympathetic motor fibers reach the pelvic plexus through the hypogastric nerve. This input is reinforced by two small sacral splanchnic nerves that arrive directly from the sacral sympathetic trunk. All preganglionic parasympathetic motor outflow into the plexus is carried in the pelvic splanchnic nerves. These leave the S_{2-4} ventral rami proximal to formation of the sacral (somatic) plexus, penetrate the parietal fascia covering piriformis, run anteromedially through the dorsal region of the parametrium in the base of the cardinal ligament, and enter the lateral surface of the pelvic plexus level with the 5th sacral vertebral segment. Visceral sensory fibers are provided by both hypogastric and pelvic splanchnic nerves.

○ *(Middle) rectal plexus.* The rectal plexus consists of a variable series of strands leaving the posteroinferior margin of the pelvic plexus. They pass medially and downward to reach the posterolateral margin of the rectum through the visceral connective tissues forming the lateral ligament of the rectum (rectal "stalk" or "pillar"). The plexus does not usually accompany the middle rectal branch of the internal iliac artery, which reaches the rectal wall just above the pelvic floor and not through the lateral ligament.[2,7] Thus, the frequently used term '*middle* rectal plexus' is a misnomer.

○ *Vesical plexus.* The vesical plexus represents the anteroinferior continuation of the pelvic plexus. It accompanies the inferior vesical branches of the internal iliac arterial system downward, medially, and forward in the visceral connective tissue forming the posterior portion

of the pubocervical ligament. The plexus courses lateral to the cervix and the vaginal vault to supply the bladder, bladder neck, and proximal urethra.

○ *Uterovaginal plexus.* The uterovaginal plexus leaves the medial aspect of the pelvic plexus in the base of the broad ligament and turns toward the midline, running with the uterine vessels in the upper portion of the cardinal ligament. The plexus contains numerous small ganglia, and occasionally a larger, "cervical" ganglion can be found. Nerve fibers are given off directly to the cervix; those to the body, fundus, and tube turn upward in the parametrial core of the broad ligament with the uterine vessels.

○ *Vaginal plexus.* The intermixture of sympathetic, parasympathetic, and visceral sensory nerve fibers destined for the vagina, urethra, and vulva turn downward with the vaginal artery. Although accounts differ slightly, there is a general consensus that the plexus consists of a series of interlacing longitudinal strands descending at first on the lateral vaginal wall and then in the groove between the vagina and the urethra.[8–10] Here they are said to occupy the 2 and 10 o'clock positions on the vaginal perimeter (12 o'clock being the ventral midline).[6] Branches fan outward from these trunks to invest the vagina. Proximally, the density of innervation is greatest on the anterior wall, but, distally, it decreases as the connective tissue plane between vagina and urethra thins markedly. Parasympathetic ganglion cells are scattered sparsely along the course of larger nerves in the adventitia. Smaller bundles of nerve fibers penetrate the vaginal wall. These traverse the muscularis, supplying vascular and nonvascular smooth muscle, and form a rich plexus in the lamina propria.[11,12] Rarely, fibers cross the basement lamina and ramify among cells of the stratified squamous vaginal epithelium.[11]

The vaginal plexus is closely associated with the vesical plexus (see above), and it distributes branches to the bladder neck and the proximal and middle portions of the urethra.[6,9] Most of the latter hug the lateral margin of the urethra and penetrate the muscle coat anterolaterally, at the 1 and 11 o'clock positions.[8] Motor fibers are destined for urethral smooth muscle, vessels, and glands while sensory fibers contribute to a plexus beneath the epithelium.

○ *Cavernous nerves.* The cavernous nerves carry visceral innervation to the erectile tissues of the vulva. Arising as downward extensions of the vaginal plexus, they descend along the posterolateral border of the proximal urethra (5 and 7 o'clock positions).[6] Gradually they incline forward onto the lateral urethral wall, upon which they pass through the perineal membrane. Below the membrane, each nerve distributes branches to the corresponding dorsal nerve of the clitoris and (presumably) to the bulb of the vestibule. The cavernous nerve ends by piercing the tunic albuginea of the corpus cavernosum just proximal to the body of the clitoris.

Neurotransmitters

The functional significance of any neural pathway depends on the nature of the neurotransmitters produced and released by its fiber types (see Chapter 5.4 in this volume).

Acetylcholine has long been recognized as the basic motor neurotransmitter in the somatic nervous system, responsible for innervation of striated, voluntary muscle. Acetylcholine is the ganglionic neurotransmitter in both sympathetic and parasympathetic systems and is an important postganglionic agent in parasympathetic regulation of cardiac muscle, smooth muscle, vessels, and glands. It also serves as the sympathetic transmitter in sweat glands of the skin.

Noradrenaline, also known as norepinephrine, is the classic sympathetic postganglionic neurotransmitter in cardiac muscle, smooth muscle, blood vessels, and glands.

Nonadrenergic, noncholinergic neurotransmitters have been identified in substantial numbers during the past 50 years. They encompass a wide variety of molecules, including amino acids, amines, peptides, purines, and even nitric oxide, which, as a potent vasodilator, has been shown to play an important role in engorgement of the erectile tissues. Neuropeptides, such as calcitonin-gene-related peptide, substance P, and vasoactive intestinal polypeptide, are now recognized as important neurotransmitters in somatic and visceral sensory nerve fibers.

Various means have been used to study the distribution of neurotransmitters in tissues. Cholinergic fibers were identified initially by a histochemical reaction to localize activity of acetylcholinesterase, the enzyme responsible for degradation of acetylcholine released at nerve terminals. Adrenergic fibers were identified by a formaldehyde-induced amine fluorescence reaction that localized noradrenaline itself. Although still in use, these techniques are cumbersome: acetylcholinesterase reactions involve the use of highly toxic inhibitors to determine the specificity of the enzyme, and formaldehyde-induced fluorescence is best carried out in freeze-dried material. Work has, however, been greatly facilitated by the development of modern immunohistochemical methods, which permit two basic strategies. In the first, antibodies are developed that recognize specific neurotransmitter molecules such as calcitonin-gene-related peptide, substance P, vasoactive intestinal polypeptide, and neuropeptide Y. In the second approach, antibodies are used to localize key enzymes or other molecules involved in the metabolism of a given neurotransmitter. Examples include tyrosine hydroxylase for noradrenaline, choline-acetyl transferase and vesicular acetylcholine transporter for acetylcholine, and nitric oxide synthase for nitric oxide. In the latter case, two different enzymes can be identified, one in neurons (neural nitric oxide synthase) and the other in vascular endothelium (endothelial nitric oxide synthase). Although neurotransmitter localizations reveal only subpopulations of neurons along a pathway or in a tissue, antibodies to protein-gene product 9.5 (PGP 9.5)[8,11,12] and to S-100 protein[6] serve as generic immunohistochemical markers for the entire population of nerve fibers and ganglion cells.

To date, a number of neurotransmitter systems have been demonstrated in nerves associated with the human female perineum and reproductive tract. These include the following:

- acetylcholine, shown by acetylcholinesterase[13] and vesicular acetylcholine transporter[6]
- noradrenaline, shown by tyrosine hydroxylase[14]
- nitric oxide, shown by neural nitric oxide synthase[6,11,15] and endothelial nitric oxide synthase[15]
- neuropeptide Y[11,14,16 18]
- substance P[6,11,14]
- calcitonin-gene-related peptide P[6,11,14]
- vasoactive intestinal polypeptide P.[11,14,16]

As summarized by Butler-Manuel et al.,[14] vasoactive intestinal polypeptide often colocalizes with cholinergic markers and is therefore considered to be a neurotransmitter in the parasympathetic system along with acetylcholine. Neuropeptide Y, on the other hand, often colocalizes with tyrosine hydroxylase and is viewed with noradrenaline as a postganglionic sympathetic agent. Calcitonin-gene-related peptide is thought to be a sensory transmitter, and substance P is associated with nociception and sensorimotor functions. Presumably, the latter activity would involve axon reflexes. Vasoactive intestinal polypeptide is also classed as a sensory neurotransmitter.[1]

Recent immunohistochemical studies have begun to plot systematically the distribution of nerve fibers and neurotransmitters in human female genital tissues,[6,11] but certain points must be considered in assessing the functional implications of any neurotransmitter localization, no matter how thorough. First, the fact that two neurotransmitters colocalize does not necessarily mean that they always will do so. Second, developmental plasticity may be a factor in evaluating results obtained in fetal material: considerable remodeling of the nervous system can occur between the second trimester of gestation and sexual maturity. Third, neurotransmitters are only part of the puzzle, for their actions depend on the spectrum of specific receptors available to them, and these may be distributed unevenly in target tissues. At present, significant gaps remain to be filled in our map of neurotransmitter distributions, little is known about the availability and especially the tissue localization of receptors for specific neurotransmitters, and the possibility that the hormonal status of women may affect the spectrum of neurotransmitters and their receptors is only now being acknowledged.

Targets of motor innervation

Skin of the perineum

Sweat glands and blood vessels in the perineal skin receive visceral, sympathetic innervation. Postganglionic fibers pass through gray rami from the sympathetic trunk to enter the ventral primary rami of lumbar, sacral, and coccygeal nerves. They are distributed to skin of the urogenital region and vulva by appropriate branches of the ilioinguinal, genitofemoral, pudendal, and lateral femoral cutaneous nerves (Fig. 4.2.1). Skin of the anal region is supplied through inferior rectal and perineal branches of the pudendal nerve and through the perineal branch of the S_4 ventral ramus. Preganglionic outflow is from lower thoracic and upper lumbar cord segments. The postganglionic neurotransmitters are noradrenaline (blood vessels) and acetylcholine (sweat glands).

Striated, voluntary muscles of the perineum

All striated muscle fibers in the region receive a somatic motor innervation that utilizes acetylcholine as the neuromuscular transmitter. Bulbospongiosus, ischiocavernosus, and transversus perinei are supplied from the S_{2-4} spinal cord segments via the sacral plexus and the perineal branch of the pudendal nerve. The external (voluntary) anal sphincter is supplied by the same cord segments. Motor fibers travel in the inferior rectal and perineal branches of the pudendal nerve to reach the posterior two-thirds and the anterior one-third of the muscle, respectively. Most sources agree that the sphincter is also innervated by the perineal branch of the 4th sacral ventral ramus, which descends through the pelvic floor. This point is of surgical interest because it means that fecal continence can be impaired by dissections involving the upper (internal) surface of the pelvic floor as well as those conducted in the ischioanal fossa. Blood vessels in all these striated muscles receive an adrenergic innervation from the sympathetic trunk; postganglionic fibers are distributed through the appropriate branches of the sacral plexus.

Although the voluntary, external urethral sphincter is a perineal muscle, its nerve supply will be described with that of the urethra (see below).

Striated, voluntary muscles of the pelvic floor
(*see Chapters 12.3 and 17.4 of this volume*)

The muscles of the pelvic diaphragm also receive cholinergic somatic motor innervation from the sacral spinal cord. This is distributed by branches of the sacral plexus that also carry adrenergic postganglionic sympathetic fibers to local blood vessels. The coccygeus is supplied on its pelvic surface by direct branches from the S_3 and S_4 ventral primary rami.[2] Anterior portions of the muscle complex collectively termed "levator ani", including pubovaginalis and puborectalis (see Chapter 4.4 of this volume), are innervated on their extrapelvic (perineal) surface by twigs from the perineal branch of the pudendal nerve (S_{2-4}). Most sources agree on the existence of an intrapelvic pathway as well, but differ in the details. It has been described as an intrapelvic branch of the pudendal nerve,[19] as a single nerve arising from the S_3 or S_4 ventral ramus,[2] as separate twigs from

the S_3 and S_4 rami,[1-3] and even as the sole motor nerve to the entire levator complex. None of these patterns lie outside the range of normal variation: the author, for instance, can remember a dissection in which the *dorsal nerve of the penis* ran forward *above* the pelvic floor, distributing fine branches to levator ani along its course. The clinical implications are clear, however: motor innervation to the levator ani can be compromised during intrapelvic as well as perineal surgical procedures.

Cervix and vagina

Smooth muscle, vessels, and glands of the lower genital and urinary tracts all receive sympathetic and parasympathetic innervation through the pelvic, uterovaginal, and vaginal visceral nerve plexuses. Sympathetic input comes from the $T_{11}-L_2$ spinal cord segments, through the superior hypogastric plexus and the hypogastric nerves; parasympathetic input is provided from the S_{2-4} cord segments through the pelvic splanchnic nerves. A wide variety of transmitters and transmitter markers have been localized to nerve fibers and/or ganglion cells in components of this network, including vesicular acetylcholine transporter,[6] vasoactive intestinal polypeptide,[14,16] neuropeptide Y,[14,16] tyrosine hydroxylase,[14] calcitonin-gene-related peptide,[6,14] substance P,[6,14] and neural nitric oxide synthase.[6] However, as will become evident, there is at present no comprehensive picture of the distribution and actions of these transmitters in the target tissues.

Blood vessels in the cervix and vagina are innervated by nerve fibers containing acetylcholine,[13] vasoactive intestinal polypeptide,[13,16] neuropeptide Y,[13,16,17] and noradrenaline. Those in the vagina also receive fibers immunoreactive for neural nitric oxide synthase and calcitonin-gene-related peptide.[11] Physiologic studies in humans and rabbits[17,18] have demonstrated that noradrenaline constricts the vessels, and vasoactive intestinal polypeptide relaxes them. Neuropeptide Y, a weak vasoconstrictor by itself, potentiates the effect of noradrenaline by inhibiting vasoactive intestinal polypeptide-induced vasodilation. Vaginal hemodynamics are of major importance because vaginal lubrication depends largely on transudation of fluid across the lining epithelium. The fact that many subepithelial capillaries are innervated is therefore of interest, and Hoyle et al.[11] have suggested that neuropeptides may regulate capillary permeability. The vaginal plexus also contains many neural nitric oxide synthase-immunoreactive nerve fibers,[6] and some of these find their way into the vaginal wall.[11] Although their targets in the vagina are unclear at present, the vascular system is a likely possibility given that nitric oxide is a potent vasodilator in erectile tissue.[15] The significance of calcitonin-gene-related peptide in regulation of vaginal blood flow is unknown.

Although the vagina itself is devoid of glands, secretory activity of cervical glands, which contribute to vaginal lubrication, is promoted by parasympathetic innervation.

Nerve fibers containing neuropeptide Y and vasoactive intestinal polypeptide have been described among fascicles of nonvascular smooth muscle in the cervix and vagina. These are indicative of innervation by sympathetic and parasympathetic systems, respectively.

Urethra

The urethra receives visceral motor nerve fibers from the vaginal plexus and somatic nerve fibers from the sacral plexus.

The "urethral continence mechanism" involves striated as well as smooth muscle. The intrinsic (involuntary) element consists of inner, longitudinal and outer, circular layers of smooth muscle fibers that are continued downward from the detrusor muscle in the bladder neck. The external sphincter (sphincter urethrae or rhabdosphincter) consists of striated muscle fibers that encircle the urethra outside the circular layer of smooth muscle, with which they are blended. The voluntary *sphincter urethrae* has long been described as a planar ring of striated muscle lying on the upper surface of the perineal membrane. This view is outdated, but although modern accounts agree that an investment of striated muscle ascends along the urethra, they disagree as to how far it extends and where it is best developed.[8,9,16]

Visceral motor outflow enters the upper and middle thirds of the urethral wall in branches of the vaginal plexus.[6,9] The intrinsic smooth muscle coat is permeated by a rich network of nerve fibers. Most are cholinergic and relatively few contain noradrenaline. This pattern resembles that of the detrusor, which is stimulated by acetylcholine and relaxed by noradrenaline. Yucel et al.[6] have traced vesicular acetylcholine transporter-immunoreactive and neural nitric oxide synthase-immunoreactive fibers from the vaginal plexus into the muscle coat of the proximal urethra, and nitric oxide has been implicated in the relaxion of human detrusor muscle and urethral smooth muscle in a variety of animals.[20] Somatic motor fibers enter the middle and lower thirds of the urethral wall through fine twigs from the perineal branch of the pudendal nerve. These are cholinergic and are destined for striated muscle of the rhabdosphincter.[6,9] A number of authors report the existence of an intrapelvic somatic motor pathway to the external sphincter as well.[8,19] These paths, all beginning in one way or another from the S_{2-4} ventral primary rami, are linked with the intrapelvic somatic innervation of levator ani. Again, they may represent normal individual variability and should not necessarily be discounted. However, recent studies employing computer-assisted 3-D reconstructions have failed to show any nerves descending from the pelvic cavity into the external sphincter.[6,9] One of these studies, that of Yucel et al.,[6] is especially telling, because the authors were able to distinguish between visceral fibers (branches of the vaginal plexus) that were neural nitric oxide synthase-immunoreactive and somatic fibers (branches of the pudendal nerve) that were not.

The human female is supplied with small periurethral glands. They are especially prevalent in the caudal third of the urethra, where, on each side, a larger group is drained by a common duct opening into the vestibule lateral to the urethral orifice. These are the paraurethral – or Skene's – glands, which are gaining recognition as the "female prostate".[21,22] Little is

usually said in the literature or in textbooks about the innervation of the urethral glands or blood vessels, but presumably they are regulated by the same mixture of adrenergic, cholinergic, and neural nitric oxide synathase-positive fiber types known to enter the urethral wall from the vaginal plexus.

The clitoris and bulbs of the vestibule

In the erectile tissues, parasympathetic stimulation results in arterial dilation leading to engorgement and erection; sympathetic stimulation, on the other hand, is thought to terminate erection by constricting local vessels.

The clitoris receives the bulk of its visceral motor innervation through descending branches of the vaginal plexus – the cavernous nerves. Vesicular acetylcholine transporter, neural nitric oxide synthase, calcitonin-gene-related peptide, and substance P all have been localized to nerves in the clitoris and in the intrapelvic visceral plexuses. Yucel et al.[6] have shown recently that neural nitric oxide synthase-immunoreactive elements are not present in proximal branches of the pudendal nerve; instead, these presumptively vasodilator fibers are conveyed from the vaginal plexus in the cavernous nerves. Many pass directly to the corpus cavernosum and proximal body of the clitoris; others are added to the dorsal nerve for distribution along the shaft and to the glans. The density of neural nitric oxide synthase-positive nerve fibers in the glans is lower than in the corpora and clitoral body, but the level of endothelial nitric oxide synthase in vascular endothelium is proportionately higher.[15] The sympathetic outflow pathway to the clitoris is less well defined. The most obvious route involves the hypogastric nerves, pelvic visceral plexuses, and cavernous nerves, but the pudendal nerve provides branches to the corpus cavernosum and body of the clitoris from the dorsal nerve. Although these may well be sensory in nature, they might also carry postganglionic sympathetic fibers added to the sacral plexus through gray communicating rami from the sympathetic chain.

Little appears to have been written about the innervation of the bulb of the vestibule, but presumably the pattern is similar to that of the clitoris. Certainly, the cavernous nerves pass very close to the bulb as they descend along the lower urethra,[6,23] and the bulb receives a twig directly from the perineal branch of the pudendal nerve, which may carry sympathetic as well as sensory fibers.

Vestibular glands

Numerous small glands open into the vestibule, and on each side the greater vestibular gland (of Bartholin) lies in the connective tissue flanking the lower vagina. It is closely related to the caudal pole of the vestibular bulb, and its duct opens into the groove between the labium minus and the hymen. The vestibule itself is innervated largely by the perineal branch of the pudendal nerve, from which the greater vestibular gland receives a separate filament. Thus, the vestibular glands might receive postganglionic fibers added to the sacral ventral primary rami through gray communicating rami from the sympathetic chain. Little additional information is available, although the proximity of the cavernous nerves is suggestive.

Sources of sensory return

Sensory input is as important as motor outflow in sexual arousal, sexual pleasure, and orgasm, and such information comes from a variety of sources in the female perineum, external genitalia, vagina, cervix, and urethra. Some of these inputs are widely recognized and well understood; others are not.

Skin

The skin and subcutaneous tissues of the perineum and external genitalia are richly provided with touch, pressure, thermal, and pain receptors. Structurally, these can be classified as free nerve endings, endings associated with the hair follicles, endings associated with specialized epithelial cells (Merkle disks), and encapsulated endings (Pacinian corpuscles, Meissner's corpuscles, Ruffini corpuscles, bulbous corpuscles of Krause, and others). The density of innervation is especially high in the prepuce and on the dorsal surface of the glans. In summarizing the distribution of various nerve endings in the vagina and external genitalia, Krantz[24] noted a near absence of organized tactile receptors in the vestibule and clitoral body. This does not necessarily mean an absence of sensation, however, for cutaneous innervation is well documented in these areas, and subpopulations of free nerve endings are known to be responsive to light touch and temperature as well as to pain.[1] As a rule, such somatic sensory input is conveyed to the spinal cord by fibers in branches of the ilioinguinal (L_1), genitofemoral (L_{1-2}), and pudendal (S_{2-4}) nerves (Fig. 4.2.1).

The skin of the clitoris, glans, prepuce, labia minora, and vestibule presents a somewhat different picture. Here, in fetal human specimens, many nerve fibers have been shown to contain neural nitric oxide synthase in addition to the sensory transmitters calcitonin-gene-related peptide and substance P. The source of the calcitonin-gene-related peptide- and substance P-containing fibers has not been made clear, but those immunoreactive for neural nitric oxide synthase probably come through the vaginal plexus and cavernous nerves. Although there is no evidence that these nerves are sensory in nature, their presence seems to distinguish the skin in this region as distinct from that in the rest of the perineum.

Erectile tissues

Numerous branches of the perineal and dorsal clitoral nerves enter the substance of the clitoris and vestibular bulb as well as the clitoral tunica albuginea. Many if not all of these fibers are assumed to be sensory, and encapsulated mechanoreceptors have been found in the erectile tissues.

Vagina, cervix, and urethra

In the region of the introitus and hymen, the vagina is supplied with somatic sensory innervation through the perineal and inferior rectal branches of the pudendal nerve, whose fibers convey information from intraepithelial free nerve endings (pain) and scattered lamellated tactile endings in the submucosa.[12,24] Above the hymen, the vagina and cervix receive visceral sensory fibers through the uterovaginal and vaginal plexuses. Numerous free nerve endings and occasional lamellar corpuscles occur in the endocervix; the vaginal portion, which is relatively insensitive to ordinary pain but not to stretch, is supplied with a smaller complement of free endings.

The degree and quality of visceral vaginal sensation is a matter of controversy. Although usually described as relatively insensitive to pain and touch, the vagina is also proposed as the site of the G-spot, alleged to be a highly erogenous zone located roughly a third of the way up the anterior vaginal wall.[21,22] It is generally agreed that intraepithelial nerve terminals are rare in the vagina and that lamellated tactile endings are absent, except near the introitus. To some, this appears to rule out the existence of an entity such as the G-spot.[21] However, there is now good evidence for a rich plexus of nerves immediately beneath the vaginal epithelium and in the lamina propria, many of which are not associated with blood vessels.[11,12] A sizeable proportion of these small fibers contain sensory neurotransmitters (calcitonin-gene-related peptide, substance P, vasoactive intestinal polypeptide),[11] and, as already mentioned, subpopulations of free nerve endings are sensitive to stretch, light mechanical touch, temperature, and pain. Therefore, pressure applied to the vaginal wall may elicit sensory return in the absence of "typical" tactile receptors. Furthermore, it has been suggested that pain may be elicited indirectly from hollow organs, such as the vagina, when shear or other mechanical stress leads to release of ATP from the lining epithelium. The purine then would diffuse across the basal lamina and bind to specific receptors on subepithelial nociceptive sensory neurons.[25]

Input from sensory endings in adjacent structures must also be considered. For example, the urethra, which is virtually embedded in the anterior vaginal wall, also possesses a submucosal network of fine nerves derived from the vaginal plexus and is encircled by its voluntary external sphincter. Like the urethra and the anal canal, the vagina itself descends through the pelvic floor into the perineum. As it does so, it is flanked closely by striated muscle fibers of the levator ani, some of which blend with its distal wall (see Chapter 4.4 in this volume). Above the levator, the vagina is invested by endopelvic visceral fascia, and the posterior wall of the vaginal vault is covered by the peritoneum of the rectouterine pouch. Thus, distention or displacement of the vagina during sexual activity could be expected to stimulate muscle spindles and other proprioceptive endings in voluntary musculature, visceral stretch and pressure receptors in the pelvic peritoneum and extraperitoneal connective tissues, and quite possibly endings in the urethra, either directly or through release of serotonin from paracrine cells in the urethral wall. (For a more detailed analysis, see Levin.[26])

Central destinations of sensory input

Cutaneous sensation from the anterior urogenital region is carried to the upper lumbar spinal cord by the ilioinguinal and genitofemoral nerves. Sensory return from the remainder of the perineum, external genitalia, lower reproductive tract, and adjoining structures is carried centrally through either the pudendal nerve or the pelvic splanchnic nerves. Thus, somatic and visceral inputs converge on the S_{2-4} cord segments, where the information plays a crucial role in spinal reflexes and is directed upward to higher centers. Animal experiments, however, indicate that there may be an extraspinal sensory pathway to the brain,[27] and this is supported by reports that in some women, conscious awareness of genital stimulation persists despite severe spinal cord injury.[28] Although the vagus nerve has been suggested as the most likely extraspinal route, there is as yet no widely accepted anatomic evidence for this assumption.

Conclusion

From the above account, it can be seen that innervation of the *human female* perineum and lower reproductive tract is already fairly well documented in its broad outlines. It is also clear that recent studies using immunohistochemistry, computer-assisted reconstruction, and modern imaging technologies have made significant advances toward a more detailed understanding. There are, however, a number of areas that warrant concerted attention.

1. Courses of the intrapelvic neural pathways, so important to nerve-sparing surgical procedures, need to be more clearly defined. Although a great deal of information is available, it is scattered throughout the literature and is made less accessible owing to a lack of settled terminology. This is nowhere more evident than in descriptions of the intrapelvic "ligaments" and fascial planes that give passage to elements of the visceral nerve plexuses.
2. Mapping of the distribution of specific nerve fiber types needs to be completed. This work is already underway, but substantial gaps remain to be filled.
3. Functions of the different neurotransmitters need to be defined with greater precision, and this will have to involve localization of specific receptors in the tissues.
4. Finally, systematic studies are needed to characterize and map the distribution of sensory nerve terminals, especially in the clitoris, vestibule, vagina, and urethra.

Acknowledgment

The author is grateful to Dr Trudy Van Houten for her generous advice and support.

References

1. Williams PL, Bannister LH, Berry MM et al. *Gray's Anatomy*, 38th British edn (rev.). New York: Churchill Livingstone, 1995.
2. Hollinshead WH. *Anatomy for Surgeons: Volume 2, The Thorax, Abdomen, and Pelvis*, 2nd edn. New York: Harper and Row, 1971.
3. Lockhart RD, Hamilton GF, Fyfe FW. *Anatomy of the Human Body*, 2nd rev. edn. London: Faber and Faber, 1969.
4. Huber GC, ed. *Human Anatomy*, 9th rev. edn. Philadelphia: JB Lippincott, 1930.
5. Shafik A, Doss S. Surgical anatomy of the somatic terminal innervation to the anal and urethral sphincters: role in anal and urethral surgery. *J Urol* 1999; 161: 85–9.
6. Yucel S, De Souza A Jr, Baskin LS. Neuroanatomy of the human female lower urogenital tract. *J Urol* 2004; 172: 191–5.
7. Tamakawa M, Murakami G, Takashima K, Kato T, Hareyama M. Fascial structures and autonomic nerves in the female pelvis: a study using macroscopic slices and their corresponding histology. *Anat Sci Int* 2003; 78: 228–42.
8. Borirakchanyavat S, Aboseif SR, Carroll PR, Tanagho EA, Lue TF. Continence mechanism of the isolated female urethra: an anatomical study of the intrapelvic somatic nerves. *J Urol* 1997; 158: 822–6.
9. Colleselli K, Stenzl A, Eder R et al. The female urethral sphincter: a morphological and topographical study. *J Urol* 1998; 160: 49–54.
10. Ball TP. The female urethral sphincter: a morphological and topographical study: editorial comment. *J Urol* 1998; 160: 54.
11. Hoyle CH, Stones RW, Robson T, Whitley K, Burnstock G. Innervation of vasculature and microvasculature of the human vagina by NOS and neuropeptide-containing nerves. *J Anat* 1996; 188: 633–44.
12. Hilliges M, Falconer C, Ekman-Ordeberg G, Johansson O. Innervation of the human vaginal mucosa as revealed by PGP 9.5 immunohistochemistry. *Acta Anat (Basel)* 1995; 153: 119–26.
13. Amenta F, Porcelli F, Ferrante F, Cavallotti C. Cholinergic nerves in blood vessels of the female reproductive system. *Acta Histochem* 1979; 65: 133–7.
14. Butler-Manuel SA, Buttery LD, A'Hern RP, Polak JM, Barton DP. Pelvic nerve plexus trauma at radical and simple hysterectomy: a quantitative study of nerve types in the uterine supporting ligaments. *J Soc Gynecol Invest* 2002 ; 9: 47–56.
15. Burnett AL, Calvin DC, Silver RI, Peppas DS, Docimo SG. Immunohistochemical description of nitric oxide synthase isoforms in human clitoris. *J Urol* 1997; 158: 75–8.
16. Blank MA, Gu J, Allen JM et al. The regional distribution of NPY-, PHM-, and VIP-containing nerves in the human female genital tract. *Int J Fertil* 1986; 31: 218–22.
17. Jorgensen JC, Sheikh SP, Forman A et al. Neuropeptide Y in the human female genital tract: localization and biological action. *Am J Physiol* 1989; 257: E220–7.
18. Jorgensen JC. Neuropeptide Y in mammalian genital tract: localization and biological action. *Dan Med Bull* 1994; 41: 294–305.
19. Hollabaugh RS, Steiner MS, Dmochowski RR. Neuroanatomy of the female continence complex: clinical implications. *Urology* 2001; 57: 382–8.

20. Zhou Y, Ling EA. Neuronal nitric oxide synthase in the neural pathways of the urinary bladder. *J Anat* 1999; 194: 481–96.

21. Hines TM. The G-spot: a modern gynecologic myth. *Am J Obstet Gynecol* 2001; 185: 359–62.

22. Zaviacic M, Ablin RJ. The G-spot. *Am J Obstet Gynecol* 2002; 187: 519–20.

23. O'Connell HE, Hutson JM, Anderson CR, Plenter RJ. Anatomical relationship between urethra and clitoris. *J Urol* 1998; 159: 1892–7.

24. Krantz KE. Anatomy of the female reproductive system. In AH DeCherney, ML Pernoll, eds. *Current Obstetric and Gynecologic Diagnosis and Treatment*, 8th edn. East Norwalk: Appleton & Lange, 1994: ch 2.

25. Burnstock G. Release of vasoactive substances from endothelial cells by shear stress and purinergic mechanosensory transduction. *J Anat* 1999; 194: 335–42.

26. Levin RJ. The mechanism of human female sexual arousal. In Bancroft J, ed. *Annual Review of Sex Research*, vol 3. Society for the Scientific Study of Sex, 1992: 1–48.

27. Guevara-Guzman R, Buzo E, Larrazolo A, de la Riva C, Da Costa AP, Kendrick KM. Vaginocervical stimulation-induced release of classical neurotransmitters and nitric oxide in the nucleus of the solitary tract varies as a function of the oestrus cycle. *Brain Res* 2001; 898: 303–13.

28. Komisaruk BR, Gerdes CA, Whipple B. 'Complete' spinal cord injury does not block perceptual responses to genital self-stimulation in women. *Arch Neurol* 1997; 54: 1513–20.

4.3 Histology and immunohistochemical studies of female genital tissue

Emmanuele A Jannini, Giulia d'Amati, Andrea Lenzi

Introduction

While the anatomy, pathophysiology, and possible therapies of male sexual response have been extensively explored in recent years, little and discordant information has been produced for the female counterpart. However, scattered but interesting reports of female functional anatomy are now being published, and useful animal models are now available.[1] This chapter considers the three anatomic structures mainly involved in sexual female arousal: the clitoris, vagina, and urethra. Discussion of histologic and immunohistochemical findings may provide important insights into female sexual pathophysiology and therapy.

In the classic Masters and Johnson description of human sexual response, the excitation phase consists of female lubrication.[2]

The clitoris

Masters and Johnson found the macroanatomy of the clitoris to be quite variable.[2] They described women with a long, thin shaft surmounted by a relatively small glans, and those with a short, thick shaft with a rather large glans, with numerous variations and combinations. A study of 200 women revealed that clitoris length varies by more than 25%,[3] demonstrating that individual differences are macroanatomic. It has only recently been clearly demonstrated by gross anatomy techniques that the clitoris consists of an erectile tissue complex surrounding the urethra and embedding the anterior vaginal wall.[4] This is of particular physiologic interest considering the role of this region in the sexual response.

The microscopic anatomy of the clitoris is consistent among different subjects. It consists of cavernous tissue, encircled by a thin fibrous capsule surrounded by large nerve trunks. Its cavernosal tissue consists of trabecular smooth and connective tissues, which encase the cavernosal sinusoidal spaces. The nerve network distribution pattern was studied by S-100 and neuron-specific enolase-immunoreactivity[5] (Fig. 4.3.1). The findings demonstrate that tissue organization in the corpora cavernosa of the clitoris is tunica albuginea and erectile tissue. There is a strong link between an increase in age and a subsequent decrease in clitoral cavernosal smooth muscle fibers with a relative increase of cavernosal connective tissue, as measured by histomorphometry.[6] Vascular risk factors and/or low estrogen levels, important in the pathophysiology of age-associated female sexual arousal disorders, may adversely affect clitoral cavernosal fibrosis.

Table 4.3.1 shows the immunohistochemical substances found in the clitoris and vagina of humans and experimental animals. Recent data from Burnett et al. showed the presence of nitric oxide-synthase isoforms in the human clitoris, suggesting that nitric oxide may be involved in its erectile physiology as a modulator of smooth muscle activity.[7] Findings of phosphodiesterase type 5 activity in human clitoral tissue support this theory (Fig. 4.3.2).[8]

The vagina

The vagina is a fibromuscular virtual tube, designed as the female copulatory organ. It extends from the vestibule, between

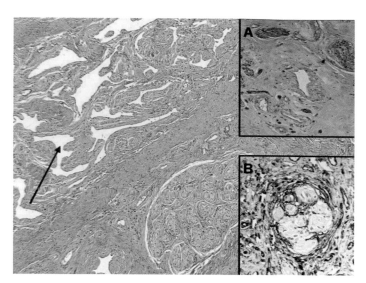

Figure 4.3.1. Human clitoris – specimens in these figures were obtained at autopsy from phenotypically normal premenopausal women aged 23–39 years. The cavernosum tissue (upper left, arrow) is surrounded by nerve fibers. Haematoxylin and eosin (HE) staining, ×5. Insert A shows immunostaining with the neuronal specific antibody to S100, demonstrating the abundant presence of nervous fibers (×10). Insert B is a section stained with the endothelial marker CD31, showing the presence of small vessels (×10). All the figures in the chapter are original, unpublished pictures obtained in our laboratory.

the labia minora, and the uterus, the anterior urethra and bladder, and the posterior anal canal and rectum.[9] Depending on rectum and bladder content, the vagina describes a 90° angle with respect to the uterus axis, ascending posterosuperiorly. Considered as a parallelepiped, the vagina is composed of a *posterior* wall, separated from the rectum by the rectouterine

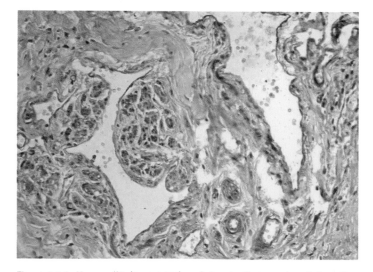

Figure 4.3.2. Human clitoris – expression of phosphodiesterase type 5. Smooth muscle cells within the vessels of the cavernous tissue show a diffuse cytoplasmic stain. To our knowledge, this original figure is the first published showing the immunohistochemical distribution of phosphodiesterase within the human clitoris. ×20. For material and methods, see [10].

pouch and from the anal canal by the fibromuscular structure of the perineal body. The *lateral* walls are the pelvic fascia and the muscle *levator ani*. From a sexologic point of view, the most important is the *anterior* vaginal wall, under the clitoris, in which the urethra and clitoral bodies are embedded.

Microscopic examination reveals that the vaginal structure comprises (1) the inner mucosal epithelial stratum, (2) a lamina propria containing thin-walled veins, (3) the intermediate muscularis stratum, and (4) the external adventitial layer. The *inner mucosal epithelial stratum* adheres strictly to the muscular stratum. Its nonkeratinized squamous epithelium is raised by two median, anterior and posterior, longitudinal ridges, between which are the *rugae* divided by sulci of variable depth, the *vaginal columns*. These conical papillae, most numerous close to the orificium and in the posterior wall, are less developed after natural parturition. Furthermore, the mucosal epithelium is hormone-dependent (estrogen) and changes during the menstrual cycle, having the potential for a basal, nonsexual, moisture. This basal lubrication is usually not sufficient for painless penetration: the vagina needs an enhancement of lubrication for coitus. The epithelium thickens after puberty and is rich in glycogen, mostly during ovulation. Glycogen is fermented by Döderlein's bacillus, lowering the vaginal pH. The *lamina propria* of the mucosa contains blood vessels contributing to the diffusion of the vaginal fluid across the epithelium, elastic fibers, lymphatic vessels, and nerves. It is a labyrinthine pathway, across which the neurogenically stimulated transudate filters during sexual arousal. An external longitudinal and an internal circular layer of nonstriated muscularis myocells, connected by oblique decussating fasciculi, make up the strong muscular stratum. The muscularis is composed of autonomically innervated smooth muscle fibers, containing a great variety of transmitters. For the majority of these compounds, the function is still unclear. The adventitia is rich in collagen and elastic fibers, giving structural support to the vaginal wall and allowing expansion during coitus and labor. The striated muscle bulbospongiosus surrounds the first third of the vagina. (Fig. 4.3.3.)

In evaluating the histology of the human vagina, three concepts should be considered: individual differences (accounting for many discrepancies in the scientific literature), locoregional differences between anterior and posterior vagina, and the fact that the vagina and its histology are hormone-dependent, and thus cyclic.

The microscopic anatomy of the human vagina's anterosuperior wall differs among subjects. The presence of pseudo-cavernous tissue (clitoral bulb) in the anterior vaginal mucosa is a frequent, but not universal finding (86%).[10] This anatomic variability should be taken in account when evaluating the physiology, pathology, and possible medical treatments of female sexual response. In the rabbit vagina, there are regional and functional differences. Adrenergic agonists in all regions can induce the contractile response, while prominent nerve-mediated relaxation can be identified only in the lower third.[11] Interestingly, this response is inhibited by the nitric oxide synthase inhibitor N-Ω-nitro-L-arginine methyl ester (NAME)

Table 4.3.1. Histologic findings in the clitoris and vagina

Factor	Tissue	Animal	Function/localization	Reference
NOS	Clitoris Vagina	Human Rabbit Mouse Pig Cow	Neurotransmission, blood flow control, and capillary permeability	19, 20, 22, 30, 33, 41
nNOS	Clitoris Vagina	Human Rat Rabbit	Nerve fibers supplying smooth muscle, perivascular nerve plexuses, lamina propria	7, 31–33, 40, 42
eNOS	Clitoris Vagina	Human Rat Rabbit	Vascular endothelium, perivascular smooth muscle	7, 31, 32, 34, 40, 41
iNOS	Vagina	Human	Production of NO under certain conditions	32
PDE5	Clitoris Vagina Skene's glands	Human Rabbit	Breakdown of cGMP. Decrease of sexual arousal	8, 10, 32, 44
CGRP	Vagina Clitoris	Human Pig	Neurotransmission, blood flow control, and capillary permeability	18, 19, 22
SP	Clitoris Vagina	Human Pig Cow	Neurotransmission, blood flow control, and capillary permeability	18, 20, 22
NPY	Clitoris Vagina	Human Pig	Neurotransmission, blood flow control, and capillary permeability	18, 19, 21, 22
Estrogen receptors	Distal vagina	Rabbit	Downregulation of NOS	39
Androgen receptors	Proximal Vagina	Rabbit	Facilitation of vaginal smooth muscle relaxation	39
TGFβ1	Vagina	Diabetic rat	Fibrosis	26
VIP	Clitoris Vagina	Human Cat Rat Guinea pig Goat Hen Pig	Smooth muscle relaxation, neurotransmission, blood flow control, and capillary permeability	14–16, 18–20, 22, 29
PSA	Skene's glands	Human	Prostatic marker	51, 52, 54, 57
PAP	Skene's glands	Human	Prostatic marker	52, 53, 57
UP1	Skene's glands	Human	Protection of uroepithelium?	59
Chromogranin	Skene's glands	Human Pig	Marker of neurosecretion	32, 58

cGMP: cyclic guanosine monophosphate; CGRP: calcitonin gene-related peptide; NO: nitric oxide; NOS: nitric oxide synthase; NPY: neuropeptide Y; PAP: prostatic acid phosphatase; PDE5: phosphodiesterase type 5; PSA: prostate-specific antigen; SP: substance P; TGF: transforming growth factor; UP1: urine protein 1; VIP: vasoactive intestinal protein.

and by D-vasoactive intestinal peptide. In the human fetal vagina, adrenergic innervation is most prominent in the cranial portion and decreases toward the vestibulum.[12] These locoregional differences have been attributed to differences in embryologic origin. In fact, the lower third of the human vagina is derived from the urogenital sinus and the Wolffian duct, while the rest arises from the Müllerian structure.[13]

Vasoactive intestinal peptide has been previously considered as involved in vaginal vasodilation, the prerequisite for vaginal lubrication.[14–16] It is present in the nerves closely applied to blood vessels in the vaginal wall, and its systemic or local administration increases vaginal blood flow and induces vaginal fluid production (see[17], and references therein). However, vasoactive intestinal peptide-ergic fibers are distributed in the clitoris[18] and

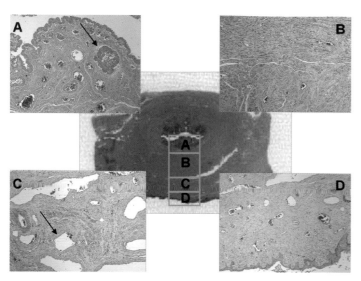

Figure 4.3.3. Human vagina – the central section is obtained by cutting the entire anterior vaginal wall. The urethra (A) was removed intact by sharp dissection. Specimens included periurethral tissue attached to the anterior vaginal mucosa (D). The vagina was then excised and opened along the posterior wall. The inserts are sections obtained at the levels indicated. Insert A: urothelium covering the lamina propria with numerous large vessels and an exocrine (Skene's) gland. Insert B: intermediate muscular stratum. Insert C: lamina propria of vagina with corpora cavenosa (clitoral bulb). Insert D: inner mucosal stratum of vagina covered by the vaginal epithelium. Inserts ×5.

in the animal[19,20] and human vagina to a lower extent than neuropeptide Y (NPY) (also present in the clitoris[21]), but more extensively than calcitonin gene-related peptide (CGRP) and substance P (SP).[22] These results imply that nerves that utilize neuropeptide Y, vasoactive intestinal peptide, or calcitonin gene-related peptide as a neurotransmitter may play a role in controlling blood flow and capillary permeability in the vagina. In fact, vasoactive intestinal peptide administration, both intravenously and by subepithelial injection in the vaginal wall, increases blood flow and induces lubrication.[15]

A possible alternative avenue for the treatment of erectile dysfunction has recently been found in the calcium-sensitizing ρ-A/Rho-kinase pathway, which, together with norepinephrine and endothelin, plays a synergistic role in cavernosal vasoconstriction to maintain penile flaccidity. In fact, in animal studies, its pharmacologic antagonism with Y-27632 results in increased corpus cavernosum pressure, initiating erection independently of nitric oxide.[23] The same compound elicits relaxation of the rabbit vaginal wall and clitoral corpus cavernosum.[24]

Diabetes may induce lack of vaginal lubrication.[25] The smooth muscle profibrotic transforming growth factor (TGF) β_1 is expressed in diabetic rats, but not in normal animals, suggesting its involvement in diabetes-induced female sexual dysfunction.[26] Receptors for TGF β have been detected in rabbit clitoral smooth muscle cell cultures along with androgen and estrogen receptors.[27]

The nitric oxide–cyclic guanosine monophosphate (cGMP)–phosphodiesterase type 5 pathway is an important, if not the primary, regulator of vaginal hemodynamics.[28] Hen,[29] mouse,[30] and rat[31] vaginal muscular wall contains abundant nitric oxide synthase-reactive nerve fibers running parallel to the smooth muscle bundles and beneath the epithelium. Nitric oxide synthase isoforms are largely distributed in the vagina of humans[10,32] and experimental animals.[33] A distinct distribution of immunoreactivity for nitric oxide synthase isoforms has been demonstrated in the human vagina.[32] In all subjects, the nerve bundles and fibers coursing within the organ were positive for the constitutive isoforms of nitric oxide synthase (neuronal and endothelial). These isoforms were also present in the endothelial lining of sinusoids and blood vessels and in the vaginal epithelium. Furthermore, neuronal (Fig. 4.3.4) and endothelial (Fig. 4.3.5) nitric oxide synthase isoforms have been found in the smooth muscle of the cavernous erectile tissue of the anterior wall of the vagina. In particular, endothelial nitric oxide synthase S has been found in the stratified squamous epithelial lining and in smooth cells, with maximum expression in experimental animals during estrus and proestrus.[34] This suggests that nitric oxide may be involved in vaginal secretion. Surprisingly, the inducible nitric oxide synthase isoform was found expressed in the human vagina, mostly in the epithelium and focally in smooth muscle.[32] To confirm this finding, the inducible nitric oxide synthase antibody was tested for in cells harvested *in vivo* from the anterior wall of a volunteer's vagina. These cells were found to be highly positive. While specific immunoreactivity for inducible nitric oxide synthase was not demonstrated within clitoridal specimens, it is present mostly in the vaginal epithelium and in the smooth muscle cells. Since inducible nitric oxide synthase is stimulated by bacterial products,[35] the presence of this inflammatory isoform may be due to normal bacterial flora in the human vagina. The presence of inducible nitric

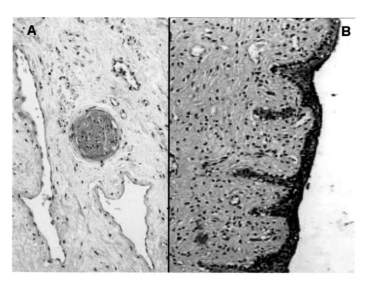

Figure 4.3.4. Human vagina (anterior wall) – staining of neuronal nitric oxide synthase with a specific commercial antibody. In panel A, a single nerve fiber is strongly positive, close to the lacunae of sinusoids. ×25. Panel B shows that the enzyme is also present in the vaginal epithelium ×10.

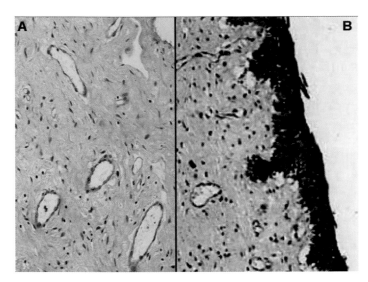

Figure 4.3.5. Human vagina (anterior wall) – staining of endothelial nitric oxide synthase with a specific commercial antibody. Endothelial lumen of sinusoids (panel A) and the vaginal epithelium (panel B) are strongly positive. ×20.

oxide synthase may imply that the human vagina can produce nitric oxide under certain conditions. Vaginal smooth muscle is stained by constitutive nitric oxide synthase, as are smooth muscle fibers of other tissues.[36] The presence of neuronal nitric oxide synthase in nerves suggests that this isoform produces nitric oxide as a postganglionic neurotransmitter mediating smooth muscle relaxation in the nitric oxide synthase-rich corpora cavernosa. The abundance of endothelial nitric oxide synthase suggests its prominent role in female sexual response. Endothelial nitric oxide synthase was mostly localized in the endothelial lining of sinusoids and blood vessels throughout the erectile tissue of the vaginal anterior wall. Both those findings mirror the anatomic scenario found in the human clitoris,[7] with some exceptions. The distribution of nitric oxide synthase isoforms partially supports the recently found relationship between the urethra and clitoris: gross anatomy techniques have demonstrated that the female perineal urethra is embedded in the anterior vaginal wall and surrounded by erectile tissue forming the bulbs of the clitoris.[4] The anterior vaginal wall thus contains the clitoral bulbs, but it is probably much richer in nitric oxide synthase than the clitoris itself.

Nitric oxide synthase expression and activity are under steroid hormone regulatory activity. In fact, androgens and female steroids modulate distinct physiologic responses in the vagina. Progesterone upregulates vaginal nitric oxide synthase.[37] Although estrogen treatment reduced total nitric oxide synthase activity in the proximal vagina, estrogens are known to enhance vaginal blood flow.[38] Androgens facilitate vaginal smooth muscle relaxation through their own receptor localized in the proximal vagina, while estrogen downregulates nitric oxide synthase activity in the distal vagina.[39]

This paradoxical observation has been explained by differential, locoregional (distal with respect to proximal vagina)

regulation of estrogen receptors. Both neuronal and endothelial nitric oxide synthase are under estrogen control. In fact, after oophorectomy, levels of both enzymes decline, with a parallel induction of apoptosis, vaginal atrophy, intramural collagen accumulation, and perivascular wall thickening.[40] However, these results have not been replicated in other experimental models.[41,42]

Treatment with sildenafil enhances intracellular cyclic cGMP synthesis and accumulation of cultured human and rabbit vaginal smooth muscle cells.[43] This suggests that vaginal smooth muscle expresses phosphodiesterase type 5. Immunoreactivity for phosphodiesterase type 5 partially followed the distribution of nitric oxide synthase isoforms. In fact, it was observed focally in the endothelial lining and smooth muscle of the anterior vaginal wall's cavernous erectile tissue, and was widespread in the vaginal epithelium. The immunocytochemistry of vaginal cells harvested in vivo confirmed the latter finding. No staining of nerve bundles was observed and, considering the vagina as a whole, phosphodiesterase type 5 expression was low, confirming the focal expression of this enzyme.[44] The colocalization of phosphodiesterase type 5 in the tissues considered as bona fide targets for nitric oxide (epithelia, exocrine glands, and muscle) may warrant the breakdown of cGMP produced locally upon nitric oxide stimulation.

The demonstrated presence of the nitric oxide synthase–phosphodiesterase type 5 machinery in the human clitoris and vagina is the anatomic rationale for the use of phosphodiesterase type 5 inhibitors in female sexual arousal disorders, defined by the Consensus Panel of the American Foundation of Urological Diseases as the persistent inability to attain or maintain sexual excitement (lubrication/swelling).[45] Sildenafil has been found capable of antagonizing the sexual discomforts induced by antidepressant drugs,[46] as well as of partially reversing sexual dysfunction in women with spinal cord injuries.[47] In a double-blind, crossover, placebo-controlled study performed in young women affected by arousal disorders, sildenafil was demonstrated to improve sexual performance significantly,[48] a result which has been subsequently replicated.[49]

The urethra

The female urethra from the bladder to the orifice is about 4 cm long, with a diameter of 6 mm. It runs anteroinferiorly behind the symphysis pubis, embedded in the anterior vaginal wall. The mucous membrane lining the lumen is a stratified epithelium under the lamina propria of fibroelastic connective tissue. Its proximal section is a transitional urothelium identical to that of the bladder neck, while the distal section changes into a nonkeratinizing, stratified squamous epithelium. The muscular coat is composed of both the striated, external urethral sphincter and an inner coat of abundant smooth muscles, oriented obliquely or longitudinally.

The female urethra is surrounded by numerous sinusoids (corpus spongiosus of urethra). However, individual differences have been found in the presence and extension of these venous/sinous channels.[10,32] In the luminal epithelium, serotonin-producing cells have been detected. Mechanical stimulation of the urinary urethra converts it into the "sexual" urethra, possibly by the releasing of 5-hydroxytryptamine (5-HT), which enhances neural afferent input from the organ.

Skene's glands

Classic anatomic textbooks fail in careful and exact description of the macro- and microanatomy of the female genital tract.[4] *Gray's Anatomy* summarily and inexactly describes the urethral glands (Fig. 4.3.6) and the minute, pit-like recesses (lacunae) opening into the urethral lumen. Some of these glands are grouped together and may open in two symmetric, paraurethral ducts, on the lateral margin of the external urethral orifice. However, numerous ducts open independently in the urethra, coming from glandular acini with both exocrinal and endocrinal activity.[50] In 1672, the Dutch anatomist Regnier de Graaf illustrated a set of glands and ducts surrounding the female urethra. Later, in 1880, Alexander Skene redirected attention to this structure, giving his name to these glands and ducts.[51]

Histomorphologically, Skene's glands (Fig. 4.3.7) strongly resemble the male prostate before puberty.[52] In many cases, they remain immature throughout life because of a lack of androgenic stimulus. However, when they appear more mature and with high secretory activity, this could be due to the absolute or relative overpresence of androgens during a certain time of life. They are surrounded by a nonglandular contractile system, composed of smooth muscle cells and/or muscolofibrosus

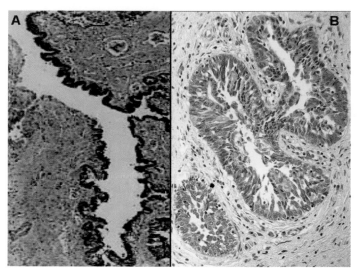

Figure 4.3.7. Skene's glands – panel A: staining with antiendothelial nitric oxide synthase antibody (×25). Panel B: staining with an anti-phosphodiesterase type 5 antibody, showing a diffuse cytoplasmatic positivity (×20).

tissue.[53] The complex Skene's glands smooth muscle is strongly stained when nitric oxide synthase and phosphodiesterase type 5 antibodies are used (Fig. 4.3.8),[10,32] suggesting that upon sexual stimuli the tonus and congestion of the complex may contribute to evacuation of the exocrine glandular product. The immunohistochemical profile of Skene's glands is similar to that of the male prostate.[54,55] These glands and ducts are embedded in a fibrous muscular stroma that is more abundant than in the male prostate, and rich in nerves and blood vessels. Skene's glands are thought to be the principal source of prostate-specific antigen (PSA) in the fluid of the so-called female ejaculate produced

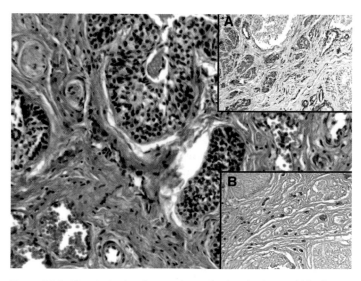

Figure 4.3.6. Skene's glands – the exocrine-endocrine glands are within the anterior vaginal wall, surrounded by fibromuscolar stroma (insert A, stained with muscular actin antibody) and vessels (insert B, stained with S100 antibody). HE staining ×10.

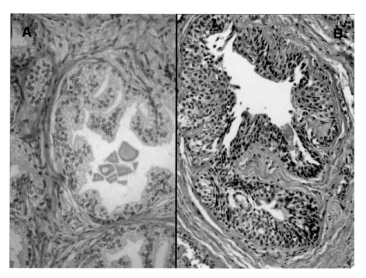

Figure 4.3.8. Prostate – comparison between histology of a male prostatic acinus (panel A) and Skene's glands (panel B). Note the microanatomic identities. HE staining ×10.

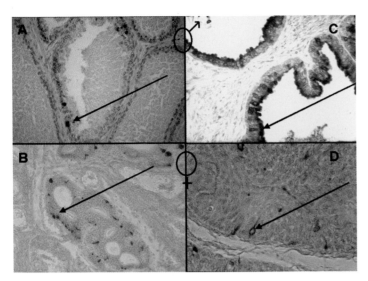

Figure 4.3.9. Prostate – expression of prostatic-specific factors in normal male prostate (panels A and C) and in Skene's glands (panels B and D). Panels A and B are stained with the neuroendocrine marker chromogranin A (arrow). Panel B shows the intense staining with prostate-specific antigen (arrow) and panel C the focal distribution of the same antigen in the Skene's glands. ×10.

during direct stimulation of the anterior vaginal wall.[56] Immunohistochemical evidence for prostatic markers, such as prostate specific antigen,[52,54,57] prostatic acid phosphatase (PAP),[52,54] bombesin, and chromogranin,[58] in Skene's glands supports this hypothesis (Fig. 4.3.9). Urine protein 1 (UP1), found throughout the male prostate, is also present at high levels in human Skene's glands.[59] Steroid hormones are the putative regulators of Skene's glands differentiation: estrogen receptor-associated protein (ER-D5) was found in the glands,[52] but the presence of androgen receptors needs to be investigated.

The ultrastructure of normal adult human Skene's glands has been studied by Zaviačiač et al.[60] Cells are tall, cylindrical, and secretory, with short stubby microvilli, a protuberance of the apical cytoplasm, and bleb formation. The glands display mature secretory and basal cells. The complexity of the biochemical apparatus and enzymatic equipment expressed in Skene's glands makes it unlikely that they are embryonic vestiges,[61] as previously supposed.

In view of their possibly embryologic origin, expression of prostatic-specific markers, and hypothesized function during female orgasm (see later), it has been proposed to rename Skene's glands as *prostata feminina*, "the female prostate", following de Graff's original definition.[62] The inference from this definition is that the same diseases of the male prostate may occur in the female, such as carcinoma,[63] prostatitis,[64] and, possibly, benign hyperplasia. In fact, the quite frequent female urethral syndrome (retropubic pressure, dyspareunia, urinary frequency, and dysuria) is often diagnosed and treated as a male prostatitis.[64] Interestingly, the microscopic anatomy of the human anterior vaginal wall, as well the presence of the female prostate, shows considerable variability among examined

subjects.[32,54] Even immunostaining for PSA and PAP has been demonstrated to vary from 67% to 83%[52,54,57] of studied cases.

Microanatomy of the "G–Spot"

Within the vaginal wall, generally considered quite insensitive, a position relatively sensitive to electric stimuli can be detected at the 12 o'clock position (the anterior vaginal wall).[65] This area has been very controversial for more than half a century. The term "G-spot" was first used by two researchers, Beverly Whipple and John D Perry, to name the sensitive area felt through the anterior vaginal wall, halfway between the back of the pubic bone and the cervix, along the course of the urethra.[66] They referred to a 1950 paper describing this area by the gynecologist Ernst Gräfemberg.[67] Sexual stimulation of the G-spot can produce a variety of initial feelings: discomfort, sensation of urination, or pleasure. With additional stimulation, the area may begin to swell, and then produce an intense orgasm, possibly together with a semen-like (although less viscous) fluid emission, the so-called female ejaculation.[66] This is thought to be the product of Skene's glands.

More than 250 papers on this issue have been published, but only a few in peer-reviewed journals. This is one reason for skepticism. The existence of the G-spot was denied by Masters and Johnson: "Female ejaculation is an erroneous but widespread concept."[2] Furthermore, in a recent (and poorly researched) review article, Hines, of the Psychology Department of Pace University, New York, described the G-spot as a "a modern gynecologic myth".[68] Another reason for skepticism is that the presence of a functional G-spot is highly variable. By studying 48 coitally experienced volunteers, Alzate and Londoño found that the large majority, but not all, reported erotic sensitivity in the upper anterior wall.[69] Indeed, most women do not ejaculate, and this cannot be exclusively due to inexperience or partner incompetence. It may be due to the large differences in vaginal microanatomy among individuals.

Conclusion

Differences in histology and immunohistochemical findings between the clitoris and vagina are only apparent. Nitric oxide is the key pathway mediating clitoral and vaginal smooth muscle relaxation. However, its role in mediating vaginal muscularis smooth muscle relaxation has been considered controversial.[70] This apparent discrepancy should be considered in light of the evidence that, while the clitoris is a relatively homogeneous erectile tissue, vagina histology changes in function of its topography, which varies according to the different levels examined. The first third of the vagina should in fact be considered as continuous with the clitoris, as the clitoral bulb, an erogenous zone expressing the same biochemical mediators of arousal, such as nitric oxide synthase, vasoactive intestinal peptide, and phosphodiesterase, is embedded in it. In contrast, the remaining two-thirds appears almost devoid of sexually responsive structures. This justifies the traditional assumption of sexologic and anatomic literature that the vagina is almost inert in sexual response. Finally, the large interindividual histologic variability may account for these discrepancies. Given its manifest behavioral and clinical consequences, this evidence needs to be more deeply studied in future.

Anatomy studies normally precede physiology. While the anatomy of the penis and the biochemical and molecular regulation of erection are largely known, the exact anatomic description of the human clitoris was produced in 1998, the taxonomy of female sexual dysfunctions classified in 1999, and the biochemistry of female excitation described only in 2002. There are various reasons for this. Female sexual physiology is much more complex than that of the male, and cultural, political, and religious considerations have discouraged the scientific study of female sexuality. However, it is now evident that modern sexology cannot be truly called sexual medicine if female sexual anatomy and the physiology of female sexual response are unknown.

References

1. Kim SW, Jeong SJ, Munnarriz R et al. An *in vivo* rat model to investigate female vaginal arousal response. *J Urol* 2004; 171: 1357–61.

2. Master WH, Johnson VE. *Human sexual response*. Boston: Little Brown, 1966.

3. Verkauf BS, Von Thron J, O'Brien WF. Clitoral size in normal women. *Obstet Gynecol* 1992; 80: 41–4.

4. O'Connell HE, Hutson JM, Anderson CR, et al. Anatomical relationship between urethra and clitoris. *J Urol* 1998; 159: 1892–1897.

5. Toesca A, Stolfi VM, Cocchia D. Immunohistochemical study of the corpora cavernosa of the human clitoris. *J Anat* 1996; 188: 513.

6. Tarcan T, Park K, Goldstein I et al. Histomorphometric analysis of age-related structural changes in human clitoral cavernosal tissue. *J Urol* 1999; 161: 940–4.

7. Burnett AL, Calvin DC, Silver RI et al. Immunohistochemical description of nitric oxide synthase isoforms in human clitoris. *J Urol* 1997; 158: 75–8.

8. Park K, Moreland RB, Goldstein I et al. Sildenafil inhibits phosphodiesterase type 5 in human clitoral corpus cavernosum smooth muscle. *Biochem Biophys Res Commun* 1998; 249: 612–19.

9. Williams PL, Warwick R, Dyson M et al., eds. The reproductive organs of the female. In: *Gray's Anatomy*. Edinburgh: Churchill Livingstone, 1989: 1422–4, 1435–50.

10. d'Amati G, di Gioia CRT, Bologna M et al. Type 5 phosphodiesterase expression in the human vagina. *Urology* 2002; 60: 191–5.

11. Oh S-J, Hong SK, Kim SW et al. Histological and functional aspects of different regions of the rabbit vagina. *Int J Impot Res* 2003; 15: 142–50.

12. Owman CH, Rosengren E, Sjöberg N-O. Adrenergic innervation of the human female reproductive organs: a histochemical and chemical investigation. *Obstet Gynecol* 1967; 30: 763–73.

13. Maizels M. Normal and anomalous development of the urinary tract. In: Walsh PC, Retik AB, Vaughan Jr ED et al., eds. *Campbell's Urology*. Philadelphia: WB Saunders, 1998: 1545–1600.

14. Larsson LI, Fahrenkrug J, Shaffalitzky et al. Vasoactive intestinal polypeptide occurs in nerves of the female genitourinary tract. *Science* 1977; 197: 1374–5.

15. Levin RJ. VIP, vagina, clitoral and periurethral glans: an update on human female genital tract. *Exp Clin Endocrinol* 1991; 98: 61–9.

16. Ottesen B, Fahrenkrug J. Vasoactive intestinal polypeptide and other preprovasoactive intestinal polypeptide–derived peptides in the female and male genital tract: localization, biosynthesis, and functional and clinical significance. *Am J Obstet Gynecol* 1995; 172: 1615–31.

17. Wagner G. Aspects of genital physiology and pathology. *Semin Neurol* 1992; 12: 87–97.

18. Hauser–Kronberg C, Cheung A, Hacker GW et al. Peptidergic innervation in the human clitoris. *Peptides* 1999; 20: 539–43.

19. Lakomy M, Happola O, Majewski M et al. Immunohistochemical localization of neuropeptides in nerve fibers of the porcine vagina and uterine cervix. *Folia Histochem Cytobiol* 1994; 32: 167–75.

20. Majewski M, Sienkiewicz W, Kaleczyc J et al. The distribution and co-localization of immunoreactivity to nitric oxide synthase, vasoactive intestinal polypeptide and substance P within nerve fibers supplying bovine and porcine female genital organs. *Cell Tissue Res* 1995; 281: 445–64.

21. Cocchia D, Rende M, Toesca A et al. Immunohistochemical study of neuropeptide Y-containing nerve fibers in the human clitoris and penis. *Cell Biol Int Rep* 1990; 14: 865–75.

22. Hoyle CHV, Stones RW, Robson T et al. Innervation of vasculature and microvasculature of the human vagina by NOS and neuropeptide-containing nerves. *J Anat* 1996; 188: 633–40.

23. Jannini EA, Lenzi A, Wagner G. New perspectives in the pharmacology of erectile dysfunction. *Idrugs* 2003; 6: 1165–72.

24. Cellek S. The Rho-kinase inhibitor Y-27632 and the soluble guanylyl cyclase activator BAY41-2272 relax rabbit vaginal wall and clitoral corpus cavernosum. *Br J Pharmacol* 2003: 138: 287–90.

25. Bultrini A, Carosa E, Colpi EM et al. Possible correlation between type 1 diabetes mellitus and female sexual dysfunction: case report and literature review. *J Sex Med* 2004; 1: 337.

26. Park K, Ryu SB, Park YI et al. Diabetes mellitus induces vaginal tissue fibrosis by TGF-b1 expression in the rat model. *J Sex Marital Ther* 2001; 27: 577–87.

27. Sedeghi-Nejad H, Moreland RB, Traish AM et al. Preliminary report on the development and characterization of rabbit clitoral smooth muscle cell culture. *Int J Impot Res* 1998; 10: 165–9.

28. Kim SW, Jeong SJ Munarriz R et al. Role of the nitric oxide-cyclic GMP pathway in regulation of vaginal blood flow. *Int J Impot Res* 2003; 15: 355–61.

29. Costagliola A, Mayer B, Vittoria A et al. NADPH-diaphorase-, nitric oxide synthase- and VIP-containing nerve structures in the hen oviduct: a histochemical and immunohistochemical study. *Arch Histol Cytol* 1997; 60: 245–56.

30. Grozdanovic Z, Mayer B, Baumgarten HG et al. Nitric oxide synthase-containing nerve fibers and neurons in the genital tract of the female mouse. *Cell Tissue Res* 1994; 275: 355–60.

31. Giraldi A, Persson K, Werkstrom V et al. Effects on neurotrasmission in rat vaginal muscle. *Int J Impot Res* 2001; 13: 58–66.

32. d'Amati G, Di Gioia CRT, Proietti-Pannunzi L *et al.* Functional anatomy of the human vagina. *J Endocrinol Invest* 2003; 26 (Suppl 3): 92–6.

33. Al-Hijji J, Batra S. Down regulation by estrogen of nitric oxide synthase activity in the female rabbit low urinary tract. *Urology* 1999; 53: 637–42.

34. Chatterjee S, Gangula PR, Dong YL et al. Immunocytochemical localization of nitric oxide synthase-III in reproductive organs of female rats during oestrus cycle. *Histochem J* 1996; 28: 715–23.

35. Bogdan C. Of microbes, macrophages and nitric oxide. *Behring Inst Mitt* 1997; 99: 58–63.

36. Fleming I, Gray GA, Schott C et al. Inducible but not constitutive production of nitric oxide by vascular smooth cells. *Eur J Pharmacol* 1991; 200: 375–8.

37. Al-Hijji J, Larsson B, Batra S. Nitric oxide synthase in the rabbit uterus and vagina: hormonal regulation and functional significance. *Biol Reprod* 2000; 62: 1387–92.

38. Traish AM, Kim NN, Huang YH et al. Sex steroid hormones differentially regulate nitric oxide synthase and arginase activities in the proximal and distal rabbit vagina. *Int J Impot Res* 2003; 15: 397–404.

39. Traish AM, Kim N, Min K et al. Role of androgens in female genital sexual arousal: receptor expression, structure, and function. *Fertil Steril* 2002; 77 (Suppl 4): S11–S18.

40. Berman JR, McCarthy MM, Kyprianou N. Effect of estrogen withdrawal on nitric oxide synthase expression and apoptosis in the rat vagina. *Urology* 1998; 51: 650–6.

41. Batra S, Al-Hijji J. Characterization of nitric oxide synthase activity in rabbit uterus and vagina: downregulation by estrogen. *Life Sci* 1998; 62: 2093–2100.

42. Yoon HN, Chung WS, Park YY et al. Effects of estrogen on nitric oxide synthase and histological composition in the rabbit clitoris and vagina. *Int J Impot Res* 2001; 13: 205–11.

43. Traish A, Moreland RB, Huang YH et al. Development of human and rabbit vaginal smooth muscle cell cultures: effects of vasoactive agents on intracellular levels of cyclic nucleotides. *Mol Cell Biol Res Commun* 1999; 2: 131–7.

44. Morelli A, Filippi S, Mancina R et al. Androgens regulate phosphodiesterase type 5 expression and functional activity in corpora cavernosa. *Endocrinology* 2004; 145: 2253–63.

45. Berman JR, Berman L, Goldstein I. Female sexual dysfunction: incidence, pathophysiology, evaluation, and treatment options. *Urology* 1999; 54: 385–91.

46. Nurnberg HG, Lauriello L, Hensley PL et al. Sildenafil for iatrogenic serotonergic antidepressant medication induced sexual dysfunction in 4 patients. *J Clin Psychiatry* 1999; 60: 33–5.

47. Spiski ML, Rosen RC, Alexander CJ et al. Sildenafil effects on sexual and cardiovascular responses in women with spinal cord injury. *Urology* 2000; 55: 812–15.

48. Caruso S, Intelisano G, Lupo L et al. Premenopausal women affected by sexual arousal disorder treated with sildenafil: a double-blind, cross-over, placebo-controlled study. *Br J Obstet Gyn* 2001; 108: 623–8.

49. Berman JR, Berman LA, Toler SM et al. Safety and efficacy of sildenafil citrate for the treatment of female sexual arousal disorder: a double-blind, placebo controlled study. *J Urol* 2003; 170: 2333–8.

50. Huffman JW. The detailed anatomy of the paraurethral ducts in the human female. *Am J Obstet Gynecol* 1948; 55: 86–101.

51. Zaviačič M, Ablin RJ. The female prostate. *J Natl Cancer Inst* 1998; 90: 713–14.

52. Wernert N, Albrect M, Sesterhenn I et al. The "female prostate": location, morphology, immunohistochemical characteristics and significance. *Eur Urol* 1992; 22: 64–9.

53. Zaviačič M. Enzime histochemistry of the adult female prostate: acid phosphatase distribution. *Mol Cell Biol Res* 1984; 30: 545–51.

54. Pollen JJ, Dreilinger A. Immunohistochemical identification of prostatic acid phosphatase and prostate specific antigen in female periurethral glands. *Urology* 1984; 23: 303–7.

55. Di Sant'Agnese AP, De Mesy JKL. Endocrine-paracrine (APUD) cells of the human female urethra and paraurethral ducts. *J Urol* 1987; 137: 1250–4.

56. Zaviačič M. *The Human Female Prostate.* Bratislava: Slovack Academic Press, 1999.

57. Tepper SL, Jagirdar J, Heath D et al. Homology between the female paraurethral (Skene's) glands and the prostate. Immunohistochemical demonstration. *Arch Pathol Lab Med* 1984; 108: 423–5.

58. Czaja K, Sienkiewicz W, Vittoria A et al. Neuroendocrine cells in the female urogenital tract of the pig, and their immunohistochemical characterization. *Acta Anat* 1996; 157: 1119.

59. Zaviačič M, Danihel L, Ruzickova M et al. Immunohistochemical localization of human protein 1 in the female prostate (Skene's gland) and in the male prostate. *Histochemical J* 1997; 29: 219–27.

60. Zaviačič M, Jakubovska V, Belosovic M et al. Ultrastructure of the normal adult human female prostate gland (Skene's gland). *Anat Embryol (Berl)* 2000; 201: 51–61.

61. Zaviačič M. The adult human female prostata homologue and the male prostate gland: a comparative enzyme-histochemical study. *Acta Histochem* 1985; 77: 19–31.

62. Zaviačič M. The human female prostate and its role in woman's life: sexology implications. *Scand J Sexol* 2001; 4: 199–211.

63. Dodson MK, Cliby WA, Keeney GL et al. Skene's gland adenocarcinoma with increased serum level of prostate-specific antigen. *Gynecol Oncol* 1994; 55: 304–7.

64. Gittes RF. Female prostatitis. *Urol Clin North Am* 2002; 29: 613–16.

65. Weijmar Schultz WCM, van de Wield HBM, Klatter JA et al. Vaginal sensitivity to electric stimuli: theoretical and practical implications. *Arch Sex Behav* 1989; 18: 87–95.

66. Perry JD, Whipple B. Pelvic muscle strength of female ejaculators: evidence in support of a new theory of orgasm. *J Sex Res* 1981; 17: 22–39.

67. Gräfemberg E. The role of urethra in the female orgasm. *Int J Sexol* 1950; 3: 145–8.

68. Hines TM. The G-spot: a modern gynecologic myth. *Am J Obstet Gynecol* 2001; 185: 359–62.

69. Alzate H, Londoño ML. Vaginal erotic sensitivity. *J Sex Marital Ther* 1984; 10: 49–57.

70. Munarriz R, Kim SW, Kim NN et al. A review of the physiology and pharmacology of peripheral (vaginal and clitoral) female genital arousal in the animal model. *J Urol* 2003; 170 (2 Pt 2): S40–4.

4.4 Anatomy of the pelvic floor and pelvic organ support system

Trudy Van Houten

Introduction

The term "pelvic organ prolapse" encompasses a spectrum of debilitating medical conditions. Weakening or failure of the pelvic organ support system can lead to uterine prolapse, including emergence of the cervix through the labia minora; protrusion of portions of the urinary bladder, urethra, small intestine, or rectum through the vaginal wall; difficulty in evacuating the bladder or rectum; and, conversely, difficulty in maintaining urinary or fecal continence. Recent studies of the impact of these conditions on sexual function have adopted widely differing methodologies and have presented conflicting results. It seems intuitively certain, however, that for many patients, the discomfort, pain, and embarrassment associated with pelvic floor disorders significantly diminishes self-esteem and sexual enjoyment, if not sexual function.

Pelvic organ prolapse is a major health concern for older women, particularly postmenopausal women, but younger women may also be affected. Nygaard and colleagues concluded that some degree of prolapse is nearly ubiquitous in older women.[1] Tarnay and Bhatia estimate that urinary incontinence alone affects 13 million women in the USA.[2] Olsen and colleagues calculated an 11.1% lifetime risk of undergoing a single operation for pelvic organ prolapse and urinary incontinence.[3] The annual direct cost of urinary incontinence in the USA (in 1995 dollars) was estimated as $16.3 billion, including $12.4 billion (76%) for women and $3.8 billion (24%) for men.[4] The actual incidence of pelvic organ prolapse may also significantly exceed the reported incidence, and the number of women affected by pelvic floor disorders is also likely to increase sharply as longevity is extended and the population of aging women increases. The single greatest risk factor for pelvic organ prolapse is vaginal birth. Mant and colleagues found that a woman was four times more likely to develop prolapse after the birth of her first child, and 11 times more likely to develop prolapse with four or more deliveries.[5]

The effectiveness of surgical treatment for pelvic organ prolapse and urinary and fecal incontinence is difficult to evaluate but overall is discouraging. Olsen and colleagues estimate that 29% of women undergoing surgery for pelvic organ prolapse will require at least one reoperation, and that the time intervals between repeat procedures decreases with each subsequent reoperation.[3] In a retrospective study, Whiteside and colleagues found that 58% of women undergoing vaginal prolapse and incontinence surgery had recurrent prolapse at 1-year follow-up.[6] This finding suggests that recurrence rates for pelvic organ prolapse may be even higher than reoperation rates. Cundiff recently stated that the number of techniques currently advocated for treatment of rectocele is "another suggestion of less than optimal effectiveness for surgical intervention".[7] Tarnay and Bhatia identified 130 operative procedures for the treatment of female urinary stress incontinence, concluding that it is "not surprising that many of the procedures have not had long-term success".[2]

Recent magnetic resonance imaging (MRI) studies and three-dimensional modeling techniques provide a powerful new method for analyzing the anatomy of the pelvic floor.[8–13] However, profound difficulties with traditional descriptions of pelvic floor anatomy, the lack of a precise standardized terminology for describing the components of the pelvic organ support system, and the exuberant proliferation of unexplained synonyms in the literature make it difficult to compare, or even interpret, the findings from different imaging studies, surgical series, and laboratory dissections. It is even more challenging to assemble the rapidly accumulating data into a reliable and consistent body of knowledge useful for understanding the anatomic basis of pelvic organ prolapse, and effectively diagnosing and treating this condition.

The present discussion is a critical review of currently available information on the anatomy of the pelvic organ support system.

Normal anatomy of the pelvic organ support system

Overview

Maintaining the pelvic organs in their normal anatomic positions requires continual resistance to the forces of gravity and to increases in intra-abdominal pressure that occur during coughing, sneezing, urination, defecation, pregnancy, and delivery. The structures supporting the pelvic organs comprise an integrated system consisting of four basic components (Fig. 4.4.1).

1. *Pelvic bones, joints, and interosseous ligaments.* The bones of the pelvis, the joints uniting the pelvic bones, and the sturdy interosseous ligaments reinforcing the pelvic joints provide a rigid articulated framework surrounding the pelvic organs. The pelvic bones, joints, and interosseous ligaments also provide attachment sites for the midline connective tissue structures of the pelvic outlet, and for the muscles of the pelvic walls, pelvic floor, and perineum.

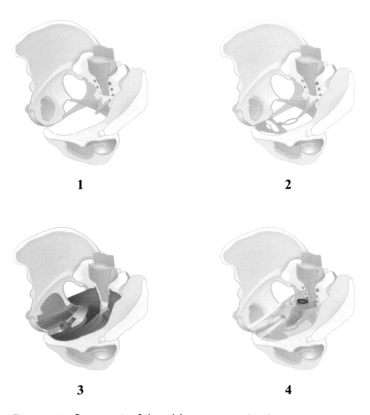

Figure 4.4.1. **Components of the pelvic organ support system.**
1 Pelvic bones, joints, and interosseous ligaments; 2 Midline connective tissue structures of the pelvic outlet; 3 Pelvic muscles and investing pelvic fascia; 4 Visceral pelvic fascia and visceral fascial ligaments.

2. *Midline connective tissue structures of the pelvic outlet.* The perineal membrane, perineal body, and anococcygeal ligament form a series of dense connective tissue structures bridging the pelvic outlet in the anteroposterior midline. The midline connective tissue structures resist downward movement of the pelvic contents and provide attachment sites for the muscles of the pelvic floor and perineum. Fibers of the muscles attaching to the midline connective tissue structures become interwoven with one another, and this web of muscle fibers reinforces the midline connective tissue structures.

3. *Pelvic muscles and investing pelvic fascia.* The muscles of the pelvic walls close apertures between the pelvic bones and ligaments, but the muscles of the pelvic floor are the active supports of the pelvic contents. The resting tone of the pelvic floor muscles supports the pelvic contents and resists their downward movement; contraction of the pelvic floor muscles helps increase intraabdominal pressure during Valsalva maneuvers. The medial muscles of the pelvic floor act in concert with the deep perineal muscles as the continence mechanisms of the urethra and vagina. The dense investing pelvic fascia invests the surfaces of the muscles of the pelvic walls and floor and blends with the periosteum of the pelvic bones. The investing pelvic fascia covering the pelvic walls condenses to form a sturdy tendinous arch that provides attachment for the muscles of the pelvic wall. The investing pelvic fascia covering the muscles of the pelvic floor condenses to form another sturdy tendinous arch that provides attachment for the visceral pelvic fascia anchoring the pelvic organs to the pelvic walls and floor. The presacral fascia covering the sacrum also anchors elements of the pelvic floor and the visceral pelvic fascia.

4. *Visceral pelvic fascia and visceral fascial ligaments.* The visceral pelvic fascia is a three-dimensional connective tissue layer, occupying the spaces between the pelvic organs, the investing pelvic fascia, and the peritoneum lining the abdominopelvic cavity. The visceral pelvic fascia forms a complex connective tissue scaffold between the pelvic organs and the pelvic walls, sacrum, and midline connective tissue structures of the pelvic outlet. The visceral pelvic fascia is highly variable in composition. In some areas, it is relatively amorphous; in other areas, it condenses into demonstrable ligaments. The rectovaginal septum has a different embryonic origin, but it forms an important part of the visceral fascial scaffold, reinforcing the posterior vaginal wall and tying the perineal body to the scaffold and to the pelvic walls and upper part of the pelvic floor.

As an integrated system, the components of the pelvic organ support system normally work together to maintain the horizontal and vertical position of the pelvic organs and to maintain alignment of the continence mechanisms. Strain resulting from defects in one component of the pelvic organ support system can initiate defects in other components of the system.

Pelvic bones, joints, and interosseous ligaments

Pelvic bones

The bony pelvis serves three primary functions: it acts as a relatively rigid cage supporting the abdominal and pelvic organs; it transmits body weight to the lower limbs when standing; and it provides attachment for the ligaments, muscles, and fascia of the trunk wall, back, pelvic floor, perineum, and lower limbs.

The bones of the pelvis form a sturdy articulated ring with the paired *os coxae* (innominate bones) anterolaterally and the sacrum and coccyx posteriorly. Each os coxae itself consists of three bones, the ilium, ischium, and pubis, which meet at the acetabulum (socket) of the hip joint (Fig. 4.4.2). Ossification of the epiphyses between the three bones is normally completed by age 22. Some important anatomic landmarks on the bony pelvis are shown in Fig. 4.4.3. The *ischial spine* is a particularly important landmark, since it provides attachment for many of the muscles and connective tissue structures of the pelvic organ support system.

The *ilium* consists of a broad flat ala superiorly, which articulates posteriorly with the sacrum, and a body inferiorly which fuses with the ischium and pubis (Fig. 4.4.3). The ilium thickens at the junction between the ala and body as an adaptation for transmitting weight from the sacroiliac joint across the

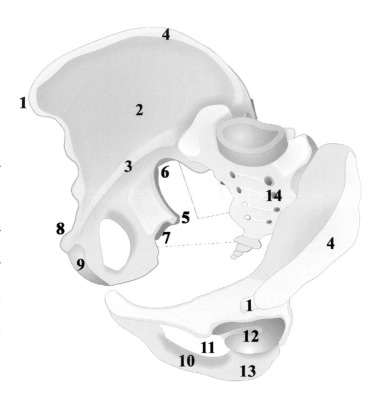

Figure 4.4.3. **Important landmarks of the pelvic bones;** lateral oblique view with left os coxae distracted.
1 Anterior superior iliac spine; 2 Iliac fossa; 3 Arcuate line; 4 Iliac crest; 5 Ischial spine; 6 Greater sciatic notch; 7 Lesser sciatic notch; 8 Pubic tubercle; 9 Symphyseal surface of the pubic bone covered with hyaline articular cartilage; 10 Ischiopubic ramus; 11 Obturator foramen; 12 Acetabulum; 13 Ischial tuberosity; 14 Anterior sacral foramina.

ilium to the *acetabulum* of the hip joint. This thickened buttress is marked by the *arcuate line* visible on radiographs of the pelvis. The superior margin of the ala widens to form the *iliac crest*. The gluteal muscles of the lower limb attach to the external surface of the ala. The pelvic surface of the ala forms a gentle concavity, the iliac fossa, which provides attachment for the iliacus muscle of the lower limb.

The *ischium* consists of a robust *body* and an *ischial ramus*. The *ischial spine* projects from the posterior margin of the ischial body, separating the *greater sciatic notch* superiorly from the *lesser sciatic notch* inferiorly (Fig. 4.4.3). The body of the ischium is very robust where it forms the prominent *ischial tuberosity*. The ischial tuberosities support the body weight when seated, provide attachment for the hamstring muscles of the lower limb, and provide the posterior attachment for structures in the perineum.

The *pubis* consists of a body and superior and inferior pubic rami. The bodies of the left and right pubic bones articulate in the anterior midline at their *symphyseal surfaces* to form the pubic symphysis (Fig. 4.4.3). The superior ramus runs posteriorly to fuse with the bodies of the ilium and ischium at the acetabulum; the inferior ramus runs posteroinferiorly to fuse with the ischial ramus, forming the *ischiopubic ramus*. The superior and inferior pubic rami, and the body of the ischium, enclose the *obturator*

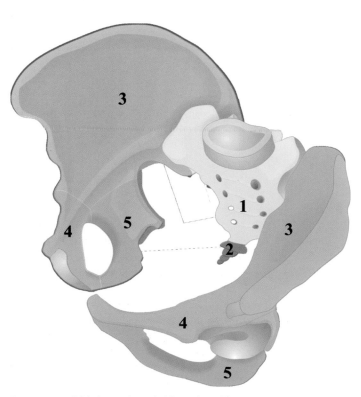

Figure 4.4.2. **Pelvic bones;** lateral oblique view with left os coxae distracted.
1 Sacrum; 2 Coccyx; 3 Ilium; 4 Pubis; 5 Ischium.
The ilium, ischium, and pubis comprise the os coxae (innominate bone).

foramen. The *pubic arch* is framed by the diverging ischiopubic rami.

The *sacrum* normally consists of five sacral vertebrae fused in a curve (Fig. 4.4.3). The pelvic surface of the sacrum is concave; the external surface is convex and bears sacral crests. Laterally, the upper portion of the sacrum widens to meet the ilium at the sacroiliac joint. The meninges and the roots of the sacral spinal nerves run within the sacral canal, which opens inferiorly at the sacral hiatus. The anterior and posterior rami of the spinal nerves leave the sacral canal through the *anterior* and *posterior sacral foramina*, respectively. The *coccyx* consists of a series of three to five small vertebrae joined to the apex of the sacrum.

Pelvic joints and ligaments

The *pubic symphysis* is a midline fibrocartilaginous joint that permits only slight angulation and rotation. The symphysis is reinforced superiorly by the superior pubic ligament and inferiorly by the inferior pubic (*arcuate*) ligament (Fig. 4.4.4).

The entire weight of the trunk, head, neck, and upper limbs is transmitted to the pelvis and lower limbs through the vertebral column and sacrum. The *anterior* and *posterior longitudinal ligaments* reinforce the vertebral column and intervertebral joints, including the joint between the fifth lumbar vertebra and

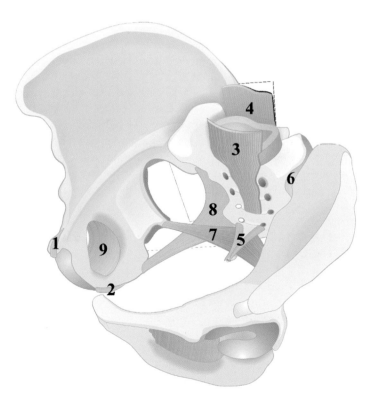

Figure 4.4.4. **Pelvic joints and ligaments;** lateral oblique view with left os coxae distracted.
1 Superior pubic ligament; 2 Inferior pubic (*arcuate*) ligament; 3 Anterior longitudinal ligament; 4 Posterior longitudinal ligament; 5 Anterior sacrococcygeal ligament; 6 Auricular surface of sacrum at sacroiliac joint; 7 Sacrospinous ligament; 8 Sacrotuberous ligament; 9 Obturator membrane.

the sacrum. *Anterior sacrococcygeal ligaments* stabilize the sacrococcygeal and intercoccygeal joints. From the sacrum, body weight is transmitted to the ilium across the broad articular surfaces of the *sacroiliac joints*. Although they are technically synovial joints, the complexly reciprocal articular surfaces of the sacroiliac joints normally permit only slight gliding. The sacroiliac joints may become fibrous, or even ossify, in older individuals. Each sacroiliac joint is reinforced by robust anterior and posterior sacroiliac ligaments, and by the interosseous sacroiliac ligament superiorly.

Each sacroiliac joint is further stabilized by two substantial, dense connective tissue ligaments that anchor the inferior part of the sacrum to the ischium (Fig. 4.4.4). The *sacrospinous ligament* extends from the sacrum to the ischial spine, separating the greater sciatic notch from the lesser sciatic notch, and completing the greater sciatic notch to form the greater sciatic foramen. The *sacrotuberous ligament* runs external to the sacrospinous ligament and extends from the sacrum to the ischial tuberosity. The sacrospinous and sacrotuberous ligaments together complete the lesser sciatic notch to form the lesser sciatic foramen. Each *obturator membrane* is a thin plate of dense connective tissue anchored to the margins of the obturator foramen and closing the foramen except for the small *obturator canal* anterosuperiorly (Fig. 4.4.4).

The pelvic joints and ligaments relax during the later stages of pregnancy, permitting greater rotation and possible sacroiliac joint subluxation.[14] Although the position of the sacrum may alter only slightly after sacroiliac rotation or subluxation, any change could conceivably increase strain on the other structures comprising the pelvic floor support system, and this would be particularly important if other components of the system had been weakened or damaged during childbirth.

In normal standing position, the ischiopubic rami are dependent and the pelvic outlet is obliquely posterior rather than directly inferior. A vertical plane passing through the *anterior superior iliac spines* intersects the *pubic tubercles*, and a horizontal plane passing through the superior surface of the pubic symphysis intersects the ischial spines and apex of the sacrum.

Pelvic apertures
Even with its joints and ligaments in place, the articulated bony pelvis forms a barred cage rather than a bowl surrounding the abdominopelvic viscera. The muscles, fasciae, and connective tissue of the abdominal walls, pelvic walls, and pelvic floor convert the pelvis from a cage to a container for the abdominopelvic viscera.

The muscles and fasciae of the abdominal walls attach along the superior surfaces of the pubis and the alae of the ilium. The flared alae and the superior part of the sacrum form the "greater pelvis" or "false pelvis", which surrounds the inferior extent of the abdominal cavity. The *pelvic inlet* (pelvic brim) is an irregularly round or oval opening bounded by the pubis anteriorly, the arcuate line of the ilium laterally, and the sacrum posteriorly (Fig. 4.4.5). The pelvic inlet is continuous superiorly with the "greater pelvis" and abdominal cavity.

The *pelvic outlet* is an irregular, diamond-shaped opening bounded by the ischiopubic rami anteriorly, the ischial tuberosity and sacrotuberous ligament laterally, and the coccyx posteriorly (Fig. 4.4.5). All landmarks of the pelvic outlet are palpable on physical examination. An imaginary line connecting the anterior surfaces of the ischial tuberosities divides the pelvic outlet into two triangles and forms the base for both the urogenital and anal triangles (Fig. 4.4.5). The apex of the *urogenital triangle* lies anteriorly at the pubic symphysis; the apex of the *anal triangle* lies posteriorly at the sacrum and coccyx. The planes of the urogenital triangle and anal triangles intersect at an angle. Baragi and colleagues found that the overall area of the pelvic outlet is 5.1% smaller in African–American women than in European–American women,[15] a fact which may partially explain the lower incidence of pelvic floor disorders in African-American women.

The *pelvic walls* include the entire bony pelvis inferior to the arcuate line, and the obturator membranes, sacrotuberous ligaments, and sacrospinous ligaments (Fig. 4.4.5). The *muscles of the pelvic wall* cover and partially close the obturator foramen, greater sciatic foramen, and lesser sciatic foramen. The pelvic walls form the lateral limits of both the pelvic cavity and the perineum. The paired *muscles of the pelvic floor* attach laterally along the pelvic walls in a continuous line from the pubis to the sacrum, converge medially around the inferior portions of the pelvic organs, and form an aponeurosis posterior to the rectum. The *pelvic cavity* ("lesser pelvis" or "true pelvis") is the anatomic region bounded by the pelvic inlet superiorly, the pelvic walls laterally, and the muscles of the pelvic floor inferiorly (Fig. 4.4.5). The pelvic cavity is occupied by the pelvic viscera and their fascial supports and peritoneal covering, and by the nerves and blood vessels of the pelvic organs and lower limbs. The *perineum* is the anatomic region bounded by the muscles of the pelvic floor superiorly; the pelvic walls laterally; the coccyx and gluteus maximus muscle posteriorly; and the skin of the vulva, inferior buttocks, and superomedial thighs inferiorly. The perineum is occupied by the urethra, vagina, and anus; the urethral and anal continence mechanisms; the external genitalia; abundant subcutaneous fat filling the ischioanal fossae in the anal triangle; the nerves and blood vessels supplying the perineal structures; and the midline connective tissue structures of the pelvic outlet.

Midline connective tissue structures of the pelvic outlet

Attachment sites for the pelvic muscles include not only the bones and sturdy interosseous ligaments of the pelvis but also the midline connective tissue structures of the pelvic outlet and the thick connective tissue covering the muscles of the pelvic wall (Fig. 4.4.6).

A series of *midline connective tissue structures* bridges the pelvic outlet from the pubis to the coccyx. The dense fibrous connective tissue of the perineal membrane, perineal body, and anococcygeal ligament (anococcygeal body) support structures superior to the pelvic outlet and provide a series of stable attachment sites for the muscles of the pelvic floor, the muscles of the urethral and anal continence mechanisms, the external genitalia, and the muscles of the external genitalia. Fibers from the pelvic and perineal muscles attaching to the midline connective tissue structures become interwoven with one another to form a substantial fibromuscular chain bridging the pelvic outlet. Continuity between the perineal body and the anococcygeal complex is provided by the dense fibrous connective tissue and muscles surrounding the anus.

The *perineal membrane* (Fig. 4.4.6) is a sheet of dense fibrous

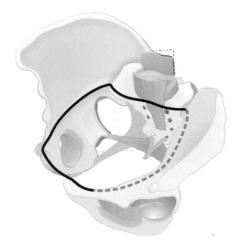 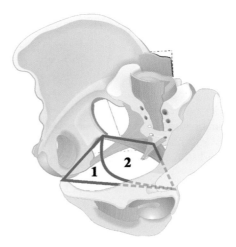

Figure 4.4.5. **Pelvic inlet (red line) and pelvic outlet (green line);** lateral oblique view with left os coxae distracted.
1 Urogenital triangle anteriorly within pelvic outlet; 2 Anal triangle posteriorly within pelvic outlet.

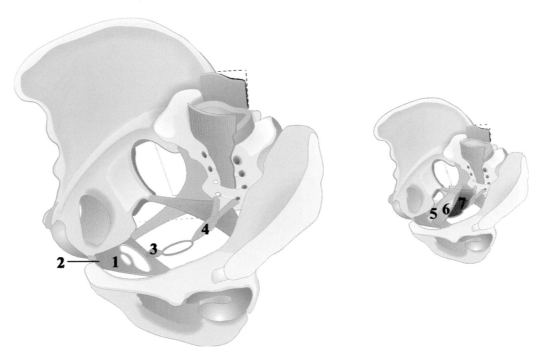

Figure 4.4.6. **Midline connective tissue structures of the pelvic outlet;** lateral oblique view with left os coxae distracted.
1 Perineal membrane; 2 Transverse perineal ligament; 3 Perineal body; 4 Anococcygeal ligament.
Inset: 5 Urethra; 6 Vagina; 7 Rectum.

connective tissue spanning the interval between the ischiopubic rami. Central openings in the perineal membrane allow passage for the terminal portions of the urethra and vagina. Connective tissue attachments between the urethra, vagina, and perineal membrane may enable the perineal membrane to function as a platform supporting the urethra and vagina.

Anterior to the urethral opening, the margin of the perineal membrane thickens to form the *transverse perineal ligament* (Fig. 4.4.6). The deep dorsal vein of the clitoris passes between the arcuate ligament and the transverse perineal ligament to enter the pelvic cavity. In the midline, the posterior margin of the perineal membrane fuses with the perineal body. The muscles of the urethral continence mechanism attach to the superior surface of the perineal membrane; the external genitalia and the muscles of the external genitalia attach to the inferior surface of the perineal membrane.

The *perineal body* (Fig. 4.4.6) is a conical node of dense fibroelastic connective tissue and interlacing muscle fibers occupying the approximate center of the perineum. The base of the perineal body lies in the plane of the perineal membrane; the apex extends superiorly for several centimeters. The perineal body is anchored anteriorly to the perineal membrane (and through the perineal membrane to the ischiopubic rami), posteriorly to the muscles and fibrous coat of the anorectum, and superiorly to the rectovaginal fascia. The rectovaginal fascia links the perineal body to the support scaffold formed by the visceral pelvic fascia and to the presacral fascia covering the sacrum. The perineal body provides direct attachment for the puboperineal fibers of the pelvic floor muscles, for the external anal sphincter, and for all perineal muscles except ischiocavernosus. All the muscles attaching to the perineal body contribute fibers to an interlacing meshwork that surrounds and reinforces it.

The *anococcygeal ligament* (anococcygeal body; Fig. 4.4.6) is a fibroelastic structure extending from the external anal sphincter and connective tissue coat of the anorectum to the coccyx and presacral fascia. Superiorly, the anococcygeal ligament lies directly parallel to the median raphe of the iliococcygeus muscle, an important muscle of the pelvic floor. The anococcygeal ligament and ilioccygeal raphe blend at their attachments to the coccyx and anorectum.

The perineal membrane is fixed by its lateral attachments to the ischiopubic rami, but the perineal body and anococcygeal ligament are more mobile, particularly the anococcygeal ligament. Contraction of the pelvic floor muscles causes upward movement of the anococygeal ligament and anus; increases in intra-abdominal pressure cause downward movement of these structures.

Pelvic muscles and investing pelvic fascia

The pelvic muscles include the muscles of the pelvic walls and the muscles of the pelvic floor.

Muscles of the pelvic walls

The *muscles of the pelvic wall* cover the large apertures framed by the bony struts and ligaments of the pelvic walls – the obturator, and greater sciatic and lesser sciatic foramina (Fig. 4.4.7). Between the pubis and the ischial spine, the dense investing pelvic fascia covering the muscles of the pelvic walls thickens conspicuously to form an attachment site for the muscles of the pelvic floor.

The *obturator internus muscle* closes both the obturator foramen and the lesser sciatic foramen (Fig. 4.4.7). Obturator internus originates from the pelvic margins of the obturator foramen and the obturator membrane, closely follows the pelvic wall posteriorly, passes through the lesser sciatic foramen, turns sharply, and inserts on the greater trochanter of the femur. Obturator internus functions as a lateral rotator of the lower limb. The nerve to obturator internus (L_5, S_1) innervates the obturator internus muscle, entering its perineal surface inferior to the pelvic floor. The internal pudendal and obturator vessels provide the vascular supply to obturator internus. The obturator canal, at the anterosuperior border of obturator internus, transmits the obturator nerves and vessels from the pelvic cavity to the muscles and skin of the medial thigh. The obturator nerve (L_{2-4}) supplies obturator externus, but not obturator internus.

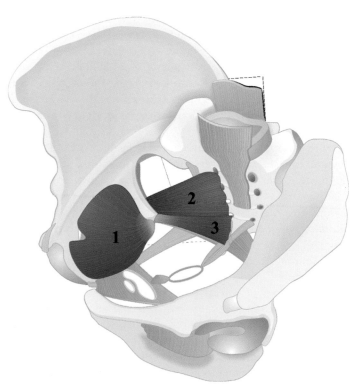

Figure 4.4.7. **Muscles of the pelvic walls and striated muscles of the urethra and anus;** lateral oblique view with left os coxae distracted.
Muscles of the pelvic walls: 1 Obturator internus; 2 Piriformis; 3 Coccygeus; 4 Tendinous arch of levator ani (condensation of investing fascia over the obturator internus muscle).
Striated muscles of the urethra and anus: 5 External urethral sphincter (sphincter urethrae); 6 Compressor urethrae; 7 Sphincter urethrovaginalis; 8 External anal sphincter.

The *piriformis muscle* closes the greater sciatic foramen (Fig. 4.4.7). Piriformis originates on the pelvic surface of the sacrum by three slips surrounding the second and third anterior sacral foramina, and then passes laterally through the greater sciatic foramen to insert on the greater trochanter of the femur. Like the obturator internus muscle, piriformis functions as a lateral rotator of the lower limb. The nerve to piriformis (L_5, $S_{1,2}$) enters the pelvic surface of the muscle. The lateral sacral and superior gluteal arteries provide the vascular supply to piriformis.

Many important neurovascular structures leave the pelvic cavity through the greater sciatic foramen, and these structures are vulnerable to injury during pelvic or perineal surgery. Structures leaving the pelvic cavity between piriformis and the muscles of the pelvic floor include the inferior gluteal nerves and vessels, sciatic nerve, posterior cutaneous femoral nerve, nerve to quadratus femoris, nerve to obturator internus, pudendal nerve, and internal pudendal vessels. As they leave the greater sciatic foramen, the last three structures make a sharp turn around the external surface of the ischial spine and enter the perineum inferior to the pelvic floor, and then run anteriorly in a fascial canal formed by the investing pelvic fascia covering the obturator internus muscle. Any of the structures leaving the greater sciatic foramen inferior to piriformis are vulnerable to injury during sacrospinous colpopexy, a surgical procedure in which the vaginal vault is suspended from the sacrospinous ligament.

The pudendal nerve (S_{2-4}) or its branches may also be injured in their perineal course over the obturator internus muscle during procedures using transvaginal or transanal surgical approaches. The *inferior rectal branch* of the pudendal nerve provides motor innervation to the external anal sphincter and conveys sensation from the anal skin and the inferior portion of the anal canal. The *perineal branch* of the pudendal nerve provides motor innervation to the urinary continence mechanism and muscles of the external genitalia, and it conveys sensation from the perineum, including the labia, lower portion of the vagina, and clitoris.[16] Welgoss and colleagues reported prolonged perineal nerve terminal latencies postoperatively, compared with baseline presurgical measurements, in 11 of 31 women undergoing bilateral sacrospinous ligament vault suspension and bilateral paravaginal cystocele repair.[17] In this study, women with perineal neuropathy were more likely to have a suboptimal surgical outcome than women without perineal neuropathy.

Parietal pelvic fascia

The term "fascia" is used in the anatomic and surgical literature to refer to any of a large number of diverse connective tissue structures with very different shapes, locations, tissue properties, and functions. A fascial structure may be a flat sheet or a thick layer; it may be a sturdy conspicuous structure or a collagenous condensation within a loose amorphous agglomeration. Unfortunately, the use of the term "fascia" to describe very disparate structures may seem to imply an unwarranted anatomic or functional similarity.

Three different fascias are found in the pelvis and perineum. The subcutaneous fat (superficial fascia, hypodermis) of the perineum and ischioanal fossa lies directly beneath the dermis of the skin, and consists of a loose network of collagen fibers containing many adipocytes. Anteriorly, the subcutaneous fat forms the bulk of the mons pubis and labia majora. Posteriorly the subcutaneous fat expands, filling the relatively large spaces between the pelvic floor, pelvic walls, anorectum, and skin, and extends anteriorly for a short distance above the perineal membrane. Colles' fascia is a recognizable condensation of collagen fibers near the internal limit of the subcutaneous fat of the perineum.

The *parietal pelvic fascia* covering the muscles of the pelvic walls, pelvic floor, and perineum is continuous with the deep investing fascia surrounding all the bones and striated muscles of the body. This dense connective tissue layer fuses with the epimysium covering individual muscles, splits to surround muscle groups, bridges the gaps between muscles, and fuses with the periosteum of bones. All muscles have a covering of deep fascia, including the muscles of the thorax, abdomen, and pelvis. The deep investing fascia covers both the external surfaces of the muscles and the internal surfaces facing the body cavities. Although the deep investing fascia forms a continuous layer, its essential continuity may be obscured by the regional names applied to it. The term "investing pelvic fascia" is used to describe the entire investing deep fascial layer covering the pelvic surfaces of the pelvic walls and floor. Specific terms, such as "obturator internus fascia", "presacral fascia", "piriformis fascia", and "levator ani fascia", describe regions of this continuous layer, and not separate structures.

The investing pelvic fascia varies greatly in thickness from a thin covering inseparable from the epimysium to robust structures capable of providing secure attachment for muscles or for other connective tissue structures. The investing pelvic fascia covering the obturator internus muscle thickens to form a substantial tendinous arch, the *tendinous arch of levator ani* (Fig. 4.4.7), which provides a sturdy attachment for the iliococcygeus muscle and part of the pubococcygeus muscle between their bony attachments. Iliococcygeus and pubococcygeus are muscles of the pelvic floor. The deep investing fascia covering iliococcygeus thickens to form another substantial tendinous arch, the *tendinous arch of the pelvic fascia* (*white line*) (Fig. 4.4.7), continued anteriorly as the *pubovesical ligament*. The visceral pelvic fascia supporting the pelvic organs blends laterally with the tendinous arch of the pelvic fascia, which anchors it to the pelvic wall. In the *Terminologia Anatomica*,[18] the term "endopelvic fascia" is listed as a synonym for "pelvic investing fascia". In the clinical literature, however, the term "endopelvic fascia" is generally used as a synonym for "visceral pelvic fascia."

The *visceral pelvic fascia* (*endopelvic fascia*) filling the spaces between the pelvic organs, pelvic walls, pelvic floor, and the peritoneum lining the abdominopelvic cavity is highly variable in terms of its tissue properties. The visceral pelvic fascia everywhere consists of smooth muscle, collagen fibers, and elastin fibers. In some regions, the collagen fibers and elastin fibers are relatively dispersed, in other regions they form demonstrable ligaments such as the cardinal and uterosacral ligament complex. The visceral pelvic fascia and the visceral fascial ligaments are described more fully in a later section.

Muscles of the pelvic floor

The clinical importance of the muscles of the pelvic floor far exceeds the clarity and accuracy of most descriptions of pelvic floor anatomy. Almost no other region of the body is so commonly described in unhelpful generalizations, confusing and overlapping terminology, and misleading metaphor. These conceptual difficulties are not mere quibbles, but real obstacles to understanding the pelvic organ support system and the role of the pelvic floor muscles within that system.

In most traditional accounts, the pelvic floor muscles are described as the "pelvic diaphragm", which consists of the coccygeus (ischiococcygeus) and levator ani muscles.[18–25] The levator ani muscle is said to consist of the iliococcygeus and pubococcygeus muscles, and pubococcygeus is said to consist of the pubourethralis and puborectalis muscles. Additional small muscles, such as the puboperinealis and puboanalis, may also be included in levator ani. The editors of the 39th British edition of Gray's *Anatomy* include ischiococcygeus (coccygeus) in levator ani.[26] The terms "pelvic diaphragm" and "levator ani muscle" are currently used more or less interchangeably in the literature with little explanation of how inclusively they are meant to be interpreted.

At every level of generalization, the structures included are nearly always described as "a muscle", although the paradoxical consequence of this description is that levator ani is a muscle comprised of other muscles, a situation unparalleled in any other region of the body. And, at every level of generalization, the function of the pelvic floor muscle or muscles is described as "supporting the pelvic viscera". The interesting and clinically important questions, however, are exactly *how* each of the muscles of the pelvic floor contributes to the support of the pelvic organs, how the failure of one pelvic floor muscle affects the other components of the pelvic organ support system, and how the intact components of the pelvic organ support system may be safely and effectively recruited, or augmented, to compensate for the failed structure. Detailed studies of the *functions of the individual muscles of the pelvic floor*, rather than studies of the functions of "levator ani" or the "pelvic diaphragm", are requisite for an adequate understanding of the normal and pathologic anatomy of the pelvic floor and the pelvic organ support system. The first step in addressing the functions of the individual muscles of the pelvic floor is a specific and consistent terminology for referring to them. Difficulties in reconciling the terms and measurement points used by different researchers and clinicians lead to difficulties in interpreting or comparing the results of their research studies or surgical series.

Recent MRI studies have elegantly documented normal pelvic floor anatomy,[12–27] identified defects in pelvic wall anatomy,[10,11] and compared pelvic wall anatomy in patients with pelvic organ prolapse and normal controls.[11,13,14,29] Several studies have attempted to identify imaging markers that can be used to diagnose pelvic floor dysfunction, to assess the severity of pelvic floor dysfunction, and to assist in treatment planning.[10,13,14] Singh and colleagues have described four patterns of change in levator ani conformation associated with pelvic floor dysfunction.[28]

These imaging studies have great potential for enhancing our knowledge of pelvic floor anatomy, and they offer the possibility of more accurate diagnosis and effective treatment of pelvic floor disorders. Their comparability and applicability, however, are limited by persistent difficulties with the terminology used to refer to the muscles of the pelvic floor, by the use of ambiguously defined reference points, and by the use of unexplained terms.

In a recent review, Kearney and colleagues summarized the conflicting terminology used by various authors to describe the levator ani muscle group.[19,29] They suggest that although there is widespread disagreement on the terminology applied to the muscles of the pelvic floor, there is basic consensus on the origins and insertions of the muscles themselves. These authors sensibly propose a standardized terminology for the pelvic floor muscles based on their attachment sites. It is worth pointing out, however, that strict application of this principle requires a terminological revision perhaps more radical than the authors intended, requiring elimination of the terms "levator ani", "iliococcygeus", and "pelvic diaphragm". Specific muscle names, based on attachments will be used throughout the following discussion.

Consideration of the origins and insertions of the muscles of the pelvic floor presents two initial difficulties for the traditional account. First, the *coccygeus (ischiococcygeus) muscle cannot actively support the pelvic viscera.* The inconstant muscle fibers of *coccygeus* (ischiococcygeus) originate on the lateral pelvic surfaces of the fifth sacral vertebra and coccyx, follow the sacrospinous ligament laterally, and insert on the ischial spine (Fig. 4.4.7). In quadrupeds, the sacrospinous ligament is absent, and coccygeus is a robust depressor and lateral flexor of the tail. In humans, the sacrospinous ligament is robust, and the muscle fibers of coccygeus are often few or absent, suggesting that, in humans, coccygeus has lost its active role as a tail muscle and is evolving into a ligament. Regardless of its evolutionary antecedents and robusticity, attachments of coccygeus to the sacrum, coccyx, and ischial spine, and lack of attachment to the pelvic viscera or midline connective tissue structures, would exclude coccygeus from any role in supporting the pelvic organs. For this reason, coccygeus is probably better included among the muscles of the pelvic wall than among the muscles of the pelvic floor. The inconstant substance of the coccygeus muscle suggests that it may not be a reliable surgical landmark or a reliably available buffer between sharp instruments and fragile neurovascular structures. Neither should the absence of a conspicuous coccygeus on MRI or other imaging studies necessarily be interpreted as a sign of pelvic floor weakness when the iliococcygeus and pubococcygeus muscles appear normal.

A second difficulty with the traditional account of the pelvic floor muscles is that *iliococcygeus has no attachment to the ilium.* Despite its name, iliococcygeus attaches laterally to the tendinous arch of levator ani and to the pelvic surface of the ischial spine (Fig. 4.4.8). This is a minor point, however, and even if its name inaccurately describes its attachments, iliococcygeus belongs among the muscles of the pelvic floor.

Consideration of the actual configuration of the pelvic floor muscles suggests that even the term "pelvic floor" is somewhat misleading, since the *pelvic floor is neither flat nor horizontal.* Instead, the paired muscles of the pelvic floor form an obliquely oriented muscular funnel, higher posteriorly than anteriorly and slanting obliquely from superior attachments relatively high on the pelvic wall toward inferior attachments on the sacrum, coccyx, midline connective tissue structures, and connective tissue coats of the anorectum and vagina (Fig. 4.4.8). *Neither is the pelvic floor shaped like a basin.* In many textbook diagrams, the muscles of the pelvic floor are depicted as forming a shallow but capacious muscular basin with sides curving gently outward away from the pelvic organs. Recent MRI studies confirm, however, that the pelvic floor is closely contiguous with the pelvic organs.[11,12] The slanting surfaces of the muscles of the pelvic floor approach the sides of the pelvic organs, as well as their inferior portions, and the pelvic floor also supports the posterior surfaces of the vagina and rectum.

Recent dynamic MRI studies conducted by Hjartardottir and colleagues suggest that, at resting tone, the pelvic floor is convex superiorly rather than inferiorly and that it is shaped like a dome, and not a basin.[30] Other MRI studies have reported similar results[31,32] Hjartardottir and colleagues also suggest that the muscles of the pelvic walls straighten during muscular contraction, and that they are basin-shaped only when downwardly displaced by intra-abdominal pressure during the Valsalva maneuver.

In the following description, the muscles of the pelvic floor will be named according to their individual attachments, except for iliococcygeus. In the absence of detailed electromyographic or other studies of the individual muscles of the pelvic floor, their functions can be inferred only from their attachments and muscle fiber orientations. These inferences are provided in the following discussion, but they are largely hypothetic and await further study.

Iliococcygeus

From fixed attachments to the tendinous arch of levator ani and the ischial spine, the paired *iliococcygeus muscles* descend in an obliquely horizontal path to converge posterior to the anorectum, where they form a strong median raphe (Fig. 4.4.8). The iliococcygeal raphe is attached anteriorly to the muscles and fibrous coat of the anorectum and to the anterior part of the anococcygeal ligament; the raphe is attached posteriorly to the coccyx and apex of the sacrum and to the posterior part of the anococcygeal ligament. The muscle fiber orientation and attachments of iliococcygeus suggest that bilateral contraction would draw the iliococcygeus raphe

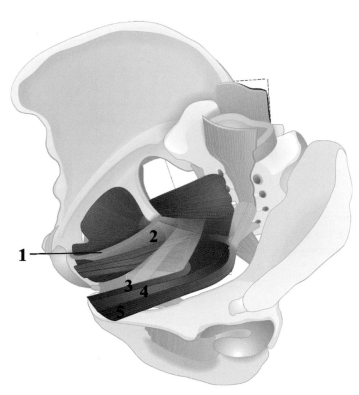

Figure 4.4.8. **Muscles of the pelvic floor;** lateral oblique view with left os coxae distracted.
1 Tendinous arch of levator ani (condensation of investing fascia over the obturator internus muscle); 2 Iliococcygeus; 3 Pubovaginalis and puboperitonealis; 4 Puborectalis; 5 Pubococcygeus; 6 Levator plate; 7 Tendinous arch of the pelvic fascia.

superiorly and anteriorly. Resting tone would support structures superior to iliococcygeus, including the levator plate, rectum, and vagina, and would help maintain the organs in their normal midline positions. Indirect effects of the bilateral contraction of iliococcygeus would be tension on any structures attached to the median raphe of iliococcygeus, such as the anus and the anococcygeal ligament.

Iliococcygeus receives its motor innervation directly from intrapelvic branches of $S_{2,3,4}$, which enter its pelvic surface. Branches of the pudendal nerve, entering its perineal surface, may also provide innervation to iliococcygeus. The internal pudendal and inferior gluteal vessels provide the vascular supply to iliococcygeus. Intrapelvic somatic branches to iliococcygeus are vulnerable to injury during pregnancy and delivery, particularly vaginal delivery, or during any pelvic surgery.

Pubococcygeus

The pubococcygeus muscle, or muscle complex, consists of lateral and medial parts (Fig. 4.4.8). The lateral pubococcygeus part extends between the pubis anteriorly and the coccyx and sacrum posteriorly. The medial part extends between the pubis anteriorly and the pelvic organs and perineal body posteriorly,

and consists of the pubovaginalis, puboperinealis, puborectalis, and puboanalis muscles.*

Pubococcygeus ascends in an obliquely vertical path from anterior attachments to the pubis and pubic symphysis to posterior attachments on the coccyx, anterior sacrococcygeal ligament, and sacrum. Posterior to the rectum, the left and right pubococcygeus muscles form a broad aponeurosis, the tendinous plate of levator ani, or *levator plate*. The presacral fascia also contributes to the formation of the levator plate. Pubococcygeus has two fixed attachments, and its isometric contraction shortens the overall length of the muscle between the pubis and sacrum. Bilateral contraction of pubococcygeus would elevate the levator plate and the rectum and vagina which recline upon its sloping surface; resting tone would support these organs.

The muscle fibers of the pubococcygeus and iliococcygeus muscles run roughly perpendicular to one another, overlapping posterior to the rectum and connected to, or resting above, the anococcygeal ligament. Although it is true that iliococcygeus and pubococcygeus "support the pelvic organs", this is a very general description of the more complex functions suggested by their attachments and muscle fiber orientations. In fact, iliococcygeus and pubococcygeus probably support the pelvic organs in several different ways.

(1) Their resting tone supports the pelvic organs lying above the levator plate of pubococcygeus and the median raphe of iliococcygeus.
(2) The attachment of iliococcygeus to the anococcygeal ligament supports the anus by reinforcing and elevating its posterior attachment to the coccyx.
(3) The balanced tone or balanced contraction of the paired iliococcygeus and pubococcygeus muscles helps stabilize the pelvic organs in their midline positions, minimizing strain on the visceral pelvic fascia anchoring them to the pelvic walls, and maintaining the vertical aligment between the pelvic organs, pelvic floor, and urinary and fecal continence mechanisms.

It is important to note that the stabilizing functions of iliococcygeus and pubococcygeus require that *both* the left and right muscles of each pair be intact and functioning. If either muscle of the pair is fibrotic, torn, avulsed from its attachment to the pelvic wall, or paralyzed from loss of its somatic motor innervation, then the intact contralateral muscle will tend to draw the iliococcygeal raphe away from the midline toward the intact side, and could conceivably place additional tension on the

*The *Terminologia Anatomica* recognizes the terms "puboprostaticus" (in males, although this muscle is more commonly referred to as "pubourethralis"), "pubovaginalis" (in females), "puboperinealis", "puboanalis", and "puborectalis".[33] The 39th British Edition of *Gray's Anatomy* recognizes "pubourethralis" (in males) "pubovaginalis" (in females), some unnamed muscle fibers from pubourethralis or pubovaginalis attaching to the perineal body, muscle fibers attaching to the anorectal junction (sometimes called "puboanalis"), and "puborectalis".

visceral pelvic fascial supports running from the organs to the pelvic walls on the affected side. Delancey and colleagues[11] found both unilateral and bilateral damage to the pubococcygeus and iliococcygeus among primiparous women, but not among nulliparous controls.

The muscle fiber orientations and attachments of the medial part of the pubococcygeus complex suggest that pubovaginalis, puboperinealis, and puborectalis support the pelvic organs in yet another way. Fibers of the paired pubovaginalis muscles run posteriorly from the pubic symphysis, decussate, and blend with fibers from the opposite side to form a muscular sling posterior to the vagina; fibers also blend with the connective tissue of the vaginal wall. Fibers of the puboperinealis muscle detach from pubovaginalis and blend with the connective tissue of the perineal body. The urethra is closely approximated to the anterior wall of the vagina, and the resting tone of the sling formed by pubovaginalis would support both the vagina and urethra. Contraction of pubovaginalis would draw the vagina and urethra anteriorly and superiorly and might also have some effect on stabilizing the perineal body.

Fibers of the paired puborectalis muscles run posteriorly from the pubic symphysis, decussate, and blend with fibers from their contralateral counterparts to form a sling posterior to the rectum. Puborectalis is a substantial muscle, extending below the level of the other muscles of the pelvic floor. The sling formed by *puborectalis* surrounds the anorectal junction, drawing it anteriorly and forming a kink, the anorectal angle, which helps maintain fecal continence. Fibers of the *puboanalis* muscle contribute to the conjoint longitudinal coat of the anus, a layer of striated and smooth muscle fibers and fibroelastic tissue between the internal and external anal sphincters, and extending inferiorly, through fibroelastic connections, to the skin of the anus. Although it is true, in a fairly trivial way, that pubovaginalis and puborectalis "support" the pelvic organs, the actual mechanisms and vectors of support are very different from those of iliococcygeus and pubococcygeus. Pubovaginalis and puborectalis also hold the urethra, vagina, and rectum together in a block, approximate their walls,[33] and maintain their vertical aligment.

Cooperation among the puborectalis, internal anal sphincter, and external anal sphincter is essential for continence, and maintaining the alignment of the rectum, puborectalis, and external and internal sphincters is essential for normal function. Relaxation of puborectalis, loss of alignment, injury to motor or proprioceptive nerve fibers supplying the rectum and its muscles, or herniation of the rectum through the posterior wall of the vagina can compromise normal bowel function. Obstetric trauma is the most common cause of external anal sphincter injury.[34]

Yucel and colleagues have suggested that the levator ani muscles do not support the proximal urethra and play no active role in continence.[35] The relationship between pubovaginalis and the urinary continence mechanism is not obvious, but an interesting speculative possibility suggests itself. The paired compressor urethrae muscles attach posteriorly to the ischiopu-

bic rami and runs anteriorly to form a sling around the urethra. The pubovaginalis sling and the compressor urethrae sling pull in opposite directions, and it is conceivable that contraction of pubovaginalis, which draws both vagina and urethra anteriorly, would increase the effectiveness of compressor urethrae, which draws the urethra posteriorly and compresses it against the anterior vaginal wall.

Pubococcygeurs, pubovaginalis, and puborectalis probably receive most of their innervation from the pudendal nerve (S_{2-4}), although some intrapelvic somatic fibers may also reach their pelvic surfaces.

Tunn and colleagues[11] found that detachment of the "pubovisceral" portion is the most common levator ani injury during vaginal delivery, but that iliococcygeus may also be injured. Injury to the puborectalis muscle would have very different consequences from injury to the iliococcygeus muscle, and the distinction between injuries to different pubovisceral muscles would be helpful.

The volume of the levator ani muscle decreases with age,[36] and fibrotic changes in the levator ani muscle of cadavers with vaginal parity have been documented.[37] The association between pelvic nerve injury and pelvic floor dysfunction has also been documented.[38,39]

Visceral pelvic fascia and visceral fascial ligaments

The muscles of the pelvic floor and the midline connective tissue structures constitute the primary supports of the pelvic organs. The visceral pelvic fascia (endopelvic fascia) and visceral pelvic ligaments surround the pelvic organs; blend with the connective tissue of the pelvic organ walls; form partitions between the organs; and tie the pelvic organs to the pelvic walls, pelvic floor, and midline connective tissue structures. The connective tissue scaffold formed by condensations within the visceral pelvic fascia maintains the pelvic organs in their central positions and customary orientations, while allowing for continual changes in their shapes and relative positions.

The *peritoneum* is the mesothelial lining of the abominopelvic cavity. It follows the contours of the pelvic walls and drapes over the superior surfaces of the pelvic organs, the visceral pelvic fascia and the visceral ligaments formed by collagenous condensations within the visceral pelvic fascia, and pelvic neurovascular structures. Where peritoneum spans the distance between two pelvic organs, or between a pelvic organ and the pelvic walls, it may double back on itself to form peritoneal folds. The space between the layers of peritoneum forming the fold is filled by loose visceral pelvic fascia and may contain neurovascular structures.

The term "ligament", as it is used in the anatomic and surgical literature, is at least as problematic as the term "fascia". In the pelvis, structures described as "ligaments" include the sturdy interosseous ligaments of the bony pelvis (such as the sacrospinous and sacrotuberous ligaments), vestiges of embryonic structures draped in peritoneal folds (such as the median ligament of the bladder and round ligament of the uterus), and neurovascular structures draped in peritoneal folds (such as the lateral ligament of the bladder and lateral ligament of the rectum). Use of the term "ligament" may suggest a degree of substance and robusticity. This implication is often misleading, however, and it is important to distinguish between the visceral pelvic ligaments tethering the pelvic organs and the peritoneal folds or ligaments adorning them. The round ligament and the broad ligament of the uterus are frequently included among the uterine supports. Although the broad and round ligaments may help to maintain uterine position, they are unlikely to contribute significantly to uterine support.

Visceral pelvic fascia

The visceral pelvic fascia (endopelvic fascia) is a three-dimensional connective tissue layer extending anteriorly to the retropubic space (space of Retzius), posteriorly to the sacrum, laterally to the tendinous arch of the pelvic fascia and pelvic walls, superiorly to the peritoneum, and inferiorly to the investing pelvic fascia covering the muscles of the pelvic floor and to the perineal membrane and perineal body.

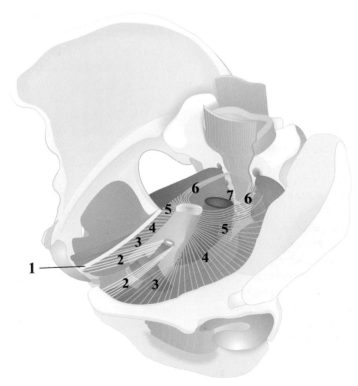

Figure 4.4.9. **Visceral pelvic fascia and visceral pelvic ligaments;** lateral oblique view with left os coxae distracted.
1 Tendinous arch of the pelvic fascia; 2 Pubovesical and pubourethral ligaments; 3 Pubocervical ligament; 4 Paracervical connective tissue; 5 Transverse cervical ligament (cardinal ligament of Mackenrodt); 6 Uterosacral ligament; 7 Posterior rectal ligament.

The visceral pelvic fascia is composed of fat cells interspersed with varying amounts of collagen, elastin and smooth muscle fibers.[7,40] In some regions, the visceral pelvic fascia functions as a relatively amorphous packing material occupying the spaces between the pelvic organs, the peritoneum, and the pelvic walls and floor. The paravesical fascia, pararectal fascia, and the parametrium within the broad ligament are all examples of loose visceral pelvic fascia that fills the spaces around organs and provides passage for the nerves and vessels supplying the organs. Loose visceral pelvic fascia also extends into the peritoneal folds.

In other regions, the collagen fibers and elastin fibers of the visceral pelvic fascia coalesce to form sheaths around neurovascular structures, or condense to form a series of demonstrable ligaments attaching the pelvic organs to the investing pelvic fascia covering the pubis, pelvic walls and floor, and sacrum. The tendinous arch of the pelvic fascia (white line) is a condensation of the iliococcygeus investing fascia which extends anteriorly as the pubovesical ligaments and posteriorly to the ischial spine, where it becomes less distinct. The visceral fascial supports of the pelvic organs attach in a line along the tendinous arch of the pelvic fascia to the ischial spine, and then continue their attachment posteriorly to the investing coccygeus fascia and presacral fascia. Less conspicuous accumulations of collagen fibers and elastin fibers probably extend from the organs to the pelvic walls and floor wherever the visceral and investing pelvic fascias lie adjacent to one another.

Visceral fascial supports of the bladder and urethra

The *pubovesical* and *pubourethral ligaments* are sturdy condensations of visceral pelvic fascia extending anteriorly to the pelvic aspect of the pubic bones and transverse perineal ligament and laterally to the anterior part of the tendinous arch of the pelvic fascia. The retropubic venous plexus lies between the paired pubovesical and pubourethral ligaments. The pubourethral ligaments consist of dense fibrous connective tissue and smooth muscle fibers.[41] MRI studies have found both thinning of the urethral striated muscle and distortion of the pubourethral ligaments in women with stress incontinence versus controls.[42]

The median ligament of the umbilicus and lateral ligament of the bladder are peritoneal folds rather than visceral fascial supports. The median umbilical ligament is a peritoneal fold surrounding the remnant of the embryonic urachus; the lateral ligament of the bladder is a peritoneal fold containing the superior vesical arteries in their course from the internal iliac artery to the superior portion of the bladder.

Visceral fascial supports of the cervix and vagina

The body of the uterus is relatively unencumbered by fascial supports, enabling it to change size and position, notably during pregnancy, or to respond to changes in the sizes and positions of the bladder and rectum on either side. All ligaments superior to the cervix are peritoneal ligaments. The uterus, uterine tubes, ovaries, and parametrium are draped in the peritoneum of the broad ligament; the ovarian and uterine vessels, lymphatics, and autonomic nerve plexuses traverse the parametrium to reach the uterus and adnexae. The uterovesical fold (anterior ligament of the uterus) and rectovaginal fold (posterior ligament of the uterus) are peritoneal folds surrounding a core of loose visceral pelvic fascia. The round ligament of the uterus, a vestigial structure containing smooth muscle and small blood vessels, passes from the uterine wall to the inguinal canal and labia majora.

The cervix and vagina are held comparatively immobile, although the vagina increases somewhat in length during sexual arousal. The vagina is a fibromuscular tube, which normally reclines obliquely on the rectum and levator plate. The urethra is virtually embedded in the anterior vaginal wall. A dense fascial condensation, the *paracervical connective tissue*, surrounds the cervix and provides reinforcement and attachment for the visceral fascial ligaments. Ligaments attaching to the paracervical connective tissue anchor the cervix to the pubis, tendinous arch of the pelvic fascia, ischial spine, coccygeus and piriformis fascia, and sacrum. The boundaries between the visceral fascial ligaments are somewhat arbitrary, and the names given the ligaments are roughly based on their attachments after development during dissection or surgery.

The *pubocervical ligaments* (anterior vaginal fascia), are sturdy condensations of endopelvic fascia extending anteriorly from the vagina and paracervical connective tissue to the tendinous arch of the pelvic fascia and pelvic surface of the pubic bones, and extending inferiorly to the perineal membrane, where they attach just lateral to the urethra. The vesical plexus runs within the pubocervical fascia.[17] The *paravaginal supports*[43–45] are condensations of endopelvic fascia extending laterally from the vagina and cervix to the tendinous arch of the pelvic fascia.

The *transverse cervical ligaments* (cardinal ligaments, ligaments of Mackenrodt) are condensations of visceral pelvic fascia running from the vagina and paracervical connective tissue posterolaterally to the tendinous arch of the pelvic fascia and ischial spine.

The uterine artery enters the base of the transverse cervical ligament as it crosses the pelvic floor between the internal iliac artery and the lateral aspect of the cervix. The ureter also enters the base of the transverse cervical ligament, running posterior and inferior to the uterine artery to reach the trigone of the bladder. Autonomic nerve fibers of the hypogastric plexus accompany the ureter and uterine artery. The nerves are vulnerable to injury during delivery or pelvic surgery, including hysterectomy and pelvic floor repair.

The *uterosacral ligaments* (rectouterine folds) are condensations of visceral pelvic fascia extending from the paracervical fascia vaginal vault, where the ligament is thickest, to

the coccygeus and piriformis parietal pelvic fascia and sacrum. The uterosacral ligament is palpable per rectum. The sacral attachment of the uterosacral ligament is, apparently, quite variable. Buller and Thompson[46] identified a sacral attachment extending over the first three sacral vertebrae and variably over the fourth, Umek et al. identified a sacral attachment in only 7% of MRI studies,[47] and Fritsch and Hotzinger[48] found no sacral attachment in plastinated sections. Buller and Thompson also described three portions of the uterosacral ligament, and adjacent anatomic structures, in order to identify the safest site for vaginal vault fixation. These authors describe important associations between the sacral portion of the uterosacral ligament and the superior gluteal vein; between the intermediate portion of the ligament, the middle rectal artery, and "nerve elements"; and between the sacral portion and the ureter. They conclude that the optimum fixation site is the intermediate part of the uterosacral ligament. Nerve fibers traveling in the uterosacral ligament may include not only autonomic fibers traveling to the rectal, cervical, and vesical plexuses, but also intrapelvic somatic fibers traveling to the iliococcygeus muscle and possibly to other muscles of the pelvic floor.

Recent discussions and publications have referred to a cardinal uterosacral complex including both the transverse cervical ligament and the uterosacral ligament,[10,44,49] and the paravaginal supports and pubocervical ligament could also be logically included in the series of visceral fascial supports extending from the cervix and vagina to the pelvic walls.

The *rectovaginal fascia* (rectovaginal septum, posterior vaginal fascia, or Denonvillier's fascia) is derived embryonically from a double-layered peritoneal fold that extended inferiorly between the cervix and vagina anteriorly and the rectum posteriorly, and that fused during development. The rectovaginal fascia forms a septum between the two organs and attaches laterally to the cardinal-uterosacral complex and inferiorly to the perineal body. The intact rectovaginal fascia forms an important posterior support for the vaginal wall and a barrier to encroachment of the rectum into the posterior vaginal wall in a rectocele.[7]

Another recent trend in the literature is to distinguish anterior and posterior compartments relative to the supports of the cervix and vagina.[10] According to this terminology, the vagina and uterus, and the visceral pelvic supports attaching them to the pelvic walls, separate the pelvis into an anterior compartment including the urethra and bladder and a posterior compartment including the anus and rectum. Failure of the uterine and vaginal visceral fascial supports can lead to descent of the cervix within the vagina or even outside the vagina (vaginal vault prolapse and procidentia). Failure of the anterior compartment supports can lead to protrusion of a portion of the bladder or urethra into the anterior vaginal wall (cystocele or urethrocele). Failure of the posterior compartment supports can lead to protrusion of a portion of the rectum or small intestine into the posterior vaginal wall. Multicompartment failures may also occur.

Visceral fascial supports of the rectum and anorectum

Condensations of the visceral pelvic fascia anchor the rectum to the pelvic surface of the sacrum and to the tendinous arch of the pelvic fascia. The posterior rectal ligaments (Waldeyer's fascia) are sturdy attachments between the fibrous coat of the anorectum and the third and fourth sacral vertebrae. The lateral rectal ligaments are usually considered as peritoneal folds surrounding the middle rectal arteries.[19] Based on cadaver dissections, Jones and colleagues have doubted the existence of substantial lateral rectal ligaments and found only small or unilaterally present middle rectal arteries.[50]

It is important to note that the visceral investing supports attach the anterior walls of the bladder and urethra to the pubic symphysis and attach the posterior walls of the rectum and anus to the sacrum. The pubocervical ligaments anchor the vagina anteriorly to the pubis but provide no barrier between the walls of the urethra and vagina; in fact, the urethra is virtually embedded in the anterior vaginal wall. The rectovaginal fascia does provide a barrier between the vagina and rectum, and defects in the rectovaginal fascia are associated with rectocele.

Conclusions

The anatomy of the pelvic organ support system is complex and defies easy characterization. Traditional anatomic descriptions of the pelvic organ support system appear to be inadequate for the rapidly accumulating body of data on normal and pathologic pelvic floor anatomy. Misconceptions about the extent and configurations of the pelvic floor, an inadequate and confusing terminology, and a proliferation of undefined synonyms and landmarks in the recent literature are all obstacles to an adequate understanding of pelvic floor anatomy. Recent technological advances offer the opportunity to study pelvic floor anatomy in powerful and exciting ways, but until conceptual and terminological difficulties are resolved, these studies cannot achieve their full potential for improving the understanding, diagnosis, and treatment of pelvic floor disorders.

The pelvic organ support system consists of four basic components:

(1) *pelvic bones, joints, and interosseous ligaments*
(2) *midline connective tissue structures of the pelvic outlet*
(3) *pelvic muscles and investing pelvic fascia*
(4) *visceral pelvic fascia and visceral fascial ligaments.*

The importance of the midline connective tissue structures is overlooked in most discussions of the pelvic organs support system.

The nearly ubiquitous idea that the pelvic floor muscles comprise a single levator ani muscle with a single function, "supporting the pelvic floor", is an impediment to more detailed study of the actual functions and dysfunctions of the muscles of the pelvic floor. Attention to the attachments and muscle fiber orientations of the individual pelvic floor muscles suggest that their functions are more complex, more interesting, and probably more clinically relevant than the description "supporting the pelvic floor" would suggest. The functions of individual muscles merit further research. Additional studies are also needed to determine how the components of the pelvic floor support system work together, their relative contributions to pelvic organ support, and the consequences of the failure of one component for other components of the pelvic floor support system.

The somatic innervation to muscles of the pelvic floor, continence mechanisms, and pelvic organs may have both intrapelvic and extrapelvic courses. These nerves are particularly vulnerable to injury in surgical procedures involving the sacrospinous ligament and uterosacral ligament.

The increasing incidence of pelvic organ prolapse and the low success rates of many very invasive surgical procedures suggest that additional clarification of the pelvic floor support system is urgently needed.

Acknowledgments

I am grateful to Dr Richard F Hoyt, for his encyclopedic knowledge of anatomy, sound judgment, and deft editorial pencil, and to David Chapin, for his superb summary of pelvic floor supports.

References

1. Nygaard I, Bradley C et al. Pelvic organ prolapse in older women: Prevalence and risk factors. *Obstet Gynecol* 2004; 104(3): 489–97.
2. Tarnay CM, Bhatia NN. Urogynecology. In DeCherney AH and Nathan L, eds. *Current Obstetric and Gynecologic Diagnosis and Treatment*, 9th edition. New York: McGraw-Hill, 2003.
3. Olsen AL, Smith VJ, Bergstrom JO, Colling JC, Clark AL. Epidemiology of surgically managed pelvic organ prolapse and urinary incontinence. *Obstet Gynecol* 1997; 89: 501–6.
4. Leslie Wilson L, Brown JS et al. Annual direct cost of urinary incontinence. *Obstet Gynecol* 2001; 98: 398–406.
5. Mant J, Painter R, Vessey M. Epidemiology of genital prolapse: observations from the Oxford Family Planning Association Study. *Br J Obstet Gynecol* 1997; 104: 579–85.
6. Whiteside JL, Weber AM et al. Risk factors for recurrent prolapse after vaginal repair. *Am J Obstet Gynecol* 2004; 191:1533–8.
7. Cundiff GW, Fenner D. Evaluation and treatment of women with rectocele: focus on associated defecatory and sexual dysfunction. *Obstet Gynecol* 2004; 104: 1403–21.
8. Strohbein K. Normal pelvic floor anatomy. *Obstet Gynecol Clin North Am* 1998; 25: 689–705.
9. Fielding JR. Practical MR imaging of female pelvic floor weakness. *Radiographics* 2002; 22: 295–304

10. Delancey JO, Kearney R et al. The appearance of levator ani muscle abnormalities in magnetic resonance images after vaginal delivery. *Obstet Gynecol* 2003; 101: 46–53.

11. Tunn R, Delancey JO. Anatomic variations in the levator ani muscle, endopelvic fascia, and urethra in nulliparas evaluated by magnetic resonance imaging. *Am J Obstet Gynecol* 2003; 188: 116–21.

12. Hoyte L. Levator ani thickness variations in symptomatic and asymptomatic women using magnetic resonance-based-3-dimensional color mapping. *Obstet Gynecol* 2004; 103: 447–51.

13. Hoyte L, Schierlitz L, Zou K, Flesh G, Fielding JR. Two- and 3-dimensional MRI comparison of levator ani structure, volume, and integrity in women with stress incontinence and prolapse. *Am J Obstet Gynecol* 2001; 185: 11–19

14. Williams PL, Bannister LH, Berry MM et al., eds. *Gray's Anatomy of the Human Body*, 38th edn. New York: Churchill Livingstone, 1995: 1842.

15. Baragi RV, Delancey JO et al. Differences in pelvic floor area between African American and European American women. *Am J Obstet Gynecol* 2002; 187: 111–5.

16. Hoyt RF. Innervation of the vagina and vulva. In Goldstein I, Meston C, Davis S and Traish A eds. Women's Sexual Function and Dysfunction, London: Taylor and Francis, 2005: 113–124.

17. Welgoss JA, Vogt VY, et al. Relationship between surgically induced neuropathy and outcome of pelvic organ prolapse surgery. *Int Urogynecol J Pelvic Floor Dysfunct* 1999; 10: 11–14.

18. Federative Committee on Anatomical Terminology. *Terminologia Anatomica*. New York: Thieme, 1998.

19. Williams PL, Bannister LH, Berry MM et al., eds. *Gray's Anatomy of the Human Body*, 38th ed. New York: Churchill-Livingstone, 1995.

20. Drake RL, Vogel W et al. *Gray's Anatomy for Students*. New York: Elsevier, 2005.

21. Rosse C, Gaddum-Rosse P, eds. *Hollinshead's Textbook of Anatomy*, 5th ed. Philadelphia: Lippincott-Raven, 1997.

22. Moore KF, Dailey AF. *Clinically Oriented Anatomy*, 4th edition. Philadelphia: Lippincott, Williams and Wilkins, 1999.

23. Snell RS. *Clinical Anatomy for Medical Students*. Boston: Little Brown and Company, 1995.

24. Putz R, Pabst R. *Sobotta's Atlas of Human Anatomy*. Philadelphia: Lippincott, Williams and Wilkins, 2000.

25. Lockhart RD, Hamilton GF, Fyfe FW. *Anatomy of the Human Body*. Philadelphia: JB Lippincott, 1965.

26. Standring S, ed. *Gray's Anatomy of the Human Body*, 39th Ed. New York: Churchill Livingstone, 2005.

27. Strohbehn K, Ellis JH et al. Magnetic resonance imaging of the levator ani with anatomic correlation. *Am J Obstet Gynecol* 1996; 87: 277–85.

28. Singh K, Jakab M, Reid WM, Berger LA, Hoyte L. Three-dimensional magnetic resonance imaging assessment of levator ani morphologic features in different grades of prolapse. *Am J Obstet Gynecol* 2003; 188: 910–15.

29. Kearney R, Sawhney R, Delancey JO. Levator ani muscle anatomy evaluated by origin-insertion pairs. *Obstet Gynecol* 2004; 104: 168–73.

30. Hjartardottir S, Nilsson J, Petersen C, Lingman G. The female pelvic floor: a dome – not a basin. *Acta Obstet Gynecol Scand* 1997; 76: 567–71.

31. Aukee P, Usenius JP, Kirkinen P. An evaluation of pelvic floor anatomy and function by MRI. *Eur J Obstet Gynecol Reprod Biol* 2004; 112: 84–8.

32. Schmeiser G, Putz R. The anatomy and function of the pelvic floor. *Radiologe* 2000; 40: 429–36.

33. Delancey JO. Structural anatomy of the posterior pelvic compartment as it relates to rectocele. *Am J Obstet Gynecol* 2004; 180: 815–23.

34. Rao SS. Pathophysiology of adult fecal incontinence. *Gastroenterology* 2004; 126 (Suppl): S14–22.

35. Yucel S, Baskin LS. An anatomical description of the male and female urethral sphincter complex. *J Urol* 2004; 171: 1890–7.

36. Copas P, Bukovsky A, Asbury B, Elder RF, Caudle MR, Estrogen, progesterone, and androgen receptor expression in levator ani muscle and fascia. *J Womens Health* 2001; (Larchmt) 10: 785–95.

37. Dimpfl T, Jaegar C, Mueller-Felber W et al. Myogenic changes of the levator ani muscle in premenopausal women: the impact of vaginal delivery and age. *Neurourol Urodyn* 1998; 17: 197–206.

38. Smith ARB, Hosker GL, Warrell DW. The role of partial denervation of the pelvic floor in the aetiology of genitourinary prolapse and stress incontinence of urine: a neurophysiological study. *Br J Obstet Gynaecol* 1989; 96: 24–8.

39. Snooks SJ, Swash M, Mathers SE, Henry MM. Effect of vaginal delivery on the pelvic floor: A 5-year follow-up. *Br J Surg* 1990; 77: 1358–60.

40. Strohbein K. Normal pelvic floor anatomy. *Obstet Gynecol Clin North Am* 1998; 25: 689–705.

41. Vazzoler N, Soulie M, Escourrou G et al. Pubourethral ligaments in women: anatomical and clinical aspects. *Surg Radiol Anat* 2002; 24: 33–7.

42. Kim JK, Kim YJ, Choo MS, Cho KS. The urethra and its supporting structures in women with stress urinary incontinence: MR imaging using an endovaginal coil. *Am J Roentgenol* 2003; 180: 1037–44.

43. Richardson AC, Edmonds PB, Williams NL. Treatment of stress urinary incontinence due to paravaginal fascial defect. *Obstet Gynecol* 1981; 57: 357–62.

44. Delancey JO. The anatomy of the pelvic floor. *Curr Opin Obstet Gynecol* 1994; 6: 313–6.

45. Delancey JO. Structural anatomy of the posterior pelvic compartment as it relates to rectocele. *Am J Obstet Gynecol* 2004; 180: 815–23.

46. Buller JL, Thompson JR. Uterosacral ligament: description of anatomic relationships to optimize surgical safety. *Obstet Gynecol* 2001; 97: 873–9.

47. Umek WH, Morgan DM et al. Quantitative analysis of uterosacral ligament origin and insertion points by magnetic resonance imaging. *Obstet Gynecol* 2004; 103: 447–51.

48. Fritsch H, Hotzinger H. Tomographical anatomy of the pelvis, visceral pelvic connective tissue, and its compartments. *Clin Anat* 1995; 8: 17–24.

49. Chapin DS. The anatomy of pelvic supports. Presentation to Applied Clinical Anatomy course, Harvard Medical School. August 2000.

50. Jones OM, Smeulders N. Lateral ligaments of the rectum: an anatomical study. *Br J Surg* 1999; 86(4): 487–9

PHYSIOLOGIC MECHANISMS

5.1 Cellular and molecular mechanisms underlying sexual arousal

Jessica A Mong, Anna W Lee, Amy Easton, Donald W Pfaff

The molecular analyses of sexual behaviors dependent on sexual arousal have benefited greatly from several strategic advantages. From the cellular and circuitry point of view, even in complex experimental animals such as mammals, simple reproductively relevant stimuli and sexual responses permit neural network analysis. From a molecular point of view, steroid hormones acting through nuclear receptors which are transcription factors invoke regulated gene expression, for example, in hypothalamic neurons.[1] In turn, these neurons control mating behavior circuits. This chapter attempts to offer basic, reductionistic principles which apply to all mammals, human patients included. We dare to be so ambitious because of the large number of mechanisms for hormone action in the central nervous system known to be conserved as we move from animal brain to human brain tissue.

Drawing hormone-regulated gene expression into the explanation of mammalian sex behavior has proceeded rapidly. Here we theoretically propose a gene network – really, a micronet – downstream of estrogen action in the forebrain responsible for courtship and lordosis behavior in quadruped females. This chapter comprises an attempt to draw different transcriptional systems into a new theoretic formulation. These efforts to explain hormone-driven behaviors have benefited from Rosenfeld's example of genetic network control over pituitary gland development.[2] Both direct and indirect causal routes are described below.

Causal routes, downstream from the genomic actions of sex hormones; a modular system emergent

The primary sex behavior of female quadrupeds, lordosis, depends on defined physical signals: cutaneous stimuli and estrogens plus progestins.[1] The neural circuit has been worked out; estrogen-dependent transcription in ventromedial hypothalamic cells allows permissive signals to the midbrain central grey, thus enabling the rest of the circuit. In the absence of fear or anxiety-provoking conditions, females under the influence of estrogens plus progestins will demonstrate courtship and then mating behaviors. During the normal female cycle, these behavioral components of reproduction are synchronized with ovulation. Thus, with the mediation of estrogens plus progestins, the neural, behavioral, and endocrine preparations for reproduction are harmonized.

Since (a) the hormone receptors discovered in neurons turned out to be transcription factors, (b) mating behaviors follow estrogen administration by more than 18h, and (c) inhibitors of RNA and protein synthesis disrupt the estrogen effect, it was natural to look for genes whose induction comprised important mechanisms for the behavioral facilitation. Below are listed gene/neuronal and gene/glial modules found so far. The wording and formulation presented here were published first in the article by Mong and Pfaff.[3]

Throughout these studies, we compare two extremely similar transcription factors, estrogen receptors alpha and beta. Likely gene duplication products, both have high affinity for estradiol and for genomic estrogen response elements in vertebrate gene promoters.[4-7] Yet, they have distinctly different neuroanatomic patterns of expression[8] and different functional consequences.

All of the genetic systems discussed below have the character that estrogen treatment turns them on *in vivo*; and that they participate in facilitating estrogen-dependent female reproductive behaviors (Fig. 5.1.1).

Direct effects, from gene induction to neural circuit to behavioral change

Hormone effects on neurotransmitter receptors in ventromedial hypothalamic neurons directly trigger the rest of the lordosis circuit to operate.

Noradrenergic alpha-1b receptors are induced[9] *in vivo* in female rats by estrogen treatment in ventromedial hypothalamic cells which govern the rest of the lordosis behavior circuit.[10,11] Noradrenergic ascending afferents synapse on ventromedial hypothalamic neurons, coming in from the ventral noradrenergic bundle, which originates in arousal-related neuronal groups A1 and A2, and signals heightened arousal upon stimulation from the male. In biophysical studies, directly applied noradrenaline increases the electrical activity of ventromedial hypothalamic neurons.[10] Beginning with Gq or G11 proteins activating phospholipase C, noradrenaline action will produce both diacylglycerol, a protein kinase C (PKC) activator, and inositol-3-phosphate, which mobilizes intracellular calcium. This signal transduction route is predicted to lead to L-type calcium channel opening as in the heart, but this needs to be established. The induction of alpha-1b receptors by estrogen treatment is consistent with the greater electrophysiologic effectiveness of noradrenaline following estrogen, but the detailed step-by-step transduction route to the channel now

provides a timely subject for analysis. Since these ventromedial hypothalamic neurons are at the top of the lordosis behavior circuit, the noradrenergic ascending afferents effect fosters reproductive behavior.

Muscarinic receptors responding to the neurotransmitter acetylcholine are also expressed in ventromedial hypothalamic neurons.[12] Estrogen treatment increases their activities as determined electrophysiologically. Inputs to ventromedial hypothalamic neurons come from, among other places, the lateral dorsal nucleus of the tegmentum. Neurons there are part of the ascending arousal pathways, and would signal stimulation from the male upon mounting the female. We note that apparent redundancy between ascending noradrenergic and muscarinic cholinergic afferents to the hypothalamus helps to guarantee that the system will not fail, and so exemplifies a design characteristic prominent in brainstem arousal system neurobiology. In any case, inducing muscarinic receptors increases the ventromedial hypothalamic cellular electrophysiologic response to acetylcholine. Whether the estrogen effect employs a membrane receptor, a signal transduction mechanism, or a classical genomic facilitation is not yet known. However, it is known that the enhanced ventromedial hypothalamic neuronal output primes lower pathways in the circuit for lordosis behavior.[13]

Indirect effects, from gene induction to downstream genes to behavioral change

Some hormone effects occur early, long before the onset of reproductive behaviors, and set the stage for later developments.

Neuronal growth

Growth promotion by estrogens in ventromedial hypothalamic neurons, in female rats, follows from the stimulation of synthesis

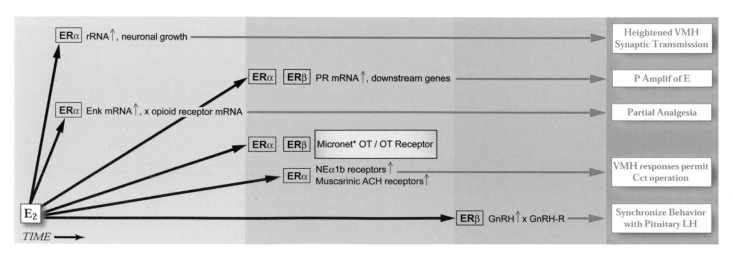

Figure 5.1.1. Genes and systems downstream from estrogen-facilitated transcription. All of these systems foster female reproductive behavior. Along the causal routes, estrogen receptor (ER) alpha-dependent inductions are signaled in red; ER alpha-dependent in blue; functional consequences in green. Time reads from left to right. Early-induced genes to the left, later to the right. Further, in some cases estrogens induce both the mRNA for a ligand and for its cognate receptor. These cases are indicated by "X". ** designates an ER-alpha/beta micronet illustrated in Fig. 5.1.2. *Abbreviations*: E2, estradiol; rRNA, ribosomal RNA; PR, progesterone receptor; Enk, enkephalin, an opioid peptide; NE, norepinephrine; ACH, acetylcholine; GnRH, gonadotropin-releasing hormone (synonym, LHRH).

of ribosomal RNA, which precedes the elaboration of dendrites and synapses on ventromedial hypothalamic neurons observed after hormonal treatment. The earliest estrogen effect is the increase of transcription of ribosomal RNA,[14] followed rapidly by morphologic effects, including those in the nucleolus itself[15] and a striking elaboration of rough endoplasmic reticulum in the cytoplasm.[16] Woolley[17] and her colleagues have shown, probably consequent to the phenomena above, a stimulatory effect of estrogen treatment on dendritic growth. In the female rat hypothalamus, Frankfurt[18] and Flanagan[19,20] have reported that estrogens foster dendritic growth and an increased number of synapses.[21]

Therefore, in ventromedial hypothalamic cells which control lordosis behavior circuitry, estrogens apparently provide the structural basis for increased synaptic activity and, therefore, greater sex-behavior-facilitating output. While the greater signaling capacity of these ventromedial hypothalamic cells thus proposed is consistent with the actual electrophysiologic activity of such cells after estrogen treatment, the causal relation of structure to function still needs direct proof.

Amplification by progesterone

Administration of progesterone 24 or 48 h after estrogen priming greatly amplifies the effect of estrogen on mating behavior. This effect requires the nuclear progesterone receptor, as it disappears after antisense DNA against progesterone receptor mRNA has been administered onto ventromedial hypothalamic neurons.[22–24] It also disappears in progesterone receptor knockout mice.[25] Since progesterone receptor itself is a transcription factor, its induction by estrogen might imply that certain downstream genes would, consequently, be upregulated. With molecular probes directed to specific genes, studied primarily in female rats, several have been revealed as upregulated by progesterone: these include neuropeptide Y receptor,[26] galanin,[27,28] oxytocin,[29] gonadotropin-releasing hormone,[30,31] mu opioid receptors,[32] pro-opiomelanocortin,[33] glutamic acid decarboxylase,[34] a glutamate receptor,[35] and tyrosine hydroxylase.[36,37] The manners in which these particular downstream genes contribute to reproductive behaviors will be exciting to explore.

Gonadotropin-releasing hormone

The physiologic importance of estrogenic elevation of gonadotropin-releasing hormone (GnRH, synonym LHRH) mRNA levels under positive feedback conditions – as well as elevation of the receptor mRNA for GnRH – would be to *synchronize* reproductive behavior with the ovulatory surge of luteinizing hormone (LH). The same GnRH decapeptide that stimulates the ovulatory release of gonadotropins also facilitates mating behavior.[38,39] In many small animals, synchrony of sex behavior with ovulation would be biologically adaptive because it eliminates unnecessary exposure to predation. In this respect, the behavioral effect of this neuropeptide is consonant with its peripheral physiologic action.

Gonadotropin-releasing hormone also brings up the unusual case of an individual gene causally related to a human social behavior. During development in vertebrates ranging from fish to humans, GnRH neurons migrate from their birth place in the olfactory placode into the brain.[40] A human with damage at the Kallmann's syndrome[41] locus on the X chromosome did not fail to express the GnRH gene in the appropriate neurons. Instead, the neurons failed to migrate out of the olfactory placode.[42] A single gene for the Kall protein[43,44] accounts for the deficit. It is for an extracellular matrix protein which is necessary for the GnRH neuronal migration and which, in fact, decorates the migration route.[45] A striking feature of the phenotype in men is important to note. They have no libido. Here is the causal route. The men have no sexual drive *because* they have little testosterone, *because* they have little luteinizing hormone and follicle-stimulating hormone circulating from the pituitary gland, *because* no GnRH is coming down the portal circulation to the pituitary from the hypothalamus, *because* there is no GnRH in the hypothalamus, *because* the GnRH neurons did not migrate during development into the brain, *because* of a mutation in the gene for the Kall protein. Therefore, we can causally connect, step-by-step, an individual gene to an important human social behavior, but at least six causal links are required. This causal route illustrates the complexity of gene/behavior relationships in humans.

Indirect effects, from gene induction to intermediate behaviors

Some of the genes affected by estrogens work by altering other behaviors which then prepare the animal for the behavior in question – in this case, mating.

Analgesia

The enkephalin gene is turned on rapidly, in female mouse and rat hypothalamic neurons, by estrogens,[46–48] within about 30 min, and this is proven by *in vitro* transcription assays to represent a hormone-facilitated transcriptional activation.[49] The route of action upon lordosis of the enkephalin gene product would theoretically be indirect, through other behaviors. That is, we propose that, through the reduction of pain, enkephalins help to allow the female to engage in mating behavior despite the mauling she receives from the male. The strong somatosensory and interoceptive stimuli, which ordinarily would be treated by the female as noxious, are now tolerable and allow successful mating to proceed.[50] Hypothetically, the ability of estrogens to also turn on genes for opioid receptors[51] has the potential of multiplying the hormone's effect on mating behavior sequences. Specificity among opioid receptors, as well as neuroanatomic site specificity, is observed in this course of action.[52–55] The indirect route of action of this multiplicative set of gene inductions is likely to allow the female to participate in sex behavior sequences.

Anxiety reduction

The oxytocin gene and the gene for its receptor are both expressed by hypothalamic neurons at higher levels in the presence of estrogens. The indirect route of action of this multiplicative set of gene inductions, on mating behavior, is likely through a behavioral link: anxiety reduction allows courtship and mating. This proposal is consistent with previous formulations: oxytocin has been conceived as protecting instinctive behaviors connected with reproduction, maternity, and other social behaviors from the disruptive effects of stress.[56] Indeed, oxytocin has an anxiolytic action in the presence of estrogens (which presumably elevate the oxytocin receptor gene product).[57]

Social recognition and aggression

The induction of the oxytocin gene by estrogens is an estrogen receptor beta-dependent,[58] behaviorally significant[59] phenomenon. This makes sense, since only estrogen receptor beta gene expression is found in oxytocinergic cells.[8] In turn, oxytocinergic projections to the amygdala are thought to be important for social recognition in mice, and this helps to prevent aggression.[60-62] Thus, the lack of social recognition by estrogen receptor beta knockout mice[63] could explain the hyperaggressiveness displayed by estrogen receptor beta knockout male mice.[64] Together, these data invoke the idea of a four-gene micronet important for social behaviors (Fig. 5.1.2).

Orchestrated genomic responses to hormones (GAPPS)

From this series of individual gene inductions by estrogens acting in the basal forebrain, and the recounting (above) of downstream genes and their physiologic routes of action, there emerges a theoretic molecular 'formula' which appears to account for some of the causal relations between sex hormones and female sex behaviors. First, there is a hormone-dependent *growth* response, which permits hormone-facilitated, behavior-directing hypothalamic neurons a greater range of input/output connections and, thus, physiologic power. Second, progesterone can *amplify* the estrogen effect, in part through the downstream genes listed above. Then, through indirect behavioral means – the reduction of anxiety and partial analgesia – the female as an organism is *prepared for* engaging in reproductive behavior sequences. Here the genes for oxytocin (and its receptor) as well as the genes for the opioid peptide enkephalin (and its receptors) are important. Next, neurotransmitter receptor induction by estradiol *permits* the neural circuit for lordosis behavior to be activated. The noradrenaline alpha-1 receptor and the muscarinic acetylcholine receptors are key here, in the ventromedial nucleus of the hypothalamus. Finally, with induction of the decapeptide that triggers ovulation, gonadotropin-releasing hormone as well as its cognate receptor acts to *synchronize* mating behavior with ovulation in a biologically adaptive fashion.

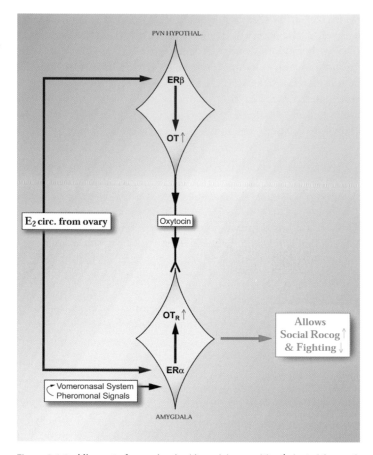

Figure 5.1.2. Micronet of genes involved in social recognition (adapted from ref. 62). These comprise part of the larger set of causal routes summarised in Fig. 5.1.1. Estradiol (E) produced in the ovaries and circulating in the bloodstream is bound by estrogen receptor (ER) β in paraventricular hypothalmic (PVN) neurons. Many of these PVN neurons express oxytocin (OT↑). Oxytocin production is thereby increased. Axons carrying oxytocin project to the amygdala. In neurons of the amygdala, estradiol is bound by cells expressing ERα. As a result, mRNA and functional protein levels of the oxytocin receptor (OT$_R$↑) are increased. The medial and cortical nuclei of the amygdala receive pheromonal inputs from the vomeronasal system. Such inputs are crucial for directing neuroendocrine events and social behavior. Oxytocinergic action there enhances social recognition among mice. For mice, this permits reproduction and reduces aggression.

This theoretic formulation is intended to tie together disparate results from several transcriptional systems into one set of modules. Even so, the genomic mechanisms uncovered so far probably represent only a subset of the full range of neurochemical steps underlying sex behaviors.

Arousal mechanisms underlying sex behaviors

Given that sex hormonal facilitation on concrete, explicit sexual behaviors can be understood in detail, what about the motivational forces which underlie the emission of reproductive responses? It is widely accepted that all motivational forces depend on the arousal of the central nervous system, the activation of behavior. Generalized arousal of the central nervous system has been defined and can be measured efficiently in experimental animals.[65] It turns out that sex hormones can influence gene expression associated with generalized arousal of the brain, and in turn that some of these gene products influence sex behavior-relevant neurons in the medial hypothalamus.

Regarding the former point, in a microarray study, we discovered that estrogen administration can significantly alter mRNA levels for the arousal-related enzyme, lipocalin-type-prostaglandin D synthase.[66] Surprisingly, the regulation was in opposite directions between the medial hypothalamus and the preoptic area: elevated mRNA levels in the hypothalamus, but decreased in the preoptic area. The arousal-related transmitters norepinephrine and histamine turn on electrical activity in the ventromedial

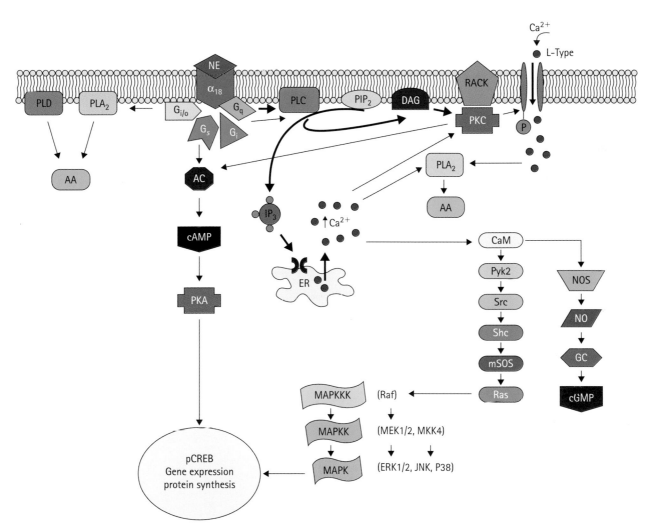

Figure 5.1.3. A cartoon derived from the literature on alpha–adrenergic signaling. Reproduced with permission from Pfaff et al., *The Physiology of Reproduction*, 3rd edn (Academic Press/Elsevier, 2005). This is important because it specifies how a generalized arousal system could influence specific, sexual arousal, in this case through norepinephrine increasing the electrical activity of the ventromedial hypothalamic neurons which control lordosis behavior. α_{1B}-Adrenergic receptors couple primarily to G_q, stimulating phospholipase C (PLC). PLC cleaves phosphatidylinositol 4,5-biphosphate (PIP$_2$), generating inositol 1,4,5-triphosphate (IP$_3$), and diacylglycerol (DAG). IP$_3$ mobilizes intracellular Ca^{2+} and DAG activates protein kinase C (PKC). The mobilization of cytoplasmic Ca^{2+} stimulates phospholipase A$_2$ (PLA$_2$), releasing arachidonic acid (AA), and activates nitric oxide synthase (NOS), producing nitric oxide (NO), guanylyl cyclase (GC), and cyclic guanosine monophosphate (cGMP). PKC has been proposed to bind to the receptor for activated C kinases (RACK) near the L-type Ca^{2+} channel, which it phosphorylates, causing an influx of Ca^{2+}. There is some evidence that α_{1B}-adrenergic receptors may also couple to G_h, leading to production of IP$_3$ and DAG; to G_s, leading to stimulation of protein kinase A (PKA); and to G$_i$/G$_o$, increasing AA through PLA$_2$ or phopholipase D (PLD). Although, the precise signaling mechanism is not known, α_{1B}-adrenergic receptors can stimulate the mitogen-activated protein kinase (MAPK) pathway. α_{1B}-adrenergic receptors can activate extracellular signal-regulated kinases (ERKs), P38, or c-Jun *N*-terminal kinases (JNKs), depending upon the particular cell line or tissue it is expressed in. AC indicates adenylyl cyclase; CaM, calmodulin; cAMP, cyclic 3',5'-adenosine monophosphate; ER, endoplasmic reticulum; NE, norepinephrine; pCREB, cAMP-responsive element binding protein. *Sources include*: A. Etgen, in *Hormones, Brain and Behavior* (Academic Press/Elsevier, 2002); K. Minneman, *Pharmacological Reviews*, 1988; G. Michelotti, *Pharmacology and Therapeutics*, 2000; T. Koshimitzu, *Biological and Pharmaceutical Bulletin*, 2002; and S. Kreda and W. Wetsel, *Endocrinology*, 2001.

hypothalamic cells that are at the top of the lordosis behavior (mating behavior) circuit in female animals. Our understanding of exactly how these transmitters work on the neurons we record is summarized very briefly in the two paragraphs following. In each case we are discerning how generalized arousal mechanisms influence the level of specifically sexual arousal.

The most important noradrenergic receptor subtype for the control of female sex behavior by hypothalamic neurons is the alpha-1b subtype. This receptor is coupled primarily with Gq proteins, which have several ways of signaling (Fig. 5.1.3). The easiest to understand is the activation of phospholipase C, which yields both calcium mobilization and diacylglycerol (DAG), which in turn activates PKC.

Histamine receptors also belong to the 7-transmembrane-spanning, G-protein receptor superfamily. Signal transduction pathways are most well defined for histamine H1 receptors, and these are likely the most important for influencing electrical activity in hypothalamic neurons controlling sex behavior. Activation of histamine H1 receptors stimulates the formation of second messengers – inositol 1,4,5-triphosphate (IP_3), diacylglycerol, and arachidonic acid (AA), via coupling with $G_{q/11}$ protein (Fig. 5.1.4). IP_3 (inositol 1,4,5-triphosphate) increases intracellular Ca^{2+} levels, which can have at least two effects: enhancing the production of histamine H2/A2 receptor-induced cyclic adenosine monophosphate and the production of cyclic guanosine monophosphate. Diacylglycerol potentiates the activity of protein kinase C, ultimately enhancing glutamate N-methyl-D-aspartate (NMDA) receptor-mediated currents. Histamine H1 receptor activation also can act to block a leak K^+ conductance, resulting in excitation of the neuron. By all of these routes, histamine, as a transmitter exquisitely associated with generalized arousal of the brain, could influence hypothalamic neurons responsible for regulating sex behavior.

Summary

In experimental animals, we can analyze, step by step, in physical detail, the mechanisms triggered by sex hormones to influence sexual arousal, which elevates sexual motivation, and permits sexual behaviors. The relative simplicity of these mechanisms in common laboratory animals has led to the primacy of cellular and molecular mechanisms for reproduction within neuroendocrinology: the discovery of sex hormone receptors in the brain, the unraveling of the first neural circuit for a vertebrate behavior (lordosis behavior), the discovery of hormone-facilitated gene expression in the brain, and the functional genomics of sex hormone receptors in the central nervous system.

Histamine receptor signal transduction pathways

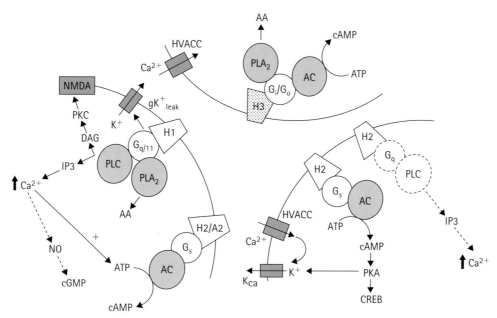

Figure 5.1.4. Schematic representation, based on the literature regarding histamine neurobiology, of membrane and cellular responses to histamine receptor activation. Reproduced with permission from Pfaff et al., *The Physiology of Reproduction*, 3rd edn (Academic Press/Elsevier, 2004). Like Fig. 5.1.3, this step-by-step formulation is important because it specifies how a generalized arousal system could influence specific, sexual arousal by increasing the electrical activity of the ventromedial hypothalamic neurons which control lordosis behavior. Figures drawn with dashed lines indicate possible, but as yet unverified, signal transduction pathways. H1 receptors, when activated, bind to the $G_{q/11}$ protein, stimulating PIP2 (phosphatidyl-4,5-biphosphate) hydrolysis, which results in the formation of inositol 1,4,5-triphosphate (IP_3) and diacylglycerol (DAG). IP_3 induces the release of calcium from intracellular stores, which can initiate the augmentation of cyclic adenosine monophosphate (cAMP) production by neighboring H2 or adenosine receptors. DAG potentiates the activity of protein kinase C (PKC), which in turn phosphorylates the N-methyl-D-aspartate (NMDA) receptor, weakening the Mg^+ block. H1 receptor activation also leads to an increase in arachidonic acid (AA) and cGMP, and the blockade of a leak K^+ conductance. CREB = cAMP-responsive element binding protein, PLA_2 = phospholipase A_2, AC = adenylyl cyclase. *Sources include*: R.E. Brown et al., *Progress in Neurobiology*, 2001; S.J. Hill, *Agents Actions* Suppl. 1991); Greene & Haas, *Neuroscience*, 1990.

However, the facts and concepts related to sexual arousal simply fit into a huge and growing body of knowledge about hormone effects in thje central nervous system (see *Hormones, Brain and Behavior*, 5 vols, Academic Press, 2002), whose main features recently have been summarized in didactic form (*Principles of Hormone/Behavior Relations*, Academic Press, 2004).

Acknowledgments

This chapter constitutes an adaptation and updating of an article, "Hormonal Symphony: Functional genetic modules for sociosexual behaviors".[3] The new experimental work was supported by NIH Grants HD-05751-31 and MH-38273-17. The authors acknowledge the help with the illustrations offered by Parthiv Parekh, of Rockefeller University.

References

1. Pfaff DW. *Drive: Neural and Molecular Mechanisms for Sexual Motivation*. Cambridge: MIT Press, 1999.

2. Scully KM, Rosenfeld MG. Pituitary development: regulatory codes in mammalian organogenesis. *Science* 2002; 295: 2231–5.

3. Mong JA, Pfaff DW. Hormonal symphony: steroid orchestration of gene modules for sociosexual behaviors. *Mol Psychiatry* 2004; 9: 550–6.

4. Jensen EV, Jacobson HI. Basic guides to the mechanism of estrogen action. *Recent Prog Horm Res* 1962; 18: 387–414.

5. Walter P, Green S, Greene G et al. Cloning of the human estrogen receptor cDNA. *Proc Natl Acad Sci USA* 1985; 82: 7889–93.

6. Kuiper CG, Enmark E, Pelto-Huikko M et al. Cloning of a novel receptor expressed in rat prostate and ovary. *Proc Natl Acad Sci USA* 1996; 93: 5925–30.

7. Nilsson S, Gustafsson JA. Biological role of estrogen and estrogen receptors. *Crit Rev Biochem Mol Biol* 2002; 37: 1–28.

8. Shughrue PJ, Lane MV, Merchanthaler I. Comparative distribution of estrogen receptor alpha and beta RNA in the rat central nervous system. *J Comp Neurol* 1997; 388: 507–25.

9. Etgen AM. Estrogen regulation of neurotransmitter and growth factor signaling in the brain. In Pfaff DW, Arnold A, Etgen A et al., eds. *Hormones, Brain and Behavior*, vol 3. New York: Academic Press, 2002: 381–440.

10. Kow L, Weesner G, Pfaff D. Alpha 1-adrenergic agonists act on the ventromedial hypothalamus to cause neuronal excitation and lordosis facilitation: electrophysiological and behavioral evidence. *Brain Res* 1992; 588: 237–45.

11. Petitti N, Karkanias GB, Etgen AM. Estradiol selectively regulates alpha 1B-noradrenergic receptors in the hypothalamus and preoptic area. *J Neurosci* 1992; 12: 3869–76.

12. Kow LM, Tsai YF, Weiland NG et al. *In vitro* electro-pharmacological and autoradiographic analyses of muscarinic receptor subtypes in rat hypothalamic ventromedial nucleus: implications for cholinergic regulation of lordosis. *Brain Res* 1995; 694(1–2): 29–39.

13. Menard CS, Dohanich GP. Physostigmine facilitation of lordosis

in naturally cycling female rats. *Pharmacol Biochem Behav* 1990; 36: 853–8.

14. Jones K, Harrington CA, Chikaraishi DM et al., Steroid hormone regulation of ribosomal RNA in rat hypothalamus: early detection using *in situ* hybridization and precursor-product ribosomal DNA probes. *J Neurosci* 1990; 10: 1513–21.

15. Cohen R, Chung S, Pfaff D. Alteration by estrogen of the nucleoli in nerve cells of the rat hypothalamus. *Cell Tissue Res* 1984; 235: 485–9.

16. Cohen R, Pfaff D. Ultrastructure of neurons in the ventromedial nucleus of the hypothalamus in ovariectomized rats with or without estrogen treatment. *Cell Tissue Res* 1981; 217: 451–70.

17. Woolley CS, Cohen RS. Sex steroids and neuronal growth in adulthood. In DW Pfaff, A Arnold, A Etgen et al., eds. *Hormones, Brain and Behavior*, vol 4. San Diego: Academic Press, 2002: 717–77.

18. Frankfurt M. Gonadal steroids and neuronal plasticity: studies in the adult rat hypothalamus. *Ann N Y Acad Sci* 1994; 743: 45–60.

19. Flanagan-Cato L. Estrogen-induced remodeling of hypothalamic neural circuitry. *Front Neuroendocrinol* 2000; 4: 309–29 (Review).

20. Flanagan-Cato LM, Calizo LH, Daniels D. The synaptic organization of VMH neurons that mediate the effects of estrogen on sexual behavior. *Horm Behav* 2001; 40: 178–82.

21. Carrer H, Aoki A. Ultrastructural changes in the hypothalamic ventromedial nucleus of ovariectomized rats after estrogen treatment. *Brain Res* 1982; 240: 221–33.

22. Pollio G, Xue P, Zanisi M et al. Antisense oligonucleotide blocks progesterone-induced lordosis behavior in ovariectomized rats. *Mol Brain Res* 1993; 19: 135–9.

23. Ogawa S, Olazabal UE, Parhar IS et al. Effects of intrahypothalamic administration of antisense DNA for progesterone receptor mRNA on reproductive behavior and progesterone receptor immunoreactivity in female rat. *J Neurosci* 1994; 14: 1766–74.

24. Mani SK, Blaustein JD, Allen JM et al. Inhibition of rat sexual behavior by antisense oligonucleotides to the progesterone receptor. *Endocrinology* 1994; 135: 1409–14.

25. Lydon JP, DeMayo FJ, Funk CR et al. Mice lacking progesterone receptor exhibit pleiotropic reproductive abnormalities. *Genes Dev* 1995; 9: 2266–78.

26. Xu M, Urban JH, Hill JW et al. Regulation of hypothalamic neuropeptide Y1 receptor gene expression during the estrous cycle: role of progesterone receptors. *Endocrinology* 2000; 141: 3319–27.

27. Brann DW, Chorich LP, Mahesh VB. Effects of progesterone on galanin mRNA levels in the hypothalamus and the pituitary: correlation with the gonadotrophin surge. *Neuroendocrinology* 1993; 58: 531–8.

28. Rossmanith WG, Marks DL, Clifton DK et al. Induction of galanin mRNA in GNRH neurons by estradiol and its facilitation by progesterone. *J Neuroendocrinol* 1996; 8: 185–91.

29. Thomas A, Shughrue PJ, Merchenthaler I et al. The effects of progesterone on oxytocin mRNA levels in paraventricular nucleus of the female rat can be altered by the administration of diazepam or RU486. *J Neuroendocrinol* 1999; 11: 137–44.

30. Cho BN, Seong JY, Cho H et al. Progesterone stimulates GnRH gene expression in the hypothalamus of ovariectomized, estrogen treated adult rats. *Brain Res* 1994; 652: 177–80.

31. Petersen SL, Ottem EN, Carpenter CD et al. Effects of estrogen and progesterone on luteinizing hormone-released hormone messenger ribonucleic acid levels: consideration of temporal and neuroanatomical variables. *Endocrinology* 1995; 136: 3604–10.

32. Petersen SL, LaFlamme KD. Progesterone increases levels of mu-opioid receptor mRNA in the preoptic area and arcuate nucleus of ovariectomized, estradiol-treated female rats. *Mol Brain Res* 1997; 52: 32–7.

33. Petersen SL, Keller ML, Carder SA et al. Differential effects of estrogen and progesterone on levels of POMC mRNA levels in the arcuate nucleus: relationship to the timing of LH surge release. *J Neuroendocrinol* 1993; 5: 643–8.

34. Unda R, Brann DW, Mahesh VB. Progesterone suppression of glutamic acid decarboxylase (GAD_{67}) mRNA levels in the preoptic area: correlation to luteinizing hormone surge. *Neuroendocrinology* 1995; 62: 562–70.

35. Gu G, Varoqueaux F, Simerly RB. Hormonal regulation of glutamate receptor gene expression in the anteroventral periventricular nucleus of the hypothalamus. *J Neurosci* 1999; 19: 3213–22.

36. Arbogast LA, Voogt JL. Progesterone reverses the estradiol-induced decrease in tyrosine hydroxylase mRNA levels in the arcuate nucleus. *Neuroendocrinology* 1993; 58: 501–10.

37. Arbogast LA, Voogt JL. Progesterone suppresses tyrosine hydroxylase messenger ribonucleic acid levels in the arcuate nucleus on proestrus. *Endocrinology* 1994; 135: 343–50.

38. Moss R, McCann S. Induction of mating behavior in rats by luteinizing hormone-releasing factor. *Science* 1973; 181: 177–9.

39. Pfaff D. Luteinizing hormone releasing factor (LRF) potentiates lordosis behavior in hypophysectomized ovariectomized female rats. *Science* 1973; 182: 1148–9.

40. Schwanzel-Fukuda M, Pfaff DW. Origin of luteinizing hormone-releasing hormone neurons. *Nature* 1989; 338: 161–4.

41. MacColl G, Quinton R, Bouloux PMG. GnRH neuronal development – insights into the mechanisms of hypogonadotropic hypogonadism. *Trends Endocrinol Metab* 2002; 13: 112–18.

42. Schwanzel-Fukuda M, Bick D, Pfaff DW. Luteinizing hormone releasing hormone (LHRH) expressing cells do not migrate normally in an inherited hypogonadal (Kallmann) syndrome. *Mol Brain Res* 1989; 6: 311–26.

43. Legouis R, Hardelin JP, Levilliers J et al. The candidate gene for the X-linked Kallmann syndrome encodes a protein related to adhesion molecules. *Cell* 1991; 67: 423–35.

44. Ballabio A, Camerino G. The gene for X-linked Kallmann syndrome: a human neuronal migration defect. *Curr Opin Genet Dev* 1992; 2: 417–21.

45. Dellovade T, Hardelin JP, Pfaff DW et al. Anosmin-I immunoreactivity during embryogenesis in a primitive eutherian mammal. *Dev Brain Res* 2003; 140: 157–67.

46. Romano GJ, Harlan RE, Shivers BD et al. Estrogen increases proenkephalin messenger ribonucleic acid levels in the ventromedial hypothalamus of the rat. *Mol Endocrinol* 1988; 2: 1320–8.

47. Zhu Y-S, Cai LQ, You X et al. Molecular analysis of estrogen induction of preproenkephalin gene expression and its modulation by thyroid hormones. *Mol Brain Res* 2001; 91: 23–33.

48. Priest CA, Eckersell CB, Micevych PE. Estrogen regulates preproenkephalin-A mRNA levels in the rat ventromedial nucleus: temporal and cellular aspects. *Mol Brain Res* 1995; 28: 251–62.

49. Vasudevan N, Zhu YS, Daniel S et al. Crosstalk between oestrogen receptors and thyroid hormone receptor isoforms results in differential regulation of the preproenkephalin gene. *J Neuroendocrinol* 2001; 13: 779–90.

50. Bodnar R, Commons K, Pfaff D. *Central Neural States Relating Sex and Pain*. Baltimore: Johns Hopkins University Press, 2002.

51. Quinones-Jenab V, Jenab S, Ogawa S et al. Estrogen regulation of mu-opioid receptor mRNA in the forerain of female rats. *Mol Brain Res* 1997: 47: 134–8.

52. Acosta-Martinez M, Etgen AM. Activation of mu-opioid receptors inhibits lordosis behavior in estrogen and progesterone-primed female rats. *Horm Behav* 2002; 41: 88–100.

53. Pfaus J, Pfaff D. m-, d- and k-opioid receptor agonists selectively modulate sexual behaviors in the female rat: differential dependence on progesterone. *Horm Behav* 1992; 26: 457–73.

54. Pfaus J, Gorzalka B. Opioids and sexual behavior. *Neurosci Biobehav Rev* 1987; 11: 1–34 (Review).

55. Pfaus JG, Gorzalka BB. Selective activation of opioid receptors differentially affects lordosis behavior in female rats. *Peptides* 1987; 8: 309–17.

56. McCarthy M, Chung S, Ogawa S et al. Behavioral effects of oxytocin: is there a unifying principle? In JR Jard, ed. *Vasopressin*. New York: INSERM/John Libbey Eurotext, 1991: 195–212.

57. McCarthy MM, McDonald CH, Brooks PJ et al. An anxiolytic action of oxytocin is enhanced by estrogen in the mouse. *Physiol Behav* 1996; 60: 1209–15.

58. Nomura M, McKenna E, Korach KS et al. Estrogen receptor-beta regulates transcript levels for oxytocin and arginine vasopressin in the hypothalamic paraventricular nucleus of male mice. *Brain Res Mol Brain Res* 2002; 109(1–2): 84–94.

59. Krezel W, Dupont S, Krust A et al. Increased anxiety and synaptic plasticity in estrogen receptor b-deficient mice. *Proc Natl Acad Sci USA* 2001; 98: 12278–82.

60. Insel T, Young L. Neuropeptides and the evolution of social behavior. *Curr Opin Neurobiol* 2000; 10: 784–9 (Review).

61. Ferguson J, Young L, Insel T. The neuroendocrine basis of social recognition. *Front Neuroendocrinol* 2002; 2: 200–24 (Review).

62. Ferguson J, Aldag JM, Insel TR et al. Oxytocin in the medial amygdala is essential for social recognition in the mouse. *J Neurosci* 2001; 21: 8278–85.

63. Choleris E, Gustafsson JA, Korach KS et al. An estrogen dependent 4-gene micronet regulating social recognition: a study with oxytocin- and estrogen receptor alpha and beta-knockout mice. *Proc Natl Acad Sci USA* 2003; 100: 6192–7.

64. Nomura M, Durback L, Chan J et al. Genotype/age interactions on aggressive behavior in gonadally intact estrogen receptor b knockout (bERKO) male mice. *Horm Behav* 2002; 41: 288–96.

65. Pfaff D. *Brain Arousal and Information Theory*. Cambridge: Harvard University Press, 2005.

66. Mong JA, Devidze N, Frail DE et al. Estradiol regulation of lipocalin-type prostaglandin D synthase transcript levels in the rodent brain: evidence from high density oligonucleotide arrays and *in situ* hybridization. *Proc Natl Acad Sci U S A* 2003; 100: 318–23.

5.2 Neuroendocrine factors in sexual desire and motivation

Lisa A Scepkowski, Michaela Georgescu, James G Pfaus

Sexual motivation is the energizing force that generates our level of sexual interest at any given time. It drives our sexual fantasies; compels us to seek out, attend to, and evaluate sexual incentives; regulates our levels of sexual arousal and desire (a process that Whalen[1] referred to as "arousability"); and enables us to masturbate, copulate, or engage in other forms of sex play. As a heuristic, sexual motivation is relatively simple to define, and can be viewed as an internal process built upon neuroendocrine mechanisms, such as alterations in brain anatomy and neurochemical function by steroid hormone actions. Sexual motivation is also tuned by our experiences and expectations, learned patterns of behavior, and underlying neural activity related to sexual arousal, desire, reward, and inhibition. In turn, these aspects of sexual function feed back on mechanisms of motivation, either to increase (as in the case of arousal, desire, or reward) or decrease (as in the case of reward or inhibition) the expression of sexual interest (Fig. 5.2.1).

Sexual desire has been more difficult to define. This stems, in part, from a lack of objective measures of desire, a lack of specific subjective measures of desire, and an association with concepts like "libido", in which desire and arousal are not clearly delineated. In the *Diagnostic and Statistical Manual of Mental Disorders* (DSM),[2] the diagnosis of hypoactive sexual desire disorder is given when "desire for and fantasy about sexual activity are chronically or recurrently deficient of absent". By converse logic, sexual desire would be the presence of desire for, and fantasy about, sexual activity. Clinicians and motivational theorists both view desire as distinct from arousal in animals and humans.[3-5] This is also apparent in the DSM categorization of arousal disorders as distinct from desire disorders, a distinction that generally reflects blood flow to the genitals and erectile tissues versus a "psychological" sexual interest in which individuals "want" or "crave" sex (with wanting and craving defined here, as in Robinson and Berridge,[6] for drugs of abuse). Despite

the fact that desire and arousal are separable processes, desire may well be informed or even confirmed by the presence of autonomic and central responses that define arousal. In fact, both women and men regard desire and arousal as parts of one another, despite being given distinct definitions.[3,7] When an individual expresses sexual desire behaviorally, it follows that attention and behavior focus on obtaining some form of positive sexual reinforcement. This can occur alone in fantasies or together with others in goal-directed social and sexual behavior. Thus, in addition to people stating colloquially that they feel "horny" (with or without corresponding arousal), desire encompasses the work people will perform to obtain sexual rewards, the excitement displayed in anticipation of such rewards, and the strength of the incentive value ascribed to a particular sexual stimulus.

Operational definitions of desire

Operational definitions of sexual desire and the methods of measuring this construct vary widely in the literature, and a particular challenge in defining desire is its intricate relationship with sexual arousal. Bancroft[8] discussed the concept of sexual arousal in terms of both sexual "appetite" and desire, and central and peripheral arousability. Sexual appetite was defined as that which motivates us to seek out sexual stimulation and is a complex interaction between cognitive processes, neurophysiologic mechanisms, and affect or mood. Bancroft also described arousal as involving an individual's capacity to respond to external sexual stimuli appropriately as mediated by the tendency to seek them out as well as the capacity to create internal sexual stimuli (e.g., fantasies). Similarly, Singer and Toates[5] compared sexual desire to appetite in an incentive-motivation model in which sexual motivation is located in the

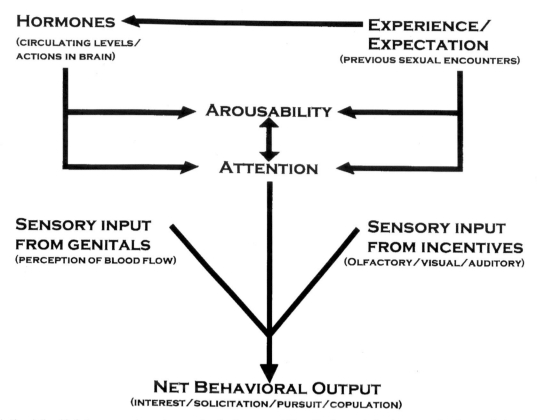

Figure 5.2.1. Hypothetic relationship between experience, hormonal activation, arousability, attention, and stimulus processing from genital sensations and external incentives on net sexual responding at any given time. Note that excitatory and inhibitory feedback can occur anywhere in this flowchart to strengthen or reduce responding. Such feedback provides moment-to-moment modulation of sexual motivation.

central nervous system, and structural changes induced by sex hormones in the central nervous system, sensory receptors, and peripheral organs (i.e., genitalia) alter sexual motivation. Thus, an interaction between central and peripheral processes may be responsible for manifestations of sexual desire. When Beck et al.[9] asked college students to indicate what most accurately reflected their degree of sexual desire, females most frequently cited genital arousal, intercourse frequency, and sexual daydreams, in that order. In contrast, the general population appears to view sexual desire as primarily psychological, as Regan and Berscheid[10] found that 98.5% of participants defined the construct by making reference to a motivational, cognitive, emotional, or subjective state. Interestingly, 7.6% of women, but only 1.5% of men, viewed sexual desire as a physiologic state such as arousal.

If women tend to view the degree of genital arousal as an index of sexual desire, difficulties with attaining adequate physical sexual arousal should have implications for subjective, motivational aspects of sexual experience. Within the past few years, there has been an impetus to examine the effects of peripherally acting agents, such as phosphodiesterase inhibitors, on female arousal. Studies have yielded varying results, ranging from no appreciable effects[11] to significant increases in self-reported sexual arousal,[12] to increases in genital arousal without a corresponding increase in subjective arousal.[13] Recently,

Basson and Brotto[14] found that in women with arousal disorder and lower vaginal pulse amplitude, sildenafil significantly increased both subjective sexual arousal and perception of genital arousal.

Hormonal influences

Steroid hormones secreted from the gonads, such as androgens, estrogens, and progestins, increase the sensitivity of an individual to sexual stimuli. In the brain this involves an increase in attention toward the incentive qualities that define the stimuli as sexual, awareness of the emotional value of the stimuli, an expectation of sexual reward, and an increase in behavioral output directed toward those stimuli, moving an individual from distal to proximal to interactive with regard to sexual incentives. In the periphery steroid actions help to prepare vaginal, clitoral, and penile tissues to be engorged with blood, enable proper lubrication, and maintain the hormonal output of the gonads themselves. In both men and women, a dynamic interplay of androgens, estrogens, and progestins does this simultaneously in the brain and periphery,[15-17] essentially changing the motivational "state" and preparing the body for action. Cues associated with sexual reward also activate hormonal output,[18,19] thus priming hormone-sensitive systems for sexual activity. Average sex steroid levels in women during the ovulatory cycle are shown in Table 5.2.1.

Much of what is known about steroid influences in female desire comes from studies in animal models, such as rats and primates.[20–23] The ovulatory cycles of rats and humans are shown in Figs 5.2.2 and 5.2.3. In rats, the cycle is approximately 4 days long, and is divided into four daily phases (diestrus 1, diestrus 2, proestrus, and estrus). Estrogen levels begin to rise during diestrus 2, and peak the morning of proestrus. Progesterone levels begin to rise the afternoon of proestrus and females typically go into "heat" a few hours later, and remain sexually interested and active for another 12 h. This state can be created in ovariectomized females by the sequential administration of estrogen 48 h before, and progesterone 4 h before, a test with sexually active male rats.[17] While in heat, females display behaviors that indicate sexual interest, including solicitations, hops, darts, and ear-wiggles.[21,24–26] After running away, which forces the male to chase her, the female will hold a lordosis posture and allow the male to mount and achieve vaginal intromission. This pattern of solicitation, runaway, and lordosis defines a bout of copulation in the female rat. After receiving

Table 5.2.1. Sex steroid levels in women during phases of the ovulatory cycle

Hormone	Phase of the cycle		
	Early follicular	Preovulatory	Midluteal
Progesterone (mg)	1.0	4.0	25.0
17-Hydroxyprogesterone (mg)	0.5	4.0	4.0
Dehydroepiandrosterone (mg)	7.0	7.0	7.0
Androstenedione (mg)	2.6	4.7	3.4
Testosterone (µg)	144.0	171.0	126.0
Estrone (µg)	50.0	350.0	250.0
Estradiol (µg)	36.0	380.0	250.0

Data from Yen SSC, Jaffe RB. *Reproductive Endocrinology* (3rd edn). San Francisco: Saunders, 1991.

multiple vaginal intromissions and ejaculations, the female begins to run away more and more, imposing more temporal distance between stimulations. The ability to pace or control the initiation and rate of copulation enhances fertility,[27] and is the

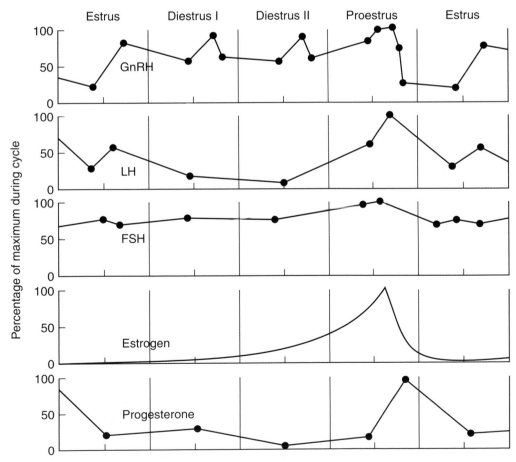

Figure 5.2.2. Ovulatory cycle of the rat. Gonadotropin-releasing hormone (GnRH) stimulates the pituitary to secrete luteinizing hormone (LH) and follicle stimulating hormone (FSH), which in turn causes a steady increase in estrogen levels until the afternoon of proestrus. A second increase in LH and FSH, along with a corresponding increase in estrogen and progesterone levels, causes ovulation. The increase in estrogen and progesterone prime hypothalamic and limbic brain structures for sexual behavior. After WF Ganong, *Review of Medical Physiology* (17th edn). Norwalk: Appleton & Lange, 1995; RJ Nelson, *An Introduction to Behavioral Endocrinology* (2nd edn). Sunderland: Sinauer, 2000.

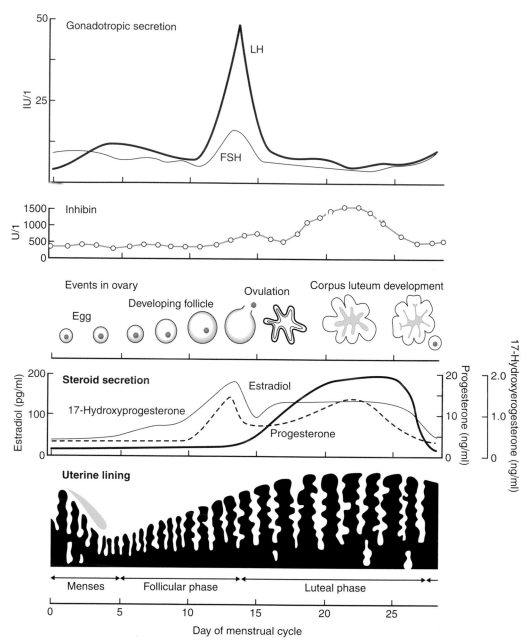

Figure 5.2.3. Ovulatory cycle of the human. FSH, follicle stimulating hormone; LH, luteinizing hormone. From RJ Nelson, *An Introduction to Behavioral Endocrinology* (3rd edn). Sunderland, MA: Sinauer, 2005.

critical feature that female rats find rewarding about copulation.[28] Thus, sexual interest is generated by the sequential actions of estrogen and progesterone, and occurs around the time of ovulation, thus linking behavior to reproduction in most mammalian females.

Although females of some primate species (including humans) can have sex any time during the ovulatory cycle, there is evidence that increased desire and female-initiated sexual activity tend to occur around the time of ovulation, for example, in humans and macaques[23,29] (Fig. 5.2.4). However, female-directed desire has not been assessed in most human studies, but rather subsumed in questions regarding overall sexual activity. Thus, studies aimed at finding the presence of a hormone-related periovulatory peak in sexual response have yielded conflicting results. Typically, these studies have used behavioral measures such as intercourse or masturbation frequency to index changes in sexual interest. Some studies have provided evidence of this midcycle peak,[30–33] while others have shown peaks in female-initiated sexual activity during the follicular phase,[34] or no difference at all across cycles regardless of hormonal or contraceptive status.[35] Some studies have shown sexual arousal to be highest during the midfollicular and late luteal phases as opposed to during ovulation. For example, studies employing self-report and psychophysiologic techniques have reported greater genital arousal during the follicular and luteal phases[36] or greater arousal during the follicular than luteal phase.[37] Meuwissen and Over[16]

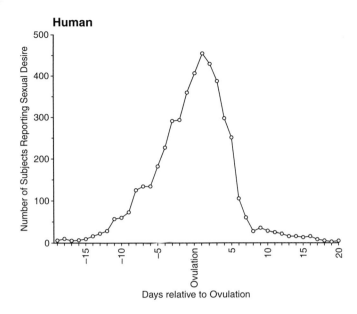

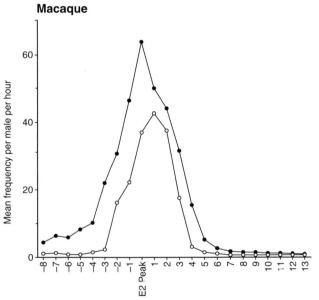

Figure 5.2.4. Measures of female-directed sexual desire in humans and rhesus macaques. Top: the number of women reporting sexual desire for the first time in their ovulatory cycle in relation to the time of ovulation (based on basal body temperature shift). Data from Stanislaw and Rice[29] and adapted from Wallen.[23] Bottom: the mean frequency of female approach (solid circles) and sexual solicitation (open circles) toward males in relation to the female's midcycle estradiol peak. Note that female approach is elevated earlier than solicitation. Data from Wallen.[23]

found that subjective sexual arousal was relatively stable across all phases of the menstrual cycle, but they also found that vaginal pulse amplitude was highest during the luteal, or premenstrual, phase. Studies relying more heavily on subjective measures of sexual desire and interest have shown a higher interest in erotic films postmenstrually,[38] with the highest reported sexual desire a

few days prior to the basal body temperature shift associated with ovulation,[29] and sexual feelings independent of mood to be highest during the midfollicular and late luteal phases, with the highest reported sexual activity during the midfollicular phase.[39] Another study found a peak in sexual interest in women with premenstrual complaints during the ovulatory phase, but women without complaints reported a peak during the follicular phase.[40] The high variability in methods used to determine menstrual cycle phase and levels of sexual arousal and desire has made it difficult to draw definitive conclusions about the relationship between hormone levels and menstrual cycle.

Estrogens and progestins

It is generally accepted that estrogens are important for maintaining the health and integrity of vaginal tissue in women, and it naturally follows that the lack of the hormones after menopause will be related to decreases in sexual functioning. However, the role of estrogen in psychologic processes related to sexual desire is less well understood. Sherwin and colleagues[41-45] have demonstrated an enhancing effect of estrogen on mood. It is speculated that estrogens enhance mood by neurochemical mechanisms associated with the activation of ascending serotonin systems. Sherwin[42] suggested that, in addition to increasing the degradation of monoamine oxidase, estrogen displaces tryptophan from binding sites to albumin, thereby allowing more free tryptophan to be available to the brain, where it is metabolized to serotonin. In addition to its effect on mood, Sherwin and colleagues found that levels of desire and arousal were highest in postmenopausal women when receiving estrogen compared with receiving both estrogen and progestin or no hormones at all. Progestins were found in that study to dampen mood and increase reported unpleasant psychologic symptoms. It is not clear whether that effect might be related to the peak or fall in plasma progesterone concentrations.

Androgens

Bancroft[46] suggested a role for androgens in stimulating sexual motivation in both men and women, involving effects on cognition and attention, and an increased tendency to respond to sexual stimuli with central arousal or excitement. A growing body of research has formed around this hypothesis. Although there has been a larger focus on androgens in male sexuality, more recent work has demonstrated the importance of androgens in female sexuality at both central and peripheral levels.

Androgens, including dehydroepiandrosterone (DHEA), dehydroepiandrosterone sulfate (DHEA-S), androstenedione (A), testosterone (T), and dihydrotestosterone (DHT) are produced by the ovaries and/or adrenal glands, and peripheral tissues in women (Table 5.2.1). Only unbound, or "free" testosterone and dihydrotestosterone are considered biologically active, as they are able to bind to androgen receptors in tissue.[47,48] However, it remains unclear whether testosterone is acting on the brain via androgen receptors or through aromatization to estrogens, as both types of receptors are present in the brain.[49,50] The majority of research investigating the effects of androgens on female sexuality has examined women with diminished androgen levels from various causes. Although androgen levels are known to decrease with age, there are a number of other causes of androgen insufficiency, including oophorectomy, premature ovarian failure, hypopituitarism, adrenal insufficiency, corticosteroid therapy, chemotherapy/radiation, and estrogen replacement therapy.[51] Women with diminished androgen levels have reported decreased sexual function, in terms of lower sexual desire, infrequent sexual fantasies, decreased sexual interest, decreased vaginal lubrication, and difficulty achieving arousal.[50] These symptoms have been treated with dehydroepiandrosterone and/or testosterone replacement therapy, with measurable degrees of success in improving sexual interest and desire,[50,51] libido, and sexual satisfaction.[52]

The mechanisms by which androgens influence cognitive processes involved in sexual desire and arousal are not well understood. As mentioned above, androgens were first proposed to facilitate central arousal mechanisms and sexual appetite. Krug et al.[53] demonstrated that visual sexual stimuli are better recognized by women around the time of ovulation (when testosterone peaks) and that in this phase the amplitude of the late positive component of event-related potentials was greater for sexual stimuli than neutral stimuli when they engaged in affective processing of the stimuli. As androgens are important for a functional genital response via physical mechanisms, they have also been shown to influence attentional aspects of sexual functioning. Alexander and Sherwin[54] used a dichotic listening task to examine selective attention for sexual stimuli in women using oral contraceptives, and found that in the group of women whose free testosterone levels were below average, there was a significant positive relationship between free testosterone and attentional bias toward sexual stimuli. The same relationship was not shown for women with levels within the normal range.

Androgens, estrogens, and sex hormone-binding globulins

Androgens and estrogens may work in concert to alter sexual desire and arousal. The most efficacious hormone-replacement therapy to restore both sexual arousal and desire in postmenopausal women has been treatment with androgens and estrogens, rather than either one alone.[41,43,49] Bancroft[10] suggested that this efficacy stems from an action of androgens on sex hormone-binding globulins and a resulting increase in bioavailable estrogens. Sex hormone-binding globulins are transport glycoproteins produced in the liver that regulate the delivery of steroid hormones to target tissues.[55] Roughly 66–78% of circulating testosterone is bound strongly to sex hormone-binding globulin, 20–33% is bound weakly to albumin, and the remaining 1–2% is unbound or free, where it is able to exert its actions on target tissues. The sex hormone-binding globulin

binding affinity for steroid hormones is dihydrotestosterone > testosterone > androstenedione > estradiol > estrone.[56] Sex hormone-binding globulin binds dehydroepiandrosterone very weakly, and does not bind dehydroepiandrosterone sulfate at all. Circulating sex hormone-binding globulin levels are reduced by testosterone, glucocorticoids, growth hormone, and insulin, and increased by estradiol and thyroxine.[57] Exogenous administration of estradiol increases sex hormone-binding globulin levels, and this in turn reduces the free fractions of both testosterone and estradiol.[58] This helps to explain why treatment with estradiol alone is relatively ineffective.

When testosterone is given in conjunction with estradiol, at least three effects serve to increase bioavailable estradiol. The first is a decrease in sex hormone-binding globulin production; the second is an increase in bound testosterone; and the third is a further increase in estradiol levels due to the aromatization of free testosterone into estradiol (this latter effect would not be likely in the case of coadministration of methyltestosterone, which inhibits aromatase activity).[59] Thus, coadministration of testosterone and estradiol should increase estradiol's actions on peripheral tissues, such as the clitoris and vagina,[60] resulting in improvements in vasomotor symptoms and vaginal dryness, and sexual satisfaction in cases of atrophic vaginitis,[45,61] in addition to its actions in the brain to stimulate sexual desire in the appropriate circumstances.

Neurochemical "mediators"

In the brain, increased estradiol levels can enhance the action of monoamine (e.g., dopamine, noradrenaline, and serotonin), small molecule [e.g., gamma-aminobutyric acid (GABA) and glutamate] and neuropeptide (e.g., opioid, gonadotropin-releasing hormone, melanocortin) neurotransmitter systems that control central arousal and excitation, mood, and incentive salience.[20,62] The activation of those systems has begun to be examined in animal models of female sexual "desire," such as solicitation and pacing, and sexual reward (e.g., sexually conditioned place or partner preference), in addition to measures of sexual receptivity such as lordosis.[21] Two promising effects have emerged with the dopamine receptor agonist apomorphine, and the melanocortin receptor agonist PT-141, stimulating sexual solicitation in ovariectomized rats treated with estradiol.[21,63]

Dopamine may play a key role in the attribution of incentive salience to external stimuli, especially those of conditional incentive value.[55] Mesolimbic dopamine transmission is stimulated by estradiol and testosterone in rat brain.[64,65] In some regions of the hypothalamus, binding of dopamine to dopamine (D1) receptors activates progestin receptors independently of the presence of progesterone.[66] In fact, such activation by dopamine-mediated second messenger cascades may be superseded if progesterone levels are high, thus decreasing the availability of progestin receptors (as progesterone binds irreversibly to its own receptor). Indeed, administration of the progestin receptor antagonist RU-486 eliminates the ability of either apomorphine or the D1-selective agonist SKF-38393 to activate lordosis after infusion to the ventromedial hypothalamus.[66]

Neuropeptides derived from proopiomelanocortin (POMC), including β-endorphin, corticotropin (ACTH), and α-melanocyte-stimulating hormone (MSH), have pronounced excitatory and inhibitory effects on the sexual behavior of female rats.[63,67–71] Estradiol regulates this system in a complex way; for example, it decreases the number and affinity of receptors for μ-opioid receptors (that inhibit female sexual behavior) and increases α-melanocyte-stimulating hormone and melanocortin receptor levels.[72–74] These factors may be intermediaries of estrogen's effects on sexual desire.

Conclusions

Sexual motivation is stimulated, maintained, and terminated by a constellation of neurotransmitter and receptor changes, induced by progestins, androgens, estrogens, and sensory feedback, that generates peripheral and central "state" changes. These changes, in turn, activate sexual arousal and desire and link them to reproductive function. Androgens may be permissive in this by allowing more estradiol to be distributed to target tissues, in addition to their own role in the activation of neurochemical systems. Progestins appear to play a dual role in females, with small amounts activating progestin receptors in key hypothalamic and limbic structures to increase sexual motivation and desire, but larger amounts leading to a faster decline in these processes. The activation of melanocortin, dopamine, and progestin receptors may be key intermediaries in the stimulation of sexual desire, incentive sexual motivation, and sexual reward, but they are by no means the entire story. Simultaneous down-regulation of neurochemical systems that inhibit sexual motivation and desire also occurs after estrogen treatment, at least long enough to ensure that sexual activity has been successful (from a reward and/or reproductive standpoint). Accordingly, these changes all come under the rubric of sexual motivation. Obviously, the expression of sexual desire in women is more than the sum of its physiologic parts. The neurochemical actions of steroid hormones stimulate sensory awareness, arousal, mood, and reward, and link them to salient features of a partner, place, and action. Neuroendocrine factors provide the instruments, whereas each individual's experience writes the songs.

Acknowledgments

The authors would like to thank Drs Kim Wallen, Lori Brotto, Julia Heiman, Irwin Goldstein, Peter Eriksson, Donald Pfaff, Raúl Paredes, and Annamaria Giraldi, for many useful discussions that have helped form the ideas expressed in this chapter. Research findings from the laboratory of JGP were funded by grants from the Natural Sciences and Engineering Research Council of Canada, Canadian Institutes for Health Research, and Palatin Technologies.

References

1. Whalen RE. Sexual motivation. *Psychol Rev* 1966; 73: 151–63.
2. American Psychiatric Association. *Diagnostic and Statistical Manual of Psychiatric Disorders IV-TR* (Text Revision). Washington, DC: APA Press, 2000.
3. Basson R. Female sexual response: the role of drugs in the management of sexual dysfunction. *Obstet Gynecol* 2001; 98: 350–3.
4. Pfaus JG. Revisiting the concept of sexual motivation. *Annu Rev Sex Res* 1999; 10: 120–57.
5. Singer B, Toates FM. Sexual motivation. *J Sex Res* 1987; 23: 481–501.
6. Robinson TE, Berridge KC. The neural basis of drug craving: an incentive-sensitization theory of addiction. *Brain Res Brain Res Rev* 1993; 18: 247–91.
7. Toledano RR, Pfaus JG. The sexual arousal and desire inventory (SADI): a multidimensional scale to assess the subjective experience of sexual arousal and desire. *Arch Sex Behav* 2005; *submitted*.
8. Bancroft J. *Human Sexuality and Its Problems*. New York: Churchill Livingstone, 1989.
9. Beck JG, Bozman AW, Qualtrough T. The experience of sexual desire: psychological correlates in a college sample. *J Sex Res* 1991; 28: 443–56.
10. Regan PC, Berscheid E. Beliefs about the state, goals, and objects of sexual desire. *J Sex Marital Ther* 1996; 22: 110–20.
11. Basson R, McInnis R, Smith M et al. Efficacy and safety of sildenafil citrate in women with sexual dysfunction associated with female sexual arousal disorder. *J Womens Health Gend Based Med* 2002; 11: 339–49.
12. Caruso S, Intelisano G, Lup L et al. Premenopausal women affected by sexual arousal disorder treated with sildenafil: a double-blind, cross-over, placebo-controlled study. *Br J Obstet Gynecol* 2001; 108: 623–8.
13. Laan E, van Lunsen RH, Everaerd W et al. The enhancement of vaginal vasocongestion by sildenafil in healthy premenopausal women. *J Womens Health Gend Based Med* 2002; 11: 357–65.
14. Basson R, Brotto LA. Sexual psychophysiology and effects of sildenafil citrate in oestrogenised women with acquired genital arousal disorder and impaired orgasm: a randomized controlled trial. *Br J Obst Gyn* 2003; 110: 1014–24.
15. Meisel RD, Sachs BD. The physiology of male reproduction. In E Knobil, JD Neil, eds. *The Physiology of Reproduction*, vol 2. New York: Raven Press, 1994: 3–105.
16. Meuwissen IM, Over R. Sexual arousal across phases of the human menstrual cycle. *Arch Sex Behav* 1992; 21: 101–19.
17. Pfaff DW. *Estrogens and Brain Function*. Berlin: Springer-Verlag, 1980.
18. Anonymous. Effects of sexual activity on beard growth in man. *Nature* 1970; 226: 869–70.
19. Graham JM, Desjardins C. Classical conditioning: induction of luteinizing hormone and testosterone secretion in anticipation of sexual activity. *Science* 1980; 210: 1039–41.
20. Pfaff DW. *Drive: Neurobiological and Molecular Mechanisms of Sexual Motivation*. Bradford: MIT Press, 1999.
21. Pfaus JG, Kippin TE, Coria-Avila G. What can animal models tell us about human sexual response? *Annu Rev Sex Res* 2003; 14: 1–63.

22. Wallen K. Desire and ability: hormones and the regulation of female sexual behavior. *Neurosci Biobehav Rev* 1990; 14: 233–41.

23. Wallen K. The evolution of female sexual desire. In PR Abramson, SD Pinkerton, eds. *Sexual Nature, Sexual Culture*. Chicago: University of Chicago Press, 1995: 57–79.

24. Erskine MS. Solicitation behavior in the estrous female rat: a review. *Horm Behav* 1989; 23: 473–502.

25. Madlafousek J, Hliòák Z. Sexual behavior of the female laboratory rat: inventory, patterning, and measurement. *Behaviour* 1978; 63: 129–73.

26. McClintock MK. Group mating in the domestic rat as a context for sexual selection: consequences for the analysis of sexual behavior and neuroendocrine responses. *Adv Stud Behav* 1984; 14: 1–50.

27. Adler NT. On the mechanisms of sexual behavior and their evolutionary constraints. In Hutchison JB, ed. *Biological Determinants of Sexual Behavior*. Chichester: Wiley, 1978: 657–95.

28. Paredes RG, Vazquez B. What do female rats like about sex? Paced mating. *Behav Brain Res* 1999; 105: 117–27.

29. Stanislaw H, Rice FJ. Correlation between sexual desire and menstrual cycle characteristics. *Arch Sex Behav* 1988; 17: 499–508.

30. Harvey SM. Female sexual behavior: fluctuations during the menstrual cycle. *J Psychosom Res* 1987; 31: 101–10.

31. Matteo S, Rissman EF. Increased sexual activity during the midcycle portion of the human menstrual cycle. *Horm Behav* 1984; 18: 249–55.

32. Morris NM, Udry JR, Khan-Dawood F et al. Marital sex frequency and midcycle female testosterone. *Arch Sex Behav* 1987; 16: 27–37.

33. Persky H, Lief HI, Strauss D et al. Plasma testosterone level and behavior of couples. *Arch Sex Behav* 1978; 7: 157–73.

34. Silber M. Menstrual cycle and work schedule: effects on women's sexuality. *Arch Sex Behav* 1994; 23: 397–404.

35. Alexander GM, Sherwin BB, Bancroft J et al. Testosterone and sexual behavior in oral contraceptive users and nonusers: a prospective study. *Horm Behav* 1990; 24: 388–402.

36. Schreiner-Engel P, Schiavi RC, Smith H et al. Sexual arousability and the menstrual cycle. *Psychosom Med* 1981; 43: 199–214.

37. Slob AK, Bax CM, Hop WCJ et al. Sexual arousability and the menstrual cycle. *Psychoneuroendocrinology* 1996; 21: 545–58.

38. Zillmann D, Schweitzer KJ, Mundorf N. Menstrual cycle variation of women's interest in erotica. *Arch Sex Behav* 1994; 23: 579–97.

39. Bancroft J, Sanders D, Davidson D et al. Mood, sexuality, hormones, and the menstrual cycle. III. Sexuality and the role of androgens. *Psychosom Med* 1983; 45: 509–16.

40. Van Goozen SH, Wiegant VM, Endert E et al. Psychoendocrinological assessment of the menstrual cycle: the relationship between hormones, sexuality, and mood. *Arch Sex Behav* 1997; 26: 359–82.

41. Sherwin BB. Affective changes with estrogen and androgen replacement therapy in surgically menopausal women. *J Affect Disord* 1988; 14: 177–87.

42. Sherwin BB. The impact of different doses of estrogen and progestin on mood and sexual behavior in postmenopausal women. *J Clin Endocrinol Metab* 1991; 72: 336–43.

43. Sherwin BB. Randomized clinical trials of combined estrogen-androgen preparations: effects on sexual functioning. *Fert Steril* 2002; 77(Suppl 4): S49–54.

44. Sherwin BB, Gelfand MM. Sex steroids and affect in the surgical menopause: a double-blind cross-over study. *Psychoneuroendocrinology* 1985; 10:.325–35.

45. Sherwin BB, Gelfand MM, Brender W. Androgen enhances sexual motivation in females: a prospective, crossover study of sex steroid administration in the surgical menopause. *Psychosom Med* 1985; 47: 339–51.

46. Bancroft J. Endocrinology of sexual function. *Clin Obstet Gynecol* 1980; 7: 253–81.

47. Lobo RA. Androgens in postmenopausal women: production, possible role, and replacement options. *Obstet Gynecol Surv* 2001; 56: 361–76.

48. Longcope C. Androgen metabolism and the menopause. *Semin Reprod Endocrinol* 1998; 16: 111–15.

49. Bancroft J. Sexual effects of androgens in women: some theoretical considerations. *Fert Steril* 2002; 77: S55–9.

50. Guay A, Davis SR. Testosterone insufficiency in women: fact of fiction? *World J Urol* 2002; 20: 106–10.

51. Apperloo MJA, Van Der Stege JG, Hoek A et al. In the mood for sex: the value of androgens. *J Sex Marital Ther* 2003; 29: 87–102.

52. Spark RF. Dehydroepiandrostenedione: a springboard hormone for female sexuality. *Fert Steril* 2002; 77: S19–25.

53. Krug R, Plihal W, Born J. Selective influence of menstrual cycle on perception of stimuli with reproductive significance: an event-related potential study. *Psychophysiology* 2000; 37: 111–22.

54. Alexander GM, Sherwin BB. Sex steroids, sexual behavior, and selection attention for erotic stimuli in women using oral contraceptives. *Psychoneuroendocrinology* 1993; 18: 91–102.

55. Pugeat M, Crave JC, Tourniaire J et al. Clinical utility of sex hormone-binding globulin measurement. *Horm Res* 1996; 45: 148–55.

56. Dunn JF, Nisula BC, Rodboard D. Transport of steroid hormones. Binding of 21 endogenous steroids to both testosterone-binding globulin and corticosteroid-binding globulin in human plasma. *J Clin Endocrinol Metab* 1981; 53: 58–68.

57. Davis SR, Burger HG. The rationale for physiological testosterone replacement in women. *Baillieres Clin Endocrinol Metab* 1998; 12: 391–405.

58. Mathur RS, Landgreebe SD, Moody LO et al. The effect of estrogen treatment on plasma concentrations of steroid hormones, gonadotropins, prolactin, and sex hormone-binding globulin in post-menopausal women. *Maturias* 1985; 7: 129–33.

59. Mor G, Eliza M, Song J et al. 17–alpha methyl testosterone is a competitive inhibitor of aromatase activity in Jar choriocarcinoma cells and macrophage-like THP-1 cells in culture. *J Steroid Biochem Mol Biol* 2001; 79: 239–46.

60. Campbell S, Whitehead M. Oestrogen therapy and the menopausal syndrome. *Clin Obstet Gynecol* 1977; 4: 31–47.

61. Studd JWW, Chakravarti S, Oram D. The climacteric. *Clin Obstet Gynecol* 1977; 4: 3–29.

62. Pfaff DW, Schwartz-Giblin S, McCarthy MM et al. Cellular and molecular mechanisms of female reproductive behaviors. In E Knobil, JD Neill, eds. *The Physiology of Reproduction*, vol 2. New York: Raven Press, 1994: 107–220.

63. Pfaus JG, Shadiack A, Van Soest T et al. Selective facilitation of sexual solicitation in the female rat by a melanocortin receptor agonist. *Proc Natl Acad Sci USA* 2004; 101: 10201–4.

64. Castner SA, Xiao L, Becker JB. Sex differences in striatal dopamine: *in vivo* microdialysis and behavioral studies. *Brain Res* 1993; 610: 127–34.

65. Du J, Hull EM. Effects of testosterone on neuronal nitric oxide synthase and tyrosine hydroxylase. *Brain Res* 1999; 836: 90–8.

66. Mani SK, Allen JM, Clark JH et al. Convergent pathways for steroid hormone- and neurotransmitter-induced rat sexual behavior. *Science* 1994; 265: 1246–9.

67. Cragnolini AB, Scimonelli TN, Celis ME et al. The role of melanocortin receptors in the sexual behavior of female rats. *Neuropeptides* 2000; 34: 211–15.

68. Gonzalez MI, Celis ME, Hole DR et al. Interaction of oestradiol, alpha-meoanotrophin, and noradrenaline within the ventromedial nucleus in the control of female sexual behavior. *Neuroendocrinology* 1993; 58: 218–26.

69. Nocetto C, Cragniolini AB, Schioth HB et al. Evidence that the effect of melanocortins on female sexual behavior in preoptic area is mediated by the MC3 receptor. Participation of nitric oxide. *Behav Brain Res* 2004; 153: 537–41.

70. Pfaus JG, Everitt BJ. The psychopharmacology of sexual behavior. In FE Bloom, DJ Kupfer, eds. *Psychopharmacology: The Fourth Generation of Progress*. New York: Raven Press, 1995: 743–58.

71. Raible LH, Gorzalka BB Short- and long-term inhibitory actions of alpha melanocyte stimulating hormone on lordosis in rats. *Peptides* 1986; 7: 581–6.

72. Medina F, Siddiqui A, Scimonelli T et al. The inter-relationship between gonadal steroids and POMC peptides, beta-endorphin and alpha-MSH, in the control of sexual behavior in the female rat. *Peptides* 1998; 19: 1309–16.

73. Watanobe H, Schioth HB, Wikberg JE et al. The melanocortin 4 receptor mediates leptin stimulation of luteinizing hormone and prolactin surges in steroid-primed ovariectomized rats. *Biochem Biophys Res Commun* 1999; 257: 860–4.

74. Wilson CA, Thody AJ, Hole DR et al. Interaction of estradiol, alpha-melanocyte-stimulating hormone, and dopamine in the regulation of sexual receptivity in the female rat. *Neuroendocrinology* 1991; 54: 14–22.

5.3 Neurophysiology of female genital sexual response

François Giuliano, Véronique Julia-Guilloteau

Introduction

Anatomic structures in the genital apparatus that are involved in the female genital response include the vestibular bulb, the vagina, the uterus and the pelvic–perineal musculature. The vulva, including the portions of the female genital apparatus that are externally visible in the perineal region, consists of the mons veneris, the labia minora and majora, the clitoris, the vestibule, the vaginal orifice, and the urethral meatus.

Female genital sexual response consists of local arousal and orgasm. Peripheral genital sexual arousal may be defined as a genital vasocongestion that is controlled by the autonomic nervous system. It involves an increase in pelvic-perineal blood flow leading to the engorgement with blood of (1) the labia; (2) the vaginal wall, resulting in lubrication; and (3) the clitoral erectile tissue.[1] From a neurophysiologic genital aspect, orgasm involves rhythmic contractions of the pelvic striated circumvaginal musculature, often with concomitant uterine and anal contractions; therefore, orgasm involves both smooth and striated muscles.[2–5]

Anatomic structures involved in female genital sexual response are innervated by autonomic and somatic nerves. These include (1) the pelvic nerve issuing from the intermediolateral cell column of S2 to S4 levels of the spinal cord, also called the parasympathetic nucleus; (2) the hypogastric and the lumbosacral sympathetic chain conveying sympathetic fibers originating from both intermediolateral cell column and dorsal gray commissure of thoracolumbar levels of the spinal cord (T12–L2); (3) the pudendal nerve (somatic) with cell bodies of the motoneurons located in Onuf's nucleus divided in the rat into dorsomedial and dorsolateral nuclei in the ventral horn of the sacral spinal cord (S2–S4); and (4) the vagus nerves issuing from the nucleus tractus solitaris.

Afferent pathways consist of pudendal, pelvic, and hypogastric nerves and the lumbosacral sympathetic chain. They relay information to the dorsal horn, medial, central, and lateral gray matter of the lumbosacral spinal cord.[6–8] In addition, vagal afferent fibers convey sensory information from the genital apparatus directly to the nucleus tractus solitaries.

During sexual genital response, the genital apparatus can be considered as an effector and a receptor. Afferent pathways play a crucial role in participating in the facilitation and/or the triggering of both peripheral arousal and orgasm. They convey sensory information from the periphery to the central nervous system through the spinal cord, which represents a relay to supraspinal sites via the spinothalamic and spinoreticular pathways.[9]

Peripheral neurophysiology

Afferent pathways/sensory innervation of the genital apparatus

There is little information available about the exact role of afferent fibers innervating the female genital tract. It appears that the sensitivity and the responses to local stimuli are variable, depending on anatomic structures, that is, the vagina, clitoris, cervix, and uterus. Different sensitivities are defined in function of the different types of stimuli: mechanosensitivity (pressure stimulus), chemosensitivity (irritant stimulus, e.g., bradykinin), and thermosensitivity (cool or warm stimulus). Afferent fibers conveying sensory information are generally divided into three types: A-beta fibers, the largest fibers, which mediate touch, mild pressure, and vibration; A-delta fibers, which mediate cold and pain sensations; and C-fibers, the smallest fibers, which mediate pain and temperature sensations. Sensitivity can be divided into somatic sensitivity for skin and articulations and visceral sensitivity for internal organs. Genital sensitivity includes both somatic and visceral sensitivities, depending on location of the anatomic structure (outer versus inner). Moreover, the distinct physiologic role of each structure, such as the clitoris, vagina, and uterus in sexual arousal, orgasm, and parturition, determines the nature of neural afferent inputs (sensation or/and nociception).

Clitoral stimulation is the main source of sensory input for eliciting orgasm.[9–12] In female cats, the afferent fibers from the clitoris travel exclusively in the pudendal nerve since pudendal nerve transection eliminates 99% of the labeled cells in the sacral dorsal root ganglia following antegrade axonal transport from the clitoris. In contrast, 40% of neural cell bodies of the S1 dorsal root ganglion whose fibers are conveyed by the pudendal nerve innervate the clitoris. In the S2 dorsal root ganglia, only 5% of neural cell bodies whose fibers are conveyed by the pudendal nerve are clitoral afferent fibers.[13] In female cats, the conduction velocity of myelinated clitoral afferent fibers ranges from 5.2 to 30 m/s but is mainly 10–15 m/s. This conduction velocity is slightly slower than skin afferent pathways,[14] suggesting that although the clitoris is an external genital organ, its sensitivity is close to that of the skin. In women, Vardi et al.[15] have characterized the clitoral sensitivity in response to different applied stimuli. Stimulation of the woman's clitoris can be induced by temperature changes (cold and warm) and vibrations.

Generally, it may be hypothesized that coital orgasm is triggered by stimulation of internal genital organs; i.e., the vagina, cervix, and uterus. The exact neurophysiologic support for the coital orgasm is less clear than for the one elicited by clitoral stimulation.

In female cats, vaginal afferents travel in the pelvic nerve.[16] In female rats, the conduction velocities of afferent units from the uterus or the vagina are always less than 2 m/s, corresponding to C-fiber conduction velocity. Low or no spontaneous activity is observed. The receptive fields of the vaginal afferent

fibers increase from the vaginal orifice to the vaginocervical junction.[17] In female rats, the hypogastric nerve afferent fibers innervate the uterus, the cervix, and the ovaries. These afferent fibers carry only noxious information[18] (Fig. 5.3.1).

The urogenital reflex intends to mimic the human orgasmic response by applying a mechanical stimulation to the urethra. An experimental model has been developed in anesthetized female rats. The urogenital reflex can be elicited only after acute spinalization of female rats. Thus, it is suggested that to observe this reflex, it is necessary to cut descending inhibitory inputs.[19] The urogenital reflex includes rhythmic contractions of the vagina, the uterus, and the anal sphincter, as well as the striated pelvic musculature. Stimulation of the urethra may mimic stimulation of the anterior wall of the vagina, which is the area with the highest "erotic" sensitivity. Indeed, the anterior wall of the vagina has a denser innervation than the posterior wall, and the distal area has more nerve fibers than the proximal.[20] In the female rat, vaginocervical stimulation induced by mechanical probing (300 g) against the vaginal cervix elicits a variety of responses, including analgesia, pupil dilation, increase in blood pressure and heart rate, flexor inhibition, and behavioral responses such as facilitation of lordosis.[21] Although this stimulation is nonphysiologic, this experimental model allowed observation of the role of pelvic, hypogastric, pudendal, and vagus nerves in the female sexual response. Indeed, bilateral transection of pelvic, hypogastric, and pudendal nerves does not affect pupil dilation and analgesia. Conversely, these two responses were reduced after transection of the vagus nerve, suggesting its role in the transmission of the messages in response to vaginocervical stimulation.

Despite the fact that the vagus nerve is involved in the transmission of sensory information from the female genital organs to the nucleus tractus solitaries, its exact role in the female genital response remains unclear. It is not known whether the vagus nerve represents a supplemental afferent pathway to the spinal system or is activated only after spinal

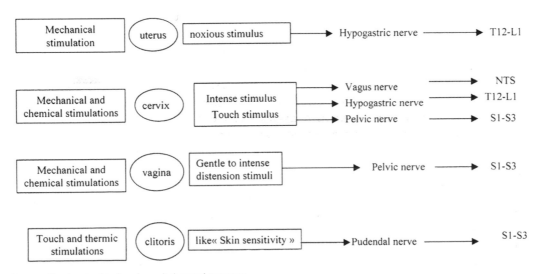

Figure 5.3.1. Afferent innervation involved in female genital sexual response.

injury. Indeed, it has been reported that in spinal cord-injured women, orgasms induced by vaginal and cervical self-stimulations can occur.[22,23] These data suggest that genital information may be sent to supraspinal centers via the vagus nerve. It is proposed that the afferent vagal pathway may be involved in the central feeling of orgasm in women with complete spinal cord transection, or may exert a facilitatory role in addition to the spinal to brain pathway in normal women. In contrast, the urogenital reflex is not abolished after transection of the vagus nerves.[24]

Overall, the pudendal nerve that conveys sensory information from the vulva and the striated pelvic-perineal musculature to the spinal cord plays a central role in the occurrence of clitoral orgasm. The pelvic and hypogastric nerves convey sensory information from the internal pelvic organs; they may have a role in "coital orgasm".

Efferent pathways

The parasympathetic pathway which innervates the genital apparatus is responsible for clitoral swelling during sexual excitation as well as vaginal congestion, and lubrication and lengthening of the vagina.[25,26] In anesthetized rabbits, electrical stimulation of the pelvic nerve elicits an increase in vaginal blood flow, wall pressure and length as well as intraclitoral pressure and clitoral blood flow. In contrast, electrical stimulation of the pelvic nerve decreases intravaginal luminal pressure.[27] In the rat, clitoral and vaginal blood flows increase after electrical stimulations of both the clitoral and pelvic nerves.[28,29]

In spinalized female rats, the urogenital reflex elicited by urethral distention comprises vaginal and uterine contractions accompanied by rhythmic contractions of the vaginal and anal orifices. The urogenital reflex implicates several efferent nerves, since firing of pelvic, hypogastric, pudendal, and cavernous nerves has been recorded during the reflex.

Activation of the sympathetic nervous system, which occurs during the later stages of sexual arousal and orgasm, is responsible for an increase in heart rate and blood pressure in women.[30] The effects of sympathetic nervous system activation on sexual arousal have been examined during exercise, which is accompanied by sympathetic nervous system activation. Meston and Gorzalka[31] have demonstrated that, in women, physiologic sexual arousal is facilitated by acute and intense exercise in the presence of an erotic stimulus. In laboratory conditions after exercise, an increase in vaginal pulse amplitude and vaginal blood volume have been observed, suggesting a facilitatory effect of sympathetic activation on physiologic sexual arousal. The time course of the facilitatory effect of sympathetic nervous system activation on sexual arousal in women has been determined: sexual arousal is not increased by immediate sympathetic activation (5 min after exercise), whereas delayed and residual sympathetic activation facilitates women's sexual arousal.[32] In female rats, peripheral administration of guanethidine (a postganglionic noradrenergic blocker) suppresses lordosis and proceptive behavior. These results suggest

that the sympathetic nervous system is implicated in female sexual behavior.[33]

The pudendal nerve innervates the striated pelvic-perineal musculature. Its recruitment is responsible for the rhythmic contractions of these muscles occurring during orgasm through a reflex arc handled at the sacral spinal cord level. The motor innervation of perineal muscles plays an additional role in the sexual response in women, because voluntary contractions of these muscles may enhance arousal and contribute to the feeling of pleasure during sexual intercourse.[34]

Central neurophysiology

Spinal cord

Genital arousal and genital physiologic events, which occur during orgasm, are processed at the spinal cord level. This theory is based on (1) clinical studies reporting that in laboratory conditions genital stimulation elicits orgasm in spinal cord-injured women when the sacral reflex arc is intact[35] and (2) the occurrence of the urogenital reflex in spinalized female rats at the T8 level of the spinal cord.[19]

The spinal cord is an integration site for afferent information from the periphery and modulation from supraspinal origin, including both excitatory and inhibitory inputs.

Using the transneuronal retrograde tracing technique with pseudorabies virus, the spinal neurons destined to the clitoris have been identified in rats.[33,36] The major input to the clitoris originates from the lumbosacral spinal cord (L5–S1), with a strong labeling present on both sides of the lateral gray in the region of the parasympathetic preganglionic neurons of the pelvic nerve and in the dorsal gray commissure. Fewer labeled cells were found in the T13–L2 spinal segments, where the sympathetic neurons of both the hypogastric nerve and the lumbosacral paravertebral sympathetic chain are located. The retrograde transneuronal tracing technique was also used to identify pathways to the cervix in rat. Retrograde transport from the cervix occurs via the hypogastric and pelvic nerves. In addition, intraspinal circuitry has been suggested between the thoracolumbar and lumbosacral levels.[37] Such an intraspinal organization is probably involved in the coordination between parasympathetic and sympathetic output to the genital apparatus. This leads to a discussion as to whether a discrete group of spinal cells, designated as the lumbar spinothalamic cells, which have been demonstrated in males as a spinal ejaculation generator,[38,39] plays a major role in females. The lumbar spinothalamic cells are not activated during vaginocervical stimulation in females,[38,39] but are activated during urogenital reflex in female rats.[24]

Ascending and descending pathways

Sensory information is relayed through the spinothalamic and spinoreticular pathways to the brain. Fast myelinated fibers travel in the dorsal columns and dorsal lateral quadrant and terminate in the thalamus. Spinoreticular fibers cross to the opposite side of the cord and travel in the lateral spinal columns, terminating in brainstem reticular formation.[40]

Descending information from the brain also travels in the dorsal and dorsolateral white matter and enters into the spinal gray matter.

Spinal interneurons

Spinal interneurons relay afferent input from the genital apparatus to the efferent somatic and autonomic spinal neurons destined to the anatomic structures participating in the female genital sexual response. They also receive projections from the supraspinal structures and may be a site for modulating the activity of the spinal nuclei controlling the peripheral events occurring during female sexual response. These interneurons are located in and around the intermediolateral cell column and in the medial gray forming a column of neurons through segments T13 to S1. In cats, electrophysiologic recordings suggested that spinal interneurons in the medial gray are involved in the mediation of pelvic and perineal stimulation.[13,41,42]

The role of the spinal cord in female sexual response has been investigated in women with spinal cord injury. It is common that women with spinal cord injury have difficulties in achieving orgasm.[43] Systemic modifications associated with orgasm, such as blood pressure, heart rate, and respiratory rate fluctuations, are similar in women with and without spinal cord injury.[44] Women with complete spinal cord injury at midthoracic level still present perceptual responses to vaginal and/or cervical self-stimulation.[22]

Overall, the spinal cord is a key structure in the control/command of the female genital response. It receives genital afferent input and contains neurons projecting to every anatomic genital element participating in the sexual response. In addition, spinal interneurons may (1) connect afferent and efferent pathways responsible for sexual response by local stimulation, suggesting that orgasm is at least partly a spinal reflex and (2) may be responsible for the coordination between various components of the sexual response. Last but not least, the spinal cord receives the inhibitory/excitatory projections from the brain.

Brain structures

Anatomic organization

Descending projections from the brainstem, pons, and hypothalamus reach the spinal nuclei controlling the genital sexual response. Thus, spinal autonomic preganglionic neurons as well as motoneurons receive direct monosynaptic inputs from a variety of nuclei in supraspinal structures. In particular, several brainstem nuclei send projections to the spinal sympathetic and parasympathetic nuclei controlling sexual functions. In rats, the thoracolumbar cell column (intermediolateral cell column), the dorsal gray commissure, the sacral parasympathetic nucleus, and the pudendal motoneurons receive abundant serotoninergic innervation from raphe nuclei.[34,45–48] The same structures are also innervated by the noradrenergic nuclei A5, A6 (locus coeruleus), and A7.[49,50] Terminal projections from the A11 dopaminergic cells group also reach the intermediolateral cell column and the dorsal gray commissure down to the sacral levels.[51] Injection of pseudorabies virus into the rat clitoris labeled neurons in the paragigantocellularis nucleus (nPGi), raphe pallidus, raphe magnus, Barrington's nucleus, ventrolateral central gray, hypothalamus and the medial preoptic area.[33,36] By the same technique, neurons in the ventrolateral nucleus of the hypothalamus are labeled after virus injection into the uterus and the vagina.[52]

Functional data

In female rats, the ventromedial nucleus of the hypothalamus has been shown to play a pivotal role in the control of lordosis, which is a supraspinal reflex leading to arching of the back and raising of the head. Lordosis is a behavioral marker for receptivity; this is a reflex activity occurring during copulation in this species. The clinical extrapolation of female rat lordosis is highly questionable. To date, there has been no demonstration that lordosis is accompanied by sexual arousal.

It was demonstrated that sexual stimulation induces c-fos gene expression within specific regions in the forebrain of female rats. Vaginocervical stimulation or copulation with intromission elicits c-fos expression in the medial preoptic area, the bed nucleus of the stria terminalis, the paraventricular hypothalamus, the ventromedial nucleus, the medial amygdala, and the ventral premammillary nuclei.[53,54]

The medial preoptic area is an important structure in controlling female sexual response. In anesthetized female rats, electrical stimulation of the medial preoptic area resulted in an increase in vaginal blood flow and wall tension.[29] Neuronal pathways from the medial preoptic area interconnect with the periaqueductal gray, which plays a facilitator role in lordosis.[53]

In contrast, the paragigantocellularis nucleus inhibits the urogenital reflex. Because this nucleus receives sensory information from the genital apparatus and sends descending projections to the spinal nuclei controlling the female genital sexual response, it is proposed that this structure inhibits female peripheral sexual function.

Brain imaging by positron emission tomography studies in humans have revealed the structures implicated in the female sexual response. During orgasm, there is enhanced activation in the paraventricular hypothalamus, the periaqueductal gray, the amygdala, the hippocampus, the striatum, the cerebellum, and different regions of cortex.[55] During self-stimulation, nucleus tractus solitaries, somatosensory and motor cortices, the thalamus, and sensory areas of the spinal medulla are activated. However, it seems that visual sexual stimulation (frequently used to evaluate female sexual arousal) does not activate the same brain structures implicated in orgasm. Several studies have reported the differences between men and women in brain structure activation in response to sexual arousal. Generally, brain imaging studies showed that during sexual arousal the amygdala and the hypothalamus are more strongly activated in men than women.[56]

Conclusion

We have attempted to summarize information regarding the neural control of the female genital sexual response to sexual stimulation. We have not discussed the crucial issue of hormonal status, which strongly interacts with the neural command of female sexuality along the entire neuraxis. Another chapter is dedicated to the key role of hormones. On the other hand, the neurochemical support of female sexuality has not been well described. There is a tremendous need for research in this area, particularly at the central nervous system level. Indeed, better knowledge of the central neurotransmitter system involved in the command of sexual response would facilitate design of pharmacologic interventions to restore impaired sexual function in women.

References

1. Levin RJ. Sex and the human female reproductive tract – what really happens during and after coitus. *Int J Impot Res* 1998;10 (Suppl 1): S14–S21.
2. Chayen B, Tejani N, Verma UL et al. Fetal heart rate changes and uterine activity during coitus. *Acta Obstet Gynecol Scand* 1986; 65: 853–5.
3. Fox CA. Some aspects and implications of coital physiology. *J Sex Marital Ther* 1976; 2: 205–13.
4. Bohlen JG, Held JP. An anal probe for monitoring vascular and muscular events during sexual response. *Psychophysiology* 1979; 16: 318–23.
5. Bohlen JG, Held JP, Sanderson MO et al. The female orgasm: pelvic contractions. *Arch Sex Behav* 1982; 11: 367–86.
6. McKenna KE, Nadelhaft I. The organization of the pudendal nerve in the male and female rat. *J Comp Neurol* 1986; 248: 532–49.
7. Thor KB, Morgan C, Nadelhaft I et al. Organization of afferent and efferent pathways in the pudendal nerve of the female cat. *J Comp Neurol* 1989; 288: 263–79.
8. Morgan C, Nadelhaft I, de Groat WC. The distribution of visceral primary afferents from the pelvic nerve to Lissauer's tract and the spinal gray matter and its relationship to the sacral parasympathetic nucleus. *J Comp Neurol* 1981; 201: 415–40.
9. Goldstein I, Graziottin A, Heiman JR et al. Female sexual dysfunction. In A Jardin, G Warner, S Khoury et al., eds. *Erectile Dysfunction*. Plymouth: Health Publications, 2004: 507–56.
10. Darling CA, Davidson JK Sr, Jennings DA. The female sexual response revisited: understanding the multiorgasmic experience in women. *Arch Sex Behav* 1991; 20: 527–40.
11. Darling CA, Davidson JK, Sr, Cox RP. Female sexual response and the timing of partner orgasm. *J Sex Marital Ther* 1991; 17: 3–21.
12. Mah K, Binik YM. The nature of human orgasm: a critical review of major trends. *Clin Psychol Rev* 2001; 21: 823–56.
13. Kawatani M, Tanowitz M, de Groat WC. Morphological and electrophysiological analysis of the peripheral and central afferent pathways from the clitoris of the cat. *Brain Res* 1994; 646: 26–36.
14. Bradley WE, Teague CT. Electrophysiology of pelvic and pudendal nerves in the cat. *Exp Neurol* 1972; 35: 378–93.
15. Vardi Y, Gruenwald I, Sprecher E et al. Normative values for female genital sensation. *Urology* 2000; 56: 1035–40.
16. Cueva-Rolon R, Munoz-Martinez EJ, Delgado-Lezama R et al. Prolonged inhibition of the flexor reflex by probing the cervix uteri in the cat. *Brain Res* 1993; 600: 27–32.
17. Berkley KJ, Hotta H, Robbins A et al. Functional properties of afferent fibers supplying reproductive and other pelvic organs in pelvic nerve of female rat. *J Neurophysiol* 1990; 63: 256–72.
18. Berkley KJ, Robbins A, Sato Y. Functional differences between afferent fibers in the hypogastric and pelvic nerves innervating female reproductive organs in the rat. *J Neurophysiol* 1993; 69: 533–44.
19. McKenna KE, Chung SK, McVary KT. A model for the study of sexual function in anesthetized male and female rats. *Am J Physiol* 1991; 261: R1276–85.
20. Hilliges M, Falconer C, Ekman-Ordeberg G et al. Innervation of the human vaginal mucosa as revealed by PGP 9.5 immunohistochemistry. *Acta Anat (Basel)* 1995; 153: 119–26.
21. Gintzler AR, Komisaruk BR. Analgesia is produced by uterocervical mechanostimulation in rats: roles of afferent nerves and implications for analgesia of pregnancy and parturition. *Brain Res* 1991; 566: 299–302.
22. Whipple B, Gerdes CA, Komisaruk BR. Sexual response to self-stimulation in women with complete spinal cord injury. *J Sex Res* 2004; 33: 231–40.
23. Komisaruk BR, Gerdes CA, Whipple B. "Complete" spinal cord injury does not block perceptual responses to genital self-stimulation in women. *Arch Neurol* 1997; 54: 1513–20.
24. Marson L, Cai R, Makhanova N. Identification of spinal neurons involved in the urethrogenital reflex in the female rat. *J Comp Neurol* 2003; 462: 355–70.
25. Weisberg M. Physiology of female sexual function. *Clin Obstet Gynecol* 1984; 27: 697–705.
26. Levin RJ. VIP, vagina, clitoral and periurethral glans – an update on human female genital arousal. *Exp Clin Endocrinol* 1991; 98: 61–9.
27. Park K, Goldstein I, Andry C et al. Vasculogenic female sexual dysfunction: the hemodynamic basis for vaginal engorgement insufficiency and clitoral erectile insufficiency. *Int J Impot Res* 1998; 10: 67–97.
28. Vachon P, Simmerman N, Zahran AR et al. Increases in clitoral and vaginal blood flow following clitoral and pelvic plexus nerve stimulations in the female rat. *Int J Impot Res* 2000; 12: 53–7.
29. Giuliano F, Allard J, Compagnie S et al. Vaginal physiological changes in a model of sexual arousal in anesthetized rats. *Am J Physiol Regul Integr Comp Physiol* 2001; 281: R140–9.
30. Fox CA, Fox B. Blood pressure and respiratory patterns during human coitus. *J Reprod Fertil* 1969; 19: 405–15.
31. Meston CM, Gorzalka BB. The effects of sympathetic activation on physiological and subjective sexual arousal in women. *Behav Res Ther* 1995; 33: 651–64.
32. Meston CM, Gorzalka BB. The effects of immediate, delayed, and residual sympathetic activation on sexual arousal in women. *Behav Res Ther* 1996; 34: 143–8.

33. Meston CM, Moe IV, Gorzalka BB. Effects of sympathetic inhibition on receptive, proceptive, and rejection behaviors in the female rat. *Physiol Behav* 1996; 59: 537–42.

34. Messe MR, Geer JH. Voluntary vaginal musculature contractions as an enhancer of sexual arousal. *Arch Sex Behav* 1985; 14: 13–28.

35. Sipski ML, Alexander CJ. Sexual activities, response and satisfaction in women pre- and post-spinal cord injury. *Arch Phys Med Rehabil* 1993; 74: 1025–9.

36. Marson L. Central nervous system neurons identified after injection of pseudorabies virus into the rat clitoris. *Neurosci Lett* 1995; 190: 41–4.

37. Lee JW, Erskine MS. Changes in pain threshold and lumbar spinal cord immediate-early gene expression induced by paced and non-paced mating in female rats. *Brain Res* 2000; 861: 26–36.

38. Truitt WA, Coolen LM. Identification of a potential ejaculation generator in the spinal cord. *Science* 2002; 297: 1566–9.

39. Truitt WA, Shipley MT, Veening JG et al. Activation of a subset of lumbar spinothalamic neurons after copulatory behavior in male but not female rats. *J Neurosci* 2003; 23: 325–31.

40. Hubscher CH, Johnson RD. Effects of acute and chronic midthoracic spinal cord injury on neural circuits for male sexual function. II. Descending pathways. *J Neurophysiol* 2000; 83: 2508–18.

41. Fedirchuk B, Song L, Downie JW et al. Spinal distribution of extracellular field potentials generated by electrical stimulation of pudendal and perineal afferents in the cat. *Exp Brain Res* 1992; 89: 517–20.

42. Honda CN. Visceral and somatic afferent convergence onto neurons near the central canal in the sacral spinal cord of the cat. *J Neurophysiol* 1985; 53: 1059–78.

43. Harrison J, Glass CA, Owens RG et al. Factors associated with sexual functioning in women following spinal cord injury. *Paraplegia* 1995; 33: 687–92.

44. Sipski ML, Alexander CJ, Rosen R. Sexual arousal and orgasm in women: effects of spinal cord injury. *Ann Neurol* 2001; 49: 35–44.

45. Hermann GE, Bresnahan JC, Holmes GM et al. Descending projections from the nucleus raphe obscurus to pudendal motoneurons in the male rat. *J Comp Neurol* 1998; 397: 458–74.

46. Loewy AD, McKellar S. Serotonergic projections from the ventral medulla to the intermediolateral cell column in the rat. *Brain Res* 1981; 211: 146–52.

47. Loewy AD. Raphe pallidus and raphe obscurus projections to the intermediolateral cell column in the rat. *Brain Res* 1981; 222: 129–33.

48. Skagerberg G, Bjorklund A. Topographic principles in the spinal projections of serotonergic and non-serotonergic brainstem neurons in the rat. *Neuroscience* 1985; 15: 445–80.

49. Westlund KN, Bowker RM, Ziegler MG et al. Noradrenergic projections to the spinal cord of the rat. *Brain Res* 1983; 263: 15–31.

50. Westlund KN, Bowker RM, Ziegler MG et al. Origins and terminations of descending noradrenergic projections to the spinal cord of monkey. *Brain Res* 1984; 292: 1–16.

51. Skagerberg G, Lindvall O. Organization of diencephalic dopamine neurones projecting to the spinal cord in the rat. *Brain Res* 1985; 342: 340–51.

52. Papka RE, Williams S, Miller KE et al. CNS location of uterine-related neurons revealed by trans-synaptic tracing with pseudorabies virus and their relation to estrogen receptor-immunoreactive neurons. *Neuroscience* 1998; 84: 935–52.

53. Pfaus JG, Pfaff DW. Mu-, delta-, and kappa-opioid receptor agonists selectively modulate sexual behaviors in the female rat: differential dependence on progesterone. *Horm Behav* 1992; 26: 457–73.

54. Pfaus JG, Kleopoulos SP, Mobbs CV et al. Sexual stimulation activates c-fos within estrogen-concentrating regions of the female rat forebrain. *Brain Res* 1993; 624: 253–67.

55. Whipple B, Komisaruk BR. Brain (PET) responses to vaginal-cervical self-stimulation in women with complete spinal cord injury: preliminary findings. *J Sex Marital Ther* 2002; 28: 79–86.

56. Canli T, Desmond JE, Zhao Z et al. Sex differences in the neural basis of emotional memories. *Proc Natl Acad Sci U S A* 2002; 99: 10789–94.

5.4 Vascular physiology of female sexual function

Annamaria Giraldi, Roy J Levin

Introduction

During sexual stimulation, the female sexual arousal response is elicited by sensory stimulation as well as central nervous system activation, resulting in increased genital blood flow and, to some extent, relaxation of genital smooth muscle structures. This culminates in a series of vasocongestive as well as neuromuscular events leading to physiologic changes, including engorgement of the labia, vaginal lubrication, and increased length and width of the clitoris.

Dickinson,[1] Kinsey et al.,[2] and Masters and Johnson[3] described the human female sexual arousal, largely phenomenologically, with few quantitative aspects. For many years, most advances in our knowledge about the human female sexual arousal response have been from methods that measure changes in genital functions, primarily giving information about physiologic mechanisms in the sexual arousal response very often from isolated organ models, and not "whole" women. The reason for the lack of studies on female sexual arousal may rely on the taboo and ethical considerations against laboratory use of women for studies on human sexual arousal. However, during the last 10 years, there has been an increased focus on studies on female sexuality and more laboratory experiments with quantitative data. Still, much of our knowledge about basal vascular and tissue physiology involved in the female sexual arousal response derives from animal models, which can help to elucidate similar mechanisms in the human but never can replace human measurements.

This chapter describes the physiologic mechanisms behind these vasocongestive and neuromuscular events during the female sexual arousal response, based on data from both animal and human studies.

Blood supply of the female genitals

The genitals have a rich arterial blood supply. The labia are supplied from the inferior perineal and posterior labial branches of the internal pudendal artery as well as from superficial branches from the femoral artery. The clitoris receives its arterial blood supply mainly via the ileohypogastric pudendal arterial bed. After the internal iliac artery has given off its last anterior branch, it transverses Alcock's canal (pudendal canal) and terminates as the common clitoral artery, which gives off the clitoral cavernosal arteries and the dorsal clitoral artery. The proximal (middle) part of the vagina is supplied by the vaginal branches of the uterine artery and the hypogastric artery. The distal part of the vagina is supplied by the middle hemorrhoidal and clitoral arteries.

During female sexual arousal, the blood flow to the genitals is increased, leading to vasocongestion, engorgement, and lubrication.[4-6] In a study on 48 pre- and post-menopausal women, Berman et al. demonstrated that sexual stimulation resulted in significant increases in clitoral, labial, urethral, and vaginal peak systolic velocity and end diastolic velocity as a measure of arterial blood flow[7] (Table 5.4.1). In addition to the increased blood flow, the venous drainage is most probably reduced, resulting in vasocongestion and genital engorgement, clitoral tumescence, and increased genital sensitivity and vaginal lubrication.[8]

The data of Table 5.4.1 objectively illustrate the physiologic changes during female sexual arousal. In the next sections, the consequences of the increased genital blood flow will be described in more detail (Fig. 5.4.1).

Vaginal lubrication, basal and during sexual arousal

Vaginal lubrication during sexual arousal is a consequence of increased vaginal blood flow to sexual stimuli. The vagina consists of a tube of smooth muscle lined on the luminal side by squamous epithelial without glands. The smooth muscle is set in a bed of the pelvic striated muscle (Fig. 5.4.1).

During sexual quiescence, the human vagina is a potential

Table 5.4.1. Mean pre- and poststimulation clitoral, labial, urethral, and vaginal arterial blood flow measurements

	Blood flow			
	Pre- stimulation		Post- stimulation	
	EDV (cm/s)	PSV (cm/s)	EDV (cm/s)	PSV (cm/s)
Clitoral	3.35 ± 2.24	12.39 ± 6.22	8.20 ± 5.68*	22.00 ± 6.22*
Left labial	4.07 ± 3.12	16.91 ± 9.52	12.58 ± 14.90*	27.18 ± 18.06*
Right labial	3.21 ± 2.20	15.20 ± 7.08	6.94 ± 4.10*	25.31 ± 12.32*
Urethral	2.74 ± 2.07	15.10 ± 7.77	7.31 ± 4.50*	29.00 ± 16.64*
Left vaginal	4.12 ± 3.30	20.33 ± 10.99	9.51 ± 5.97*	39.96 ± 20.69*
Right vaginal	5.56 ± 4.60	18.32 ± 10.31	9.70 ± 5.60*	31.41 ± 12.80*

PSV = peak systolic velocity; EDV = end diastolic velocity. * Statistically significant increases in PSV and EDV from pre- to post-stimulation at the $p < 0.05$ level.
Modified from Berman et al.[7]

space with an H-shaped transverse cross-section and an elongated S-shaped longitudinal section. The anterior and posterior walls of the vagina are normally collapsed and touch each other. Nevertheless, they do not adhere, as they are covered with a thin layer of basal fluid allowing them to separate easily. No glandular elements have ever been identified in the normal human vagina. The fluid is a mixture of secretions from the whole female genital tract, mainly a vaginal plasma transudate mixed with desquamated cervical and vaginal cells and cervical secretion (see reviews[8–10]). The vaginal fluid is a transudate formed from the blood circulating through the capillaries supplying the vaginal epithelium. A plasma filtrate from the blood leaks out of the capillaries into the interstitial tissue space. In the vagina, the fluid then passes through the epithelium. In the sexually unstimulated state, the vaginal fluid has a higher K^+ and lower Na^+ concentration than plasma throughout the phases of the menstrual cycle.[11,12] The basal transudate that percolates through the epithelium is modified by the cells' capacity to reabsorb Na^+ ions.[13] During nonsexual stimulation, the slow passage through the epithelium results in sufficient contact time, making the cells capable of reabsorbing Na^+ by the vaginal epithelium and acting as the main determinant of reabsorption of vaginal fluid through the mechanism of ionic driving force. This leads to a condition in the basal condition where the vagina is just moist, but not lubricated enough to allow penetration without pain. The circulation to the nonsexually aroused vagina is low,[8] resulting in a hypoxic lumen with a low oxygen tension.[8,9] During sexual arousal, the blood flow to the vaginal epithelium is rapidly increased as a consequence of neural innervation via the sacral anterior nerves (S2–S4).[14,15] The

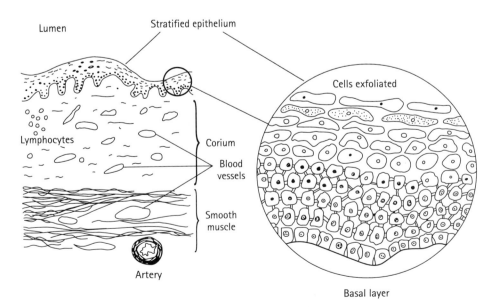

Figure 5.4.1. Vaginal wall showing main structural features. With permission from Wagner et al.[9]

increased flow results in an increased ultrafiltrate percolating between the vaginal epithelial cells and saturating their limited reabsorptive Na$^+$ transfer capacity. As a consequence of this, the fluid accumulates on the vaginal surface as a clear, slippery, and smooth lubricant, moistening the vagina so painless penile penetration and thrusting is possible. In addition to the increased blood flow, the venous drainage is most probably reduced, enhancing the vasocongestion.[8] When the sexual stimulus stops, the neural stimuli for the vasodilation also stop, leading to a slow return to basal level of the vaginal blood flow and transudation.

Clitoral engorgement during arousal

The clitoris is an erectile organ similar to the penis. It consists of three parts: the outermost glans, the middle corpus, and the innermost paired crura. The paired crura are homologous to the male corpora cavernosa. They are composed of trabecular smooth muscle and collagen connective tissue forming a sinusoidal structure surrounded by a fibrous sheath, the tunica albuginea.[16] During sexual arousal, the blood flow to the clitoris is increased, the trabecular smooth muscle in the clitoris is relaxed, and thereby the intracavernous clitoral pressure rises. As the tunica albuginea in the clitoris is unilaminar, in contrast to the penis with a bilaminar structure, the fascia is more elastic and thus no mechanism for venous occlusion occurs in the clitoris. Consequently, the clitoris shows increased tumescence and becomes engorged, but has not a true "erection" (stiffness) during arousal, as has been elegantly shown by Maravilla and coworkers, using magnetic resonance imaging (MRI) to visualize the engorgement of the genitalia during sexual arousal.[4–6]

Preferential innervation of importance for the female genital arousal response

The neurotransmitters that modulate vaginal, clitoral, and vascular smooth muscle tone are currently under study. The neural control regulating the female genital response is poorly investigated, and is therefore less understood than in the male. Most of the investigations examining the neural control have been done in animals; primarily rodents, and only few human studies exist. Studies on mechanisms of genital arousal include: the regulation of vaginal blood flow; clitoral, labial, and vestibular bulb engorgement; and studies on contraction and relaxation of the vaginal smooth muscle wall. The role of contraction and relaxation of the vaginal smooth muscle wall in the genital arousal response is still debatable. Many *in vitro* studies have focused on vaginal tone and its regulation, as it is an easy end organ to study and exhibits basal smooth muscle properties, which may be comparable with that of smooth muscle in the genital vasculature and clitoris.

Autonomic neurotransmitters in the female genital arousal response

Acetylcholine and noradrenaline

Adrenergic and cholinergic neurotransmitters have been identified in the postganglionic fibers to the vagina and the clitoris, primarily in animal models,[17–23] just as alpha-adrenergic receptors have been demonstrated biochemically and functionally in the rabbit vagina.[20,21]

Limited data exist on the presumed inhibitory effect of adrenergic stimulation on the female sexual genital response. *In vitro* experiments on rat and rabbit vaginal and rabbit clitoral smooth musculature show contractile response to adrenergic stimulation.[24–26] In a pilot study, oral phentolamine was administrated to postmenopausal women with female sexual arousal disorder. The results indicated a moderate effect on subjective and objective parameters of sexual arousal.[27] Unfortunately, it was impossible to discriminate between peripheral and central effects in the study. Meston and colleagues interpreted their photoplethsymographic evidence for a facilitatory role of peripheral adrenergic activation on genital arousal in women. Ephedrine (50 mg), an alpha- and beta-adrenergic agonist, facilitated vaginal photoplethysmograph measures of sexual arousal in a randomized, controlled trial on 20 women.[28]

The role of noradrenaline (norepinephrine) in the control of clitoral tumescence is indirect and illustrated only by case reports on treatment of so-called "clitoral priapism" with injection of adrenergic agonists.[29,30]

Despite the rich cholinergic innervation, the role of acetylcholine is uncertain. In the *in vivo* animal model described by Giuliano et al.,[31] intravenous injection of atropine only slightly decreased the vaginal blood engorgement induced by stimulation of the pelvic nerve. In the same model, intravenous atropine decreased vaginal smooth muscle contractions, also induced by pelvic nerve stimulation. In a small uncontrolled study on six women, intravenous injection of atropine had no effect on vaginal blood flow during masturbation.[32]

Nonadrenergic, noncholinergic neurotransmitters/mediators

A great variety of nonadrenergic, noncholinergic neurotransmitters/mediators have been identified in the female genital tract, mainly in animal models. In animal studies on the vagina and its vasculature, vasoactive intestinal polypeptide, nitric oxide synthase (producing nitric oxide), neuropeptide Y, calcitonin gene-related peptide, substance P, pituitary adenylate cyclase-activating polypeptide, helospectine, and peptide histidine methionine have all been identified and localized.[19,20,23,25,33–40]

In humans, vasoactive intestinal polypeptide, neuropeptide Y, adenylate cyclase-activating polypeptide, nitric oxide synthase, and calcitonin gene-related peptide immunoreactive nerves have also been identified and localized in the vagina.[41–45]

In the tissue from pre- and post-menopausal women, Hoyle et al.[44] demonstrated a dense innervation of the vaginal vasculature (arteries, veins, and subepithelial plexuses); most abundant were neuropeptide Y and vasoactive intestinal polypeptide immunoreactive fibers, and less abundant were nitric oxide synthase, calcitonin gene-related peptide and substance P fibers. In the postmenopausal tissue, little or no nitric oxide synthase was found. Human studies are crucial. The major drawback of these studies is the fact that the tissues have been obtained from women undergoing hysterectomy, and therefore represent tissue from the proximal part of the vagina, which is the less innervated and of different embryologic origin from the denser innervated distal part,[46] which may be of more importance in the physiologic sexual arousal response. An exception is the study of Jorgensen et al., who demonstrated neuropeptide Y immunoreactivity in both the proximal and distal part of the human vagina as plexuses of nerve fibers beneath the vaginal epithelium in relationship to the small vessels.[41]

In the human clitoris, immunohistochemical studies on a few subjects have demonstrated vasoactive intestinal polypeptide, peptide histidine methionine, neuropeptide Y, calcitonin gene-related peptide, and substance P immunoreactive nerves,[47] and one human case study demonstrated nitric oxide-containing nerves in the clitoris.[48]

Other signal transduction systems have been investigated. In cell cultures from human and rabbit vaginal smooth muscle, the signal transduction molecules, cyclic adenosine monophosphate and cyclic guanosine monophosphate have been studied. In the vaginal smooth muscle cells, cyclic adenosine monophosphate was increased by prostaglandin E_1, and isoproterenol and cyclic guanosine monophosphate by sodium nitroprusside, a nitric oxide donor, suggesting that these signal transduction pathways are of importance for regulation of vaginal smooth muscle tone. Furthermore, sildenafil enhanced the intracellular accumulation of cyclic guanosine monophosphate in the human and rabbit vaginal smooth muscle cells.[49]

In the human vagina, phosphodiesterase type 5 expression has been demonstrated in the anterosuperior vaginal wall.[50]

The role of nonadrenergic, noncholinergic transmitters in the arousal response

Very little is known about the role of these neurotransmitters/mediators in the regulation of the genital arousal response in females, as the demonstration of their existence in the genital tract gives no information as to their functional roles in the physiology and pathophysiology of the genital arousal.

Vasoactive intestinal polypeptide

Vasoactive intestinal polypeptide has traditionally been considered to be the most important neurotransmitter in the regulation of human vaginal blood flow in the sexual arousal response. This assumption is based on (1) the high concentration of vasoactive intestinal polypeptide in the tissue of the genital tract, (2) the close association with the genital vasculature and vasoactive intestinal polypeptide-containing nerve fibres, (3) the observation that sexual arousal in women increases the level of vasoactive intestinal polypeptide in the plasma and (4) that intravenous and subepithelial administration of vasoactive intestinal polypeptide was able to increase vaginal blood flow in women.[51] However, these are only indirect evidence, and further clinical studies have to be performed in order to obtain more information. The role of vasoactive intestinal polypeptide in the physiologic arousal response still needs to be investigated further.

Nitric oxide

During the last few years, the role of nitric oxide in the arousal phase has been studied with more interest, partly based on the knowledge from males, where it is known to play a crucial role for the erectile response. New *in vivo* models on rats, rabbits, and dogs have made it possible to investigate vaginal and clitoral blood flow, vaginal oxygen tension, and temperature and vaginal luminal pressure as indices of sexual arousal.[31,52–56] In the *in vivo* animal models, pelvic nerve stimulation increases vaginal blood flow and temperature as well as clitoral blood flow.[31,53,56] Stimulation of the paravertebral sympathetic chain reversed the pelvic nerve stimulation-induced effect in the rat.[31] In both the rabbit and dog model, the phosphodiesterase type 5-inhibitors sildenafil and vardenafil, respectively, enhanced the pelvic nerve stimulation-induced vaginal and clitoral blood flow, indicating that the nitric oxide/cyclic guanosine monophosphate pathway is involved in the physiologic mechanism of female genital arousal.[57,58]

A role of the nitric oxide/cyclic guanosine monophosphate system on clitoral tumescence is further indicated by *in vitro* animal experiments. In rabbit clitoral corpus cavernosum, inhibition of nitric oxide synthase dramatically abolishes electrically stimulated relaxations, whereas sildenafil augments the relaxations.[24,59,60] In human clitoral tissue, sildenafil has been demonstrated to inhibit phosphodiesterase type 5,[61] and immunohistochemical studies have identified nitric oxide synthase immunoreactive nerve bundles within the glans and corpora cavernosa of the clitoris.[62] Clinically, sildenafil has been shown to enhance vaginal engorgement measured by photoplethysmography during erotic stimulus in healthy women without sexual dysfunction.[63] Clinical trials have been performed in order to investigate a possible role of sildenafil in treatment of female sexual dysfunction,[64–66] but the efficacy of sildenafil in the treatment of female sexual dysfunction is still under debate, as the results were not very promising.

There are several indications of a role of the nitric oxide/cyclic guanosine monophosphate system in the genital arousal response, but the exact role in the normal arousal response still needs to be investigated further.

Pathophysiologic factors that may influence the physiologic genital arousal response

Diabetes

In rat models it has been shown that diabetes mellitus (type 1) induces vaginal fibrosis, measured as transforming growth factor beta expression in collagen connective tissue, fibroblasts, and smooth muscle fibers,[67] and that the nitrergic-dependent relaxation of vaginal tissue is impaired during the diabetic state.[25] Park and colleagues also have demonstrated that type 1 diabetes mellitus, in the *in vivo* rabbit model, produces significant adverse effects on the hemodynamic mechanism of clitoral engorgement and leads to diffuse clitoral cavernous fibrosis.[68]

Arteriosclerosis

In the rabbit, experimentally induced arteriosclerosis resulted in decreased pelvic nerve stimulation-induced vaginal blood flow and vaginal wall pressure.[55]

Conclusions

During sexual stimulation, the physiologic female sexual arousal response is elicited by sensory stimulation as well as central nervous system activation, resulting in increased genital blood flow and, to some extent, relaxation of genital smooth muscle structures. This culminates in a series of vasocongestive as well as neuromuscular events leading to physiologic changes, including engorgement of the labia, vaginal lubrication, and increased length and width of the clitoris, as well as increased sensitivity of the genitals, all representing the physiologic sexual arousal response in women. Modulation of vaginal and clitoral engorgement, vasocongestion, and vaginal lubrication may be antagonistically regulated by parasympathetic and sympathetic components of the autonomic nervous system of the female genitalia. Vasoactive intestinal polypeptide and nitric oxide may be the primary facilitators, and noradrenaline and neuropeptide Y the primary inhibitors, of the genital arousal response. There is still a need to expand our current understanding of the physiologic mechanisms responsible for the arousal response.

References

1. Dickinson RL. *Human Sex Anatomy*, 2nd edn. London: Baillière, Tindal & Cox, 1949.
2. Kinsey AC, Pomeroy WB, Martin CE et al. *Sexual Behavior in the Human Female*. Philadelphia: WB Saunders, 1953.
3. Masters WH, Johnson VE. *Human Sexual Response*. Boston: Little, Brown, 1966.
4. Deliganis AV, Maravilla KR, Heiman JR et al. Female genitalia: dynamic MR imaging with use of MS-325 initial experiences evaluating female sexual response. *Radiology* 2002; 225: 791–9.
5. Maravilla KR, Heiman JR, Garland PA et al. Dynamic MR imaging of the sexual arousal response in women. *J Sex Marital Ther* 2003; 29 (Suppl 1): 71–6.
6. Maravilla KR, Cao Y, Heiman JR et al. Serial MR imaging with MS-325 for evaluating female sexual arousal response: determination of intrasubject reproducibility. *J Magn Reson Imaging* 2003; 18: 216–24.
7. Berman JR, Berman LA, Werbin TJ et al. Clinical evaluation of female sexual function: effects of age and estrogen status on subjective and physiologic sexual responses. *Int J Impot Res* 1999, 11 (Suppl 1): S31–8.
8. Levin RJ. The mechanisms of human female sexual arousal. *Annu Rev Sex Res* 1992; 3: 1–48.
9. Wagner G, Levin RJ. Vaginal fluid. In E Hafez, T Evans, eds. *The Human Vagina*. Amsterdam: Elsevier/North-Holland Biomedical Press, 1978: 121–37.
10. Levin RJ. The ins and outs of vaginal lubrication. *Sex Relats Ther* 2003; 18: 509–13.
11. Wagner G, Levin RJ. Electrolytes in vaginal fluid during the menstrual cycle of coitally active and inactive women. *J Reprod Fertil* 1980; 60: 17–27.
12. Wagner G. Vaginal transudation. In F Beller, G Schumacher, eds. *The Biology of the Fluids in the Female Genital Tract*. Amsterdam: Elsevier North Holland, 1979: 25–34.
13. Levin RJ. Actions of spermicidal and virucidal agents on electrogenic ion transfer across human vaginal epithelium *in vitro*. *Pharmacol Toxicol* 1997; 81: 219–25.
14. Levin RJ, Macdonagh RP. Increased vaginal blood flow induced by implant electrical stimulation of sacral anterior roots in the conscious woman: a case study. *Arch Sex Behav* 1993; 22: 471–5.
15. Giuliano F, Rampin O, Allard J. Neurophysiology and pharmacology of female genital sexual response. *J Sex Marital Ther* 2002; 28 (Suppl 1): 101–21.
16. Tarcan T, Park K, Goldstein I et al. Histomorphometric analysis of age-related structural changes in human clitoral cavernosal tissue. *J Urol* 1999; 161: 940–4.
17. Rosengren E, Sjoberg NO. The adrenergic nerve supply to the female reproductive tract of the cat. *Am J Anat* 1967; 121: 271–83.
18. Owman C, Sjoberg NO. Adrenergic innervation of the female genital tract of the dog. *J Reprod Med* 1972; 8: 63–6.
19. Papka RE, Cotton JP, Traurig HH. Comparative distribution of neuropeptide tyrosine-, vasoactive intestinal polypeptide-, substance P-immunoreactive, acetylcholinesterase-positive and noradrenergic nerves in the reproductive tract of the female rat. *Cell Tissue Res* 1985; 242: 475–90.
20. Giraldi A, Alm P, Werkstrom V et al. Morphological and functional characterization of a rat vaginal smooth muscle sphincter. *Int J Impot Res* 2002; 14: 271–82.
21. Kim NN, Min K, Huang YH et al. Biochemical and functional characterization of alpha-adrenergic receptors in the rabbit vagina. *Life Sci* 2002; 71: 2909–20.
22. Adham N, Schenk EA. Autonomic innervation of the rat vagina,

cervix, and uterus and its cyclic cariation. *Am J Obstet Gynecol* 1969; 104: 508–16.

23. Lakomy M, Kaleczyc J, Majewski M et al. Peptidergic innervation of the bovine vagina and uterus. *Acta Histochem* 1995; 97: 53–66.

24. Cellek S, Moncada S. Nitrergic neurotransmission mediates the non-adrenergic non-cholinergic responses in the clitoral corpus cavernosum of the rabbit. *Br J Pharmacol* 1998; 125: 1627–9.

25. Giraldi A, Persson K, Werkstrom V et al. Effects of diabetes on neurotransmission in rat vaginal smooth muscle. *Int J Impot Res* 2001; 13: 58–66.

26. Ziessen T, Moncada S, Cellek S. Characterization of the non-nitrergic NANC relaxation responses in the rabbit vaginal wall. *Br J Pharmacol* 2002; 135: 546–54.

27. Rosen RC, Phillips NA, Gendrano NC III et al. Oral phentolamine and female sexual arousal disorder: a pilot study. *J Sex Marital Ther* 1999; 25: 137–44.

28. Meston CM, Heiman JR. Ephedrine-activated physiological sexual arousal in women. *Arch Gen Psychiatry* 1998; 55: 652–6.

29. Brodie-Meijer CC, Diemont WL, Buijs PJ. Nefazodone-induced clitoral priapism. *Int Clin Psychopharmacol* 1999; 14: 257–8.

30. Pescatori ES, Engelman JC, Davis G et al. Priapism of the clitoris: a case report following trazodone use. *J Urol* 1993; 149: 1557–9.

31. Giuliano F, Allard J, Compagnie S et al. Vaginal physiological changes in a model of sexual arousal in anesthetized rats. *Am J Physiol Regul Integr Comp Physiol* 2001; 281: R140–9.

32. Wagner G, Levin RJ. Effect of atropine and methylatropine on human vaginal blood flow, sexual arousal and climax. *Acta Pharmacol Toxicol (Copenh)* 1980; 46: 321–5.

33. Huang WM, Gu J, Blank MA et al. Peptide-immunoreactive nerves in the mammalian female genital tract. *Histochem J* 1984; 16: 1297–1310.

34. Steenstrup BR, Ottesen B, Jorgensen M et al. Pituitary adenylate cyclase activating polypeptide induces vascular relaxation and inhibits non-vascular smooth muscle activity in the rabbit female genital tract. *Acta Physiol Scand* 1994; 152: 129–36.

35. Lakomy M, Happola O, Majewski M et al. Immunohistochemical localization of neuropeptides in nerve fibers of the porcine vagina and uterine cervix. *Foli Histochem Cytobiol* 1994; 32: 167–75.

36. Grozdanovic Z, Mayer B, Baumgarten HG et al. Nitric oxide synthase-containing nerve fibers and neurons in the genital tract of the female mouse. *Cell Tissue Res* 1994; 275: 355–60.

37. Blank MA, Gu J, Allen JM et al. The regional distribution of NPY-, PHM-, and VIP-containing nerves in the human female genital tract. *Int J Fertil* 1986; 31: 218–22.

38. Majewski M, Sienkiewicz W, Kaleczyc J et al. The distribution and co-localization of immunoreactivity to nitric oxide synthase, vasoactive intestinal polypeptide and substance P within nerve fibres supplying bovine and porcine female genital organs. *Cell Tissue Res* 1995; 281: 445–64.

39. Fahrenkrug J, Hannibal J. Pituitary adenylate cyclase activating polypeptide innervation of the rat female reproductive tract and the associated paracervical ganglia: effect of capsaicin. *Neuroscience* 1996; 73: 1049–60.

40. Al Hijji J, Larsson B, Batra S. Nitric oxide synthase in the rabbit

uterus and vagina: hormonal regulation and functional significance. *Biol Reprod* 2000; 62: 1387–92.

41. Jorgensen JC. Neuropeptide Y in mammalian genital tract: localization and biological action. *Dan Med Bull* 1994; 41: 294–305.

42. Polak JM, Bloom SR. Localisation and measurement of VIP in the genitourinary system of man and animals. *Peptides* 1984; 5: 225–30.

43. Steenstrup BR, Alm P, Hannibal J et al. Pituitary adenylate cyclase-activating polypeptide: occurrence and relaxant effect in female genital tract. *Am J Physiol* 1995; 269 (1 Pt 1): E108–17.

44. Hoyle CH, Stones RW, Robson T et al. Innervation of vasculature and microvasculature of the human vagina by NOS and neuropeptide-containing nerves. *J Anat* 1996; 188 (Pt 3): 633–44.

45. Helm G, Ottesen B, Fahrenkrug J et al. Vasoactive intestinal polypeptide (VIP) in the human female reproductive tract: distribution and motor effects. *Biol Reprod* 1981; 25: 227–34.

46. Forsberg J, Kalland T. Embryology of the genital tract in humans and rodents. In A Herbst, H Bern, eds. *Developmental Effects of Diethylstilbestrol (DES) in Pregnancy.* New York: Thieme-Stratton, 1981: 4–25.

47. Hauser-Kronberger C, Cheung A, Hacker GW et al. Peptidergic innervation of the human clitoris. *Peptides* 1999; 20: 539–43.

48. Creigton SM, Crouch NS, Foxwell NA et al. Functional evidence for nitreregic neurotransmission in a human clitoral corpus cavernosum: a case study. *Int J Impot Res* 2004; 16: 319–24.

49. Traish A, Moreland RB, Huang YH et al. Development of human and rabbit vaginal smooth muscle cell cultures: effects of vasoactive agents on intracellular levels of cyclic nucleotides. *Mol Cell Biol Res Commun* 1999; 2: 131–7.

50. D'Amati G, di Gioia CR, Bologna M et al. Type 5 phosphodiesterase expression in the human vagina. *Urology* 2002; 60: 191–5.

51. Levin RJ. VIP, vagina, clitoral and periurethral glans – an update on human female genital arousal. *Exp Clin Endocrinol* 1991; 98: 61–9.

52. Beharry R, Hale T, Wilson E et al. Evidence for centrally initiated genital vasocongestive engorgement in the female rat: findings from a new model of female sexual arousal response. *Int J Impot Res* 2003; 15: 122–8.

53. Min K, Munarriz R, Berman J et al. Hemodynamic evaluation of the female sexual arousal response in an animal model. *J Sex Marital Ther* 2001; 27: 557–65.

54. Min K, O'Connell L, Munarriz R et al. Experimental models for the investigation of female sexual function and dysfunction. *Int J Impot Res* 2001; 13: 151–6.

55. Park K, Goldstein I, Andry C et al. Vasculogenic female sexual dysfunction: the hemodynamic basis for vaginal engorgement insufficiency and clitoral erectile insufficiency. *Int J Impot Res* 1997; 9: 27–37.

56. Vachon P, Simmerman N, Zahran AR et al. Increases in clitoral and vaginal blood flow following clitoral and pelvic plexus nerve stimulations in the female rat. *Int J Impot Res* 2000; 12: 53–7.

57. Min K, Kim NN, McAuley I et al. Sildenafil augments pelvic nerve-mediated female genital sexual arousal in the anesthetized rabbit. *Int J Impot Res* 2000; 12 (Suppl 3): S32–9.

58. Angulo J, Cuevas P, Bischoff E et al. Vardenafil enhances clitoral

and vaginal blood flow response to pelvic nerve stimulation in female dogs. *Int J Impot Res* 2003; 15: 137–41.

59. Vemulapalli S, Kurowski S. Sildenafil relaxes rabbit clitoral corpus cavernosum. *Life Sci* 2000; 67: 23–9.

60. Park JK, Kim JU, Lee SO et al. Nitric oxide-cyclic GMP signaling pathway in the regulation of rabbit clitoral cavernosum tone. *Exp Biol Med (Maywood)* 2002; 227: 1022–30.

61. Park K, Moreland RB, Goldstein I et al. Sildenafil inhibits phosphodiesterase type 5 in human clitoral corpus cavernosum smooth muscle. *Biochem Biophys Res Commun* 1998; 28: 249.

62. Burnett AL, Calvin DC, Silver RI et al. Immunohistochemical description of nitric oxide synthase isoforms in human clitoris *J Urol* 1997; 158: 75–8.

63. Laan E, van Lunsen RH, Everaerd W et al. The enhancement of vaginal vasocongestion by sildenafil in healthy premenopausal women. *J Womens Health Gend Based Med* 2002; 11: 357–65.

64. Basson R, McInnes R, Smith MD et al. Efficacy and safety of sildenafil citrate in women with sexual dysfunction associated with female sexual arousal disorder. *J Womens Health Gend Based Med* 2002; 11: 367–77.

65. Caruso S, Intelisano G, Lupo L et al. Premenopausal women affected by sexual arousal disorder treated with sildenafil: a double-blind, cross-over, placebo-controlled study. *Br J Obstet Gynaecol* 2001; 108: 623–8.

66. Berman JR, Berman LA, Toler SM et al. Safety and efficacy of sildenafil citrate for the treatment of female sexual arousal disorder: a double-blind, placebo controlled study. *J Urol* 2003; 170(6 Pt 1): 2333–8.

67. Park K, Ryu SB, Park YI et al. Diabetes mellitus induces vaginal tissue fibrosis by TGF-beta 1 expression in the rat model. *J Sex Marital Ther* 2001; 27: 577–87.

68. Park K, Ahn K, Chang JS et al. Diabetes induced alteration of clitoral hemodynamics and structure in the rabbit. *J Urol* 2002; 168: 1269–72.

5.5 Modulation of female genital sexual arousal by sex steroid hormones

Abdulmaged M Traish, Noel N Kim

Introduction

The important role of sex steroids in modulating sexual function in women has been recognized for many years. However, the great majority of investigative efforts have focused on the regulation of female reproductive function by sex steroid hormones. Correspondingly, knowledge in this area has contributed significantly to successful clinical management of contraception, infertility, and gynecologic disorders by the use of sex steroid hormones or synthetic hormone analogs as therapeutic agents. In contrast, the physiology of peripheral genital sexual arousal and its regulation by sex steroid hormones has received limited attention. Receptors for sex steroid hormones (estrogens, progestins, and androgens) are widely expressed in the brain and genital tissues, suggesting that steroid hormones may modulate sexual function at both central and peripheral levels. It should be noted that most of the studies with sex steroid hormones have focused on the effects of androgens on female sexual desire, and little attention was paid to female sexual arousal response.[1,2]

With regard to sex steroid hormones, critical evaluation of the literature points to the fact that sexual function studies in women are almost entirely clinical in nature and that, in some instances, the data remain controversial. There is a great deal of skepticism regarding the therapeutic value of sex steroid hormones in treating female sexual dysfunction, especially peripheral genital arousal dysfunction in women. Unfortunately, an accurate appraisal of the usefulness of sex steroid hormones in the management of female sexual dysfunction remains elusive due to the paucity of objective clinical criteria and the limited

preclinical and clinical studies investigating the underlying pathophysiology. Employment of objective criteria of biologic effectiveness, together with clinical observations, are needed in order to have a critical and effective appraisal of the role of sex steroid hormones in modulating sexual function in women. Thus, caution must be exercised when interpreting clinical studies, especially when objective criteria are not available and since most of the work in the literature is anecdotal. Furthermore, preclinical studies are needed to develop reliable measures for evaluating objective physiologic parameters to be tested in response to sex steroid treatments. This requires development of experimental models and validating the physiologic responses to be measured. In this chapter we discuss the critical role of steroid hormones in regulating female genital arousal. There is a vast literature on sex steroid hormones and human physiology, and this chapter is not intended to cover such literature, but to focus on sex steroid and peripheral sexual arousal function and dysfunction. To this end, we present historical highlights in investigation of the relationship between sex steroids and sexual function in women, review the biochemistry of steroid metabolism, and summarize recent research efforts.

Historical perspective

It has been known for quite some time that while estrogens have little or no effect on sexual interest, they are important and necessary for the maintenance of structural and functional integrity of genital organs. The action of androgens in sexual interest was noted as an incidental finding in studies on the effects of androgens on menopause.[3] Loeser reported that all female patients who were treated with testosterone had experienced an enlargement of the clitoris and increased sexual drive.[4] The author suggested that androgens play a key role in enhancing libido in women. This observation was further confirmed by several investigators.[5–9] To this end, it was thought that the effects of androgens on increasing libido were universal observations. It was further suggested that a combination of estrogens and androgens exerted optimal effects on libido and sexual response. The increased libido and sexual response were attributed in part to changes in the external genitalia (increased sensitivity to engorgement and hypertrophy of the clitoris and the vulva) and increased sensation secondary to sexual stimulation.

It should be noted that stimulation of sex drive in women by estrogen is not commonly encountered in clinical experience in spite of the fact that sexual receptivity in the female of lower animals is controlled by estrogens. However, administration of androgens in females intensifies sexual interest.[10] As early as 1938, Shorr et al. observed that libido and sexual responses were greater when testosterone was administered together with estrogen rather than administering estrogen alone.[3] Along with reported heightened sexual desire, easier attainment of orgasm and heightened satisfaction during intercourse were also observed. It was not clear whether the effects of androgens were at the central nervous system or at the genital level or both.

In 1943, Salmon and Geist suggested that androgens have threefold action in women: (a) increased susceptibility to psychosexual stimulation, (b) increased sensitivity of the external genitalia, and (c) greater intensity of sexual gratification.[8] The authors suggested that endogenous androgens in the normal mature woman may act as the physiologic sensitizer of both the psychic and somatic components of the sexual mechanism. The authors further suggested that dryness of the vagina occurring during androgen treatment may lead to dyspareunia and might be ameliorated by estrogen administration.[8]

At present, with the exception of local vaginal administration of estrogen, there is no established and accepted scientific rationale for pharmacologic management of women with sexual dysfunction by sex steroid hormones or hormone analogs. In fact, doubts have been cast on the potential usefulness of sex steroid therapy in light of the data from the hormone replacement study that was conducted in the USA as part of the Women's Health Initiative (WHI). The trials with estrogen therapy alone did not show increased risk of breast cancer and decreased risk of colon cancer and osteoporosis coupled with decreased fracture risk, and no change in heart disease was noted as opposed to estrogen and progesterone trials in postmenopausal women. These trials with estrogen plus progesterone and estrogen alone therapy were prematurely terminated when the data indicated increased risk of stroke and general lack of benefit.

Nevertheless, a number of studies suggest that steroid hormones are important in modulating the physiology of genital organs and sexual response in women. Bachmann et al.[11] reported that estrogen deficiency associated with the postmenopausal state resulted in: (1) loss of collagen and adipose tissue in the vulva; (2) attenuated maturation of vaginal epithelial cells; (3) thinning and loss of elasticity of the vaginal wall with loss of premenopausal ridges; (4) bleeding and ulceration of the vaginal epithelium, even with minor trauma; (5) delayed onset of lubrication with sexual stimulation; and (6) increased vaginal pH leading to heightened vulnerability to urogenital pathogens and flora. In a series of studies, Sarrel and co-workers[12–15] reported that women with plasma estradiol levels less than 50 pg/ml had significantly more complaints of vaginal dryness and increased frequency and intensity of dyspareunia and burning than women with estradiol values greater than 50 pg/ml. Several investigators have shown that treatment with estradiol increases vaginal blood flow and lubrication, improves epithelial maturation indices, normalizes vaginal pH, and prevents vaginal atrophy.[15–17]

Androgen insufficiency, in women who are treated with adequate doses of estrogens, is also associated with sexual dysfunction.[13,18–22] When supraphysiologic doses are used, androgen replacement in women with sexual dysfunction is associated with changes in the external genitalia, including increased sensitivity, engorgement and hypertrophy of the clitoris, and vulvar hyperemia.[6,7,9] It has been reported that women with higher levels of testosterone exhibit significantly greater increases in vaginal blood flow in response to erotic stimuli than those with lower levels of testosterone.[23,24] Moreover, exogenous administration of androgens has significantly increased subjective ratings of sexual arousal in postmenopausal women.[25–27] In a limited study (nine patients), Tuiten et al.[27] showed that arousal response in young women given testosterone undecanoate orally and allowed to watch erotic video resulted in marked arousal response, albeit delayed by several hours after treatment. In oophorectomized women treated with testosterone, those who had a higher ratio of testosterone to sex hormone-binding globulin had greater sexual arousal response.[19] In a recent review, Sherwin suggested that combined estrogen and testosterone therapy enhances sexual desire, interest, and sometimes the frequency of intercourse.[1] In addition, the overall quality of life was improved in naturally and surgically menopausal women on this combined treatment. Even more compellingly, administration of transdermal testosterone improved sexual function and psychologic well-being in women who had undergone oophorectomy and hysterectomy.[28,29] Treatment of women with adrenal insufficiency with dehydroepiandrosterone also improved overall well-being and sexual function.[30,31] In separate studies, androgen replacement therapy with dehydroepiandrosterone in pre- and post-menopausal women with sexual dysfunction and androgen insufficiency significantly decreased sexual distress, significantly increased sexual function in the domains of desire, arousal, lubrication, satisfaction, and orgasm, and normalized androgen blood levels to values within the physiologic range.[32]

Thus, there is growing evidence that an imbalance in the sex steroid hormonal milieu may be responsible for some of the sexual complaints in women. It is well recognized that sex steroid hormones play an important role in reproductive function and sexual desire. However, their role in modulating genital arousal is poorly understood. Insufficiency in sex steroid hormones may not only alter sexual desire at the level of the central nervous system, but also modify peripheral genital tissues, resulting in decreased blood flow and lubrication, altered mucification and smooth muscle contractility, and adverse effects on clitoral and vaginal arousal. It is our view that basic and clinical research in the next decade will shed light not only on the mechanisms of hormonal regulation of female sexual arousal but also on therapeutic values of androgens and estrogens in the management of female sexual arousal dysfunction.

Biosynthesis and metabolism of sex steroid hormones in women

Biosynthesis of androgens in the ovaries and adrenals

Androgen hormones are a class of C-19 steroids, produced by the gonads and the adrenals.[33-35] Steroids with androgenic activity include testosterone, 5α-dihydrotestosterone (5α-DHT), Δ4-androstenedione, Δ5-androstenediol, 5α-androstane-3β, 17β-diol, dehydroepiandrosterone (DHEA), and 3α-hydroxyandrosterone (Fig. 5.5.1). Approximately 25% of androgen biosynthesis takes place in the ovaries, 25% is produced by the adrenal gland, and the remaining 50% is produced in the periphery.[33,34,36] In women, essentially all of the androgens detected in the urine are of adrenal origin.[10] In Addison's disease, the output of urine androgens in the female approaches zero.

In the ovaries, cholesterol is metabolized to pregnenolone, which serves as the precursor for the synthesis of sex steroids.

Biosynthesis of testosterone from pregnenolone proceeds via participation of several key enzymes in two interrelated pathways, namely, the Δ5 and Δ4 pathways (Fig. 5.5.2). In the Δ5 pathway, hydroxylation of pregnenolone by 17α-hydroxylase and subsequent cleavage of the C-17,20 side chain by the C-17,20-lyase produces dehydroepiandrosterone. The latter is converted to Δ5-androstenediol via 17β-hydroxysteroid dehydrogenase (17β-HSD). This derivative is converted into testosterone by the enzyme complex, 3β-hydroxy-Δ5-steroid dehydrogenase (3β-HSD), Δ4,5-isomerase. In the Δ4 pathway, pregnenolone is converted first into progesterone by 3β-HSD, Δ4,5-isomerase. Progesterone is then hydroxylated at the C17 position by the 17α-hydroxylase and becomes the substrate for the C-17,20-lyase, which converts 17α-hydroxyprogesterone to Δ4-androstenedione. This last product is metabolized to testosterone by the action of the 17β-hydroxysteroid dehydrogenase.

In the adrenal gland, cholesterol is metabolized to pregnenolone, which serves as the precursor for the synthesis of glucocorticoids and androgens. Similar to the ovarian synthetic pathway, pregnenolone is converted to dehydroepiandrosterone by the actions of 17α-hydroxylase and C-17,20-lyase (Fig. 5.5.2). At this stage, dehydroepiandrosterone is converted to Δ4-androstenedione via the enzyme complex, 3β-hydroxysteroid dehydrogenase, Δ4,5-isomerase, and this product is then metabolized to testosterone by the action of the 17β-hydroxysteroid dehydrogenase.

Biosynthesis of estrogens in the ovaries

Synthesis of estrogen from androgens in the ovary is thought to involve both the thecal layer and the granulosa. The theca cells have a rich blood supply, and steroids synthesized in the theca can readily pass into the circulation. In contrast, the granulosa

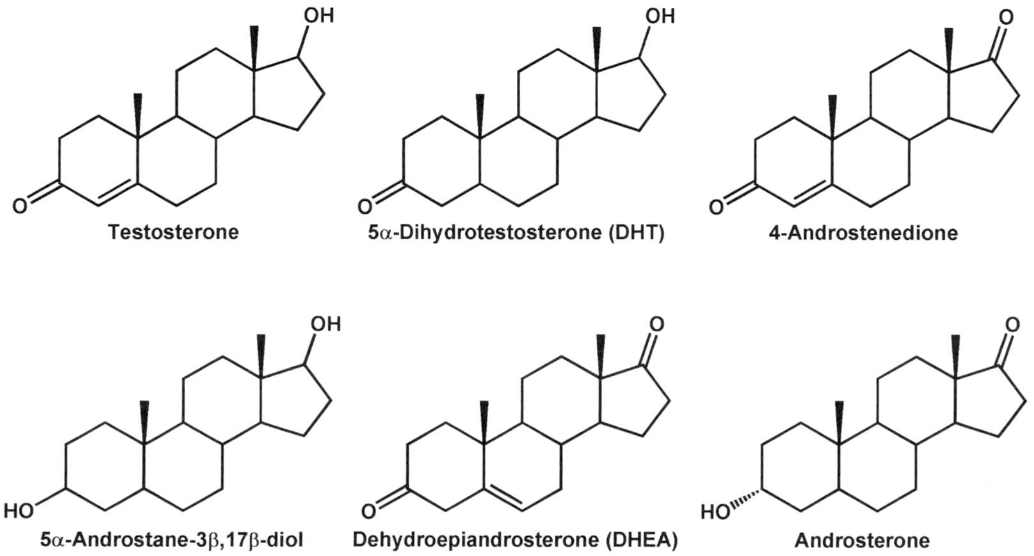

Figure 5.5.1. Structures of steroid hormones with androgenic activity.

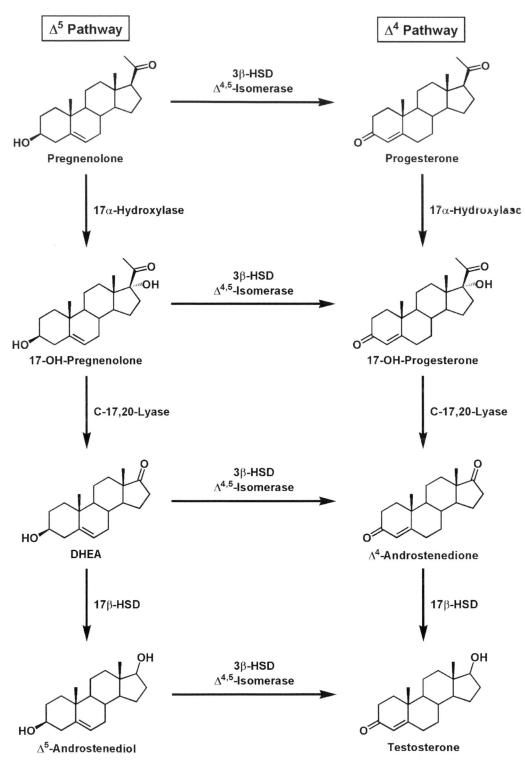

Figure 5.5.2. Biosynthesis of progesterone and androgenic steroid hormones. DHEA, dehydroepiandrosterone; 3β-HSD, 3β-hydroxy-Δ5-steroid dyhydrogenase; 17β-HSD, 17β-hydroxy-Δ5-steroid dehydrogenase.

cell layer is relatively avascular, and steroids formed in these cells cross into the theca interna in order to enter the circulation. Both the theca and the granulosa express the aromatase enzyme systems for synthesis of estrogens (Fig. 5.5.3). In the theca cells, androstenedione and estradiol are derived from 17-hydroxypregnenolone (Δ5 pathway). In the granulosa, pregnenolone is readily converted into progesterone, suggesting that the primary mechanism of synthesis is through the Δ4 pathway. Estradiol is the major steroid detected in ovarian venous blood.

The synthesis of estrogens from androgens is regulated by the

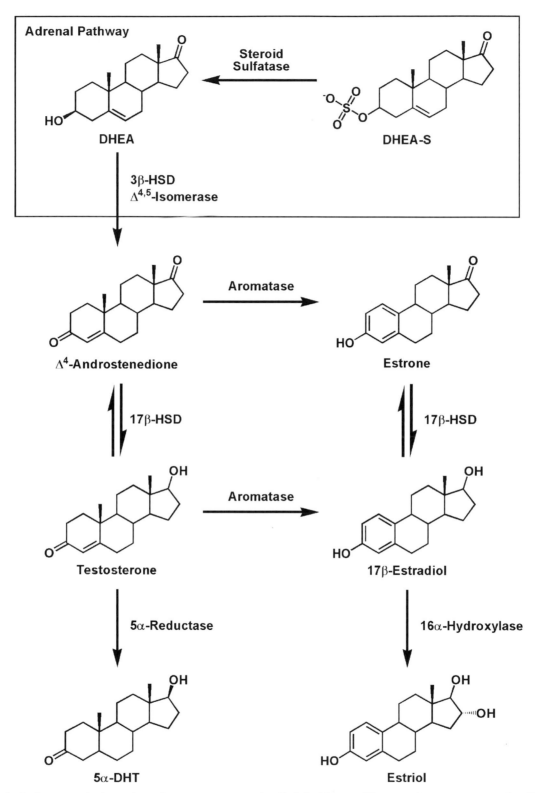

Figure 5.5.3. Biosynthesis of estrogens. In the ovaries, androgen precursors are primarily derived from 17-OH-pregnenolone or progesterone (see Fig. 5.5.2). Conversion of dehydroepiandrosterone (DHEA) sulfate or DHEA to androgens primarily takes place in the adrenals or other peripheral target tissues. 3β-HSD, 3β-hydroxy-Δ5-steroid dehydrogenase; 17β-HSD, 17β-hydroxy-Δ5-steroid dehydrogenase.

gonadotrophic hormones luteinizing hormone (LH) and follicle-stimulating hormone (FSH). Follicle-stimulating hormone acts mainly on the granulosa cells, while luteinizing hormone acts on multiple sites, including the theca, stroma, luteum, and granulosa. The theca interna expresses luteinizing hormone receptors that regulate androgen biosynthesis, mainly androstenedione and testosterone. Androgens ($\Delta 4$-androstenedione and testosterone) produced by the thecal compartment diffuse into the follicular fluid, where they are converted into estrogens by the granulosa cells or released into the ovarian vein. The granulosa cells express follicle-stimulating hormone receptors, and an increase in follicle-stimulating hormone levels upregulates the number of follicle-stimulating hormone receptors due to increased granulosa cell number. Furthermore, follicle-stimulating hormone upregulates aromatase activity in the granulosa, thus increasing conversion of androgens into estrogens. Estradiol via autocrine or paracrine mechanisms increases the mitogenic activity, independent of that of follicle-stimulating hormone. Estradiol augments the activity of follicle-stimulating hormone in increasing aromatase activity and increasing the conversion of androgens to estrogens. In menopause, serum levels of follicle-stimulating hormone and luteinizing hormone rise,[37] probably due to the loss of feedback mechanism. However, the increased levels of follicle-stimulating hormone and luteinizing hormone may explain the temporarily early rise in androgen levels in postmenopausal women due to the activity of these hormones on the interstitial cells. Eventually, the loss of expression of receptors for follicle-stimulating hormone and luteinizing hormone in ovaries of postmenopausal women and inactivation of steroidogenic enzymes result in loss of synthesis of androgens and estrogens in the ovaries.[38] This suggests that the adrenals become the major source of androgens in the circulation in postmenopausal women.[38]

Peripheral conversion of androgens in target tissues

Conversion of precursor steroids, derived from adrenal or ovarian origin, into active androgens in peripheral tissues is an important pathway of androgen metabolism.[35] Thus, dehydroepiandrosterone and $\Delta 4$-androstenedione may be converted into testosterone and 5α-DHT in target tissues.[34,36] Labrie and his colleagues suggested that in postmenopausal women almost 100% of active sex hormones are derived from peripheral conversion of the steroid precursor dehydroepiandrosterone and dehydroepiandrosterone sulfate (DHEA-S) into active estrogens and androgen hormones.[34,38] This concept suggests that active androgen hormones could be made on demand by the target tissues from precursors of ovarian or adrenal origin. This would also suggest that conversion of dehydroepiandrosterone and $\Delta 4$-androstenedione from adrenal or ovarian origin to testosterone and estradiol may take place in many tissues.

The conversion of dehydroepiandrosterone and $\Delta 4$-androstenedione into specific metabolites in the peripheral target tissues is catalyzed by tissue-specific, unidirectional 17β-hydroxysteroid dehydrogenases.[36] A family of several enzymes have been cloned and characterized to date. These enzymes may play an important role in providing target tissues with active sex steroid hormones, via a well-controlled intracellular pathway. Thus, local conversion of dehydroepiandrosterone or dehydroepiandrosterone sulfate into $\Delta 4$-androstenedione (via 3β-HSD) or $\Delta 5$-androstenediol (via 17β-hydroxysteroid dehydrogenase) leads to production of testosterone. Testosterone may be converted locally into 5α-dihydrotestosterone (via 5α-reductase) or into estradiol (via aromatase enzyme). $\Delta 4$-Androstenedione may be converted locally into estrone via the aromatase and into estradiol via 17β-hydroxysteroid dehydrogenase.[36] Since different target tissues express specific and selective isoforms of 17β-hydroxysteroid dehydrogenase, it is likely that conversion of the adrenal androgen precursors into active androgen derivatives is regulated by a given tissue's specific physiologic requirement.

Effects of plasma binding proteins on availability of bioactive androgens and estrogens

Plasma sex steroid binding proteins act as depot storage and transport sex steroid hormones from the site of synthesis to the target tissue. It is presumed that the free fraction of sex steroid hormone that enters the cells elicits the biologic response. Thus, the availability of bioactive hormone is dependent on the levels of plasma binding proteins and the affinity of these steroids for the protein. Since the free hormone also acts on the pituitary to regulate further synthesis of steroids and the free hormone is preferentially inactivated by the hepatic metabolism, plasma proteins play an important role in regulating the bioavailable steroids in the plasma. However, it remains unclear what role plasma binding proteins play in modulating the physiologic response. It is possible that changes in the levels of sex hormone-binding globulin may contribute significantly to androgen insufficiency in women. Sex hormone-binding globulin binds testosterone and estradiol with high affinity but does not bind androstenedione or estrone, neither does it bind dehydroepiandrosterone except for negligible amounts. The concentration of sex hormone-binding globulin increases in response to estrogens and increases fivefold during pregnancy. Sex hormone-binding globulin synthesis is influenced not only by estrogens but also by thyroid hormones.

Modulation of female genital arousal by sex steroid hormones

Estrogens are important in regulating the development, growth, and maintenance of many organs and tissues in women. In addition to their critical role in reproductive function, estrogens are important as metabolic regulators and modulate the development and growth of the mammary gland, genital tissue, bone, and skin. The role of estrogens in sexual behavior in rodents is well studied and well recognized.[39,40] However, their role in human sexual behavior and sexual function is not well understood. The decline in circulating estrogen levels associated with menopause is thought to be responsible for many of the sexual complaints seen in postmenopausal women.[41,42] Preclinical and clinical studies suggest that estrogens modulate genital hemodynamics and are critical for maintaining structural and functional integrity of vaginal tissues.[11,15,43,44] Estrogen deprivation may lead to decreased pelvic blood flow, resulting in diminished vaginal lubrication, clitoral fibrosis, thinning of the vaginal wall, and decreased vaginal submucosal vasculature.[42] In addition, estrogen deficiency leads to involution and atrophy of the genital organs, adversely affecting cervical, endocervical, and glandular mucin production. In contrast, estrogen replacement in postmenopausal women increases pelvic blood flow, re-establishing vaginal integrity and lubrication.[42]

Androgens modulate the function of many organs and tissues in women, including the pituitary, bone, adipose tissue, kidney, skeletal muscle, blood, ovaries, uterus, vagina, oviduct, clitoris, and mammary gland, and they regulate secondary sex characteristics.[10] Androgens are not only essential for the development of reproductive function in women and hormonal homeostasis, but also represent the immediate precursors for the biosynthesis of estrogens. Androgens affect sexual desire, bone density, adipose tissue distribution, mood, energy, and well-being. Consequently, an imbalance in androgen biosynthesis or metabolism in women may have undesirable effects on general health and on sexual and reproductive functions.[45] Although clinical studies have indicated that androgens modulate sexual arousal responses,[6,18–21,28–32,46] no investigations have addressed the mechanisms by which androgens facilitate such responses.

Recent work has suggested that progesterone is an important signaling molecule in peripheral nerves, where it promotes myelin sheath formation by activating expression of specific hormone-sensitive genes.[47] However, the role of progesterone on peripheral vaginal arousal is poorly understood. In the following section, we provide a brief discussion of the experimental data published to date on sex steroid hormones in modulating physiologic parameters of genital arousal as well as recent observations from our laboratory and others. Specifically, we will discuss the role of steroid hormones in modulating tissue structure, blood flow, lubrication and mucification, neurotransmitter biosynthesis and function, smooth muscle contractility, and expression of sex steroid receptors in genital tissue.

Effects of androgens and estrogens on vaginal tissue structure

Estrogens are crucial in maintaining tissue structure. In rat studies, it has been noted that ovariectomy caused considerable changes in vaginal epithelium and, to a limited extent, the muscularis and lamina propria. Estradiol treatment restored the

changes in tissue structure as determined by histologic assays (M. A. Pessina et al., unpublished observations). The thickness of the vaginal epithelium was dramatically reduced by ovariectomy and was restored by estrogen administration (Fig. 5.5.4). Similar observations were noted when estradiol was coadministered with testosterone or progesterone. However, administration of testosterone alone or progesterone alone did not normalize the vaginal epithelium to that observed in intact control rats.

In intact animals, the muscularis layer is comprised of circular and longitudinal smooth muscle fibers. The muscle fibers are most notable in the upper layer of the vagina. Ovariectomy reduced the volume of the muscularis layer (M. A. Pessina et al., unpublished observations), and it was noted that there was considerable deposition of connective tissue between muscle bundles. Estradiol treatment of ovariectomized animals resulted in increased cross-sectional area of the muscularis, but compared with control animals, individual muscle fibers appeared enlarged, and there was less connective tissue between the muscle bundles. Testosterone treatment resulted in restoration of the muscularis fiber bundles, but not to the same extent as that noted for estradiol. Clearly, the effects of estradiol alone or testosterone alone on the fine structure of the muscularis need to be examined in more detail. Treatment of ovariectomized rats with progesterone did not have any significant effects on the muscularis layer. When ovariectomized rats were treated with estradiol plus testosterone or estradiol plus progesterone, the muscularis fiber bundle was restored with an appearance similar to that of control intact animals (Pessina et al., unpublished observation).

Examination of blood vessel density in the lamina propria confirmed that there is a rich vascular network of blood vessels. Interestingly, we (Pessina et al., unpublished data) observed no

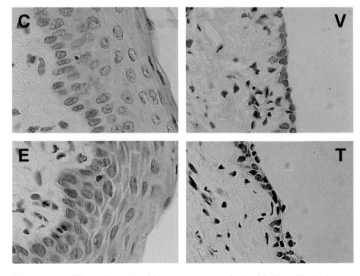

Figure 5.5.4. Effect of sex steroid hormones on vaginal epithelium. Vaginal tissue was obtained from intact control rats (C) or ovariectomized rats infused with vehicle (V) or physiologic concentrations of estradiol (E) or testosterone (T). Fixed tissue sections were stained with Gill's hematoxylin and photographed at ×200 magnification to highlight the epithelial layers.

differences in vaginal tissues from intact and ovariectomized animals at 4 weeks. It is possible that the short period after ovariectomy does not produce sufficient changes in the lamina propria and that longer periods of time may be needed to observe such changes.

Modulation of genital blood flow by estrogens and androgens

In studies with animal models, hormone depletion by ovariectomy resulted in a significant reduction in vaginal blood flow after pelvic nerve stimulation when compared to controls.[43,48,49] Estradiol or estradiol plus testosterone treatment of ovariectomized animals increased pelvic nerve-stimulated genital blood flow when compared to controls. Treatment of ovariectomized animals with testosterone alone did not result in increased genital blood flow in the rabbit,[50] but was effective in increasing blood flow in the rat (Stankovic et al., unpublished observations). These observations suggest that estrogens and androgens regulate the vascular components of genital tissues.

Evidence suggests that sex steroid hormones may modulate blood flow by regulating the activities of vasoactive intestinal polypeptide (VIP) and neural and endothelial nitric oxide synthase (NOS) in the vagina.[51-58] In ovariectomized rabbits, treatment with sex steroids had no effect on vasoactive intestinal polypeptide content. However, the binding affinity of vasoactive intestinal polypeptide to tissues of the genital tract was greatest in ovariectomized rabbits treated with estrogen and progesterone.[55] Furthermore, administration of vasoactive intestinal polypeptide to postmenopausal women receiving no hormone replacement failed to increase vaginal blood flow, whereas those receiving hormone replacement exhibited increases in blood flow that were comparable to premenopausal women.[56] In both rats and rabbits, total nitric oxide synthase in the vagina has been observed to be downregulated by estrogen and upregulated by progesterone.[51-54] When specific isoforms of nitric oxide synthase are considered, estrogen has been reported to upregulate endothelial nitric oxide synthase in the rat vagina when assessed by immunohistochemistry.[59] Using Western blot analyses, we have also corroborated these findings in ovariectomized rats replaced with estradiol (Traish et al., unpublished observations). However, other studies in rabbits have shown that ovariectomy increases both endothelial and neural nitric oxide synthase in the clitoris and vagina.[57] Using an ovariectomized rabbit model, our studies indicate that neural nitric oxide synthase protein and enzyme activity in the vagina is downregulated by estrogen but upregulated by androgens.[58]

While the consistency and significance of these data remain unresolved, there appears to be differential regulation of nitric oxide synthase isoforms by various sex steroids, and this regulation may be cell type and species specific. In addition, while the regulation of phosphodiesterase (PDE) type 5 in female genital tissues by sex steroid hormones has not been examined, the sensitivity of the nitric oxide pathway to sex steroids may provide a partial explanation for the inconsistent results of several clinical studies with sildenafil in women in which both positive and negative results were obtained.[60-64] It is possible that the endocrine status (sex steroid hormone insufficiency) of the patient may play an important role in determining whether phosphodiesterase type 5 inhibitors will be effective in facilitating the genital arousal response.

Modulation of vaginal lubrication by estrogens and androgens

Vaginal lubrication is an indicator of tissue health and increases significantly during genital sexual arousal, facilitating sexual intercourse. Production of vaginal fluid transudate and glycoproteins (such as mucin) contributes to the overall lubrication process. In estrogen-deprived animals, production of vaginal transudate, as measured by fluid weight absorbed by cotton swabs, was markedly decreased compared with controls and was restored by estrogen treatment.[50] However, treatment with testosterone alone did not improve vaginal transudate production.[48]

Vaginal mucin production, assessed by tissue sialic acid content, has been reported to be stimulated by low doses of estrogen and reduced by high doses of estrogen.[65-67] We have observed a significant decrease in vaginal sialic acid concentration in ovariectomized, vehicle-treated animals compared with the intact control group. Further decreases in vaginal sialic acid concentration were noted in the animals treated with high doses of estradiol, whereas testosterone treatment restored sialic acid to that of the vehicle treated group (Traish et al., unpublished observations). With regard to testosterone, these data are consistent with the findings of Kennedy and Armstrong, who have shown that androgens increase vaginal mucification in the rat.[68,69] Treatment of ovariectomized rats with topical dehydroepiandrosterone resulted in complete reversal of vaginal atrophy and stimulated proliferation and mucification of the vaginal epithelium.[70]

While vaginal fluid transudate production is dependent on genital blood flow and development of pressure within the vascular bed of the lamina propria, it remains unclear whether the synthesis and secretion of glycoproteins are modulated by acute hemodynamic events. Genital atrophy, in conjunction with diminished genital blood flow, secondary to estrogen deprivation, may bring about structural and functional changes in the genital tissues that negatively affect lubrication. Thus, while some effects of steroid hormones on vaginal lubrication have been noted, their exact roles and the mechanisms by which they act remain incompletely characterized.

Effects of androgens and estrogens on vaginal smooth muscle contractility

Genital sexual arousal induces changes in the tissue properties of the vaginal canal that are in part regulated by the tone of the smooth muscle within the muscularis layer. We have demonstrated that ovariectomy reduces smooth muscle relaxation to electric field stimulation and to exogenous vasoactive intestinal polypeptide in organ bath studies.[71] Estrogen treatment of ovariectomized animals reduced the relaxation response. In contrast, androgen treatment facilitated vasoactive intestinal polypeptide-induced relaxation, suggesting that androgens may modulate neurotransmitter function. These observations suggest that androgens facilitate vaginal smooth muscle relaxation while estrogens attenuate this response. However, it should be stressed that these studies were performed with supraphysiologic levels of hormones. Future studies using plasma concentrations that approximate the physiologic range are required to corroborate these findings.

Effects of sex steroid hormones on vaginal neurotransmitters and innervation

Aside from the effects of sex steroids on nitric oxide production and vasoactive intestinal polypeptide receptors (see previous section on genital blood flow), it has been known for almost 40 years that adrenergic nerves of the female genital tract are sensitive to changes in the hormonal milieu.[72,73] In animal studies, estrogen treatment increased the norepinephrine content of adrenergic nerves. In addition, administration of a mixture of estradiol and progesterone to ovariectomized pigs caused an increase in vaginal norepinephrine content.[74] In contrast to the effects of estrogen on adrenergic neurotransmitter content, a recent report indicates that the density of innervation (assessed by the panneuronal marker PGP 9.5) increased in the rat vagina subsequent to ovariectomy and was reduced by estrogen administration.[75] These changes were attributed to true axonal proliferation, rather than altered tissue volume, and consisted of adrenergic, cholinergic, and calcitonin gene-related peptide-containing nerves, which can mediate vasoconstriction and nociception. It was suggested that similar changes may explain the sensitivity and hyperalgesia of the vagina in postmenopausal women.

In our own studies using rats, we found no significant changes in vaginal nerve distribution or density after ovariectomy or with estradiol or progesterone replacement. In contrast, testosterone significantly increased the density of adrenergic nerve fibers, and this effect was attenuated when estradiol was coadministered with testosterone (Pessina et al., unpublished observations). These observations suggest differential regulation of vaginal innervation by sex steroid hormones. Clearly, additional studies undertaking detailed analyses of vaginal nerve fiber density and distribution are necessary to assess the effects of various hormones, alone or in combination, on vaginal histology and function.

Effects of steroid hormones on estrogen and androgen receptor expression in the vagina

Several studies have shown the presence of steroid receptors in the vagina by biochemical and immunochemical assays.[76–83]

While the effects of steroid hormones on the regulation of estrogen and progesterone receptors in reproductive organs have been extensively investigated,[84] there are limited studies on the regulation of expression of sex steroid hormone receptors in the vagina. Steroid receptors are regulated differentially in different target tissues by sex steroid hormones. It has recently been reported that expression of the beta isoform of the estrogen receptor (ER) is diminished or lost in the vagina of postmenopausal women, suggesting that the loss of physiologic response may be mediated by this receptor isoform.[83] Since hormone replacement therapy is used to treat various symptoms in postmenopausal women, it will be important to determine how sex steroids regulate the expression of vaginal steroid hormone receptors. Moreover, these studies will be invaluable in correlating the changes in receptor expression with changes in neurotransmitter function and modulation of the physiologic parameters of vaginal arousal (vaginal blood flow, lubrication, mucification, and smooth muscle contractility).

We have investigated the regulation of expression of estrogen and androgen receptors in the rat vagina under various endocrine manipulations.[49] Since intact animals undergo an estrous cycle, a variation in estrogen receptor concentration is expected because of the changing levels of estradiol in the serum. After 4 weeks, ovariectomized animals exhibited increased levels of estrogen receptor in the total vaginal extract, whereas estradiol replacement (at physiologic concentrations) downregulated vaginal estrogen receptor. These changes in estrogen receptor were confirmed by radioligand binding and Western blot analyses. Ovariectomized animals treated with a physiologic dose of testosterone exhibited no change in estrogen receptor levels. Immunohistochemical data (unpublished observations) supported these biochemical data. For these reasons, we believe that estrogen receptor is negatively regulated by estradiol in the vagina, but unaffected by testosterone. Interestingly, treatment of ovariectomized rats with a subphysiologic dose of estradiol did not decrease estrogen receptor levels when compared with ovariectomized rats receiving no hormone.[49] This suggests that a critical level of estrogen is required to downregulate its own receptor in the vagina. We suggest that downregulation of estrogen receptor by estrogen in the vagina is a mechanism that may be important to impart a refractory phase to attenuate the effect of estradiol surges during the estrus cycle.

In preliminary radioligand binding studies, we have observed androgen receptor levels in rat vaginal tissue to increase after ovariectomy and be down-regulated with estrogen treatment but unaltered by testosterone (unpublished observations). Similarly, progesterone receptor levels in rat vaginal tissue increased after ovariectomy and were down-regulated with estrogen treatment but unaltered by testosterone. Immunohistochemical and Western blot analyses yielded inconsistent trends with regard to androgens and with progesterone receptors, suggesting that detection limits of the antibody may be compromised by stability of the androgen receptor and progesterone receptor due to loss of a specific epitope on the protein in ovariectomized animals. The inconsistency between ligand binding studies and immunochemical assays may be attributed to partial proteolysis of the receptor in the absence of ligand. Pelletier et al. have shown that androgen receptor mRNA expression in mice is downregulated by ovariectomy and upregulated by estradiol administration.[85] These studies investigated the early temporal relationship of androgen receptor expression 3–12 h after estradiol injection.

Summary and conclusions

Sex steroid hormones are critical in maintaining the structural and functional integrity of genital tissues and therefore are critical for genital arousal (genital blood flow, lubrication, mucification, and sensation). While the effect of androgens on sexual desire is well established, the role of sex steroid hormones in genital sexual arousal is not well understood and remains a subject of debate and controversy. Better understanding of the role of sex steroid hormones in modulating female sexual function requires investigation of the biochemical, cellular, and physiologic mechanisms by which sex steroid hormones modulate sexual function in general and genital sexual arousal in particular in experimental models. Future investigative efforts will benefit from the establishment of a host of experimental models and the advancement in biochemical and molecular biologic approaches for preclinical research. With the emerging consensus on female sexual dysfunction and sex steroid insufficiency, it is anticipated that the coming years will bring new advancement toward better understanding and management of female sexual dysfunction with sex steroid hormones.

References

1. Sherwin BB. Randomized clinical trials of combined estrogen-androgen preparations: effects on sexual functioning. *Fertil Steril* 2002; 77 (Suppl 4): S49–S54.
2. Burger HG, Hailes J, Menelaus M et al. The management of persistent menopausal symptoms with oestradiol-testosterone implants: clinical, lipid and hormonal results. *Maturitas* 1984; 6: 351–8.
3. Shorr E, Papanicolaou GN, Stimmel BF. Neutralization of ovarian follicular hormone in women by simultaneous administratin of male sex hormone. *Proc Soc Exp Biol Med* 1938; 38: 759–62.
4. Loeser A. Subcutaneous implantation of female and male hormone in tablet from in women. *BMJ* 1940; 1: 479–82.
5. Greenblatt RB, Wilcox EA. Hormonal therapy of fibromyomas of the uterus. *South Surg* 1941; 10: 339–46.
6. Greenblatt RB, Mortara F, Torpin R. Sexual libido in the female. *Am J Obstet Gynecol* 1942; 44: 658–63.
7. Salmon U. Rationale for androgen therapy in gynecology. *J Clin Endocrinol* 1941; 1: 162–79.
8. Salmon U, Geist SH. Effects of androgens upon libido in women. *J Clin Endocrinol* 1943; 3: 235–8.

9. Carter AC, Cohen EJ, Shorr E. The use of androgens in women. *Vitam Horm* 1947; 5: 317–91.
10. Dorfman RI, Shipley RA. *Androgens: Biochemistry, Physiology and Clinical Significance.* New York: Wiley, 1956: 152–217.
11. Bachmann GA, Ebert GA, Burd ID. Vulvovaginal complaints. In Lobo RA, ed. *Treatment of the Postmenopausal Woman: Basic and Clinical Aspects.* Philadelphia: Lippincott Williams & Wilkins 1999: 195–201.
12. Sarrel PM. Sexuality in the middle years. *Obstet Gynecol Clin North Am* 1987; 14: 49–62.
13. Sarrel PM. Ovarian hormones and vaginal blood flow: using laser Doppler velocimetry to measure effects in a clinical trial of postmenopausal women. *Int J Impot Res* 1998; 10 (Suppl 2): S91–3.
14. Sarrel PM. Effects of hormone replacement therapy on sexual psychophysiology and behavior in postmenopause. *J Womens Health Gend Based Med* 2000; 9 (Suppl 1): S25–S32.
15. Sarrel PM, Wiita B. Vasodilator effects of estrogen are not diminished by androgen in postmenopausal women. *Fertil Steril* 1997; 68: 1125–7.
16. Semmens JP, Wagner G. Estrogen deprivation and vaginal function in postmenopausal women. *JAMA* 1982; 248: 445–8.
17. Utian WH, Shoupe D, Bachmann G et al. Relief of vasomotor symptoms and vaginal atrophy with lower doses of conjugated equine estrogens and medroxyprogesterone acetate. *Fertil Steril* 2001; 75: 1065–79.
18. Sherwin BB, Gelfand MM. The role of androgen in the maintenance of sexual functioning in oophorectomized women. *Psychosom Med* 1987; 49: 397–409.
19. Sherwin BB, Gelfand MM, Brender W. Androgen enhances sexual motivation in females: a prospective, crossover study of sex steroid administration in the surgical menopause. *Psychosom Med* 1985; 47: 339–51.
20. Davis SR, McCloud P, Strauss BJ et al. Testosterone enhances estradiol's effects on postmenopausal bone density and sexuality. *Maturitas* 1995; 21: 227–36.
21. Davis SR, Burger HG. The rationale for physiological testosterone replacement in women. *Baillieres Clin Endocrinol Metab* 1998; 12: 391–405.
22. Bachmann G, Bancroft J, Braunstein G et al. Female androgen insufficiency: the Princeton consensus statement on definition, classification, and assessment. *Fertil Steril* 2002; 77: 660–5.
23. Schreiner-Engel P, Schiavi RC, Smith H et al. Sexual arousability and the menstrual cycle. *Psychosom Med* 1981; 43: 199–214.
24. Schreiner-Engel P, Schiavi RC, White D et al. Low sexual desire in women: the role of reproductive hormones. *Horm Behav* 1989; 23: 221–34.
25. Hackbert L, Heiman JR. Acute dehydroepiandrosterone (DHEA) effects on sexual arousal in postmenopausal women. *J Womens Health Gend Based Med* 2002; 11: 155–62.
26. Tuiten A, van Honk J, Verbaten R et al. Can sublingual testosterone increase subjective and physiological measures of laboratory-induced sexual arousal? *Arch Gen Psychiatry* 2002; 59: 465–6.
27. Tuiten A, Van Honk J, Koppeschaar H et al. Time course of effects of testosterone administration on sexual arousal in women. *Arch Gen Psychiatry* 2000; 57: 149–53.

28. Shifren JL, Braunstein GD, Simon JA et al. Transdermal testosterone treatment in women with impaired sexual function after oophorectomy. *N Engl J Med* 2000; 343: 682–8.

29. Shifren JL. The role of androgens in female sexual dysfunction. *Mayo Clin Proc* 2004; 79 (Suppl): S19–S24.

30. Arlt W, Callies F, van Vlijmen JC et al. Dehydroepiandrosterone replacement in women with adrenal insufficiency. *New Engl J Med* 1999; 341: 1013–20.

31. Arlt W, Callies F, Allolio B. DHEA replacement in women with adrenal insufficiency – pharmacokinetics, bioconversion and clinical effects on well-being, sexuality and cognition. *Endocr Res* 2000; 26: 505–11.

32. Munarriz R, Talakoub I., Flaherty E et al. Androgen replacement therapy with dehydroepiandrosterone for androgen insufficiency and female sexual dysfunction: androgen and questionnaire results. *J Sex Marital Ther* 2002; 28 (Suppl 1): 165–73.

33. Abraham GE. Ovarian and adrenal contribution to peripheral androgens during the menstrual cycle. *J Clin Endocrinol Metab* 1974; 39: 340–6.

34. Labrie F, Diamond P, Cusan L et al. Effect of 12-month dehydroepiandrosterone replacement therapy on bone, vagina, and endometrium in postmenopausal women *J Clin Endocrinol Metab* 1997; 82: 3498–3505.

35. Labrie F, Luu-The V, Lin S et al. Role of 17beta-hydroxysteroid dehydrogenases in sex steroid formation in peripheral intracrine tissues. *Trends Endocrinol Metab* 2000; 11: 421–7.

36. Luu-The V, Dufort I, Pelletier G et al. Type 5 17beta-hydroxysteroid dehydrogenase: its role in the formation of androgens in women. *Mol Cell Endocrinol* 2001; 171: 77–82.

37. Landgren BM, Collins A, Csemiczky G et al. Menopause transition: annual changes in serum hormonal patterns over the menstrual cycle in women during a nine-year period prior to menopause. *J Clin Endocrinol Metab* 2004; 89: 2763–9.

38. Couzinet B, Meduri G, Lecce MG et al. The postmenopausal ovary is not a major androgen-producing gland. *J Clin Endocrinol Metab* 2001; 86: 5060–6.

39. Mani S. Emerging concepts in the regulation of female sexual behavior. *Scand J Psychol* 2003; 44: 231–9.

40. Erskine MS, Lehmann ML, Cameron NM et al. Co-regulation of female sexual behavior and pregnancy induction: an exploratory synthesis. *Behav Brain Res* 2004; 153: 295–315.

41. Notelovitz M. Management of the changing vagina. *J Clin Pract Sex* 1990; Special Issue: 16–17.

42. Bachmann GA. The impact of vaginal health on sexual function. *J Clin Pract Sex* (Special Issue) 1990; 18–21.

43. Park K, Ahn K, Lee S et al. Decreased circulating levels of estrogen alter vaginal and clitoral blood flow and structure in the rabbit. *Int J Impot Res* 2001; 13: 116–24.

44. Park K, Ryu SB, Park YI et al. Diabetes mellitus induces vaginal tissue fibrosis by TGF-beta 1 expression in the rat model. *J Sex Marital Ther* 2001; 27: 577–87.

45. Breuer H. Androgen production in the woman. In Hammerstein J, Lachnit-Fixson U, Neumann F, Plewig G, eds. *Androgenization in Women.* Princeton: *Excerpta Medica* 1980: 21–39.

46. Sherwin BB. The impact of different doses of estrogen and progestin on mood and sexual behavior in postmenopausal women. *J Clin Endocrinol Metab* 1991; 72: 336–43.

47. Schumacher M, Guennoun R, Mercier G et al. Progesterone synthesis and myelin formation in peripheral nerves. *Brain Res Brain Res Rev* 2001; 37: 343–59.

48. Min K, Munarriz R, Kim NN et al. Effects of ovariectomy and estrogen and androgen treatment on sildenafil-mediated changes in female genital blood flow and vaginal lubrication in the animal model. *Am J Obstet Gynecol* 2002; 187: 1370–6.

49. Kim SW, Kim NN, Jeong Seong-Joo et al. Modulation of rat vaginal blood flow and estrogen receptors by estradiol. *J Urol* 2004; 172: 1538–43.

50. Min K, Munarriz R, Kim NN et al. Effects of ovariectomy and estrogen replacement on basal and pelvic nerve stimulated vaginal lubrication in an animal model. *J Sex Marital Ther* 2003; 29 (Suppl 1): 77–84.

51. Batra S, Al-Hijji J. Characterization of nitric oxide synthase activity in rabbit uterus and vagina: downregulation by estrogen. *Life Sci* 1998; 62: 2093–3010.

52. Al-Hijji J, Batra S. Down regulation by estrogen of nitric oxide synthase activity in the female rabbit lower urinary tract. *Urology* 1999; 53: 637–41.

53. Al-Hijji J, Larsson B, Batra S. Nitric oxide synthase in the rabbit uterus and vagina: hormonal regulation and functional significance. *Biol Reprod* 2000; 62: 1387–92.

54. Al-Hijji J, Larsson I, Batra S. Effect of ovarian steroids on nitric oxide synthase in the rat uterus, cervix and vagina. *Life Sci* 2001; 69: 1133–42.

55. Ottesen B, Pedersen B, Nielsen J et al. Vasoactive intestinal polypeptide (VIP) provokes vaginal lubrication in normal women. *Peptides* 1987; 8: 797–800.

56. Palle C, Bredkjaer HE, Ottesen B et al. Vasoactive intestinal polypeptide and human vaginal blood flow: comparison between transvaginal and intravenous administration. *J Clin Exp Pharm Physiol* 1990; 17: 61–8.

57. Yoon HN, Chung WS, Park YY et al. Effects of estrogen on nitric oxide synthase and histological composition in the rabbit clitoris and vagina. *Int J Impot Res* 2001; 13: 205–11.

58. Traish AM, Kim NN, Huang YH et al. Sex steroid hormones differentially regulate nitric oxide synthase and arginase activities in the proximal and distal rabbit vagina. *Int J Impot Res* 2003; 15: 397–404.

59. Berman JR, McCarthy MM, Kyprianou N. Effect of estrogen withdrawal on nitric oxide synthase expression and apoptosis in the rat vagina. *Urology* 1998; 51: 650–6.

60. Basson R, McInnes R, Smith MD et al. Efficacy and safety of sildenafil citrate in women with sexual dysfunction associated with female sexual arousal disorder. *J Womens Health Gend Based Med* 2002; 11: 367–77.

61. Caruso S, Intelisano G, Farina M et al. The function of sildenafil on female sexual pathways: a double-blind, cross-over, placebo-controlled study. *Eur J Obstet Gynecol Reprod Biol* 2003; 110: 201–6.

62. Caruso S, Intelisano G, Lupo L et al. Premenopausal women affected by sexual arousal disorder treated with sildenafil: a double-

blind, cross-over, placebo-controlled study. *Br J Obstet Gynaecol* 2001; 108: 623–8.

63. Laan E, van Lunsen RH, Everaerd W et al. The enhancement of vaginal vasocongestion by sildenafil in healthy premenopausal women. *J Womens Health Gend Based Med* 2002; 11: 357–65.

64. Berman JR, Berman LA, Toler SM et al. Sildenafil Study Group. Safety and efficacy of sildenafil citrate for the treatment of female sexual arousal disorder: a double-blind, placebo controlled study. *J Urol* 2003; 170: 2333–8.

65. Carlborg L. Comparative action of various oestrogenic compounds on mouse vaginal sialic acids. II. *Acta Endocrinol (Copenh)* 1969; 62: 663–70.

66. Galletti F, Gardi R. Effect of ovarian hormones and synthetic progestins on vaginal sialic acid in the rat. *J Endocrinol* 1973; 57: 193–8.

67. Nishino Y, Neumann F. The sialic acid content in mouse female reproductive organs as a quantitative parameter for testing the estrogenic and antiestrogenic effect, antiestrogenic depot effect, and dissociated effect of estrogens on the uterus and vagina. *Acta Endocrinol Suppl (Copenh)* 1974; 187: 3–62.

68. Kennedy TG. Vaginal mucification in the ovariectomized rat in response to 5alpha-pregnane-3,20-dione, testosterone and 5alpha-androstan-17beta-ol-3-one: test for progestogenic activity. *J Endocrinol* 1974; 61: 293–300.

69. Kennedy TG, Armstrong DT. Induction of vaginal mucification in rats with testosterone and 17beta-hydroxy-5alpha-androstan-3-one. *Steroids* 1976; 27: 423–30.

70. Sourla A, Flamand M, Belanger A et al. Effect of dehydroepiandrosterone on vaginal and uterine histomorphology in the rat. *J Steroid Biochem Mol Biol* 1998; 66: 137–49.

71. Kim NN, Min K, Pessina MA et al. Effects of ovariectomy and steroid hormones on vaginal smooth msucle contractility. *Int J Impot Res* 2004; 16: 43–50.

72. Rosengren E, Sjoberg NO. Changes in the amount of adrenergic transmitter in the female genital tract of rabbit during pregnancy. *Acta Physiol Scand* 1968; 72: 412–24.

73. Sjoberg NO. Increase in transmitter content of adrenergic nerves in the reproductive tract of female rabbits after oestrogen treatment. *Acta Endocrinol (Copenh)* 1968; 57: 405–13.

74. Kaleczyc J. Effect of estradiol and progesterone on noradrenaline content in nerves of the oviduct, uterus and vagina in ovariectomized pigs. *Folia Histochem Cytobiol* 1994; 32: 119–26.

75. Ting AY, Blacklock AD, Smith PG. Estrogen regulates vaginal sensory and autonomic nerve density in the rat. *Biol Reprod* 2004; 71: 1397–1404.

76. MacLean AB, Nicol LA, Hodgins MB. Immunohistochemical localization of estrogen receptors in the vulva and vagina. *J Reprod Med* 1990; 35: 1015–16.

77. Hodgins MB, Spike RC, Mackie RM et al. An immunohistochemical study of androgen, oestrogen and progesterone receptors in the vulva and vagina. *Br J Obstet Gynaecol* 1998; 105: 216–22.

78. Chen GD, Oliver RH, Leung BS et al. Estrogen receptor alpha and beta expression in the vaginal walls and uterosacral ligaments of premenopausal and postmenopausal women. *Fertil Steril* 1999; 71: 1099–1102.

79. Blakeman PJ, Hilton P, Bulmer JN. Oestrogen and progesterone receptor expression in the female lower urinary tract, with reference to oestrogen status. *Br J Urol Int* 2000; 86: 32–38.

80. Mowa CN, Iwanaga T. Differential distribution of oestrogen receptor-alpha and -beta mRNAs in the female reproductive organ of rats as revealed by *in situ* hybridization. *J Endocrinol* 2000; 165:59–66.

81. Schwartz PE. The oestrogen receptor (ER) in vulva, vagina and ovary. *Eur J Cancer* 2000; 36 (Suppl 4):S31–S32.

82. Wang H, Eriksson H, Sahlin L. Estrogen receptors alpha and beta in the female reproductive tract of the rat during the estrous cycle. *Biol Reprod* 2000; 63:1331–1340.

83. Gebhart JB, Rickard DJ, Barrett TJ et al. Expression of estrogen receptor isoforms alpha and beta messenger RNA in vaginal tissue of premenopausal and postmenopausal women. *Am J Obstet Gynecol* 2001; 185:1325–1330.

84. Clark JH, Peck EJ Jr. Female sex steroids: receptors and function. *Monogr Endocrinol* 1979; 14:I–XII, 1–245.

85. Pelletier G, Luu-The V, Li S et al. Localization and estrogenic regulation of androgen receptor mRNA expression in the mouse uterus and vagina. *J Endocrinol* 2004; 180:77–85.

5.6 Animal models in the investigation of female sexual function and dysfunction

Kwangsung Park

Introduction

Female sexuality has many components, including physiologic, psychologic, social, and emotional factors. Female sexual dysfunction is an important health issue that affects the quality of life of many women. There have been, however, a limited number of investigations studying the physiology of female sexual function and dysfunction, primarily because of a lack of reliable experimental models and tools. An historical difficulty was the notion that female sexual dysfunction consists primarily of problems related to orgasm, and thus the only appropriate model for study was the human.[1] Recently, several experimental models have been introduced to assess genital hemodynamics,[2,3] genital smooth muscle contractility,[4,5] vaginal lubrication,[6,7] and the pharmacology of female genital sexual response.[8,9]

Female sexual dysfunction is defined as a disorder of sexual desire, arousal, orgasm, and/or sexual pain, and it is estimated to affect 20–50% of women.[10–12] The prevalence of female sexual dysfunction has been shown to increase with age and be associated with the presence of vascular risk factors (e.g. diabetes mellitus, atherosclerosis) and the development of menopause.[13] In addition, traumatic injury to the iliohypogastric/pudendal arterial bed from pelvic fractures or blunt trauma can result in sexual dysfunction.[14–16] Investigation of female sexual dysfunction requires establishment of appropriate animal models to elucidate the pathophysiologic mechanisms. Recently, several animal models have been introduced to evaluate sexual dysfunction associated with menopause, atherosclerosis, and diabetes mellitus. This chapter will review animal models that help to elucidate female sexual function and dysfunction.

Models for female sexual arousal response

In vivo studies

Female sexual arousal is characterized by genital swelling and vaginal lubrication responses resulting from increased clitoral and vaginal blood flow. Animal models are valuable in investigating vaginal and clitoral hemodynamics, as they are able to mimic genital arousal in response to sexual stimulation. Recently, several objective methods were introduced that use experimental models to measure clitoral and vaginal blood flow. A rabbit model was first introduced by Park et al.[2] to investigate the physiology and pathophysiology of female sexual arousal. In the New Zealand white female rabbit, vaginal wall blood flow and clitoral intracavernosal blood flow can be measured by laser Doppler flow probes that are placed in the vaginal wall and the clitoral corporal bodies, respectively (Fig. 5.6.1).[2] The laser Doppler flowmeter (Transonic Systems, Ithaca, NY, USA) is calibrated against an internal standard to yield flow in units of ml/min per 100 g tissue. The branches of the pelvic nerve that serve the vagina and clitoris can be identified under the perivesical fat on the posterolateral aspect of the vagina as the nerve emerges from its associations with the rectum, bladder, and uterus.[2] Pelvic nerve stimulation causes an increase in vaginal blood flow, vaginal wall pressure, and vaginal length, as well as clitoral blood flow and clitoral intracavernosal pressure. One of the drawbacks of laser Doppler flowmetry is its sensitivity to motion artifacts. As an alternative approach, Min et al.[17]

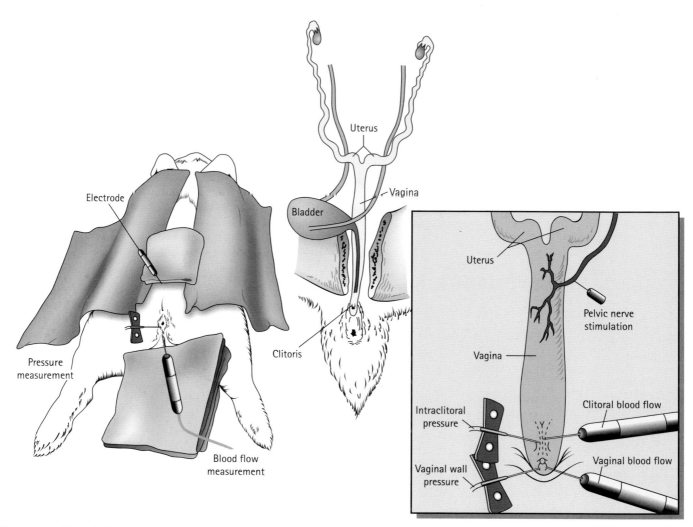

Figure 5.6.1. Schematic diagram showing female rabbit genitalia and experimental model. The symphysis pubis is dissected to expose the vaginal tube and uterus. Experimental setup for the measurement of vaginal and clitoral blood flow and pressure is shown within the box. Reproduced from Park et al.[2] with permission.

introduced laser oximetry, which can measure genital blood flow in the rabbit. As laser oximetry measures tissue hemoglobin content rather than rate of blood flow, it may be useful for measuring tissue engorgement during sexual arousal.

Although the rabbit is a good model for hemodynamic studies of the vagina and clitoris, the limitation of this model is that rabbits, being induced ovulators, have endocrine physiology that is very different from human.[18] The rabbit vagina is also anatomically different from the human. It has two distinct anatomic regions, a proximal region that represents 2/3 of the length of the vagina with a single layer of columnar epithelium, and a distal region that serves coital functions and is characterized by squamous epithelium.[19]

The female rat is another good model for the study of female sexual function and dysfunction. The female rat has a regular estrous cycle similar to women; in addition, the human and rat vaginas have a similar histologic structure. Vachon et al.[20] first developed a rat model for the study of physiology, pharmacology, and sexual dysfunction relating to blood flow to

clitoral and vaginal tissue. Recently, Kim et al.[3] introduced an improved rat model to investigate female vaginal arousal. Kim et al. recommended a longer duration of pelvic nerve stimulation (30 s instead of 5 s). They also suggested that an alternative to determining peak vaginal blood flow magnitudes might be measurement of the area under the curve of flowmetry recordings. The area under the curve measures the perfusion intergrated over time, to get a more accurate reflection of blood flow. In contrast to the rabbit, the pelvic nerve in female rats is buried in fragile fatty tissue overlying the lateral vaginal wall (Fig. 5.6.2). Therefore, careful dissection is recommended to avoid inadvertent injury to the nerve.[3] Giuliano et al.[21] also described a rat model of sexual arousal in which they assessed vaginal vascular events with oximetry and temperature measurements in addition to laser Doppler flowmetry. In this study, pelvic nerve stimulation induced reproducible increases in various vaginal parameters. However, concomitant electrical stimulation of the paravertebral sympathetic chain inhibited vaginal response induced by pelvic nerve stimulation.

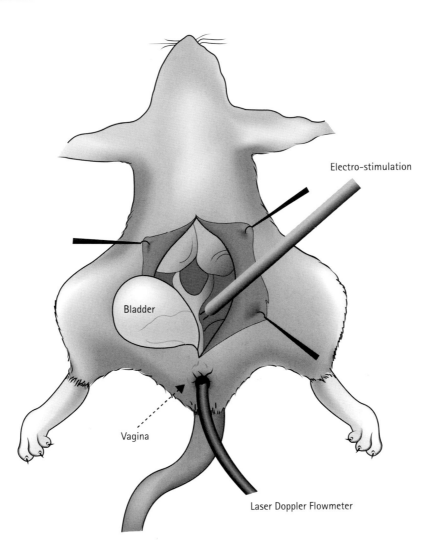

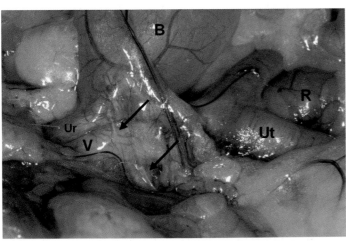

Figure 5.6.2. Female rat model. Upper: diagrammatic representation measuring vaginal blood flow with laser Doppler flowmeter during pelvic nerve stimulation. Lower: magnified figure showing pelvic anatomy of female rat. The pelvic nerve branches are identified under the fragile fatty tissue overlying the lateral vaginal wall (arrows). V, vagina; Ur, urethra; B, bladder; R, rectum; Ut, uterus.

Vaginal lubrication is one of the indicators of genital arousal and tissue integrity. In the basal state, the vaginal epithelium reabsorbs sodium from the submucosal capillary plasma transudate. During arousal, a dramatic increase in capillary inflow in the submucosa overwhelms sodium reabsorption, leading to 3–5 ml of vaginal transudate, and enhancing lubrication essential for pleasurable coitus.[6] Vaginal lubrication can be measured by use of a preweighed, cotton-tipped swab in rabbits.[7] After insertion of the cotton swab into the distal vaginal canal, the pelvic nerve is stimulated for 1 min, and the swab is left in place for an additional 5 min. Vaginal lubrication is assumed to be proportional to the weight of the fluid absorbed by the cotton swab.

Beharry et al.[22] introduced a rat model of female sexual arousal response for centrally initiated genital vasocongestive engorgement, using a video monitoring system. Low doses of apomorphine were administered to the conscious female rat, resulting in reproducibly induced behavioral and genital responses. They also demonstrated that the apomorphine-induced genital arousal responses were hormonally regulated in this model.

Animal models of sexual behavior have also been used to study human sexual behavior and its neurobiologic bases.[23] Tong et al.[24] used infrared-light-illuminated video recording to study behavioral aspects of the sexual activities of rats. This dark-cycle video recording method has been successfully applied to study sexual arousal and copulation-ejaculatory responses in rat. When a male rat encounters a female in estrous, it explores her genital area and initiates copulatory acts. During mounting, the female rat displays a concave dorsiflexion, extending her hind legs and moving the tail to the side (lordosis posture).[23–24] Recently, Agmo and Ellingsen[23] reviewed the relevance of non-human animal studies to the understanding of human sexuality. They commented that two striking similarities between humans and other mammals are the hormone dependency of sexual motivation and the bisexual potential of sexual behaviors. The specific gonadal hormone involved in sexual motivation varies among species, even though the general principles remain constant.[23,25] There have been limited studies on sexual climax in female nonhuman primates. Behavioral and physiologic evidence of sexual climax was observed in the female stump-tailed macaque.[26]

Organ bath studies

Functional studies of isolated tissues in organ baths are necessary to understand various local regulatory mechanisms that modulate tone in the clitoral erectile tissue and vaginal smooth muscle. Female New Zealand white rabbits are usually chosen for these studies.[7,27] Cellek and Moncada[4] demonstrated that nitrergic neurotransmission mediates the nonadrenergic, non-cholinergic relaxation responses in the clitoral corpus cavernosum of the rabbit. Pretreatment of clitoral corpus cavernosum strips with sildenafil (100 nM) enhanced the electrical field stimulation-induced relaxation both in magnitude and duration.[28] Therefore, the nitric oxide (NO) cyclic guanosine monophosphate pathway seems critical for smooth muscle relaxation in the clitoris. However, nonnitrergic, nonadrenergic, noncholinergic relaxation responses seem to be involved in the rabbit vaginal wall.[29] Ziessen et al.[29] showed that non-adrenergic, noncholinergic relaxation was partly mediated by nitric oxide in the rabbit vagina, and the remaining part may be mediated by a non-nitrergic component that was not associated with any known neuropeptides or purines.

In contrast, the rat vagina shows a different relaxation response from rabbit. Giraldi et al.[30] reported that electrical field

stimulation elicits nonadrenergic, noncholinergic relaxation of the vaginal smooth muscle tissue, and these relaxations were mediated by the nitrergic system, since they were blocked by inhibitors of the nitric oxide–cyclic guanosine monophosphate pathway. This finding is supported by the large number of nerves that contain nitric oxide synthase in the vaginal sphincter (the distal part of the vagina).[30] Therefore, the role of the nitric oxide-cyclic guanosine monophosphate pathway in the vagina needs further investigation. Vasoactive intestinal peptide also induces vaginal smooth muscle relaxation, but its functional role remains to be determined.[31,32]

The smooth muscle contractility of the clitoris and vagina is regulated by the balance between vasoconstrictors and smooth muscle relaxants. Exogenously added norepinephrine caused a dose-dependent contraction of the vaginal and clitoral tissues, and this contraction was attenuated by alpha-1 and alpha-2 adrenergic receptor antagonists.[27] This finding implies that adrenergic nerves mediate the contraction of clitoral and vaginal smooth muscle through alpha-adrenergic receptors. In addition, the Rho-kinase signaling pathway seems to be involved in the regulation of angiotensin II-induced contraction in the clitoral cavernosal smooth muscle. Park et al.[33] suggested that the RhoA/Rho-kinase pathway acts in angiotensin II-induced contraction independently of the nitric oxide pathway in rabbit clitoral cavernosal smooth muscle. The role of other vasoconstrictors (e.g., endothelin or eicosanoids) in regulating the smooth muscle tone of the clitoris and vagina remains to be determined.

Animal models of female sexual dysfunction

Surgical menopausal models

Estrogen is thought to have a major role in the maintenance of the functional integrity of the female genitalia.[34] The decline in the circulating level of estrogen is a major physiologic change during natural menopause. It has been reported that female sexual arousal function correlates negatively with menopausal symptoms such as hot flashes.[35]

Park et al.[36] investigated the effects of estrogen deprivation and replacement on genital hemodynamics by laser Doppler flowmetry. They showed that the decline in circulating levels of estrogen adversely affected the hemodynamic mechanism of vaginal and clitoral engorgement in the rabbit. Decreased levels of circulating estrogen also produced marked changes in the structure of the vaginal and clitoral tissues, leading to thinning of the vaginal epithelial layers, decreased vaginal submucosal vasculature, and diffuse clitoral cavernosal fibrosis.

Using laser oximetry, Min et al.[7] investigated the effects of ovariectomy and androgen and estrogen treatment on genital blood flow and vaginal lubrication. In contrast to the observations made by Park et al.,[36] ovariectomy did not significantly affect genital blood flow in the rabbit model. The difference between these two studies may be the length of time after ovariectomy. Park et al.[36] performed data collection 6 weeks after ovariectomy, whereas Min et al.[7] collected data after 2 weeks. It is possible that the longer period of estrogen deprivation may have produced changes in the tissue structure of the clitoris and vagina. Because the female rabbit remains in continuous diestrus until mounted, serum estrogen levels are normally low (32–39 pg/ml), and ovariectomy produces only a small decrease (22–25 pg/ml).[7,36]

Estradiol or estradiol plus testosterone treatment of ovariectomized rabbits increased genital blood flow after pelvic nerve stimulation compared with controls.[7,36] However, treatment of ovariectomized rabbits with testosterone alone did not result in increased genital blood flow. These results suggest that estrogens, but not androgens, modulate the vascular component of the female genital organs. Min et al.[37] also showed that vaginal lubrication was reduced in ovariectomized animals, but returned to normal after estrogen treatment.

Estrogen plays an important role in regulating vaginal and clitoral nitric oxide synthase expression. Studies with the rat model have shown that the decrease in circulating levels of estrogen induced by ovariectomy downregulates nitric oxide synthase expression and increases apoptosis in nerves, smooth muscle, vascular endothelium, and epithelium of the rat vagina.[38] Using an imaging analyzer, Dundar et al.[39] reported the effect of estrogen-replacement therapy on clitoral-cavernosal tissue in oophorectomized rats. Although there was a tendency for the untreated group to have a higher collagen fiber content, no statistically significant difference was found among groups.

There have been discrepancies in data reported for nitric oxide synthase regulation by estrogen in the vagina, and these discrepancies may be due to differences either in species or in methods for assessment of nitric oxide synthase expression and activity.[40] Vaginal nitric oxide synthase activity was significantly reduced by estrogen treatment in castrated rabbit.[41,42] However, vaginal endothelial nitric oxide synthase and neural nitric oxide synthase expression increased significantly after estrogen replacement in castrated rat.[38]

Diabetic models

Diabetes mellitus causes female sexual dysfunction.[43,44] Diabetic women may experience less sexual desire, less sexual arousal, inadequate lubrication, difficulty achieving orgasm, and dyspareunia.[43] To investigate the pathophysiologic mechanism of diabetes mellitus in female sexual dysfunction, Park et al.[45] introduced a streptozotocin-induced diabetic rat model. They used a single high dose of intravenous streptozotocin (50 mg/kg) and found that 3 or 4 weeks was enough to develop a diabetic model.[45] Giraldi et al.[46] made a diabetic rat model by an intraperitoneal injection of streptozotocin (45 mg/kg), and then leaving the animals untreated for 8 weeks. The indicators that confirm the development of diabetes are weight loss, glucosuria,

and increase in blood glucose levels. In diabetic animals, vaginal tissue revealed reduced epithelial layers and decreased vaginal submucosal vasculature, and also showed a dense and distorted arrangement of the collagen connective tissue compared with control animals (Fig. 5.6.3). In functional studies, diabetes interfered with adrenergic-, cholinergic-, and nonadrenergic, noncholinergic-neurotransmitter mechanisms in the smooth muscle of the rat vagina.[46] In an insulin-controlled diabetic rat model, Park et al.[47] reported that hyperglycemia causes alteration of vaginal blood flow and structure.

A diabetic rabbit model was established by an intravenous injection of alloxan hydrochloride (100 mg/kg).[48] However, diabetes developed in only 25% of cases, as determined by serum glucose greater than 200 mg/dl after 12 weeks. In this study, diabetes mellitus produced significant adverse effects on the hemodynamic mechanism of clitoral engorgement and led to diffuse clitoral cavernous fibrosis.

Atherosclerotic models

The prevalence of female sexual arousal disorders increases with age and vascular risk factors.[13] A female New Zealand White rabbit model was developed to examine hemodynamic function in the presence of pelvic atherosclerotic vascular disease of the ilio–hypogastric–pudendal arterial bed.[2] This model was induced by repeated aortofemoral balloon de-endothelialization followed by feeding the rabbits a 0.5% cholesterol diet for 16 weeks. In this study, atherosclerosis inhibited vaginal and clitoral engorgement and elongation, and led to diffuse vaginal wall and clitoral cavernosal smooth muscle fibrosis.

Model for neurogenic female sexual dysfunction

Central nervous system disorders have a significant impact on female sexuality and sexual response.[49] There have been a few animal models for the study of the central nervous system, including spinal cord lesion. McKenna et al.[50] introduced a model for experimental study of the neural mechanisms of sexual function. They measured the urethrogenital reflex, which is produced by a spinal pattern generator and is under tonic descending inhibition from the brainstem. This model has been used to study sexually relevant genital responses in females. The role of the hypothalamus has been extensively studied for sexual behavior with particular attention to lordosis in the female rat. The medial preoptic area has been shown to be involved in the expression of lordosis. Furthermore, the medial preoptic area may have an important role in the control of the female sexual response. Giuliano et al.[21,51] showed that electrical stimulation of the medial preoptic area induced a significant increase in vaginal blood flow and a corresponding decrease in vaginal vascular resistance in female rats, suggesting that sexual genital arousal may be triggered by medial preoptic area activation.

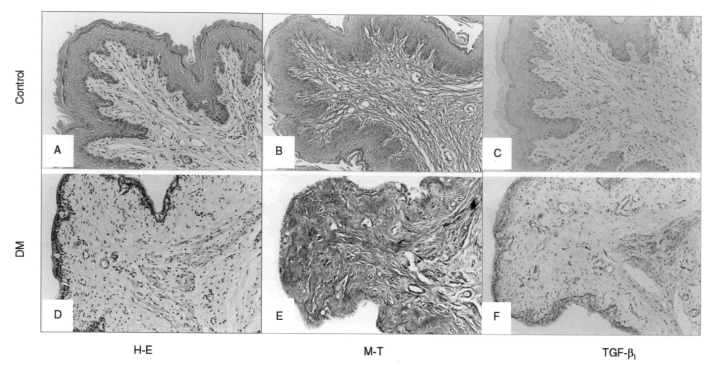

Figure 5.6.3. Histology of vaginal tissue in control (A, B, C) and diabetic rat (D, E, F). The vaginal wall in the control rat showed a typical cornified mucosa with seven to eight epithelial layers and a normal structure of smooth muscle, connective tissue, and vasculature. In the diabetic rat, the vaginal epithelium was reduced and the submucosal vasculatures were decreased (D). The size and number of collagen bundles increased, and collagen fibers showed an irregular, distorted arrangement (E). The immunoreactivity of transforming growth factor β_1 (TGF-β_1) was prominent in the collagen connective tissue, fibroblast, and smooth muscle fibers (F). H-E: H&E stain; M-T: Masson's trichrome stain; TGF-β_1: immunohistochemical stain for TGF-β_1. Reduced from ×180. Reproduced from Park et al.[45] with permission.

Future research directions

Animal model studies have provided a better understanding of the physiology and pharmacology of both central and peripheral (vaginal and clitoral) female sexual arousal by allowing assessments of genital hemodynamics, vaginal lubrication, and regulation of genital smooth muscle contractility. However, research on women's sexual health is still in its early phases compared with that of men's sexual health. The role of neurotransmitters and their signaling mechanisms in the clitoris and vagina needs further investigation. Although the nitric oxide-cyclic guanosine monophosphate system seems to have a key role in the regulation of clitoral cavernosal smooth muscle relaxation, there is still a lack of knowledge about the neurotransmitters regulating vaginal smooth muscle contractility. Steroid sex hormones significantly influence female sexual function and dysfunction. Although the effect of androgens on sexual desire is widely acknowledged, the role of steroid sex hormones on genital sexual arousal is not well understood. Animal models such as rat and rabbit have some limitations in the investigation of sexual desire and orgasmic function. Nevertheless, animal models of sexual behavior have proven to be useful for studying human sexual behavior and its neurobiologic bases. Investigation of female sexual dysfunction requires establishment of appropriate animal

models to elucidate the pathophysiologic mechanisms. Recently, several animal models have been introduced to evaluate the pathologic mechanisms of menopause, atherosclerosis, and diabetes mellitus. However, further efforts are needed to develop a model for hypercholesterolemia, smoking, and other cardiovascular risk factors. In addition, future research is needed to develop an animal model to determine the impact of various central nervous system disorders and neuroanatomic sites of injury on sexual function.

References

1. Levin R. The mechanisms of human female sexual arousal. *Annu Rev Sex Res* 1992; 3: 1–48.
2. Park K, Goldstein I, Andry C et al. Vasculogenic female sexual dysfunction: the hemodynamic basis for vaginal engorgement insufficiency and clitoral erectile insufficiency. *Int J Impot Res* 1997; 9: 27–37.
3. Kim SW, Jeong SJ, Munarriz R et al. An *in vivo* rat model to investigate female vaginal arousal response. *J Urol* 2004; 171: 1357–61.
4. Cellek S, Moncada S. Nitrergic neurotransmission mediates the non-adrenergic non-cholinergic responses in the clitoral corpus cavernosum of the rabbit. *Br J Pharmacol* 1998; 125: 1627–9.

5. Munarriz R, Kim SW, Kim NN et al. A review of the physiology and pharmacology of peripheral (vaginal and clitoral) female genital arousal in the animal model. *J Urol* 2003; 170(2 Pt 2): S40–4; discussion S4–5.

6. Munarriz R, Kim NN, Goldstein I et al. Biology of female sexual function. *Urol Clin North Am* 2002; 29: 685–93.

7. Min K, Munarriz R, Kim NN et al. Effects of ovariectomy and estrogen and androgen treatment on sildenafil-mediated changes in female genital blood flow and vaginal lubrication in the animal model. *Am J Obstet Gynecol* 2002; 187: 1370–6.

8. Tarcan T, Siroky MB, Park K et al. Systemic administration of apomorphine improves the hemodynamic mechanism of clitoral and vaginal engorgement in the rabbit. *Int J Impot Res* 2000; 12: 235–40.

9. Min K, Kim NN, McAuley I et al. Sildenafil augments pelvic nerve-mediated female genital sexual arousal in the anesthetized rabbit. *Int J Impot Res* 2000; 12 (Suppl 3): S32–9.

10. Laumann EO, Paik A, Rosen RC. Sexual dysfunction in the United States: prevalence and predictors. *JAMA* 1999; 281: 537–44.

11. Rosen RC, Taylor JF, Leiblum SR et al. Prevalence of sexual dysfunction in women: results of a survey study of 329 women in an outpatient gynecological clinic. *J Sex Marital Ther* 1993; 19: 171–88.

12. Basson R, Berman J, Burnett A et al. Report of the international consensus development conference on female sexual dysfunction: definitions and classifications. *J Urol* 2000; 163: 888–93.

13. Sadeghi-Nejad HMR, Traish A, Azadzoi K et al. Impotence is a couple's disease: studies in female sexual dysfunction. *J Urol* 1996; 155: 677A.

14. Berman JR, Bassuk J. Physiology and pathophysiology of female sexual function and dysfunction. *World J Urol* 2002; 20: 111–18.

15. Goldstein MK, Teng NN. Gynecologic factors in sexual dysfunction of the older woman. *Clin Geriatr Med* 1991; 7: 41–61.

16. Slob AK, Koster J, Radder JK et al. Sexuality and psychophysiological functioning in women with diabetes mellitus. *J Sex Marital Ther* 1990; 16: 59–69.

17. Min K, O'Connell L, Munarriz R et al. Experimental models for the investigation of female sexual function and dysfunction. *Int J Impot Res* 2001; 13: 151–6.

18. Hilliard J, Eaton LW Jr. Estradiol-17 beta, progesterone and 20-alpha-hydroxypregn-4-en-3-one in rabbit ovarian venous plasma. II. From mating through implantation. *Endocrinology* 1971; 89: 522–7.

19. Barberini F, Correr S, De Santis F et al. The epithelium of the rabbit vagina: a microtopographical study by light, transmission and scanning electron microscopy. *Arch Histol Cytol* 1991; 54: 365–78.

20. Vachon P, Simmerman N, Zahran AR et al. Increases in clitoral and vaginal blood flow following clitoral and pelvic plexus nerve stimulations in the female rat. *Int J Impot Res* 2000; 12: 53–7.

21. Giuliano F, Allard J, Compagnie S et al. Vaginal physiological changes in a model of sexual arousal in anesthetized rats. *Am J Physiol Regul Integr Comp Physiol* 2001; 281: R140–9.

22. Beharry RK, Hale TM, Wilson EA et al. Evidence for centrally initiated genital vasocongestive engorgement in the female rat:

findings from a new model of female sexual arousal response. *Int J Impot Res* 2003; 15: 122–8.

23. Agmo A, Ellingsen E. Relevance of non-human animal studies to the understanding of human sexuality. *Scand J Psychol* 2003; 44: 293–301.

24. Tong YC, Hung YC, Lin SN et al. Dark-cycle video surveillance of sexual performances of normal and diabetic rats. *Urol Int* 1996; 56: 207–10.

25. Sherwin BB, Gelfand MM, Brender W. Androgen enhances sexual motivation in females: a prospective, crossover study of sex steroid administration in the surgical menopause. *Psychosom Med* 1985; 47: 339–51.

26. Goldfoot DA, Westerborg-van Loon H, Groeneveld W et al. Behavioral and physiological evidence of sexual climax in the female stump-tailed macaque (*Macaca arctoides*). *Science* 1980; 208(4451): 1477–9.

27. Kim NN, Min K, Huang YH et al. Biochemical and functional characterization of alpha-adrenergic receptors in the rabbit vagina. *Life Sci* 2002; 71: 2909–20.

28. Vemulapalli S, Kurowski S. Sildenafil relaxes rabbit clitoral corpus cavernosum. *Life Sci* 2000; 67: 23–9.

29. Ziessen T, Moncada S, Cellek S. Characterization of the non-nitrergic NANC relaxation responses in the rabbit vaginal wall. *Br J Pharmacol* 2002; 135: 546–54.

30. Giraldi A, Alm P, Werkstrom V et al. Morphological and functional characterization of a rat vaginal smooth muscle sphincter. *Int J Impot Res* 2002; 14: 271–82.

31. Ottesen B, Ulrichsen H, Fahrenkrug J et al. Vasoactive intestinal polypeptide and the female genital tract: relationship to reproductive phase and delivery. *Am J Obstet Gynecol* 1982; 143: 414–20.

32. Ottesen B. Vasoactive intestinal polypeptide as a neurotransmitter in the female genital tract. *Am J Obstet Gynecol* 1983; 147: 208–24.

33. Park JK, Lee SO, Kim YG et al. Role of rho-kinase activity in angiotensin II-induced contraction of rabbit clitoral cavernosum smooth muscle. *Int J Impot Res* 2002; 14: 472–7.

34. Laan E, van Lunsen RH. Hormones and sexuality in postmenopausal women: a psychophysiological study. *J Psychosom Obstet Gynaecol* 1997; 18: 126–33.

35. McCoy N, Culter W, Davidson JM. Relationships among sexual behavior, hot flashes, and hormone levels in perimenopausal women. *Arch Sex Behav* 1985; 14: 385–94.

36. Park K, Ahn K, Lee S et al. Decreased circulating levels of estrogen alter vaginal and clitoral blood flow and structure in the rabbit. *Int J Impot Res* 2001; 13: 116–24.

37. Min K, Munarriz R, Kim NN et al. Effects of ovariectomy and estrogen replacement on basal and pelvic nerve stimulated vaginal lubrication in an animal model. *J Sex Marital Ther* 2003; 29 (Suppl 1): 77–84.

38. Berman JR, McCarthy MM, Kyprianou N. Effect of estrogen withdrawal on nitric oxide synthase expression and apoptosis in the rat vagina. *Urology* 1998; 51: 650–6.

39. Dundar M, Kocak I, Erkus M et al. The effect of estrogen-replacement therapy on clitoral-cavernosal tissue in oophorectomized rats: a histo-quantitative study by image analyzer. *Urol Res* 2001; 29: 317–20.

40. Traish AM, Kim NN, Huang YH et al. Sex steroid hormones differentially regulate nitric oxide synthase and arginase activities in the proximal and distal rabbit vagina. *Int J Impot Res* 2003; 15: 397–404.

41. Yoon HN, Chung WS, Park YY et al. Effects of estrogen on nitric oxide synthase and histological composition in the rabbit clitoris and vagina. *Int J Impot Res* 2001; 13: 205–11.

42. Al-Hijji J, Batra S. Downregulation by estrogen of nitric oxide synthase activity in the female rabbit lower urinary tract. *Urology* 1999; 53: 637–41.

43. Enzlin P, Mathieu C, Vanderschueren D et al. Diabetes mellitus and female sexuality: a review of 25 years' research. *Diabet Med* 1998; 15: 809–15.

44. Meeking D, Fosbury J, Cradock S. Assessing the impact of diabetes on female sexuality. *Community Nurse* 1997; 3: 50–2.

45. Park K, Ryu SB, Park YI et al. Diabetes mellitus induces vaginal tissue fibrosis by TGF-beta 1 expression in the rat model. *J Sex Marital Ther* 2001; 27: 577–87.

46. Giraldi A, Persson K, Werkstrom V et al. Effects of diabetes on neurotransmission in rat vaginal smooth muscle. *Int J Impot Res* 2001; 13: 58–66.

47. Park K, Ahn K, Kim MK et al. Effect of hyperglycemia on vaginal blood flow and structure in the streptozotocin-induced diabetic rat. *J Urol* 2003; 169: 310S.

48. Park K, Ahn K, Chang JS et al. Diabetes induced alteration of clitoral hemodynamics and structure in the rabbit. *J Urol* 2002; 168: 1269–72.

49. Sipski ML. Central nervous system based neurogenic female sexual dysfunction: current status and future trends. *Arch Sex Behav* 2002; 31: 421–4.

50. McKenna KE, Chung SK, McVary KT. A model for the study of sexual function in anesthetized male and female rats. *Am J Physiol* 1991; 261(5 Pt 2): R1276–85.

51. Giuliano F, Rampin O, Allard J. Neurophysiology and pharmacology of female genital sexual response. *J Sex Marital Ther* 2002; 28 (Suppl 1): 101–21.

PATHOPHYSIOLOGIC MECHANISMS: DESIRE, AROUSAL, ORGASM & PAIN

6.1 Mechanisms involved in desire and arousal dysfunction

Rossella E Nappi, Francesca Ferdeghini, Franco Polatti

Introduction

In the last few years, increasing knowledge has been achieved in the field of female sexual function from both a biologic and a psychosocial standpoint. However, despite the high prevalence of sexual complaints and problems in women (see Chapters 2.1–2.4 of this volume), our understanding of the pathophysiology of female sexual dysfunction is limited, mainly owing to methodological difficulties associated with the multidimensionality of the sexual response cycle. Animal models have been extremely helpful in understanding the neuroanatomic and neuroendocrine mechanisms that underlie sexual desire and arousal (see Chapters 5.1–5.6), but it is still very difficult to translate this growing body of basic research into the practical management of women with sexual symptoms. The inadequacy of our clinical approach is, indeed, confirmed by the paucity of available treatments specifically designed for female sexual dysfunction.[1]

This chapter will attempt to report the most relevant data currently available in order to understand the biologic mechanisms involved in desire and arousal dysfunction in women.

Libido and arousal

Physiologic sexual function (that is, briefly, an intact libido and the capacity to achieve satisfactory intercourse) is guaranteed by the integrity of (1) neural (autonomic, somatosensory, and somatomotor) and muscular substrates, (2) vascular supplies (arterial and venous), (3) hormonal environment, and (4) modulating mechanisms depending on cortical and hypothalamic–limbic structures. An impairment of both peripheral and central pathways involved in the sexual response cycle may lead to female sexual dysfunction, which includes disorders of libido, arousal and orgasm, and sexual pain[2] (see Chapter 9.1).

Sexual desire or libido is the physical and mental need to behave sexually in order to experience a sense of reward. It may be activated by endogenous and/or exogenous stimuli, and it is very much a result of integrated biologic, psychosocial, and cultural factors. Multiple neuroendocrine messages are basically involved in promoting the instinctual component of libido (lust) modulated by emotional (attraction) and cognitive (attachment) aspects. A complex interplay among these factors gives rise to passion (see Chapter 3.3), affection, and commitment.[3–5]

The most recent definition of women's sexual desire disorder, hypoactive sexual desire disorder, is "absent or diminished feelings of sexual interest or desire, absent sexual thoughts or fantasies and a lack of responsive desire. Motivations (reasons, incentives, etc.) for attempting to become sexually aroused are scarce or absent. The lack of interest is considered to be beyond a normative lessening with life cycle and relationship duration."[6]

Such a definition introduces the concept of sexual arousal, a critical step in the woman's sexual response cycle, which has been elegantly described as a mixture of subjective physical and mental feelings of sexual excitement and of objective awareness of genital sensations due to vulvovaginal engorgement and lubrication.[6] Very briefly, it is most likely that women, by mentally feeling motivations to be sexually intimate, may activate desire and arousal or be responsive to sexual stimulation and become physically aware of peripheral genital tension and excitement. Thus, three subtypes of arousal disorders are described. The first includes subjective sexual arousal disorders defined as "absence of or markedly diminished feelings of sexual arousal (sexual excitement and sexual pleasure), from any type of sexual stimulation. Vaginal lubrication or other signs of physical response still occur." The second subtype is genital sexual arousal disorder defined as "complaints of absent or impaired genital sexual arousal. Self-report may include minimal vulvar swelling or vaginal lubrication from any type of sexual stimulation and reduced sexual sensations from caressing genitalia. Subjective sexual excitement still occurs from nongenital sexual stimuli." The third subtype includes combined genital and subjective sexual arousal disorder, defined as "absence of or markedly diminished feelings of sexual arousal (sexual excitement and sexual pleasure), from any type of sexual stimulation as well as complaints of absent or impaired genital sexual arousal (vulvar swelling, lubrication)" (see Chapter 9.1). Less common, but highly distressing, are the so-called persistent sexual arousal disorders. These are defined as "the spontaneous, intrusive and unwanted genital arousal (e.g. tingling, throbbing, pulsating) in the absence of sexual interest and desire". There is also sexual aversion disorder, which indicates "the extreme anxiety and/or disgust at the anticipation of/or attempt to have any sexual activity"[6] (see Chapter 16.9).

Libido and arousal are tightly connected but may also be independent. Both may be positive, nondysfunctional perceptions of pleasure and satisfaction. Both may be mentally and physically present when subjective and objective sexual responses follow the same track.

Key sexual organs for women's libido and arousal

The brain

The nervous system produces a vast array of cognitive, emotional, physical, and behavioral responses that are critical to sexual function. The cerebral cortex is the coordinating and controlling center, interpreting what sensations are to be perceived as sexual and issuing appropriate commands to the rest of the nervous system. In particular, the brain creates sexual fantasies and by recalling them it may generate erotically stimulating sensations in women's bodies. Mental awareness is important both to live out sexual experiences and to provide sexual satisfaction.

The mechanical stimulation of external genitalia by means of pressure, touch, and attrition provokes the excitation of sensorial receptors of several kinds, located in the skin, mucosa, and subcutaneous tissue. This excitation travels through the sensory nerves of the lower abdomen to the sacral spinal cord and triggers numerous autonomic reflexes (both sympathetic and parasympathetic). These reflexes control the selective afflux of blood to these regions, glandular secretion, and the contraction of smooth muscles in the sexual organs. The sensory cortex and limbic system, in addition to their signaling functions, excite the hypothalamus and other structures that control the autonomic nervous system. The result is that the spinal cord reflexes accompanying coitus are even more stimulated, creating a kind

of self-perpetuating cycle. The neuroendocrine environment affects the integrity and the sensitivity of both the local and the central levels involved in the sexual response. At the same time, the mass of sensorial impulses emitted by the genitalia, in response to touch and to the local responses (i.e., genital engorgement), travel up the spinal cord to the brain, to the sensory cortex, and to the limbic system, where they elicit conscious perception and reactions of pleasure.

The main areas within the central nervous system modulating genital reflexes are brainstem structures (nucleus paragigantocellularis locus ceruleus and midbrain periaqueductal gray); hypothalamic structures (medial preoptic area, ventromedial nucleus and paraventricular nucleus); and forebrain structures (amygdala and hyppocampus)[6–9] (see Chapters 5.1–5.3).

The genitals

The genitals play a critical role in the hemodynamic process of arousal, involving the peripheral neurovascular complex and the pelvic floor muscles. Arousal is modulated by sexual stimulation, hormonal milieu, and ascending/descending neurologic pathways. Thus, the genitals are directly responsible for the perception of objective activation in response to sexual stimuli, and their adequate functioning leads to orgasmic tension and sexual pleasure.[10–15]

The breasts

The breasts are one of the most predominate features of a woman and stand out as a symbol of womanliness and livelihood. They are relevant to sexual pleasure in both sexes, but erotic sensitivity varies enormously. Sex hormone changes affect the glandular composition; thus, the tenderness of the breasts may vary during the menstrual cycle, hormonal treatments, pregnancy, and menopause. During the sexual response, the breasts become engorged with blood, and a pink/red rush is common. The nipples are supplied with many nerve endings that make them highly sensitive to sexual stimulation, while thin muscle fibers enable them to become erect during arousal. The stimulation of the nipple and areola may lead directly to orgasm.[16,17]

The skin

The skin, the largest sexual organ, is woven with an intricate system of nerves that are responsive to changes in temperature, touch, and texture. Common areas identified as erogenous zones are very sensitive and responsive to stimulation, thus causing sexual arousal and pleasure. Erogenous zones include the neck, earlobes, mouth, lips, nipples, genitalia, buttocks, inner thighs, anus, backs of knees, fingers, and toes. However, erogenous zones are unique to each individual and virtually any part of the body can be erogenous, independent of the high concentration of nerves. The skin also represents an important part of a woman's identity, being a symbol of beauty and sex appeal, and it is an important target for hormones that influence both the appearance and the threshold of sensitivity to external stimuli.[16,18]

Key sexual systems for women's libido and arousal

The peripheral neurovascular complex

The precise location of autonomic neurovascular structures related to the uterus, cervix, and vagina is still a matter of debate. Uterine nerves arise from the inferior hypogastric plexus formed by the union of hypogastric nerves (sympathetic T10–L1) and the splanchnic fibers (parasympathetic S2–S4). This plexus, which has three portions: the vesical plexus, the rectal plexus, and the uterovaginal plexus (Frankenhauser's ganglion), lies at the base of the broad ligament, dorsal to the uterine vessels, and lateral to the uterosacral and cardinal ligament. This plexus provides innervation via the cardinal ligament and uterosacral ligaments to the cervix, upper vagina, urethra, vestibular bulbs, and clitoris. At the cervix, sympathetic and parasympathetic nerves form the paracervical ganglia. The larger one is called the uterine cervical ganglion, and it is probably at this level that injury to the autonomic fibers of the vagina, labia, and cervix may occur during hysterectomy. The pudendal nerve (S2–S4) reaches the perineum through Alcock's canal and provides sensory and motor innervation to the external genitalia. The arterial supply into the genitals comes from the internal and external pudendals, with extensive anastomoses, and follows the course of the nerves. Spinal cord reflex mechanisms produce sexual response at genital and nongenital level. The afferent reflex arm is primarily via the pudendal nerve. The efferent reflex arm consists of coordinated somatic and autonomic activity. One spinal sexual reflex is the bulbocavernosus reflex involving sacral cord segments S2–4 in which pudendal nerve stimulation results in pelvic floor muscle contraction. Another spinal sexual reflex involves vaginal and clitoral cavernosal autonomic nerve stimulation, resulting in clitoral, labial, and vaginal engorgement[19] (see Chapters 4.1–4.3).

The pelvic floor muscles

Among the muscles forming the pelvic diaphragm, the levator ani muscle seems the most relevant to sexual function. It forms the floor of the pelvis and the roof of the perineum, and is divisible into three portions: the iliococcygeus, the pubococcygeus, and the puborectalis. The levator ani muscle fixes the vesical neck, anorectal junction, and vaginal fornices to the side wall of the pelvis by means of the suspensory sling and hiatal ligament. On contraction, it shares in the mechanism of evacuation (urination and defecation). During the sexual act, vaginal distention by the erect penis evokes the vaginolevator and vaginopuborectalis reflexes, with a resulting levator ani muscle contraction. The levator ani muscle also contracts upon stimulation of the clitoris or cervix uteri, an action mediated through clitoromotor and cervicomotor reflexes. The levator ani muscle contraction leads to upper vagina ballooning, which acts as a receptacle for semen collection, to uterine elevation and straightening, and to elongation and narrowing of the vagina. These actions enhance the sexual response and facilitate reproductive function. The levator ani dysfunction is associated with parity, and it is more common in women with a history of a prolonged second stage of labor. Muscles of external genitalia, such as the bulbocavernosus (BC) and ischiocavernosus (IC) muscles, take an active part in the process leading to clitoral engorgement and vaginal lubrication[20–22] (see Chapter 4.4).

Key sexual mediators for women's libido and arousal

Sex steroids

Sex steroids exert both organizational and activational effects that are relevant to sexual function, and their actions are mediated by nongenomic as well as direct and indirect genomic pathways. Androgens are essential for the development of reproductive function and the growth and maintenance of secondary sex characteristics directly or throughout their conversion to estrogens. In addition, they are crucial to secure libido in both sexes. Estrogens also play a critical role in maintaining the physiologic function of many tissues, including the central nervous system and the genital apparatus, and of organs relevant to general health.[23,24]

The importance of adequate estrogen levels in preserving vaginal receptivity and preventing dyspareunia has long been established. Women with a level of estradiol of less than 50 pg/ml reported vaginal dryness, increased frequency and intensity of dyspareunia, pain with penetration and deep insertion, and burning. Women with higher estradiol levels had no complaints related to sexual desire, response, or satisfaction. Indeed, estradiol levels below 35 pg/ml are associated with reduced coital frequency, and decline in estradiol is related to a decline in sexual function.[25,26]

Data derived from *in vivo* animal models indicates that estrogen modulates genital blood flow, peripheral nerve function, vaginal tissue structural integrity, and, therefore, the process of lubrication.[27] Within the nervous system, estradiol plays a permissive role in sexual receptivity by acting on its own estrogen receptor-alpha[28] and by increasing the progesterone receptor expression that takes part in sexual response.[29] In addition, estradiol stimulates oxytocin release and expression of its receptor,[30] and facilitates the lordosis reflex by stimulating noradrenaline alpha-1 receptor.[31] Some neurosteroids, such as allopregnanolone, a derivative of progesterone, are involved in the lordosis reflex at hypothalamic levels. Allopregnanolone may interfere with gamma-aminobutyric acid function, a major inhibitory neurotransmitter in the central nervous system.[32] In addition, progesterone and its metabolites may indirectly influence sexual receptivity by modulating mood and cognition together with estrogens and androgens.[33] The role of progesterone in peripheral vaginal arousal is poorly understood, even though the use of progestins seems to blunt the positive effect on vaginal dryness and dyspareunia exerted by estrogen, an action that seems highly dependent on biochemical properties of progestins.[34]

The most potent androgen, testosterone, is secreted by the adrenal zona fasciculata (25%) and the ovarian stroma (25%), while the remaining amount (50%) derives from peripheral conversion of circulating androstenedione. Plasma testosterone levels are in the range 0.2–0.7 ng/ml (0.6–2.5 nmol/l), with significant fluctuations related to the phase of the menstrual cycle, being highest at ovulation, lowest during the early follicular phase, and higher during the luteal phase with respect to the early follicular phase. In addition, testosterone shows circadian variations, with a peak in the early morning hours. Testosterone is converted to dihydrotestosterone, but it can also be aromatizable to estradiol, in target tissues. Dihydrotestosterone is the principal ligand to androgen receptors. Other androgens in women include dehydroepiandrosterone sulfate, dehydroepiandrosterone, and androstenedione, which are considered to be proandrogens because they convert to testosterone.[35]

While estrogen decreases sharply at menopause, plasma testosterone levels fall slowly with age. At physiologic menopause, the cessation of follicular activity is characterized by a significant decline of ovarian production of androstenedione, more than testosterone. The progressive fall of plasma testosterone concentrations is the consequence of the reduced peripheral conversion from its major precursor and from dehydroepiandrosterone and dehydroepiandrosterone sulfate, which decline with age. Indeed, plasma testosterone and androstenedione levels at 60 are about half those in women aged 40 years. As far as surgical menopause is concerned, bilateral oophorectomy, both premenopausally and postmenopausally, leads to a sudden 50% fall in circulating testosterone levels. Low androgens are associated with significant deterioration of sexual desire in premenopausal and postmenopausal women. There is, however, no consensus regarding the cutoff level for a normal range of testosterone because of the difficulties with sensitive assays of total and free testosterone in women and the fluctuations during the menstrual cycle and different ages.[36,37]

Testosterone, directly or through aromatization to estradiol within the central nervous system, contributes to initiation of sexual activity and permission for sexual behavior.[38] A further nongenomic action by testosterone metabolites on sexual receptivity has been described at the hypothalamic level.[39] Experimental data suggest that androgens directly modulate vaginal and clitoral physiology by influencing the muscular tone of erectile tissue and of vaginal walls. Androgens facilitate vaginal smooth muscle relaxation, especially in the proximal vagina, producing distinct physiologic responses in comparison with estradiol. In addition, testosterone being converted to estradiol, may enhance lubrication.[40,41]

Prolactin

Prolactin levels have been found to increase significantly after orgasm.[42] An inhibitory action of prolactin on sexual desire and arousal has been demonstrated in hyperprolactinemic states and pharmacologic manipulations with psychoactive drugs.[43] Such an effect is probably mediated by the interference with androgen biosynthesis and by the abnormal release of oxytocin. Amenorrhea and/or menstrual abnormalities, which are very common in hyperprolactinemic women, may contribute to an altered vaginal receptivity as a consequence of the hypoestrogenic state.

Oxytocin

Oxytocin has been strictly related to sexual behavior and may work synergistically with sex steroids to facilitate orgasm during sexual stimulation. The actions of oxytocin range from modulating neuroendocrine reflexes to establishing complex social and bonding behaviors related to the reproduction and care of offspring. The intensity of muscular contractions during orgasm in both men and women are highly correlated with oxytocin plasma levels.[44] In addition, plasma oxytocin fluctuations throughout the menstrual cycle correlate with lubrication in fertile women with normal sexual activity, further supporting the role of this neurohormone in peripheral activation of sexual function.[45]

Endogenous opioids

Endogenous opioids and their receptors relate to a wide range of functions and behaviors, including the control of sexual behavior leading to intercourse, directly or through the modulation of several neurotransmitters and other neuropeptides. Opioids play an important role in female receptivity, but their involvement is quite complex, affecting differently anticipatory and contact components of sexual behavior.[46]

Classical neurotransmitters

The effects of several neurotransmitters on sexual function have been characterized within the central nervous systems by means of pharmacologic tools. Briefly, dopamine plays an excitatory role, promoting the craving for continued sexual activity once sexual stimulation has started, directly or though inhibiting prolactin release or stimulating oxytocin secretion. Even noradrenaline has a stimulating action on sexual behavior, while serotonin plays an inhibitory role on central desire and arousal by reducing the dopaminergic and noradrenergic activity.[8,47] The function of the adrenergic/sympathetic and cholinergic/parasympathetic systems in peripheral sexual function is still confusing and needs further investigation. Despite a rich cholinergic innervation to the vaginal arteries, acetylcholine plays a minor role in the regulation of the vaginal blood flow. Some data are in agreement with regard to the inhibitory effect of noradrenaline on the female sexual genital response. However, vaginal and clitoral smooth muscle contraction seems to be the result of activation of alpha-adrenergic receptors by noradrenaline released from adrenergic nerves. A facilitatory role of peripheral adrenergic activation on sexual arousal in women has been reported. The role of noradrenaline in the control of clitoral erection is indirectly supported by successful treatment of clitoral priapism by an alpha adrenergic agonist. Serotonin seems to exert a negative effect on sexual response by inhibiting the spinal sexual reflex at the periphery.[48,49]

Nonadrenergic, noncholinergic (NANC) neurotransmitters/neuromodulators

A great variety of nonadrenergic, noncholinergic neurotransmitters/neuromodulators have been identified in the female genital tract in animal models and humans, and are regulated by sex steroids. Nitric oxide synthase is present in the deep arteries, veins, and capillaries of the vagina and in nerve fibers within the glans and corpora cavernosa of the clitoris. Phosphodiesterase type 5 expression has been demonstrated in the clitoris and in the anterosuperior wall of the human vagina.[50] After sexual stimulation, neurogenic and endothelial release of nitric oxide plays an important role in clitoral cavernosal artery and helicine arteriolar smooth muscle relaxation. This leads to a rise in clitoral cavernosal artery inflow, an increase in clitoral intracavernosal pressure, and clitoral engorgement. The result is extrusion of the glans clitoris and enhanced sensitivity. Nitric oxide and vasoactive intestinal peptide are highly present and released in order to modulate vaginal vascular and nonvascular smooth muscle relaxation and to enhance vaginal blood flow, lubrication, and secretions. However, while the crucial role of the nitric oxide/cyclic guanosine monophosphate system is strongly supported by increasing experimental evidence, no conclusive experimental data of functional involvement of vasoactive intestinal peptide has been forthcoming. Even neuropeptide Y has been identified in the human vagina and clitoris as having vasoconstrictive activity, along with calcitonin-gene related peptide, substance P, pituitary adenylate cyclase-activating peptides, and peptide histidine methionine, with unclear effects.[13,51–53]

To summarize the current conception of vaginal vasocongestion and increased lubrication during objective arousal, it is likely that vaginal arteriolar dilation from vasoactive intestinal peptide, nitric oxide and other unknown neurotransmitters, and neuropeptide Y-associated venoconstriction leads to increased interstitial fluid formation from vaginal submucosal capillaries. Neurogenic fluid filters through epithelial cells onto lumen with less potassium and more sodium than in the nonarousal state. Similarly, labia minora are able to release a transudate with the same modalities, while nitric oxide plays a dominant androgen- and estrogen-dependent role in vasocongestion of the clitoral cavernous bodies by regulating, together with prostaglandins, clitoral smooth muscle tone[13] (see Chapter 5.4).

In clinical practice, the inadequate hormonal-dependent vaginal receptivity is the precipitating factor of dyspareunia that may cause other sexual symptoms and contribute to pain amplification during coital activity. It is extremely common to observe a lack of arousal and a decline of libido after a history of sexual pain; the consequent reduction of orgasmic capacity may reduce sexual satisfaction, negatively influencing sexual motivation, activity, and ultimately the couple's relationship. This model explains the high degree of comorbidity of sexual symptoms in women, particularly throughout the climacteric period when hormonal imbalance is highly dominant.[54]

Conclusion

From this short summary of the biologic mechanisms involved in desire and arousal, it is fairly clear that every organic condition is able to impair the anatomic and physiologic substrates of a women's sexual response cycle and may be a potential source of dysfunction. Endocrine, reproductive, urogenital, and surgical factors (see Chapter 16.7), as well as vascular, muscular, nervous, general health, drugs, lifestyle, and partner's health and sexual function-related factors (see Chapters 8.1 and 8.2) should always be thoroughly investigated for appropriate management of women's sexual dysfunctions.

References

1. Lue TF, Basson R, Rosen R et al., eds. *Sexual Medicine – Sexual Dysfunctions in Men and Women*. Paris: Editions 21, 2004.
2. Basson R, Berman J, Burnett A et al. Report of the international consensus development conference on female sexual dysfunction: definitions and classifications. *J Urol* 2000; 163: 888–93.
3. Levine SB. The nature of sexual desire: a clinician's perspective. *Arch Sex Behav* 2003; 32: 279–85.
4. Wallen K. The evolution of female sexual desire. In PR Abramson, SD Pirkerton, eds. *Sexual Nature, Sexual Culture*. Chicago: University of Chicago Press, 1995: 57–9.
5. Graziottin A. Libido. In J Studd, ed. *Yearbook of RCOG*. London: RCOG Press, Parthenon, 1996: 235–43.
6. Basson R, Leiblum SL, Brotto L et al. Definitions of women's sexual dysfunctions reconsidered: advocating expansion and revision. *J Psychosom Obstet Gynecol* 2003; 24: 221–9.
7. Master WH, Johnson VE, Kolodny RC. *Heterosexuality*. Glasgow: HarperCollins, 1994.
8. Meston CM, Frohlich PF. The neurobiology of sexual function. *Arch Gen Psychiatry* 2000; 57: 1012–30.
9. Pfaff DW. *Drive: Neurobiological and Molecular Mechanisms of Sexual Motivation*. Bradford: MIT Press, 2001.

10. Berman JR, Berman LA, Werbin TJ et al. Female sexual dysfunction: anatomy, physiology, evaluation and treatment options. *Curr Opin Urol* 1999; 9: 563–8.

11. Berman JR, Adhikari SP, Goldstein I. Anatomy and physiology of female sexual function and dysfunction: classification, evaluation and treatment options. *Eur Urol* 2000; 38: 20–9.

12. Meston CM. Aging and sexuality. *West J Med* 1997; 167: 285–90.

13. Munarriz R, Kim NN, Goldstein I et al. Biology of female sexual function. *Urol Clin North Am* 2002; 29: 685–93.

14. Hines TM. The G-spot: a modern gynecological myth. *Am J Obstet Gynecol* 2001; 185: 359–62.

15. Schultz WW, van Andel P, Sabelis I et al. Magnetic resonance imaging of male and female genitals during coitus and female sexual arousal. *BMJ* 1999; 319: 1596–1600.

16. Master WH, Johnson VE. *Human Sexual Response.* Boston: Little Brown, 1966.

17. Kohout E. The breast in female sexuality. *Int J Psychoanal* 2004; 85: 1235–8.

18. Fink B, Grammer K, Thornhill R. Human (*Homo sapiens*) facial attractiveness in relation to skin texture and color. *J Comp Psychol* 2001; 115: 92–9.

19. Degroat WC. Neural control of the urinary, bladder and sexual organs. In Mathias JJ, Bannister R, eds. *Autonomic Failure: A Textbook of Clinical Disorders of the Autonomic Nervous System*, 4th edn. New York: Oxford University Press, 1999.

20. Shafik A. Vagino-levator reflex: the description of a reflex and its role in the sexual performance. *Eur J Obstet Gynecol Reprod Biol* 1994; 60: 161–3.

21. Shafik A. The role of the elevator ani muscle in evacuation, sexual performance and pelvic floor disorders. *Int Urogynecol J* 2000; 11: 361–76.

22. Barber MD, Bremer RE, Thor KB et al. Innervation of the female levator ani muscles. *Am J Obstet Gynecol* 2002; 197: 64–71.

23. McEwen BS. Clinical review 108: the molecular and neuroanatomical basis for estrogen effects in the central nervous system. *J Clin Endocrinol Metab* 1999; 84: 1790–7.

24. Davis S, Tran J. Testosterone influences libido and well-being in women. *Trends Endocrinol Metab* 2001; 12: 33–7.

25. Cutler WB, Garcia CM, McCoy N. Perimenopausal sexuality. *Arch Sex Behav* 1987; 16: 225–34.

26. Dennerstein L, Randolph J, Taffe J et al. Hormones, mood, sexuality, and the menopausal transition. *Fertil Steril* 2002 ; 77: S42–8.

27. Min K, Munarriz R, Kim NN et al. Effects of ovariectomy and estrogen and androgen treatment on sildenafil-mediated changes in female genital blood flow and vaginal lubrication in the animal model. *Am J Obstet Gynecol* 2002; 187: 1370–6.

28. Ogawa S, Chan J, Chester AE et al. Survival of reproductive behaviours in estrogen receptor beta gene-deficient male and female mice. *Proc Natl Acad Sci USA* 1999; 96: 12887–92.

29. Etgen AM. Estrogen induction of progestin receptors in the hypothalamus of male and female rats which differ in their ability to exhibit cyclic gonadotropin secretion and female sexual behavior. *Biol Reprod* 1981; 25: 307–13.

30. Bale TL, Pedersen CA, Dorsa DM. CNS oxytocin receptor mRNA expression and regulation by gonadal steroids. *Adv Exp Med Biol* 1995; 395: 269–80.

31. Kow LM, Weesner GD, Pfaff DW. Alpha 1–adrenergic agonists act on the ventromedial hypothalamus to cause neuronal excitation and lordosis facilitation: electrophysiological and behavioral evidence. *Brain Res* 1992; 588: 237–45.

32. Frye CA, Bayon LE, Pursnani NK et al. The neurosteroids, progesterone and 3α,5α-THP, enhance sexual motivation, receptivity, and proceptivity in female rats. *Brain Res* 1998; 808: 72–83.

33. Sherwin BB. The impact of different doses of estrogen and progestin on mood and sexual behavior in postmenopausal women. *J Clin Endocrinol Metab* 1991; 72: 336–43.

34. Sarrel PM. Androgen deficiency: menopause and estrogen-related factors. *Fertil Steril* 2002; 77: S63–7.

35. Rosen R, ed. Androgen Insufficiency in Women: the Princeton Conference. *Fertil Steril* 2002; 77 (Suppl 4): S1–99.

36. Davis SR, Burger H. Androgen and postmenopausal women. *J Clin Endocrinol Metab* 1996; 81: 2759–63.

37. Nappi RE, Abbiati I, Ferdeghini F et al. Androgen-insufficiency syndrome and women's sexuality. In AR Genazzani, ed. *Hormone Replacement Therapy and the Brain.* London: Parthenon, 2003: pp 107–14.

38. Nappi RE, Detaddei S, Ferdeghini F et al. Role of testosterone in feminine sexuality. *J Endocrinol Invest* 2003; 26: 97–101.

39. Frye CA. The role of neurosteroids and non-genomic effects of progestins and androgens in mediating sexual receptivity of rodents. *Brain Res Rev* 2001; 37: 201–22.

40. Traish AM, Kim N, Min K et al. Role of androgens in female genital sexual arousal: receptor expression, structure and function. *Fertil Steril* 2002; 77: S11–S18.

41. Munarriz R, Kim SW, Kim NN et al. A review of the physiology and pharmacology of peripheral (vaginal and clitoral) female genital arousal in the animal model. *J Urol* 2003; 170: S40–4.

42. Kruger TH, Haake P, Hartmann U et al. Orgasm-induced prolactin secretion: feedback control of sexual drive? *Neurosci Biobehav Rev* 2002; 26: 31–44.

43. Bloom FE, Kupfer D, eds. *Psychopharmacology.* New York: Raven Press, 1995.

44. Anderson-Hunt M, Dennerstein L. Oxytocin and female sexuality. *Gynecol Obstet Invest* 1995; 40: 217–21.

45. Salonia A, Nappi RE, Pontillo M et al. Menstrual cycle-related changes in plasma oxytocin are relevant to normal sexual function in healthy women. *Horm Behav* 2005; 47: 164–9.

46. Bodnar RJ, Klein GE. Endogenous opiates and behavior: 2003. *Peptides* 2004; 25: 2205–56.

47. Clayton AH. Sexual function and dysfunction in women. *Psychiatr Clin N Am* 2003; 26:673–682.

48. Giuliano F, Rampin O, Allard J. Neurophysiology and pharmacology of female genital sexual response. *J Sex Marital Ther* 2002; 28 (Suppl 1): 101–21.

49. Meston CM. Sympathetic nervous system activity and female sexual arousal. *Am J Cardiol* 2000; 86: 30F–34F.

50. D'Amati G, di Gioia CR, Proietti Pannunzi L et al. Functional anatomy of the human vagina. *J Endocrinol Invest* 2003; 26(Suppl 3): 92–6.

51. Meston CM, Frohlich PF. Update on female sexual function. *Curr Opin Urol* 2001; 11: 603–9.

52. Levine RJ. Sex and the human female reproductive tract, what really happens during and after coitus. *Int J Impot Res* 1998; 10: S14–S21.

53. Goldstein I. Female sexual arousal disorder: new insights. Int J Impot Res 2000; 12: S152–7.

54. Nappi RE, Baldaro Verde J et al. Self-reported sexual symptoms in women attending menopause clinics. *J Obstet Gynecol Invest* 2002: 53: 181–7.

6.2 Pathophysiologic mechanisms involved in genital arousal dysfunction

Noel N Kim, Abdulmaged M Traish

Introduction

Female sexual dysfunction consists of multiple disorders classified into the diagnostic categories of desire, arousal, orgasm, and pain (Fig. 6.2.1). Each of these categories involves both psychologic and physiologic aspects and requires subjective as well as objective assessments. However, this discussion will be limited to peripheral physiologic mechanisms that directly affect the genital organs and can be objectively assessed. In its most general terms, arousal disorder is defined as "the persistent or recurrent inability to attain or maintain sufficient sexual excitement that causes personal distress".[1] The normal female genital arousal response is manifested by engorgement and swelling of genital tissues and production of lubricating mucus and fluid transudate from the cervix, periurethral glands, and vagina (see Chapters 4.1–4.4, 5.1–5.6, and 6.1 of this volume). These physiologic events are dependent upon the structural integrity of the genital tissues and the function of neural, endocrine, and vascular systems that regulate and coordinate the genital arousal response. Women diagnosed with "sexual arousal disorder" may have sexual complaints of diminished vaginal lubrication, increased time for arousal, diminished vaginal and clitoral sensation, and difficulty with orgasm (see Chapter 9.4). These clinical conditions may exist, in part, due to disruptions in the normal vascular, neural, and/or endocrine/paracrine regulatory mechanisms with concomitant changes in genital tissue structure or cellular organization. It is reasonable to hypothesize that chronic disease states (e.g., hypertension, atherosclerosis, diabetes), physical trauma, endocrine imbalances, or medications that adversely affect genital blood flow or sensation contribute to genital arousal dysfunction. There is an increased awareness of the role of physiologic factors mediating female sexual arousal and a new appreciation for the role of organic pathophysiologic conditions resulting in female sexual arousal disorders. However, the cellular and molecular mechanisms responsible for disruptions in normal genital arousal remain unknown. Thus, building upon the previous sections of this textbook on genital tissue anatomy and physiology, this chapter focuses on established and *postulated* peripheral mechanisms within the genital tissues that may contribute to female genital arousal dysfunction (Fig. 6.2.2).

Vascular insufficiency

Vascular insufficiency states have been associated with disorders and diseases of the heart, brain, eye, and bladder, as well as arousal disorders in men.[2–5] However, the association between vascular insufficiency and arousal disorders in women has been made only recently.[6] Genital vasocongestion and vaginal lubrication responses result from increased blood flow to the clitoris, vagina, and labia. These hemodynamic processes are regulated by the tone of the vascular smooth muscle of the erectile tissue and blood vessels within the genital tissues. There is limited understanding of local regulatory mechanisms modulating clitoral, vaginal, and labial smooth muscle tone and how these mechanisms are altered by disease states. However, recent studies using animal models (see Chapter 5.6) of several different species indicate that the nitric oxide/cyclic guanosine

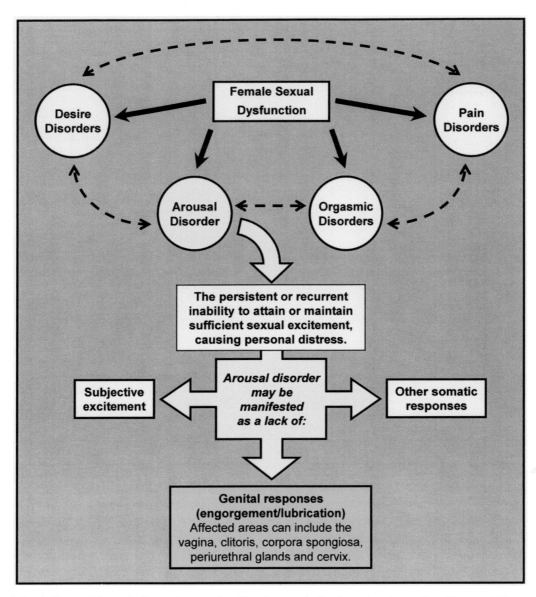

Figure 6.2.1. "Arousal disorder" is one of four main diagnostic categories of female sexual dysfunction and can be manifested in several different ways. Engorgement and lubrication of the genital tissues may be decreased or absent in women with arousal disorder.

monophosphate pathway is an important regulator of clitoral and vaginal blood flow.[7-11]

A developing hypothesis is that diminished arterial inflow after sexual stimulation is a major factor contributing to impaired "genital arousal", as manifested by inadequate genital engorgement. While animal models of disease that exhibit genital arousal dysfunction are generally lacking, several recently published studies provide insight into some potential pathophysiologic mechanisms. Laboratory studies that have demonstrated various conditions leading to vascular insufficiency and attenuated genital arousal are discussed in the following sections in the broader context of vascular disease. Relevant hypothesized mechanisms from the field of cardiovascular research are also discussed.

Atherosclerosis and fibrosis

In the female rabbit model, Park et al. induced atherosclerosis of the ilio-hypogastric-pudendal arterial bed by injuring the intima with a balloon catheter and maintaining the rabbits on a high-cholesterol diet for 16 weeks.[12] When compared with control animals, rabbits with atherosclerotic lesions had significantly diminished vaginal and clitoral blood flow after pelvic nerve stimulation, as well as reduced development of pressure in vaginal and clitoral tissues.[12] Upon histologic examination, clitoral and vaginal tissues from atherosclerotic animals exhibited diffuse fibrosis. In a separate study, clitoral corpus cavernosum tissue from atherosclerotic animals was found to have significantly decreased smooth muscle content with a concomitant increase in connective tissue.[13]

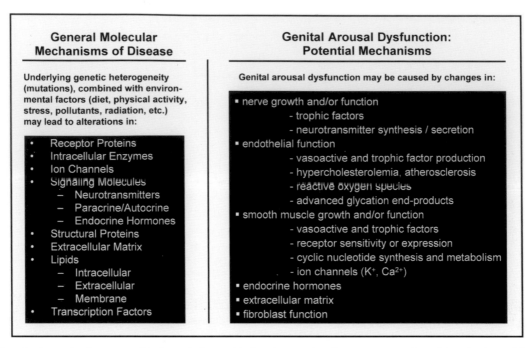

Figure 6.2.2. Specific molecular mechanisms responsible for genital arousal dysfunction remain unknown at present. Potential mechanisms of disease, derived from the study of other vascular systems, are presented.

While specific pathophysiologic processes have yet to be explicitly demonstrated in vaginal or clitoral tissues, it seems likely that the development of atherosclerotic plaques within the blood vessels feeding the genital tissues and the progression of disease would be similar to what has been described in the heart and coronary vessels. This process includes: (1) the accumulation of lipoprotein particles on the intimal surface; (2) entry of lipoprotein into the subendothelial space and subsequent modification (e.g., oxidation); (3) stimulation of inflammatory response by oxidized lipoproteins; (4) expression of adhesion molecules on the endothelial surface and attraction of monocytes via production of chemokines; (5) entry of monocytes into the blood vessel wall and differentiation into foam cells.[14] In addition, the production of various cytokines and chemoattractants stimulates the proliferation of vascular smooth muscle cells and their movement into the intimal layer. Smooth muscle cells in both the medial and intimal layers synthesize greater amounts of extracellular matrix, contributing to the establishment of atherosclerotic lesions.

Atherosclerotic blood vessels that have developed significant stenosis may not maintain sufficient perfusion, such that female genital tissues are exposed to chronic ischemia and hypoxia. In penile cavernosal tissue, profibrotic mechanisms related to decreased perfusion and oxygenation have been postulated.[15] These mechanisms are based on the concept that tissue oxygen tension regulates the local production of vasoactive factors, growth factors, and cytokines that can modulate extracellular matrix metabolism. An important cytokine mediator of tissue fibrosis that is sensitive to changes in oxygen tension is transforming growth factor beta$_1$. In tissue culture experiments, messenger RNA for transforming growth factor beta$_1$ increased two- to three-fold when penile cavernosal smooth muscle cells were exposed to low oxygen tension ($PO_2 = 30$ mmHg) for 18–24 h.[16] Similar studies in human penile cavernosal smooth muscle cells and rabbit penile cavernosal tissue have also demonstrated that prostanoid synthesis is suppressed at low oxygen tension and positively correlated with intracellular accumulation of cyclic adenosine monophosphate.[17–19] In separate studies, agents that increase intracellular cyclic adenosine monophosphate levels, such as prostaglandin E$_1$ or forskolin, were shown to inhibit transforming growth factor beta$_1$ and collagen synthesis in penile cavernosal smooth muscle.[18,20]

Thus, in vaginal and clitoral tissues, chronic hypoxia secondary to ischemia may induce transforming growth factor beta$_1$ and inhibit the synthesis of prostaglandins, stimulating the accumulation of perivascular and interstitial collagen that is the hallmark of tissue fibrosis. It is also likely that other aspects of extracellular matrix metabolism are altered with ischemic hypoxia. These may include changes in the signaling or synthesis of trophic factors, such as connective tissue growth factor, vascular endothelial growth factor, fibroblast growth factor, insulin-like growth factor, platelet-derived growth factor, tumor necrosis factor alpha, endothelins, and interleukins, all of which have been linked to tissue fibrosis. Furthermore, matrix metalloproteinases are enzymes that break down fibrillar collagen while tissue inhibitors of matrix metalloproteinases are endogenous inhibitors of matrix metalloproteinases. Each of these two families of proteins can modulate signaling molecules, as well as actively regulate the rate at which collagen is deposited in or removed from the extracellular space. In addition, tissue inhibitors of matrix metalloproteinases and matrix metalloproteinases may themselves be induced or suppressed by different trophic factors. Thus, an imbalance in the normal types, amounts, or activity of matrix metalloproteinases and tissue inhibitors of matrix metalloproteinases can dramatically change the content of extracellular matrix within any given tissue. As the knowledge gained from the field of connective tissue research indicates, tissue fibrosis is a complex process that can involve numerous other biologic mediators. The specific mediators of female genital tissue fibrosis remain to be elucidated.

Endothelial dysfunction

The clitoral and labial erectile tissue and the vaginal lamina propria are all highly vascular structures that contain endothelial cells (see Chapter 5.4). The endothelium consists of a monolayer of cells that forms a single, continuous surface lining the vascular compartment throughout the body. The total mass of the endothelium has been estimated to be 500 g in the average adult human, the majority of which is contained in the pulmonary vasculature.[21] Much like skin, the endothelium may be considered a single organ with multiple functions and differential responses that are dependent upon both the systemic and local environments. Among other functions, a healthy endothelium serves to provide an antithrombotic, anti-inflammatory, and antiatherogenic surface while also regulating vascular tone and permeability. Diseased or damaged endothelium may be a major contributor to vascular insufficiency of female genital tissues. Endothelium-dependent relaxation of blood vessels has been shown to be compromised in animal models of atherosclerosis, hypertension, diabetes, aging, smoking, and renal failure.[21–24] While it remains unclear whether endothelial dysfunction is a cause or a consequence of any of these disease states, its existence as a common pathologic state warrants consideration and further investigation.

The most commonly observed type of endothelial dysfunction is that of reduced endothelium-dependent relaxation of vascular smooth muscle. For the purposes of this discussion, this impairment is the most relevant. The endothelium produces many vasoactive compounds that can influence the contractile, trophic or synthetic function of vascular smooth muscle cells. Among the factors that cause relaxation are nitric oxide, endothelium-derived hyperpolarizing factor, prostacyclin, and endothelin (through endothelin B receptors). Among the factors that cause contraction are endoperoxides, thromboxane A_2, superoxide anions, and endothelin (through endothelin A receptors). Dysfunctional endothelium may produce decreased amounts of relaxing factors and/or increased amounts of constricting factors. More specifically, attenuated endothelium-dependent relaxation may be caused by: (1) impaired signal transduction mechanisms within the endothelial cell; (2) changes in substrate availability for the production of specific vasoactive factors; (3) increased inactivation of relaxing factors; (4) impaired diffusion of substances to the smooth muscle;

(5) increased release of constricting factors; and (6) decreased sensitivity of smooth muscle to vasoactive substances.[23]

Although many of the mechanisms listed in the previous paragraph have been demonstrated in animal models of disease, it should be stressed that conflicting data do exist and that some findings may depend on the specific vascular bed or tissue used for study. In rat retina, diabetic conditions resulted in downregulation and structural modification of G-proteins.[25] One of the more novel proposed mechanisms of dysfunctional endothelial signaling involves a decrease in the number of caveolae on the surface of endothelial cells. Caveolae are invaginated microdomains of plasma membrane that are rich in endothelial nitric oxide synthase and the family of transmembrane structural proteins known as caveolins, as well as cholesterol, sphingolipids, and glycosylphosphatidylinositol-linked proteins. In addition, caveolae contain numerous other signaling proteins such as receptors with seven-transmembrane domains, G-proteins, adenylyl cyclase, phospholipase C, protein kinase C, calcium pumps, and calcium channels. Thus, these specialized signaling regions have been termed "transductosomes".[26] In rabbits that were maintained for 8 weeks on a hypercholesterolemic diet, regions of aortic endothelium that were infiltrated by fatty streaks exhibited lower numbers of caveolae transductosomes, as well as decreased clustering density.[26] These cellular changes were correlated with attenuated endothelium-dependent relaxation.

With regard to substrate availability and increased inactivation of relaxing factors, the well-studied example of nitric oxide will be used to illustrate such mechanisms. It is debatable whether significantly different plasma levels of L-arginine (a cosubstrate for nitric oxide synthase) occur in disease states. However, L-arginine supplementation has been shown to improve parameters of cardiovascular function, reduce myocardial ischemia, and lower systemic blood pressure and renal vascular resistance in various patient populations that smoked cigarettes or those that were diagnosed with coronary artery disease, hypertension, or hypercholesterolemia.[27] In addition, accumulating evidence suggests that asymmetric dimethylarginine, an endogenous competitive inhibitor of nitric oxide synthase, plays an important role in endothelial dysfunction. Elevated levels of asymmetric dimethylarginine have been positively correlated with a variety of clinical conditions, including hypercholesterolemia, hypertriglyceridemia, hypertension, chronic renal failure, chronic heart failure, and diabetes mellitus type II.[28,29] Alternatively, nitric oxide production may remain unchanged or even transiently increased in disease states, but there may also be increased inactivation. Particularly in diabetes, oxidative stress has been implicated as an important pathogenic mechanism. The addition of antioxidants and superoxide dismutase has been shown to improve endothelium-dependent relaxation in animal models of atherosclerosis and diabetes.[23] Increased formation of free radicals and/or impairment in normal antioxidant mechanisms (e.g., superoxide dismutase, catalase, glutathione, ascorbic acid) can lead to accumulation of reactive oxygen species and superoxide anions that scavenge nitric oxide. The reaction between nitric oxide and superoxide may also progress to form peroxynitrite, which can modify key proteins, such as prostacyclin synthase and superoxide dismutase, and inactivate them.

While impaired diffusion of endothelium-derived relaxing factors and decreased sensitivity of vascular smooth muscle to these factors remain plausible mechanisms, far fewer studies have focused on these aspects and will not be discussed here, since they are not, in and of themselves, forms of endothelial dysfunction. The remaining mechanism of increased release of constricting factors by the endothelium has been reported in animal models of diabetes. Increased production of vasoconstricting prostanoids has been observed in pial arterioles and aorta of diabetic rats.[30–32] Evidence to support abnormally high production of nonprostanoid constricting factors, such as endothelins, remains inconclusive.

Thus, endothelial dysfunction can occur through various mechanisms, and it is likely that more than one mechanism is associated with a given disease state. Given the vascular nature of genital tissue and the importance of blood flow during the genital arousal response, perturbations in endothelial function are likely to be important mechanisms mediating genital arousal dysfunction.

Endocrine pathophysiology

There is growing evidence that alterations in the sex steroid hormonal milieu may, in part, contribute to sexual dysfunction (see Chapters 6.1 and 6.3). Imbalances in sex steroid hormones (estrogens, androgens, and progestins) may alter nerve function, synthesis or activity of growth factors, tissue composition and structure, and smooth muscle contractility. These changes may lead to decreases in genital blood flow and sensation. Since other chapters in this book address the physiology and pathophysiology of sex steroid hormones in greater detail, this section presents only a general hypothesized mechanism relating to genital arousal dysfunction.

Sex steroid hormones may regulate distinct cellular processes within the multiple layers and components of the vagina, clitoris, and labia. Each of these direct cellular interactions may influence specific processes such as growth and function of neurons, blood vessels, smooth muscle, endothelium, and epithelial cells. These changes may include alterations in: (1) the synthesis, secretion, and reuptake of neurotransmitters; (2) vascular and nonvascular smooth muscle contractility; (3) production of autocrine or paracrine vasoactive/trophic factors; (4) synthesis, deposition, and degradation of extracellular matrix components; and (5) mucification, keratinization, and/or permeability of vaginal epithelium. The additive, synergistic or antagonistic interactions of such cellular processes will ultimately determine the overall physiologic responses manifested as genital blood flow, vaginal lubrication, tissue compliance, or sensation.

Diabetes

Diabetes is known to cause multiple medical complications, affecting vascular, neural, and endocrine mechanisms (see Chapter 7.3). However, the effects of diabetes on sexual function in women have received limited attention in basic and clinical research.[33–35] The most common sexual dysfunction in women with diabetes is decreased genital arousal with inadequate lubrication.[33,36,37] Women with diabetes were also determined to have decreased sensation at both genital and extragenital sites.[38] In addition, diabetic women may have decreased physiologic arousal responses to erotic stimuli when compared with nondiabetic women.[39]

In laboratory studies, vaginal tissue from diabetic rats exhibited attenuated contractile responses to exogenous norepinephrine as well as diminished relaxation to exogenous nitric oxide or calcitonin gene-related peptide.[40] Further, both neurogenic contraction and relaxation responses elicited by electrical stimulation were inhibited in vaginal tissue from diabetic animals when compared with control responses. However, the mechanisms responsible for the observed changes remain unclear. In separate studies, vaginal tissues from diabetic rats were observed to have decreased epithelial thickness, decreased overall wall thickness, and atrophic submucosal vasculature.[41] Moreover, the cross-sectional area of connective tissue and immunostaining for transforming growth factor beta[1] was significantly higher in vaginal tissue from diabetic animals. Subsequent studies using female rabbits have indicated that the diabetic state inhibits both baseline and nerve-stimulated clitoral blood flow and causes diffuse clitoral cavernosal fibrosis.[42] Recent investigations have measured the vaginal blood flow response to pelvic nerve stimulation in diabetic rats and have shown that vaginal blood flow is also significantly attenuated when compared with responses in control animals (A. Traish et al., unpublished observations; K. Park et al., personal communication).

Thus, the diabetic condition may cause a state of vascular insufficiency that leads to adverse changes in tissue structure. However, as the clinical findings suggest, there are most certainly other aspects that need to be explored. In general, diabetic complications are thought to arise from increased oxidative stress, which is associated with an array of hyperglycemia-induced alterations. These changes include protein kinase C activation, formation of advanced glycation end-products, and increased activity of the polyol and hexoseamine pathways.[43] While the consequences of these individual pathways in various tissues have been extensively investigated, recent work suggests that enhanced superoxide generation within the mitochondria is the underlying mechanism that directly or indirectly stimulates these metabolic pathways. Nevertheless, the mechanisms by which diabetes modulates female genital arousal responses are not well understood and require further investigation.

Antidepressant medications

Antidepressants have long been associated with adverse effects on sexual function[44–46] (see Chapter 16.2). However, the ability to draw conclusions from the data from most clinical studies has been limited for several reasons. First, the already high prevalence of sexual dysfunction in patients diagnosed with clinical depression makes it difficult to distinguish an increased prevalence or severity of sexual dysfunction due to treatment with antidepressants. Second, validated rating scales are often not used to assess sexual dysfunction. Moreover, the manner in which the prevalence of sexual dysfunction is determined (i.e., direct interview versus self-report) can affect the data collected. Sexual dysfunction in patients has been shown to be significantly lower by spontaneous reporting than with direct patient interview by physicians.[44] Finally, many studies examining the relative effects of different antidepressants on sexual function are not done by direct comparison and lack placebo controls.

Angulo et al. have performed laboratory studies to investigate the effects of various antidepressants on vaginal and clitoral blood flow.[47] In female rabbits, acute administration of venlafaxine (5 mg/kg) and duloxetine (1 mg/kg), mixed inhibitors of serotonin and norepinephrine reuptake, significantly inhibited the increase in genital blood flow that is normally observed after pelvic nerve stimulation. The specific serotonin reuptake inhibitor paroxetine (5 mg/kg) also inhibited the genital blood flow response after pelvic nerve stimulation. Interestingly,

serotonin itself or the highly selective inhibitor of serotonin reuptake escitalopram did not appreciably affect the genital blood flow response. Thus, it seems unlikely that the inhibitory effect on genital blood flow caused by venlafaxine, duloxetine, and paroxetine results from increased serotonin levels. In the same study, administration of L-arginine completely blocked the inhibitory effect of paroxetine on genital blood flow, while the alpha-adrenergic antagonist phentolamine prevented the inhibitory effect of venlafaxine. The inhibitory effect of duloxetine was partially attenuated by either L-arginine or phentolamine, and completely blocked by the combination of L-arginine and phentolamine. These data suggest that some serotonin reuptake inhibitors can also inhibit the production of nitric oxide in genital tissues and thereby attenuate genital blood flow, while others may increase the availability of norepinephrine in the genital vascular bed and cause vasoconstriction. While this initial study provides some insight, further elucidation of the mechanisms responsible for the inhibitory effects of antidepressants on sexual function is required. In addition to the roles of the nitric oxide, serotonin, and alpha-adrenergic signaling pathways, it also remains important to distinguish between the central and peripheral effects of various antidepressant drugs.

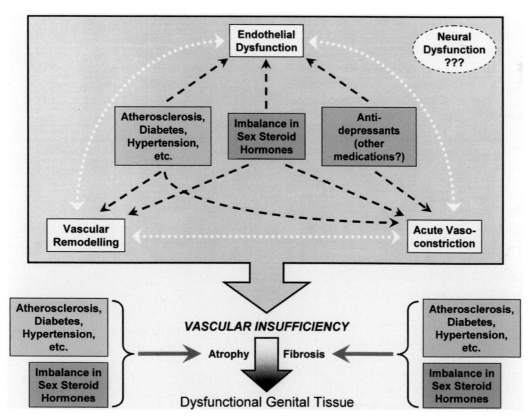

Figure 6.2.3. Hypothetic mechanisms of genital arousal dysfunction. Cardiovascular disease, deficient levels of sex steroid hormones, or medication (e.g., antidepressants) may all cause vascular insufficiency states of genital tissue, resulting in genital arousal dysfunction. Alternatively, vascular disease and/or sex steroid hormone deficiency may directly cause genital tissue atrophy and/or fibrosis. While many of the pathophysiologic states that are shown in the figure affect neuronal function, their associations with vascular mechanisms have been delineated much more clearly. It is likely that multiple mechanisms contribute to dysfunctional genital arousal.

Summary and conclusions

The physiology of genital arousal is highly dependent on the structural and functional integrity of the tissue, involving complex neurovascular processes modulated by numerous local neurotransmitters, vasoactive agents, sex steroid hormones, and growth factors. As discussed in this chapter, the vascular nature of genital tissue lends itself to many parallel comparisons from the already established field of cardiovascular biology (Fig. 6.2.3). However, it is also well known that different vascular beds can yield diverse responses to the same disease state. Thus, there are probably mechanisms that are unique to the genital tissues and their vasculature. For example, Δ-5-androstenediol, a steroid hormone possessing both androgenic and estrogenic activity, binds to a unique nuclear receptor that may be preferentially expressed in the vagina.[48,49] In addition, the alpha-adrenergic and purinergic signaling systems, the neurotransmitter vasoactive intestinal polypeptide, and the enzyme arginase have all been shown to regulate the genital arousal response. Whether any of these mediate genital arousal dysfunction remains to be seen. Thus, although there is much to learn about the normal physiologic mechanisms of genital arousal, additional understanding of the cellular and molecular mechanisms of pathogenesis will help to identify potential points of intervention for the treatment of female genital arousal dysfunction.

Acknowledgment

This work was supported by grants DK56846 (AMT) and DK02696 (NNK) from the National Institute of Diabetes and Digestive and Kidney Diseases.

References

1. Basson R, Berman J, Burnett A et al. Report of the international consensus development conference on female sexual dysfunction: definitions and classifications. *J Urol* 2000; 163: 888–93.

2. Lusis AJ. Atherosclerosis. *Nature* 2000; 407: 233–41.

3. Bhardwaj A, Alkayed NJ, Kirsch JR et al. Mechanisms of ischemic brain damage. *Curr Cardiol Rep* 2003; 5: 160–7.

4. Flammer J, Orgul S, Costa VP et al. The impact of ocular blood flow in glaucoma. *Prog Retin Eye Res* 2002; 21: 359–93.

5. Azadzoi KM. Effect of chronic ischemia on bladder structure and function. *Adv Exp Med Biol* 2003; 539: 271–80.

6. Goldstein I, Berman JR. Vasculogenic female sexual dysfunction: vaginal engorgement and clitoral erectile insufficiency syndromes. *Int J Impot Res* 1998; 10 (Suppl 2): S84–S101.

7. Cellek S, Moncada S. Nitrergic neurotransmission mediates the non-adrenergic non-cholinergic responses in the clitoral corpus cavernosum of the rabbit. *Br J Pharmacol* 1998; 125: 1627–9.

8. Min K, Kim NN, McAuley I et al. Sildenafil augments pelvic nerve-mediated female genital sexual arousal in the anesthetized rabbit. *Int J Impot Res* 2000; 12 (Suppl 3): S32–9.

9. Kim SW, Jeong SJ, Munarriz R et al. Role of the nitric oxide-cyclic GMP pathway in regulation of vaginal blood flow. *Int J Impot Res* 2003; 15: 355–61.

10. Kim SW, Jeong SJ, Munarriz R et al. An *in vivo* rat model to investigate female vaginal arousal response. *J Urol* 2004; 171: 1357–61.

11. Angulo J, Cuevas P, Cuevas B et al. Vardenafil enhances clitoral and vaginal blood flow responses to pelvic nerve stimulation in female dogs. *Int J Impot Res* 2003; 15: 137–41.

12. Park K, Goldstein I, Andry C et al. Vasculogenic female sexual dysfunction: the hemodynamic basis for vaginal engorgement insufficiency and clitoral erectile insufficiency. *Int J Impot Res* 1997; 9: 21–37.

13. Park K, Tarcan T, Goldstein I et al. Atherosclerosis-induced chronic arterial insufficiency causes clitoral cavernosal fibrosis in the rabbit. *Int J Impot Res* 2000; 12: 111–16.

14. Plutzky J. The vascular biology of atherosclerosis. *Am J Med* 2003; 115: 55S–61S.

15. Moreland RB. Is there a role of hypoxemia in penile fibrosis: a viewpoint presented to the Society for the Study of Impotence. *Int J Impot Res* 1998; 10: 113–20.

16. Moreland RB, Watkins MT, Nehra A et al. Oxygen tension modulates transforming growth factor β_1 expression and PGE production in human corpus cavernosum smooth muscle cells. *Mol Urol* 1998; 2: 41–7.

17. Daley JT, Brown ML, Watkins T et al. Prostanoid production in rabbit corpus cavernosum. I. Regulation by oxygen tension. *J Urol* 1996; 155: 1482–7.

18. Moreland RB, Gupta S, Goldstein I et al. Cyclic AMP modulates TGF-beta 1-induced fibrillar collagen synthesis in cultured human corpus cavernosum smooth muscle cells. *Int J Impot Res* 1998; 10: 159–63.

19. Moreland RB, Albadawi H, Bratton C et al. O₂-dependent prostanoid synthesis activates functional PGE receptors on corpus cavernosum smooth muscle. *Am J Physiol* 2001; 281: H552–8.

20. Moreland RB, Traish A, McMillin MA et al. PGE₁ suppresses the induction of collagen synthesis by transforming growth factor-beta 1 in human corpus cavernosum smooth muscle. *J Urol* 1995; 153: 826–34.

21. Triggle CR, Hollenberg M, Anderson TJ et al. The endothelium in health and disease – a target for therapeutic intervention. *J Smooth Muscle Res* 2003; 39: 249–67.

22. Frohlich ED. Fibrosis and ischemia: the real risks in hypertensive heart disease. *Am J Hypertens* 2001; 14: 194S–9S.

23. De Vriese AS, Verbeuren TJ, Van de Voorde J et al. Endothelial dysfunction in diabetes. *Br J Pharmacol* 2000; 130: 963–74.

24. Matz RL, Schott C, Stoclet JC et al. Age-related endothelial dysfunction with respect to nitric oxide, endothelium-derived hyperpolarizing factor and cyclooxygenase products. *Physiol Res* 2000; 49: 11–18.

25. Sobrevia L, Mann GE. Dysfunction of the endothelial nitric oxide signaling pathway in diabetes and hyperglycaemia. *Exp Physiol* 1997; 82: 423–52.

26. Darblade B, Caillaud D, Poirot M et al. Alteration of plasmalemmal caveolae mimics endothelial dysfunction observed in atheromatous rabbit aorta. *Cardiovasc Res* 2001; 50: 566–76.

27. Tapiero H, Mathe G, Couvreur P et al. I. Arginine. *Biomed Pharmacother* 2002; 56: 439–45.

28. Böger RH. The emerging role of asymmetric dimethylarginine as a novel cardiovascular risk factor. *Cardiovasc Res* 2003; 59: 824–33.

29. Tran CT, Leiper JM, Vallance P. The DDAH/ADMA/NOS pathway. *Atheroscler Suppl* 2003; 4: 33–40.

30. Mayhan WG, Simmons LK, Sharpe GM. Mechanisms of impaired responses of cerebral arterioles during diabetes mellitus. *Am J Physiol* 1991; 260: H319–26.

31. Shimizu K, Muramatsu M, Kakegawa Y et al. Role of prostaglandin H_2 as an endothelial-derived contracting factor in diabetic state. *Diabetes* 1993; 42: 1246–52.

32. Tesfamariam B, Jakubowski JA, Cohen RA. Contraction of diabetic rabbit aorta caused by endothelium-derived PGH_2-TxA_2. *Am J Physiol* 1989; 257: H1327–33.

33. Enzlin P, Mathieu C, Vanderschueren D et al. Diabetes mellitus and female sexuality: a review of 25 years' research. *Diabet Med* 1998; 15: 809–15.

34. Enzlin P, Mathieu C, Van den Bruel A et al. Sexual dysfunction in women with type 1 diabetes: a controlled study. *Diabetes Care* 2002; 25: 672–7.

35. Koch PB, Young EW. Diabetes and female sexuality: a review of the literature. *Health Care Women Int* 1988; 9: 251–62.

36. Meeking D, Fosbury J, Cradock S. Assessing the impact of diabetes on female sexuality. *Community Nurse* 1997; 3: 50–2.

37. Meeking DR, Fosbury JA Cummings MH et al. Sexual dysfunction and sexual health concerns in women with diabetes. *Sex Dysfunct* 1998; 1:83–7.

38. Erol B, Tefekli A, Sanli O et al. Does sexual dysfunction correlate with deterioration of somatic sensory system in diabetic women? *Int J Impot Res* 2003; 15: 198–202.

39. Wincze JP, Albert A, Bansal S. Sexual arousal in diabetic females: physiological and self-report measures. *Arch Sex Behav* 1993; 22: 587–601.

40. Giraldi A, Persson K, Werkström V et al. Effects of diabetes on neurotransmission in rat vaginal smooth muscle. *Int J Impot Res* 2001; 13: 58–66.

41. Park K, Ryu SB, Park YI et al. Diabetes mellitus induces vaginal tissue fibrosis by TGF-β_1 expression in the rat model. *J Sex Marital Ther* 2001; 27: 577–87.

42. Park K, Ahn K, Chang JS et al. Diabetes induced alteration of clitoral hemodynamics and structure in the rabbit. *J Urol* 2002; 168: 1269–72.

43. Brownlee M. Biochemistry and molecular cell biology of diabetic complications. *Nature* 2001; 414: 813–20.

44. Montejo-Gonzalez AL, Llorca G, Izquierdo JA et al. SSRI-induced sexual dysfunction: fluoxetine, paroxetine, sertraline, and fluvaoxamine in a prospective, multicenter, and descriptive clinical study of 344 patients. *J Sex Marital Ther* 1997; 23: 176–94.

45. Clayton AH. Female sexual dysfunction related to depression and antidepressant medications. *Curr Womens Health Rep* 2002; 2: 182–7.

46. Montgomery SA, Baldwin DS, Riley A. Antidepressant medications: a review of the evidence for drug-induced sexual dysfunction. *J Affect Disord* 2002; 69: 119–40.

47. Angulo J, Cuevas P, Cuevas B et al. Mechanisms for the inhibition of genital vascular responses by antidepressants in a female rabbit model. *J Pharmacol Exp Ther* 2004; 310: 141–9.

48. Shao TC, Castaneda E, Rosenfield RL et al. Selective retention and formation of a Δ5-androstenediol-receptor complex in cell nuclei of the rat vagina. *J Biol Chem* 1975; 250: 3095–3100.

49. Traish AM, Huang YH, Min K et al. Binding characteristics of [^{3}H]Δ(5)-androstene-3β,17β-diol to a nuclear protein in the rabbit vagina. *Steroids* 2004; 69: 71–8.

6.3 Pathophysiology of sex steroids in women

André T Guay, Richard Spark

Biogenesis of sex steroid hormones

In women, the biogenesis of sex steroid hormones from cholesterol occurs in the ovaries and the adrenal glands via distinct and overlapping Δ4 and Δ5 metabolic pathways[1] (Fig. 6.3.1). The Δ4 pathway yields progesterone, 17-OH progesterone, androstenedione, and testosterone, while the Δ5 pathway produces pregnenolone, 17-OH pregnenolone, dehydroepiandrosterone (DHEA), and Δ5 androstenediol, and the latter can be converted into testosterone. As can be seen in Fig. 6.3.2, the Δ4 and Δ5 pathways are represented in both organs, but the Δ4 pathway predominates in the ovaries and the Δ5 pathway predominates in the adrenal glands.[2] Moreover, the majority of dehydroepiandrosterone is converted into dehydroepiandrosterone

sulfate (DHEA-S), in the adrenal glands by a sulfotransferase.[3] Thus, dehydroepiandrosterone sulfate is considered an adrenal hormone and is converted back to dehydroepiandrosterone on demand by the sulfatase enzyme. Approximately one-half of the testosterone in the plasma in women is derived directly from precursors in the ovaries and the adrenal glands. The other half is the result of peripheral conversion of androgenic precursors to testosterone in various target tissues.[2]

Progesterone

Progesterone, which is produced cyclically during the menstrual cycle, is a critical hormone during the reproductive years, as it is

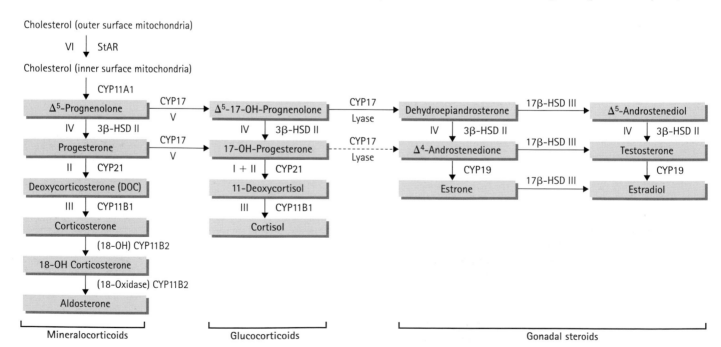

Figure 6.3.1. Steroid metabolism pathways in the female ovary and adrenal glands, emphasizing the Δ4 and Δ5 pathways. CYP = Human Cytochrome P450. HSD = hydroxysteroid dehydrogenase. StAR = Steroidogenic Acute Regulatory protein. Reprinted with permission from Grumbach and Conte.[1]

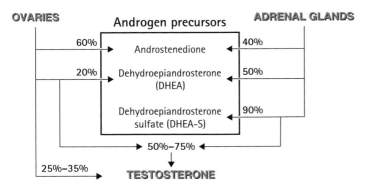

Figure 6.3.2. The Δ4 and Δ5 metabolic pathways of androgenic hormones and their precursors in women during the reproductive years. From Davis.[3]

a prerequisite for normal menstrual cycling and for achieving pregnancy. This cyclical production of progesterone is lost after menopause, but progesterone is still detected in serum and in the brain.[4] Animal studies have shown that estrogen and progesterone act in the hypothalamus to regulate neuronal networks that control female sexual behavior.[5] A similar effect in humans is inferred but has yet to be proven, although there is a suggestion that progesterone, when given to postmenopausal women, does have some effect on mood and sexual behavior.[6]

Progesterone is an important sex steroid intermediate in the Δ4 pathway, but does not appear to have any appreciable conversion to either estrogen or an effective androgen when administered orally or transdermally.[7] No apparent effectiveness in sexual function was noted when progesterone was given in a clinical trial.[8] One important clinical aspect is that progestins have little effect on sex hormone-binding globulin (SHBG) levels and may minimize the ability of estrogens to raise sex hormone-binding globulin.[9] This would minimize any effect of estrogen in lowering free testosterone levels. Another view is that progesterone may exert androgenic effects by displacing testosterone from sex hormone-binding globulin, thereby allowing increased conversion to its high-affinity active metabolite 5α-dihydrotestosterone (5α-DHT).[10] Ovarian dysfunction will primarily affect progesterone levels, but adrenal disorders can further decrease circulating amounts.

Dehydroepiandrosterone and androstenedione

Dehydroepiandrosterone is converted to androstenediol and then directly to testosterone in the biosynthetic organs, the adrenal glands and the ovaries, but most of the conversion to other sex steroids occurs in the peripheral tissues. Depending on the specific enzymes in the various target tissues, dehydroepiandrosterone may be converted to androgens and subsequently to estrogens, depending on the target tissue.[2] In addition to conversion to estradiol, estrone, or testosterone, dehydroepiandrosterone may be converted to the very potent androgen, Δ5 androstanediol,[11] which may have unique and dual function in genital tissue.[11]

Androstenedione, a weaker androgen, is produced in more significant quantities in the ovaries than the adrenal glands, and has several distinctive features.[12] It is the only circulating androgen that is higher in premenopausal women than in men and, like dehydroepiandrosterone, less than 4% of this steroid is bound to sex hormone-binding globulin. Its androgenic potency is approximately 10% that of testosterone, while that of dehydroepiandrosterone is 5%. Serving as a prohormone, androstenedione is readily converted to testosterone and/or estrone, and both steroids are precursors for estradiol via aromatization.

Estrone

Estradiol is the potent estrogen in women and may be the more important estrogen in the premenopausal state, while estrone is less potent and more predominant in the postmenopausal state.[14] Estrone can be derived from androstenedione as well as from estradiol. Both estradiol and estrone may be the product of aromatization of testosterone, directly or indirectly. Therefore, factors which contribute to estradiol or testosterone deficiency would equally contribute to estrone deficiency.

Estrogen and androgen deficiency

Conversion of androgens to estrogens via the enzyme aromatase occurs both peripherally and in the various sex steroid-producing glands. We have evaluated the relationship between female sex steroids (Table 6.3.1) and symptoms of female sexual dysfunction.

Table 6.3.1. Symptom-related laboratory evaluation of female sexual dysfunction

Symptom	Consider	Measure
Diminished libido	Androgen deficiency	Testosterone Free testosterone by dialysis SHBG Free testosterone index DHEA-S
Dyspareunia	Estrogen deficiency	FSH Estradiol
Sexual apathy	Depression Hypothyroidism	Beck index TSH
Menstrual irregularity	Pituitary-ovarian dysfunction	Estradiol Prolactin FSH
Galactorrhea	Pituitary adenoma Drug effect	Prolactin Review medication list

DHEA-S, dehydroepiandrosterone sulfate; FSH, follicle stimulating hormone; SHBG, sex hormone-binding globulin; TSH, thyroid stimulating hormone.

Symptoms of female sexual dysfunction are observed mainly with deficiencies in estradiol and testosterone rather than excesses in these steroids. Since estradiol is derived from testosterone (Figs 6.3.1 and 6.3.2),[14] the deficiencies are often simultaneous, although more attention has been given over the past few decades to estrogen deficiency. Research in testosterone deficiency in women is in its infancy owing to a multiplicity of causes. One is the limited sensitivity of current testosterone assays to measure the low levels of testosterone present in women.[15] The other is the paucity of data outlining normal ranges of testosterone by age in women. It is known that testosterone levels, and those of their precursors, decline with age in men and women.[16] Several attempts have been made to determine normal levels of dehydroepiandrosterone and testosterone in premenopausal women.[17] A decrease in dehydroepiandrosterone with age has been well established (Fig. 6.3.3);[16,18–21] however, clinical correlations with sexual function have rarely been made, even though plasma assays for dehydroepiandrosterone are reproducible, not controversial, and fairly accurate even in the lower ranges.

Symptoms of estrogen and androgen deficiency

Common symptoms of estrogen (Table 6.3.2), and testosterone deficiency (Table 6.3.3) in women share some similarities. There are also certain similarities between the symptoms of testosterone deficiency in men and women. Androgen deficiency-related symptoms are more reliably ascribed in women if such patients had adequate physiologic levels premenopausally or were treated with estrogen postmenopausally.[22] Varying combinations of these signs and symptoms are seen in women with

Table 6.3.2. Common symptoms of estrogen deficiency, and associated medical conditions

Vasomotor instability
Hot flashes and night sweats
Effects on cognition, mood, motivation
    Specific effects on sexual desire and sexual behavior
    Question of increased incidence of Alzheimer's disease
Vaginal dryness (loss of lubrication)
    Vaginal atrophy
    Vaginal infections
    Dyspareunia
Loss of skin elasticity
Muscle and joint aches
Decrease in the size of the uterus and breasts
    Decreased uterine fibroid tumors
Postmenopausal osteoporosis
Question of an increase in cardiovascular disease
Question of an increase in colon cancer

sex steroid deficiency from a variety of causes, necessitating a search of one or more of the possible etiologies that are noted in Table 6.3.4.

Potential causes of sex steroid deficiency

If the sources of production of estrogens and androgens, and of their precursors, are the adrenal glands and the ovaries, any condition that impairs the anatomy or function of these glands will lead to a deficiency of both androgens and estrogens.

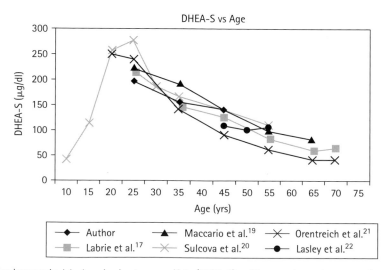

Figure 6.3.3. Relationship between the decrease in dehydroepiandrosterone sulfate (DHEA-S) and increase in age in women. From Guay et al.[18] Copyright 2004. *International Journal of Impotence Research.* Reproduced with permission.

Table 6.3.3. Common symptoms ascribed to androgen deficiency

Decreased sexual desire
  Decreased sexual fantasies and dreams
Decreased energy (increased fatigue)
  Decreased sense of well-being
Decreased muscle strength
  Decreased lean muscle mass
Decreased sexual arousability
  Decreased vaginal lubrication
Decreased orgasmic ability
  Decreased bone density
Decreased pubic hair

Ovarian pathology

The ovaries produce androgens and estrogens, directly and via the sex steroid precursors dehydroepiandrosterone and androstenedione. The most common cause is natural menopause, although surgical removal will produce the same results, albeit more acutely.[23] Premature menopause occurs earlier with more severe symptoms. There is some debate about the ability of the postmenopausal ovary to produce sex steroids. A commonly held theory is that the elevated gonadotropin levels during the menopause stimulate estradiol and testosterone production, especially from ovarian interstitial cells.[24] Recently, Couzinet[25] made an excellent argument for a lack of testosterone production in the menopause due to lack of hormone, enzymes, and receptors in ovarian tissue homogenates. The difference of opinion may be explained by the fact that Couzinet's study was performed in women further along in menopause. In addition, about 50% of ovarian testosterone production is from dihydroepiandrosterone sulfate and Couzinet's study was undertaken in women with adrenal insufficiency who therefore had low dihydroepindrosterone sulfate levels.

Varying degrees of ovarian hormone production can be seen with destruction from chemotherapy and radiation therapy. Suppression of steroid production from estrogen therapy is more complicated, whether it is from the use of oral contraceptives in younger women or from estrogen replacement during the menopause. In these cases, not only does estrogen therapy suppress estradiol and testosterone production from the ovary, but sex hormone-binding globulin production is stimulated from the liver, causing an increased binding of testosterone, and to a lesser extent estradiol, preventing them from being available to peripheral target tissues.[26]

Sexual difficulties with ovarian pathology

With loss of ovarian function from any cause, there is a decrease in both androgens and estrogens. A decrease in sexual function occurs, ranging from a decrease in sexual desire and mood

Table 6.3.4. Some major causes of sex steroid (estradiol and testosterone) deficiency

Ovarian
Menopause
  Natural
  Surgical (oophorectomy)
Premature ovarian failure
Destruction of ovarian tissue
  Chemotherapy
  Radiation therapy
Drug suppression of ovarian function
  Oral contraceptive agents
  Hormone replacement therapy in menopause

Adrenal
Adenalectomy
Addison's disease
Polyendocrine deficiency syndrome
Drug suppression of adrenal function
  Cortisone therapy
  Cortisone excess in Cushing's syndrome
Severe stress and illnesses

Pituitary and hypothalamus
Pituitary disease
  Idiopathic hypopituitarism
  Lymphocytic hypophysitis
  Pituitary adenoma
    Pituitary apoplexy
  Sheehan's postpartum necrosis
  Other pituitary tumors
    Parasellar meningiomas and other primary tumors
    Metastatic tumors
  Medications
    Gonadotropin releasing hormone (GnRH) therapy
    Estrogen therapy
      Postmenopausal replacement
      Oral contraceptive agents
Hypothalamic disease
  Hypothalamic functional amenorrhea
    Anxiety stress
    Acute illness
    Chronic illnesses, especially catabolic conditions
      acquired immune deficiency syndrome (AIDS) wasting, for example
      Medications (especially those affecting the central nervous system)
  Craniopharyngiomas and other suprasellar tumors

Miscellaneous
Increase in sex hormone-binding globulin (SHBG)
Idiopathic
  Premenopausal women

disturbances to a decrease in receptivity and arousability. Since estrogens are derived from androgens, it has long been debated whether symptoms and benefit with therapy should be attributed to the particular androgen or estrogen. It is debated as to whether aging or decreased ovarian function contributes more to sexual dysfunction, especially in older women during the perimenpausal years.

Longitudinal studies are preferable to cross-sectional ones in evaluating changes in hormones and symptoms. Burger[27] studied women during these transitional years and found a decrease in sexual function. The declining sexual function seemed to relate more to declining estradiol levels than to androgen levels. The investigators were also able to compare changes caused by aging and changes due to the menopause. Sexual responsivity was adversely affected by both aging and the menopause. However, other aspects of sexuality, especially sexual frequency and libido, were more related to the postmenopausal state.

There is no doubt that estrogen therapy improves vasomotor and other general symptoms[28,29] after the loss of ovarian function. The common menopausal findings of decreased vaginal lubrication and genital atrophy respond very nicely to systemic or local estrogen therapy.[30] The fact that estrogen therapy helps sexual receptivity and satisfaction may, however, be more related to relief of sexual discomfort, than to any direct effect of the estrogen.[29,31] Androgen therapy is thought by some to be more important in sexual desire and receptivity.[32] One limitation is the observation that when supraphysiologic levels of estrogens are used, there seems to be a definite link to fantasy, libido, and sexual satisfaction.[33]

Sexual difficulties with adrenal pathology

The adrenal glands also produce androgens via the precursors dehydroepiandrosterone and androstenedione, but the Δ5 steroid pathway predominates, through the production of pregnenolone and dehydroepiandrosterone. Sulfation of dehydroepiandrosterone occurs exclusively in the adrenal glands, so that dehydroepiandrosterone sulfate is considered an adrenal androgen. Clinical measurement of dehydroepiandrosterone is generally ordered through dehydroepiandrosterone sulfate because of its more stable serum levels due to a much longer half-life.

Adrenalectomy decreases androgen levels, especially dehydroepiandrosterone, dehydroepiandrosterone sulfate, and testosterone.[34] The loss of estrogen with the loss of the adrenal glands is minimal and comes mostly from the loss of those estrogens that are converted in peripheral tissues. Symptomatology will involve more loss of sexual desire, but decreased lubrication and arousability, making orgasmic ability difficult, are also seen with the loss of adrenal hormones. The levels of androgens are lower than those seen with the normal decline in these androgen levels with age that have been reported by numerous authors[35,36] (Fig. 6.3.3).

Adrenal insufficiency, either as an isolated organ failure, or as part of a polyendocrine deficiency syndrome, will produce a deficiency of adrenal androgens as well as a deficiency of cortisol.[35–37] Estrogens are a minor factor here also, as many women

with adrenal deficiency maintain normal menstrual cycles. Blocking adrenal androgen production by the use of cortisol medication will also decrease androgen production.[38,39] Excess cortisol from Cushing's syndrome will have the same effect.[40] Severe systemic illnesses, including anorexia nervosa,[41,42] and even acute stress[43] will also affect androgen production. It is felt that the body, in trying to conserve energy to survive, will decrease the production of reproductive hormones in favor of the life-saving corticosteroids and mineralocorticoids.

Sexual difficulty with pituitary pathology

If pituitary function is compromised, functions of both the ovaries and the adrenal glands will be affected. Therefore, a substantial or a total loss of estrogen and androgen hormones will be seen. This fact has been well outlined in both premenopausal and postmenopausal women, both with and without estrogen replacement[44] (Fig. 6.3.4).

Decreased pituitary function, causing decreased or absent gonadotropins, luteinizing hormone, and follicle-stimulating hormone, as well as decreased adenocorticotropic hormone, can be caused by a variety of conditions (Table 6.3.4). Destruction of the pituitary gland may occur from pituitary adenomas and other tumors, both primary and metastatic. Tumors may become so large that they impinge on their blood supply, creating autodestruction of the tumor and destruction of surrounding normal pituitary tissue, a condition termed pituitary apoplexy, which usually presents with acute symptoms of headache, nausea, vomiting, and visual impairment. A similar condition, called Sheehan's postpartum pituitary necrosis, may occur during pregnancy. Enlargement of the pituitary gland occurs normally during pregnancy, but damage can occur at the time of delivery when complications, such as excessive bleeding and hypotension, occur. Autoimmune destruction of the pituitary gland may occur as an isolated phenomenon or as part of a multiple endocrine syndrome. Lymphocytic hypophysitis is a variation of autoimmune destruction, which is now known to occur in men, but which has been described mostly in women during the peripartum period.[45]

Sexual symptoms with hypothalamic pathology

Pituitary function is dependent on hormonal and neural stimulation emanating from the hypothalamus. Therefore, diseases or destruction of the hypothalamus will cause a decrease in pituitary function that will then affect hormonal production of the ovaries and the adrenal glands. The most common cause of hypothalamic malfunction is a functional suppression due to stress from anxiety, acute illness, chronic illness, or medications.[46,47] Some chronic illnesses, but mostly acute illnesses,

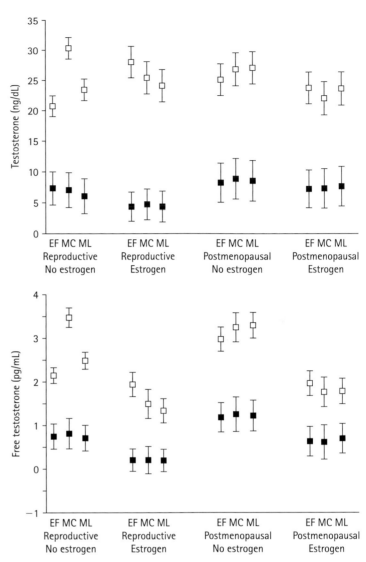

Serum testosterone levels in four groups
of hypopituitary women compared with controls:
(1) women of reproductive age, (2) women of reproductive
age receiving estrogen, (3) women of postmenopausal age,
and (4) women of postmenopausal age receiving estrogen
at three time points during a month.
■, Women with hypopituitarism; □, healthy controls;
EF, early follicular phase; MC, midcycle; ML, mid-luteal
phase. $p \leq 0.0003$ for all comparisons between women
with hypopituitarism and controls.

Serum free testosterone levels in four groups
of hypopituitary women compared with controls:
(1) women of reproductive age, (2) women of reproductive
age receiving estrogen, (3) women of postmenopausal age,
and (4) women of postmenopausal age receiving estrogen
at three time points during a month.
■, Women with hypopituitarism; □, healthy controls;
EF, early follicular phase; MC, midcycle; ML, mid-luteal
phase. $p < 0.03$ for all comparisons between women
with hypopituitarism and controls.

Figure 6.3.4. Testosterone levels in women with pituitary disease, outlined by menopausal status and by presence or absence of estrogen replacement. Reproduced with permission.[44]

cause suppression of gonadotropin-releasing hormone and subsequently the pituitary gonadotrophs, luteinizing hormone and follicle-stimulating hormone.[48] Similar medications that suppress the pituitary, ovaries, and adrenal glands, i.e., cortisone products and estrogen preparations, will also suppress hypothalamic function, as feedback androgen and estrogenic receptors are found in both the hypothalamus and the pituitary gland. The adrenal androgens are affected by acute disease stress, but cortisol production is either not affected or is increased, so that total adrenal insufficiency is rarely seen in these conditions.[49] Many chronic illnesses, such as metastatic cancer and acquired immune deficiency syndrome wasting, can cause chronic suppression of the hypothalamic hormones.[50] The central nature of this suppression has been demonstrated by a positive response of ovarian hormone to human chorionic gonadotropin stimulation.[26] At times, tumors can destroy hypothalamic tissue,

especially those that have a predilection for the suprasellar area, such as craniopharyngionoma.

Miscellaneous situations

Increase in sex hormone-binding globulin

Sex hormone-binding globulin is closely related to sex steroids because many forms of estrogen increase its biosynthesis in the liver and increase its plasma levels. The free, active, or bioavailable levels of sex steroids are determined by the equilibrium between binding and dissociation from sex hormone-binding globulin. Thus, increased plasma levels of sex hormone-binding globulin will bind sex steroids and reduce the bioavailable, and vice versa. Sex hormone-binding globulin may be considered as a measure of estradiol or testosterone clearance from the body. The binding affinity for steroids by sex hormone-binding globulin is dihydrotestosterone > testosterone > androstenediol > estradiol > estrone. Dehydroepiandrosterone is weakly bound, but dehydroepiandrosterone sulfate is not bound at all.[51] The availability of testosterone to the tissues is clinically more relevant in the discussion of sex hormone-binding globulin metabolism. Under normal physiologic conditions in women, only 1–2% of the total circulating testosterone is free or immediately bioavailable. The rest is bound, 66% bound tightly to sex hormone binding globulin and 30% bound loosely to albumin.[52]

Oral administration of estrogens, whether as postmenopausal therapy or premenopausal oral contraception, will elevate sex hormone-binding globulin, which will bind more sex steroids, causing less to be available to the tissues.[53] Oral androgen therapy will decrease sex hormone-binding globulin, and allow more hormones to act on the peripheral tissues. Parenteral delivery of sex steroids will affect sex hormone-binding globulin much less, and therefore will allow the delivery of more hormones to target tissues. An important difference is the oral contraceptive patch containing norelgestromin and ethinyl estradiol, which raises sex hormone binding globulin markedly (Ortho-McNeil Pharmaceutical, Inc.

In addition to oral estrogen therapy, sex hormone-binding globulin may be increased by pregnancy, cirrhosis or other forms of liver disease, hyperthyroidism, anorexia nervosa, or antiepileptic drugs. Apart from oral androgen therapy, sex hormone-binding globulin levels may be decreased by hypothyroidism, obesity, hyperinsulinemia, and growth hormone.[54] Several authors have found a clear-cut fall in sex hormone-binding globulin related to the menopause,[28,55] but not all.[56] Thus far, no difference in sex hormone-binding globulin levels has been noted during the premenopausal years.[17,56]

Miscellaneous or idiopathic?

Diagnosis of premenopausal women with sex hormone insufficiency is extremely difficult and controversial, especially in the absence of usual causes such as drug therapy or medical or surgical ovariectomy. Estrogen deficiency is diagnosed readily in most cases due to cessation or irregularity of menstrual periods. Any moderately severe and acute illness may cause this to happen.[42] A confusing observation is that catabolic illnesses may also be observed in women who still have regular menses.[57]

There is early evidence that premenopausal women with regular menses may have symptoms of sexual dysfunction along with androgen deficiency. Guay et al. studied healthy young women who had no identifiable cause for sex steroid deficiency, but who had symptoms of sexual dysfunction. They had significantly lower Δ5 adenal androgens and precursors than an age-matched control group.[58] These androgen levels were distinctly lower than the range of normal androgens described in a previous healthy population of premenopausal women screened for the lack of sexual dysfunction symptoms.[17] A study by Goldstat

et al. evaluated the results of androgen treatment in healthy premenopausal women, with regular menses, complaining of decreased libido.[59] The authors reported a significant improvement in well-being, mood, and sexual function with testosterone therapy over that of placebo. Doubt has been expressed about the supraphysiologic levels of androgens reached in the study.[60] If the data are compared with a normal population of premenopausal women screened for sexual dysfunction reported by decade,[17] the free androgen index of Goldstat's patients is seen to be low at 2.0 nmol/l, as compared with the low-normal value of 2.04 nmol/l reported for women in their thirties, the mean age of Goldstat's patients. Using the same normal criteria, the post-treatment free androgen index was only slightly elevated at 5.5 nmol/l, where the upper normal free androgen index for women in their twenties was found to be 4.96 nmol/l. Normal ranges of androgens in women are still to be considered estimates until more data are determined.

Measuring androgen levels in men and women

Total testosterone and free testosterone levels

Considerable energy has been devoted to determining what is the best way to determine whether a woman is capable of producing sufficient testosterone for her physiologic needs. In the woman, testosterone is partly of gonadal origin, i.e., produced within the ovarian theca cells and released into the circulation, and partly of adrenal origin. In women, testosterone is tightly bound to sex hormone-binding globulin and loosely bound to albumin. Free testosterone is that fraction of testosterone that actually interacts with androgen receptors. Measuring free testosterone has proven to be difficult. Several different free testosterone assays are now available, some with greater and others with less reliability (Table 6.3.5).

The free testosterone assays

Several free testosterone assays are currently available:

(1) free analog testosterone assay (free testosterone)
(2) free testosterone by equilibrium dialysis (free testosterone by dialysis)
(3) bioavailable testosterone (BT)
(4) free testosterone index (FTI)
(5) free testosterone by mass action–Sodergard equation

Which free testosterone assay is best and most reliable?

In an academic setting, the free testosterone by dialysis has emerged as the reference standard, the assay to which all other

Table 6.3.5. Comparison of normal ranges of testosterone (T) provided by assay vendors and observed in clinical practice. Adapted with permission from Miller KK, Rosner W, Lee H et al. Measurement of free testosterone in women with androgen deficiency: comparison of methods.. Adapted from ref 61.

Assay	Normal range provided	Normal range observed
Total T by RIA nM after column chromatography	0.35–1.91	0.14–0.98
Total T by direct RIA nM	0.35–2.77	0.35–1.23
Free T by dialysis pM	3.82–21.6	1.73–8.67
Free T analog	1.56–11.0	1.73–8.67
SHBG RIA nM	30–95	26.1–63.4

assays are compared. The free testosterone by dialysis assay may be too expensive and time-consuming, and is unlikely to provide the rapid turnaround clinicians have come to expect from their laboratories.

For clinicians who want a cost-effective test that correlates well with the free testosterone by dialysis in women, the free androgen index may be more readily available. For clinicians, the free androgen index (FAI) may be the most readily available and reliable assay to provide an estimate of female androgen sufficiency or insufficiency.

FAI = Total testosterne in ng/dL × 0.347 × 100/SHBG in nmol\L (normal range in premenopausal women found in ref. 17)

What is a normal hormone level?

For a few hormone measurements, such as prolactin and follicle-stimulating hormone, there is a general consensus of what is a below normal and excessive hormone level, so that the diagnosis of hormone sufficiency or insufficiency is relatively easy. Unfortunately, this is not the case with many of the hormones important for normal female sexual function, so the diagnosing and treating physician must rely on a package of tests to determine whether a disruption in hormone secretion is contributing to the patient's sexual distress. The patient is then at the mercy of the local laboratory that has "purchased a normal range" from the vendor supplying the materials needed to perform the specific hormone assay. When these assays are " field tested" in women of known age and medical status, the reported normal range provided by assay vendors does not always correlate with clinical observations.

Compare, for example the differences between normal ranges provided by assay vendors and actual levels of total testosterone, free testosterone, and sex hormone-binding globulin levels (Table 6.3.5). In all instances, the hormones of importance for female sexual function conform to a narrower normal range than previously suspected. When studies are expanded to include women who do or do not have sexual dysfunction, the normal range can be even more precisely defined.

For the clinician confronted with a woman with complaints of sexual dysfunction, a focused examination, as well as a symptom-specific checklist followed by targeted laboratory tests (Table 6.3.1), is the most efficient way to determine whether a treatable hormone abnormality is present and responsible for her sexual distress.

Conclusion

Sex steroid hormone deficiency in women occurs as a result of pathophysiologic changes in the ovaries, adrenal glands, or peripheral organs. Such pathophysiologic changes may be attributed to either destruction of endocrine glands and organs, or changes in the function of the hypothalamus and pituitary that regulate the biosynthesis of sex steroid hormones via protein and peptide hormones such as adrenocorticotropic hormone, luteinizing hormone, and follicle-stimulating hormone.

Similarly, the loss of function of sex steroid hormone-producing organs may be manifested by infection, medication, and illnesses or by severe emotional stress. Furthermore, factors that affect the synthesis and plasma level of sex hormone-binding globulin may also modify the bioavailability of estrogens and androgens, and this also alters their function. It has been suggested that healthy, premenopausal women, not taking medications, may also exhibit symptoms of androgen deficiency. These initial observations remain to be confirmed and related to sexual function. One key hurdle to assessment of sex steroid hormones in women, especially androgens, is the lack of analytic bioassays with reliable, sensitive, and valid measures to detect low levels of testosterone and other androgen metabolites on routine clinical and laboratory bases.

References

1. Grumbach MM, Conte FA. Disorders of sex differentiation. In JD Wilson, DW Foster, HM Kronenburg et al., eds. *Williams Textbook of Endocrinology*, 9th edn. Philadelphia: WB Saunders, 1998: 1303–1425.

2. Labrie F, Belanger A, Cusan L et al. Physiological changes in dehydroepiandrosterone are not reflected by serum levels of active androgens and estrogens but of their metabolites: intracrinology. *J Clin Endocrinol Metab* 1997; 82: 2403–9.

3. Davis SSR. Androgen treatment in women. *Med J Aust* 1999; 170: 545–9.

4. Bixo M, Andersson A, Winblad B et al. Progesterone, 5α-pregnane-3,20-dione and 3α-hydroxy-5α-pregnan-20-one in specific regions of the human female brain in different endocrine states. *Brain Res* 1997; 764: 173–8.

5. Mani S, Blaustein J, O'Malley BW. Progesterone receptor function from a behavioral perspective. *Horm Behav* 1997; 31: 244–55.

6. Sherwin BB. The impact of different doses of estrogen and progestin on mood and sexual behavior in postmenopausal women. *J Clin Endocrinol Metab* 1991; 72: 336–43.

7. Ojeda SR. Female reproductive function. In: E Griffen, SR Ojeda, eds, *Textbook of Endocrine Physiology*. New York: Oxford University Press, 1992: pp 134–68.

8. Wren B. Champion S. Willetts K et al. Transdermal progesterone and its effect on vasomotor symptoms, blood lipid levels, bone metabolic markers, moods, and quality of life for postmenopausal women. *Menopause* 2003; 10: 13–18.

9. Darney PD. The androgenicity of progestational agents. *Am J Med* 1995; 98: 104S–110S.

10. Phillips A, Hahn DW, McGuire JL. Relative binding affinity of norgestimate and other progestins for human sex hormone-binding globulin. *Steroids* 1990; 55: 373–5.

11. Legrain S, Massien C, Lahlou N et al. Dehydroepiandrosterone replacement administration: pharmacokinetic and pharmacodynamic studies in healthy elderly subjects. *J Clin Endocrinol Metab* 2000; 85: 3208–17.

12. Yen SSC. (Chapter 18) Chronic anovulation caused by peripheral endocrine disorders. In SSC Yen, RB Jaffe, RL Barbieri RL, eds. *Reproductive Endocrinology: Physiology, Pathophysiology, and clinical Management*, 4th edn. Philadelphia: WB Saunders, 1999: 479–515.

13. Lobo R. Absorption and metabolic effects of different types of estrogens and progestogens. *Obstet Gynecol Clin North Am* 1987; 14: 143–67.

14. Simpson ER. Aromatization of androgens in women: current concepts and findings. *Fertil Steril* 2002; 77 (S4): S6–S10.

15. Guay AT. Screening for androgen deficiency in women: methodological and interpretive issues. *Fertil Steril* 2002; 77 (S4): S83–8.

16. Labrie F, Belanger A, Cusan L et al. Marked decline in serum concentrations of adrenal C19 sex steroid precursors and conjugated androgen metabolites during aging. *J Clin Endocrinol Metab* 1997; 82: 2396–2402.

17. Guay A, Munarriz R, Jacobson J et al. Serum androgen levels in healthy premenopausal women with and without sexual dysfunction. Part A. Serum androgen levels in women aged 20–49 years with no complaints of sexual dysfunction. *Int J Impot Res* 2004; 16: 112–20.

18. Maccario M, Mazza E, Ramunni J et al. Relationships between dehydroepiandrosterone-sulfate and anthropometric, metabolic and hormonal variables in a large cohort of obese women. *Clin Endocrinol (Oxf)* 1999; 50: 595–600.

19. Sulcova J, Hill M, Hampl A et al. Age and sex-related differences in serum levels of unconjugated dehydroepiandrosterone and its sulfate in normal subjects. *J Endocrinol* 1997; 154: 57–62.

20. Orentreich N, Brind JL, Rizer RL et al. Age changes and sex differences in serum dehydroepiandrosterone sulfate concentrations throughout adulthood. *J Clin Endocrinol Metab* 1984; 59: 551–5.

21. Lasley B, Santoro N, Randolf J et al. The relationship of circulating dehydroepiandrosterone, testosterone and estradiol to stages of the menopausal transition and ethnicity. *J Clin Endocrinol Metab* 2002; 87: 3760–7.

22. Braunstein GD. Androgen insufficiency in women: summary of critical issues. *Fertil Steril* 2002; 77 (S4): S94–S100.

23. Judd HL, Lucas WE, Yen SSC. Effect of oophorectomy on circulating testosterone and androstenedione levels in patients with endometrial cancer. *Am J Obstet Gynecol* 1994; 118: 793–8.

24. Judd HL, Judd G, Lucas WE et al. Endocrine function of the postmenopausal ovary. Concentrations of androgens and estrogens in ovarian and peripheral venous blood. *J Clin Endocrinol.* 1974; 39: 1020–5.

25. Couzinet B, Meduri G, Lecce MG, et al. The postmenopausal ovary is not a major androgen producing gland. *J Clin Endocrinol Metab* 2001; 86: 5060–5.

26. Dunn JF, Nisula BC, Rodboard D. Transport of steroid hormones. Binding of 21 endogenous steroids to both testosterone-binding globulin and cortico-steroid binding globulin in human plasma. *J Clin Endocrinol Metab* 1981; 53: 58–68.

27. Burger HG, Dudley EC, Cui J et al. A prospective longitudinal study of serum testosterone, dehydroepiandrosterone sulfate, and sex hormone-binding globulin levels through the menopausal transition. *J Clin Endocrinol Metab* 2000; 85: 2832–8.

28. Dennerstein L, Randolph J, Taffe J et al. Hormones, mood, sexuality, and the menopausal transition. *Fertil Steril* 2002; 77 (Suppl 4): S42–8.

29. Dennerstein L, Dudley E, Burger H. Are changes in sexual functioning during midlife due to aging or menopause? *Fertil Steril* 2001: 76: 456–60.

30. Utian WH. The true clinical features of postmenopausal oophorectomy and their response to estrogen replacement therapy. *S Afr Med J* 1972; 46: 732–7.

31. Campbell S, Whitehead M. Oestrogen therapy and the menopausal syndrome. *Clin Obstet Gynecol* 1977; 4: 31–47.

32. Cardozo L, Bachmann GA, McClish D et al. Meta-analysis of estrogen therapy in the management of urogenital atrophy in postmenopausal women: second report of the Hormones and Urogenital Therapy Committee. *Obstet Gynecol* 1998; 92: 722–7.

33. Sherwin BB, Gelfand MM, Brender W. Androgen enhances sexual motivation in females: a prospective, crossover study of sex steroid administration in surgical menopause. *Psychosom Med* 1985; 47: 339–51.

34. Davis SR, McCloud PI, Strauss BJG et al. Testosterone enhances estradil's effects on postmenopausal bone density and sexuality. *Maturitas* 1995; 21: 227–36.

35. Abraham GE, Chakmakjian ZH. Serum steroid levels during the menstrual cycle in a bilaterally adrenalized woman. *J Clin Endocrinol Metab* 1973; 37: 581–7.

36. Zumoff B, Strain GW, Miller LK et al. Twenty-four hour mean plasma testosterone concentration declines with age in normal premenopausal women. *J Clin Endocrinol Metab* 1995; 80: 1429–30.

37. Arlt W, Callies F, Van Vlijmen JC et al. Dehydroepiandrosterone replacement in women with adrenal insufficiency. *N Engl J Med* 1999; 341: 1013–20.

38. Hunt P, Gurnell E, Huppert F. Improvement in mood and fatigue after dehydroepiandrosterone replacement in Addison's disease in a randomized, double blind trial. *J Clin Endocrinol Metab* 2000; 85: 4650–6.

39. Abraham GE. Ovarian and adrenal contribution to peripheral androgens during the menstrual cycle. *J Clin Endocrinol Metab* 1974; 39: 340–6.

40. Cunningham SK, McKenna TJ. Dissociation of adrenal androgens and cortisol secretion in Cushing's syndrome. *Clin Endocrinol (Oxf)* 1994; 41: 795–800.

41. Parker LN, Levin ER, Lifrat ET. Evidence for adrenocortical adaptation to severe illness. *J Clin Endocrinol Metab* 1985; 60; 947–52.

42. Parker LM, Eugene J, Farber D et al. Dissociation of adrenal androgen and cortisol levels in acute stress. *Horm Metab Res* 1985; 17: 209–12.

43. Zumoff B, Walsh B, Katz J. Subnormal plasma dehydroepiandrosterone to cortisol ratio in anorexia nervosa: a second hormone parameter of ontogenic regression. *J Clin Endocrinol Metab* 1983; 56: 668–72.

44. Miller KK, Sesmilo G, Schiller A et al. Androgen deficiency in women with hypopituitarism. *J Clin Endocrinol Metab* 2001; 86: 561–7.

45. Guay AT, Agnello V, Tronic BC et al. Lymphocytic hypophysitis in a man. *J Clin Endocrinol Metab* 1987; 64: 631–4.

46. Miller K. Androgen deficiency in women. *J Clin Endocrinol Metab* 2001; 86: 2395–2401.

47. Tuiten A, Laan E, Panhuysen G et al. Discrepancies between genital responses and subjective sexual function during progesterone substitution in women with hypothalamic amenorrhea. *Psychosom Med* 1996; 58: 234–41.

48. Gebhart SP, Watts NB, Clark R et al. Reversible impairement of gonadotropin secretion in critical illness. *Arch Int Med* 1989; 149: 1637–41.

49. Miller K, Corcoran C, Armstrong C. Transdermal testosterone administration in women with acquired immunodeficiency syndrome wasting: a pilot study. *J Clin Endocrinol Metab* 1998; 83: 2717–5.

50. Grinspoon S, Corcoran C, Stanley T et al. Mechanisms of androgen deficiency in human immunodeficiency virus-infected women with the wasting syndrome. *J Clin Endocrinol Metab* 2001; 86: 4120–6.

51. Davis SR, Guay AT, Shifren JL et al. Endocrine aspects of female sexual dysfunction. In: Lue TF, Basson R, Rosen R, Giuliano F, Khoury S, Montorsi F eds. Sexual Medicine: Sexual Dysfunctions in Men and Women. Paris: Health Publications, 2004: 749–781.

52. Mather RS, Landgrebe SC, Moody LO, et al. The effect of estrogen treatment on plasma concentrations of steroid hormones, gonadotropins, prolactin and sex steroid-binding globulin in postmenopausal women. *Maturitas* 1985; 7: 129–33.

53. Guay A, Davis SR. Testosterone insufficiency in women: fact or fiction? *World J Urol* 2002; 20: 106–10.

54. Rannevik G, Jeppsson S, Johnell O. A longitudinal study of the perimenpausal transition: altered profiles of steroid and pituitary hormones, SHBG and bone mineral density. *Maturitas* 1986; 8: 189–96.

55. Bancroft J, Cawood EHH. Anadrogens and the menopause: a study of 40–60 year old women. *Clin Endocrinol* 1996; 45: 577–87.

56. Davis S, Schneider H, Donarti-Sarti C et al. Androgen levels in normal and oophorectomized women. *Climacteric* 2002; Proceedings of the 10th International Congress on the Menopause, Berlin.

57. Dolan S, Wilkie S, Aliabadi N et al. Effects of testosterone administration in human immunodifficiency virus – infected women with low weight. *Arch Int Med* 2004; 164: 897–904.

58. Guay A, Jacobson J, Munarriz R et al. Serum androgen levels in healthy premenopausal women with and without sexual dysfunction. Part B. Reduced serum androgen levels in healthy premenopausal women with complaints of sexual dysfunction. *Int J Impot Res* 2004; 16: 121–9.

59. Goldstat R, Briganti E, Tran J et al. Transdermal testosterone therapy improves well-being, mood, and sexual function in premenopausal women. *Menopause* 2003; 10: 390–8.

60. Shifren JL. The role of androgens in female sexual dysfunction. *Mayo Clin Proc* 2004; 79 (Suppl): S19–S24.

6.4 The physiology and pathophysiology of the female orgasm

Roy J Levin

Introduction

While males have little or no difficulty in having and identifying their orgasms, this cannot be said for a significant proportion of women. Two topics of female sexuality and its dysfunctions, the difficulty in inducing orgasm, especially through coitus, and recognizing that an orgasm has occurred, have been discussed at length.

It is often stated that for men orgasm is the hoped-for goal whenever they initiate a sexual scenario, but that this is not the case with women. Women, it is claimed, value the "afterglow" of the sexual arousal and the physical intimacy of being cuddled as much as the orgasm.[1,2] In one survey, admittedly questioning self-selected women subjects, affection, love, and intimacy were given as the major reasons for liking coitus, with the act of penetration rather than orgasm *per se* as their favorite sexual experience.[3] These American studies were undertaken some 30 years ago, and, as the sexual perceptions and attitudes of individuals and societies change, their conclusions may not now be valid. In fact, orgasm and its difficulties have been claimed as the second most reported sexual problem for women.[4] A study conducted in 1992 looked at the relationship between sexual enjoyment and orgasm in couples attending university.[5] It was reported that "nothing in the data supports the cultural stereotype that orgasms are more important to men than to women." When asked whether "sex without orgasm cannot really be satisfying" in a recent, statistically valid, national survey of British sexual behavior, approximately half of the men (48.7%) agreed that orgasm was necessary to male sexual satisfaction, and when women were asked, some 43% also agreed that this was so for men.[6] When the question was asked in relation to women, 37% of men agreed, while 29% of women also agreed with the statement. Thus, nearly a third of women, a highly significant percentage, do think orgasm is important. Apart from the obvious reward of its ecstatic pleasure, the physiology of female sexual arousal may be the reason for women desiring orgasm. Sexual arousal creates hyperemia and vasocongestion in a wide number of female pelvic structures (uterus, vagina, clitoris, urethra, labia, pelvic ligaments, and even possibly the fallopian tubes and ovaries), giving rise to an uncomfortable feeling of "pelvic fullness" (see Chapters 5.1– 5.6, 6.1, and 6.2). Its dissipation is very slow, even with orgasm, which facilitates the action, although a single orgasm does not usually cause complete dissipation.[7] Orgasms, however, are the natural and pleasant means to ameliorate the pelvic discomfort.

Objective specific indices of the female orgasm

"How does an orgasmic-naive woman know that an orgasm has occurred?" Levin[8] discussed the problem by asking, "Who defines what an orgasm is?" The subjective experience of orgasm (ecstasy, euphoria, and extreme pleasure) is normally accompanied by physiologic body changes, a number of which have been used to indicate that an orgasm is impending, is occurring, or has occurred. The descriptions of many of these changes come from the classic observations of Masters and Johnson[7] nearly 40 years ago, but a few newer ones have been added since. These specific objective indicators which occur either just before, during, or after the female orgasm are listed in Table 6.4.1. They have been discussed critically and fully in a recent review on the female orgasm.[9] The most quoted physical indicator for the occurrence of an orgasm is that of contractions of the vaginal/pelvic striated muscles (see Chapter 4.4 in this volume), but some women say they have orgasms without experiencing such contractions, although they may be weak and thus women are unaware of them.[9,10]

Table 6.4.1. Specific objective indicators of the female orgasm

Those indicating impending orgasm (prospective)
(i)   Colour changes of the labia minora (pink to deep red)

Those occurring during the orgasm (current)
(i)   Vaginal contractions (induced by rhythmic pelvic striated muscle contractions)
(ii)   Uterine contractions
(iii) Anal sphincter contractions
(iv)   Release of prolactin

Those occurring after orgasm (retrospective)
(i)   Areolar decongestion (rapid, causes corrugation of areolae)
(ii)   Raised and maintained prolactin levels in the plasma
(iii) Increase vaginal pulse amplitude (VPA) as measured by a vaginally inserted, free, indwelling photoplethsymograph.

Typologies of female orgasm

Early psychoanalytic opinion about the female orgasm (see Chapters 1.1, 3.1, and 11.1) proposed a dual typology; because they were easier to obtain, those obtained by stimulation of the clitoris were regarded as "less mature", the only authentic orgasms being those obtained through vaginal coitus.[11] This duality developed into the concept that female orgasms were obtained from either clitoral or vaginal stimulation. The literature abounds with descriptions and discussion of vaginal as opposed to clitoral orgasms.[7] Anecdotal reports from women revealed that those obtained from the clitoris used descriptions employing the words "warm", "ticklish", "electrical", and "sharp" whereas those from vaginal stimulation were more often referred to as "throbbing", "deep", "soothing", and "comfortable".[12] Kinsey et al.[13] and Masters and Johnson[7] reported that the vagina had few sensory receptors and that some clitoral stimulation would occur from penile thrusting during coitus. Moreover, according to Ingelman-Sundberg,[14] the vagina acts like a hummock around the urethra, so that during vaginal coitus, the penis stretches two of the ligaments inserted around the base of the clitoris (see Chapters 4.1–4.4). Thus, coitus should always create a mixture of vaginal and clitoral stimulations. If this is true, the anatomic basis of the different feelings is puzzling unless we accept that, mentally and emotionally, coitus (where the vagina is distended) and stimulation of the clitoris *per se* are likely to be appreciated differently.[10,15] Masters and Johnson[7] posed the question: are clitoral and vaginal orgasms truly separate anatomic entities? Their answer was an unequivocal "no". They stated "from an anatomic point of view there is absolutely no difference in the responses of the pelvic viscera to effective sexual stimulation regardless of whether the stimulation occurs as a result of the clitoral-body or mons area manipulation, natural or artificial coition, or, for that matter, specific stimulation of any other erogenous area of the female body". Most of their changes that supported this statement came from direct observations with few physiologic measurements. More recent physiologic recordings of uterine smooth muscle and pelvic striated muscle contractions during orgasms induced by stimulating either the anterior vaginal wall (G spot) or the clitoris have revealed different patterns of contractions of these muscles, suggesting that there may well be objective evidence of at least two types of orgasmic response created by the stimulation of different genital sites. A set of these myographic recordings by John Perry is shown by Levin.[16]

A frequently quoted typology is that of Singer,[17] a philosopher without any experience in laboratory studies, who proposed three types of orgasm from published descriptions: (1) "vulval", showing rhythmic contractions of the vagina activated by clitoral or coital stimulation; (2) "uterine", without vaginal contractions but accompanied by apnea and gasping activated during coitus and largely due to penis–cervix contact; and (3) "blended", containing elements of both vulval and uterine orgasms activated by coitus and accompanied by apnea.

Singer's evidence for this typology relied on remarkably limited scientific observations obtained from a very few subjects, and he used a novelist's description (see Levin[16] for extended critical discussion). The importance of cervical stimulation by the thrusting penis in this typology was not about stimulating the organ *per se*, but of its displacement, causing it to rub against the peritoneal membrane claimed to be "a highly sensitive structure".[18] However, a recent review of the cervix in sexual arousal concluded that the evidence for or against its involvement in orgasm was weak and that observational studies could not answer the question.[19]

John Perry and Beverly Whipple, in *The G-Spot and Other Recent Discoveries About Human Sexuality*, proposed an interesting "continuum schema or typology" for the female orgasm that incorporated Singer's categories but added those originating from the G-spot (anterior vaginal wall) stimulation.[20] At one end were orgasms produced by clitoral stimulation that created rhythmic contractions of the pelvic muscles (mainly mediated through the pudendal nerve), while at the other end were those produced from stimulation of the G-spot (mainly mediated through the pelvic and hypogastric nerves), which expressed uterine contractions (see previous description above of Perry's myographic data). In the middle were the two types of orgasm that probably occur most often. This "continuum" typology, however, did not catch on.

The most recent typology for female orgasms was developed by Bohlen et al.[21], using the different types of vaginal contractions recorded during laboratory studies of orgasm. They divided orgasms into those that had regular rhythmic contractions (mean duration of orgasm about 13 s), those that had regular contractions with later irregular ones (mean duration 51 s), and those that had no regular rhythmic contractions during their orgasms (mean duration of orgasm 24 s). The differences in the duration of these orgasms are remarkably large: Levin and Wagner, who timed the orgasms of their 26 laboratory subjects, recorded a mean (± SD) duration of 19.9 ± 12 s.[22] Unfortunately, only 11 nulliparous subjects were studied by Bohlen et al.[21], and no other confirmatory studies have been published. A general classification of female orgasm built on such a limited number of subjects must remain *sub judice*. Mah and Binik[23] have discussed the variability of human orgasmic expression in terms of typologies.

Functional imaging of the brain at orgasm

One of the more recent and exciting technological advances in sexual arousal studies has been the use of functional brain imaging to identify which areas are activated or inhibited by sexual behaviors. A number of studies on sexual arousal and orgasm (ejaculation) have been carried out in men, but few so far in women. Holstege et al.[24] used blood oxygenation level-dependent positron emission tomography to record the various parts of the brain involved in ejaculation (and thus orgasm) in men during an observational window of some 60 s (see Chapter 10.2). A large number of sites were found to be highly active – the mesodiencephalic transition zone, including the ventral tegmental area, midbrain lateral and central field, zona incerta, subparafaccicular nucleus, thalamic nuclei (ventral, posterior midline, and intralaminar), cerebellum, lateral putamen, and claustrum – while there was neocortical activity in Brodman's areas 7/40, 18, 21, 23, and 47. Two sites were deactivated, the amygdala and the entorhinal cortex, while the hypothalamus showed (during the short period of observation) no activity (see Chapters 5.2 and 5.3). The reason for detailing these sites in men is that Holstege,[25] at a recent conference, reported that the pattern of activation of these sites was similar during orgasm in women except for two outstanding differences: first, the amygdala was active in women and not deactivated; second, the periaqueductal gray area was activated, but this was not seen in men.

One of the difficulties in interpreting these data is that many of the brain areas apparently involved in arousal/orgasm are also known to be involved in other body functions. The amygdala, for example, is involved among other things in anxiety, fear, and anger, while the periaqueductal gray area receives input from the amygdala, lateral stria terminalis, hypothalamus (medial and lateral), preoptic region, and parts of the prefrontal cortex. It sends its outputs to the spinal cord directly and indirectly, and these are involved in nociception control, micturition, vocalization, and pupil dilation. The most interesting of these, perhaps, is the nociception control, with the stimulation of periaqueductal gray area creating an analgesic effect. Vaginal self-stimulation has been claimed to raise the pain threshold in women, while the induction of orgasm further raised it, both without changing tactile sensitivity.[26] Thus, activation of the periaqueductal gray area during female orgasm may well be through this mechanism.

Development of pleasure from orgasms

Two opposing views of obtaining orgasmic release are that it is simply a reflex involving a stimulus–response reaction,[27] or

that the sensations of orgasm have no immanent meaning attached to them and that they are identified by women as "orgasm" because of the situation in which they occur rather than due to specific connection between sensory inputs and the brain. It is thus a "learned" activity.[28] Mead observed, "the human female's capacity for orgasm is to be viewed more as a potentiality that may or may not be developed by a given culture" and "the capacity to learn a total orgasmic response is present differentially in all women."[29] Certainly, the pleasure associated with coitus and its orgasms appears to be a learned activity.[10]

Why do women, but not men, have multiple serial orgasms?

One obvious difference between orgasms in men and women is that women can have multiple serial orgasms,[10] with the latter ones being as good as or even better than the first. Most males have a post-ejaculatory refractory time. It has been proposed that the release of prolactin at the time of orgasm causes the post-ejaculatory refractory time in men, but women do not experience this. Presumably, prolactin released at orgasm acts differently in women.[30]

The arousal sites to trigger orgasm

The induction of female orgasm can occur from a variety of anatomic sites. These include the major ones of the clitoris (especially the glans) and the vagina (especially the anterior wall that includes Halban's fascia, the urethra, and the G-spot), but orgasm can be obtained by stimulation of the periurethral glans area (the area surrounding the urethral meatus), mons, or breasts/nipples by mental imagery or fantasy, or even by hypnotic suggestion. Kinsey et al.[13] reported that orgasm could occur even from bizarre stimulations such as that of the teeth or blowing on the hair of subjects. Consciousness is not a requirement, as orgasm is known to occur during sleep.

Putative roles of orgasm in reproduction

In no other area of the female orgasm has so much been attributed with so little scientific evidence. Time and again authors repeat the mantra that the contractions of the uterus induced at orgasm will facilitate sperm transport by increasing the rate at which they will be moved along the female genital tract. This faster transport, it is then said, will aid fertility. The reality, however, is that the fastest sperm transport in the female genital tract is observed in the nonaroused female! This has been shown experimentally.[31] Rapid sperm transport during coitus has been inferred from the results of Settlage et al., who actually studied their transport in anesthetized women during surgery.[32] While their findings have been equated to what occurs during coitus in the sexually aroused women, the two conditions are entirely different and cannot be compared. Levin has described the differences and why the conclusions from the experiments are physiologically invalid.[33] In fact, as the women in the Settlage et al.[32] experiments were anesthetized and thus could not be sexually excited, they would indeed have shown the rapid transport of sperm as expected. The scenario during coitus is quite different. Sexual arousal causes vaginal tenting to occur, elevating the cervix well away from the vaginal posterior wall and the ejaculate. Under these conditions, uterine contractions would have no effect on sperm transport because the cervix is not in contact with the semen. Only when resolution of the sexual arousal occurs does the cervix get immersed into the now liquefied seminal pool. Levin has described this scenario in detail and the importance to reproduction that delaying the sperm transport creates.[34] Orgasm, by hastening the descent of the cervix into the seminal pool, may not be the most facilitatory factor in fertilization. There is, however, some evidence that after arousal/orgasm the female genital tract has an inhibited motility.[34]

Baker and Bellis[35] made a number of provocative suggestions, based on their studies of the amount of leakage of semen from the vagina (termed "flowback"), about how the occurrence and timing of female orgasm in relation to copulation and male ejaculation influenced the number of sperm retained at both the current and next copulation.

Orgasms were claimed to generate a "blow–suck" mechanism that could take sperm or acid vaginal contents into the cervical fluid, thus affecting sperm viability. A chosen orgasm strategy could be used to facilitate pregnancy from a particular desired partner, not necessarily the husband. These suggestions and conclusions are controversial and have yet to be accepted or confirmed by others.[34]

Why do women have contractions of their pelvic muscles at orgasm?

Males need striated muscle contractions to forcefully eject their semen.[36] Many women, although not all, experience striated pelvic muscle contractions at orgasm, but their function is unknown. The contractions may cause the pleasure experienced at orgasm, but simply contracting muscles voluntarily does not yield ecstasy. The contractions may dissipate the pelvic vasocongestion induced by arousal, but multiple orgasms would be needed to evacuate the blood congestion. The contractions may be for expressing the female urethral expulsions. Not all females have urethral expulsions (from the periurethral glands), and in those that do, the volume expelled is normally around 0.5 ml. Powerful striated contractions are hardly necessary for such a volume. However, it is possible that the contractions serve a "housekeeping" function, "sweeping" out any residual or buildup of secretions in the urethra, although subsequent urination would suffice. It is possible the

contractions serve to excite the male to ejaculate during coitus, thus capturing his sperm. This would be a reproductive function, but most males have ejaculated before females have their coital orgasm. Finally, the contractions could simply be an example of a "biological spandrel"[37] – a mechanism, function, or structure that has no apparent function in one sex but is present because it is essential in the other. The striated musculature of the pelvis stems from a common fetal prototype. While its contractions at orgasm may have no function in the female, they do no harm.

Vocalizations at coitus and orgasm

Both males and females make involuntary sounds during high levels of sexual arousal and at orgasm, conveying the acceptance, the effectiveness of the sexual arousal, the pleasure induced, and the approach and arrival of orgasm.[38] These erotic sounds made by the female are highly exciting to males and enhance their arousal, thus facilitating ejaculation and the capture of the semen. Apart from this, Passie et al.[39] have suggested that the groaning and hyperventilation can create hypocapnia (lowered plasma partial pressure of carbon dioxide) that reduces cerebral blood flow mainly in the neocortex gray matter rather than in the limbic structures. The imbalance may intensify the emotional states of the sexual experience.

Arousal and orgasm in nonconsenting subjects

When both parties are willing to partake in sexual stimulation, the outcome of sexual arousal and orgasm is usually welcome. Thus, the mental state of the parties is one of happy acceptance of the arousal and the orgasm(s) to come. Without this state, it is often thought that arousal and orgasm would be difficult to achieve. What happens, then, in the case of nonconsenting women subjected to sexual stimulation through force, fear, or an impaired state of consciousness (sleep, drug, alcohol, or hypnotically induced)? Levin and van Berlo[40] posed the question of whether or not the female can experience sexual arousal and orgasm involuntarily or even against her will. Upon review of the topic and its limited literature, Levin and van Berlo[40] concluded that such stimulation can and does lead to unwanted arousal and even orgasm, but that such outcomes cannot be used as a sexual assault defense to imply that the subject consented to the stimulation.

The pathophysiology of female orgasm

Nosology and terminology

The nosology of women's sexual disorders is formalized in the American Psychiatric Association's *Diagnostic and Statistical*

Manual of Mental Disorders (DSM), fourth edition (DSM-IV-TR),[41] and in the International Statistical Classification of Diseases and Related Health Problems (ICD-10).[42] The diagnostic criteria in relation to orgasmic dysfunction are shown in Table 6.4.2 from the DSM, and from the ICD-10 classification of mental and behavioral disorders diagnostic for research by the World Health Organization. Both rely on the sexual response cycle as described by Masters and Johnson[7,43] and modified by Kaplan.[27]

There has been increasing criticism of this nosology and even a recent attempt to modify the definitions of female sexual dysfunction by a 17-member international consensus committee,[44] who stated: "Orgasmic disorder is the persistent or recurrent difficulty, delay in, or absence of attaining orgasm following sufficient sexual stimulation and arousal which causes personal distress." Even the deliberations of this group failed to satisfy the critics.[45] More recently, a second, self-selected group, comprising seven of the previous one with six new participants, have made further suggestions to revise the previous revision in the light of a burgeoning evidence-based movement. However, as they state, many of the suggested revisions and expansions will need to be tested for validity and usefulness in the clinical setting. The methodological difficulties of characterizing female sexual dysfunction in relation to definitions (see previous comment), assessment (use of self-reported data), and type of population (selection bias, prevalence, and incidence estimates) have been discussed at length in another committee report published in 2000,[46] and they will not be repeated here. One difficulty with the diagnostic criteria of DSM-IV is that if a woman is diagnosed as having an orgasmic disorder, it precludes her from having a sexual arousal disorder, but, in reality, many women with orgasmic disorders also have arousal disorders.[47] Indeed, comorbidity seems to be the usual condition of female sexual dysfunction(s) rather than its being isolated into the specific diagnostic categories.[48] Other complications involve terms such as "lifelong versus acquired" and "generalized versus situational circumstances". It is not always clear whether a secondary disorder is acquired under any circumstances. There are serious problems with the whole concept of female sexual dysfunctions, even to the extent that some authors claim that they are influenced too much by the needs of the pharmaceutic industry.[49,50]

The assessment and subsequent treatment of orgasmic dysfunction by Masters and Johnson[43] was a milestone. They diagnosed a woman as having "primary orgasmic dysfunction" if she reported lack of orgasm during her entire life span, whatever the method used to try to induce an orgasm. If a woman had experienced at least one instance of orgasm, regardless of the method of stimulation used, she was classified as having "situational orgasmic dysfunction". Three arbitrary categories of this dysfunction were defined further: masturbatory orgasmic inadequacy, where the woman is unable to achieve orgasm by masturbation even though it has occurred during coital activity; coital orgasmic inadequacy, where the woman is unable to achieve orgasm through coitus, although she is orgasmic through masturbation by herself or her partner; and random orgasmic inadequacy, where the woman has had coital and/or masturbatory orgasms, but they are rare and usually unexpected.

While the term "primary orgasmic dysfunction" has remained in the clinical literature, the situational dysfunction has been renamed "secondary orgasmic dysfunction". The term "frigidity" has disappeared from the literature,[51] but the term "anorgasmia" is used for persistent and recurring difficulty in achieving orgasm.

Prevalence of impaired orgasm

The prevalence of orgasmic dysfunction in a statistically valid sample of the general female population has been difficult to ascertain. Recently, Bancroft et al. undertook a national telephone survey of female distress about sex in their heterosexual relationships over an age range of 20–65 years.[52] They reported

---

Table 6.4.2. Diagnostic criteria for orgasmic dysfunction from DSM-IV and ICD-10

DSM-IV: Female orgasmic dysfunction (302.73)
1. Persistent or recurrent delay in, or absence of, orgasm following a normal sexual excitement phase, Women exhibit wide variability in the type of intensity of stimulation that triggers orgasm the diagnosis of female orgasmic disorder should be based on the clinician's judgment that the woman's orgasmic capacity is less than would be reasonable for her age, sexual experience, and the adequacy of sexual stimulation that she receives.
2. The disturbance causes a marked distress or interpersonal difficulty.
3. The orgasmic dysfunction is not better accounted for by another Axis 1 disorder (other than a sexual dysfunction) and is not due exclusively to the direct physiological effects of a substance (e.g., a drug of abuse, a medication) or a general medical condition.

CD-10: Orgasmic dysfunction (F32.3)
1. The general criteria for sexual dysfunction (F52) must be met.
2. There is orgasmic dysfunction (either absence or marked delay of orgasm) which takes one of the following forms:
   (i) orgasm has never been experienced in any situation
   (ii) orgasmic dysfunction has developed after a period of relatively normal response
       (a) general orgasmic dysfunction occurs in all situations and with any partner;
       (b) situational for women, orgasm does occur in certain situations (e.g., when masturbating or with certain partners).

that 9.3% of their sample had "impaired orgasm" (not specifically defined), and they compared this with four other surveys undertaken in 1988–99, which quoted a prevalence of "impaired orgasms" of 16–27%. Thus, orgasm difficulties, as reported by the women's own assessments, are probably around 9–27%.

Causes of orgasmic dysfunction

It is said that 90% of female orgasmic difficulties arise from psychologic/sociologic causes: poor sexual communication and knowledge, inadequate or unsuitable stimulation, poor relationships, traumatic early sexual experiences, and mental conditions (mood disorders or mental illness). Some of other possible causes of orgasmic dysfunction are listed in Table 6.4.3 (see Chapter 9.4).

Treatments

Although disorders of orgasm have been treated by a variety of methods,[53] extensive empirical outcome research for controlled and uncontrolled studies is available mainly for cognitive behavioral approaches and less so for pharmacologic approaches (see Chapter 11.4).[54] These will be described briefly. In general, the hierarchy of successful treatment is that it is greatest with self-induced orgasm, less with partner-induced orgasm by manual or oral stimulation, and least with coitus without any other stimulation. Outcome is also better for women who have never had an orgasm than for those with a desire to increase orgasms with partner sex.

For a review of the field of sex therapy, the analysis of Schover and Leiblum is very critical as it claimed that the field was in the doldrums.[55] In the case of the treatment for female orgasmic disorder, they argued that all the major components were present in the 1970s and few new treatments had been added. Furthermore, outcome research, especially long term, was conspicuously absent.

Directed masturbation

Directed masturbation is used in a variety of contexts including group, individual, couples therapy, and bibliography. It is highly successful for treating primary anorgasmia.[56]

Extended foreplay and intromission did not enhance female coital response.[57]

Anxiety reduction techniques

The treatment originating from Masters and Johnson[43] is their "sensate focus" that involves a graded (step-by-step), hierarchic sequence of body touching routed through nondemand genital touching by partner, guidance by female of genital manual and penile stimulation, and using coital positions to enhance pleasurable stimulation. Most studies now use this in combination with adjuvants such as sexual technique training, sex and communication education, bibliography, and pelvic exercises (Kegel exercises).

Miscellaneous techniques

The concept that protracted foreplay and coitus will significantly increase the probability of the woman's attaining coital orgasm is not substantiated by empirical data.[53] Kegel reported that his pelvic exercises for prevention of stress incontinence appeared to improve the sexual pleasure and orgasms of the women who practiced them. Other studies, however, could not show this improvement (see Levin[58] for brief review). Techniques for educating women about their anatomy and for enhancing communication skills have been effective in facilitating orgasmic ability.[59]

The coital alignment technique, a positional method (pelvic male override in the missionary position) to create stimulation of the clitoris during coital penile thrusting and thus enhance sexual arousal, is claimed to bring about female coital orgasm only if given the proper time to be learned and practiced correctly.[60] It was found, however, to create more improvements in orgasmic ability than simply using directed masturbation.[61]

Pharmacologic treatments

At present, no pharmacologic agent has been proven to be better than placebo in facilitating orgasmic function in women. Open-label trials without benefit of comparison with placebo often give false hopes. It is surprising how many researchers and investigators appear to forget that the human mind, given appropriate cues, is capable of either facilitating or inhibiting sexual

Table 6.4.3. Some nonpsychologic causes of female orgasmic dysfunction

1. **Neurological disorders**
   Damage to sacral/pelvic nerves, multiple sclerosis, Parkinson's disease, narcolepsy, epilepsy, spina bifida, amytrophic lateral sclerosis

2. **Surgical conditions**
   Obstetrical trauma, hysterectomy complications, scarring from episiotomy, radical cystectomy

3. **Genital dysfunctions**
   Clitoral adhesions, vulvodynia

4. **Endocrine/medical disorders**
   Diabetes mellitus, hypothalamo–pituitary disorders, Sickle cell anaemia

5. **Drugs/medication**
   Antidepressants, antipsychotics, antihypertensives, antiepileptics, alpha blockers, recreational drugs (chronic use)- heroin (& methadone), cocaine
   cancer chemotherapy
   3,4-methyfenedioxymethamphatamine (MDMA or ecstacy)- orgasmic delay

arousal and orgasm. Meston et al. stress the importance of using a placebo based on the results of their study with ephedrine.[9]

Conclusion

An orgasm in the human female is a variable, transient peak sensation of intense pleasure creating an altered state of consciousness, usually with an initiation accompanied by involuntary, rhythmic contractions of the pelvic striated, circumvaginal musculature. There are often concomitant uterine and anal contractions and myotonia that resolve the sexually induced vasocongestion (sometimes only partially) and myotonia usually with an induction of well-being and contentment.[62] More simply, while sexual arousal creates hyperemia and vasocongestion in female pelvic structures, orgasms may be considered as the natural and pleasant means to ameliorate the pelvic discomfort. Clinically, orgasmic dysfunction is a common source of distress, and treatments require more evidence-based safety and efficacy data. More research is needed in the physiology of orgasm and the pathophysiology of orgasmic dysfunction in women.

References

1. Hollender MH. The need or wish to be held. *Arch Gen Psychiatry* 1970; 22; 445–53.
2. Schaefer LC. *Women and Sex*. London: Hutchinson, 1974.
3. Hite S. *The Hite Report: A Nationwide Study of Female Sexuality*. New York: Dell, 1976.
4. Lauman, EO, Gagnon JH, Michael RT et al. *The Social Organisation of Sexuality: Sexual Practices in the United States*. Chicago: University of Chicago, 1994.
5. Waterman CK, Chiauzzi EJ. The role of orgasm in male and female sexual enjoyment. *J Sex Res* 1992: 18: 146–59.
6. Wellings K, Field, J, Johnson AM et al. *Sexual Behaviour in Britain*. London: Penguin Books, 1994.
7. Masters WH, Johnson VE. *Human Sexual Response*. Boston: Little, Brown, 1966.
8. Levin RJ. An orgasm is … who defines what an orgasm is? *Sex Relatsh Ther* 2004; 19: 101–7.
9. Meston C, Hull E, Levin RJ, Sipski M. Women's orgasm. In TF Lue, R Basson, R Rosen et al., eds. *Sexual Medicine: Sexual Dysfunctions in Men and Women*. Paris: Health Publications, 2004: 783–850.
10. Levin RJ. The female orgasm – a current appraisal. *J Psychosom Res* 1981; 25: 119–33.
11. Shainess N. Authentic feminine orgastic responses. In ET Adelson, ed. *Sexuality and Psychoanalysis*. New York: Brunner/Mazel, 1975: 145–60.
12. Fisher S. *The Female Orgasm*. New York: Basic Books, 1973.
13. Kinsey AC, Pomeroy WB, Martin C et al. *Sexual Behaviour in the Human Female*. Philadelphia: WB Saunders, 1953.
14. Ingelman-Sundberg A. The anterior vaginal wall as an organ for the transmission of active forces to the urethra and clitoris. *Int Urogynecol J Pelvic Floor Dysfunct* 1997; 8: 50–1.
15. Levin RJ. Is prolactin the biological "off-switch" for human sexual arousal? *Sex Relatsh Ther* 2003; 18: 282–7.
16. Levin RJ. Sexual desire and the deconstruction and reconstruction of the human female sexual response model of Masters and Johnson. In W Everaerd, E Laan & S Both, eds. *Sexual Appetite, Desire and Motivation: Energetics of the Sexual System*. Amsterdam: Royal Netherlands Academy of Arts and Science, 2001.
17. Singer I. *The Goals of Human Sexuality*. London: Wildwood House, 1973: pp 72–5.
18. Singer J, Singer I. Types of female orgasm. *J Sex Res* 1972; 8: 255–67.
19. Grimes DA. Role of the cervix in sexual response. Evidence for and against. *Clin Obstet Gynecol* 1999; 42: 972–8.
20. Ladas AK, Whipple B, Perry J. *The G-Spot and Other Recent Discoveries About Human Sexuality*. New York: Holt, Rinehart & E Winston, 1982: 149–51.
21. Bohlen G, Held JP, Sanderson MO et al. The female orgasm: pelvic contractions. *Arch Sex Behav* 1982; 11: 367–86.
22. Levin RJ, Wagner G. Orgasm in women in the laboratory – quantitative studies on duration, intensity, latency, and vaginal blood flow. *Arch Sex Behav* 1985; 14: 439–49.
23. Mah K, Binik YM. The nature of the human orgasm: a critical review of major trends. *Clin Psychol Rev* 2001; 21: 823–56.
24. Holstege GG, Geiorgiadis JR, Paans AM et al. Brain activation during human male ejaculation. *J Neurosci* 2003; 33: 9185–9.
25. Holstege GG. The central nervous system control of female orgasm. *International Society for the Study of Women's Sexual Health. Annual Meeting, Amsterdam, The Netherlands*. 2003; Abstract, 179.
26. Whipple B, Komisaruk BR. Elevation of pain threshold by vaginal stimulation in women. *Pain* 1985; 21: 357–67.
27. Kaplan H. *The New Sex Therapy: Active Treatment of Sexual Dysfunctions*. New York: Brunner-Mazel, 1974.
28. Eysenck HJ, Wilson G. *The Psychology of Sex*. London: JM Dent, 1979.
29. Mead M. *Male and Female*. New York: William Morrow, 1949.
30. Levin RJ. Do women gain anything from coitus apart from pregnancy? Changes in the human female genital tract activated by coitus. *J Sex Marital Ther* 2003; 29: 59–69.
31. Kunz G, Beil D, Deininger H et al. The dynamics of rapid sperm transport through the female genital tract: evidence from vaginal sonography of uterine peristalsis and hysterosalpingoscintigraphy. *Hum Reprod* 1996; 11: 627–32.
32. Settlage DSF, Motoshima M, Tredway DR. Sperm transport from the external cervical os to the fallopian tube in women; a time and quantitation study. *Fertil Steril* 1973; 24: 655–61.
33. Levin RJ. Sex and the human female reproductive tract – what really happens during and after coitus. *Int J Impot Res* 1998; 10(Suppl 1): S14–S21.
34. Levin RJ. The physiology of sexual arousal in the human female: a recreational and procreational synthesis. *Arch Sex Behav* 2002; 31: 405–11.
35. Baker RR, Bellis MA. *Human Sperm Competition, Copulation, Masturbation and Infidelity*. London: Chapman & Hall, 1995.

36. Gerstenberg TC, Levin RJ, Wagner G. Erection and ejaculation in man. Assessment of the electromyographic activity of the bulbocavernosus and ischiocavernosus muscles. *Br J Urol* 1990; 65: 395–402.

37. Gould SJ, Lewontin RC. The spandrels of San Marco and the Panglossian paradigm: a critique of the adaptionist programme. *Proc R Soc Lond B Biol Sci* 1979; 205: 581–98.

38. Levin RJ. The mechanisms of human female sexual arousal. *Annu Rev Sex Res* 1992; 3: 1–48.

39. Passie T, Hartman U, Schneider U et al. On the function of groaning and hyperventilation during sexual intercourse: intensification of sexual experience by altering brain metabolism through hypocapnia. *Med Hypotheses* 2003; 60: 660–3.

40. Levin RJ, van Berlo W. Sexual arousal and orgasm in subjects who experience forced or non-consensual sexual stimulation – a review. *J Clin Forensic Med* 2004; 11: 82–8.

41. American Psychiatric Association. *DSM-IV-TR: Diagnostic and Statistical Manual for Mental Disorders*, 4th edn. Washington, DC: American Psychiatric Press, 2000.

42. World Health Organization. *ICD-10 – International Classification of Diseases and Related Health Problems*. Geneva: World Heath Organization, 1992.

43. Masters WH, Johnson VE. *Human Sexual Inadequacy*. Boston: Little, Brown, 1970.

44. Basson R, Berman J, Burnett A et al. Report of the International Consensus Development Conference on Female Sexual Dysfunction: Definitions and Classifications. *Urology* 2000; 163: 889–93.

45. Segraves RT. Editor's comments. *J Sex Marital Ther* 2001; 27: 81.

46. Goldstein I, Graziottin A, Heiman JR et al. Female sexual dysfunction. In A Jardin, G Wagner, S Khoury et al., eds. *Erectile Dysfunction*. Plymouth: Plymbridge Distributors, 2000: 507–56.

47. Meston C. Validation of the female sexual function index (FSFI) in women with female orgasmic disorder and in women with hypoactive sexual desire disorder. *J Sex Marital Ther* 2003; 29: 39–46.

48. Basson R, Leiblum S, Brotto L et al. Definitions of women's sexual dysfunction reconsidered: advocating expansion and revision. *J Psychosom Obstet Gynaecol* 2003; 24: 221–9.

49. Tiefer L. The medicalization of sexuality: conceptual, normative, and professional issues. *Annu Rev Sex Res* 1996; 7: 252–82.

50. Moynihan R. The making of a disease: female sexual dysfunction. *BMJ* 2003; 326: 45–7.

51. O'Gorman ERC. The treatment of frigidity: a comparative study of group and individual desensitization. *Br J Psychiatry* 1978; 132: 580–4.

52. Bancroft J, Loftus J, Scott Long J. Distress about sex: a national survey of women in heterosexual relationships. *Arch Sex Behav* 2003; 32: 193–208.

53. Heiman JR. Orgasmic disorders in women. In SR Leiblum, R Rosen, eds. *Principles and Practices of Sex Therapy*, 3rd edn. New York: Guilford Press, 2000.

54. Heiman JR, Meston CM. Empirically validated treatment for sexual dysfunction. *Annu Rev Sex Res* 1997; 8: 148–94.

55. Schover LR, Leiblum SR. Commentary: the stagnation of sex therapy. *J Psychol Hum Sex* 1994; 6: 5–30.

56. McMullen S, Rosen RC. Self-administered masturbation training in the treatment of primary orgasmic dysfunction. *J Consult Clin Psychol* 1979; 47: 912–18.

57. Huey CJ, Kline-Graber G, Graber B. Time factors and orgasmic response. *Arch Sex Behav* 1981; 10: 111–18.

58. Levin RJ. Measuring female genital functions- a research essential but still a clinical luxury. *Sex Relat Ther* 2004; 19: 191–200.

59. Everaaerd W, Dekker J. Treatment of secondary orgasmic dysfunction: a comparison of systematic desensitisation and sex therapy. *Behav Res Ther* 1982; 20: 269–74.

60. Pierce AP. The coital alignment technique (CAT): an overview of studies. *J Sex Marital Ther* 2000; 26: 257–68.

61. Hurlbert DF, Apt C. The coital alignment technique and directed masturbation: a comparative study on female orgasm. *J Sex Marital Ther* 1995; 21: 21–9.

6.5 Sexual pain disorders: pathophysiologic factors

Caroline F Pukall, Marie-Andrée Lahaie, Yitzchak M Binik

Introduction

The sexual pain disorders included in the *Diagnostic and Statistical Manual of Mental Disorders* (DSM)[1] – dyspareunia and vaginismus – have long been classified as sexual dysfunctions (see Chapter 9.1 of this volume), despite recent research indicating that sexuality is just one aspect affected in these conditions and that other factors should be given equal importance.[2] The purpose of this chapter is to give an overview of etiologic factors involved in the development and maintenance of these conditions (see Chapters 12.1–12.6).

Dyspareunia

Classification

The fourth edition of the DSM (DSM-IV-TR)[1] has continued the tradition started in the third edition (DSM-III-R)[3] of including dyspareunia as a sexual pain disorder, defining it as a "recurrent and persistent genital pain associated with sexual intercourse". This definition, based on interference with sexual intercourse, is understandable, given that this is what brings many women to clinical attention. However, this focus has drawn attention away from the major clinical symptom of pain. One major reason for the classification of dyspareunia as a sexual dysfunction is the lack of a known physical basis for the pain; however, the presence of physical findings is not an important criterion for defining a pain syndrome. For example, 85% of patients with back pain present without identifiable pathology,[4] yet they still receive the diagnosis of back pain.

The DSM-IV-TR[1] reinforces the outdated view that pain is either physical *or* psychologic. For example, it mentions post-menopausal dyspareunia but classifies it as a sexual dysfunction due to a general medical (i.e., physical) condition, despite the fact that there is very little systematic research evidence to support a strong link between physical factors and dyspareunia in this age group.[5] Deep dyspareunia, the most common symptom associated with pelvic pathology and chronic pelvic pain[6], is similarly classified. While the distinction between dyspareunia due to psychologic versus physical factors seems intuitively useful from a classification standpoint, it does not reflect the reality of the pain experience. Therefore, we have adopted a pain perspective of dyspareunia,[7] which views pain as a multidimensional experience, including both physical and psychologic factors. Adopting this approach necessitates that pain is the major focus of assessment and treatment; psychosocial, psychologic, and sexual factors are also ascribed great importance since they play a crucial role in the disability resulting from the pain, and in pain perception and control.

Consistent with this approach, the International Society for the Study of Vulvovaginal Disease proposed a new classification of vulvodynia based on pain location: generalized and localized. Each of these is subdivided into provoked, unprovoked, or mixed pain presentations; both sexual and nonsexual situations can elicit pain. This classification, based on pain characteristics, is in line with viewing dyspareunia as a vulvar pain problem.[8] However, as this classification is new and has not yet been adopted in research, we will standardize our use of the terminology in this chapter as follows: "dyspareunia" denotes any form of recurrent or chronic genital pain that interferes with, but may not be limited to, sexual activity in women of any age. Dyspareunic pain can be experienced in a number of different genital locations and can be characterized by different pain qualities and patterns. "Vulvar vestibulitis syndrome" refers to pain experienced in the vulvar vestibule upon contact,[9] and the term "vulvodynia" denotes generalized and chronic vulvar pain that occurs in the absence of external stimulation. This part of the chapter will focus on vulvar vestibulitis syndrome and vulvodynia.

Etiologic factors

Vulvar vestibulitis syndrome

Vulvar vestibulitis syndrome is the most common form of dyspareunia in premenopausal women,[1] affecting an estimated 12% in the general population.[11] Women with vulvar vestibulitis typically experience a severe burning pain at the entrance of the vagina in response to contact during both sexual and nonsexual activities.[10,12] Friedrich[9] proposed the following diagnostic criteria for vulvar vestibulitis syndrome: (1) severe pain upon vestibular touch or attempted vaginal entry; (2) tenderness to pressure localized within the vulvar vestibule; and (3) physical findings limited to vestibular erythema of various degrees. While the last criterion has not proven to be a reliable diagnostic indicator of vulvar vestibulitis,[12] its diagnosis of vulvar vestibulitis syndrome is relatively easy to make via the cotton-swab test, which consists of the application of a cotton swab to various areas of the vulvar vestibule.

Yeast infections

Numerous etiologic theories exist regarding what initiates the increase in sensitivity of the vulvar vestibule in sufferers.[13] One of the most consistently reported findings associated with the onset of vulvar vestibulitis is a history of repeated yeast infections.[14] However, it is not clear whether the culprit is the yeast itself, the treatments undertaken, which can sensitize the vestibular tissue, or an underlying sensitivity already present in the tissue.[15] Since not all women with vulvar vestibulitis syndrome report a history of repeated yeast infections, many researchers have recently begun to examine the properties of vestibular tissue in controlled studies.

Physical findings in the vulva

While early, uncontrolled studies concluded that inflammation played a role in vulvar vestibulitis, recently published controlled studies suggest that inflammatory infiltrates are common in the vestibule.[16,17] Other investigations suggest that altered tissue properties play a role in the development and/or maintenance of the pain in vulvar vestibulitis syndrome. Evidence for this includes heightened innervation of intraepithelial nerve fibers,[18,19] increase in vanilloid receptor 1 expression (i.e., a receptor present in pain fibers),[20] increase in blood flow,[21] presence of calcitonin gene-related peptide (a peptide found in pain nerves),[22] lowered tactile and pain thresholds,[23] and nociceptor sensitization.[24] These properties would lead to a heightened sensitivity in response to vestibular pressure, consistent with the clinical picture of provoked pain in women with vulvar vestibulitis.

In addition to abnormalities present in the vestibule, controlled studies have found that women with vulvar vestibulitis syndrome exhibit an increase in pelvic floor muscle tension,[25,26] possibly representing a protective reaction against, or a condi-

tioned response to, vulvar pain. While there has been much advancement in terms of pain-related findings at the local (i.e., genital) level, other research indicates that there may be more generalized abnormalities in women with vulvar vestibulitis.

Genetic factors and generalized sensitivity

Gerber et al.[27] conducted a series of studies examining genetic factors in women with vulvar vestibulitis syndrome. They demonstrated that affected women were more frequently homozygous at allele 2 of the interleukin-1 receptor antagonist gene and at allele 2 of the interleukin-1 beta gene than nonaffected women. Each of these alleles has been associated with a severe and prolonged proinflammatory immune response.[28] Consistent with this finding, they demonstrated that the immune systems of women with vulvar vestibulitis syndrome are not effective in terminating the inflammatory process. Based on these findings, they proposed that, in some women with vulvar vestibulitis syndrome, there is a genetic susceptibility to development of a chronic localized inflammation in the vestibule after an initial inflammatory response has been triggered (as after yeast infections). The prolonged and intensified inflammation could then trigger other events that may result in increased pain sensitivity due to chronic inflammation in both genital and nongenital areas of the body. Although this is just beginning to be examined, controlled studies support the implication of higher sensitivity in nongenital body areas in women with vulvar vestibulitis: they are more sensitive to nongenital touch, pain, pressure, and heat pain[23,29] and report more somatic pain-related complaints[23,30] than nonaffected women.

Hormonal factors

Hormonal factors are also associated with vulvar vestibulitis syndrome in controlled studies. Bazin et al.[31] and Bouchard et al.[32] found that women who used oral contraceptives, especially those who started at a young age, had an increased risk of developing vulvar vestibulitis syndrome later in life. Early menarche and dysmenorrhea were also associated with increased risk.[11,31] In addition, one recently published controlled study found that women with vulvar vestibulitis have significantly decreased estrogen receptor-alpha expression.[33] These findings suggest that hormonal factors may play a role in vulvar vestibulitis syndrome, but the question of how hormones are involved remains to be elucidated (see Chapter 12.4).

Psychosocial factors

Elevated levels of psychologic distress, anxiety, depression, shyness, harm avoidance, hypervigilance to pain stimuli, pain catastrophization, and somatization, as well as low sexual self-esteem,[23,29,30,34–36] have been found in women with vulvar vestibulitis syndrome. Not surprisingly, women with vulvar vestibulitis report lower frequencies of intercourse; lower levels of sexual desire, arousal, and pleasure; and less orgasmic success than nonaffected women.[10,37,38] Despite the significant effects on sexuality, the examination of relationship factors has been limited. In addition, while uncontrolled reports imply that sexual abuse is common in women with vulvar vestibulitis syndrome,[13,39] controlled studies of sexual abuse[10,37,40] show no difference between affected and nonaffected women.

Vulvodynia

Vulvodynia is a noncyclic, chronic vulvar discomfort extending to the urethral and rectal areas, characterized by the patient's complaint of burning, stinging, irritation, or rawness.[41] Light touch of the vulvar area often exacerbates the ongoing pain; however, dyspareunia is not always reported. Vulvodynia affects 6–7% of women in the general population, with a higher prevalence in women over the age of 30.[11] The diagnosis of vulvodynia is a diagnosis of exclusion; hence, a careful physical examination to rule out all potential causes (e.g., dermatologic conditions, yeast infections) must precede the diagnosis.[42] The onset of vulvodynia is sometimes linked to episodes of local treatments, such as vulvar cream application, laser surgery for genital wart or malignancy removal, or vulvar injury.

Vulvodynia as a neuropathic pain syndrome

McKay[42] proposed that the pain of vulvodynia results from altered cutaneous perception, as in neuropathic pain syndromes. This perspective has gained support; vulvodynia patients report symptom reduction when they are treated with medications typically prescribed for neuropathic pain (e.g., amitriptyline).[43] Neuropathic pain states originate with an injury to the nervous system itself; this leads to the transmission of pain signals even when acute injury is no longer present. Neuropathic pain in the vulva can result from damage to sensory nerves during surgery, or damage to the pudendal nerve due to sports trauma (e.g., horseback riding), childbirth, or vaginal surgery.[44] Another potential cause of vulvodynia is the condition of referred pain (i.e., when injury in one area causes pain in a different body area); any injury or orthopedic condition affecting muscles (e.g., pubococcygeus) or joints (e.g., sacroiliac) can refer pain to the perineal, vaginal, and rectal areas. In addition, injuries to the spinal cord (e.g., ruptured disk) and other conditions (e.g., varicella zoster) may manifest as vulvodynia.[44]

Pelvic floor muscle abnormalities and psychosocial factors

Women with vulvodynia exhibit abnormalities in pelvic floor contractile amplitudes of tonic, phasic, and endurance contractions as compared with nonaffected women.[45] Rehabilitation of the pelvic floor muscles via surface electromyography has been found successful in reducing pain and increasing sexual interest (see Chapter 4.4), pleasure, and activity.[46] Vulvodynia is not associated with depression[47,48] or with higher than normal instances of sexual abuse.[40,49] It is unfortunate that so little research has been conducted in the physical, psychosocial, and sexual realms of vulvodynia; more research is needed.

Discussion

It is likely that multiple etiologies for vulvar vestibulitis syndrome and vulvodynia exist, and that these vary from woman to woman. Spending much time trying to determine what initially "caused" the pain will not be particularly helpful since a vicious cycle of pain has already been put into motion, involving physical, muscular, psychologic, sexual, behavioral, and relationship factors. What is important is managing the pain and its consequences; many areas of these women's lives must be addressed simultaneously in order to achieve therapeutic success. We believe the same to be true for vaginismus.

Vaginismus

Classification

Vaginismus made its first appearance in the DSM-III-R[3] and has been present in all versions of the DSM since then, including the most recent.[1] Vaginismus is defined as a "recurrent or persistent involuntary spasm of the musculature of the outer third of the vagina that interferes with intercourse" (p. 558). However, several problems exist with this definition. Perhaps the most damaging evidence against it is that the occurrence of vaginal muscle spasms is neither exclusive nor specific to vaginismus.[26] Nevertheless, the criterion of the vaginal muscle spasm remains the hallmark of the definition of vaginismus; this can be seen in other classification systems.[50]

In addition, although vaginismus is classified as a sexual pain disorder in the DSM, the experience of pain is not required for its diagnosis, and no information is provided on the location, intensity, duration, or quality of the pain experienced by vaginismic women. Related to this point is the confusion about whether the pain should be considered a consequence of the vaginal muscle spasm or whether the spasm is a reaction to the pain experience.[51] Another important limitation is that vaginismus is reported to interfere solely with sexual intercourse, despite indications that spasms can occur when vaginal insertion is attempted with tampons and during gynecologic examinations. These difficulties with the current definition of vaginismus have led us to propose a reappraisal, with the major focus on the phobic, muscular, and pain aspects of vaginismus.

Etiologic factors

Vaginismus

There are no epidemiologic studies investigating the prevalence of vaginismus; however, in clinical settings, the rates range from 12% to 17%.[52,53] Moreover, there are no standardized assessment protocols for vaginismus. It is not uncommon for vaginismus to be diagnosed based on a single report of difficulties with penetration[54] and without a gynecologic examination.[55] The diagnosis is typically made by health professionals who have little experience in the assessment and treatment of muscle problems; physical therapists are rarely consulted.

Vaginal muscle spasm

It has long been suggested that lack of control over the pelvic floor muscles can contribute to vaginismus. According to Barnes et al.,[56] women with vaginismus have difficulty in evaluating vaginal muscle tone and differentiating between a relaxed state and a spasm. Since the early 1940s, acquiring greater control over pelvic floor muscles has been an important component in the treatment of vaginismus. While two well-controlled studies comparing women with and without vaginismus on voluntary control of the pelvic floor muscles found no differences between the groups in terms of baseline measures[57] or in response to physically or sexually threatening film segments[58] via a vaginal surface electromyography device, Reissing et al.[26] demonstrated – by pelvic floor physical therapy techniques – that women with vaginismus display higher vaginal/pelvic muscle tone and lower muscle strength than both women with vulvar vestibulitis syndrome and a control group. In addition, they found that the presence of vaginal muscle spasm did not differentiate among the groups, indicating that this criterion should not be used as the defining characteristic for women with vaginismus. While the muscle component plays a role in vaginismus, further research is needed to clarify whether it is a cause, a symptom, or a consequence of vaginismus.

Dyspareunia

While dyspareunia has frequently been found to play a role in the development of vaginismus,[37,59] the relationship between dyspareunia and vaginismus remains unclear, with some researchers arguing that chronic dyspareunia results in vaginismus and others reporting that the spasms cause pain.[60] It has been proposed that chronic dyspareunia as a result of physical disorders, such as hymeneal and congenital abnormalities, is likely to result in vaginismus,[51] leading some researchers to propose that vaginismus and dyspareunia are difficult, if not impossible, to differentiate.[61,62] In support of this, Reissing et al.[26] found no differences in the reported quality and intensity of the pain experienced during attempted vaginal penetration between women with vaginismus and vulvar vestibulitis syndrome. Although pain seems to be an important component of vaginismus, further investigation is needed to clarify its role in the development and/or maintenance of this condition.

Psychosocial factors, such as a penetration fear/phobia, negative sexual attitudes, lack of sexual knowledge, sexual abuse, and relationship factors, have also been implicated in the etiology of vaginismus (see Chapters 3.1–3.3 and 11.1–11.5).

Penetration phobia

Numerous reports in the literature suggest that vaginismus results from fear of pain, of vaginal penetration, or of sexual intimacy. As early as 1909, Walthard[63] suggested that vaginismus is a phobic reaction to an excessive fear of pain. This idea was reiterated by Kaplan,[64] who perceived vaginismus as a reflexive or phobic reaction to the anticipation of pain, resulting in the avoidance of intercourse. In concordance with these claims, a survey study found fear of pain to be the primary reason reported by women with vaginismus for their abstinence.[65] Although fear of pain has been reported by some to be an etiologic factor associated with vaginismus, others suggest that fear of pain should be perceived as a symptom rather than a cause of vaginismus.[66]

It has also been suggested that vaginismus be considered a sexual phobia;[67] however, women with vaginismus avoid not only sexual situations involving penetration but also vaginal penetrative situations such as tampon insertion and gynecologic examinations. Moreover, some women with vaginismus engage in and enjoy sexual activities that do not involve penetration; this would not be the case if vaginismus were a purely "sexual" phobia. On the other hand, the strong behavioral reactions to penetration observed in women with vaginismus may be related specifically to a vaginal penetration phobia, regardless of the situation (i.e., sexual or nonsexual). In support of this, women with vaginismus behave in ways consistent with those of a phobic who is exposed to the feared stimulus. Reissing et al.[26] found women with vaginismus to be characterized by intense emotional and behavioral reactions to attempted vaginal penetration, active avoidance of intercourse, and chronic hypertonicity of the pelvic floor muscles. Some authors have proposed a reconceptualization of vaginismus as a specific phobia of vaginal penetration.[26] The phobic element in vaginismus should be further investigated.

Negative sexual attitudes and lack of sexual knowledge/education

Vaginismus has been associated with a lack of sexual education and knowledge.[68] One study showed that vaginismic women believed that "being brought up to believe that sex was wrong" played a major role in the development of their condition. Consistent with this finding, Basson[69] found that the majority of women with vaginismus in her study held negative views about sexuality. Furthermore, Leiblum[59] reported that it is not uncommon for women with vaginismus to have received negative messages about men and sexual pleasure, resulting in negative attitudes toward sex and penile penetration. Masters and Johnson[70] found that a large proportion of vaginismic women reported a strict religious upbringing involving strong taboos regarding sexuality. However, two well-controlled studies demonstrated no differences in the level of sexual knowledge and education between a group of vaginismic women and controls.[37,71] However, Reissing et al.[37] found that although women with vaginismus do not hold more negative sexual self-views than women with vulvar vestibulitis syndrome and control women, they have less positive sexual self-schemas. With this in mind, the role of negative sexual attitudes and lack of sexual knowledge in the development of vaginismus still remains to be determined.

Sexual abuse

The belief about the relationship between sexual abuse and the development of vaginismus has had a long history;[55,59] yet, in general, well-controlled empirical studies have found no evidence of a higher prevalence of sexual abuse in women with vaginismus.[61,72] While Reissing et al.[37] reported that women with vaginismus were twice as likely to report a history of negative sexual experiences in childhood than a control group, they were not more likely to report a history of childhood or adulthood physical abuse, or a history of negative sexual experiences in adulthood, than women with vulvar vestibulitis syndrome and a control group. According to current studies, sexual abuse does not seem to be an important etiologic factor in the development of vaginismus (see Chapter 3.4).

Couple and relationship factors
While vaginismus has frequently been stated to result from marital problems and poor communication,[55,73] only a few empirical studies have investigated the role of couple factors in the etiology of vaginismus. They report no differences between women with vaginismus and control women on marital adjustment,[37,74] leading investigators to examine patterns related to behaviors, personality, and sexuality in male partners of vaginismic women. For instance, it has been reported that partners of vaginismic women are more likely to suffer from sexual problems, such as premature ejaculation and erectile dysfunction,[70,75,76] and from lack of self-confidence, passivity, dependency, and fear of failure[73,77] than partners of nonaffected women. Given the significance of the effects of vaginismus on relationship and couple factors, more research in this area is needed (see Chapter 3.1).

Discussion

It is difficult to examine the various etiologic factors involved in the development and maintenance of vaginismus when we do not have a clear understanding of what this disorder entails. Is it a sexual dysfunction? A phobia? A pain disorder? Or a combination of these? There is significant need for empirical studies to investigate the different aspects of vaginismus. In particular, exploring the similarities and differences between women with vulvar vestibulitis syndrome and women with vaginismus could prove fruitful, as many authors suggest they are part of the same disorder. Given that women with vaginismus and those with dyspareunia both suffer from pain and hypertonic pelvic floor muscles, the difference between these two disorders might be one of degree rather than kind,[51,78] with vaginismic women exhibiting more fear of pain and/or penetration than dyspareunic women.

Future directions

It is interesting to note that much research concerning vulvar vestibulitis syndrome has focused on physical factors, such as innervation and genetics, with relatively little research examining relationship or psychosocial factors despite their importance in the development and maintenance of this condition. With vaginismus, it appears to be the opposite case, and with respect to vulvodynia, not much research has been done in either realm. It is clear that all subtypes of dyspareunia and vaginismus

need to be examined from a multidisciplinary perspective; therefore, we suggest a reappraisal of the "sexual pain disorders". We suggest that dyspareunia and its subtypes be seen as pain disorders, focusing on psychologic, relational, cognitive, sexual, and behavioral aspects involved in pain perception and control, and that the investigation of vaginismus focus on the pain, muscular, and phobic components.

We will continue to adopt a multidisciplinary perspective to examine dyspareunia and vaginismus in order to support the reclassification of these conditions. For example, current studies in our laboratory are investigating baseline superficial blood flow in the vestibule and how this changes over time after the application of a painful stimulus, the effects of sexual arousal on pain perception, hypnosis as a treatment in women with vulvar vestibulitis syndrome, and genital pain in postmenopausal women. In terms of examining the phobic aspect in women with vaginismus, we plan to investigate the pain aspect by psychophysical methods, the muscular component by pelvic floor physical therapy, and the phobic aspect through psychophysiologic, behavioral, and self-report measures. These studies will provide valuable information regarding the interplay of different factors in both conditions, as well as similarities between the two.

Acknowledgments

We thank Samir Khalifé, the gynecologist on our research team, for the countless gynecologic examinations he has performed over the years and for his endless insight and enthusiasm. We extend much gratitude to Rhonda Amsel, the statistical expert on our research team, for her patience, wit, and ability to help us with any statistical issue, no matter how obscure. We extend a heartfelt thank-you to Katherine Muldoon, our full-time research assistant, who helped us in countless ways over the last year, and the members of our McGill laboratory: Nicole Flory, Alina Kao, Tuuli Kukkonen, and Kimberley Payne. The research performed in our laboratory could not have been done without the help of the following granting agencies: the Canadian Institutes of Health Research (CIHR), Health Canada, and Pfizer Canada, Inc. Caroline F. Pukall was supported by the Fonds pour la formation de Chercheurs et l'Aide à la Recherche (FCAR), the Lloyd Carr-Harris McGill Majors Fellowship, and the McGill University Health Center Post-Doctoral Fellowship; Marie-Andrée Lahaie was supported by the Fonds pour la formation de Chercheurs et l'Aide à la Recherche (FCAR) and the McGill University Health Center Doctoral Fellowship.

References

1. American Psychiatric Association. *Diagnostic and Statistical Manual of Mental Disorders*, 4th edn, text revision. Washington, DC: 2000.

2. Binik YM. Should dyspareunia be classified as a sexual dysfunction in DSM-V? A painful classification decision. *Arch Sex Behav* 2005; 34: 11–21.

3. American Psychiatric Association. *Diagnostic and Statistical Manual of Mental Disorders,* 3rd edn, (rev.) Washington, DC: 1987.

4. Deyo RA. Early diagnostic evaluation of low back pain. *J Gen Intern Med* 1986; 1: 328–38.

5. Laan E, van Lunsen RHW. Hormones and sexuality in post-menopausal women: a psychophysiological study. *J Psychosomat Obstet Gynecol* 1997; 18: 126–33.

6. Bachmann GA, Phillips NA. Sexual dysfunction. In Steege JF, Metzger DA, Levy BS, eds. *Chronic Pelvic Pain: An Integrated Approach.* London: W.B. Saunders, 1988: 77–90.

7. Binik YM, Reissing ED, Pukall CF et al. The female sexual pain disorders: genital pain or sexual dysfunction? *Arch Sex Behav* 2002; 31: 425–9.

8. Foster DC. Chronic vulval pain. In AB MacLean, RW Stones, S Thornton, eds. *Pain in Obstetrics and Gynecology.* London: RCOG Press, 2001: 198–208.

9. Friedrich EG Jr. Vulvar vestibulitis syndrome. *J Reprod Med* 1987; 32: 110–14.

10. Meana M, Binik YM, Khalifé S et al. Biopsychosocial profile of women with dyspareunia. *Obstet Gynecol* 1997; 90: 583–9.

11. Harlow BL, Wise LA, Stewart, EG. Prevalence and predictors of chronic lower genital tract discomfort. *Am J Obstet Gynecol* 2001; 185: 545–50.

12. Bergeron S, Binik YM, Khalifé S et al. Reliability and validity of the diagnosis of vulvar vestibulitis syndrome. *Obstet Gynecol* 2001; 98: 45–51.

13. Bergeron S, Binik Y, Khalifé S et al. Vulvar vestibulitis syndrome: a critical review. *Clin J Pain* 1997; 13: 27–42.

14. Mann MS, Kaufman RH, Brown D et al. Vulvar vestibulitis: significant clinical variables and treatment outcome. *Obstet Gynecol* 1992; 79: 122–5.

15. Goetsch MF. Vulvar vestibulitis: prevalence and historic features in a general gynecologic practice population. *Am J Obstet Gynecol* 1991; 164: 1609–16.

16. Chadha S, Gianotten WL, Drogendijk AC et al. Histopathologic features of vulvar vestibulitis. *Int J Gynecol Pathol* 1998; 17: 7–11.

17. Bohm-Starke N, Falconer C, Rylander E et al. The expression of cyclooxygenase 2 and inducible nitric oxide synthase indicates no active inflammation in vulvar vestibulitis. *Acta Obstet Gynecol Scand* 2001; 80: 638–44.

18. Bohm-Starke N, Hilliges M, Falconer C et al. Increased intraepithelial innervation in women with vulvar vestibulitis syndrome. *Gynecol Obstet Invest* 1998; 46: 256–60.

19. Weström LV, Willén R. Vestibular nerve fiber proliferation in vulvar vestibulitis syndrome. *Obstet Gynecol* 1998; 91: 572–6.

20. Tympanidis P, Casula MA, Yiangou Y et al. Increased vanilloid receptor VR1 innervation in vulvodynia. *Eur J Pain* 2004; 8: 129–33.

21. Bohm-Starke N, Hilliges M, Blomgren BO et al. Increased blood flow and erythema in the posterior vestibular mucosa in vulvar vestibulitis. *Obstet Gynecol* 2001; 98: 1067–74.

22. Bohm-Starke N, Hilliges M, Falconer C et al. Neurochemical characterization of the vestibular nerves in women with vulvar vestibulitis syndrome. *Gynecol Obstet Invest* 1999; 48: 270–5.

23. Pukall CF, Binik YM, Khalifé S et al. Vestibular tactile and pain thresholds in women with vulvar vestibulitis syndrome. *Pain* 2002; 96: 163–75.

24. Bohm-Starke N, Hilliges M, Brodda-Jansen G et al. Psychophysical evidence of nociceptor sensitization in vulvar vestibulitis syndrome. *Pain* 2001; 94: 177–83.

25. Glazer HI, Rodke G, Swencionis C et al. Treatment of vulvar vestibulitis syndrome with electromyographic biofeedback of pelvic floor musculature. *J Reprod Med* 1995; 40: 283–90.

26. Reissing ED, Binik YM, Khalifé S et al. Vaginal spasm, pain, and behavior: an empirical investigation of the diagnosis of vaginismus. *Arch Sex Behav* 2004; 33: 5–17.

27. Gerber S, Bongiovanni AM, Ledger WJ et al. Interleukin-1B gene polymorphism in women with vulvar vestibulitis syndrome. *Eur J Obstet Gynecol Reprod Biol* 2003; 107: 74–7.

28. Witkin SS, Gerber S, Ledger WJ. Influence of interleukin-1 receptor antagonist gene polymorphism on disease. *Clin Infect Dis* 2002; 34: 204–9.

29. Granot M, Friedman M, Yarnitsky D et al. Enhancement of the perception of systemic pain in women with vulvar vestibulitis. *Br J Obstet Gynecol* 2002; 109: 863–6.

30. Danielsson I, Eisemann M, Sjöberg I et al. Vulvar vestibulitis: a multi-factorial condition. *Br J Obstet Gynecol* 2001;108:456–61.

31. Bazin S, Bouchard C, Brisson J et al. Vulvar vestibulitis syndrome: an exploratory case-control study. *Obstet Gynecol* 1994; 83: 47–50.

32. Bouchard C, Brisson J, Fortier M et al. Use of oral contraceptives and vulvar vestibulitis: a case-control study. *Am J Epidemiol* 2002; 156: 254–61.

33. Eva LJ, MacLean AB, Reid W et al. Estrogen receptor expression in vulvar vestibulitis syndrome. *Am J Obstet Gynecol* 2003; 189: 458–61.

34. Payne KA, Binik YM, Amsel R et al. When sex hurts, anxiety and fear orient attention towards pain. *Eur J Pain* 2005; 9: 427–36.

35. van Lankveld JJ, Weijenborg, PT, Ter Kuile MM. Psychologic profiles of and sexual function in women with vulvar vestibulitis and their partners. *Obstet Gynecol* 1996; 88: 65–70.

36. Gates EA, Galask RP. Psychological and sexual functioning in women with vulvar vestibulitis. *J Psychosom Obstet Gynecol* 2001; 22: 221–8.

37. Reissing ED, Binik YM, Khalifé S et al. Etiological correlates of vaginismus: sexual and physical abuse, sexual knowledge, sexual self-schema, and relationship adjustment. *J Sex Marital Ther* 2003; 29: 47–59.

38. Reed BD, Advincula AP, Fonde KR et al. Sexual activities and attitudes of women with vulvar dysesthesia. *Obstet Gynecol* 2003; 102: 325–31.

39. Jantos M, White G. The vestibulitis syndrome: medical and psychosexual assessment of a cohort of patients. *J Reprod Med* 1997; 42: 145–52.

40. Dalton VK, Haefner HK, Reed BD et al. Victimization in patients with vulvar dysesthesia/vestibulodynia: is there an increased prevalence? *J Reprod Med* 2002; 47: 829–34.

41. McKay M. Vulvodynia versus pruritus vulvae. *Clin Obstet Gynecol* 1985; 28: 123–33.

42. McKay M. Vulvodynia. In JF Steege, DA Metzger, BS Levy, eds. *Chronic Pelvic Pain: An Integrated Approach.* London: W.B. Saunders, 1988: 188–96.

43. McKay M. Dysesthetic ("essential") vulvodynia: treatment with amitriptyline. *J Reprod Med* 1993; 38: 9–13.

44. Stewart EG. Vulvodynia: diagnosing and managing generalized dysesthesia. *OBG Manag* 2001; 13: 48–57.

45. Glazer HI, Jantos M, Hartmann EH et al. Electromyographic comparisons of the pelvic floor in women with dysesthetic vulvodynia and asymptomatic women. *J Reprod Med* 1998; 43: 959–62.

46. Glazer HI. Dysesthetic vulvodynia: long term follow-up after treatment with surface electromyography-assisted pelvic floor muscle rehabilitation. *J Reprod Med* 2000; 45: 798–802.

47. Bodden-Heinrich R, Küppers V, Beckmann MW et al. Psychosomatic aspects of vulvodynia: comparison with the chronic pelvic pain syndrome. *J Reprod Med* 1999; 44: 411–16.

48. Aikens JE, Reed BD, Gorenflo DW et al. Depressive symptoms among women with vulvar dysesthesia. *Am J Obstet Gynecol* 2003; 189: 462–6.

49. Edwards L, Mason M, Phillips M et al. Childhood sexual and physical abuse: incidence in patients with vulvodynia. *J Reprod Med* 1997; 42: 135–9.

50. American College of Obstetricians and Gynecologists, ACOG technical bulletin: sexual dysfunction. *Int Gynecol Obstet* 1995; 51: 265–77.

51. Reissing ED, Binik YM, Khalifé S. Does vaginismus exist? A critical review of the literature. *J Nerv Ment Dis* 1999; 187: 261–74.

52. Spector I, Carey M. Incidence and prevalence of the sexual dysfunctions: a critical review of the empirical literature. *Arch Sex Behav* 1990; 19: 389–96.

53. Hirst JF, Baggaley MR, Watson JP. A four year survey of an inner city psychosexual problems clinic. *Sex Marital Ther* 1996; 11: 19–36.

54. Harrison CM. Le vaginisme. *Contraception Sex Fertil* 1996; 24: 223–8.

55. Biswas A, Ratnam SS. Vaginismus and outcome of treatment. *Ann Acad Med* 1995; 24: 755–8.

56. Barnes J, Bowman EP, Cullen J. Biofeedback as an adjunct to psychotherapy in the treatment of vaginismus. *Biofeedback Self Regul* 1984; 9: 281–9.

57. van der Velde J, Everaerd W. Voluntary control over pelvic floor muscles in women with and without vaginismic reactions. *Int Urogynecol J Pelvic Floor Dysfunct* 1999; 10: 230–6.

58. van der Velde J, Laan E, Everaerd W. Vaginismus, a component of a general defensive reaction: an investigation of pelvic floor muscle activity during exposure to emotion inducing film excerpts in women with and without vaginismus. *Int Urogynecol J Pelvic Floor Dysfunct* 2001; 12: 328–31.

59. Leiblum SR. Vaginismus: a most perplexing problem. In SR Leiblum, RC Rosen eds. *Principles and Practice of Sex Therapy*, 3rd edn. New York: Guilford, 2000: pp 181–202.

60. Abramov L, Wolman I, Higgins MP. Vaginismus: an important factor in the evaluation and management of vulvar vestibulitis syndrome. *Gynecol Obstet Invest* 1994; 38: 194–7.

61. van Lankveld JJDM, Brewaeys AMA, Ter Kuile MM et al. Difficulties in the differential diagnosis of vaginismus, dyspareunia and mixed sexual pain disorder. *J Psychosom Obstet Gynecol* 1995; 16: 201–9.

62. Kaneko K. Penetration disorder: dyspareunia exists on the extension of vaginismus. *J Sex Marital Ther* 2001; 27: 153–5.

63. Walthard M. Die psychogene Ätiologie und die Psychotherapie des Vaginismus. *Munch Med Wochenschr* 1909; 56: 1997–2000.

64. Kaplan HS. *The New Sex Therapy.* New York: Brunner/Mazel, 1974.

65. Ward E, Ogden J. Experiencing vaginismus – sufferers' beliefs about causes and effects. *J Sex Marital Ther* 1994; 9: 33–45.

66. Dawkins S, Taylor R. Non-consummation of marriage: a survey of seventy cases. *Lancet* 1961; 280: 1029–33.

67. Rachman SJ. *Fear and Courage.* New York: WH Freeman, 1978.

68. Ellison C. Psychosomatic factors in the unconsummated marriage. *J Psychosom Res* 1968; 12: 61–5.

69. Basson R. Lifelong vaginismus: a clinical study of 60 consecutive cases. *J Soc Gynecol Obstet Can* 1996; 3: 551–61.

70. Masters WH, Johnson VE. *Human Sexual Inadequacy.* Boston: Little & Brown, 1970.

71. Duddle M. Etiological factors in the unconsummated marriage. *J Psychosom Res* 1977; 21: 157–60.

72. Hawton K, Catalan J. Sex therapy for vaginismus: characteristics of couples and treatment outcome. *Sex Marital Ther* 1990; 5: 39–48.

73. van de Wiel HBM, Jaspers JPM, Weijmar Schultz WCM et al. Treatment of vaginismus: a review of concepts and treatment modalities. *J Psychosom Obstet Gynecol* 1990; 11: 1–18.

74. Rust J, Golombok S, Collier J. Marital problems and sexual dysfunction: how are they related? *Br J Psychiatry* 1988; 152: 629–31.

75. Lamont JA. Vaginismus. *Am J Obstet Gynecol* 1978; 131: 632–6.

76. Steege JF. Dyspareunia and vaginismus. *Clin Obstet Gynecol* 1984; 27: 750–9.

77. Freidman LJ. *Virgin Wives: A Study of Unconsummated Marriages.* London, Tavistock Publications, 1962.

78. de Kruiff ME, ter Kuile MM, Weijenborg PThM et al. Vaginismus and dyspareunia: is there difference in clinical presentation? *J Psychosom Obstet Gynecol* 2000; 21: 149–55.

SPECIAL ISSUES CONCERNING ETIOLOGY OF FEMALE SEXUAL DYSFUNCTION

Aging issues

Richard D Hayes, Lorraine Dennerstein

Introduction

Aging comprises a number of facets, each of which has the potential to affect a woman's sexual function and dysfunction. Hormonal (see Chapter 5.5 in this volume) and physiologic changes (see Chapters 3.1–3.4) take place over the course of a woman's life. Testosterone levels decline from a woman's early 20s (see Chapter 6.3) and estrogen declines most rapidly during the menopausal transition (see Chapter 7.2). During puberty, pregnancy and postpartum hormonal and physiologic changes are particularly pronounced. Having and raising children, and relationship factors, including the presence of a partner, the partner's age and sexual functioning, and the length of the relationship, each influence sexual activities (see Chapter 3.1). Her health and that of her partner will inevitably decline with age, and this will affect their sexual experiences. The use of medication tends to increase with age, resulting in a higher risk of side effects that may lead to sexual problems. Emotional and psychologic changes also occur with age. A woman's priorities may alter, as may her feelings for her partner. The importance of sex in her life and level of distress she feels if she suffers from sexual dysfunction may also differ as a consequence of her age. The era in which a woman was born also has an impact, affecting her values and attitudes toward sexuality and her experiences.

Methodological issues

Information on the sexual changes that occur as women age can be drawn from both cross-sectional and longitudinal studies (see Chapters 2.1–2.4). Each methodology has advantages and limitations. Cross-sectional studies have the advantage of allowing a broad range of ages to be investigated with relative ease. However in cross-sectional studies, the effects of age and cohort membership are inevitably confounded. For example, a Danish study investigated 625 women who were born in 1958, 1936, or 1910 and found the percentage of women who never experienced an orgasm was greatest in the oldest cohort, while the percentage of women who had experienced spontaneous desire or desire after stimulation, or had ever masturbated was highest in the youngest cohort.[1] We would expect that the longer a woman has lived, the greater the chances she would have had these experiences at some point in her life. Here we see the reverse trend, a result of social or other factors relating to the era in which the older women grew up.

Longitudinal studies are useful since they allow us to examine both aggregate trends and intraindividual patterns of change. We can see that in a given sample of women, patterns of constant, declining, and increasing sexual functioning are usually present. We can look at events that have precipitated these changes and see when they occurred. By being able to separate suspected causes and effects in time, we have stronger evidence for causation. One of the main problems in the literature on sex and aging is just how few longitudinal investigations there are. For many studies that purport to be longitudinal, either the recording or analysis of data relating to aging is cross-sectional rather than longitudinal.[2] For practical reasons, the length of follow-up is usually limited, so it can be difficult to establish whether the change in sexual functioning is an exception or is consistent with the overall pattern of sexual functioning in a woman's life. Many longitudinal studies in this area focus on the menopausal transition, and often the age range included is very limited for this reason, or the data are analysed by menopausal status rather than age.

Cross-sectional studies

Sexual activities

The vast majority of studies indicate a decline in the frequency of sexual activities with age.[3–10] A community study of 9578 women aged 16–59 years who were sexually active (in masturbation or with partner) found that the frequency of sexual activities with a regular sexual partner was less in older women.[11] On average, women in their late teens and 20s engaged in sexual activities 2.2 times a week, in contrast to 1.3 times per week reported by women in their 50s. There is also evidence that in the 60–85 year age group, this decline continues.[6,7] In the older age groups, there is also a smaller number of women who remain sexually active. In a national study in the USA, the number of women who report sexual activity with a partner peaked at 93% for women in their late 20s, gradually declined to 82% for women in their early 50s, and then declined more rapidly to 60% for women in their late 50s.[8] In a British study of 2045 women aged 55–85 years, the number of women who reported being still sexually active was 46% for women in their late 50s to early 60s, and declined to 4% for those in their late 70s to early 80s.[9] Kinsey et al.[3] investigated differences in the frequency of sexual activities with age and noted differences between married and unmarried women (these differences are described in detail in the 'Partner age, health, and sexual function' section of this chapter). Most investigators do not distinguish between women of different relationship status when reporting differences in sexual activities with age. Research investigating women's masturbation frequency indicates that the frequency of masturbation increases from the teen years through to the early 20s, after which it plateaus until around the mid-40s and 50s, when it starts to decline.[8,10,12] Masturbation has also been found to be more common in women without a regular partner.[12]

Sexual functioning

In cross-sectional studies, although findings vary, the overall pattern of a woman's sexual functioning is one of decline with increasing age. It is difficult to identify when this decline in sexual functioning begins. Most studies investigating sexual function do not include women under the age of 35,[4,5,7,10,13,14] and those which do include younger women use broad age categories to analyze their data.[15,16] The most we can conclude is that a woman's sexual function starts to decline sometime between her late 20s and late 30s. There is general agreement in the literature that with age there is a decline in desire[1,16] and sexual interest.[4,5,15,17] In addition, when older subjects were asked to compare their current level of sexual interest with that of their younger years, the majority reported a decline.[7,18] A small increase in sexual interest in women in their late 60s and early 70s has been reported, but this was still in the context of an overall decline in sexual interest with age.[4] A number of studies have demonstrated that the frequency with which women experience orgasm also decreases with age (see Chapter 6.4).[5,16,18] Hallstrom[5] specifically investigated orgasm associated with sexual intercourse, but usually the type of sexual activity involved is not reported.[16,18] Research into changes in arousal with age is very limited. Arousal incorporates psychologic arousal, such as the subjective feeling of sexual excitement; nongenital arousal, which may be expressed as increase in blood pressure, flushing, or other somatic responses; and genital arousal, such as increased blood flow to the genitals and increased vaginal lubrication.[19–21] Of these aspects, more often than not, it is only vaginal lubrication that is investigated. There are reports of arousal both decreasing with age[16] and remaining constant.[10]

Sexual difficulties and dysfunction

For the most part, the number of sexual difficulties and dysfunctions women report remains fairly constant with increasing age, the exception being sexual pain, which appears to decrease. There are a few reports of sexual desire problems either increasing[22,23] or decreasing[24] with age. However, most community-based studies which ask specifically about problems with sexual desire or interest show no relationship with age,[2,25–28] even though, collectively, these studies span an age range of 18–96 years. This is surprising, since, as noted above, there is good evidence that sexual desire decreases with age,[1,4,5,15–17] so one might expect problems of sexual desire to increase with age as a result. Studies where difficulties in achieving orgasm are investigated consistently show no association with age,[22,24–29] with only a rare exception breaking this trend.[23] When arousal problems are investigated, most studies focus on problems with lubrication, neglecting other aspects of arousal. The data on arousal problems are ambiguous, with a similar number of studies reporting an increase in problems,[22,23] and no change with increasing age.[15,17,26] Surprisingly, perhaps, most studies report that problems with pain during intercourse decrease with age[9,10,23,26,28,29] or at least remain constant.[24,27,30] Relatively few studies have investigated changes in vaginismus with age. One such study of women aged 18–65 years found no significant relationship between age and the proportion of women reporting vaginismus.[27]

Longitudinal studies

Frequency of intercourse and sexual interest/desire are the main outcomes considered in longitudinal studies which investigate the effects of age. Stability over time is the most commonly observed pattern for frequency of intercourse[31,32] and for sexual interest or desire.[31–33] There are also, however, reports of sexual frequency and desire declining with age.[34,35] Studies which report patterns of stability also report patterns of increase and decline but in smaller percentages of the sample. Longitudinal studies also show that partner factors play an important role in changes in sexual frequency and desire over time.[31–34]

Factors associated with decline in sexual functioning with age

Length of relationship

The effect of increasing age on women with partners is confounded by the increasing length of the relationship. This is important because the amount of time a couple has been together has significant consequences for sex in the relationship. In 1981, William James investigated the rate of decline of coital rates with duration of marriage and identified a "honeymoon effect": a rapid decline in the rate of intercourse during the first year of marriage.[36] This was found to be true at least in couples who had no premarital sex. In this and a later study,[37] James reported frequency of sexual intercourse halving in the first 12 months of a relationship, then halving again over the next 20 years. There is also evidence that some aspects of sexual functioning may decline with increasing length of relationship. The Fugl-Meyers'[22] reported that sexual desire and interest decreased with length of relationship for women in their late teens to early 30s, and sexual desire decreased with length of relationship for women in their early 50s to mid-60s.

Partner age, health, and sexual function

In 1953, Kinsey et al. reported that the frequency of sexual activities remained constant in unmarried women up to age 55 years.[3] In men, he found that sexual activities declined steadily from puberty onward. Married women, however, were found to have a similar pattern of decline to men. Kinsey concluded that declining frequency of intercourse and orgasm in marriage does not prove that the sexual capacity of a woman is influenced by her aging, but instead could be the result of her husband's aging. In heterosexual couples, the effect of male aging on the relationship is enhanced by the fact that, on average, men are older than their partners.[11] This is almost certainly the main reason that the frequency of intercourse reported is higher in males than females of the same age.[32] As the woman ages, so, too, does her partner. As he ages, his health will inevitably decline. His use of medications will increase, as will the risk of negative side effects of these on his sexual functioning. His risk of developing a sexual dysfunction generally will increase as they both age.[38] All of this will also happen to the female partner as she ages, but because, on average, he is older, it is most likely to happen to the male partner first. The era in which a woman's partner was born will affect her partner's attitudes toward sex and also influence their sex life together.[18] These issues may help explain why women report significantly lower levels of sexual interest than their male peers.[4,32]

Reasons for ceasing sexual activities

Factors relating to a woman's partner and the relationship as a whole are as important as her own sexual functioning in dictating when sexual activities in a relationship end. In some early investigations, men and women were asked why sexual activities had ended in their relationships. The majority of women blamed their husbands, and the majority of men blamed themselves.[4,31,32] More recently, Blumel et al.[39] conducted a clinically based study of 534 Chilean women aged 40–64 years and found that the reasons for ending sexual activities varied with age. The most common reason given for ending sexual activities was partner erectile dysfunction in women younger than 45 years, low sexual desire in women 45–59, and lack of a partner for women older than 60.

Other factors associated with decline in sexual functioning

There are a range of other factors which can affect a women's sexual functioning and activities as she ages. In a study by Deeks

and McCabe in 2001,[38] sexual communication, measured on a scale designed by the authors, was shown to decrease with age. The scale used to assess sexual communication in this study incorporated a range of questions, including how active the woman is in sexual activity, how well a woman's partner tunes in to what she likes, and how caring her partner is as a lover. There is also evidence that a woman's feelings toward her partner may change with certain hormonal conditions which occur during her life, such as the menopausal transition.[40] Reproductive changes and the menopausal transition have major influences on a woman's sexual functioning and sexual dysfunction. These topics are discussed elsewhere in this text and are not the focus of this chapter, except to mention that reproductive changes and different menopausal states are inherently confounded with aging.

Factors associated with periods of improvement in sexual functioning with age

Although the exception rather than the rule, improvements in sexual functioning with age have been noted in both longitudinal and cross-sectional studies. Usually, a small percentage of women (5–15%) in longitudinal studies show an improvement in sexual frequency or functioning with age. It should be noted that the periods of time we are considering are very short. For practical reasons, longitudinal studies rarely have long periods of follow-up, so these improvements are not ones spanning youth to old age but more likely represent short periods of improvement in a general pattern of decline. Most studies suggest those who report increasing sexual interest are small in number and become steadily fewer with age.[5] Caution should also be exercised in how we interpret these data to ensure that we are observing a real increase in sexual frequency or functioning, and not simply a shift in attitudes over time.

The effect of the novelty of a new relationship

Just as sexual frequency declines with length of a relationship, the forming of a new relationship usually results in an increase in sexual frequency. This positive effect of novelty on sexual frequency seems to be quite robust. In a community-based, cross-sectional study of 2001 women aged 45–55, 7% of women reported increased sexual interest compared with 12 months previously. This increase in sexual interest was most commonly associated with a new partner.[41]

Regression toward the mean

A longitudinal study in Sweden conducted in 1968–75 found that an increase in sexual desire was predicted by weak desire at first interview, reports of negative marital relations prior to first interview, and mental disorder at first interview.[34] In a sample of 108 married women aged 46–71 years, 5% reported an increase in sexual activity over the 6 years of follow-up, but half of these had resumed sexual activities after a period of cessation.[32] Why should these ostensibly negative experiences predict an increase in sexual functioning? One reason for the increase may simply be regression toward the mean. A further decline in functioning experienced by a woman who reports the lowest level on a scale will not be detected, and it is likely that at some point the factors contributing to her being at the lowest end of the spectrum will change. The result is an improvement in a woman's sexual functioning to bring it more in accord with the majority of women her age. The regression toward the mean also works in the reverse direction, with high levels of sexual functioning predicting a decline over time.[34]

Healthy survivor effects

Interestingly in the oldest age groups, an increase in sexual functioning has occasionally been reported.[4] This is most likely due to a survival effect, with sick, sexually inactive women dying and so no longer being included in the cohort, or their partners dying and renewed sexual activity taking place with a new partner.

Reasons for stability over time

As noted, stability over time is the most commonly observed pattern for frequency of sexual activities and for sexual interest or desire in longitudinal studies.[31–33] Why should this be the case, given that the majority of cross-sectional studies[1,4,5,7,15–18] and some longitudinal studies[34,35] report that sexual activities and sexual functioning decline with age? For practical reasons, the length of follow-up is rarely much longer than 10 years. This restricts the ability of longitudinal studies to detect small changes that occur over larger periods of time and may mean that these changes are detectable only in some women. Most studies which report patterns of stability over time also report patterns of increase and decline in small percentages of the sample. Discrepancies between studies may also relate to the sensitivity of the instruments used. In addition, in older cohorts, a large proportion of those who show no change in sexual frequency or desire over time are women who are no longer sexually active or feel no desire.[31] There is further evidence, however, that sexual activities and sexual functioning may be relatively resistant to change. Koster and Garde[33] found current frequency of desire to be correlated with former sexual activity. More recently, Dennerstein and Lehert[42] found that prior level of sexual functioning was the most important predictor of current sexual functioning. It is reasonable to conclude that for most women sexual function and activities are relatively stable over the short term, any changes taking place being quite small and difficult to detect.

The presence of a regular partner

A woman's sexual activities are significantly influenced by the availability of a regular partner (see Chapters 8.1 and 8.2). In 1953, Kinsey et al. (see Chapter 1.1) investigated changes in sexual frequency with age and reported differences between married and unmarried women.[3] In an investigation of 250 Caucasian and African-American men and women aged 60–93 years, Newman and Nichols[43] found that 54% of respondents who were married were sexually active compared with only 7% of respondents who were single, divorced, or widowed. In 1990, Diokno reported similar findings for women aged 60–85 years. Feelings of desire and enjoyment of sexual activities are also affected by the availability of a partner, although studies disagree whether this is a positive or negative relationship. Koster and Garde[33] found that the frequency of desire a woman experienced was positively correlated with partner availability. Conversely, in a study of woman aged 35–55 years, Mansfield and co-workers[13] found that a decrease in desire for sexual activity was associated with being married, but not with current age, and a decrease in enjoyment of sexual activities was associated with increasing age and being married. The effect of other factors, such as the length of the relationship and changes in feeling for one's partner, may be responsible for these conflicting results.

Sexual satisfaction, personal distress, and the importance of sex

Recognition that personal distress plays an important role in sexual dysfunction has increased in recent years (see Chapter 2.4). New definitions of sexual dysfunctions have developed which include personal distress as part of the definitions for vaginismus, desire, arousal, and orgasmic disorders.[21] Only recently have validated instruments for assessing sexually related distress been developed.[44] Thus, validated measures of sexual distress have rarely been included in epidemiologic studies. However, age-related changes in some aspects of sexual anxiety and distress have been investigated. Bancroft and co-workers explored distress about the relationship and one's own sexuality in a group of 987 women aged 20–65 years.[15] In selected comparisons, both forms of distress increased slightly with age; however, for the most part, there was no significant relationship with age. Laumann et al.[26] found that anxiety about sexual performance decreased with age, and Richters et al.[45] found that while anxiety during sex remained constant with age, worrying about attractiveness decreased.

Since most of the evidence points to sexual functioning declining with age,[1,4,5,7,15–18] it is surprising that the proportion of women experiencing anxiety and distress does not rise with age in response to this. Some light may be shed on this by studies of changes in the importance of sex with age. There is evidence that as women get older the relative importance of sex may decrease.[7,46] This age-related decline in the importance of sex may help explain why older women are not more distressed by poor sexual functioning and may also explain why the number of women who are motivated to report sexual difficulties does not increase with age.

Unlike sexual distress and sexual dysfunction, age-related changes in the levels of sexual satisfaction are more in line with changes observed in sexual functioning. Sexual satisfaction appears to decrease[16,22,38,47] or at least remain at the same level with age.[10,17,25]

Conclusions

Overall, the number of women reporting sexual difficulties or dysfunctions remains fairly constant with advancing age. The exception to this is sexual pain disorders, which appear to decline with age. Sexual functioning and the frequency of sexual activities have been observed to decline with age in most cross-sectional studies. In longitudinal studies, this decline has also been detected, but patterns of stability and improved sexual functioning with age have also been observed for short periods of time. A variety of factors influence the changes in sexual functioning and frequency of sexual activities that occur with age. Among these, the length of relationship, partner health, partner sexual functioning, and feelings for partner are particularly important. While many women may become less sexually satisfied as sexual function declines with age, the decrease in the relative importance of sex with age may be one of the factors which allows them to be less distressed by these changes and less inclined to report sexual difficulties.

References

1. Lunde I, Larsen G, Fog E et al. Sexual desire, orgasm and sexual fantasies: a study of 625 Danish women born in 1910, 1936 and 1958. *J Sex Educ Ther* 1991; 17: 111–15.

2. Gracia CR, Sammel MD, Freeman EW et al. Predictors of decreased libido in women during the late reproductive years. *Menopause* 2004; 11: 144–50.

3. Kinsey A, Pomeroy W, Martin C et al. *Sexual behaviour in the human female.* Philadelphia: WB Saunders, 1953.

4. Pfeiffer E, Verwoerdt A, Davis GC. Sexual behavior in middle life. *Am J Psychiatry* 1972; 128: 1262–7.

5. Hallstrom T. Sexuality in the climacteric. *Clin Obstet Gynaecol* 1977; 4: 227–39.

6. Diokno AC, Brown MB, Herzog AR. Sexual function in the elderly. *Arch Intern Med* 1990; 150: 197–200.

7. Bergstrom-Walan M, Neilsen H. Sexual expression among 60–80 year old men and women: a sample from Stockholm, Sweden. *J Sex Res* 1990; 27: 289–95.

8. Laumann E, Gagnon J, Michael R et al. *The Social Organization of Sexuality. Sexual Practices in the United States.* Chicago: University of Chicago Press, 1994.

9. Barlow DH, Cardozo L, Francis R et al. Urogenital ageing and its effect on sexual health in older British women. *Br J Obstet Gynaecol* 1997; 104: 87–91.

10. Cain V, Johannes C, Avis N et al. Sexual functioning and practices in a multi-ethnic study of midlife women: baseline results from SWAN. *J Sex Res* 2003; 40: 266–76.

11. Rissel CE, Richters J, Grulich AE et al. Sex in Australia: selected characteristics of regular sexual relationships. *Aust N Z J Public Health* 2003; 27: 124–30.

12. Richters J, Grulich AE, de Visser RO et al. Sex in Australia: auto-erotic, esoteric and other sexual practices engaged in by a representative sample of adults. *Aust N Z J Public Health* 2003; 27: 180–90.

13. Mansfield PK, Voda A, Koch PB. Predictors of sexual response changes in heterosexual midlife women. *Health Values* 1995; 19: 10–19.

14. Cawood EH, Bancroft J. Steroid hormones, the menopause, sexuality and well-being of women. *Psychol Med* 1996; 26: 925–36.

15. Bancroft J, Loftus J, Long JS. Distress about sex: a national survey of women in heterosexual relationships. *Arch Sex Behav* 2003; 32: 193–208.

16. Cayan S, Akbay E, Bozlu M et al. The prevalence of female sexual dysfunction and potential risk factors that may impair sexual function in Turkish women. *Urol Int* 2004; 72: 52–7.

17. Hunter M, Whitehead M. *Psychological Experience of the Climacteric and Postmenopause.* In C Hammond, FP Haseltime, I Schiff, eds. *Menopause: Evaluation, Treatment and Health Concerns.* New York: Alan R Liss, 1989: pp 211–24.

18. Adams CG, Turner BF. Reported change in sexuality from young adulthood to old age. *J Sex Res* 1985; 21: 126–41.

19. Masters WH, Johnson AM. *Human Sexual Response.* Boston: Little, Brown, 1966.

20. Zuckerman M. Physiological measures of sexual arousal in the human. *Psychol Bull* 1971; 75: 297–329.

21. Basson R, Berman J, Burnett A et al. Report of the international consensus development conference on female sexual dysfunction: definitions and classifications. *J Urol* 2000; 163: 888–93.

22. Fugl-Meyer AR, Fugl-Meyer K. Sexual disabilities, problems and satisfaction in 18–74 year old Swedes. *Scand J Sexol* 1999; 2: 79–105.

23. Richters J, Grulich AE, de Visser RO et al. Sex in Australia: sexual difficulties in a representative sample of adults. *Aust N Z J Public Health* 2003; 27: 164–70.

24. Kadri N, McHichi Alami KH, McHakra Tahiri S. Sexual dysfunction in women: population based epidemiological study. *Arch Women Ment Health* 2002; 5: 59–63.

25. Ventegodt S. Sex and the quality of life in Denmark. *Arch Sex Behav* 1998; 27: 295–307.

26. Laumann E, Paik A, Rosen R. Sexual dysfunction in the United States. *JAMA* 1999; 281: 537–44.

27. Fugl-Meyer K. Women's sexual dysfunctions and dysfunctional distress: a Swedish report. In *ISSWSH.* Amsterdam: 2003.

28. Johnson S, Phelps D, Cottler L. The association of sexual dysfunction and substance use among a community epidemiological sample. *Arch Sex Behav* 2004; 33: 55–63.

29. Najman J, Dunne M, Boyle F et al. Sexual dysfunction in the Australian population. *Aust Fam Physician* 2003; 32: 951–4.

30. Boulet MJ, Oddens BJ, Lehert P et al. Climacteric and menopause in seven south-east Asian countries. *Maturitas*. 1994; 19: 157–76.

31. Pfeiffer E, Verwoerdt A, Wang HS. Sexual behavior in aged men and women. I. Observations on 254 community volunteers. *Arch Gen Psychiatry* 1968; 19: 753–8.

32. George LK, Weiler SJ. Sexuality in middle and late life. The effects of age, cohort, and gender. *Arch Gen Psychiatry* 1981; 38: 919–23.

33. Koster A, Garde K. Sexual desire and menopausal development. A prospective study of Danish women born in 1936. *Maturitas* 1993; 16: 49–60.

34. Hallstrom T, Samuelsson S. Changes in women's sexual desire in middle life: the longitudinal study of women in Gothenburg. *Arch Sex Behav* 1990; 19: 259–68.

35. Dennerstein L, Randolph J, Taffe J et al. Hormones, mood, sexuality, and the menopausal transition. *Fertil Steril* 2002; 77: S42–8.

36. James WH. The honeymoon effect on marital coitus. *J Sex Res* 1981; 17: 114–23.

37. James WH. Decline in coital rates with spouses' ages and duration of marriage. *J Biosoc Sci* 1983; 15: 83–7.

38. Deeks AA, McCabe MP. Sexual function and the menopausal woman: the importance of age and partners' sexual functioning. *J Sex Res* 2001; 38: 219–25.

39. Blumel JE, Castelo-Branco C, Cancelo MJ et al. Impairment of sexual activity in middle-aged women in Chile. *Menopause* 2004; 11: 78–81.

40. Dennerstein L, Dudley E, Burger H. Are changes in sexual functioning during midlife due to aging or menopause? *Fertil Steril* 2001; 76: 456–60.

41. Dennerstein L, Smith AM, Morse CA et al. Sexuality and the menopause. *J Psychosom Obstet Gynaecol* 1994; 15: 59–66.

42. Dennerstein L, Lehert P. Modelling mid-aged women's sexual functioning: a prospective, population-based study. *J Sex Marital Ther* 2004; 30: 173–83.

43. Newman G, Nichols CR. Sexual attitudes in older persons. *JAMA* 1960; 173: 33–5.

44. Derogatis L, Rosen R, Leiblum S et al. The Female Sexual Distress Scale (FSDS): initial validation of a standardized scale for assessment of sexually related personal distress in women. *J Sex Marital Ther* 2002; 28: 317–30.

45. Richters J, Grulich AE, de Visser RO et al. Sex in Australia: sexual and emotional satisfaction in regular relationships and preferred frequency of sex among a representative sample of adults. *Aust N Z J Public Health* 2003; 27: 171–9.

46. Bretschneider JG, McCoy NL. Sexual interest and behavior in healthy 80 to 102 year olds. *Arch Sex Behav* 1988; 17: 109–29.

47. Spira A, Bajos N. *Sexual Behaviour and AIDS*. Aldershot: Avebury, 1994.

7.2 Sexual function in the menopause and perimenopause

Manjari Patel, Candace S Brown, Gloria Bachmann

Introduction

Just as pain syndromes or cancers have many etiologies, so do female sexual dysfunctions that women report during the peri- and postmenopausal years (see Chapters 13.1–13.3 in this volume). That is, not all of the sexual complaints that a woman in this stage of her life cycle reports to her clinician are due to gonadal hormone insufficiency. Rather, sexual function depends on an intact neurologic and vascular system in addition to endocrinologic integrity. Any deviation in one of these systems will cause dysfunction affecting sexual health[1] (see Chapters 3.1–3.4 and 6.1–6.5). In addition, nonmedical factors also affect the sexual health of the menopausal patient, which may either act by themselves (care of an elderly parent living in the home) or exacerbate the condition already caused by the hormonal changes (sleep deprivation from night sweats caused by diminished estrogen) or disease (diabetes mellitus). Family structure [children leaving home, financial difficulties, dysfunctional partner (see Chapters 8.1 and 8.2)], social environment (stigma of menopause associated with aging and loss of feminine allure), religious beliefs (sexual activity solely for the purpose of reproduction), previous personal sexual experience (never having had a rewarding sexual life and onset of menopause the excuse to stop engaging in coital activity), and a history of past or current sexual abuse and domestic violence (from an alcoholic or unemployed partner; see Chapter 3.4) are all important contributors to female sexual dysfunction.

Although the hormonal changes from the menopause transition itself can be overwhelming and have a markedly negative effect on sexual health, the sexual distress that these changes trigger in the menopausal woman may not have as great an impact on her quality of life compared with the younger woman. A woman during the menopausal years may be married to a partner with declining sexual health, and so a premium may not be placed on optimal sexual function. Moreover, at this point in the life cycle, most women have completed the pregnancies they desire and therefore fertility is no longer an issue. In comparison, the reproductive-aged woman with a sexual problem who has a functional partner and who has not yet fulfilled childbearing desires will experience a greater decline in quality of life than the older woman. Nonetheless, although the impact may not be as great on personal and interpersonal relationships, female sexual dysfunctions that occur with the menopausal transition frequently lead to a deterioration in the relationship between the partners, a loss of the woman's self-esteem, and a diminution in her quality of life. For affected menopausal women, female sexual dysfunction can be physically disconcerting, emotionally distressing, and socially disruptive.[1] Another negative aspect of female sexual dysfunction in the menopausal woman is that the sexual problem is usually progressive. The lactating woman who experiences vaginal dryness and dyspareunia after childbirth has a reversible condition. The menopausal women who experiences vaginal dryness and dyspareunia from urogenital atrophy due to loss of estrogen has neither a reversible etiology nor one that decreases in intensity over time. On the contrary, vaginal dryness and pain symptoms will become more severe over time.[2] Since female sexual dysfunctions increase dramatically with menopause, offering early intervention to affected women should be the goal of all clinicians who treat this cohort of women.

Definition

Female sexual dysfunction is a multidimensional and multifactorial problem, and often all contributors to the complaint may not be obvious at the first visit in which they are addressed (see Chapter 9.1). However, for many climacteric women, having their sexual concerns addressed by the physician and being offered education and counseling is often an effective first step, regardless of whether the woman consents to pharmacologic therapy, such as estrogen or androgen treatment, or sexual counseling. The World Health Organization's *International Statistical Classification of Diseases and Related Health Problems* (ICD-10) defines sexual dysfunction as "the various ways in which an individual is unable to participate in a sexual relationship as he or she would wish".[3] Today, there are no upper limits of age at which sexual health issues should not be addressed. However, for all women, especially menopausal woman, the key to offering intervention rests with whether the sexual complaint causes personal distress. According to the *Diagnostic and Statistical Manual of Mental Disorders*, fourth edition (DSM-IV), sexual dysfunctions are "disturbances in sexual desire and in the psychophysiologic changes that characterize the sexual response cycle and cause marked distress and interpersonal difficulty"[4] (Table 7.2.1). It bears repeating that all of the sexual complaints seen in the reproductive-aged female also occur (but with greater frequency) in the menopausal woman. Each of these diagnoses is subtyped as (i) lifelong versus acquired type, (ii) generalized versus situational type, and (iii) etiologic origin (organic, psychogenic, mixed, and unknown).[4] For menopausal women, sexual complaints that begin at the time of ovarian decline are more amenable to treatment with hormones and/or counseling than sexual complaints that commence premenopausally. In fact, menopausal women reporting sexual complaints that began long before the menopausal transition should be offered referral to a sex therapist in addition to hormonal and or pharmacologic intervention.

Many women may have more than one female sexual dysfunction (such as loss of sexual desire and pain with vaginal intercourse) and more than one etiology that contributes to the complaint(s). This aspect of multiple etiologies is often overlooked in the menopausal patient when defining successful intervention. That is, when a full response is not seen with estrogen or estrogen/androgen therapy, it is often assumed that the intervention was not effective. However, since female sexual dysfunction is multifactorial, and, frequently, an overlap

Table 7.2.1. American Psychiatric Association[4] classification of sexual dysfunctions

I. Sexual desire disorder
    a. Hypoactive sexual desire disorder
    b. Sexual aversion disorder

II. Sexual arousal disorder

III. Orgasmic disorder

IV. Sexual pain disorder
    a. Dyspareunia
    b. Vaginismus
    c. Other sexual pain disorders

[1]Subtypes: lifelong vs acquired type; generalized vs situational type; due to psychologic factors vs due to combined factors.

of the disorders can be observed, the estrogen therapy intervention may have treated only one of the etiologies (the urogenital atrophy), but not the relationship issues.[2]

Epidemiology

Female sexual disorders affect 20–50% of women in the USA, affecting not only midlife and older women, but also the younger population (see Chapters 2.1–2.4). Data clearly show that sexual dysfunction affects men and women throughout the adult life cycle, but becomes more prevalent with menopause in the female and with aging in both men and women.[5,6] For example, hypoactive sexual desire disorder, more commonly reported in females than men (with a female to male ratio of approximately 2–3:1), becomes more prevalent at age 60 years and older in both sexes.[7] Moreover, according to the National Health and Social Life Survey studies, approximately 20% of women aged 18–59 years report having difficulty in lubrication during sexual stimulation,[5] whereas this number jumps to 44.2% for postmenopausal women.[8] This same pattern is seen with orgasmic dysfunction. According to the National Health and Social Life Survey studies, although there is no relationship between orgasmic dysfunction and race, socioeconomic status, and educational or religious background,[5,9] there seems to be a higher prevalence of anorgasmia in single women than married women,[5] and in postmenopausal women than reproductive-aged ones.[10] Dyspareunia is the sexual dysfunction associated most closely with menopausal status and is the most frequent sexual complaint that aging women report to their gynecologist.[5,8] With anticipation of vaginal pain, many women with dyspareunia will develop vaginismus over time, although in the general population other etiologies such as previous sexual abuse and trauma may lead to this sexual dysfunction. Up to 17% of women with vaginismus may ultimately present for intervention.[11]

Physiology

Masters and Johnson, who first detailed the female sexual response cycle, depicted a linear pattern of sexual response for both premenopausal and postmenopausal subjects. Although the four successive phases, starting with excitement and then progressing from plateau to orgasm and finally to resolution, do not change with aging, there are marked alterations that occur with loss of gonadal stimulation in each of these phases.[12] For example, the excitement phase is dependent on both the activation of central nervous system and an environment of adequate ovarian hormones to achieve genital vasocongestion, increased blood flow, smooth muscle relaxation, and ultimately transudation of vaginal wall secretions. The labia increase in size, the clitoris engorges, the vagina expands, and the uterus elevates. With inadequate estrogen, the excitement phase is prolonged, and vasocongestion may be inadequate to produce the anatomic changes and the vaginal secretions necessary for comfortable coital activity. During the plateau phase, there is further engorgement of the labia, retraction of the clitoris, increased bartholin gland secretion, congestion of the outer third of the vagina, and expansion of the upper two-thirds of the vagina. Plateau is also attenuated in an environment of estrogen insufficiency. With orgasm, the intensity and number of vaginal and uterine contractions may also decrease in the menopausal woman. The final phase of resolution, characterized by gradual, pleasant diminishment of sexual tension and response, is similar in pre- and post-menopausal women.

In 1979, Kaplan proposed a three-phase model consisting of desire, arousal, and orgasm, with the same adverse changes described in the menopausal woman as with the Masters and Johnson model. It was also noted that desire for sexual exchange may be more adversely affected in the surgically menopausal patient than the naturally menopausal one because of the complete cessation of gonadal androgens.[13] This three-phase model of sexual response is the basis for DSM-IV definitions of female sexual dysfunction. The reclassification system proposed by the American Foundation of Urologic Disease Consensus Panel in October 1998 is also based on this three-phase model.[14] Another sexual function model, described as a circuit with four main domains of libido, arousal, orgasm, and satisfaction, may more accurately describe the female sexual response cycle. In this model, sexual response is thought of as a circular rather than a linear response, such that each of the four domains may overlap with each other, and each domain can give positive or negative feedback on the remaining three domains. This model explains modification of sexual response under many circumstances (situational loss of sex desire due to a teenage child studying with friends in the next room) and with many inputs affecting ultimate sexual satisfaction.

Because of the complexity of the female sexual response and the hormonal changes that occur in the aging woman with the onset of menopause, the many biologic, physiologic, psychologic, and sociocultural factors that influence sexual response are often exacerbated. Therefore, it is necessary to evaluate all contributors to sexual health in addition to hormonal ones before making treatment recommendations.[15] Use of pharmacotherapy after evaluation of only biologic or physiologic components of the dysfunction may not achieve satisfactory treatment outcomes: that is, treating vaginal atrophy with vaginal estrogen may not correct the dyspareunia if the woman is living in a household in which there is ongoing domestic violence.

Etiology – factors affecting normal sexual function

Hormonal changes

Estrogen

In otherwise healthy women, estrogen levels are well maintained until the perimenopause. Estrogen deficiency causes cellular dysfunction in the urogenital tissue, leading to vaginal atrophy. The hypoestrogenic vaginal vault shifts from an acidic pH to an alkaline pH, which contributes not only to a shift in the vaginal flora, but also to more infections, leading to discharge and odor.[16] With chronic lack of estrogen over time, vascular, muscular, and connective tissues also atrophy, and the vaginal vault becomes pale in appearance with loss of rugation and tissue friability. When coital exchange is attempted after years of estrogen loss and abstinence, the marked shortening and narrowing of the vaginal vault may make this type of sexual exchange extremely painful or impossible to achieve. Estrogen loss also affects the bladder, and complaints of urinary frequency, urgency, nocturia, dysuria, incontinence, and postcoital infection are common. The clitoris may also get fibrosed over time with loss of estrogen and decreased blood flow. Although not anatomically visible, lack of estrogen has also been shown to decrease touch perception, diminish vibratory sensation, and slow nerve impulses, causing delays in reaction time[17] (see Chapters 9.2–9.5).

The correlation of low estradiol levels with vaginal atrophy and dyspareunia is very high. Significantly more women with an estradiol level of less than 50 pg/ml report vaginal dryness, dyspareunia, and pain than women with an estradiol level of more than 50 pg/ml, and women with an estradiol level of less than 35 pg/ml report reduced coital activity.[18] Estradiol has been reported to have a stronger relationship than testosterone with declining female sexual function across the menopausal transition.[19]

Androgens

Data from both men and women show that testosterone is very important in maintaining sexual integrity as well as for maintaining libido and orgasm. Androgens also contribute to other nonsexual physiologic functions, including bone metabolism, cognition, and feeling of well-being. Total testosterone and androstenedione start to decline in the young reproductive years, and circulating levels continue to decrease with advancing age[20] (Table 7.2.2). Androgen levels peak around age 25 years and begin their gradual age-related decline during the mid-30s[21] (see Chapter 6.3).

However, surgical menopause appears to be a major contributor not only to decreased libido and impaired sexual functioning, but also to muscle wasting, osteoporosis, loss of energy, changes in mood, and depression. Before menopause, most of the decline is from the adrenals, but after menopause, the decline has contributors in both the adrenal cortex and the ovaries. Dehydroepiandrosterone, dehydroepiandrosterone sulfate, androstenedione, and testosterone[22–26] diminish in quantity. In addition, sex hormone-binding globulin, which binds with testosterone, may increase in postmenopausal women who are treated with oral estrogen therapy, thus reducing the amount of free testosterone. A major difficulty in androgen evaluation is the lack of sensitive assays to assess the low testosterone levels founds in women, as discussed in detail elsewhere.[27]

Table 7.2.2. Mean steroid levels in women (converted to pg/ml)[1]

Hormone	Reproductive age	Natural menopause	Surgical menopause
Estradiol	100–150	10–15	10
Testosterone	400	290	110
Androstenedione	1900	1000	700
DHEA	5000	2000	1800
DHEA-S	3,000,000	1,000,000	1,000,000

DHEA = dihydroepiandrosterone; DHEA-S = dihydroepiandrosterone sulfate.
From Lobo.[20]

Psychosocial factors

Along with obvious hormonal factors, psychologic and social factors also play a role in a woman's sexual health. Unfortunately, most of the changes in these factors at the time of menopause adversely affect sexual function. Not only do these changes in the female affect sexual function, but, for heterosexual women, changes in the male partner also contribute to the woman's sexual problems. Sexual changes in the male, the most common being erectile dysfunction and a prolonged preorgasmic plateau phase leading to delayed arousal and delayed orgasm, occur in the 50s and 60s. These occur at a time when religious and cultural beliefs frequently dictate that the woman's feminine role is over since she can no longer get pregnant. Considering that women usually marry men older than they are, sexual problems in both partners often surface at the same point in the relationship. Moreover, the greater longevity of women leads to a shortage of male partners later in life, which also contributes to abstinence in many older women. Adverse changes in mental health, such as depression, mood disorders, and other psychologic disorders, also have a significant impact on sexual health during the menopausal years.[5]

Medical issues

Medical conditions, although they can occur at any point in a person's life, are more prevalent at the time of the menopause. Acute and chronic illness may have both reversible and non-reversible effects on female sexual dysfunction. Medical illnesses that often commence at the time of the menopause are coronary artery disease and arthritis, which may affect arousal and orgasm capability. Neurologic diseases, such as multiple sclerosis, Parkinson's disease, or diabetes with progressive microvascular disease, also play a role, but usually a decade or so after menopause.[5]

Medications

Medications affect female sexual dysfunction in many ways, such as altering blood flow (e.g., antihypertensive medications), or affecting the central nervous system (e.g., psychotropic drugs) (Table 7.2.3)[28] Moreover, the drug effects may not be as detrimental in the younger woman as they are in the menopausal woman. For example, drying of the mucus membranes by antihistaminics may not be very troublesome to a

Table 7.2.3. Common classes of medications causing sexual dysfunction

Class	Examples
Antihypertensive drugs	α_1- and α_2-adrenergic antagonists (clonidine, reserpine, prazosin) β-adrenergic antagonists (metoprolol, propranolol) Calcium channel antagonists (diltiazem, nifedipine) Diuretics (hydrochlorothiazide)
Chemotherapeutic drugs	Alklylating agents (busulfan, chorambucil, cyclophosphamide)
CNS drugs	Acetycholine receptor antagonists (diphenhydramine) Antiepileptic drugs (carbamazepine, phenobarbital, phenytoin) Antidepressants (MAOIs, TCAs, SSRIs) Antipsychotics (phenothiazines, butyrophenones) Opioids (oxycodone) Sedatives/anxiolytics (benzodiazepines)
Drugs affecting hormones	Antiandrogens (cimetidine, spironolactone) Antiestrogens (tamoxifen, raloxifene) Oral contraceptives

MAOIs = monoamine oxidase inhibitors; TCA = tricyclic antidepressants; SSRI = selective serotonin reuptake inhibitors.
From Walsh and Berman.[28]

reproductive-aged woman. However, the additive drying effect of the drug on the already atrophied vaginal vault will be very detrimental to the older woman. One major class of drugs that has a serious impact on sexuality in the menopausal woman, since women in this age category often use them, are the selective serotonin reuptake inhibitors. In fact, selective serotonin reuptake inhibitors are frequently prescribed for perimenopausal depression. Of the antidepressant class of drugs, bupropion has been shown to have the most favorable profile in sexual function.[29]

Surgical issues

As women progress through the menopause, the likelihood increases they will need a surgical procedure that affects their sexual self. Breast and genital tract procedures have the greatest negative influence on sexuality, but not in all cases. For example, after simple hysterectomy without excision of the ovaries for the treatment of pelvic prolapse or chronic bleeding, women usually report an improvement in sexual function (see Chapter 16.7). When hysterectomy is accompanied by oophorectomy, there is a high probability that sexual dysfunction will result, especially hypoactive sexual desire disorder.[30] Data show that adverse changes in libido and orgasmic response are more likely in women who have had an oophorectomy than in those who retain their ovaries, and they are less likely to report improvements than women who have had hysterectomy without oophorectomy (55% compared with 74%).[31] They are also more likely to experience decreased positive psychologic well-being. Compared with an age-matched normative population of partnered women, the surgically menopausal woman has significantly reduced sexual thoughts and desire, arousal, frequency of activity, receptivity and initiation, pleasure and orgasm, and relationship satisfaction.[32] Preservation of the cervix may help to avoid adverse changes in sexual response when hysterectomy is needed, but data are not conclusive. The woman and her partner should be offered preoperative counseling for potential sexual changes, better or worse, that might follow the surgery.

Nonpelvic surgery, such as coronary bypass for a woman or her partner, also may lead to physical and emotional decline.

Clinical evaluation: assessment and diagnosis

Clinicians caring for menopausal women should introduce the topic of sexual dysfunction during both the medical history and the pelvic examination, especially if urogenital atrophy is noted. Menopausal women may not discuss the topic of sexual problems themselves without direct questioning, since many come from an era when these concerns were not openly talked about. Moreover, even though a gonadal hormonal profile may be ordered in some cases, there is no consensus on this practice

for all cases, and for most women sexual history alone is sufficient to uncover hormonal insufficiency etiologies and to commence treatment with estrogens and androgens.

Sexual history should evaluate sexual interest, arousal, orgasm, and pain (Table 7.2.4)[33] (see Chapter 9.4). Treatment is offered if the woman is distressed because of the sexual change or problem. As part of the sexual history, medication use, including over-the-counter, prescription, and street drugs, should be recorded, as menopausal women are often on more medications than younger ones and there is a higher probability of their being on a drug that will affect sexual function.

Physical evaluation

A pelvic examination is essential in the menopausal woman to assess vaginal atrophy, dryness, trauma, infection, muscle tone, and pain-triggering spots (see Chapter 9.5). An important measurement is vaginal pH. A pH of more than 5 indicates atrophy, even in the younger perimenopausal women, if no other infective agent is responsible for the basic environment. The clinician should also perform a complete physical examination to rule out other comorbid conditions that might be causing sexual dysfunction.

An endocrine evaluation with measurement of the serum follicle-stimulating hormone, leuteinizing hormone, serum estradiol, dehydroepiandrosterone, total testosterone, free testosterone, sex hormone-binding globulin, and prolactin levels may be indicated in women with sexual dysfunction.[2]

Table 7.2.4. Guidelines for taking a general sexual history

General sexual history

I. Current sexual activity
  a. With partner(s) (regardless of marital status)
    i.   Orientation (e.g., heterosexual, homosexual, bisexual)
    ii. Number of sexual partners in past year
    iii. Contraceptive use
    iv. Pain
    v. Sexually transmitted diseases (STDs)
    vi. Specific concerns/questions
  b. With self (masturbation)
    i. Satisfaction
    ii. Specific concerns

II. Adequacy of sexual responses
  a. Desire (i.e., too much, too little, too different – level of interest differs from partner)
  b. Arousal (lubrication, subjective excitement)
  c. Orgasm (frequency, ease of attainment)
  d. Satisfaction

III. History of STDs (which ones, how treated)
IV. History of sexual abuse (current, past)
V. Medical conditions that may affect sexual function or behavior (e.g., pregnancy, menopause, surgeries, cancer, arthritis, medications)

From Leiblum.[33]

Psychosocial/psychosexual assessment

Psychosocial factors have great impact on female sexual dysfunction for both younger and older women (see Chapter 9.3). Social issues, past sexual beliefs, and emotional aspects and other psychiatric disorders should always be ruled out.[34]

Many subjective and objective measures have been used in clinical trials in an attempt to standardize definitions and outcomes. The clinical assessment of female sexual dysfunction in the menopausal patient does not include many objective measures except obvious changes on pelvic examination and vaginal pH. Objective research measures include (1) genital blood flow (measuring clitoral, labial, urethral, and vaginal peak systolic velocities and end-diastolic velocities by duplex Doppler ultrasonography); (2) vaginal lubrication measurements and vaginal pH; (3) vaginal compliance and elasticity (pressure volume changes); and (4) genital sensation (vibration and temperature perception thresholds).[35]

Subjective measures are primarily used in research and include self-rated questionnaires, daily diaries, and event logs. Self-report measures have been developed that are reliable, well-standardized, validated, inexpensive, and easy to administer and score, and have normative values for both clinical and nonclinical populations. The most common self-rated questionnaires measure desire, arousal, orgasm, and sexual pain; they include the Brief Sexual Function Index for Women,[36] the Female Sexual Function,[37] and the Derogatis Interview for Sexual Functioning.[38] Daily diaries and event logs quantify the frequency of sexual activity, attempts at intercourse, and other forms of sexual activity.[35]

Management

Accurate assessment of the menopausal patient leads to an optimal management plan. Treatment plans should always include all facets affecting sexual dysfunction, including proper education about normal anatomy and physiology, as well as endocrine factors, such as changes in androgen and estrogen levels. Women should be asked to avoid medications that may have influence on sexual function, and encouraged to avoid alcohol and to stop smoking. Maintaining optimal health and correcting reversible medical problems are important steps to optimize sexual function.[2]

Nonpharmacologic therapy

Lifestyle changes such as drinking more water, smoking cessation, and aerobic exercises all have positive impacts on sexuality by maintaining the stamina to perform sex, increase libido, decrease depression, enhance body image, and increase testosterone levels. Communicating sexual likes and dislikes between partners, and reviewing sex videos and erotic literature can broaden sexual techniques. Increased tactile stimulation can increase arousal and desire, while communication and spending time together improves intimacy. Specific treatment strategies are illustrated in Table 7.2.5.

Pharmacologic therapy

Even though there are many suggested treatment options available, there is no single intervention that will be effective in all peri- and post-menopausal women.

Estrogen therapy

Decreased sexual function in postmenopausal women is due in part to estrogen depletion after menopause. The estrogen decline associated with menopause is a major cause of climacteric signs and symptoms, such as vaginal atrophy, hot flashes, dyspareunia, and nocturnal awakening. One controlled and two open-label trials have shown reduced vaginal symptoms after estrogen therapy (Table 7.2.6). Lower doses of conjugated equine estrogen (0.45 and 0.3 mg) with and without medroxyprogesterone acetate (2.5 mg, 1.5 g) reduced vaginal atrophy compared with placebo in 2673 healthy menopausal women.[39] A 12-week, randomized clinical trial found that among 194 postmenopausal women with urogenital atrophy, a continuous, low-dose, estradiol-releasing vaginal ring provided relief comparable to conjugated equine estrogen vaginal cream, but was more acceptable than the cream.[40] Similarly, a 24-week comparative study of 159 menopausal women found that 25-μg 17-β estradiol vaginal tablets and 1.25 mg conjugated equine estrogen vaginal cream were equally efficacious in relieving atrophic vaginitis, but the vaginal tablets produced less endometrial proliferation or hyperplasia, and were more favorable than the cream.[41]

Several clinical trials have reported improved sexual desire in healthy postmenopausal women receiving estrogen therapy[42–46] (Table 7.2.6), but only one placebo-controlled trial has been conducted in postmenopausal women with sexual dysfunction.[47,48] In this 12-month trial, a significant improvement in mood, sexual desire, enjoyment, and orgasmic frequency, apart from vaginal symptoms, was reported in 49 ovariectomized women receiving ethinyl estradiol (50 μg) compared with levonorgestrol (250 μg/day), a combination of these two substances, or placebo.[47,48] No differences were found between groups in coital rate. Thus, while the literature shows that estrogen is effective in postmenopausal women with vaginal atrophy, which may impede sexual function, there are few data to suggest that estrogen improves sexual desire, enjoyment, and orgasmic frequency.

Testosterone therapy

Studies of testosterone use have been conducted in postmenopausal women for over half a century. The studies are difficult to compare because of different methodologies, pooling of diverse cohorts (oophorectomized and nonoophorectomized women), varied definitions of sexual dysfunction, and a nonoverlapping range of inclusion criteria.

The first androgen studies combined estrogen with testosterone pellets of 50[49,50] or 100 mg,[51] or intramuscular injections

Table 7.2.5. Common psychosocial contributions to female sexual difficulties and potential psychotherapeutic treatment options[1]

Contributing factors or maintaining factors	Treatment strategies
Developmental influences: Sexual myths and misconceptions; negative sexual upbringing	Education and bibliotherapy; cognitive restructuring; clarification of the impact of emotions on sexual functioning (psychodynamic therapy)
Negative emotions (anxiety, aversion, anger, disgust, guilt, shame, etc.)	Permission giving and validation, education, desensitization (readings, pictures, masturbation and nondemand touching exercises); psychodynamic exploration
Performance anxiety (i.e., arousal- and pleasure-interfering cognitions and worries)	Refocus the woman's attention on pleasurable sensations (nondemand touching exercises); cognitive restructuring and positive sexual fantasies
Body image concerns	Body image desensitization; eliminating appearance preoccupied rituals; cognitive restructuring
Relationship factors: Relationship or marital distress	Couple therapy
Secrets; sexual orientation; extrarelationship affairs; undisclosed abuse history or unconventional sexual behaviors	Treatment approach is case specific
Poor sexual technique (client or partner)	Psychoeducation; instructional and erotic videos; nondemand touching; sexual communication training
Environmental factors: stress, fatigue, inadequate time together, insufficient childcare, etc.	Enhancing conditions for sexual activity; communication training; time management skills training; clarification and exploration of priorities
Trauma and comorbid Axis I disorders: History of sexual abuse, sexual assault or other traumatic physical experiences	EMDR; Exposure-based cognitive behavioral therapy; or referral (where appropriate)
Anxiety, depression, or other Axis I disorder	Empirically supported treatment or best practice guidelines
Substance use disorder (drugs and alcohol)	Referral or substance abuse therapy
Compulsive use of Internet erotica	Stimulus control and relapse prevention; referral for psychopharmacology (SSRI)

EMDR = eye movement desensitization and reprocessing; SSRI = selective serotonergic reuptake inhibitor.
[1]From Leiblum and Wiegel.[34]

(150 mg).[52,53] Both unblinded[50,52,53] and blinded[49,51] studies showed improvement in mood and sexual functioning. However, supraphysiologic doses were often used, and intramuscular injections showed erratic absorption. Two blinded studies found that oral methyltestosterone (2.5 mg) with estrogen (Estratest)[54,55] improved sexual functioning at physiologic doses.

Transdermal patches or gels, which are more consistently absorbed and avoid first pass through the liver, are being studied for safety and efficacy in reducing sexual symptoms associated with testosterone insufficiency. Recently, transdermal testosterone patches (150 µg and 300 µg) were compared with placebo in 75 estrogenized women who had undergone oophorectomy and hysterectomy.[56] The study results showed that the 300-µg testosterone patch was significantly more effective than the 150-µg patch or placebo in improving frequency of sexual activity, pleasure, and fantasy during a 12-week period. There are no safety or efficacy data available on topical preparations in women, so their effects on sexual function are not known.

Possible adverse effects of testosterone include weight gain, clitoral enlargement, increased facial hair, voice deepening, and decreases in high-density lipoprotein cholesterol, which are dose dependent. The risks and benefits of androgen therapy are described in Table 7.2.7.[57] Testosterone dosage formulations that have been used but are not US Food and Drug Administration approved are listed in Table 7.2.8.[57,58] Safety and efficacy data are not available on off-label uses. Table 7.2.8 also provides information on how they are prescribed. There is no consensus on the value of androgen levels to predict which women will respond to androgens and at what level a response occurs.

Dehydroepiandrosterone
Dehydroepiandrosterone, which is both an ovarian and adrenal androgen precursor hormone, provides hormonal substrate for conversion to testosterone and dehydrotestosterone, which then interacts with androgen receptors.[59] Because dehydroepiandrosterone is classified as a "dietary supplement" rather than a drug, it is not under the control of the Food and Drug Administration, and thus there is no standardization of potency.

Table 7.2.6. Trials of pharmacologic agents in treating sexual dysfunction

Drug	Ref.	Design	N	Regimen	Measure	Outcome
Estrogen	39	OL	194	Vag Ring; Vag Crm	Vaginal atrophy	Vag Ring = Vag Crm
	40	OL	159	E2 Vag Tab; CEE Vag Crm	Vaginal atrophy	Vag Tab = Vag Crm
	41	RCT	2,673	CEE/MPA; PB	Vaginal atrophy	All CEE/MPA > PB
	44, 45	RCT	49	EE (50 µg); LVN (250 µg); PB	Sexual activity	EE >EE + LVN = PB
Estrogen–androgen combinations	46	RCT	20	E2 (40 µg) + T (50 mg) PT; PB	Sexual activity	E2/T > PB
	47	OL	34	E2 (50 µg) + T (50 mg) PT	Sexual activity	E2/T50 > PB
	48	RCT	17	E2 (40 µg) + T (100 mg) PT; PB	Sexual activity	E2/T > PB
	49	OL	44	E2 (8.5–10 µg) + T (150 mg) IM; PB	Sexual activity	E2/T ⌐ PB
	50	OL	53	E2 (8.5 µg) + T (150 mg) IM	Sexual activity	E2/T > PB
		RCT	75	CEE + TT (150 or 300 µg); PB	Sexual activity	CEE/TT > PB
	51	RCT	218	EE (0.625 mg) + MT (2.5 mg); PB	Sexual activity	EE/MT > PB
	52	RCT	20	EE (1.25 mg) + MT (2.5 mg); PB	Sexual activity	EE/MT > PB
Sildenafil	58	RCT	781	S (10–100 mg); PB	Sexual activity	All S = PB
	59	RCT	34	S (50 mg); PB	Erotic video;	S > PB (erotic video);
					sexual activity	S = PB (sexual activity)
	60	OL	33	S (50 mg)	Sexual activity	Effective
Tibilone	63	RCT	38	T (2.5 mg); PB	Sexual activity	T > PB
	64	RCT	28	T (2.5 mg); PB	Sexual activity	T > PB
	65	COMP	437	T (2.5 mg), E2 (2 mg) + NE	Sexual activity	T > E2/NE
DHEA	57	RCT	60	DHEA (50 mg); PB	Sexual activity	DHEA = PB
Arginine-Yohimbine	66	RCT	24	AG/Y; Y; PB	Erotic video	AG/Y > Y = PB
Phentolamine	67	RCT	6	PH (40 mg); PB	Erotic video	PH > PB
Alprostadil	68	RCT	79	A (100 µg); PB	Sexual activity	A > PB

AG = arginine; CEE = conjugated equine estrogen; COMP = comparative study; CRM = cream; DHEA, dehydroepiandrosterone; E2 = estradiol; EE = ethinyl estradiol; IM = intramuscular; LVN = levonorgestrel; OL = open label; MPA = medroxyprogesterone; MT = methyltestosterone; NE = norethindrone; P = patch; PH = phentolamine; PT = pellet; PB = placebo, RCT = randomized placebo-controlled trial, Ref = reference; S = sildenafil; T = testosterone; Vag = vaginal; Y = yohimbine.

One 3-month, placebo-controlled study of dehydroepiandrosterone (50 mg/day) in 60 perimenopausal women with complaints of altered mood and well-being, found that the active treatment produced changes in hormone levels (242% increase in dehydroepiandrosterone, 95% increase in testosterone, and 13% decline in cortisol compared with baseline), but was no more effective than placebo in improving perimenopausal symptoms, mood, dysphoria, libido, cognition, memory, or well-being.[60]

Selective phosphodiesterase type 5 inhibitors

Selective phosphodiesterase type 5 inhibitors are used for the treatment of male erectile dysfunction. They work by decreasing the catabolism of the cyclic nucleotide, cyclic guanosine monophosphate, the second messenger in the nitric oxide-mediated pathway, thus promoting smooth muscle relaxation and vascular engorgement. Theoretically, selective phosphodiesterase type 5 inhibitors should also enhance the vaginal engorgement and lubrication response in women, especially menopausal ones, through smooth muscle relaxation.[28]

Research on the use of selective phosphodiesterase type 5 inhibitors in postmenopausal women with sexual arousal disorder has shown mixed results. In a large randomized, placebo-controlled trial, 577 estrogenized and 204 estrogen-deficient women receiving a selective phosphodiesterase type 5 inhibitor (10–100 mg/day) showed no overall improvement in sexual response.[61] Selective phosphodiesterase type 5 inhibitors (50 mg/day) improved subjective arousal during visualization of an erotic video in 34 estrogenized postmenopausal women with acquired genital disorder and impaired orgasm, but it was no

Table 7.2.7. Androgen therapy: risks versus benefits

Benefits	Risks
Development or maintenance of secondary sex characteristics	Fluid retention
	Acne/oily skin
Improves libido and sexual function	Clitoromegaly
Increases muscle mass and strength	Male-pattern baldness
Increases bone mineral density	Lowered voice
Decreases body and visceral fat	Increases hematocrit
Increases hematocrit	Decreases HDL-cholesterol
Improves mood	Sleep apnea
Positive effect on cognition (?)	Aggressive behavior
Positive effect on quality of life (?)	
Assertive behavior	

HDL, high-density lipoprotein.
Adapted from Swerdloff and Wang.[57]

Table 7.2.8. Testosterone therapy regimens currently used for treatment of disorders of desire[1]

Baseline lipid profile, liver enzyme levels, mammography, Pap smear (may consider free and total testosterone levels[2] in select cases)

Initiate therapy[3]

Oral:
    Combination product
        Estratest (esterified estrogen 1.25 mg/methyltestosterone 2.5 mg)
        Estratest HS (esterified estrogen 0.625 mg/methyltestosterone 1.25 mg)
    Methyltestosterone (android 1.25–2.5 mg daily)
    Micronized oral testosterone, 5 mg twice daily

Topical:
    Testosterone propionate 2% in petroleum applied q.d. to q.o.d.

Injectable:[4]
    Testosterone cypionate/enanthate 50–400 mg IM q 2–4 weeks (female dose?)

Pellet:[4]
    Testosterone SQ implantation 150–450 mg q 3–6 months (female dose?)

Transdermal:[5]
    Androderm or AndroGel 1 patch delivers 5 gm/d
    (Apply ¼ patch to abdomen 2–4 times/week for women)

Reevaluation at 3–4 months

Repeat lipid profile, and liver enzyme levels (and possibly testosterone levels)

Monitor symptoms, side effects

Continued therapy

Taper to lowest effective dosage[6]

Monitor lipid levels and liver enzyme levels once or twice yearly

Routine Pap smear and mammography schedule

[1]From Swerdloff and Wang[57] and Phillips.[58]
[2]No testosterone therapy regimen is currently approved by the US Federal Drug Administration (FDA) for the treatment of women with desire disorders.
[3]Many authors recommend that total levels remain in "normal" range for premenopausal women
[4]None of these medications are labeled by the FDA for treatment of desire disorders.
[5]FDA approved male doses for hypogonadism.
[6]Alternate daily combined with estrogen-only pill, take testosterone pill every other day, 5 days a week, etc. (not shown in studies to be safer or have fewer side effects).
HS = take the medication at night; SQ = take the medication subcutaneously.

more effective than placebo in improving sexual arousal or orgasm.[62] Changes in vaginal lubrication and clitoral sensitivity were reported in an open-label study of selective phosphodiesterase type 5 inhibitor (50 mg) in 33 postmenopausal women with sexual dysfunction, but there was no overall improvement in sexual function.[63] Other selective phosphodiesterase type 5 inhibitors have not undergone clinical trails in postmenopausal women with sexual complaints.[28]

Tibolone

Tibolone is a synthetic steroid that is available in Europe and Asia for the management of climacteric symptoms and the prevention of osteoporosis. Recent evidence suggests that tibolone may improve mood and libido in postmenopausal women because it has androgenic as well as progestogenic and estrogenic effects.

It is thought to bind to androgen receptors, increase circulating free testosterone, and lower sex hormone-binding globulin levels.[64,65] There are a few small clinical trials that have shown an improvement in sexual desire and arousability in tilolone (2.5 mg/day) as compared with placebo and to estradiol;[66,67] tibolone (2.5 mg/day) was reported more efficacious than estradiol (2 mg) plus norethisterone acetate in increasing sexual frequency, sexual satisfaction, and enjoyment in 437 postmenopausal women in a 48-week multicenter trial.[68] More data are needed to evaluate fully tibolone's effect on postmenopausal women with low sexual desire.

Arginine and yohimbine

Arginine is an amino acid precursor to the formation of nitric oxide, and promotes relaxation of smooth muscle. Sold as a component in many herbal supplements, preliminary studies have found it to be promising in erectile disorder.[28] Yohimbine is an α_2-adrenoceptor antagonist that acts as a vasodilator.[28] One randomized, double-blind study found that the combination of arginine and yohimbine increased vaginal and subject response to an erotic film compared with yohimbine alone or placebo in 24 postmenopausal women.[69]

Phentolamine

Phentolamine is a nonspecific adrenoceptor antagonist causing vascular smooth muscle relaxation and subsequent vasodilation. It has been previously studied in men for the treatment of erectile dysfunction.[28] One study found oral phentolamine (40 mg) more effective than placebo in improving subjective arousal and vaginal blood flow in six postmenopausal women with poor arousal and lack of lubrication.[70]

Alprostadil

Alprostadil is a naturally occurring form of the hormone prostaglandin E_1 and a potent vasodilator. It was approved by the Food and Drug Administration in 1995 for the treatment of erectile dysfunction in men and is available in both injection and intraurethral suppository forms.[28] One study found topical alprostadil (400 μg) to be more effective than alprostadil (100 μg) or placebo in improving level of sexual arousal and satisfaction in 79 postmenopausal women with a sexual arousal disorder.[71]

Other products

Androgenic dietary supplements, dopamine receptor antagonists (apomorphine), α-melanocyte stimulating hormone analogs, and vasoactive intestinal peptide have been studied in erectile disorder, but have not been studied in postmenopausal women.[72]

Summary

In summary, many new and promising interventions are on the horizon for the pharmacologic treatment of sexual problems. The role of over-the-counter and herbal products used in the treatment of postmenopausal women with sexual dysfunction is based on a few, small, short-term trials, so that there is a lack of efficacy and safety data. Hormonal therapies with estrogens and androgens have been more thoroughly studied, with efficacy observed in the treatment of dyspareunia (estrogen) and hypoactive sexual desire disorder (androgen). Both systemic and topical estrogens – which is the preferred route of administration – are effective for postmenopausal women with vaginal dryness or atrophic changes causing dyspareunia, but do not appear to improve sexual desire, enjoyment, and orgasmic frequency. The use of androgens to improve sexual desire in postmenopausal women is supported by placebo-controlled studies of combined oral estrogen-testosterone, combined estrogen-testosterone pellets, combined estrogen-testosterone intramuscular injection, and transdermal testosterone in estrogenized

women. All studies showed improvement in sexual desire with the active compared with placebo groups. Further research on gonadal hormone preparations, as well as other pharmacologic and herbal interventions, is necessary for the treatment of postmenopausal sexual dysfunction.

Conclusion

Sexuality is an integral part of healthy human life and does not abruptly come to an end with the onset of menopause. The first step in treating older women is taking a comprehensive medical and sexual history to learn whether the sexual problems began before or after the onset of declining gonadal hormone levels. With menopausal women, proper knowledge of different cultural beliefs and social structure helps to understand what role menopause plays in the woman's overall sexual health and function. Newer definitions and classifications, and inclusion of the psychosocial aspect have led to important changes in approach to female sexual dysfunction in all women, including the menopausal woman. Female sexual dysfunction is complex with varied etiologies, and comprehensive history is important to reach appropriate etiologies. Researchers have developed multiple types of questionnaires that help to explore different domains of female sexual dysfunction. Many modalities of treatment options have been suggested for menopausal female sexual dysfunction, including nonpharmacologic measures, psychosocial therapies, and behavioral modifications. Many drugs are under clinical trial to help treat female sexual dysfunction with sound safety profiles and efficacy. Even though extensive work has been done to understand the impact of menopause on female sexual dysfunction, many research questions still remain, and as further clinical trials are undertaken, expanded pharmacologic therapies will be added to the interventions clinicians can use for their menopausal patients with female sexual dysfunction.

References

1. Basson R, Berman J, Derogatis L et al. Report of the international consensus development conference on female sexual dysfunction: definitions and classifications. *J Urol* 2000; 163: 888–93.
2. Lightner DJ. Female sexual dysfunction. *Mayo Clin Proc* 2002; 77: 698–702.
3. World Health Organization. *ICD-10: International Statistical Classification of Diseases and Related Health Problems.* Geneva: World Health Organization, 1992.
4. American Psychiatric Association. *DSM-IV: Diagnostic and Statistical Manual of Mental Disorders*, 4th edn. Washington, DC: American Psychiatric Press, 1994.
5. Laumann EO, Paik A, Rosen RC. Sexual dysfunction in the United States: prevalence and predictors. *JAMA* 1999; 281: 537–44.
6. Rosen RC. Prevalence and risk factors of sexual dysfunction in men and women. *Curr Psychiatry Rep* 2000; 2: 189–95.

7. Rosen RC, Leiblum SR. Treatment of sexual disorders in the 1990's: an integrated approach. *J Consult Clin Psychol* 1995; 63: 877–90.

8. Anastasiadis AG, Davis AR, Ghafar MA et al. The epidemiology and definition of female sexual disorders. *World J Urol* 2002; 20: 74–8.

9. Heimann JR, Grafton-Becker V. *Orgasmic Disorders in Women*. New York: Guilford Press, 1989.

10. Rosen RC, Taylor JF, Leiblum SR et al. Prevalence of sexual dysfunction in women. *J Sex Marital Ther* 1993; 19: 171–88.

11. Spector IP, Carey MP. Incidence and prevalence of the sexual dysfunctions: a critical review. *Arch Sex Behav* 1990; 19: 389–409.

12. Masters WH, Johnson VE. *Human Sexual Response*. Boston: Little Brown, 1966.

13. Kaplan HS. *The New Sex Therapy*. New York: Brunner/Mazel, 1974.

14. Berman JR, Berman L, Goldstein I. Female sexual dysfunction: incidence, pathophysiology, evaluation, and treatment options. *Urology* 1999; 54: 385–91.

15. Basson R. Female sexual response: the role of drugs in the management of sexual dysfunction. *Obstet Gynecol* 2001; 98: 350.

16. Semmens JP, Wagner G. Estrogen deprivation and vaginal function in postmenopausal women. *JAMA* 1982; 248: 445.

17. Marks LE. Sensory perception and ovarian secretions. In F Naftolein, AH DeCherey, JN Gutmann et al., eds. *Ovarian Secretions and Cardiovascular and Neurological Function*. New York: Raven Press, 1999: p 223.

18. Cutler WB, Garcia CR. McCoy N. Perimenopausal sexuality. *Arch Sex Behav* 1987; 16: 225–34.

19. Dennerstein L, Randolph J, Taffe J et al. Hormones, mood, sexuality and the menopausal transition. *Fertil Steril* 2002; 77(Suppl): S42–S8.

20. Lobo T. *Treatment of Postmenopausal Women*. Boston: Lippincott, 1999.

21. Longcope C, Johnston CC Jr. Androgen and estrogen dynamics: stability over a two-year interval in peri-menopausal women. *J Steroid Biochem* 1990; 35: 91.

22. Davis S, Burger H. Clinical review: androgens and the postmenopausal women. *J Clin Endocrinol Metab* 1996; 81: 1759–63.

23. Sarrel P. Psychosexual effects of menopause: role of androgens. *Am J Obstet Gynecol* 1999; 180: 319–24.

24. Sherwin B. Use of combined estrogen-androgen preparations in the postmenopause: evidence from clinical studies. *Int J Fertil Womens Med* 1998; 43: 98–103.

25. Slater C, Souter I, Zhang C et al. Pharmacokinetics of testosterone after percutaneous gel or buccal administration. *Fertil Steril* 2001; 1: 32–7.

26. Basson R. Androgen replacement for women. *Can Fam Physician* 1999; 45: 2100–7.

27. Miller KK. Androgen deficiency in women. *J Clin Endocrinol Metab* 2001; 86: 2395–2401.

28. Walsh KE, Berman JR. Sexual dysfunction in the older woman: an overview of the current understanding and management. *Drugs Aging* 2004; 21: 665–75.

29. Ashton AK, Rosen RC. Bupropion as an antidote for serotonin reuptake inhibitor-induced sexual dysfunction. *J Clin Psychiatry* 1998; 59: 112.

30. Rhodes JC, Kjerulff KH, Langenberg PW et al. Hysterectomy and sexual functioning. *JAMA* 1999; 282: 1934.

31. Nathorst-Boos J, Wiklund I, Mattson LA et al. Is sexual life influenced by transdermal estrogen therapy? A double blind placebo controlled study in postmenopausal women. *Acta Obstet Gynecol Scand* 1993; 72: 656–60.

32. Mazer NA, Leiblum SR, Rosen RC. The brief index of sexual functioning for women (BISF-W): a new scoring algorithm and comparison of normative and surgically menopausal populations. *Menopause* 2000; 7: 350–63.

33. Leiblum SR. Taking a sexual history: assessing disease risk and managing sexual concerns. *Female Patient* 1994; April: 133–6.

34. Leiblum SR. Wiegel M. Psychotherapeutic interventions for treating female sexual dysfunction. *World J Urol* 2000; 20: 127–36.

35. Rosen RC. Assessment of female sexual dysfunction: review of validated methods. *Fertil Steril* 2002; 77 (Suppl 4): S89–93.

36. Taylor JE, Rosen RC, Leiblum SR. Self-report assessment of female sexual function: psychometric evaluation of the Brief Index of Sexual Functioning for Women. *Arch Sex Behav* 1994; 23: 627–43.

37. Rosen RC, Brown C, Heiman J et al. The Female Sexual Function Index (FSFI): a multidimensional self-report instrument for the assessment of female sexual function. *J Sex Mar Ther* 2000; 26: 91–208.

38. Derogatis LR. The Derogatis Interview for Sexual Functioning (DISF/DISF-R): an introductory report. *J Sex Mar Ther* 1997; 23: 291–6.

39. Utian WH, Shoupe D, Bachmann G et al. Relief of vasomotor symptoms and vaginal atrophy with lower doses of conjugated equine estrogens and medroxyprogesterone acetate. *Fertil Steril* 2001; 75: 1065–79.

40. Ayton RA, Darling GM, Murkies AL et al. A comparative study of safety and efficacy of continuous low dose oestradiol released from a vaginal ring compared with conjugated equine oestrogen vaginal cream in the treatment of postmenopausal urogenital atrophy. *Br J Obstet Gynaecol* 1996; 103: 351–8.

41. Rioux JE, Devlin C, Gelfand MM et al. 17beta-Estradiol vaginal tablet versus conjugated equine estrogen vaginal cream to relieve menopausal atrophic vaginitis. *Menopause* 2000; 7: 156–61.

42. Sherwin BB. The impact of different doses of estrogen and progestin on mood and sexual behavior in postmenopausal women. *J Clin Endocrinol Metab* 1991; 72: 336–43.

43. Utian WH. The true clinical features of postmenopause and oophorectomy, and their response to oestrogen therapy. *S Afr Med J* 1972; 46: 732–7.

44. Coope J. The effect of "natural" oestrogen replacement therapy on menopausal symptoms. *Postgrad Med J* 1976; 52: 27.

45. Miller M, Franklin K. Theoretical basis for the benefit of postmenopausal estrogen substitution. *Exp Gerontol* 1999; 34: 587–604.

46. Hilditch J, Lewis J, Ross A et al. A comparison of the effects of oral conjugated equine estrogen and transdermal estradiol-17 beta combined with an oral progestin on quality of life in postmenopausal women. *Maturitas* 1996; 24: 177–84.

47. Dennerstein L, Burrows GD, Hyman GJ, Sharpe K. Hormone therapy and affect. *Maturitas* 1979; 1: 247–59.

48. Dennerstein L, Burrows GD, Wood C et al. Hormones and sexuality: effect of estrogen and progestogen. *Obstet Gynecol* 1980; 56: 316–22.

49. Burger H Hailes J, Nelson J et al. Effect of combined implants of oestradiol and testosterone on libido in postmenopausal women. *Br Med J (Clin Res Ed)* 1987; 294: 936–7.

50. Davis SR, McCloud P, Strauss BJ et al. Testosterone enhances estradiol's effects on postmenopausal bone density and sexuality. *Maturitas* 1995; 21: 227–36.

51. Burger HG, Hailes J, Menelaus M et al. The management of persistent menopausal symptoms with oestradiol-testosterone implants: clinical, lipid and hormonal results. *Maturitas* 1984; 6: 351–8.

52. Sherwin BB, Gelfand MM. Differential symptom response to parenteral estrogen and/or androgen administration in the surgical menopause. *Am J Obstet Gynecol* 1985; 151: 153–60.

53. Sherwin BB, Gelfand MM, Brender W. Androgen enhances sexual motivation in females: a prospective, crossover study of sex steroid administration in the surgical menopause. *Psychosom Med* 1985; 47: 339–51.

54. Lobo RA, Rosen RC, Yang HM et al. Comparative effects of oral esterified estrogens with and without methyltestosterone on endocrine profiles and dimensions of sexual function in postmenopausal women with hypoactive sexual desire. *Fertil Steril* 2003; 79: 1341–52.

55. Sarrel P, Dobay B, Witta B. Estrogen and estrogen-androgen replacement in postmenopausal women dissatisfied with estrogen-only therapy: sexual behavior and neuroendocrine responses. *J Reprod Med* 1998; 43: 847–56.

56. Shifren JL, Braunstein GD, Simon JA et al. Transdermal testosterone treatment in women with impaired sexual function after oophorectomy. *N Engl J Med* 2000; 343: 682–8.

57. Swerdloff RS, Wang C. The testis and male sexual function. In L Goldman, JC Bennett, eds. *Cecil Textbook of Medicine*, 21st edn. Philadelphia: WB Saunders, 2000.

58. Phillips NA. Female sexual dysfunction: evaluation and treatment. *Am Fam Physician* 2000; 62: 127–36, 141–2.

59. Hormone therapy, sexual dysfunction. *Obstet Gynecol* 2004 (Suppl 4): 86S-91S.

60. Barnhart KT, Freeman E, Grisso JA et al. The effect of dehydroepiandrosterone supplementation to symptomatic perimenopausal women on serum endocrine profiles, lipid parameters, and health-related quality of life. *J Clin Endocrinol Metab* 1999; 84: 3896–902.

61. Basson R, McInnes R, Smith MD et al. Efficacy and safety of sildenafil citrate in women with sexual dysfunction associated with female sexual arousal disorder. *J Womens Health Gend Based Med* 2002; 11: 367–77.

62. Basson R, Brotto LA. Sexual psychophysiology and effects of sildenafil citrate in oestrogenised women with acquired genital arousal disorder and impaired orgasm: a randomized controlled trial. *Br J Obstet Gynaecol* 2003; 110: 1014–24.

63. Kaplan SA, Reis RB, Kohn IJ et al. Safety and efficacy of sildenafil in postmenopausal women with sexual dysfunction. *Urology* 1999; 53: 481–6.

64. Kloosterboer H. Tibolone: a steroid with tissue-specific mode of action. *J Steroid Biochem Mol Biol* 2001; 76: 231–8.

65. Doren M, Rubig A, Coelingh Bennink HJ et al. Differential effects on the androgen status of postmenopausal women treated with tibolone and continuous combined estradiol and norethindrone acetate replacement therapy. *Fertil Steril* 2001; 75: 554–9.

66. Laan E, van Lunsen RH, Everaerd W. The effects of tibolone on vaginal blood flow, sexual desire and arousability in postmenopausal women. *Climacteric* 2001; 4: 28–41.

67. Palacios S, Mendez C, Jurado AR et al. Changes in sex behavior after menopause: effects of tibolone. *Maturitas* 1995; 22: 155–61.

68. Nathorst-Boos J, Hammar M. Effect on sexual life: a comparison between tibolone and continuous estradiol-norethisterone acetate regimen. *Maturitas* 1997; 26: 15–20.

69. Meston CM, Worcel M. The effects of L-arginine and yohimbine on sexual arousal in postmenopausal women with female sexual arousal disorder. International Academy of Sexual Research, 21–24 June 2000; Paris.

70. Rosen RC, Phillips NA, Gendrano NC. Oral phentolamine and female sexual arousal disorder: a pilot study. *J Sex Marital Ther* 1999; 25: 137–44.

71. Islam A, Mitchel JT, Rosen R et al. Topical alprostadil in the treatment of female sexual arousal disorder: a pilot study. *J Sex Marital Ther* 2001; 27: 541–9.

72. Fourcroy JL. Female sexual dysfunction: potential for pharmacotherapy. *Drugs* 2003; 63: 1445–7.

Medical conditions associated with female sexual dysfunction

Andrea Salonia, Alberto Briganti, Patrizio Rigatti, Francesco Montorsi

Introduction

According to the National Health and Social Life Survey, approximately 43% of American women suffer from sexual disorder.[1] Prevalence data on female sexual dysfunction in Europe and other parts of the world are reviewed in Chapters 2.2–2.4 of this volume. Female sexual dysfunction is frequently an unrecognized medical condition causing personal distress with a significant impact on women's health.

Sexual dysfunction in women is a multifactorial condition with several medical, psychologic, and social components. While it is becoming more recognized that potentially all medical conditions and their treatments may have an impact on women's quality of life and sexuality, unfortunately, well-designed, random-sample, community-based clinical and epidemiologic investigations of medical conditions associated with female sexual dysfunction are limited.

The chapter has been subdivided into four major sections evaluating female sexual dysfunction and (1) urogynecologic conditions (see Chapter 17.4); (2) endocrinologic and metabolic disorders (see Chapters 13.1–13.3); (3) psychiatric (see Chapters 16.2 and 17.3 and systemic neurologic disorders (see Chapters 16.5–16.6); and (4) cardiovascular disorders (see Chapters 5.4, 6.1, 14.1, and 14.2).

Female sexual dysfunction and urogynecologic conditions

Urinary incontinence and lower urinary tract symptoms

Urinary incontinence in women is a highly prevalent condition, both in the stress and the urge subtypes.[2,3] Lower urinary tract symptoms are also commonly reported by the women population.[4,5] Abnormalities of sexual function have been associated with urinary incontinence and pelvic organ prolapse.[6-8] Little is known either about the prevalence of female sexual dysfunction in various subsets of patients with micturition disorders, or about the potential correlation between those female patients most frequently seen by urologists (i.e., those with urinary incontinence and/or lower urinary tract symptoms). Recently, Shaw[9] reported the results of a Medline and PsychInfo review of peer-reviewed papers in English from 1980 to 2001, including all primary epidemiologic papers reporting the prevalence of urinary incontinence and its effects on sexual function in women. Although the studies concerning the impairment in sexual function were varied and methodologically heterogeneous, they reported a prevalence of female sexual dysfunction of 0.6–64%.[9] Interestingly, in a more recent evaluation of the reliability and validity of a new quality-of-life index in both men and women with urinary incontinence, Stothers[10] showed that 61% of the male patients, but only 7% of women, complaining of urinary incontinence reported a high level of impact in the sexuality domain of the index itself.

We have recently published our data regarding a cohort of 227 consecutive Caucasian women (mean age 52 years; age range 19–66 years) complaining of urinary incontinence and/or recurrent or persistent lower urinary tract symptoms.[11] After a detailed clinical and urodynamic multichannel evaluation, all patients have completed the Female Sexual Function Index[12] to standardize the interview regarding the patient's sexual life. Two hundred and sixteen patients were eligible for sexual function investigation because 11 (5%) out of 227 would not answer questions regarding their own sexuality, and were thus excluded from the final evaluation results. According to the analysis of sexual history and Female Sexual Function Index scores, female sexual dysfunction was diagnosed in 99 (46%) out of the 216 patients eligible for the investigation on sexual function. Four subgroups of sexual dysfunction were identified (namely, sexual desire disorder, sexual arousal disorder, orgasmic disorder, and sexual pain disorder), in accordance with the female sexual dysfunction classification proposed by the International Consensus Development Conference on Female Sexual Dysfunction.[13] Thirty-four out of 99 patients (34%) had hypoactive sexual desire disorder. Twenty-one (62%) of these were in menopause. Those patients reporting both urge incontinence and hypoactive sexual desire disorder mentioned uninterest in sexual intercourse because of a strong increase in the desire to void, with a subsequent frequent leakage of urine during such attempts. Twenty-three per cent (23 patients) had a sexual arousal disorder and complained of either subjective lack of, or reduced, vaginal sensitivity and lack of, or severely reduced, genital localized pleasure, during both noncoital sex and/or sexual intercourse, associated, at times, with reduction of vaginal lubrication. Seven (30%) of these women were in menopause, but three out of seven (47%) reported that they had poor genital arousal even prior to menopause. Eleven patients (11%) had an orgasmic phase disorder, with delayed orgasm in six patients and complete anorgasmia in the remaining five patients. Five of these women (45%) were in menopause.

Lastly, 44 patients (44%) had a history of sexual pain disorders. Thirty-seven (84%) of these women reported recurrent or persistent genital pain following sexual intercourse. We identified all these patients as having dyspareunia, in accordance with the categories described by the consensus panel on definition of female sexual dysfunction.[13] Vulvar vestibulitis syndrome with sharp, burning/cutting pain highly localized in the vulvar vestibule and elicited primarily via pressure applied to the area, as defined by Bergeron et al.,[14] was demonstrated in seven out of these 44 patients (16%); these women complained of both dyspareunia and noncoital sexual pain, and all of them suffered from recurrent bacterial cystitis. A total of 21 women complained of more than one sexual dysfunction. Sexual pain disorders represented the most frequent concomitant complaint, mostly in women suffering from recurrent bacterial cystitis.

The second part of this cross-sectional study was then dedicated to the direct comparison of the sexual function of the 216 patients, as described by the Female Sexual Function Index score, with the score of a group of 102 healthy, age-matched women (mean age 54; age range 19–63; $p = 0.61$), assessed in a yearly routine gynecologic evaluation for cancer prevention, and not complaining of urinary symptoms (i.e., urinary incontinence and/or lower urinary tract symptoms). The comparison of the median score of the Female Sexual Function Index demonstrated that patients reported significantly lower desire ($p < 0.01$), lubrication ($p = 0.01$), and sexual satisfaction ($p < 0.01$) than controls. Moreover, these patients also showed a higher ($p < 0.001$) sexual pain rate than controls.

Finally, our survey[11] revealed that 168 (74%) out of the

overall 227 patients evaluated had never undergone an interview concerning their sexual life or sexual activity. All 99 patients suffering from sexual dysfunction felt that they needed to verbalize their sexual problems and wished to have them treated.

Urogynecologic pelvic surgery

Radical cystectomy for urologic malignancies

Genitourinary cancers are commonly associated with treatment-related sexual dysfunction, varying from mild to severe. However, limited peer-reviewed papers have been dedicated to the evaluation of women's sexual function after major urologic surgery for bladder cancer.[15–22] Sexual problems may occur as a result of any aspect of cancer disease and cancer treatment. Sexual function is sensitive to the effects of trauma, both physical and emotional. This is particularly the case for patients whose cancer affects their genital organs.

Marshall et al. found that anterior exenteration in women can be performed accurately with a disciplined anatomic approach.[18] Women undergoing cystectomy with the simultaneous removal of uterus, ovaries, and parts of the vaginal wall face had distress regarding their femininity as well as doubts about future sexual functioning. Excision of the uterus, a portion of the vagina, and the urethra seems to reduce the potential for pelvic recurrence, but vaginal reconstruction and continent urinary diversion provide better quality of life with maintenance of sexual function and urinary continence. Original data have been reported by Bjerre et al.,[19] who evaluated the sexual profile after urinary diversion in 17 women who underwent radical cystectomy with the continent Kock reservoir and 20 women with the ileal-conduit diversion. Data from only 33 patients were eligible for analysis, but no significant differences between the groups were found. The authors found that coital frequency remained unchanged or increased among 44% of patients with a continent reservoir and among 18% of ileal-conduit patients, and did not show any statistically significant difference ($p = 0.11$). Among those reporting other than unchanged/increased activity, almost one-third indicated physical problems or decreased desire as the reason, and 30% felt less sexually attractive, cystectomized patients reporting a higher percentage than others. A higher frequency of dyspareunia among patients with a continent reservoir was an unexpected finding ($p = 0.06$).

Nordstrom and Nyman[20] reported that in their cohort of patients, five out of the six preoperatively sexually active women treated by cystectomy because of bladder cancer or incontinence/bladder dysfunction reported either a decrease or cessation of coital sexual activity postoperatively. The main problems were a decrease in sexual desire, dyspareunia, and vaginal dryness. One woman reported the inability to experience orgasm after surgery. Compared with women with bladder cancer, patients with incontinence/bladder dysfunction were more likely to have an active sexual life after urostomic surgery. Interestingly, seven women in this group, of whom four were sexually inactive before surgery, increased their sexual activity after the operation. For these women, the conduit operation removed the need to use incontinence pads or indwelling catheters.

Hautmann et al.[21] presented data about nerve-sparing cystectomy with orthotopic bladder replacement in women. Their interesting paper showed detailed data concerning urinary continence and voiding dysfunction, emphasizing that urethral support and nerve-sparing cystectomy, with the ileal neobladder as a reservoir, guarantee excellent continence in all patients. However, authors have been unable to demonstrate any advantage of the nerve- and urethral-support-sparing cystectomy technique as far as micturition is concerned. More recently, Horenblas et al.[22] reported their preliminary results of modified sexual function-preserving cystectomy in both men and women, called sexuality-preserving cystectomy and neobladder. Women's sexuality-preserving cystectomy and neobladder consisted of pelvic lymph node dissection followed by cystectomy alone with preservation of all internal genitalia. An ileal neobladder was thus anastomosed to the urethra. Three women aged 38–71 years (mean age 55 years) were enrolled in this protocol, and all these patients reported normal vaginal lubrication throughout sexual activity.

Curiously, very recently, a case of clitoral priapism causing clitoromegaly has been described in association with the localization of a transitional cell carcinoma with papillary squamous component at the clitoral site.[23]

Hysterectomy and sexual function

Many studies have explored sexuality after hysterectomy. The overall estimation of the percentage of women reporting deterioration of their sexual life and sexual activities after hysterectomy is 13–37%[15,24–32] (see Chapter 16.7).

In a very elegant study, Jensen et al.[31] reported the results of a prospective study evaluating the longitudinal course of self-reported sexual function after radical hysterectomy in 173 patients with lymph node-negative, early-stage cervical carcinoma as compared with an age-matched control group from the general population. This case-control study showed that radical hysterectomy had a persistent and negative impact on patients' sexual interest and vaginal lubrication, whereas the majority of other sexual and vaginal problems disappeared over time. Indeed, patients experienced severe orgasmic problems and uncomfortable sexual intercourse due to a reduced vaginal size during the first 6 months after radical hysterectomy, severe dyspareunia during the first 3 months, and sexual dissatisfaction during the 5 weeks after radical hysterectomy. A persistent lack of libido and lubrication were reported throughout the first 2 years after radical hysterectomy. Long-term lack of sexual interest and insufficient vaginal lubrication were confirmed by the patient's self-reported changes 12 months after radical hysterectomy compared with before the cancer diagnosis and by a pre/post comparison within patients. Interestingly, 91% of the patients who were sexually active before their cancer diagnosis were sexually active again 12 months after surgery, but with a decrease in sexual frequency reported.

Gimbel et al.[32] compared the impact of radical hysterectomy and subtotal hysterectomy on several clinical outcome measures in more than 300 women suffering from benign uterine diseases. No clinically important differences regarding satisfaction with sexual life were found between the two hysterectomy methods. Similarly, Zobbe et al.[33] prospectively compared the impact of an abdominal radical hysterectomy and a subtotal abdominal hysterectomy. These authors showed that no significant differences were observed at the 1-year follow-up in women's sexual desire, frequency of intercourse, frequency of orgasm, quality of orgasm, localization of orgasm, satisfaction with sexual life, and dyspareunia. Moreover, none of these sexual variables changed significantly from entry to the 1-year follow-up; on the contrary, dyspareunia was significantly ($p = 0.009$) reduced in both groups.

Rako[34,35] underlined that the ovaries are a critical source not only of estrogen but also of testosterone; thus, on removal of the uterus, even after ovary-sparing procedures, their function can be jeopardised. The lack of a physiologic level of testosterone in women after hysterectomy can also decrease quality of life in terms of sexual libido, sexual pleasure, and sense of well-being. A review analysis by Cutler et al.[36] strictly correlated the hormonal deficit impact on sexuality and overall quality of life in hysterectomized women. The combination of radical hysterectomy and a surgical bilateral oophorectomy may certainly worsen the clinical and quality-of-life picture. Indeed, owing to the fact that the ovaries provide approximately half of the circulating testosterone in premenopausal subjects, many women after surgery after surgery report impaired sexual functioning despite estrogen replacement. Thus, vaginal dryness and sexual arousal difficulties are important issues in women undergoing hysterectomy. Vaginal dryness has been associated with the estrogen deficiency which characterizes premenopausal hysterectomy with bilateral oophorectomy.[29,37] Nevertheless, several reports seem to demonstrate that vaginal dryness may be peculiar also after premenopausal simple hysterectomy, owing to potential ovarian damage and failure subsequent to the surgery itself.[38–40]

Surgical damage to the pelvic autonomic nerves during radical hysterectomy is thought to be responsible for considerable morbidity, including impaired bladder function, defecation problems, and sexual dysfunction. Therefore, surgical preservation of the pelvic autonomic nerves in both laparoscopic and traditional radical hysterectomy deserves consideration in the quest to improve both cure and quality of life in both chronic benign conditions and cervical cancer patients.[22–24] Well-designed prospective studies are of paramount importance to evaluate the real impact of this kind of common surgery on overall sexual function in both premenopausal and postmenopausal women.

Conversely, in a comprehensive review article, Carlson reported that in women undergoing hysterectomy for nonmalignant conditions there is a marked improvement in symptoms and quality of life during the early years after surgery.[47] Rhodes et al.,[29] for instance, recently published the results of a 2-year prospective study which longitudinally examined measures of sexual function in women undergoing radical hysterectomy. These authors showed that, in a cohort of 1101 patients, both sexual desire and frequency of sexual relations significantly ($p < 0.001$) increased after hysterectomy and throughout the follow-up period. Similarly, orgasm frequency significantly increased after surgery ($p < 0.001$), and the strength of orgasm also rose dramatically after hysterectomy ($p < 0.001$). The total amount of women reporting vaginal dryness prior to surgery also improved after hysterectomy ($p < 0.001$).

Endocrine alterations

Hypothyroidism and hyperthyroidism

To the best of our knowledge, there are no peer-reviewed papers evaluating sexual function and dysfunction in women complaining of either hypothyroidism or hyperthyroidism. We[48] had reported a few preliminary data about sexual function of 48 dysthyroidal women (namely, 30 hypothyroidal women: mean age 40.3 years; range 24–63 years; and 18 hyperthyroidal subjects: mean age 42.5; range 21–66 years), compared with a control group of healthy, age-matched women asking for a routine checkup at the gynecology clinic. Those preliminary results showed an overall response rate to the study of 82% for the control group and of 98% among dysthyroidal women. The Mann–Whitney U Test for direct comparison of the median demonstrated that women complaining of dysthyroidism had significantly worse scores for both the lubrication ($p < 0.001$) and the orgasm ($p < 0.001$) domain of the Female Sexual Function Index than the control group. Similarly, dysthyroidal women reported a significantly ($p < 0.001$) higher genital pain during both coital and noncoital sexual activity than controls. When comorbidities were evaluated, a high rate of depression was found (37%) in dysthyroidal women, and the Spearman correlation analysis showed that the Beck Depression Inventory[49] score was significantly correlated with the desire ($r = -0.78$; $p < 0.01$), the arousal ($r = -0.62$; $p = 0.003$), and the satisfaction domain ($r = -0.83$; $p < 0.001$). Higher rate of depression was also correlated with greater rate of sexual distress, as shown by the Spearman correlation analysis between the Beck Depression Inventory and the Female Sexual Distress Scale [50] ($r = 0.60$; $p = 0.02$). Similarly, when the Female Sexual Distress Scale was correlated with the different Female Sexual Function Index domains, a significant correlation was found between women's sexual distress and overall sexual satisfaction ($r = -0.83$; $p < 0.05$).

Hyperprolactinemia

Hyperprolactinemia, which is considered the most common endocrine disorder of the hypothalamic–pituitary axis,[51] occurs more commonly in women, with a prevalence ranging from 0.4% in an unselected normal adult population to as high as 9–17% in women with reproductive disorders. Hyperprolactinemia is

associated with pronounced reductions of both sexual motivation and function. Elevated levels of prolactin inhibit gonadotropin-releasing hormone pulsatility.[52] Although some experimental evidence suggests that hyperprolactinemia suppresses physiologic reproductive functions while maintaining sexual drive, other studies clearly indicate that chronic prolactin elevation also negatively affects sexual libido[53] (see Chapter 6.1).

Hulter and Lundberg,[54] assessing both sexual function and sexual appreciation in a comprehensive interview of 48 women with well-defined hypothalamo-pituitary disorders, showed that 38 (79.2%) of the women had developed a lack of or a considerable decrease in sexual desire. Moreover, problems with lubrication or orgasm were reported by 31 (64.6%) and 33 (68.7%) of the women, respectively. In this series, interestingly, normal menstrual pattern, young age, and intrasellar tumor growth correlated better with normal sexual desire and sexual functions than did normal prolactin levels and normal testosterone levels. In a previous study,[55] the same authors investigated sexuality in 109 women (aged 20–60 years) with morphologically verified hypothalamo-pituitary disorders, finding that 62.4% of them had noticed a decrease in sexual desire, especially ($p < 0.001$) in those who had hyperprolactinemia.

Great attention has been paid to the potential correlation between hyperprolactinemia and antidepressive, antipsychotic, and neuroleptic drugs. Several drugs are known to induce negative effects on the sexual function, including psychoactive drugs (opiates), hypotensive drugs, and antihistamines.[56] Antipsychotic and neuroleptic drugs also produce a pronounced reduction in sexual drive, which appears to be at least partially the result of the marked hyperprolactinemia produced by drug administration. Indeed, typical neuroleptics are commonly associated with hyperprolactinemia, which, in turn, leads to sexual dysfunction promoting both loss of libido and anorgasmia.[56-61] The mechanism of action underlying this clinical phenomenon seems to be mediated by the dopamine-blocking action of typical antipsychotic medications, which results in excessive prolactin secretion and secondary effects on gonadal function.[60] Indeed, neuroleptic-induced hyperprolactinemia can cause menstrual disorders, impaired fertility, galactorrhea, and sexual dysfunction, as well as hypoestrogenism secondary to disruption of the hypothalamic–pituitary–ovarian axis.

The new antidepressant agents, such as selective serotonin reuptake inhibitors, may also induce hyperprolactinemia.[62] Although, to our knowledge, no research has accurately reported the prevalence and the characteristics of this phenomenon in women, this so-called secondary hyperprolactinemia induces symptoms ranging from decreased sexual drive to orgasmic disturbances such as anorgasmia and delayed orgasm.[62,63]

Diabetes mellitus

The incidence of sexual dysfunction in men with diabetes mellitus approaches 50%, and this is only slightly lower in diabetic women.[64-66] Neuropathy, vascular impairment, and psychologic problems have been closely implicated in the high rate of decreased libido, slow arousability, decreased vaginal lubrication, orgasmic dysfunction, and dyspareunia in women with diabetes mellitus.[65,67-68]

Different types of diabetes seem to influence women's sexual function differently.[69-71] Schiel and Muller[72] reported data about the prevalence of sexual disorders in a selection-free diabetic population. These authors showed that the overall prevalence of women's sexual dysfunctions was 18% among 127 diabetes mellitus type I patients, and 42% among 117 type II diabetes mellitus patients.

More recently, Enzlin et al.[73] reported data of a case-control study of the prevalence and characteristics of sexual dysfunction in a total of 120 women with type I diabetes mellitus (mean age±SD: women without diabetic complications: 34.4 ± 8.5 years; women with diabetic complications: 39.6 ± 11.3 years), as compared with an age-matched control group of 180 healthy women attending an outpatient gynecologic clinic for routine checkup. Enzlin showed that significantly more women with diabetes (27%) than age-matched controls (15%) reported sexual dysfunction ($\chi^2 = 4.5$, df = 1; $p = 0.04$). Diabetic women presented a higher prevalence of sexual arousal dysfunction ($\chi^2 = 3.8$, df=1; $P = 0.05$) and of decreased lubrication ($\chi^2 = 6.5$, df = 2; $p = 0.04$) than healthy women. On the contrary, despite a high prevalence of reduced libido in diabetes mellitus women both with and without diabetic complications (16.3% and 17%, respectively), the direct comparison did not show any significant differences in the decrease of desire ($\chi^2 = 3.2$, df = 1; $p = 0.09$), orgasmic phase disorders ($\chi^2 = 0.5$, df = 1; $p = 0.52$), and sexual pain disorders ($\chi^2 = 2.4$, df = 1; $p = 0.15$) compared with the controls. Interestingly, sexual problems were not isolated in occurrence; indeed, 11% in the studied group and 75 among controls reported two or three sexual problems ($\chi^2 = 0.16$, df = 2; $p = 0.92$). It is interesting to note that this analysis did not show any statistically significant correlation between sexual complaints and age, body-mass index, length of disease, hemoglobin A1C values, peripheral neuropathy, autonomic neuropathy, nephropathy, and retinopathy.[73,74] However, a significant association was found between the number of complications and the number of sexual complaints; thus, women suffering from more complications also reported more sexual disorders ($\chi^2 = 30.9$, df = 12; $p = 0.002$). Moreover, while the statistical analysis did not demonstrate any significant evidence due to the menopausal status ($p = 0.59$) or the use of hormone replacement therapy or oral contraceptive pill ($p = 0.37$), diabetic women reported more depressive symptoms than controls ($p = 0.01$) in accordance with the Beck Depression Inventory score. According to the defined cutoff for clinically significant depression of the Beck Depression Inventory, twice as many diabetic women (24%) were depressed as were controls (11%) ($\chi^2 = 6.8$, df = 1; $p = 0.01$). More recently, Enzlin[74] concluded that sexual dysfunction in women, but not in men, was related to depression and the quality of the relationship with the partner.

Prevalence and predictors of sexual dysfunction in diabetes mellitus type II women have been reported by Erol et al.[71] A direct comparison of the FSFI questionnaire showed a mean ± SD

overall score of 29.3 ± 6.4 in 72 diabetic type II women versus 37.7 ± 3.5 in 60 age-matched, healthy controls ($p < 0.05$). Of the diabetic cohort, 77% reported reduced libido; diminished clitoral sensation was reported by 62.5% of the diabetes mellitus women, while 37.5% complained of vaginal dryness, 41.6% described vaginal discomfort, and 49% complained of orgasmic dysfunction.

We reported the preliminary results of a cross-sectional study aiming at evaluating prevalence and predictors of sexual dysfunction in both diabetes mellitus type I and type II women.[75] Among 72 diabetic women (mean ± SE age: 42.6 ± 13.6 years), 42 (58.3%) with type I and 30 (41.7%) with type II diabetes mellitus, the Mann–Whitney U Test for direct comparison of the median demonstrated that patients had worse scores for the desire ($p < 0.001$), the lubrication ($p < 0.001$), and the orgasm ($p < 0.001$) domains of the Female Sexual Function Index than a healthy, age-matched control group. Similarly, diabetic women reported significantly higher sexual pain at the genitalia level ($p < 0.001$) (both coital and noncoital sexual activity) than controls. Depression was as frequent as in 48% of diabetic women, as documented by the Beck Depression Inventory. The Beck Depression Inventory score was significantly ($r = -0.54$, $p = 0.003$) correlated with the arousal domain, the orgasm domain ($r = -0.39$, $p < 0.05$) as well as the satisfaction domain of the Female Sexual Function Index ($r = -0.48$, $P = 0.04$). Moreover, the Spearman correlation analysis was also statistically significant between Beck Depression Inventory and Female Sexual Distress Scale scores: ($r = -0.47$, $p = 0.02$). A significant correlation was also found in our series of patients between aging and reduced desire ($r = -0.47$, $p = 0.04$) and between aging and lubrication ($r = -0.55$, $p = 0.001$).

While the results of studies confirm that sexual dysfunction is highly prevalent in diabetic women, investigations aimed at better understanding the real contribution of both the psychologic and diabetes-related somatic factors in inducing and characterizing sexual disorders in these women are needed.

Chronic renal failure

Sexual dysfunction is a highly prevalent problem in both men and women with chronic renal failure, with significant impact on their overall quality of life. The genesis of sexual dysfunction is multifactorial, including physiologic, psychologic, and organic factors. Common disturbances include erectile dysfunction in men, menstrual abnormalities in women, and decreased libido and fertility in both sexes.[77,78] These abnormalities are primarily organic in nature and are related to uremia as well as the other comorbid conditions that frequently occur in the chronic renal failure patient. Fatigue and psychosocial factors related to the presence of a chronic disease are also contributory factors. Disturbances in the hypothalamic–pituitary–gonadal axis can be detected before the need for dialysis, but continue to worsen once both hemodialysis or continuous ambulatory peritoneal dialysis is initiated.[79-81] Apparently, impaired gonadal function is prominent in uremic men, whereas the disturbances in the hypothalamo-pituitary axis are more subtle. By contrast, central disturbances are more prominent in uremic women.

In a case-control study, Toorians et al.[82] attempted to determine whether the mode of treatment (namely, hemodialysis, continuous ambulatory peritoneal dialysis, or kidney transplantation), as well as biochemical and endocrine variables and neuropathy, may affect sexual functioning. They reported that transplanted patients suffered significantly less from hypoactive sexual desire disorder than the other three groups; the prevalence of other sexual dysfunctions did not differ between the groups. Moreover, genital responses during psychophysiologic assessment had no relationship to the duration of renal replacement treatment, biochemical/endocrine variables, or the presence/ absence of neuropathy. A high prevalence of loss of sexual interest, subjectively ascribed to fatigue, was also found in women on both hemodialysis and continuous ambulatory peritoneal dialysis.

During the early 1980s, some studies reported on the correlation between hyperprolactinemia and sexual disturbances among uremic women on hemodialysis.[83,84] Mastrogiacomo et al. reported that the rate of sexual intercourse and the ability to reach orgasm among 99 women on maintenance hemodialysis were significantly lower than in age-matched control women.[83] Eighty per cent declared a reduction in their sexual desire, and the frequency of intercourse was also lower than in the period prior to dialysis. Ageing, acting as an unmodifiable risk factor, decreased sexual activity in both the ill and healthy population, but in uremic patients sexual activity ended at an earlier age. Patients with hyperprolactinemia reported lower frequencies of intercourse as well as lower percentages of orgasm than normoprolactinemic ones.

Neurologic and psychiatric disorders

Spinal cord injury

Peer-reviewed literature has reported that women's desire for sexuality and sexual activities seems to decrease after injury in women with spinal cord injury.[85-88] Several authors, indeed, have shown a significantly higher level of hypoactive sexual desire disorder after injury.[89,90] Interestingly, a decrease in the frequency of self-masturbation in these women has been reported,[91] with preferred sexual activities after spinal cord injury reported to be kissing, hugging, and touching.[89]

From a pathophysiologic point of view, the influence of spinal cord injury on sexual response strictly depends on the degree and location of injury in the spinal cord. In women with complete upper motor neuron injuries affecting the sacral segments, the ability for reflex, but not psychogenic, lubrication of the vagina should be maintained.[92-94] On the contrary, in women with incomplete upper motor neuron injuries affecting the sacral segments, data seem to demonstrate the ability to maintain both the capacity for reflex and psychogenic lubrication.

Women with higher ability to perceive a combination of light touch and pinprick sensation in the T11–L2 dermatomes seem also to have a greater likelihood of achieving psychogenic lubrication.[88] Historically, only 55% of spinal cord injury women were able to reach orgasm after injury.[87,95] These authors demonstrated that spinal cord injury subjects were significantly less likely to achieve orgasm than controls ($\chi^2 = 14.3$; $p = 0.001$). Similarly, these results showed that the possibility to achieve orgasm is less likely (17%) if women have a complete lower motor neuron injury affecting the sacral segments than if they have any other levels and degrees of injury.[95]

Multiple sclerosis

Sexual dysfunction has been described as high as 72% among women suffering from multiple sclerosis.[96-99] Moreover, sexual activity ceases or is significantly unsatisfactory in 39% of multiple sclerosis women.[96] Symptoms reported include fatigue in 68%, reduced sensation in 48%, reduced vaginal lubrication and difficulty with arousal in 35%, difficulty reaching orgasm or anorgasmia in 72%, and dyspareunia and other typologies of sexual pain disorder.[97-98,100]

In a case-control study, Zorzon et al.[101] found that the number of multiple sclerosis patients who reported a reduction in sexual desire was higher than in both patients suffering from a chronic disease (namely, rheumatoid arthritis, systemic lupus erythematosus, psoriatic arthritis, and ankylosing spondylitis) and healthy subjects. Moreover, in this series, multiple sclerosis women reported significantly ($p < 0.001$) decreased vaginal lubrication compared with healthy controls; changes in vaginal sensation were also very common (27.1%), and more common in patients than in both chronic disease controls and healthy subjects ($p < 0.01$). Similar data have been previously shown by other researchers.[100,102] More frequent and severe changes in sexual function seemed characteristic of women complaining of advanced multiple sclerosis (i.e., median Expanded Disability Status Scale[104] score 6.5).[105] Sexual dysfunction was significantly correlated with relapsing-remitting multiple sclerosis ($r = -0.33$, $p = 0.0106$), but not with both the primary-progressive ($p = 0.06$) and the secondary progressive type ($p = 0.08$). A significant correlation was found between sexual and physical disorders ($r = 0.42$, $p = 0.0017$), sphincteric and bladder dysfunction ($r = 0.39$, $p = 0.0025$ and $r = 0.37$, $p = 0.0035$, respectively), fatigue score ($r = 0.30$, $p = 0.0284$), and both cognitive deterioration ($r = 0.30$, $p = 0.0280$) and the overall neurologic impairment ($r = 0.28$, $p = 0.0306$), as assessed by the Expanded Disability Status Scale.

More recently, the same group reported that Spearman's rank correlation analysis showed a relationship between symptoms of sexual dysfunction and patient's age ($r = 0.73$, $p < 0.0001$), cognitive performances ($r = -0.63$, $p < 0.0001$), level of independence ($r = -0.63$, $p < 0.0001$), disability ($r = 0.56$, $p < 0.001$), symptoms of anxiety ($r = 0.55$, $p < 0.001$) and depression ($r = 0.50$, $p < 0.005$), disease duration ($r = 0.42$, $p < 0.02$), and parenchymal atrophy in the pons ($r = -0.38$, $p = 0.031$), as detected by cranial and cervical spinal cord magnetic resonance imaging.[106] In multiple regression analysis, sexual dysfunction was predicted only by T1 lesion load of the pons.

Nortvedt et al.[107] also reported a significant reduction in the quality of life in multiple sclerosis patients with both sexual disorders and bladder dysfunction. A similar correlation was also demonstrated between sexual dysfunction and low educational level ($r = 0.37$, $p = 0.0040$) and a high value for either depression ($r = 0.40$, $p = 0.0018$) or anxiety ($r = 0.40$, $p = 0.0017$).[105] Interestingly, men reported at least one sexual dysfunction more frequently than women, both at the start and at the end of the study ($p = 0.002$). However, when both men and women were considered altogether, in a univariate analysis, changes in sexual function throughout time correlated with modifications in bladder function ($r = 0.47$, $p < 0.0001$) and Expanded Disability Status Scale score ($r = 0.41$, $p < 0.0001$). After removing the effect of psychologic aspects, only changes in bladder function maintained a significant correlation with fluctuations in sexual function ($r = 0.36$, $p = 0.003$). Very recently, a new magnetic resonance imaging study found a relationship between sexual dysfunction and pontine atrophy, and confirmed the correlation of sexual dysfunction with bladder dysfunction, while also highlighting the role of psychologic factors in determining sexual dysfunction.[108]

Curiously, Hennessey et al.[109] reported the results of a survey regarding urinary, fecal, and sexual dysfunction in 68 men and 106 multiple sclerosis women, and found that, although sexual problems occurred in 52% (55/106) of multiple sclerosis women enrolled, 65/106 (61%) were satisfied with their sexual activity. Coping strategies and levels of cognitive functioning were important predictors of sexual satisfaction, sexual dysfunction, and relationship satisfaction for women with multiple sclerosis.[110,111]

Interestingly, in a multiple sclerosis population, the acceptance of disability and perceived impairment increase significantly over time for both men and women. For men, however, being married was associated with a greater acceptance of disability and less perceived impairment; moreover, men were more concerned than women about how multiple sclerosis affected their sexual relationships.[112]

Depression and antidepressants

Chronic depression, which is more common in women than in men, represents an important public health concern in the former group[113,114] (see Chapter 16.2). Major depression is certainly underrecognized and undertreated, and it is associated with significant functional impairment and high rates of comorbidity. Women may experience illness onset at an early age and experience more severe psychosocial impairment than men.[113]

Female sexual dysfunction associated with major depression has been described in 48–70% of patients.[115–118] Indeed, changes in sexual interest/satisfaction and loss of libido are frequently and consistently related to major depression.[118,119] Nevertheless, a good sex life is regarded by 70% of general population and by

as many as 75% of depressed patients as a fundamental to quality of life.[120] In a large cross-sectional population survey, Dunn et al.[121] reported that in women the predominant association with arousal, orgasmic, and enjoyment problems was marital difficulties, but all female sexual dysfunction were associated with anxiety and depression.

Interestingly, Cyranowski et al.[122] separately examined the effects of depression, selective serotonin reuptake inhibitors treatment, and sexual partner availability on women's sexual function. Random regression models assessing changes in sexual function were conducted. Controlling for the other variables, depressive symptoms were associated with decrements in sexual desire, sexual cognition/fantasy, sexual arousal, orgasmic function, and global evaluations of sexual function. On the other hand, treatment with selective serotonin reuptake inhibitors was associated with orgasmic difficulty only. The availability of a sexual partner was associated with increased sexual arousal, orgasmic function, and sexual behaviour. Moreover, depression seems to be an independent risk factor (odds ratio 3.4; 95% confidence interval, 1.9–6.1) for decreased libido in the late reproductive years.[123] Depression was also shown to increase pain during sexual intercourse.[124]

Antidepressant drugs and medications can exacerbate preexisting sexual dysfunction or even induce new sexual disorders.[63,115,125–129] Sexual dysfunction has been reported to be associated with all classes of antidepressants (monoamine oxidase inhibitors, tricyclic antidepressants, selective serotonin reuptake inhibitors, serotonin and norepinephrine reuptake inhibitors, selective serotonin reuptake inhibitor, and new-generation antidepressants) in patients with depression and various anxiety disorders.[130]

The negative effects of selective serotonin reuptake inhibitors on sexual function appear strongly dose-related. Men taking selective serotonin reuptake inhibitors report higher rates of sexual side effects than women taking them; however, women seem to experience more severe sexual dysfunction.[126] Absent or delayed orgasm is the sexual side effect most commonly associated with selective serotonin reuptake inhibitors.[128] Sexual desire and arousal disorders are also frequently reported.[63] Frequently, sexual dysfunction which lasts during long-term administration of antidepressants becomes a major problem and may even result in treatment discontinuation.[129,131] This places patients at increased risk of recurrence, relapse, chronicity, and death (e.g., suicide).

Very recently, Nappi et al.[132] demonstrated that depression may be bimodally related to women's sexual dysfunction. In a cross-sectional study, the frequency of self-reported sexual symptoms in women ($n = 355$; age range 46–60 years) attending menopausal clinics was investigated and related to other vasomotor, psychologic, physical, and genital complaints. As expected, sexual complaints were significantly more frequent with age and years since menopause. Moreover, examining the intensity of sexual symptoms according to the presence of other complaints, these authors found that physical, psychologic, and genital well-being significantly affect components of sexual response after the menopause, and that depressive symptoms are more common in women with sexual complaints.[132]

Lastly, depression is an important cofactor in many diseases that are potentially associated with sexual dysfunction in women. For instance, very recently, some authors underlined its role in worsening the quality of life and the sexual function in multiple sclerosis patients.[108,133] Janardhan and Bakshi. demonstrated that depression and fatigue were independently associated with impaired quality of life in multiple sclerosis, after accounting for physical disability. In other words, after accounting for disability and fatigue, depression was associated with lower quality of life with respect to health perception ($p = 0.02$), sexual dysfunction ($p = 0.03$), health distress ($p = 0.03$), mental health ($p = 0.006$), overall quality of life ($p = 0.006$), emotional dysfunction ($p = 0.04$), and limitations due to emotional dysfunction ($p = 0.03$).[133]

Cardiovascular diseases

Hypertension and antihypertensive drugs

Little is available in peer-reviewed literature about sexual dysfunction in hypertensive women or in women taking antihypertensive drugs.[134-140] Burchardt et al.,[138] for instance, reported data on 67 women with hypertension (mean age of 60.4 years), revealing highly prevalent untreated sexual dysfunction of long duration. Of their cohort of patients, 81.3% had a sex partner; 42.6% had untreated sexual dysfunction with a duration of more than 5 years in 70.9% of them, and a duration of more than 10 years in 41.7%. Whereas 54.8% reported sexual activity as important, only 5.3% initiated sexual activity, while 36.6% reported less sexual activity than desired. Duncan et al.[140] reported that women with hypertension had more difficulty than did healthy controls in achieving lubrication and orgasm. Moreover, formal Spearman correlation analysis suggested that hypertensive women might have an overall impaired physiologic sexual response.[140] Hanon et al.,[139] analyzing 459 hypertensive subjects (aged 59 ± 12 years) living in France and referred to hypertension specialists, reported that sexual disturbance was declared by 38% of the subjects (148/390), but the prevalence rate was significantly higher in men than women (49% vs 18%; $p < 0.01$). In women, the interest in sexuality was decreased in 41% of subjects but unchanged for 59%; similarly, sexual pleasure was decreased for 34% and unchanged for 66% of patients. Logistic regression analysis indicates that gender ($p < 0.001$), greater number of antihypertensive tablets ($p < 0.01$), prescription of diuretics ($p = 0.03$), and presence of coronaropathy ($p = 0.01$) were independent determinants for sexual disturbance in treated hypertensive patients.

A few interesting studies have also been published regarding the potential actual impact of antihypertensive treatments over women's sexual function.

Ten premenopausal and eight postmenopausal women with mild hypertension and unimpaired sexual function were recruited by Hodge et al.[134] in a crossover, active-drug controlled pilot study using self-administered daily diaries. By analysis of variance, no significant difference in the levels of sexual function of women receiving placebo, clonidine, and prazosin was found. However, of the women who received clonidine first, fewer were receptive to partner approach during medication therapy (49%) than during placebo (61%). Moreover, a smaller number of women wished for their partners to approach them (WISH) during therapy (41% and 53% for clonidine and prazosin, respectively) than during placebo (60%). In the group that received prazosin first, WISH was affected (32% for prazosin, 31% for clonidine, 45% for placebo).

The Treatment of Mild Hypertension Study,[135] a double-blind, randomized, controlled trial, provided an excellent opportunity for examination of sexual function and effects of treatment on sexual function in 557 men and 345 women with stage I diastolic hypertension and treated with placebo or one of five active drugs (acebutolol, amlodipine maleate, chlorthalidone, doxazosin maleate, or enalapril maleate), because of the number of drug classes studied, the double-blind study design, and the long-term follow-up. Sexual function was ascertained by physician interviews at baseline and annually during follow-up. At baseline, 4.9% of women reported a problem with sexual function; 2.0% of women reported difficulties in having an orgasm. Interestingly, the rate of reported sexual problems in hypertensive women was similar, regardless of the type of drug suggested.

Coronary artery disease

While erectile dysfunction is a common and well-known problem in men suffering from coronary artery disease, and it may herald a systemic vasculopathic state, such as ischemic heart disease, to our knowledge, investigations of sexual function and dysfunction in women with coronary artery disease are fewer and rarely complete.

For better evaluation of chronologic, epidemiologic, and etiologic correlations between women's sexual dysfunction and coronary artery disease, we enrolled 60 consecutive women, from February 2001, presenting with angina pectoris at the emergency unit of our institution.[141] A total number of 30 (50%) out of the 60 patients presenting with angina pectoris (mean ± SE age: 56 ± 1.66 years) were ultimately enrolled in this still ongoing cross-sectional study, and underwent morphologic and functional evaluation of the coronary arteries by coronary angiography. Their Female Sexual Function Index results were thus compared with those of 102 age-matched, consecutive women assessed at a yearly routine checkup at the gynecology clinic. The overall prevalence of sexual dysfunction among these coronary artery disease women was 30% (9/30). Seventy-seven per cent (7/9) of the coronary artery disease women complained of female sexual arousal disorder, while a low lubrication score was reported by eight (88.9%) out of these nine women. The direct comparison of the Female Sexual Function Index scores showed that the total index value was significantly higher

($p = 0.02$) for controls than for women suffering from coronary artery disease. Patients also reported a significantly higher amount of sexual arousal ($p = 0.002$) as well as lubrication ($p = 0.10$) disorders. Moreover, patients also had significantly lower ($p = 0.01$) scores on the orgasmic phase domain of the Female Sexual Function Index. The Beck Depression Inventory demonstrated that 33% (10/30) suffered from mild depression, while severe depression affected three (10%) out of the patients. Beck's Depression Inventory score was significantly correlated with the Female Sexual Function Index desire domain ($p = 0.008$, $r = -0.48$) as well as with the arousal domain ($p = 0.0005$, $r = -0.64$), the lubrication domain ($p = 0.0008$, $r = -0.63$), the orgasm domain ($p = 0.0004$, $r = -0.66$), and the overall sexual satisfaction domain ($p = 0.0007$, $r = -0.63$). Interestingly, female sexual dysfunction became evident prior to symptoms of ischemic heart disease in seven (23%) out of the 30 patients. Therefore, seven (78%) out of nine patients in this series developed the sexual disorders before (median of 51 months; range: 12–96 months) angina or myocardial infarction. Although these findings need to be confirmed in a larger patient population, this preliminary report suggested that sexual dysfunction is an important health issue in women with coronary artery disease.

Conclusions

There are several scientific observations that female sexual dysfunctions are age-related, progressive, highly prevalent, and strongly associated with medical conditions exactly like erectile dysfunction in the male population. However, little is known about the impact on women's sexual life of many of the more common medical diseases. Thus, data from clinical prospective studies are needed to clarify the pathophysiologies of female sexual dysfunction.

A new outlook should be available to the doctor attending an everyday clinical practice, in order to avoid comments such as the following in the future: "I am a 62-year-old woman who had a heart attack last year. Overall, my medical care has been excellent, and my doctors answer most of my questions even before I ask them. The one exception is any question about sexual activity. I want to know if it is dangerous and whether the medications I'm taking will affect my sex drive. Why won't my doctors address these issues?"[142]

References

1. Laumann EO, Paik A, Rosen RC. Sexual dysfunction in the United States. Prevalence and predictors. JAMA 1999; 281: 537–44.
2. Diokno AC. Epidemiology and psychosocial aspects of incontinence. Urol Clin North Am 1995; 22: 481–5.
3. Hampel C, Wienhold D, Benken N et al. Definition of overactive bladder and epidemiology of urinary incontinence. Urology 1997; 50(Suppl 6A): 4–14.
4. Carr LK, Webster GD. Bladder outlet obstruction in women. Urol Clin North Am 1996; 23: 385–91.
5. Bump RC, Norton PA. Epidemiology and natural history of pelvic floor dysfunction. Obst Gyn Clin North Am 1998; 25: 723–46.
6. Field SM, Hilton P. The prevalence of sexual problems in women attending for urodynamic investigation. Int Urogynecol J 1993; 4: 212.
7. Haase P, Skibsted L. Influence of operations for stress incontinence and/or genital descensus on sexual life. Acta Obstet Gynecol Scand 1988; 67: 659–61.
8. Barber MD, Visco AG, Wyman JF et al. Sexual function in women with urinary incontinence and pelvic organ prolapse. Obstet Gynecol 2002; 99: 281–9.
9. Shaw C. A systematic review of the literature on the prevalence of sexual impairment in women with urinary incontinence and the prevalence of urinary leakage during sexual activity. Eur Urol 2002; 42: 432–40.
10. Stothers L. Reliability, validity, and gender differences in the quality of life index of the SEAPI-QMM incontinence classification system. Neurourol Urodyn 2004; 23: 223–8.
11. Salonia A, Zanni G, Nappi RE et al. Sexual dysfunction is common in women with lower urinary tract symptoms and urinary incontinence: results of a cross-sectional study. Eur Urol 2004; 45: 642–8.
12. Rosen RC, Brown C, Heiman J et al. The Female Sexual Function Index (FSFI): a multidimensional self-report instrument for the assessment of female sexual function. J Sex Marital Ther 2000; 26: 191–208.
13. Basson R, Berman J, Burnett A et al. Report of the international consensus development conference on female sexual dysfunction: definitions and classifications. J Urol 2000; 163: 888–93.
14. Bergeron S, Binik YM, Khalife S et al. Vulvar vestibulitis syndrome: a critical review. Clin J Pain 1997; 13: 27–42.
15. Salonia A, Munarriz RM, Naspro R et al. Women's sexual dysfunction: a pathophysiological review. BJU Int 2004; 93: 1156–64.
16. van Driel MF, Weymar Schultz WC, van de Wiel HB et al. Female sexual functioning after radical surgical treatment of rectal and bladder cancer. Eur J Surg Oncol 1993; 19: 183–7.
17. Ofman US. Preservation of function in genitourinary cancers: psychosexual and psychosocial issues. Cancer Invest 1995; 13: 125–31.
18. Marshall FF, Treiger BF. Radical cystectomy (anterior exenteration) in the female patient. Urol Clin North Am 1991; 18: 765–75.
19. Bjerre BD, Johansen C, Steven K. A questionnaire study of sexological problems following urinary diversion in the female patient. Scand J Urol Nephrol 1997; 31: 155–60.
20. Nordstrom GM, Nyman CR. Male and female sexual function and activity following ileal conduit urinary diversion. Br J Urol 1992; 70: 33–9.
21. Hautmann RE, Paiss T, de Petriconi R. The ileal neobladder in women: 9 years of experience with 18 patients. J Urol 1996; 155: 76–81.
22. Horenblas S, Meinhardt W, Ijzerman W et al. Sexuality preserving cystectomy and neobladder: initial results. J Urol 2001; 166: 837–40.

23. DiGiorgi S, Schnatz PF, Mandavilli S et al. Transitional cell carcinoma presenting as clitoral priapism. *Gynecol Oncol* 2004; 93: 540–2.

24. Dodds DT, Potgieter CR, Turner PJ et al. The physical and emotional results of hysterectomy: a review of 162 cases. *S Afr Med J* 1961; 35: 53–4.

25. Craig GA, Jackson P. Sexual life after vaginal hysterectomy. *BMJ* 1975; 3: 97.

26. Dennerstein L, Wood C, Burrows GD. Sexual response following hysterectomy and oopherectomy. *Obstet Gynecol* 1977; 49: 92–6.

27. Nathorst-Boos J, van Schoultz B. Psychological reactions and sexual life after hysterectomy with and without oophorectomy. *Gynecol Obstet Invest* 1992; 34: 971–1101.

28. Helstrom L, Lundberg PO, Sorbom D et al. Sexuality after hysterectomy: a factor analysis of women's sexual lives before and after subtotal hysterectomy. *Obstet Gynecol* 1993; 81: 357–62.

29. Rhodes JC, Kjerulff KH, Langenberg PW et al. Hysterectomy and sexual function. *JAMA* 1999; 282: 1934–41.

30. Meston CM. The effects of hysterectomy on sexual arousal in women with a history of benign uterine fibroids. *Arch Sex Behav* 2004; 33: 31–42.

31. Jensen PT, Groenvold M, Klee MC et al. Early-stage cervical carcinoma, radical hysterectomy, and sexual function. A longitudinal study. *Cancer* 2004; 100: 97–106.

32. Gimbel H, Zobbe V, Andersen BM et al. Randomised controlled trial of total compared with subtotal hysterectomy with one-year follow up results. *Br J Obstet Gynaecol* 2003; 110: 1088–98.

33. Zobbe V, Gimbel H, Andersen BM et al. Sexuality after total vs. subtotal hysterectomy. *Acta Obstet Gynecol Scand* 2004; 83: 191–6.

34. Rako S. Testosterone deficiency: a key factor in the increased cardiovascular risk to women following hysterectomy or with natural aging? *J Womens Health* 1998; 7: 825–9.

35. Rako S. Testosterone supplemental therapy after hysterectomy with or without concomitant oophorectomy: estrogen alone is not enough. *J Womens Health Gend Based Med* 2000; 9: 917–23.

36. Cutler WB, Genovese-Stone E. Wellness in women after 40 years of age: the role of sex hormones and pheromones. *Dis Mon* 1998; 44: 421–546.

37. Bellrose SB, Binik YM. Body image and sexuality in oophorectomized women. *Arch Sex Behav* 1993; 38: 781–90.

38. Siddle N, Sarrel P, Whitehead M. The effect of hysterectomy on the age at ovarian failure: identification of a subgroup of women with premature loss of ovarian function and literature review. *Fertil Steril* 1986; 47: 94–100.

39. Kaiser R, Kursche M, Wurz H. Hormone levels in women after hysterectomy. *Arch Gynecol Obstet* 1989; 244: 169–73.

40. Oldenhave A, Jaszmann LJB, Everaerd W et al. Hysterectomized women with ovarian conservation report more severe climacteric complaints than do normal climacteric women of similar age. *Am J Obstet Gynecol* 1993; 168: 765–71.

41. Butler-Manuel SA, Buttery LD, A'Hern RP et al. Pelvic nerve plexus trauma at radical hysterectomy and simple hysterectomy: the nerve content of the uterine supporting ligaments. *Cancer* 2000; 89: 834–41.

42. Kuwabara Y, Suzuki M, Hashimoto M et al. New method to prevent bladder dysfunction after radical hysterectomy for uterine cervical cancer. *J Obstet Gynaecol Res* 2000; 26: 1–8.

43. Yabuki Y, Asamoto A, Hoshiba T et al. Radical hysterectomy: an anatomic evaluation of parametrial dissection. *Gynecol Oncol* 2000; 77: 155–63.

44. Murakami G, Yabuki Y, Kato T. A nerve-sparing radical hysterectomy: guidelines and feasibility in Western patients. *Int J Gynecol Cancer* 2002; 12: 319–21.

45. Querleu D, Narducci F, Poulard V et al. Modified radical vaginal hysterectomy with or without laparoscopic nerve-sparing dissection: a comparative study. *Gynecol Oncol* 2002; 85: 154–8.

46. Quinn MJ, Kirk N. Differences in uterine innervation at hysterectomy. *Am J Obstet Gynecol* 2002; 187: 1515–19.

47. Carlson KJ. Outcomes of hysterectomy. *Clin Obstet Gynecol* 1997; 40: 939–46.

48. Salonia A, Lanzi R, Nappi RE et al. Sexual dysfunction in dysthyroidal women. *Int J Impot Res* 2002; 14(Suppl 4): 52.

49. Beck A, Beamersderfer A. Assessment of depression: the depression inventory. *Mod Probl Pharmacopsychiatry* 1974; 7: 151–69.

50. Derogatis LR, Rosen RC, Leiblum S et al. The Female Sexual Distress Scale (FSDS): initial validation of a standardized scale for assessment of sexually related personal distress in women. *J Sex Marital Ther* 2002; 28: 317–30.

51. Biller BM, Luciano A, Crosignani PG et al. Guidelines for the diagnosis and treatment of hyperprolactinemia. *J Reprod Med* 1999; 44(12 Suppl): 1075–84.

52. Sauder SE, Freger M, Case GD et al. Abnormal patterns of pulsatile luteinizing hormone secretion in women with hyperprolactinemia and amenorrhea: responses to bromocriptine. *J Clin Endocrinol Metab* 1984; 59: 941–8.

53. Koppelman MCS, Parry BL, Hamilton JA et al. Effect of bromocriptine on affect and libido in hyperprolactinemia. *Am J Psychiatry* 1987; 144: 1037–41.

54. Hulter B, Lundberg PO. Sexual function in women with hypothalamo-pituitary disorders. *Arch Sex Behav* 1994; 23: 171–83.

55. Lundberg PO, Hulter B. Sexual dysfunction in patients with hypothalamo-pituitary disorders. *Exp Clin Endocrinol* 1991; 98: 81–8.

56. Kruger THC, Haake P, Hartmann U et al. Orgasm-induced prolactin secretion: feedback control of sexual drive? *Neurosci Behav Rev* 2002; 26: 31–44.

57. Dickson RA, Seeman MV, Corenblum B. Hormonal side effects in women: typical versus atypical antipsychotic treatment. *J Clin Psychiatry* 2000; 61(Suppl 3):10–5.

58. Compton MT, Miller AH. Antipsychotic-induced hyperprolactinemia and sexual dysfunction. *Psychopharmacol Bull* 2002; 36: 143–64.

59. Maguire GA. Prolactin elevation with antipsychotic medications: mechanisms of action and clinical consequences. *J Clin Psychiatry* 2002; 63(Suppl 4): 56–62.

60. Smith S. Effects of antipsychotics on sexual and endocrine function in women: implications for clinical practice. *J Clin Psychopharmacol* 2003; 23(3 Suppl 1): S27–32.

61. Smith SM, O'Keane V, Murray R. Sexual dysfunction in patients

taking conventional antipsychotic medication. *Br J Psychiatry* 2002; 181: 49–55.

62. Montejo-Gonzalez AL, Llorca G, Izquierdo JA et al. SSRI-induced sexual dysfunction: fluoxetine, paroxetine, sertraline, and fluvoxamamine in a prospective, multicenter, and descriptive clinical study of 344 patients. *J Sex Marital Ther* 1997; 23: 176–94.

63. Rosen RC, Lane RM, Menza M. Effects of SSRI on sexual function: a critical review. *J Clin Psychopharmacol* 1999; 19: 67–85.

64. Guay AT. Sexual dysfunction in the diabetic patient. *Int J Impot Res* 2001; 13(Suppl 5): S47–S50.

65. Enzlin P, Demyttenaere K, Vanderschueren D et al. Diabetes and female sexuality: a review of 25 years' research. *Diabetic Med* 1998; 15: 809–15.

66. Jackson G. Sexual dysfunction and diabetes. *Int J Clin Pract* 2004; 58: 358–62.

67. Erol B, Tefekli A, Sanli O et al. Does sexual dysfunction correlate with deterioration of somatic sensory system in diabetic women? *Int J Impot Res* 2003; 15: 198–202.

68. Duby JJ, Campbell RK, Setter SM et al. Diabetic neuropathy: an intensive review. *Am J Health Syst Pharm* 2004; 61: 160–73.

69. Schreiner-Engel P, Schiavi RC, Vietorisz D et al. The differential impact of diabetes type on female sexuality. *J Psychosom Res* 1987; 31: 23–33.

70. Arshag D, Mooradian MD, Greiff V. Sexuality in older women. *Arch Intern Med* 1990; 150: 1033–8.

71. Erol B, Tefekli A, Ozbey I et al. Sexual dysfunction in type II diabetic females: a comparative study. *J Sex Marital Ther* 2002; 28(Suppl 1): 55–62.

72. Schiel R, Muller UA. Prevalence of sexual disorders in a selection-free diabetic population (JEVIN). *Diabetes Res Clin Pract* 1999; 44: 115–21.

73. Enzlin P, Mathieu C, Van den Bruel A et al. Sexual dysfunction in women with type 1 diabetes. *Diabetes Care* 2002; 25: 672–7.

74. Enzlin P, Mathieu C, Van Den Bruel A et al. Prevalence and predictors of sexual dysfunction in patients with type 1 diabetes. *Diabetes Care* 2003; 26: 409–14.

75. Salonia A, Lanzi R, Gatti E et al. Sexual dysfunction in Italian diabetic women. *Int J Impot Res* 2002; 14(Suppl 3): S27.

76. Palmer BF. Sexual dysfunction in men and women with chronic kidney disease and end-stage kidney disease. *Adv Ren Replace Ther* 2003; 10: 48–60.

77. Palmer BF. Sexual dysfunction in uremia. *J Am Soc Nephrol* 1999; 10: 1381–8.

78. Leavey SF, Weitzel WF. Endocrine abnormalities in chronic renal failure. *Endocrinol Metab Clin North Am* 2002; 31: 107–19.

79. Iacovides A, Fountoulakis KN, Balaskas E et al. Relationship of age and psychosocial factors with biological ratings in patients with end-stage renal disease undergoing dialysis. *Aging Clin Exp Res* 2002; 14: 354–60.

80. Camsari T, Cavdar C, Yemez B et al. Psychosexual function in CAPD and hemodialysis patients. *Perit Dial Int* 1999; 19: 585–8.

81. Steele TE, Wuerth D, Finkelstein S et al. Sexual experience of the chronic peritoneal dialysis patient. *J Am Soc Nephrol* 1996; 7: 1165–8.

82. Toorians AW, Janssen E, Laan E et al. Chronic renal failure and sexual functioning: clinical status versus objectively assessed sexual response. *Nephrol Dial Transplant* 1997; 12: 2654–63.

83. Mastrogiacomo I, De Besi L, Serafini E et al. Hyperprolactinemia and sexual disturbances among uremic women on hemodialysis. *Nephron* 1984; 37: 195–9.

84. Weizman R, Weizman A, Levi J et al. Sexual dysfunction associated with hyperprolactinemia in males and females undergoing hemodialysis. *Psychosom Med* 1983; 45: 259–69.

85. Whipple B, Komisaruk BR. Sexuality and women with complete spinal cord injury. *Spinal Cord* 1997; 35: 136–8.

86. Westgren N, Hultling C, Levi R et al. Sexuality in women with traumatic spinal cord injury. *Acta Obstet Gynecol Scand* 1997; 76: 977–83.

87. Sipski ML, Alexander CJ, Rosen RC. Sexual arousal and orgasm in women: effects of spinal cord injury. *Ann Neurol* 2001; 49: 35–44.

88. Benevento BT, Sipski ML. Neurogenic bladder, neurogenic bowel, and sexual dysfunction in people with spinal cord injury. *Phys Ther* 2002; 82: 601–12.

89. Charlifue SW, Gerhart KA, Menter RR et al. Sexual issues of women with spinal cord injuries. *Paraplegia* 1992; 30: 192–9.

90. Sipski ML, Alexander CJ. Sexual activities, response and satisfaction in women pre- and post-spinal cord injury. *Arch Phys Med Rehabil* 1993; 74: 1025–9.

91. Sipski ML. Spinal cord injury and sexual function: an educational model. In ML Sipski, CJ Alexander, eds. *Sexual Function in People with Disability and Chronic Illness.* Gaithersburg: Aspen, 1997: 149–76.

92. Berard EJJ. The sexuality of spinal cord injured women: physiology and pathophysiology. A review. *Paraplegia* 1989; 27: 99–112.

93. Sipski ML, Alexander CJ, Rosen RC. Physiological parameters associated with psychogenic sexual arousal in women with complete spinal cord injuries. *Arch Phys Med Rehabil* 1995; 76: 811–18.

94. Geiger RC. Neurophysiology of sexual response in spinal cord injury. *Sex Disabil* 1979; 2: 257–66.

95. Sipski ML, Alexander CJ, Rosen RC. Orgasm in women with spinal cord injuries: a laboratory-based assessment. *Arch Phys Med Rehabil* 1995; 76: 1097–1102.

96. Litwiller SE, Frohman EM, Zimmern PE. Multiple sclerosis and the urologist. *J Urol* 1999; 161: 743–57.

97. DasGupta R, Fowler CJ. Bladder, bowel and sexual dysfunction in multiple sclerosis. Management strategies. *Drugs* 2003; 63: 153–66.

98. DasGupta R, Fowler CJ. Sexual and urological dysfunction in multiple sclerosis: better understanding and improved therapies. *Curr Opin Neurol* 2002; 15: 271–8.

99. McDougall AJ, McLeod JG. Autonomic nervous system function in multiple sclerosis. *J Neurol Sci* 2003; 215: 79–85.

100. Lillius H, Valtonen C, Wilkstrom J. Sexual problems in patients suffering from multiple sclerosis. *J Chron Dis* 1976; 19: 643–7.

101. Zorzon M, Zivadinov R, Bosco A et al. Sexual dysfunction in multiple sclerosis: a case-control study. I. Frequency and comparison of groups. *Mult Scler* 1999; 5: 418–27.

102. Stenager E, Stenager EN, Jensen K. Sexual function in multiple sclerosis. *Ital J Neurol Sci* 1996; 17: 67–9.

103. Hulter BM, Lundberg PO. Sexual function in women with advanced multiple sclerosis. *J Neurol Neurosurg Psych* 1995; 59: 83–6.

104. Kurtzke JF. Rating neurologic impairment in multiple sclerosis: an expanded disability status scale (EDSS). *Neurology* 1983; 33: 1444–52.

105. Zivadinov R, Zorzon M, Bosco A et al. Sexual dysfunction in multiple sclerosis: a case-control study. II. Correlation analysis. *Mult Scler* 1999; 5: 428–31.

106. Zivadinov R, Zorzon M, Locatelli L et al. Sexual dysfunction in multiple sclerosis: a MRI, neurophysiological and urodynamic study. *J Neurol Sci* 2003; 210: 73–6.

107. Nortvedt M, Riise T, Myhr K et al. Reduced quality of life among multiple sclerosis patients with sexual disturbance and bladder dysfunction. *Mult Scler* 2001; 7: 231–5.

108. Zorzon M, Zivadinov R, Locatelli L et al. Correlation of sexual dysfunction and brain magnetic resonance imaging in multiple sclerosis. *Mult Scler* 2003; 9: 108–10.

109. Hennessey A, Robertson NP, Swinger R et al. Urinary, faecal and sexual dysfunction in patients with multiple sclerosis. *J Neurol* 1999; 246: 1027–32.

110. McCabe MP. Relationship functioning and sexuality among people with multiple sclerosis. *J Sex Res* 2002; 39: 302–9.

111. McCabe MP, McKern S, McDonald E et al. Changes over time in sexual and relationship functioning of people with multiple sclerosis. *J Sex Marital Ther* 2003; 29: 305–21.

112. Harrison T, Stuifbergen A, Adachi E et al. Marriage, impairment, and acceptance in persons with multiple sclerosis. *West J Nurs Res* 2004; 26: 266–85.

113. Kornstein SG. Chronic depression in women. *J Clin Psychiatry* 2002; 63: 602–9.

114. Mazure CM, Maciejewski PK. The interplay of stress, gender and cognitive style in depressive onset. *Arch Women Ment Health* 2003; 6: 5–8.

115. Clayton AH. Female sexual dysfunction related to depression and antidepressant medications. *Curr Womens Health Rep* 2002; 2: 182–7.

116. Baldwin DS. Depression and sexual dysfunction. *Br Med Bull* 2001; 57: 81–99.

117. Clayton AH. Recognition and assessment of sexual dysfunction associated with depression. *J Clin Psychiatry* 2001; 62(Suppl 3): 5–9.

118. Zajecka J, Dunner DL, Gelenberg AJ et al. Sexual function and satisfaction in the treatment of chronic major depression with nefazodone, psychotherapy, and their combination. *J Clin Psychiatry* 2002; 63: 709–16.

119. Phillips RL Jr, Slaughter JR. Depression and sexual desire. *Am Fam Physician* 2000; 62: 782–6.

120. Baldwin RC. Prognosis of depression. *Curr Opin Psychiatry* 2000: 13: 81–5.

121. Dunn KM, Croft PR, Hackett GI. Association of sexual problems with social, psychological, and physical problems in men and women: a cross sectional population survey. *J Epidemiol Community Health* 1999; 53: 144–8.

122. Cyranowski JM, Frank E, Cherry C et al. Prospective assessment of sexual function in women treated for recurrent major depression. *J Psychiatr Res* 2004; 38: 267–73.

123. Gracia CR, Sammel MD, Freeman EW et al. Predictors of decreased libido in women during the late reproductive years. *Menopause* 2004; 11: 144–50.

124. Abdo CH, Oliveira WM Jr, Moreira ED Jr et al. Prevalence of sexual dysfunctions and correlated conditions in a sample of Brazilian women – results of the Brazilian study on sexual behavior (BSSB). *Int J Impot Res* 2004; 16: 160–6.

125. Balon R. Emotional blunting, sexual dysfunction and SSRIs. *Int J Neuropsychopharmacol* 2002; 5: 415–16.

126. Hensley PL, Nurnberg HG. SSRI sexual dysfunction: a female perspective. *J Sex Marital Ther* 2002; 28(Suppl 1): 143–53.

127. Kanaly KA, Berman JR. Sexual side effects of SSRI medications: potential treatment strategies for SSRI-induced female sexual dysfunction. *Curr Womens Health Rep* 2002; 2: 409–16.

128. Ekselius L, von Knorring L. Effect on sexual function of long-term treatment with selective serotonin reuptake inhibitors in depressed patients treated in primary care. *J Clin Psychopharmacol* 2001; 21: 154–60.

129. Peuskens J, Sienaert P, DeHert M. Sexual dysfunction: the unspoken side effects of antipsychotics. *Eur Psy* 1998; 13(Suppl 1): 23–30.

130. Montgomery SA, Baldwin DS, Riley A. Antidepressant medications: a review of the evidence for drug-induced sexual dysfunction. *J Affect Disord* 2002; 69: 119–40.

131. Nurnberg HG, Hensley PL. Selective phosphodiesterase type-5 inhibitor treatment of serotonergic reuptake inhibitor antidepressant-associated sexual dysfunction: a review of diagnosis, treatment, and relevance. *CNS Spectr* 2003; 8: 194–202.

132. Nappi RE, Verde JB, Polatti F et al. Self-reported sexual symptoms in women attending menopause clinics. *Gynecol Obstet Invest* 2002; 53: 181–7.

133. Janardhan V, Bakshi R. Quality of life in patients with multiple sclerosis: the impact of fatigue and depression. *J Neurol Sci* 2002; 205: 51–8.

134. Hodge RH, Harward MP, West MS et al. Sexual function of women taking antihypertensive agents: a comparative study. *J Gen Intern Med* 1991; 6: 290–4.

135. Grimm RH Jr, Grandits GA, Prineas RJ et al. Long-term effects on sexual function of five antihypertensive drugs and nutritional hygienic treatment in hypertensive men and women. Treatment of Mild Hypertension Study (TOMHS). *Hypertension* 1997; 29(1 Pt 1): 8–14.

136. Rosen RC. Sexual dysfunction as an obstacle to compliance with antihypertensive therapy. *Blood Press Suppl* 1997; 1: 47–51.

137. Lewis C, Duncan LE, Ballance DI et al. Is sexual dysfunction in hypertensive women uncommon or understudied? *Am J Hypertens* 1998; 11(6 Pt 1): 733–5.

138. Burchardt M, Burchardt T, Anastasiadis AG et al. Sexual dysfunction is common and overlooked in female patients with hypertension. *Sex Marital Ther* 2002; 28: 17–26.

139. Hanon O, Mounier-Vehier C, Fauvel JP et al. [Sexual dysfunction in treated hypertensive patients. Results of a national survey]. *Arch Mal Coeur Vaiss* 2002; 95: 673–7.

140. Duncan LE, Lewis C, Smith CE et al. Sex, drugs, and hypertension: a methodological approach for studying a sensitive subject. *Int J Impot Res* 2001; 13: 31–40.

141. Salonia A, Briganti A, Montorsi P. Sexual dysfunction in women with coronary artery disease. *Int J Impot Res* 2002; 14(Suppl 4): S80.

142. Lee TH. Ask the doctor. *Harv Heart Lett* 2004; 14: 8.

7.4 Breast cancer and its effect on women's body image and sexual function

Alessandra Graziottin

Introduction

Body image is a concept cited extensively in the literature.[1-11] It may be defined as a multifactorial mental construct, dynamically reshaped throughout life, and rooted both in the biologic and psychologic domain.[12] Neurobiologic/somatic, psychologic/affective, and context-related factors contribute to perceptions of body image across the life span.

Body image is a critical dimension of sexual identity.[8,12] Body image may modulate sexual function and response through the complex physical and emotional interactions during sexual activity, and may be modified in turn by the quality of past and current sexual experiences.[8,12] The sexual relationship is the most intimate of the interpersonal factors that contribute to body image perception and, specifically, to the erotic meaning of the breast in adulthood.

Breast cancer affects 8–10% of women in their lifetime; 25% are premenopausal when diagnosed.[13] The beauty and appearance of the breast are important for a woman's sense of femininity, body image, self-esteem, self-confidence, and eroticism.[1-5,8,12] Female sexual identity, sexual function, and the sexual relationship may be adversely affected by the many changes and challenges facing the woman when diagnosis and treatment of breast cancer disrupts her life and that of her family.[1-11] These changes are often accompanied by changes in body image that are brought about by psychologic and iatrogenic factors.

This chapter will discuss the impact of breast cancer on women's sexuality with respect to body image by: (1) describing biologic and psychosocial contributions; (2) reviewing the key literature on the impact of breast cancer on body image and sexuality in cancer patients; (3) focusing on factors and coping strategies that may improve body image of cancer survivors after treatment; and (4) considering the impact on body image of genetic screening and prophylactic mastectomy for women at high risk of breast cancer.

Body image contributors

Biologic and psychosocial factors that contribute to body image are summarized in Table 7.4.1.

In the biologic domain, body image is influenced by sensory information such as sight, touch, smell, sound, taste, and proprioception. This sensory information contributes to the body schema, a major contributor to body image that integrates the sensorimotor aspects of the woman's body. Visceral and autonomic components of body image are less frequently considered, although they may contribute to mood, a sense of

Table 7.4.1. Factors contributing to body image

Psychologic	Biologic
• Cognitive	• Multisensorial
• Affective	• Motor/proprioceptive
• Emotional	• Hormonal
• Cosmetic	• Autonomic
• Sexual	• Disease-related
• Social	

well-being, fatigue, illness, and the ultimate perception of body image.[12]

From the psychosocial point of view, cognitive, affective, emotional, sexual, cosmetic, and social factors further interact with physical issues in modulating body image.[12] The comprehensive emotional and unconscious perception of the body is a major contributor to the private body consciousness, a psychoanalytic concept of more complex body image factors (see Chapters 3.1–3.4).

Body image and sexuality in breast cancer patients

Breast cancer diagnosis and treatment may modify the woman's body image and sexuality through several modalities. Factors dependent upon the illness, the context, and the individual interact to contribute to the woman's body image and sexual outcome.[8] Major illness-dependent and iatrogenic factors influencing body image and sexuality include stage of cancer, type of breast surgery, lymphedema, hair loss, iatrogenic premature menopause, and age at diagnosis (Table 7.4.2).

Stage of cancer

The stage of breast cancer affects body image, as it determines the extent of radical surgery; the need for lymph node removal; the presence and severity of lymphedema; the need for adjuvant chemotherapy, with the risk of iatrogenic premature menopause, and/or radiotherapy with consequent local and systemic symptoms; and the perception of the risk of death. In a study of 303 women with early stage breast cancer and 200 with advanced breast cancer, Kissane et al.[9] found an overall prevalence of mood disorders, and depression and anxiety disorders,

Table 7.4.2. Major factors affecting body image and sexuality in breast cancer survivors

1. Cancer related
   - Age at diagnosis
   - Type of cancer, stage and prognosis
   - Recurrences
   - Conservative vs radical treatment
   - Adjuvant chemotherapy and/or radiotherapy
   - Treatment impact on ovarian function (sexual hormone production and infertility)
2. Woman dependent
   - Life cycle stage and fulfillment of stage-related goals
   - Coping strategies
   - Pretreatment sexual experience, and its quality
   - Premorbid personality and psychiatric status
3. Context dependent
   - Family dynamics and couple dynamics and marital status
   - Support network (friends, colleagues, relatives, self-help groups)
   - Quality of relationship with health-care providers

as defined by the *Diagnostic and Statistical Manual of Mental Disorders*, fourth edition (DSM-IV), of 45% and 42%, respectively, Women with advanced breast cancer were significantly less distressed by hair loss, but were more dissatisfied with body image and had higher rates of lymphedema and hot flushes, than the early-stage women. The rates of psychosocial distress were similarly high in both groups, although the illness-related causes of distress were different.

Depression is significantly associated with lower sexual desire and arousal difficulties[1-8] (see Chapter 16.2). Women with higher depression scores report more cancer-related distress pertaining to body image, fear of recurrence, post-traumatic stress disorder, and sexual problems. Those with long-term medical sequelae, such as lymphedema, have poorer adjustment than those who do not.[14]

Breast surgery

The visual and tactile sensations and perceptions of the breast are affected differently according to the type of breast surgery performed.[1-7] Important factors influencing sexual outcomes include lumpectomy versus mastectomy, immediate or delayed reconstruction of the breast, the need for adjuvant radiotherapy or chemotherapy, and presence and severity of side effects.

In a recent prospective study of 990 breast cancer patients followed for 5 years,[11] mastectomy patients had significantly poorer body image and lower role and sexual function scores than patients undergoing breast-conserving therapy. Body image, sexual function and lifestyle disruptions did not improve over time.[11] Accordingly, breast-conserving therapy, when oncologically appropriate, should be encouraged for patients in all age groups. However, conservative treatment does not guarantee a more positive physical outcome. A cross-sectional study of women 1 year after treatment suggested that, because of the need for adjuvant therapies, women treated by breast conservation have better body image but poorer physical function, particularly younger patients.[15] Negative physical and sexual symptoms may be secondary to the premature iatrogenic menopause and/or to local sensory side effects of radiotherapy.

Lymphedema

Except for breast carcinoma recurrence, no event is more dreaded than the development of lymphedema.[16-18] The surgical removal of axillary nodes may impair lymphatic drainage from the arm. As a result, the arm becomes swollen, causing pain, progressive fibrosis, sensory distortion, discomfort, and disability[18] "Arm problems" are cited by 26–72% of breast cancer patients.[5,6] Fibrosis and lymphedema in the connective tissue and the muscular and functional impairment of the affected arms and fingers deeply affect the physical and psychologic dimensions of body image. When severe, it may impair body image even more than breast surgery. The clinician who, focusing on the risk of carcinoma recurrence, trivializes the nonlethal nature of lymphedema[18] and may hinder adjustment to these symptoms. While the mastectomy can be hidden easily in social contexts, the disfigured arm/hand is a constant reminder of the breast cancer[18] and may contribute to sexual difficulties.

Hair loss

Although limited to the period of chemotherapy, hair loss may be perceived as a major insult to body image, particularly in younger patients. Vulnerability to hair loss-related distress decreases with the progression of the disease.[8,9]

Iatrogenic premature menopause

Chemotherapy may cause ovarian failure and associated autonomic disturbances. Hot flushes, night sweats, night tachycardia, insomnia, arthralgia, mood changes, and general body shape changes associated with iatrogenic premature menopause may further alter body image. The effects of menopause on sexuality (see Chapter 9.2) are even more complex if the onset is premature[19,20] (see Chapters 13.1–13.3).

Age

Age moderates body image in breast cancer patients and survivors irrespective of illness- and treatment-related factors. Women diagnosed with breast cancer at a younger age often have sexual and psychosocial concerns that are less common among older women. A cross-sectional survey of 204 women diagnosed during the past 3.5 years with breast cancer at age 50 or younger indicated that: (a) mastectomy was associated with poorer body image and lower interest in sex; (b) chemotherapy was associated with greater sexual dysfunction; (c) sexual function (e.g., lubrication, sexual pain) was a greater problem than lack of sexual interest; (d) concerns about premature menopause and fertility were rated as the most problematic issues facing this group[10] (see Chapter 7.1).

While the ramifications of age on body image among breast cancer patients vary by individual and by reproductive goals,[8,21–25] this does not mean that elderly women are less vulnerable to issues of body image from breast surgery. In Engel's 5-year prospective study, body image, sexual function, and lifestyle disruption scores did not improve over time, indicating that sexual vulnerability persists or increases over time.[11] This finding was substantiated in the prospective study by Ganz et al.[4]

Cognitive

Ultimately, the woman judges her body image by integrating the visible results of surgery, the personal and cultural context of oncologic breast surgery, and the threat of death. An especially sensitive issue is the decision regarding whether or not to perform breast reconstruction at the time of the mastectomy. Attitudes of physicians toward conservative (in younger patients) or radical treatment (in older patients) may influence the patient's decision, with possible regrets later.[26]

A feeling of helplessness, hopelessness, or resignation is reported to be significantly associated with depression and vulnerability to body image impairments.[9,26–28] Cognitive deficits secondary to chemotherapy seem to be independent of depression and anxiety and independent of menopausal status.[28]

Affective

Affective factors seem to change the vulnerability of body image. Love is one of the most powerful shapers of body image, able to lessen the impact of major physical impairments and changes. An increase in affection and intimacy reduces the negative impact of cancer surgery on body image and sexual satisfaction. At the opposite end, frustration with love and need for attachment can impair body image perception even in healthy people with no alterations in physical appearance. After breast cancer, the women most vulnerable to poor body image are younger and either single or in troubled relationships.[1,2,10]

Emotional

Mood, anxiety, and positive or negative emotions shape the inner perception of body image. Depression and anxiety, whether pre-existent or triggered by the cancer diagnosis and treatment, and made worse in the case of premature iatrogenic menopause, may lead to a poorer body image outcome. Depression and anxiety may affect body image and sexual function via nonhormonal pathways, as reported in an average of 17–25% of breast cancer patients, and may specifically contribute to the loss of libido.[27]

Cosmetic

The primary variable affecting cosmetic outcome of breast cancer surgery is surgical skill,[11] while taking into account the oncologic need for radical surgery. However, cosmetic results of surgery may be enhanced by maintaining the integrity of pleasurable sensations from the nipple and the skin, or may be impaired by loss of sensations or unwanted sensations (paresthesia, "pins and needles," etc.).[4,5,8]

Sexual

Breast cancer may dramatically impair sexuality for the woman and the couple, from both the biologic and psychosexual points of view. Sexual identity may be harmed,[8] becoming more vulnerable with more radical surgery,[1,2,4,6,7] lymphedema,[8,16–18] premature iatrogenic menopause,[24] and chemotherapy-induced hair loss. The women most vulnerable to these effects are single, younger, in troubled relationships, have lower income, and have poor overall social support.[1,2,10]

Sexual function may be impaired as well. Sexual desire and mental arousal are diminished in a significant percentage of breast cancer patients[1–8] (see Chapters 6.1–6.5). The breast is a major sign of femininity. Breast foreplay may stimulate and trigger sexual arousal, desire, and even orgasm. The pleasure felt from breast kissing and caressing contributes to the erotic meaning of this part of the body. After breast surgery, many women report impaired, distorted, or unpleasant physical sensations. A total of 44% of women with partial mastectomy and 83% of those with breast reconstruction report that pleasure from breast caresses had decreased.[1] Loss of breast sensitivity may contribute to further loss of sexual desire and of mental and peripheral nongenital arousal.[8] Uneasiness at being naked increases the tendency to keep the breast covered while making love, and to avoid any further breast stimulation.

Vaginal dryness and dyspareunia are identified as problems by 35–60% of normal, postmenopausal women due to lack of estrogen[20] (see Chapter 7.2). Pre-existing arousal disorders may be made worse by the menopausal loss of estrogen and loss of libido after breast cancer. A second biologic cause of arousal difficulties is the spasm of the pubococcygeal muscle secondary to vaginal dryness and dyspareunia.[8] Attention to hypertonic conditions of the pelvic floor secondary to dyspareunia is important in breast cancer patients. Teaching relaxation of the levator ani muscle and encouraging self-massage with a medicated oil may effectively relieve dyspareunia and arousal disorders secondary to hypoestrogenism, when the woman is unable to receive estrogen treatment because of the risk of breast cancer recurrence.[8,29] Controversy still exists regarding the use of hormonal therapy after breast cancer. Topical vaginal estrogen treatments are considered safe by many oncologists; however, the decision must be made with the patient being informed of the risks and benefits. Patients with good libido and genital arousal disorders may have some clinical improvement with vasoactive drugs, such as selective phosphodiesterase type-5 inhibitors,[30] that are not contraindicated in breast cancer patients. Considering the high prevalence of dyspareunia in breast cancer patients, the viability of nonhormonal alternative treatments needs to be evaluated.

Quality-of-life impairment secondary to iatrogenic factors and/or menopause may harm the woman's sense of eroticism.[10–13] In a prospective, longitudinal study conducted by Ganz et al.,[5] 61% of breast cancer patients reported difficulty with sexual arousal and 57% reported difficulty with lubrication. Interestingly, the group attained maximum recovery from the physical and psychologic trauma of cancer treatment within 1 year of surgery. A number of aspects of quality of life, including sexuality, significantly worsened after that time. Another study reported that women who received chemotherapy tended to have less frequent desire, more vaginal dryness, more dyspareunia, less frequent sex, and reduced ability to reach orgasm through intercourse; overall, sexual satisfaction was significantly decreased.[1] Postmenopausal breast cancer survivors were more likely to report vaginal dryness and tightness, as well as genital pain, with sexual activity.[1] Loss of ovarian androgens secondary to chemotherapy may contribute to loss of libido.[20,28]

Orgasmic difficulties may be the end point of a number of biologic as well as motivational-affective and cognitive factors (see Chapter 6.4). Difficulty in reaching orgasm was reported in 55% of patients in the study by Ganz et al.,[5] with a significant decrease in sexual function over the 3-year follow-up. In a retrospective study by Schover et al.,[1] the ability to reach orgasm through intercourse tended to be significantly reduced in women who received chemotherapy, although their ability to reach orgasm through noncoital caressing did not differ from control women. The inhibitory effect of dyspareunia on vaginal orgasm might explain this difference, together with the effect of androgen-dependent nitric oxide pathways on clitoral response, and estrogen-dependent vasoactive intestinal peptide on vaginal response.[31,32]

Sexual satisfaction, which includes both physical and emotional aspects, should be investigated separately. Pain and disappointing sexual experiences might be responsible for the significantly reduced satisfaction reported by breast cancer survivors.[2] A prospective study indicated that sexual satisfaction remained significantly reduced in breast cancer survivors (compared to age-matched controls) 8 years after primary treatment.[6] Objective parameters to quantify and qualify sexual satisfaction are at present undefined. The diagnosis of cancer places a strain on both the couple and the family.[1,2,9,33] Young women and young couples may be particularly vulnerable, as studies indicate that younger women experience more emotional distress than older women, and younger husbands report more difficulty in fulfilling domestic roles and feel more vulnerable to life stresses.[34] When breast cancer is diagnosed, the demands of the illness supersede the normal demands of family life, and the impact on the family may vary depending on the phase of the family life cycle at the time of cancer diagnosis.[34]

Social

Social factors may be divided into two major categories: the "social mirror", which is determined by the culturally based importance of the breast and its aesthetics; and the "social network", which encompasses the woman's resources for support. Health-care providers and self-help groups may represent an important resource for body image concerns. However, one study reported that 62% of breast cancer patients found it easier to discuss their sexual problems during their illness with their partner than with physicians and psychologists, and only 15% of breast cancer patients openly expressed their concerns to health-care professionals.[35]

Coping strategies to improve body image after breast cancer

Family and psychologic support, self-help groups, and good relationships between the patient and her health-care providers may all contribute to reducing the distress associated with the diagnosis and treatment of breast cancer. Regular exercise is an effective coping strategy that deserves special emphasis for its positive effects, its consistency over time, and its low cost.

Indeed, studies have shown that breast cancer survivors who exercise regularly, in comparison with sedentary women, have significantly more positive attitudes toward their physical condition and sexual attractiveness, as well as significantly less confusion, fatigue, depression, and mood disorder, regardless of age. The positive impact of regular exercise on body image, body schema, and self-image lessens the specific impact of breast changes. Due to the positive effects of exercise on mood, sexual desire may be less impaired and sexual arousal facilitated.

Psychosexual functioning after bilateral prophylactic mastectomy

Women with a strong family history of breast cancer, or a BCRA1 or BCRA2 mutation (markers of significantly higher vulnerability to developing breast cancer in their lifetime), are encouraged to undergo bilateral prophylactic mastectomy. Metcalfe et al.[36] examined psychosocial outcomes related to this procedure. While the vast majority (97%) were satisfied with their decision to have the surgery, younger women (< 50 years) were less likely to report satisfaction than older women. Breast reconstruction was associated with higher levels of body satisfaction. Van Geel[37] reported that prophylactic mastectomy decreased women's anxiety about developing breast cancer but had a negative impact on their sexual lives. Appropriate sexual counseling should be offered to women at high risk of breast cancer before and after surgery to ease the impact of this distressing decision.

Conclusion

Breast cancer may have a strong effect on a woman's body image and impair her sexual identity, sexual function, and sexual relationship. The impact of breast cancer on the sexuality of the individual woman is dependent upon the cancer, the woman, and the context. The issues of body image and sexuality after breast cancer become increasingly important with increasing time after surgery. The vulnerability of body image and sexuality is reduced in women with early-stage breast cancer who undergo conservative breast surgery, have limited side effects, enjoy a strong network of family and social support, and exercise regularly. The vulnerability of both body image and sexuality is higher in those who have advanced breast cancer, need adjuvant treatment, have lymphedema, are sedentary, have poor family and social support, and/or are single or in unstable relationships. The fact that overall adjustment and quality of life of breast cancer survivors are positive in an average of 70–80% of cases should not mask the fact that outcomes are frequently less favorable for body image, sexual function, and physical satisfaction.

Breast cancer survivors and their partners may need sexual counseling during and after cancer treatment. Psychologic counseling is available in most hospitals in North America and Europe. Unfortunately, the opportunity for sexual counseling is rarely offered by oncologic services. Competent sexual support could greatly improve the quality of intimacy, body image, and sexual relationships in cancer patients, cancer survivors, and their partners.

References

1. Schover LR, Yetman RJ, Tuason LJ et al. Partial mastectomy and breast reconstruction. A comparison of their effects on psychosocial adjustment, body image, and sexuality. Cancer 1995; 75: 54–64.
2. Schover LR. Sexuality and body image in younger women with breast cancer. J Natl Cancer Inst Monogr 1994; 16: 177–82.
3. Andersen BL, Anderson B, de Prosse C. Controlled prospective longitudinal study of women with cancer. I. Sexual functioning outcomes. J Consult Clin Psychol 1989; 75: 683–91.
4. Ganz PA, Shag AC, Lee JJ et al. Breast conservation versus mastectomy: is there a difference in psychological adjustment or quality of life in the year after surgery? Cancer 1992; 69: 1729–8.
5. Ganz PA, Coscarelli A, Fred C et al. Breast cancer survivors: psychosocial concerns and quality of life. Breast Cancer Res Treat 1996; 38: 183–99.
6. Dorval M, Maunsell E, Deschenes L et al. Long term quality of life after breast cancer: comparison of 8 years survivors with population controls. J Clin Oncol 1998; 16: 487–94.
7. Dorval M, Maunsell E, Deschenes L et al. Type of mastectomy and quality of life for long term breast carcinoma survivors. Cancer 1998; 83: 2130–8.
8. Graziottin A, Castoldi E. Sexuality and breast cancer: a review. In J Studd, ed. The Management of the Menopause. The Millennium Review. New York: Parthenon, 2000: 211–20.
9. Kissane DW, Grabsch B, Love A et al. Psychiatric disorders in women with early stage and advanced breast cancer: a comparative analysis. Aust N Z J Psychiatry 2004; 38: 320–6.
10. Avis NE, Crawford S, Mamuel J. Psychosocial problems among younger women with breast cancer. Psychooncology 2004; 13: 295–308.
11. Engel J, Kerr J, Schlesinger-Raab A et al. Quality of life following breast-conserving therapy or mastectomy: results of a 5-year prospective study. Breast J 2004; 10: 223–31.
12. Graziottin A. Immagine corporea e sessualità in perimenopausa AA. In Proceedings of the 76th National Congress of the Italian Society of Obstetricians and Gynecologists. Naples, 4–7 June 2000. Rome: CIC Edizioni Internazionali, 2000: 29–40.
13. Bloom JR, Stewart SL, Chang S et al. Then and now: quality of life of young cancer survivors. Psychooncology 2004; 13: 147–60.
14. Kornblith AB, Ligibel J. Psychosocial and sexual functioning of survivors of breast cancer. Semin Oncol 2003; 30: 779–813.
15. Kenny P, King MT, Shiell A et al. Early stage breast cancer: costs and quality of life one year after treatment by mastectomy or conservative surgery and radiation therapy. Breast 2000; 9: 37–44.
16. Paci E, Cariddi A, Barchielli A et al. Long term sequelae of breast cancer surgery. Tumori 1996; 82: 321–4.

17. Runowicz CD. Lymphedema: patients and provider education – current status and future trends. *Cancer* 1998; 83: 2874–6.

18. Petrek JA, Heelan MC. Incidence of breast-carcinoma related lymphedema. *Cancer* 1998; 83: 2776–81.

19. Graziottin A. Libido. In J Studd, ed. *Yearbook of the Royal College of Obstetricians and Gynaecologists*. London: RCOG Press–Parthenon, 1996: 235–43.

20. Graziottin A, Basson R. Management of sexual dysfunction in women with premature menopause. *Menopause* 2004; **in press**.

21. Lamb MA. Effects of cancer on the sexuality and fertility of women. *Semin Oncol Nurs* 1995; 11: 120–7.

22. Collichio FA, Agnello R, Staltzer J. Pregnancy after breast cancer: from psychosocial issues through conception. *Oncology (Huntingt)* 1998; 12: 759–65, 769; discussion: 770, 773–5.

23. Danforth D. How subsequent pregnancy affects outcome in women with a prior cancer. *Oncology* 1991; 5: 23–30.

24. Dow KH, Harris JR, Roy C. Pregnancy after breast conserving surgery and radiation therapy for breast cancer. *Natl Cancer Inst Monogr* 1994; 16: 131–7.

25. Kroman N, Jensen MB, Melbye M et al. Should women be advised against pregnancy after breast cancer treatment? *Lancet* 1997; 350: 319–22.

26. Harcourt D, Rumsey N. Mastectomy patients decision-making for or against immediate breast reconstruction. *Psychooncology* 2004; 13: 106–15.

27. Andersen BL. Sexual functioning morbidity among cancer survivors. Current status and future research directions. *Cancer* 1985; 55: 1835–42.

28. Schagen SB, van Dam FSAM, Muller MJ et al. Cognitive deficits after postoperative adjuvant chemotherapy for breast carcinoma. *Cancer* 1999; 85: 640–50.

29. Baker PK. Musculoskeletal origins of chronic pelvic pain. Diagnosis and treatment. *Obstet Gynecol Clin North Am* 1993; 20: 719–42.

30. Park K, Moreland RB, Goldstein I et al. Sildenafil inhibits phosphodiesterase type 5 in Human clitoral corpus cavernosum smooth muscle. *Biochem Biophys Res Commun* 1998; 249: 612–17.

31. Levin RJ. The mechanisms of human female sexual arousal. *Ann Rev Sex Res* 1992; 3: 1–48.

32. Levin RJ. The physiology of sexual arousal in the human female: a recreational and procreational synthesis. *Arch Sex Behav* 2002; 31: 405–11.

33. Northouse LL. Breast cancer in younger women: effects on interpersonal and family relations. *Monogr Natl Cancer Inst* 1994; 16: 183–90.

34. Haddad P, Pitceathly C, Maguire P. Psychological morbidity in the partners of cancer patients. In L Baider, CL Cooper, A Kaplan de-Nour, eds. *Cancer and the Family*. Chichester: Wiley, 1996: 414–20.

35. Barni S, Mondin R. Sexual dysfunction in treated breast cancer patients. *Ann Oncol* 1997; 8: 149–53.

36. Metcalfe KA, Esplen MJ, Goel VN et al. Psychosocial functioning in women who have undergone bilateral prophylactic mastectomy. *Psychooncology* 2004; 13: 14–25.

37. Van Geel AN. Prophylactic mastectomy: the Rotterdam experience. *Breast* 2003; 12: 357–61.

7.5 Pregnancy, childbirth and the postpartum period

Kirsten von Sydow

Introduction

The sexual relations of expectant and young parents are of great medical and psychologic significance – sexual activity during pregnancy might harm the fetus, and pregnancy, birth, and breast-feeding might also impair maternal sexual health. Sexuality can become a problem within the relationship of (expectant) parents, but becoming a mother or a father can also strengthen sexual health and interpersonal relationships.

This chapter will include information on the following: (1) sexual function during pregnancy and the first year postpartum; (2) maternal sexual activity throughout pregnancy; (3) the epidemiology and etiology of sexual problems in both genders during pregnancy and the postpartum period; (4) the diagnosis and treatment options of sexual problems; (5) research implications. This review is founded on a systematic meta-content-analysis of 59 studies on parental sexuality during pregnancy and the postpartum period, published between 1950 and 1996,[1] on new reviews,[2–5] and on new publications identified through research in medical and psychologic databases and through cross-references. The data presented here refer to only adult (not teenage) pregnancy.

Sexual function during pregnancy and the first year postpartum

Genital physiology and sexual responsiveness

During sexual excitement, genital vasocongestion is intensified in the first and second trimesters of pregnancy (see Chapters 4.1–4.4 and 5.1–5.6 of this volume). In the third trimester, vasocongestion generally is strong and barely influenced by sexual excitement. Lubrication and orgasm are intensified in pregnancy, but climax may sometimes be accompanied by cramps. In the third trimester, vaginal contractions are weaker, and sometimes tonic muscle spasms occur. Postorgasmic contractions usually disappear after about 15 min.[1,4]

In the first 6–8 weeks postpartum and during breast-feeding, the sexual excitability of mothers is physiologically reduced, the walls of the vagina are thinner, and orgasm is less intense. Breast-feeding women may ejaculate milk during climax. After about 3 months or cessation of breast-feeding, these changes regress. Some women then experience orgasm more intensely than before. On resumption of intercourse, women mostly perceive their vaginal tension as unchanged or tighter. At 3–4 months postpartum, vaginal tension is mostly unchanged, although vaginal tension is slacker in about 20%. At 6–12 months after the birth, sexual responsiveness is reduced in 40–50% of the mothers and in about 20% of the fathers.[1]

Sexual interest, initiative, and attitudes

Female sexual interest or desire (see Chapters 5.1–5.6) throughout pregnancy remains unchanged or slightly decreased in the first trimester and decreases sharply by the end of the third trimester, but, altogether, it is remarkably variable, especially in the second trimester.[5] Male sexual interest remains mostly unchanged until the end of the second trimester, and then decreases sharply. Female interest in tenderness remains unchanged in pregnancy, or increases. The preferred erotic and sexual activities tend to be unchanged throughout pregnancy and after birth, but vaginal stimulation becomes less important in the second and third trimester.[1] Compared with the time before pregnancy, female sexual interest is reduced in most cases at 3–4 months postpartum, but subsequently is very variable. It seems that men are more often sexually uninterested postpartum than women.[1]

In most couples, men show more sexual initiative before, during, and after pregnancy than women.[1] Female coital activity during pregnancy and postpartum is sometimes motivated by concerns about the partner (e.g., concern about his sexual satisfaction and faithfulness).[1,6]

Most pregnant women think that intercourse should be practiced entirely throughout pregnancy (attitudes). If intercourse has to be avoided for medical reasons, they plead for mutual petting, stimulation of the male part (12%), and sexual abstinence (6%) – none for stimulation of the female part. Some African women think that sexual activity during pregnancy might be helpful for mother and baby (e.g. widening the vagina and facilitating labor)[1] (see Chapter 16.8).

Sexual activity

Coital activity in pregnancy declines slightly in the first trimester, is variable in the second trimester, and declines sharply in the third trimester. Up to month 7 of pregnancy, most couples practice intercourse; in month 8, about half to three-quarters; and in month 9, around one-third. The last coitus occurs about 1 month before delivery. About 10% of the women abstain from coitus once pregnancy is confirmed. The use of the male superior position declines during pregnancy, while the female superior position (only in the second trimester), the side-by-side position, or the rear entry position are practiced more often. The variability of coital positions generally decreases during pregnancy. In the second trimester of pregnancy, sexual intercourse occurs about four or five times per month.[1,7,8]

In Europe and the USA, intercourse is resumed, on average, 6–8 weeks after birth of the child (Nigeria: 16.5 weeks). In month 2 postpartum, 66–94% of the couples practice intercourse; in month 3, 88–95%; in month 7, 95–100%; and in month 13, 97%. Compared with the prepregnancy period, coital frequency is reduced in most couples during the first year after the birth. Data concerning coital activity postpartum are variable due to the variable patterns of breast-feeding and cultural differences. A total of 84–90% of the couples use contraceptives postpartum, mostly birth-control pills or condoms.[1,7–9]

Nongenital physical tenderness by both partners remains unchanged throughout the first two trimesters of pregnancy and decreases continuously from month 6 of pregnancy until 3 years postpartum. On average, noncoital sexual contact is resumed 3 weeks after having given birth, usually before intercourse is resumed. Anal intercourse during pregnancy is practiced by only a minority (1–13%). The course of most heterosexual activities (e.g., coital activity, French kissing, manual genital stimulation of woman or man) and female masturbation mostly follows a "standard pattern" and is characterized by a decrease throughout pregnancy (especially during the third trimester), and no or very low activity in the first trimester postpartum, followed by a slight increase. During late pregnancy and the first weeks postpartum, fellatio is practiced more often than cunnilingus. The frequency of male masturbation remains stable throughout pregnancy and the postpartum period. Homosexual activities have not yet been researched in this context.[1,7,8]

Sexual enjoyment and orgasm

Before pregnancy, 76–79% of the women enjoyed intercourse (7–21% not at all), in the first trimester 59%, in the second 75–84%, and in the last 40–41% report enjoyment of sexual intercourse. No data could be found concerning the sexual enjoyment of men during their spouse's pregnancy. More than half of the women enjoy sexual intimacy with their partner in the first year after having given birth, 18–20% partially, and 24–30% not at all. Data reported by the fathers are comparably alike.[1]

Before pregnancy, or in women aged 30 years, the cumulative incidence of orgasm is 51–87%, while 10–26% of all women remain nonorgasmic during their entire lives. Several studies have explored female orgasm during pregnancy, but results are contradictory. In the third trimester, 54% of the sexually active women report orgasm with the last coitus.[1] The first orgasm after giving birth occurs, on average, after 7 weeks postpartum (range: 2–18 weeks). During the first coitus postpartum, only 20% of the women reach a climax; 3–6 months after childbirth, three-quarters reach orgasm (about as many as before pregnancy). The preferred methods for reaching orgasm mostly remain unchanged. Both genders prefer manual stimulation, oral stimulation, intercourse, and masturbation.[1]

Erotic aspects of the parent–infant relationship

Touching is necessary for the baby and is considered mostly pleasurable for both baby and mother (no data are available on fathers). The physical contact with the baby can be accompanied by erotic feelings, especially during breast-feeding (Leboyer: "faire l'amour").[1] One-third to one-half of mothers describe breast-feeding as an erotic experience. One-quarter express feelings of guilt due to their sexual excitement. Few women ever reach orgasm during breast-feeding – others stop nursing because of fear of the sexual stimulation.[1]

Does maternal sexual activity during pregnancy harm the fetus or the mother?

Coital and orgasmic activity during pregnancy have been associated with negative effects on baby health. The mechanisms discussed include: (1) uterine contractions through female orgasm or nipple stimulation, both of which might trigger oxytocin release, or through male orgasm due to prostaglandins in sperm; (2) sexually transmitted infections; (3) "mechanical" stress through intercourse; and (4) emotional or physical stress of mother, which might induce uterine contractions. These studies suffer from small samples and incomplete confounder control. Large and representative studies have observed no overall association between birth complications (perinatal mortality, preterm birth, premature rupture of the membranes, and low birth weight) and either coital activity or orgasmic frequency. Nevertheless, the male superior intercourse position and intercourse practiced by women suffering from certain genital infections are associated with an elevated risk of preterm delivery.[1,4,10-16]

In healthy women, no significant relationship between frequency of intercourse and genital infections can be found. Pregnant women with sexually transmitted disease-infected partners, partners with extramarital heterosexual or homosexual relationships, and partners injecting drugs should use condoms (see Chapter 7.7). Unfortunately, they usually do *not* use them.[4] Two studies (*n* = 16) associate cunnilingus during pregnancy with the very rare complication of venous air embolism, which might develop if air is blown into the vagina.[4,17,18]

Sexual problems: epidemiology and etiology

Epidemiology

The fear of harming the baby inhibits about one-quarter to one-half of the expectant mothers and fathers (who are sometimes afraid of hurting their partner as well) from performing sexual intercourse during pregnancy. Dyspareunia (painful intercourse) is experienced by 22–50% of pregnant women (prior to pregnancy: 12%). In the third trimester, a substantial proportion of women are also irritated by orgasmic uterine contractions (6–62%), positional difficulties (12–20%), a perceived lack of attractiveness (4–20%), or worry about the sexual satisfaction of the spouse (35–88%). Data regarding male perceptions have not yet become available for further scientific research.[1,19,20]

Only 12–14% of both partners report not experiencing sexual problems postpartum. However, 40–64% of the mothers and 19–64% of the fathers are afraid to resume intercourse. A total of 40% of the women report having problems with their first intercourse postpartum. Of those women with problems, 64% subsequently avoid intercourse. More than half of all women experience pain during their first intercourse after birth. At 3 and 6 months postpartum, 41% and 22%, respectively, still suffer from dyspareunia. At 13 months postpartum, 22% are still having problems. A total of 57% of the wives are worried about the sexual satisfaction of their spouses. One-fifth of the couples report problems with contraception or (in breast-feeding mothers) milk leakage. In the long run, the sexual relationship of at least one-third of all couples worsens. Sexual problems are most pronounced 3–4 years postpartum. Yet, one-quarter of all mothers report an intensification of their sexual lives after having given birth.[21] Pregnancy and birth lead to short-term

weight increase for more than half of all mothers. One year after birth of the child, 7% of the mothers still weigh 5 kg more than before pregnancy. No data are available on female attractiveness postpartum or male attractiveness.[1]

Women rarely have extramarital relationships during pregnancy and the first months postpartum, but 4–28% of all fathers report starting a new or continuing a pre-existing affair. In West Africa, postnatal marital coital abstinence is associated with increased risk of male extramarital affairs and increased risk of unprotected extramarital sex.[1,22,23]

Etiology of sexual problems and dysfunctions

It seems obvious that female sexual problems and decline in sexual activity, interest, and enjoyment during pregnancy and the postpartum period are related to the physical processes of pregnancy, delivery, and breast-feeding. But only a part of the observable changes can be attributed to physiologic processes.

The effects of time have already been described. On average, sexual interest and activity decline throughout pregnancy and increase after the birth. Not surprisingly, during pregnancy and the postpartum period, several sexual factors are correlated (e.g., interest and activity).[1] Some other influences shall be discussed in more detail.

The effect of parenthood: parents versus childless couples

Few studies compare the sexual situation of (expectant) parents with that of childless couples. Their results are contradictory. Coital activity, tenderness, and sexual satisfaction generally decline with increasing duration of the relationship, possibly independently of parenthood, or even more so in parents.[1]

Sex/gender

The few results on sex/gender effects during pregnancy and the postpartum period are mixed. It seems that men are sexually more inhibited during pregnancy than women, and that women's sexual self-acceptance is generally higher. Sexual satisfaction postpartum is identical. During the first 3 years postpartum, women describe a stronger decline in their partner's tenderness, but they still describe their partners as behaving more tenderly than men perceive their wives' behavior.[1]

Sociodemographic and work-related variables

Several sociodemographic variables (e.g., education, nationality, duration of relationship, socioeconomic data) are not significantly or consistently related to sexual variables in pregnancy and postpartum. But marital status, age, religious affiliation, and culture and ethnicity are associated with sexual behavior. More tenderness and sexual activity are found in nonmarital relationships, in younger, less religion-affiliated subjects, and in European and Australian (than US) parents (at least, participants stated this). Older mothers suffer more from dyspareunia.[1,7,8]

The overall number of hours of employment of both genders is not associated with sexual outcome for wives or husbands, but both genders' work-role quality is a predictor of sexual outcomes, especially of sexual satisfaction.[24]

Physical health, reproductive history, and delivery data

The results concerning parity and sexuality during pregnancy and postpartum remain inconsistent. But experienced parents feel more secure about sexual activity postpartum.[1]

Women who tried to conceive for a longer period of time practice intercourse less frequently during pregnancy and 3 months postpartum. Prior miscarriages have no effect on coital activity or interest throughout pregnancy and postpartum in either spouse. Expectant mothers with few or no pregnancy symptoms and less weight gain practice intercourse more often during and after pregnancy, and are coitally more interested, and their partners are sexually more contented.[1]

There are no significant correlations between the severity of birth pain and postpartum sexuality.

The degree of perineal trauma is strongly related to postnatal dyspareunia in a dose–response manner (no perineal damage: 11% coital pain; unstitched tears: 15%; stitched tears: 21%; episiotomy: 40%), and it is also associated with sexual behavior postpartum. The highest risk of developing post-birth dyspareunia is found for women with assisted vaginal deliveries (vacuum extractor or forceps); the risk is intermediate for women with spontaneous vaginal deliveries and lowest after cesarean section. Women with cesarean section resume intercourse somewhat earlier than women delivering vaginally.[1,2,7,9,21,25–28]

Postpartum tenderness between the spouses declines most if mothers suffered from birth complications and their deliveries were prolonged.[1]

The spouse's presence at birth seems to have no effect on subsequent coital activity or female sexual enjoyment.[1]

Several postpartum health factors (estrogen and prolactin status, time of cessation of lochial loss, and time of resumption of menstruation) are not related to sexual variables. Female sexual interest, but not activity, is related to testosterone levels. Kegel exercises of the vaginal muscles help to regain vaginal tonicity. Maternal fatigue (which is equally strong in employed women and in homemakers) is related to a postnatal lack of coital interest.[1,9,24,29] Potential influences of male physical and mental health factors have not yet been researched.[1]

Psychologic health and biography

Mental symptoms (depressed mood or emotional lability) during pregnancy and the postpartum period are negatively related to sexual interest, enjoyment, coital activity, and the perceived tenderness of the partner (see Chapters 3.1–3.4). Depressed women experience more sexual problems postpartum. Psychotherapy experiences are associated with heightened female sexual interest and enjoyment during pregnancy.[1,9,29,30]

Nonreproductive biographic factors have been neglected in research up to now, although strong evidence exists that interindividual and intercouple variability in sexual variables is high during the entire transition to parenthood, as in any other phase of the life cycle. Several studies reveal a remarkable intraindividual/intracouple constancy as well: the relative levels of sexual interest and activity of individual women remain constant from the time before pregnancy up to 1 year postpartum. Pregnant women and their partners reporting a good childhood (and current) relationship with their fathers (and possibly with their mothers as well) experience less decline in coital interest and activity than those with a childhood (and current) relationship exclusively focused on their mothers. If a woman reported sexual aversion before pregnancy, her coital interest declines more sharply in the first trimester. Prepregnancy sexuality is positively correlated with coital activity during pregnancy and postpartum. Prebirth dyspareunia is related to postbirth dyspareunia[1,7,1,31] (see Chapter 6.5).

Partnership variables (including attractiveness)

Relationship satisfaction is related to sexual satisfaction during pregnancy in both genders and to (female) postbirth sexual interest. In men, marital quality is also associated with coital activity and tenderness during pregnancy and postpartum.[29,32] Marital conflict at the beginning of pregnancy is not related to female coital activity or enjoyment during and after pregnancy. Pregnant women's attractiveness (self and partner evaluation) correlates positively to coital activity and sexual enjoyment, and negatively to coital pain. Mothers who trust their method of contraception experience a higher degree of sexual adjustment, but there is no effect on men.[1]

Not only do partnership variables influence sexual behavior, but the reverse is true as well: sexual activity and enjoyment throughout pregnancy are associated with subsequent (higher) evaluations of relationship stability, tenderness, and communication at 4 months and 3 years postpartum.[1,33]

Attributes of the infant, breast-feeding, and parent–child relationship

Whether a pregnancy is planned or not is not related to coital activity during pregnancy and postpartum; results concerning the (negative) effects on sexual interest in women during pregnancy are mixed, yet there is no effect on men or on postpartum women. Feelings about the pregnancy are not related to coital activity, but to sexual interest and enjoyment. Worry that the fetus could be hurt during intercourse is related to decreased interest in men.[1]

Babies' birth weight, size, and Apgar score are not related to mothers' coital activity. The baby's gender has no influence on postpartum coital activity, sexual interest, or enjoyment in women, but it seems that mothers of male babies practice intercourse less often during pregnancy and are perceived by their partners as less tender during the postpartum months than mothers of female babies. Marital tenderness decreases most in mothers with a rigid and overprotective relationship with their babies.[1]

Breast-feeding (at months 1–4 postpartum) is accompanied by reduced coital activity, reduced sexual desire, and reduced sexual satisfaction in women and their male partners. Long-time breast-feeding mothers resume intercourse at a later time, are slightly less sexually interested, suffer more often from coital pain, and enjoy intercourse to a lesser degree. The cessation of breast-feeding has a positive effect on sexual activity, but no effect on sexual responsiveness or orgasm. The negative impact of breast-feeding on maternal (and paternal) sexuality results from changes in mothers' hormone status, which influences desire and lubrication, and to the changed "meaning" of the breasts (nutritional versus sexual) for both partners.[1,7,9,21,34]

Diagnosis of sexual problems and dysfunctions, and their prevention and treatment

Gynecologic/obstetric intervention and advice

The use of episiotomy should be further reduced and strongly restricted to specified fetal-maternal indications, because it is strongly related to postbirth dyspareunia – more so than spontaneous perineal tears.[1,27]

Although the majority of gynecologists report that they spontaneously talk about sexuality to their pregnant patients, two-thirds of all women in various industrialized countries do *not* remember their gynecologist talking to them about sexuality in pregnancy. A total of 76% of the women who had not discussed these issues with their doctors felt they should have been discussed. Of those who talked to their doctor about sexuality in pregnancy, 49% raised this issue first, with 34% feeling uncomfortable in bringing up the topic themselves. A total of 45% of the young Israeli mothers rated the information about sex during pregnancy given by their physician or the hospital staff as insufficient. Women who do not dare to ask their gynecologist sexual questions during pregnancy more often experience intensification of their sexual feelings than women who dare, because doctors often give restrictive advice (such as coital abstinence for certain periods). Alternative coital positions or alternatives to intercourse (such as mutual hand stimulation) are very rarely mentioned by doctors. None of the doctors mentioned that sex could improve during pregnancy. Yet, only 8–10% of women stopped intercourse completely after medical advice to abstain.[1,4,19,35]

Intercourse and/or orgasm should be avoided by expectant mothers who suffer from such pregnancy complications as bleeding, abdominal pains, ruptured membranes, premature dilation of the cervix, or heightened risk of premature labor, placenta previa, placental insufficiency, incompetent cervix, and – possibly – twin pregnancy.[4] Infection by sexually transmitted disease,[4] including human immunodeficiency virus, can lead to miscarriage or stillbirth, or otherwise harm the embryo/fetus. But there is no reason to "forbid" sex to the majority of healthy, pregnant women and their partners in general, not even in the last weeks before birth.[1]

Many gynecologists seem to be uncertain about sexual advice with regard to potential pregnancy problems. Nearly all agree on the necessity of avoidance of intercourse during and after bleeding, but there is no such agreement on the question of how much bleeding should lead to how many days or weeks of coital abstinence. Similarly, recommendations vary with regard to the sexual consequences of premature contractions. Some doctors do not even give restrictive advice when seemingly necessary (e.g., incompetent cervix or vaginal infection). There is a lack of medical knowledge regarding the management of pregnancy complications, especially concerning the question of what conditions allow the ban on intercourse to be reversed, as when vaginal bleeding has stopped. Medical textbooks do not specify this.[4,19] Uncertainty and lack of training in couple/sexual counseling might be one reason that doctors avoid this topic altogether. Discussions concerning sexual questions are not included in the routine antenatal care. If they occur, the male partner is usually *not* included.[1,4]

Postbirth maternal and child health services in Europe and the USA focus more on the child than the mother. Health professionals do not always show the awareness, knowledge, and skills to deal with postnatal sexual problems.[25] Postbirth medical advice on sexuality usually focuses only on contraception, which is discussed in 76% of the 6-week postnatal checks – but the topics of intercourse, perineal problems, pain, and sexual interest are not mentioned and not recognized in the great majority of postnatal checks.[25] In total, 22% of young mothers seek medical advice for perineal or coital problems; 8% of these feel that they have not received adequate help. Three-quarters who need help actively seek it – one-quarter dare not do so.[9] Many couples wish to receive more information about bodily changes and sexuality postpartum, and 30% report that sexual counseling might have been helpful.[1]

Practical recommendations concerning medical advice about sexuality during pregnancy and postpartum should include the following:[1,4]

● Offer the chance to talk about the current emotional, marital, and sexual situation and signal that the doctor is open to the information needs of the patient and her partner (e.g., could sexual intercourse during pregnancy harm the baby?). Postpartum sexuality is more than contraception! Open questions about sexual interest, behavior, and potential problems with coital pain or incontinence can be helpful.

● Give information about the variability of female and male sexuality and the normality of fluctuations during the transition to parenthood. Erotic feelings evoked by breast-feeding can be mentioned and their normality articulated. Young mothers have to be informed that vaginal dryness and/or loss of libido may be associated with breast-feeding and that use of lubricants might help.

● Acknowledge patients' and partners' fears and uncertainties and respect their inner limitations. The aim is not a maximum of sexual activity, but a sexual life that allows both partners, and – from the medical and the parental point of view – the baby, a form of contentedness. This also includes the option of sexual abstinence.

- Give technical advice concerning the range of sexual options during pregnancy and postpartum: tenderness, non-coital sexual activities (e.g., manual and oral stimulation, masturbation) and alternative coital positions (female superior, rear entry/"spoon", use of pillows).
- Instruct the patient in self-help (postbirth self-inspection of vulva with a hand mirror and insertion of a finger to test for healing; vaginal muscle toning/Kegel-exercises).
- Show sensitivity regarding sexual and nonsexual domestic violence. At least 2–8% of pregnant women have had a history of sexual abuse during childhood or adulthood. This can lead to mental as well as gynecologic and obstetric problems, but it does not affect pregnancy outcome.[36,37] But health-care providers often seem rather oblivious to this problem.[38]

Health-care policy and prevention

At the final 6–8-week postnatal checkup, only about half of all new mothers have resumed sexual intercourse. Women's sexual health problems extend well into the first postnatal year and sometimes even longer.[1,25,26] Consequently, a 6-month postbirth checkup including questions about sexuality (Did you already resume intercourse? How did it feel? Do you have any perineal problems?) and other taboo topics (Do you have any problems with incontinence?) would help to identify the full range of problems women may experience after childbirth.

A new prenatal program designed to decrease the potentially negative effects of parenthood on the quality of marital relationships has positive effects on postpartum satisfaction with the sexual aspects of marriage compared with a traditional prenatal education program.[39]

Counseling, psychotherapy, and prevention

If sexual problems persist after gynecologic treatment has been successfully completed (e.g., coital pain from episiotomy scars) and the woman has terminated breast-feeding, a closer look at the psychologic situation and the relationship of both partners becomes inevitable. It is helpful if doctors or midwives can assess the psychosocial and sexual situation of the patient as well as the medical side, and that they know mental health professionals to whom they can refer patients for marital counseling or psychotherapy. Not least is this in the interest of the newborn baby, whose life will be more burdened if its parents have an unhappy relationship or divorce.

Research implications

The following research implications are concluded:[1]

- Research still is split into a medical branch and a social sciences branch. Therefore, scientists should take more notice of the publications of both branches.

- Sampling: more studies including male partners and more studies focusing on representative samples are needed.
- Designs: prospective studies going beyond month 3 to the years 1, 3, 5, or 10 postpartum are lacking. Comparisons with childless couples are scarce.
- Sexual dimensions researched: more descriptive research is needed about noncoital sexual activities (e.g., tenderness, masturbation, sexual initiative, and sexual agency) and the subjective sexual experience of women and men (e.g. enjoyment, orgasm).[40]
- Validity and reliability: reports on participation rates, dropouts, cross-method reliability, intraspouse reliability with regard to sexual activity,[7,8] nonresponse rates for certain questions, the management of terminological problems in questionnaire studies (e.g. participants who do not understand the word "orgasm"), or attributes of the interviewer (gender!) are almost nonexistent.[1,8,41]
- Data analysis: because coital activity is not the best measure of female sexual interest,[1] more analyses of the relationships between sexual interest, masturbation, enjoyment, or orgasm and biographic data, data about the marital relationship, physical and mental health data, physiologic data (e.g. episiotomy, hormonal status, vaginal tonicity postpartum), and sex/gender effects are needed.
- In most studies, the theoretic background is unexplained; some studies ignore central psychosocial context variables (e.g. marital conflicts, cultural norms about motherhood) and biographic conditions (e.g. sexuality before pregnancy). Research should be theoretically guided, as by the developmental psychology of the life span.

Important medical questions about the risks of sexual activities in expectant mothers have been answered. Therefore, one might ask whether more research is really needed. The answer is yes, because sexuality is the most vulnerable area of the relationships of young parents, the majority of couples have sexual problems immediately postpartum, and at least one-third of couples develop serious, long-lasting, psychosexual disturbances after the birth of their first baby. More research is needed – research focusing on both partners' psychosexual and social adaptation to parenthood, which generally takes much longer than the physical adaptation to motherhood, and on the complex interplay of physical, psychologic, and relational factors.

An important new question arises from the relatively recent trend that fathers in industrialized countries are strongly expected to be present and participate in their children's birth. What are the implications of this drastic historic change for fathers' mental health, mothers' birth experience, their relationship as a couple, and their subsequent sexual relationship? Another emerging research topic is the implications of the increase in assisted parenthood (e.g. the sexuality of mothers expecting twins, *in vitro* fertilization pregnancies, etc.).

Because sexuality still is a taboo topic, it is methodologically difficult to research. Therefore, research pluralism is needed. We need psychologic in-depth explorations of complex emotional and sexual issues and their longitudinal development with selected samples (the majority are not willing to participate in such studies), as well as large, representative medical and health studies which gather some partnership and sexual data.[1]

In summary, sex is of little relevance to most new, breast-feeding mothers during the first 3 months postpartum, since adaptation to motherhood takes up their entire energy and involves profound psychosocial and hormonal changes and a lack of sleep. Male sexual activity is also reduced throughout this phase of life, but to a lesser degree. While this seems to be universal, there is remarkable variation in female and male sexual behavior during all other periods of time researched here, namely, during the entire course of pregnancy and months 4–12 postpartum. On average, all heterosexual activities tend to decline throughout pregnancy and reach a point near zero in the immediate postpartum period, and then slowly start to increase again.

References

1. von Sydow K. Sexuality during pregnancy and after childbirth: a meta-content-analysis of 59 studies. *J Psychosom Res* 1999; 47: 27–49.

2. Barrett G, Victor C. Incidence of postnatal dyspareunia. *Br J Sex Med* 1996; 9/10: 6–8.

3. Hobbs K, Bramwell R, May K. Sexuality, sexual behavior and pregnancy. *Sex Marital Ther* 1999; 14: 371–83.

4. Leeners B, Brandenburg U, Rath W. Sexualität in der Schwangerschaft: Risiko oder Schutzfaktor? [Sexual activity during pregnancy: risk factor or protection?]. *Geburtshilfe Frauenheilkd* 2000; 60: 536–43.

5. Regan PC, Lyle JL, Otto AL et al. Pregnancy and changes in female sexual desire: a review. *Soc Behav Pers* 2003; 31: 603–11.

6. Orji EO, Ogunlola IO, Fasubaa, OB. Sexuality among pregnant women in South West Nigeria. *J Obstet Gynaecol* 2002; 22: 166–8.

7. Hyde JS, DeLamater JD, Plant EA et al. Sexuality during pregnancy and the year postpartum. *J Sex Res* 1996; 33: 143–51.

8. von Sydow K, Ullmeyer M, Happ N. Sexual activity during pregnancy and after childbirth: results from the Sexual Preferences Questionnaire. *J Psychosom Obstet Gynecol* 2001; 22: 29–40.

9. Glazener CMA. Sexual function after childbirth: women's experiences, persistent morbidity and lack of professional recognition. *BJOG* 1997; 104: 330–5.

10. Naeye RL. Coitus and associated amniotic-fluid infections. *N Engl J Med* 1979; 301: 1198–1200.

11. Mills JL, Harlap S, Harley EE. Should coitus late in pregnancy be discouraged? *Lancet* 1981; ii: 136–8.

12. Klebanoff MA, Nugent RP, Rhoads GG. Coitus during pregnancy: is it safe? *Lancet* 1984; ii: 914–17.

13. Read JS, Klebanoff MA, the VIP Study Group. Sexual intercourse during pregnancy and preterm delivery: effects of cervicovaginal microflora (Abstract). *Paediatr Perinat Epidemiol* 1996; 7: A1–A2.

14. Read JS, Klebanoff MA. Sexual intercourse during pregnancy and preterm delivery: effects of vaginal microorganisms. *Am J Obstet Gynecol* 1993; 168: 514–19.

15. Berghella V, Klebanoff M, McPherson C et al. Sexual intercourse association with asymptomatic bacterial vaginosis and *Trichomonas vaginalis* treatment in relationship to preterm birth. *Am J Obstet Gynecol* 2002; 187: 1277–82.

16. Ekwo EE, Gosselink CA, Woolson R et al. Coitus late in pregnancy – risk of preterm rupture of amniotic sac membranes. *Am J Obstet Gynecol* 1993; 168(pt 1): 22–31.

17. Bray P, Myers R, Cowley RA. Orogenital sex as a cause of nonfatal air embolism in pregnancy. *Obstet Gynecol* 1983; 61: 653–7.

18. Hill BF, Jones JS. Venous air embolism following orogenital sex during pregnancy. *Am J Emerg Med* 1993; 11: 155–7.

19. Bartellas E, Crane JM, Daley M et al. Sexuality and sexual activity in pregnancy. *BJOG* 2000; 107: 964–8.

20. Oruc S, Esen A, Lacin S et al. Sexual behavior during pregnancy. *Aust N Z J Obstet Gynecol* 1999; 39: 48–50.

21. Signorello LB, Harlow BL, Chekos AK et al. Postpartum sexual functioning and its relationship to perineal trauma: a retrospective cohort study of primiparous women. *Am J Obstet Gynecol* 2001; 184: 881–90.

22. Ali MM, Cleland JG. The link between postnatal abstinence and extramarital sex in Côte d'Ivoire. *Stud Fam Plan* 2001; 32: 214–19.

23. Onah HE, Ilobachie GC, Obi SN et al. Nigerian male sexual activity during pregnancy. *Int J Obstet Gynecol* 2002; 76: 219–23.

24. Hyde JS, DeLamater JD, Hewitt EC. Sexuality and the dual-earner couple: multiple roles and sexual functioning. *J Fam Psychol* 1998; 12: 354–68.

25. Barrett G, Victor C. Postnatal sexual health (Letters). *BMJ* 1994; 309: 1584–5.

26. Barrett G, Victor C. Postnatal sexual health. *Br J Gen Pract* 1996; January: 47–8.

27. Klein MC, Gauthier RJ, Robbins JM et al. Relationship of episiotomy to perineal trauma and morbidity, sexual dysfunction, and pelvic floor relaxatation. *Am J Obstet Gynecol* 1994; 171: 591–8.

28. Wenderlein JM, Merkle F. Beschwerden infolge Episiotomie: Studie an 413 Frauen mit komplikationsloser Spontangeburt [Complaints caused by episiotomy: Study of 413 women with spontaneous complication-free labor]. *Geburtshilfe Frauenheilkd* 1983; 43: 625–8.

29. De Judicibus MA, McCabe MP. Psychological factors and the sexuality of pregnant and postpartum women. *J Sex Res* 2002; 39: 94–103.

30. Morof D, Barrett G, Peacock J et al. Postnatal depression and sexual health after childbirth. *Obstet Gynecol* 2003; 102: 1318–25.

31. Bogren LY. Changes in sexuality in women and men during pregnancy. *Arch Sex Behav* 1991; 20: 35–45.

32. Miller WE, Friedman S. Male and female sexuality during pregnancy: behavior and attitudes. *J Psychol Hum Sexuality* 1988; 1: 17–37.

33. Heinig L, Engfer A. Schwangerschaft und Partnerschaft [Pregnancy and partnership]. *Rep Psychol* 1988; 13: 56–9.

34. Avery MD, Duckett L, Frantzich CR. The experience of sexuality during breastfeeding. *J Midwifery Womens Health* 2000; 45: 227–37.

35. Leeners B, Neumaier-Wagner P, Schierbaum V et al. Beratung werdender Eltern zur Sexualität in der Schwangerschaft [Sexual counseling during pregnancy by gynecologists-obstetricans working in a private office]. *Geburtshilfe Frauenheilkd* 2002; 62: 60–5.

36. Johnson JK, Haider F, Ellis K et al. The prevalence of domestic violence in pregnant women. *BJOG* 2003; 110: 272–5.

37. Stenson K, Heimer G, Lund C et al. Lifetime prevalence of sexual abuse in a Swedish pregnant population. *Acta Obstet Gynecol Scand* 2003; 82: 529–36.

38. Widding Hedin L, Janson PO. The invisible wounds: the occurrence of psychological abuse and anxiety compared with previous experience of physical abuse during the childbearing year. J Psychosom Obstet Gynecol 1999; 20: 136–44.

39. Kermeen P. Improving postpartum marital relationships. *Psychol Rep* 1995; 76(3 pt 1): 831–4.

40. Sydow K von. Sexual enjoyment and orgasm postpartum: sex differences and perceptual accuracy concerning partners' sexual experience. *J Psychosom Obstet Gynecol* 2002; 23: 147–55.

41. Sayle AE, Savitz DA, Williams JF. Accuracy of reporting sexual activity during late pregnancy. *Paediatr Perinat Epidemiol* 2003; 17: 143–7.

7.6 Oral contraceptives and sexuality

Anne R Davis, Paula M Castaño

Introduction

In women, sexuality and contraception are tightly linked. In the USA, the average age of initiating sexual activity is 17.8 years,[1] and the average age of menopause is 51.4 years.[2] A typical fertile and sexually active woman with two children might spend only about 3 years seeking pregnancy and being pregnant. Therefore, she would use contraception for about 29 years of her life.

In the USA, oral contraceptives are the most widely used reversible contraceptive method. In 1995, current oral contraceptive use was reported by 27% of all contracepting women aged 15–44 years, and 45% of those aged 15–30 years.[1] Stated another way, about 10 000 000 US women described themselves as current oral contraceptive users. Rates of use in European countries are even higher.

Several characteristics make oral contraceptives well suited for use by most women. First, oral contraceptives are very effective and completely reversible. Perfect oral contraceptive use is associated with annual pregnancy rates of less than 1% and typical oral contraceptive use with rates of approximately 7%. Second, oral contraceptives have a well-established safety profile. Third, oral contraceptive use is associated with health benefits, including decreased risk of ovarian cancer, uterine cancer, benign ovarian cysts, endometriosis, and pelvic inflammatory disease. Oral contraceptive use is also associated with desirable changes in the menstrual cycle, including improved cycle control, decreased menstrual cramps, decreased volume of menstrual blood, and fewer days of menstrual bleeding. Oral contraceptives are also an effective treatment for acne vulgaris and even hirsutism.

Most research has focused on the safety and efficacy of oral contraceptives. Little research has examined the effects of oral contraceptive use on sexuality. Reducing the fear of unwanted pregnancy is one potential positive effect. In a recent focus group study, women reported that fear of pregnancy had a very negative impact on sexual arousal, especially when the partner did not share this concern.[3] Oral contraceptive-mediated improvements of painful gynecologic conditions such as endometriosis, dysmenorrhea (painful menstrual cramps), and ovarian cysts may also improve sexual functioning. Changes in bleeding patterns during oral contraceptive use could also improve sexual functioning. Many couples avoid intercourse and other sexual behaviors during vaginal bleeding or spotting due to cultural custom, fear of infection, or hygienic reasons.[4,5] By decreasing the days and amount of menstrual bleeding, oral contraceptive use could increase the times when couples are willing to engage in sexual behaviors. Finally, oral contraceptives are approved by the US Food and Drug Administration for the treatment of acne vulgaris. Improved appearance associated with decreased acne could indirectly benefit sexual functioning. In one study, an improvement in acne was associated with decreased embarrassment and social inhibition.[6]

Oral contraceptives could also exert negative effects on sexual function. Early literature invoked psychologic mechanisms such as women feeling less interested in sex because of not being fertile, or "missing the element of risk" while on contraceptives.[7] Some authors hypothesized that oral contraceptives indirectly, affect sexual functioning by causing negative changes in mood or weight. Such negative changes are often accepted as known side effects of oral contraceptives. However, little well-conducted research, including appropriate control groups, has examined mood or weight effects in detail. Data from a few large, placebo-controlled oral contraceptive studies suggest that large effects on mood or weight attributable to oral contraceptives are unlikely, since subjects on oral contraceptives and placebos reported similar rates of mood changes and weight gain.[8,9] However, these studies were not designed to measure effects on mood or weight and therefore did not use appropriate psychometric or physical measurement techniques.

The impact of oral contraceptives on sexual desire, or libido, has received more study than any other possible effect of oral contraceptives on women's sexual functioning. Physiologic changes associated with oral contraceptive use make an oral contraceptive-mediated effect on libido biologically plausible. Combination oral contraceptive pills consist most commonly of 21 days of tablets that contain ethinyl estradiol and a synthetic, orally active progestin, followed by 7 days of inert or placebo tablets. Their main mechanism of contraceptive action is prevention of ovulation through inhibition of gonadotropin release from the pituitary, an effect which interferes with the normal cascade of events that leads to ovulation.

In addition to these changes, oral contraceptive use also causes an important reduction in androgens via several mechanisms[10] (see Chapters 5.5 and 6.3 in this volume). First, the estrogen in oral contraceptives causes an increase in hepatic production of serum hormone-binding globulin, one of the two main proteins binding testosterone in the serum. Due to increases in sex hormone-binding globulin, levels of free testosterone decrease by about 50% during oral contraceptive use. Second, oral contraceptives decrease production of androgens by the ovaries and adrenal glands. Third, oral contraceptives inhibit the enzyme 5-alpha reductase, which converts testosterone into dihydrotestosterone, the form that binds to cellular receptors.[11] The decreased androgenic environment associated with oral contraceptive use is therapeutically useful; both acne and hirsuitism improve during oral contraceptive use.

The reduced androgen environment caused by oral contraceptives is often cited as the mechanism by which oral contraceptives decrease sexual interest in women. In order to assess evidence related to whether or not oral contraceptives affect libido in women, we conducted a search of the medical literature from 1966 until 2004.

Retrospective, uncontrolled studies

In these retrospective uncontrolled studies, women compared their libido before and after initiation of oral contraceptives. Table 7.6.1 summarizes results from these studies. Changes in libido attributed to oral contraceptives were highly variable; with women reporting large increases in libido to modest decreases. Several factors could account for these results. Studies conducted in the 1960s found larger increases in libido than later studies. Large increases in libido in the early studies may indicate that women had a new opportunity to be sexually active without the fear of pregnancy. Variability in measurement may also account for inconsistent results. Women were directly questioned about libido in some studies, while in others investigators relied on spontaneous reports. In studies where the questions were explicitly stated, more women reported increases than decreases in libido.[7,13,14]

In summary, these retrospective studies found that most women experienced an improvement or no change in libido during oral contraceptive use, with a minority reporting negative effects. However, numerous methodological limitations make conclusions from these data difficult. In a retrospective study, participant reports may not be accurate when subjects are asked to recall the state of their libido especially at a distant time. Moreover, results from high-dose oral contraceptives used in these studies may not apply to modern low-dose pills.

Prospective, uncontrolled studies

The three prospective, uncontrolled studies measured libido at baseline before oral contraceptive use and then measured it during oral contraceptive use. Results from these studies are summarized in Table 7.6.2. In the Nilsson study,[26] women were randomized to four different pills and interviewed five times. Most described their libido as "marked" at baseline, and there were no changes in the proportions describing their libido as "marked, weak, or frigid" during any point in the study. There were also no differences in libido by oral contraceptive type. In the Cullberg et al. study,[27] libido was measured twice. On a visual analog scale, "no significant change" in libido occurred during the study compared to baseline; however, no data were given. The authors also stated that 5% of participants reported that their libido diminished. In the Sanders et al. study,[28] the authors used validated questionnaires to measure libido (frequency of sexual thoughts) four times during 1 year. More women reported decreases than increases in libido, but most experienced no change. Decreased libido was more common among those discontinuing than continuing oral contraceptives.

These prospective studies indicate that most women had stable libido during oral contraceptive use, with smaller proportions experiencing increases or decreases. These prospective studies provide a more accurate assessment of libido changes than the retrospective studies; comparing changes to baseline decreases effects of restrospective recall. However, two of the three studies used oral contraceptives containing much higher doses than today's oral contraceptives and were conducted more than 30 years ago.

The lack of a comparison control group in these uncontrolled studies makes it impossible to determine whether changes in libido observed during oral contraceptive use were due to oral contraceptive use or other factors. Among respondents in the National Health and Social Life Survey, a representative sample of the US population, lack of interest in sex during the past year was reported by approximately 30% of women aged 18–44 years.[29] Some of these women reporting low libido were probably oral contraceptive users. However, the high prevalence of low libido suggests that substantial numbers of women experience negative changes in libido whether on oral contraceptives or not.

Prospective and cross-sectional controlled studies

This type of study compares libido in oral contraceptive users with libido in a control group of women not using oral contraceptives. The results of these studies are summarized in Table 7.6.3. In the study by Herzberg et al.,[30] women starting three different oral contraceptives were compared with a group of intrauterine device users. Scores on a libido scale were collected at baseline and at subsequent clinic visits. Intrauterine device

Table 7.6.1. Retrospective studies

Author, year	Population, country	n	Age years (mean, and/or range given)	Measurement technique	Libido increase	Libido decrease	Libido no change
Pincus et al, 1959[12]	ND, Haiti, Puerto Rico	830	ND	Interview	20%	58%	22%
Goldzieher et al., 1962[13]	FPC, USA	210	16–40	Interview	30–50%	0%	50–70%
Ringrose, 1965[14]	ND, Canada	100	20–44	Questionnaire	22%	13%	55% (10% no opinion)
Bakker et al., 1966[15]	ND, USA	100	28	Questionnaire interview "	"Subjects in our study did not indicate that their basic interest in sexual relations had changed"		
Nilsson et al., 1967[16]	All prescribed Anovid, Sweden	313	20–38	Mailed questionnaire	2%	21%	28% (49% reported other sexual changes)
Boffa, 1971[17]	Suburban general practice, UK	140	ND	Questionnaire	4%	36% (54% slight, 32% moderately severe, 14% severe)	ND
Fortin et al., 1972[18]	Private practice and FPC Canada	70	ND	Interview, semistructured and open	39%	29%	33%
Bull, 1973[19]	One practice, UK	476	ND	Interview ("volunteered or elicited")	ND	10%	ND
Hall and Hall, 1973[7]	FPC UK	198	Less than 20 to over 35	Interview	53%	15%	32%
Gambrell et al., 1976[20]	FPC USA	211		Interview	15%	20%	65%
Hunton, 1976[21]	Private practice, UK	1090	Less than 20 to over 40	Chart review	ND	4%	ND
James and Karoussos, 1980[22]	ND, Switzerland	36	16–35	Interview	ND	11%	ND
Schellen, 1980[23]	ND, Netherlands	104	31, 18–48	ND	5%	20%	75%
Yabur et al., 1989[24]	ND, Venezuela	56	18–33	Interview	1%	1%	ND
Erkkola et al., 1990[25]	PCO patients, Finland	162	20–40	Interview	ND	1%, 5% on diff. OC	ND

FPC = family planning clinic, ND = no data given, OC = oral contraception, PCO = polycystic ovary syndrome.

users experienced a modest increase in libido, those continuing oral contraceptives experienced no change in libido, and those discontinuing experienced a modest decrease. The independent effect of oral contraceptives on libido is difficult to determine from this study. The measure of libido also included scores on orgasm and intercourse, and the oral contraceptive and intrauterine device groups were different at baseline on factors such as parity and depressive symptoms, which can also affect libido.

Table 7.6.2. Prospective uncontrolled studies

Author, year	Population, Country	n	Age years (mean, and/or range given)	Question format	Libido increase	Libido decrease	Libido no change
Nilsson, 1967[26]	FPC, Sweden	159	25	Interview	No change in proportions reporting "frigid, weak, or marked" libido		
Cullberg et al., 1969[27]	FPC, Sweden	99	24	Interview and questionnaire	ND	ND	"No significant change"
Sanders et al., 2001[28]	FPC, University Health Center, USA	107	22	Interview and questionnaire	17%	39%	44%

FPC = family planning clinic, ND = no data given.

Another study comparing continuing oral contraceptive and intrauterine device users reported that more women in the oral contraceptive group experienced decreases in libido than in the intrauterine device group.[31] However, no details on the ascertainment of change in libido were given.

Bancroft et al.[32,33] used a cross-sectional design to compare oral contraceptive users with non-oral contraceptive users; a small subgroup was followed prospectively for 1 month during which serum androgens and desire were measured. The oral contraceptive users had higher sexual motivation ($p < 0.01$) and sexual desire ratings ($p < 0.01$) and *lower* free testosterone levels than the non-oral contraceptive users. However, oral contraceptive users were more likely to have a partner, reported more premarital sexual activity, and reported "more permissive attitudes towards premarital sexual contacts". Since oral contraceptive users were so different from nonusers, the independent effect of oral contraceptives on libido is very difficult to estimate. Large differences in attitudes and behavior between the groups could obscure hormonally mediated differences.

Randomized, placebo–controlled trials

A control group is essential in order to determine the independent effects of oral contraceptives on libido. However, finding an appropriate control group for an observational study is difficult. As demonstrated by the studies reviewed above, oral contraceptive users may differ in many ways from women not using oral contraceptives. The randomized, controlled trial provides the most efficient study design, since both known and unknown potential confounders are controlled for by the randomization process. We identified four randomized trials that examined the effects of oral contraceptives on libido by comparing an oral contraceptive with placebo or another oral contraceptive. Results of the placebo-controlled studies are summarized in Table 7.6.4.

In the earliest study by Cullberg,[34] participants were randomized to one of three oral contraceptives or a placebo. After

Table 7.6.3. Prospective and cross-sectional controlled studies

Author, year	Population, country	n	Age years (mean, and/or range given)	Measurement technique	Libido increase	Libido decrease	Libido no change
Herzberg et al., 1971[30]	FPC, UK	218 OC 54 IUD	< 24 to > 40	Interview, questionnaire	Those staying on OCs no change Those discontinuing OCs decreased IUD users increased		
Barnard-Jones, 1973[31]	All patients continuing OC or IUD, UK	100 OC 100 IUD	OC 25 IUD 28	ND	OC 16% IUD 33%	33% 11%	ND ND
Bancroft et al., 1991[32,33]	Student volunteers, Canada	55 OC 55 non-OC	18–28	Validated questionnaires, Leikert scale	OC group higher sexual motivation than non OC group. OC group higher sexual desire scores than non OC group.		

FPC = family planning clinic, IUD = intrauterine device, ND = no data given, OC = oral contraception.

Table 7.6.4. Randomized, placebo-controlled trials

Author, year	Population, country	n	Age years (mean, and/or range given)	Measurement technique	Libido increase	Libido decrease	Libido no change
Cullberg 1972[34]	Contracepting women, Sweden	320, 80 in each OC group	27	Interview	OC 1 9% OC 2 6% OC 3 10% Placebo 9%	12% 5% 14% 11%	ND ND ND ND
Leeton et al., 1978[35]	OC users undergoing sterilization	20	35, 27–46	Sexual response score	Mean sex score higher during placebo than OC use.		
Graham, 1993[36]	Women with PMS, Canada	20 OC 25 placebo	29	VAS	In two of four menstrual phases, OC group had decreased interest compared with baseline, no change in other phases. No change in interest from baseline in any menstrual phase in placebo group.		
Graham et al., 1995[37]	Sterilized women or partners, Scotland and Manila	150, 50 OC 50 POP 50 placebo	32	Standardized interview, questionnaire, daily ratings	Interest in sex decreased in OC group compared with placebo or POP in Scottish women. No change in interest in sex in OC, POP or placebo in Philippine women.		

ND = no data given, OC = oral contraception, PCO = polycystic ovary syndrome, POP = progesterone only pill, VAS = visual analog scale.

2 months, participants were questioned about changes in libido, using the format listed in the Table 7.6.4. With this simple measure, most reported no change. Small and similar proportions of participants reported increases and decreases in libido during the study in all groups, and there were no statistically significant differences between the oral contraceptive groups or between the oral contraceptive and placebo groups.

In a much smaller study, Leeton et al.[35] examined the sexual effects of oral contraceptives in women undergoing surgical sterilization. Established oral contraceptive users were randomized to receive either an oral contraceptive for 1 month and then placebo for the next month or the same treatments in reverse order. During both months, participants answered questions related to frequency, enjoyment, and orgasm as well as interest and thoughts about sex. In this crossover design, participants were asked to compare their current experience with the previous month. "Sex scores" were lower (indicating worse functioning) during oral contraceptive use than during placebo use. However, effects on libido specifically cannot be determined; scores combined responses for the other measures of sexual functioning as well as libido. These results may also underestimate any negative effect of oral contraceptives on libido, since the study included only satisfied, stable oral contraceptive users, who may not be as susceptible to negative effects.

In a more recent study, Graham and Sherwin[36] examined the effects of oral contraceptives on sexuality as a subanalysis of a trial designed to examine efficacy of oral contraceptives for treatment of premenstrual syndrome. At baseline and over 3 months, participants were asked to rate their daily levels of sexual interest. Participants were randomized to receive oral contraceptive or placebo. Attrition in this study was high; of the 82 enrolled, 23 withdrew. In the oral contraceptive group, sexual interest ratings decreased during the menstrual and postmenstrual phases compared with baseline, but not during other phases of the cycle. No changes from baseline were observed in the placebo group. These results suggest decreased sexual interest was caused by oral contraceptive use. However, high discontinuation could lead to over- or under-estimation of the true effect.

The most recent study, also conducted by Graham et al.,[37] has several important strengths. This study was the only randomized clinical trial designed to examine effects of oral contraceptive use on libido as a primary outcome and had a much lower discontinuation rate (4/150) than other studies. This study also included women from a country other than the USA, Canada, or Europe. Sterilized women or women with sterilized partners were randomized to receive either a combined oral contraceptive, a progesterone-only pill, or a placebo for 4 months. Standardized, structured interviews and questionnaires were used to assess sexual function.

Baseline characteristics and effects on sexual interest were different in the two groups of women. The Manila women were less educated, had more children, were more likely to work as unskilled laborers, and reported less interest in and enjoyment of sex than the Scottish women. Among the Scottish women, but not the Philippine women, ratings of sexual interest and sexual activity declined in the oral contraceptive group, but not in the progesterone-only pill or placebo groups.

The authors postulated that the differential effect of oral contraceptive versus progesterone-only pill among Scottish women could be attributed to oral contraceptive-mediated changes in testosterone that do not occur on progesterone-only pills. These results also highlight how reactions to oral contraceptives may depend on user characteristics. Changes in sexuality associated with oral contraceptive use were greater among women with a more positive experience of their sexuality at baseline than among women with a more negative experience of their sexuality.

Conclusion

Most women spend decades of their lives avoiding pregnancy, and oral contraceptives provide an effective, safe contraceptive option. Oral contraceptives are the most widely used hormonal method, and oral contraceptive-mediated effects on sexual functioning, whether positive or negative, could affect large numbers of women. Published research exploring the impact of oral contraceptives on sexuality has focused on libido. Such an effect is biologically plausible; oral contraceptives significantly decrease circulating androgens.

Most studies examining oral contraceptive-mediated effects on libido were retrospective and uncontrolled, used non-standardized methods to measure libido, and were conducted decades ago when much higher-dose oral contraceptives were in use. These studies suggest oral contraceptive use was more often associated with stable or increased rather than decreased libido. The few prospective, uncontrolled studies found that oral contraceptive use was associated with stable libido among the vast majority of users, with small numbers experiencing increases or decreases.

Controlled, observational studies have compared oral contraceptive users with nonusers and users of other contraceptive methods such as the intrauterine device. Oral contraceptive users in these studies had both higher and lower libido than nonusers. However, users and nonusers were different in many respects. Additionally, in cross-sectional studies, there is no way to determine whether oral contraceptive use increased libido, or whether those with increased libido were more likely to use oral contraceptives. When oral contraceptive users were compared with intrauterine device users, the effect of oral contraceptives was difficult to determine because the groups were different on many factors which can affect libido (age, parity).

Results from the four randomized, placebo-controlled trials identified were mixed. In the largest trial, changes in libido were uncommon and similar among the oral contraceptive and placebo groups. A small trial among women with premenstrual syndrome found that oral contraceptive use was associated with a decrease in sexual interest compared with placebo. A small study of sterilized women found that sexual functioning was worse in the oral contraceptive than placebo group, but effects on libido were not assessed independently. In the most recent randomized, clinical trial, oral contraceptive use was associated

with decreased libido in sterilized women compared with placebo or a progesterone-only pill. However, this effect was limited to women with high baseline sexual functioning; no decreases in libido occurred among women with worse baseline sexual functioning. None of these studies meet the criteria for high-quality randomized clinical trials specified by groups such as CONSORT.[38]

When oral contraceptives became widely available in the 1960s, researchers postulated that determining the effect of oral contraceptives on libido would be difficult. As of 2004, no well-conducted randomized clinical trial has adequately addressed this question. Existing evidence suggests that libido is usually stable on oral contraceptives, but that decreases or increases may occur in some women. The social context of oral contraceptive use may determine the clinical importance of small effects on libido. For instance, increased contraceptive security or improvement in acne with oral contraceptive use may cause an increase in libido that overrides a hormonally driven decrease. In other populations, such as women who are sterilized and derive no contraceptive benefit from oral contraceptives, users may be sensitive to hormonally driven negative effects on libido.

Women and health-care providers often overestimate the negative effects of oral contraceptives and underestimate the positive effects. Better research is needed to provide a clear message to women on how oral contraceptive use affects libido. Until then, providers must be cautious in attributing negative experiences to oral contraceptives, and be willing to explore other explanations for the common experience of decreased libido. Ways in which oral contraceptives could positively affect sexuality, such as decreased risk of pregnancy, decreased bleeding, decreased pain, or improved acne and hirsutism, remain unexplored.

References

1. Abma J, Chandra A, Mosher W et al. Fertility, family planning, and women's health: new data from the 1995 National Survey of Family Growth. National Center for Health Statistics. *Vital Health Stat 23* 1997; 23.
2. McKinlay SM, Bifano NL, McKinlay JB. Smoking and age at menopause in women. *Ann Intern Med* 1985; 103: 350–6.
3. Graham CA, Sanders SA, Milhausen R et al. Turning on and off: a focus group study of the factors that affect women's sexual arousal. *Arch Sex Behav* 2004; 33: 527–38.
4. Tanfer K, Aral SO. Sexual intercourse during menstruation and self-reported sexually transmitted disease history among women. *Sex Transm Dis* 1996; 23: 395–401.
5. Davis AR, Nowygrod S, Shabsigh R et al. The influence of vaginal bleeding on the sexual behavior of urban, Hispanic women and men. *Contraception* 2002; 65: 351–5.
6. Krowchuk DP, Stancin T, Keskinen R et al. The psychosocial effects of acne on adolescents. *Pediatr Dermatol* 1991; 8: 332–8.
7. Hall DM, Hall SM. Side effects of the pill. *BMJ* 1973; 3: 105.

8. Gallo MF, Grimes DA, Schulz KF et al. Combination estrogen-progestin contraceptives and body weight: systematic review of randomized controlled trials. *Obstet Gynecol* 2004; 103: 359–73.

9. Redmond G, Godwin AJ, Olson W et al. Use of placebo controls in an oral contraceptive trial: methodological issues and adverse event incidence. *Contraception* 1999; 60: 81–5.

10. American College of Obstetricians and Gynecologists. Hyperandrogenic chronic anovulation. *ACOG Tech Bull* 202, 1995.

11. Rabe T, Kowald A, Ortman J et al. Inhibition of skin 5 alpha-reductase by oral contraceptive progestins *in vitro*. *Gynecol Endocrinol* 2000; 14: 223–30.

12. Pincus G, Garcia CR, Rock J et al. Effectiveness of an oral contraceptive. *Science* 1959: 81–3.

13. Goldzieher JW, Moses LE, Ellis LT. Study of norenthindrone in contraception. *JAMA* 1962; 180; 359–61.

14. Ringrose CAD. The emotional responses of married women receiving oral contraceptives. *Can Med Assoc J* 1965; 92: 1207–9.

15. Bakker CB, Dightman CR. Side effects of oral contraceptives. *Obstet Gynecol* 1966; 28: 373–9.

16. Nilsson Å, Jacobson L, Ingemanson C-A. Side-effects of an oral contraceptive with particular attention to mental symptoms and sexual adaptation. *Acta Obstet Gynecol Scand* 1967; 46: 537–56.

17. Boffa PS. The incidence of side-effects with a low-oestrogen contraceptive pill. *Practitioner* 1971; 206(232): 263–5.

18. Fortin JN, Wittkower ED, Paiement J et al. Side effects of oral contraceptive medication: a psychosomatic problem. *Can Psychiatr Assoc J* 1972; 17: 3–9.

19. Bull MJV. Side effects of the pill. *Br Med J* 1973; 1(5848): 295–6.

20. Gambrell RD, Bernard DM, Sanders BI et al. Changes in sexual drives of patients on oral contraceptives. *J Reprod Med* 1976; 17: 165–71.

21. Hunton M. A retrospective survey of over 1000 patients on oral contraceptives in a group practice. *J R Coll Gen Pract* 1976; 26: 538–46.

22. James A, Karoussos K. Experiences with the new oral contraceptive Ovysmen. *J Int Med Res* 1980; 8: 86–9.

23. Schellen AMCM. Preliminary experience with a "sub-50" combined oral contraceptive, containing 35 μg ethinyl oestradiol and 1 mg norethisterone ("NeoCon"). *Pharmatherapeutica* 1980; 2: 412–15.

24. Yabur JA, Alvarado M, Brito V. Clinical evaluation of a new combined oral contraceptive desogestrel – ethinyl estradiol. *Adv Contracep* 1989; 5: 57–70.

25. Erkkola R, Hirvonen E, Luikku J et al. Ovulation inhibitors containing cyproterone acetate or desogestrel in the treatment of hyperandrogenic symptoms. *Acta Obstet Gynecol Scand* 1990; 69: 61–5.

26. Nilsson L, Sölvell L. Clinical studies on oral contraceptives – a randomized, double-blind, crossover study of 4 different preparations (Anovlar® mite, Lyndiol® mite, Ovulen®, and Volidan®). *Acta Obstet Gynecol Scand* 1967; 46(Suppl 8): 3–31.

27. Cullberg J, Gelli MG, Jonsson CO. Mental and sexual adjustment before and after six months' use of an oral contraceptive. *Acta Psychiatr Scand* 1969; 45: 259–76.

28. Sanders SA, Graham CA, Bass JL et al. A prospective study of the effects of oral contraceptives on sexuality and well-being and their relationship to discontinuation. *Contraception* 2001; 64: 51–8.

29. Laumann EO, Gagnon JH, Michael RT et al. *The Social Organization of Sexuality*. Chicago: University of Chicago Press, 1994.

30. Herzberg BN, Draper KC, Johnson AL et al. Oral contraceptives, depression, and libido. *BMJ* 1971; 3: 495–500.

31. Barnard-Jones K. A study of two forms of contraception in general practice. *J R Coll Gen Pract* 1973; 23: 658–62.

32. Bancroft J, Sherwin BB, Alexander GM et al. Oral contraceptives, androgens, and the sexuality of young women. I. A comparison of sexual experience, sexual attitudes, and gender role in oral contraceptive users and nonusers. *Arch Sex Behav* 1991; 20: 105–19.

33. Bancroft J, Sherwin BB, Alexander GM et al. Oral contraceptives, androgens, and the sexuality of young women. II. The role of androgens. *Arch Sex Behav* 1991; 20: 121–35.

34. Cullberg J. Mood changes and menstrual symptoms with different gestagen/estrogen combinations. *Acta Psychiatr Scand Suppl* 1972; 236: 1–65.

35. Leeton J, McMaster R, Worsley A. The effects of sexual response and mood after sterilization of women taking long-term oral contraception: results of a double-blind cross-over study. *Aust N Z J Obstet Gynaecol* 1978; 18: 194–7.

36. Graham CA, Sherwin BB. The relationship between mood and sexuality in women using an oral contraceptive as a treatment for premenstrual symptoms. *Psychoneuroendocrinology* 1993; 18: 273–81.

37. Graham CA, Ramos R, Bancroft J et al. The effects of steroidal contraceptives on the well-being and sexuality of women: a double-blind, placebo-controlled, two-centre study of combined and progestogen-only methods. *Contraception* 1995; 52: 363–9.

38. Moher D, Schultz KF, Altman DG. The CONSORT statement: revised recommendations for improving the quality of reports of parallel group randomized trials. *Lancet* 2001; 357: 1191–4.

7.7 Sexual function and urinary tract infections, sexually transmitted diseases and human immunodeficiency virus infection

Lucia F O'Sullivan, Kimberly D Hearn

Introduction

Rates of genital tract infections are currently at their highest levels in the USA and many other Western countries.[1] Women in all societies have higher rates of sexually transmitted diseases than men, primarily because infections are more easily transmitted from men to women, especially young women.[2] Moreover, greater proportions of women tend to be asymptomatic when infected and thus go undiagnosed and untreated. They are also more likely to experience severe health complications from infection. It is increasingly clear that female sexual dysfunction can occur secondary to medical problems (see Chapters 7.1–7.6 and 16.3–16.9 of this volume), such as urinary tract infections, sexually transmitted diseases, and human immunodeficiency virus infection.[3–6] In this chapter, we summarize the current body of knowledge regarding sexual function and urinary tract infections, sexually transmitted diseases, and human immunodeficiency virus infection, in relation to disorders of desire, arousal,

orgasm, and sexual pain. We then provide some treatment guidelines for health-care professionals interested in promoting sexual health among women.

Psychosocial and relational context

The *Diagnostic and Statistical Manual of Mental Disorders*, fourth edition (DSM-IV), of the American Psychiatric Association requires that a diagnosis of female sexual dysfunction be given if the disturbance "causes marked distress" and "interpersonal difficulty" (see Chapter 9.1). This criterion is particularly pertinent to women because, with relatively few exceptions, emotional and relational dynamics take on the most profound significance in diagnosing and treating urinary tract infections, sexually transmitted diseases, and human immunodeficiency virus infection and concomitant sexual dysfunctions. Although urinary tract infections appear to have more benign effects on female sexual dysfunction, women report considerable shame and degradation from diagnoses of sexually transmitted diseases, particularly human immunodeficiency virus.[7,8] This connection between infections and female sexual dysfunction is related to the close associations with often socially undesirable activities and public or private acknowledgement of violations of societal expectations of sexual conduct. Furthermore, women are more susceptible to the repressive effects of such social constraints on sexuality than men.[9] Women may be at risk of emotional, physical, or verbal abuse in their primary relationships upon disclosure of their infection or breakup once infection is discovered[10,11] (see Chapter 3.4). Generally, women across societies tend to be penalized more severely on the basis of their sexual conduct and reproductive capacity than men, and so women suffer greater stigma and abuse as a result of infection[10,11] (see Chapters 3.1–3.3).

Depression, shame, relationship conflict, and medical illness upon disclosure of infection within a relationship may make sexual interactions distressing and uncomfortable, leading at times to a diagnosis of sexual dysfunction.[6] Emotional and relational issues significantly affect sexual arousal.[12] Self-esteem, body image, and the quality of the relationship with a partner affect a woman's ability to respond sexually.[12] However, as key elements in the diagnosis of female sexual dysfunction are the persistent personal distress or interpersonal difficulties associated with these infections, the diagnosis of female sexual dysfunction is not appropriate in cases where disturbances occur inconsistently[13] (see Chapters 9.2–9.5). For example, transient pain from intercourse during an outbreak of genital ulcers or a temporary aversion to sexual intercourse during peak infection with a bacterial sexually transmitted disease would not in themselves warrant a diagnosis of female sexual dysfunction.

Urinary tract infections

Urinary tract infection is one of the most common bacterial infections encountered in clinical practice in Western countries. In the USA, an estimated 34% of adults (20 or older) report at least one lifetime occurrence of urinary tract infection.[14] Urinary tract infections are more common among women than among men (with a ratio of men to women of 1:3.9), although prevalence in elderly women and men is similar.[15] Presentation can include different forms of cystitis, pyelonephritis, and urethral syndrome, with the most common complaints being dysuria and flank or back pain.[16] Although there are a number of potential causes of urinary tract infection in women, risk factors include sexual intercourse, use of spermicidal products, and diaphragm use.[17] For adolescents, urinary tract infections are frequently used as markers for sexual activity.[18] Among older women, obstructing lesions, estrogen deficiency, and antibiotic exposure are more common causes.[15] Uropathogenic *Escherichia coli* is the causative agent in the majority of cases. The urinary tract is armed with several specialized defenses against bacterial colonization, including

glycosamines, low pH, and salts and urea that eliminate bacteria.[19] However, significant proportions of patients have recurrent urinary tract infections, possibly linked to a persistent quiescent bacterial reservoir that establishes itself within the bacterial mucosa.[20]

One-third of women with an initial urinary tract infection have a recurrence, a third of these within the first 6 months.[21] These women are believed to have an increased susceptibility to vaginal colonization with uropathogens, with a greater propensity for uropathogenic coliforms to adhere to uroepithelial cells.[17] New approaches to prevent current urinary tract infection include the use of probiotics and vaccines. However, in a study of the *E. coli* urinary isolates from men with female partners suffering from urinary tract infection, urinary isolates were identical to the *E. coli* found in the urine or vagina of their sex partners.[22] In fact, *E. coli* that caused urinary tract infection was nine times more likely than other *E. coli* to be shared by sex partners. Moreover, sharing was twice as likely if the couple had engaged in oral sex. Because sexual abstinence is unlikely among most women, particularly for those in an established sexual relationship, some place themselves at risk of recurrent infection. For women presenting a first urinary tract infection by *E. coli*, vaginal intercourse increased the risk of a second urinary tract infection with both a different and same uropathogen, as did using a diaphragm, cervical cap, and spermicide.[23] These findings emphasize the importance of considering the context of sexual interactions and/or involving sexual partners and/or in developing a treatment plan.

Women experiencing urinary tract infections frequently experience dysuria, which is pain, burning, or discomfort on urination. They are likely to avoid sex before and during the treatment of a urinary tract infection because of severe discomfort or pain. Treatment typically comprises administration of antibiotics, though estrogen replacement therapy has been used in the past for postmenopausal women.[24] Fortunately, treatment is typically rapid and highly effective. Intercourse while infected is often avoided at the recommendation of health-care providers until treatment is completed and because pelvic thrusting during sexual intercourse causes dyspareunia,[12] potentially leading to an aversion to sexual experiences[25] and strife between sexual partners. Educating and testing the patient and her partner or partners may go far to fortify treatment efforts and forestall the development of a chronic sexual dysfunction.

Sexually transmitted diseases

Clinical trial research on links between sexually transmitted diseases and female sexual dysfunction is in the earliest stages or nonexistent. There is some suggestion of links between sexually transmitted disease infection and sexual aversion disorder, which involves the persistent or recurrent phobic aversion to and avoidance of sexual contact with a partner.[13] Sexual pain disorders may also be a logical link with sexually transmitted disease infection. Although there are a large number of asymptomatic cases, the most commonly presented symptoms among women with sexually transmitted diseases include lower abdominal pain, abnormal vaginal discharge, pain during sexual intercourse, painful micturition, vaginal itching, and genital ulcers. Each of these symptoms has clear implications for female sexual dysfunction, as described below.

For simplicity, sexually transmitted diseases can be classified as bacterial infections (gonorrhea, chlamydia, syphilis, and chancroid) and viral infections [herpes simplex virus (HSV), human papillomavirus, hepatitis B virus, and human immunodeficiency virus]. We briefly consider each of these in the sections below in terms of links to female sexual dysfunction. We consider the case of human immunodeficiency virus separately.

Bacterial infections

Gonorrhea

Rates of gonorrheal infection in the USA are the highest of all industrialized countries. Approximately 650 000 cases occur each year.[1] Rates declined steadily from the mid-1970s to 1990s, but increased again from 1997 through today. Infection is caused by the bacterium *Neisseria gonorrhoeae* and can lead to infection of the urethra, cervix, rectum, and throat. It invades epithelial cells, leaving the genital tract prone to infection by opportunistic aerobic and anaerobic bacteria.[26] This sexually transmitted disease has an equal estimated male to female ratio.[27] Gonorrhea is a major cause of pelvic inflammatory disease, infertility, and ectopic pregnancy among women. It also facilitates human immunodeficiency virus transmission.[1] Although most infected women are asymptomatic, symptoms for women may include unusual vaginal discharge, painful and urgent urination, pain and bleeding during and after intercourse, and abdominal and pelvic pain. All of these symptoms can disrupt women's sexual functioning.

Chlamydia

Chlamydia is the most commonly reported infectious disease in the USA, with three million cases each year.[28] It is caused by the bacterium *Chlamydia trachomatis*. Pathogenesis may be linked to a host cell-mediated immune response to a chlamydial heat-shock protein.[26] From 1987 through 2002, the reported rate of chlamydial infection among women increased from 78.5 cases per 100 000 to 455.5,[29] though, probably as a result of improved screening and testing procedures. Reported 1995 rates reflected a male to female ratio for chlamydia infection of 1:5.6.[2] Although easily treated with antibiotics, 75% of cases among women present no symptoms, and so the majority of these are left untreated.[1] Clinical manifestations may be related to particular serovars: in one review, women who reported abdominal pain and/or dyspareunia were more often infected with serovar F.[30] Forty per cent of women with untreated chlamydia develop pelvic inflammatory disease, with 20% of these women becoming infertile. Symptoms of chlamydia may include unusual vaginal discharge, bleeding after intercourse, abdominal pain,

and dysuria. Chlamydia is also associated with ectopic pregnancy, inflamed rectum, and chronic pelvic pain,[31] which can produce serious medical and psychologic consequences for women and their partners, and again disrupt sexual functioning.

Syphilis

Syphilis is a genital ulcerative disease caused by the bacterium *Treponema pallidum*, which appears to act by invading the intercellular junctions of endothelial cells. Rates of syphilis are at their lowest since 1941 (2.4 per 100 000 population), although occasional spikes in recent years have been noted in association with human immunodeficiency virus coinfection among men.[1] The male to female ratio is currently 3.5:1. Untreated syphilis can lead to cardiovascular and neurologic diseases, blindness, death, and perinatal death in 40% of cases among pregnant women. Syphilis is easily misdiagnosed because chancres in the primary stages may be painless and overlooked by the infected individual. Secondary syphilis involves a host of symptoms that may disappear and reappear over the first 2 years of the disease, including rash, fever, fatigue, hair loss, and swollen lymph glands. Early stages of infection are unlikely to interfere significantly with sexual function, especially if undiagnosed; however, later stages produce serious physical complications that must be treated medically to ensure survival.

Chancroid

Chancroid is caused by infection with the bacterium *Haemophilus ducreyi*, which produces a hemolysin implicated in the invasion of epithelial cells.[32] Periodic outbreaks of chancroid have occurred in the USA, although this form of sexually transmitted disease is relatively rare outside of tropical and subtropical countries. In 1995, there were only seven new cases.[14] Infection begins with the appearance of painful sores on the genitals and is sometimes accompanied by swelling of lymph nodes in the groin.[14] Among women, symptoms are typically limited to painful urination or defecation, painful intercourse, rectal bleeding, or vaginal discharge. Chancroid lesions are sometimes mistaken for genital ulcers from herpes simplex virus or syphilis infection, and, like these infections, are associated with increased risk of human immunodeficiency virus infection unless treated.[33] These symptoms, coupled with the distress of a chancroid outbreak, can interfere with sexual functioning.

Viral infections

As a family of infections, viral forms are the most serious in many respects, as they are treatable, but not curable. For sexually active individuals, there are almost no established methods of prevention beyond the condom, which is far less effective with viral forms than with bacterial forms of sexually transmitted diseases.[34] It is important to note that, although condoms are the best-known means of preventing infection with sexually transmitted diseases, other than total abstinence, use requires the cooperation of the male partner. Yet, the majority of men report resisting its use,[35] and studies consistently reveal incomplete or inaccurate use throughout intercourse,[36] reducing its prophylactic utility.

Herpes simplex virus

Genital herpes-herpes simplex virus type two (herpes simplex virus 2) infects one million people in the USA each year, most often adolescents and young adults.[1] After the patient recovers from the primary infection, the virus remains latent in sensory ganglia of the peripheral nervous system[37] and can cause disease by reactivation.[38] This disease can be fatal among newborns and those with human immunodeficiency virus.[1] Although approximately 25% of US women and 20% of US men test positive for herpes, less than 10% of those infected are aware that they are infected.[1] Like the bacterial infections, herpes simplex virus can make the patient more susceptible to human immunodeficiency virus infection, and it makes human immunodeficiency virus-infected individuals more infectious to those not yet infected – an issue of particular importance in serodiscordant couples. Prompt treatment can abort painful genital herpes simplex virus reactivation episodes, once individuals learn to recognize the onset of symptoms.[39] Superficial pain from genital herpes outbreaks[12] and the stigma attached to this infection[40] (which is considerable) may contribute to the development of female sexual dysfunction. In particular, individuals report strained relationship dynamics when partners have to abstain from sexual interactions during periodic outbreaks.[41]

Human papillomavirus

In 1999, 5.5 million people in the USA acquired human papillomavirus,[1] making it the most common sexually transmitted disease in the country. Recent Centers for Disease Control and Prevention research found that 72% of adolescent women at a public, sexually transmitted disease clinic had high-risk human papillomavirus strains;[42] these strains have caused considerable concern because of their links to cervical cancer.[43,44] Human papillomavirus sometimes causes genital warts, but in many cases is asymptomatic. Genital warts can be treated and cured, but subclinical human papillomavirus infection is much more common and is incurable at this time. Human papillomaviruses are intraepithelial pathogens.[45] They induce benign lesions on mucocutaneous surfaces that are chronic persistent growths, some of which may progress to malignancy. Infection with human papillomavirus is strongly associated with experience of vulvar vestibulitis syndrome, a disorder characterized by extreme vaginal pain and pain during intercourse.[46]

Hepatitis B virus

The incidence rate of acute hepatitis B in 2001 was 2.8/100 000 in the population, with a male to female ratio of 1.8:1.[1] Unlike the other sexually transmitted diseases, infection is likely to occur through means other than sexual contact; most cases of hepatitis B virus infection are acquired through intravenous drug use. It remains one of the most serious forms of sexually transmitted diseases, however. Although the pathogenesis of this virus remains unclear, infection with hepatitis B virus is clearly implicated in liver pathogenesis. Death from chronic liver disease occurs in 15–25% of infected persons. In addition, chronic hepatitis B virus infection has a high risk of hepatocellular carcinoma.[47] Although a vaccine is available, there are a number of barriers to its uptake, including low awareness of its availability, high cost, and few recommendations for its use by health-care providers.[48] Approximately 30% of infected persons have no symptoms, although symptoms can include jaundice, fatigue, abdominal pain, joint pain, nausea, and vomiting.[1] Implications for female sexual dysfunction relate most directly to the seriousness of medical complications associated with infection.

Human immunodeficiency virus

Organic causes of sexual dysfunctions are generally temporary and easily treatable, compared with psychologic causes such as intrapersonal and interpersonal conflict. However, human immunodeficiency virus represents a notable exception by virtue of being a chronic infection that may lead to acquired immune deficiency syndrome, and which until the recent advent of antiretroviral treatment programs meant the eventual death of the infected person. The reduction in acquired immune deficiency syndrome rates due to advances in treatment has led many to conclude mistakenly that human immunodeficiency virus rates are also drastically reduced. In fact, rates of human immunodeficiency virus infection have been steadily increasing, especially among women.[49] For example, in a prospective study of human immunodeficiency virus serodiscordant couples, women were 17.5 times more likely to seroconvert than comparably exposed seronegative men.[50] Use of highly active antiretroviral therapy has led to an increase in the pool of surviving human immunodeficiency virus-infected individuals.[51] With unprotected sexual intercourse between women and men the predominant mode of transmission,[52] the implications for the field of sexual health cannot be understated.

Infection occurs when human immunodeficiency virus binds to the T-lymphocyte surface antigen CD4 and enters the cell.[53] Viral RNA undergoes reverse transcription, which produces double-stranded viral DNA that is then incorporated into the host DNA. Viral replication results in a reduced CD4 count and eventual defeat of the individual's immune system. Today, infection with human immunodeficiency virus requires close medical supervision and often complicated treatment regimens that may help to extend the life of an individual indefinitely. Not all people infected with human immunodeficiency virus, however, have access to these treatments or adhere properly to them if available (introducing the possibility of the emergence of resistant strains[54]). Oddly, despite widespread media coverage and educational programs associated with the onset of the human immunodeficiency virus epidemic, most individuals believe that they personally are at little to no risk of infection or are reluctant to be tested, in large part because of the emotional impact of the diagnosis.[55]

There are important links between the broader family of

sexually transmitted diseases and human immunodeficiency virus. Risk of infection by human immunodeficiency virus and other sexually transmitted diseases increases as the number of sexual partners and frequency of unprotected sex increase. Sexually transmitted diseases also place women at greater risk of human immunodeficiency virus infection than men.[56] In a study comparing human immunodeficiency virus-positive and human immunodeficiency virus-negative women, those infected with human immunodeficiency virus were more likely to report a history of other types of sexually transmitted diseases.[57] Both human immunodeficiency virus status and CD4 lymphocyte count were associated with evidence of genital ulcers, genital warts, and vaginal candidiasis. Moreover, CD4 lymphocyte depletion was closely related to chronic viral infections.

As with studies of other types of sexually transmitted diseases, clinical trial research and reports on the medical management of infection and sexual dysfunction center almost exclusively on men.[58]

Studies directly assessing relationships between human immunodeficiency virus infection and sexual dysfunction are relatively rare, and those that exist typically do not include women.[59] However, there are notably more studies than those addressing other sexually transmitted diseases. The most common sexual dysfunctions in women generally (loss of desire, anorgasm, and dyspareunia) are also the most common among human immunodeficiency virus-infected women.[58,60–62] Hypoactive sexual desire disorder emerged as the most prevalent psychiatric diagnosis in a study of human immunodeficiency virus-seropositive women.[63] The symptoms were not a subset of mood or anxiety disorders, and most described significant negative effects on their quality of life and intimate relationships. Moreover, candidal and herpetic vulvovaginitis is common among infected women, as is pelvic inflammatory disease, leading to deep dyspareunia, and thus further avoidance of sexual intimacy. Human immunodeficiency virus-positive women may also have altered body image, as a result either of weight loss or redistribution of fat associated with lipodystrophy, or of the fatigue, wasting, and pain that are associated with advanced stages of the disease.[58]

Psychologic distress (e.g., depression, anxiety) secondary to the infection may exacerbate sexual dysfunction[64] (see Chapter 16.2). Newly diagnosed individuals cite a decrease in sexual interest and avoidance of sexual intimacy for fear of transmitting human immunodeficiency virus to their sexual partners.[65] Sexual dysfunction that is associated with medication regimens for acquired immune deficiency syndrome and/or depression may also occur. Several researchers have reported that the use of protease inhibitors is associated with a decrease in sexual desire and arousal.[61,62,66] For example, in a study of 904 human immunodeficiency virus-positive women and men receiving antiretroviral therapy, 29% of the women in the sample reported a decrease in sexual interest.[62] The reported decrease in sexual interest was significantly higher in those individuals whose treatment included protease inhibitors than in those not receiving protease inhibitors. Declining sexual interest was also associated with symptomatic versus asymptomatic human immunodeficiency virus infection.

Conclusions

Because of the high rates of genital tract infections among women, inquiries about female sexual health should be integrated into routine gynecologic care. Although women infected with urinary tract infections, sexually transmitted diseases, and possibly human immunodeficiency virus may present with gynecologic, urologic, or obstetric issues, there are often clear psychologic and relational implications in the forefront of these diagnoses. The psychologic and interpersonal domains may interact with the physical and biologic to hinder early diagnosis and intervention while complicating treatment options, compliance, and ultimately prognosis.

Although female sexual disorders are broadly conceptualized to encompass disorders of desire, arousal, or orgasm, as well as pain, many women present special concerns that center on problems of experience and expression of passion, communication, nongenital touching, and affection.[67] These should be considered integral components of the female sexual function evaluation, as should an individual's experience of her sexuality, self-esteem, and body image.[3] Women presenting common symptoms relating to genital tract infections, namely, vaginal discharge, genital lesions, and abdominal or pelvic pain, are probably first seen at primary health care and family planning clinics. Although the clinical picture and pathology of these infections are well known, the profound impact of these diseases on women's sexual health, and ultimately their physical and psychologic well-being, especially their self- and sexual self-esteem, needs further investigation.

To improve women's sexual health, physicians should receive formal training in sexual functioning to become competent in the first-level medical diagnosis of both gynecologic problems and female sexual dysfunction, and in developing treatment and prevention protocols. This approach should include obtaining a complete patient history, conducting a physical examination, applying treatment, providing education, and offering appropriate referrals.[68] If possible, a comprehensive evaluation of both the woman and her sexual partner or partners should be conducted before formulating a treatment plan,[69] as long as this puts the woman's safety at no risk. Ideally, a comprehensive approach involving education and reassurance in a collaboration between physician and therapist would help provide a complete treatment addressing both the medical and psychosocial consequences of infection.[12,70]

References

1. Centers for Disease Control and Prevention (CDC). *Tracking the Hidden Epidemics 2000: Trends in STDs in the United States* (accessed 30 April 2004 at www.cdc.gov/nchstp/od/news/).

2. Aral SO, Gorbach PM. Sexually transmitted infections. In GM Wingood, RJ DiClemente, eds. *Handbook of Women's Sexual and Reproductive Health.* New York: Kluwer Academic/Plenum, 2002: 255–79.

3. Goldstein I. Female sexual arousal disorder: new insights. *Int J Impot Res* 2000;12(Suppl 4): S152–7.

4. Berman LA, Berman JR, Chhabra S et al. Novel approaches to female sexual dysfunction. *Expert Opin Investig Drugs* 2001; 10: 85–95.

5. Morley JE, Kaiser FE. Female sexuality. *Med Clin North Am* 2003; 87: 1077–90.

6. Shifren JL. The role of androgens in female sexual dysfunction. *Mayo Clin Proc* 2004; 79(Suppl 4): S19–24.

7. Lee RS, Kochman A, Sikkeman KJ. Internalized stigma among people living with HIV-AIDS. *AIDS Behav* 2002; 6: 309–19.

8. Rotheram-Borus M. Variations in perceived pain with emotional distress and social identity in AIDS. *AIDS Patient Care STDS* 2000; 14: 659–65.

9. Bancroft J. The medicalization of female sexual dysfunction: the need for caution. *Arch Sex Behav* 2002; 31: 451–5.

10. El-Bassel N, Gilbert L, Rajah V et al. Fear and violence: raising the HIV stakes. *AIDS Educ Prev* 2000; 12: 154–70.

11. El-Bassel N, Witte SS, Gilbert L et al. HIV prevention for intimate couples: a relationship-based model. *Fam Sys Health* 2001; 19: 379–95.

12. Berman JR, Bassuk J. Physiology and pathophysiology of female sexual function and dysfunction. *World J Urol* 2002; 20: 111–18.

13. Basson R, Berman J, Burnett A et al. Report of the International Consensus Development Conference on female sexual dysfunction: definitions and classifications. *J Urol* 2000; 163: 888–93.

14. NIH. *Health matters: STDs.* Issued by the National Institute of Allergy and Infectious Disease (accessed 22 April 2004 at www.niaid.nih.gov/factsheets/stdother.htm).

15. Harrington RD, Hooton TM. Urinary tract infection risk factors and gender. *J Gend Specif Med* 2000; 3: 27–34.

16. Abrahamsson K, Hansson S, Jodal U et al. *Staphylococcus saprophyticus* urinary tract infections in children. *Eur J Pediatr* 1993; 152: 69–71.

17. Hooton TM. Recurrent urinary tract infections in women. *Int J Antimicrob Agents* 2001; 17: 259–68.

18. Weir M, Brien J. Adolescent urinary tract infections. *Adoles Med State Art Rev* 2000; 11: 293–313.

19. Kucheria R, Sheerin NS, Dasgupta P et al. Urinary tract infections: advances and new therapies. *BJU Int* 2004; 93: 690–1.

20. Mulvey MA, Joel SD, Hultgren SJ. Establishment of a persistent *Escherichia coli* reservoir during the acute phase of a bladder infection. *Infect Immun* 2001; 69: 81–90.

21. McLaughlin SP, Carson CC. Urinary tract infections in women. *Med Clin North Am* 2004; 88: 417–29.

22. Foxman B, Manning SD, Tallman P et al. Uropathogenic *Escherichia coli* are more likely than commensal *E. coli* to be shared between heterosexual sex partners. *Am J Epidemiol* 2002; 156: 1133–40.

23. Foxman B, Gillespie B, Koopman J et al. Risk factors for second urinary tract infections among college women. *Am J Epidemiol* 2000; 151: 1194–1205.

24. Stapleton A, Stamm WE. Prevention of urinary tract infection. *Infect Dis Clin North Am* 1997; 11: 719–33.

25. Arcos B. Female sexual function and response. *J Am Osteopath Assoc* 2004; 104(Suppl 1): S16–20.

26 Mann SN, Smith JR, Barton SE. Pelvic inflammatory disease. *Int J STD AIDS* 1996; 7: 315–21.

27. Aral SO, Holmes KK. Social and behavioral determinants of the epidemiology of STDs: industrialized and developing countries. In Holmes KK, Sparling PF, Mardh PH et al., eds. *Sexually Transmitted Diseases.* New York: McGraw-Hill, 1999: 39–76.

28 Cates W. Estimates of the incidence and prevalence of sexually transmitted diseases in the United States. *Sex Transm Dis* 1999; 26(Suppl 4): S2–7.

29. Centers for Disease Control and Prevention. *Sexually Transmitted Disease Surveillance 2002 Supplement Report: Chlamydia Prevalence Monitoring Project.* Division of STD Prevention, October 2003.

30. Geisler WM, Suchland RJ, Whittington WL et al. The relationship of serovar to clinical manifestations of urogenital *Chlamydia trachomatis* infection. *Sex Transm Dis* 2003; 30: 160–5.

31. Cohen CR, Brunham RC. Pathogenesis of *Chlamydia*-induced pelvic inflammatory disease. *Sex Transm Infect* 1999; 75: 21–4.

32. Wood GE, Dutro SM, Totten PA. Target cell range of *Haemophilus ducreyi* hemolysin and its involvement in invasion of human epithelial cells. *Infect Immun* 1999; 67: 3740–9.

33. Lewis DA. Chancroid: from clinical practice to basic science. *AIDS Patient Care STDs* 2000; 14: 19–36.

34. Wilson TE, Jaccard J, Levinson RA et al. Testing for HIV and other sexually transmitted diseases: implications for risk behavior in women. *Health Psychol* 1996; 15: 252–60.

35. VanOss Marin B, Tschann JM, Gomez CA et al. Self-efficacy to use condoms in unmarried Latino adults. *Am J Community Psychol* 1998; 26: 53–71.

36. Lee DJ, Clarke J. Cover it up or cool it? Sexual intercourse during therapy for bacterial sexually transmitted infections – a discussion for evidence for efficacy of condom use preventing transmission during an acute bacterial STI. *Int J STD AIDS* 2004; 15: 285–8.

37. Blondeau JM, Embil JA, McFarlane ES. Herpes simplex virus infections in male and female mice following pinna inoculation: responses to primary infection and artificially induced recurrent disease. *J Med Virol* 1989; 29: 320–6.

38. Steiner I, Kennedy PG. Herpes simplex virus latent infection in the nervous system. *J Neurovirol* 1995; 1: 19–29.

39. Strand A, Patel R, Wulf HC et al. Aborted genital herpes simplex virus lesions: findings from a randomized controlled trial with valaciclovir. *Sex Transm Infect* 2002; 78: 435–9.

40. Lee JD, Craft, EA. Protecting one's self from a stigmatized disease … once one has it. *Deviant Behav* 2002; 23: 267–99.

41. Mirotznik J, Shapiro RD, Steinhart JE et al. Genital herpes: an investigation of its attitudinal and behavioral correlates. *J Sex Res* 1987; 23: 266–72.

42. Samoff E. Incidence, clearance and persistence of HPV in a cohort of female adolescents. Paper presented at the 2004 National STD Prevention Conference, March, 2004.

43. Phillips Z, Johnson S, Avis M et al. Human papillomavirus and the

value of screening: young women's knowledge of cervical cancer. *Health Educ Res* 2003; 18: 318–28.

44. Waller J, McCaffery KJ, Forrest S et al. Human papillomavirus and cervical cancer: issues for biobehavioral and psychosocial research. *Ann Behav Med* 2004; 27: 68–79.

45. Stanley M, Coleman N, Chambers M. The host response to lesions induced by human papillomvirus. *Ciba Found Symp* 1994; 187: 21–32.

46. Sarma AV, Foxman B, Bayirli B et al. Epidemiology of vulvar vestibulitis syndrome: an exploratory case-control study. *Sex Transm Infect* 1999; 75: 320–6.

47. He QY, Lau GK, Zhou Y et al. Serum biomarkers of hepatitis B virus infected liver inflammation: a proteomic study. *Proteomics* 2003; 3: 666–74.

48. Ganguly R, Banerji M. Hepatitis B virus infection and vaccine acceptance among university students. *Am J Health Behav* 2000; 24: 96–107.

49. UNAIDS. *2004 Report on the global AIDS epidemic*. Geneva: Joint United Nations Program on HIV/AIDS, July 2004.

50. Padian N, Shiboski S, Jewell N. Female-to-male transmission of human immunodeficiency virus. *JAMA* 1991; 266: 1664–7.

51. Palella FJ, Delaney KM, Moorman AC. Declining morbidity and mortality among patients with advanced human immunodeficiency virus infection. HIV Outpatient Study Investigators. *N Engl J Med* 1998; 338: 853–60.

52. World Health Organization. *The World Health Report 2004 – Changing History*. Geneva: World Health Organization, May 2004 (*accessed* 22 June 2004 at www.who.int/whr).

53. Lee LK, Dinneen MD, Ahmad S. The urologist and the patient infected with human immunodeficiency virus or with acquired immunodeficiency syndrome. *BJU International* 2001; 88: 500–10.

54. Leigh Brown AJ, Frost SD, Mathews WC et al. Transmission fitness of drug-resistant human immunodeficiency virus and the prevalence of resistance in the antiretroviral-treated population. *J Infect Dis* 2003; 187: 683–6.

55. Steinbrook R. The AIDS epidemic in 2004. *N Engl J Med* 2004: 351: 115–17.

56. Fleming DT, Wasserheit JN. From epidemiological synergy to public health policy and practice: the contribution of other sexually transmitted diseases to sexual transmission of HIV infection. *Sex Transm Infect* 1999; 75: 3–17.

57. Greenblatt RM, Bacchetti P, Barkan S et al. Lower genital tract infections among HIV-infected and high-risk uninfected women: findings of the Women's Interagency HIV Study (WIHS). *Sex Transm Dis* 1999; 26: 143–51.

58. Hijazi L, Nandwani R, Kell P. Medical management of sexual difficulties in HIV-positive individuals. *Int J STD AIDS* 2002; 13: 587–92.

59. Collazos J, Martinez E, Mayo J et al. Sexual dysfunction in HIV-infected patients treated with highly active antiretroviral therapy. *J Acquir Immune Defic Syndr* 2002; 31: 322–6.

60. Brown GR, Kendall S, Ledsky R. Sexual dysfunction in HIV-seropositive women without AIDS. *J Psychol Human Sex* 1995; 7: 73–97.

61. Nusbaum MRH, Hamilton C, Lenahan P. Chronic illness and sexual functioning. *Am Fam Physician* 2003; 67: 347–54.

62. Schrooten W, Colebeunders R, Youle M et al. Sexual dysfunction associated with protease inhibitor containing highly active antiretroviral treatment. *AIDS* 2001; 15: 1019–23.

63. Brown GR, Rundell JR. A prospective study of psychiatric aspects of early HIV disease in women. *Gen Hosp Psychiatry* 1993; 15: 139–47.

64. Anastasiadis AG, Davis AR, Ghafar MA et al. The epidemiology and definition of female sexual disorders. *World J Urol* 2002; 20: 74–8.

65. Green G. The reproductive careers of a cohort of men and women following HIV-positive diagnosis. *J Biosoc Sci* 1994; 26: 409–15.

66. Martinez E, Collazos J, Mayo J et al. Sexual dysfunction with protease inhibitors. *Lancet* 1999; 353: 810–11.

67. Leiblum SR. Definition and classification of female sexual disorders. *Int J Impot Res* 1998; 10(Suppl 2): S104–6.

68. Phillips NA. Female sexual dysfunction: evaluation and treatment. *Am Fam Physician* 2000; 62: 127–36.

69 Leiblum SR, Weigel, M. Psychotherapeutic interventions for treating female sexual dysfunction. *World J Urol* 2002; 20: 127–36.

70. Berman JR, Goldstein I. Female sexual dysfunction. *Urol Clin North Am* 2001; 28: 405–16.

SPECIAL ISSUES CONCERNING COUPLES

Sexual function in women with women: lesbians and lesbian relationships

Margaret Nichols

Introduction

Since the American Psychiatric Association officially declassified homosexuality as a mental illness in 1973, most health-care professionals have gradually accepted the view that being gay or lesbian is a sexual variation rather than a disease.

Many are also recognizing that gay patients often have unique needs and concerns. While most doctors and therapists have at least an occasional homosexual patient, some practitioners find that gays comprise a noticeable portion of their patient load. Gays are concentrated more heavily in urban areas[1] and higher educational groups, and lesbian activity is common on college campuses.[2] Lesbians are heavy users of mental health services: a national survey of lesbian health[3] showed that nearly three-quarters of respondents had at some point been in therapy or counseling, and two-thirds of this lesbian sample preferred female practitioners. So, for example, female gynecologists and sex therapists located near college campuses or in urban settings may find that a significant number of their patients are women who have sex with other women.

This chapter outlines some of the unique features of lesbian sex and lesbian sexual relationships that might concern the health-care professional. The material presented here has been compiled from the relatively meager selection of research oriented toward lesbian sexuality, from the clinical experience of the author and colleagues who work with lesbian clients, and from an Internet-based study of lesbian, bisexual, and heterosexual women's sexual behavior conducted in 2003–4 at the Institute for Personal Growth, a psychotherapy center in New Jersey serving the gay, lesbian, and bisexual community. The latter data, collected by the author and her colleagues, will be referred to as the Institute for Personal Growth Internet Study results.[4]

Sensitivity: the "heterosexual assumption"

Before discussing lesbian sexuality, it is worth noting that it is more important for a doctor or therapist to have an open, aware attitude to lesbian patients than to have a wealth of knowledge about sexual minorities. Ryan and Bradford's lesbian health survey[3] established that the single biggest complaint of the respondents was that health and mental health practitioners had an inherent heterosexual bias, an automatic assumption that everyone is "straight". These assumptions are usually unconscious. For example, when a gynecologist reflexively asks about birth control, when the office intake form asks for "marital status: single/married/divorced/widowed", when the provider asks "are you sexually active?" and means "are you having heterosexual sexual intercourse", many lesbians will be offended and/or conclude that the provider is insensitive or prejudiced towards gays. Ryan and Bradford found that as many as 27% of the lesbians interviewed reported that the most common problem with their health-care practitioner was the assumption of being heterosexual. While some women are able to correct the care practitioner and reveal their sexual orientation, others find this assumption to be one more obstacle in their coming-out process. In fact, approximately 17% of the participants reported they would not reveal their sexual orientation to their health-care practitioner even though that information might be critical for treatment. Thus, the "gay-affirmative" health-care professional must approach each female patient as though she may have feelings, history, or current behavior that is homosexual. The provider must demonstrate openness to the possibility of female–female sexual experience in each woman in order to gain the trust of the lesbian patient.

Special features of lesbian sexuality

Identity versus behavior; sexual fluidity

In a culture that stigmatizes same-sex behavior, as ours still does, one would expect the incidence of same-sex attractions to be higher than the incidence of same-sex behavior, and both should be higher than the number of people who self-label as gay. Indeed, every study from Kinsey to the present day has found this. Virtually all studies from the 1950s[5] to the present[6] have found that the vast majority of self-identified lesbians, 80–90%, have had at least one male sexual partner.

However, the reality is more complicated. Recent evidence suggests that women may be physiologically "wired" for bisexuality.[7] When presented with lesbian and heterosexual visual erotica, women of all orientations show physiologic arousal to both, whereas men's arousal is "targeted": heterosexual men respond to heterosexual erotica and gay men respond to gay male erotica. This confirms what a number of theorists already believe, that women may have a more fluid sexual orientation than men.[8–12] Diamond[2] found that a significant number of lesbian-identified college women change their self-labeling to bisexual or heterosexual over a 5-year period. Moreover, these women do not "disavow" their former lesbian identity and are open to the possibility of sexual change in their futures.

The Institute for Personal Growth Internet Study reveals an even more complex picture. Of the 231 self-identified lesbians, 75% had had one or more male sex partners, and 63% reported sexual attraction to men; three of them were in relationships with men at the time they completed the survey. Moreover, 52% of the 132 self-identified heterosexual women reported sexual attraction to women, 22% had at least one female sexual partner, and one was currently in a relationship with a woman. If one were to define sexual orientation in terms of capacity for sexual attraction, the majority of these self-labeled lesbian and heterosexual women would technically be bisexual.

However, bisexuality as a personal identity is a relatively new phenomenon, emerging only within the last 20 years.[12,13] Women who self-label as bisexual – as opposed to those who simply exhibit bisexual attractions – may be a distinct and unique subgroup within what is now commonly known as the lesbian, bisexual, gay, and transgendered community. The Institute for Personal Growth Internet Study found that the 152 survey respondents who self-labeled as bisexual had some sexual behaviors that set them apart from either lesbian or heterosexual women. Bisexual

women masturbated more than ($p < 0.001$), thought about sex more than ($p < 0.003$), and had nearly twice the number of lifetime sex partners as their gay or straight counterparts ($p < 0.02$). In addition, they were far more likely to identify also with the "kink" community – women engaging in some form of dominance–submission sex play ($p < 0.001$) – and the 'polyamory' community – women with multiple concurrent sexual/relationship partners ($p < 0.001$).

In practical terms, it is clear that self-identification is at best an incomplete description of self-orientation, making it imperative that a sexual health practitioner not make any assumptions about the sexual behavior of a client without taking a careful history that includes questions about contact with both men and women regardless of the patient's expressed identity.

Gender identity and "gender bending"

At the peak of the lesbian feminist movement in the 1970s, it was unacceptable to identify someone as "butch" or "femme"; androgyny was the only "politically correct" choice. However, that has changed dramatically, so much so that female to male transsexuals are much more visible in the lesbian community.[14,15] Some of the established professional definitions of transsexualism are being challenged, as more and more women identify themselves as being part of the "transgender continuum". For example, "trannie boys" are lesbians who take male hormones, may or may not have "top surgery" on their breasts, and retain their female genitalia; "bois" are gay women with completely female bodies who dress and comport themselves like men, use male pronouns to identify themselves, and often appear in public "packing" – wearing a strap-on dildo under their pants. The Internet study allowed women to identify their gender as "female" or "other". Five per cent of lesbians identified as "other", while virtually none of the bisexual or heterosexual women did so ($p < 0.001$). Asked to describe "other", these women used words like "transgendered", "gender queer", "butch", or "ftm (female-to-male)". We also asked women to identify where they fell on a "butch–femme" continuum, and while 26% of the lesbians labeled themselves "butch", only a handful of bisexual and heterosexual women did so ($p < 0.001$).

The phenomenon described above suggests it may be time for a paradigm shift in our concepts of gender identity and sexual orientation. For three decades, both gay rights activists and sexuality experts have encouraged us to think that these two core self-concepts are separate, in part because sexology has long been dominated by the social constructivist view of gender identity. Moreover, we have come to think of "lesbianism" as a uniform sexual orientation, rather than as a label describing a broad range of behaviors and feelings. Increasingly, we are recognizing that there are substantial differences in sexual behavior among self-labeled lesbians: some women have never been attracted to men, others have strong attractions and history of involvement with men. For some, the identity will be constant throughout their lifetime; for others, it may be more fluid. We also notice the lesbian community itself returning to butch–femme dichotomies, but with new twists. Perhaps this means it is time to reconsider a biologic basis, at least for women who label themselves butch or bois, as well as for female-to-male transsexuals, who frequently have identified as lesbian before coming to a "trans" identity. Some studies have shown that girls born with congenital adrenal hyperplasia show more male-typical behavior as children, more dissatisfaction with female sex role assignment, and less heterosexual interest than noncongenital adrenal hyperplasia girls,[16] And at least one study of lesbians who identify as "butch" found that "butches" recalled more childhood gender-atypical behavior and had higher waist-to-hip ratios, higher saliva testosterone levels, and less desire to give birth than either "femme" lesbians or heterosexual women.[17] The Internet study found self-labeled "butch" women to be less attracted to males ($p < 0.05$) than other lesbians, but with no difference in their number of male partners.

For the health-care provider working with lesbian patients, this implies a need to loosen rigid definitions of gender and to change the currently marked distinction between "transsexuals" and "everybody else". In the future, the health-care community may be forced to deal with, for example, women who ask their doctors for hormones without desiring full "transition" to the opposite gender; it is not unrealistic to think that even the esteemed Harry Benjamin Standards of Care for transsexuals may need revision.

Sexually transmitted infections

Despite scant research, some of the most consistent findings regarding lesbian sexuality have been in the area of sexually transmitted infections (see Chapter 7.7). Roberts et al.[6] reviewed 10 studies, including their own, that all showed lesbians having fewer sexually transmitted infections than bisexual or heterosexual women. In particular, gonorrhea, syphilis, human immunodeficiency virus, and hepatitis B are less common among lesbians, as are abnormal Pap smears. The Institute for Personal Growth Internet Study

found significant differences in the total number of lifetime sexually transmitted infections between lesbian, bisexual, and heterosexual women, and a strong correlation ($p < 0.001$) between the total number of sexually transmitted infections and the total number of male sex partners. Looking at individual sexually transmitted infections (Table 8.1.1), we found lower rates for lesbians for each sexually transmitted infection. However, the only significant difference for an individual sexually transmitted infection was for the incidence of abnormal Pap smears: lesbians had the lowest rates, and then bisexuals, and heterosexual women had the most abnormal Pap smears ($p < 0.01$). The data on abnormal Pap smears corroborates the many studies that have shown nuns to have a low incidence of cervical cancer; the differentiating variable probably is the male penis and number of different male partners, not sexual activity alone.

It is important to note that although a number of studies show that lesbians have fewer sexually transmitted infections than heterosexual women, that finding seems to be related to the number of male partners a woman has, and we know from a multitude of sources that most lesbians have had at least one male sex partner. This is yet another reason why there is no substitute for the taking of a detailed sexual history; one cannot rely upon self-identification alone.

The nature of lesbian sexual relationships: "lesbian bed death" and other myths

The "common knowledge" about lesbian relationships

In 1983, the highly regarded book *American Couples*[18] compared heterosexual married, heterosexual cohabiting, gay male, and

Table 8.1.1. Frequency of sexually transmitted infections (STI)/conditions in lesbian, bisexual, and heterosexual women

Type of STI/condition	Lesbian %"yes"	Bisexual % "yes"	Hetero % "yes"	Total Sample % "yes"
Abnormal Pap smear	13	20	25	18*
Chlamydia	4	8	6	6
Gonorrhea	0	2	1	1
Hepatitis	3	0	2	5
Hepatitis B	6	10	11	9
Herpes	5	11	9	8
HIV	0	0	1	0
Pelvic inflammatory disease	2	2	3	2
Syphilis	0	0	0	0
Vaginitis	5	8	5	6

*Significant at $p < 0.01$; results based on the Personal Growth Internet Study; lesbian women $n = 231$; bisexual women $n = 152$; heterosexual women $n = 132$; % "yes" indicates the percentage of women who responded "yes" to the question, "Have you ever had this condition/infection?"; HIV, human immunodeficiency virus.

lesbian relationships, and found lesbian couples to have the least frequent sexual contact. Other work written from a clinical perspective also noted the existence of lesbian couples who had little or no genital contact.[19–21] By the end of the 1980s, the term "lesbian bed death" was in common usage in the gay community and eventually became part of a stereotype: the lesbian as a sensual-but-not-sexual woman. Two explanations were often given for this phenomenon; internalized shame associated with homophobia, and the "unmitigated female sexuality" of a two women together (i.e., a union in which both partners had relatively low sex drive, low sexual assertiveness, and a high degree of intimacy).[22,23] Both lesbian and gay male relationships are often viewed as being shorter than heterosexual relationships, although Blumberg and Schwartz made it quite clear in their study that longevity was related to legal marital status far more than sexual orientation.[18] That is, cohabitating heterosexual couples have relationships as short as gay and lesbian couples, and heterosexual married couples stay together significantly longer than any other type of partnership.

In recent years, some sexologists have criticized mainstream sexual theory as being phallocentric and heterosexist.[24–26] They have argued against the traditional definition of sex as genital contact directed toward orgasm and suggested an expansion to include mutual, sensual physical contact not focused on orgasm. Others have questioned using sexual frequency as an indicator of sexual health. For example, some studies have shown that lesbians spend more time on the average sexual encounter than do heterosexuals; using the measure of time spent on sex rather than sexual frequency, lesbians might be "healthier" than their straight counterparts.[27] Still others[28] contend that sex is not necessary for healthy relationship function. In particular, lesbian relationships, which some view as more egalitarian and intimate than the average heterosexual marriage,[29] may not "need" genital sex for connection – sex may be in effect, "redundant". From this point of view, sex therapy for a non-genitally sexual lesbian couple might include encouraging them to question why they feel a need to be sexual.

Some lesbian psychotherapists argue that "lesbian bed death" is a myth based on insufficient data. Matthews et al.[30] found no differences between the sexual frequency rates of heterosexual and lesbian women, and Iazenza[31] found lesbians to be more sexually arousable and more sexually assertive than heterosexual women.

Meanwhile, the lesbian community itself has become more sexual in the last two decades.[32,33] Lesbian-owned and -oriented erotica magazines, sex toy stores, and erotic video companies have proliferated. Lesbian clubs like Meow Mix in New York advertise "Pussy Galore" and "I Love Pussy" nights and brag about the "action" in the bathrooms. Lesbian "kink" organizations exist in most major US cities, and polyamory is becoming more common.[34]

Results of Institute for Personal Growth Internet Study

Data from this study of 231 self-identified lesbians, 152 bisexual women, and 132 heterosexual women were analyzed in two ways: by self-identified orientation and, for women currently in relationships, by whether the participant was involved with a woman or a man. First, like Blumberg and Schwartz,[18] we found lesbian relationships to be of shorter duration than heterosexual relationships – 4 years average compared with 8 years ($p < 0.001$), but this difference disappeared when we compared only unmarried women. Among both single and coupled women, lesbians had less sex in the year preceding the survey ($p < 0.05$) but did not differ from heterosexual women in their frequency of masturbation or how often they thought about sex.

Our primary analyses compared women in relationships with other women versus women with men. Overall, women with men had slightly more frequent sex than women with other women ($p < 0.05$), and this difference was independent of length of time in relationship. The presence of children was not a predictive factor of frequency of sexual activities; there was no difference in the number of children living with women with women versus women with men. Additionally, no difference was observed between the groups in the percentage of women who never had sex, thus casting suspicion on the notion that lesbians are more likely to have nonsexual relationships.

Looking at other aspects of sexuality, the women with women spent more time engaging in sexual activities ($p < 0.001$), had more non-penis-oriented sexual acts as part of their typical repertoire ($p < 0.001$), and were less likely to have sex because their partner wanted it ($p < 0.001$). Most significantly, women with women were more likely to have orgasms during sex with their partner than were women with men regardless of marital status or length of relationship ($p < 0.001$). The tendency to orgasm during partner sex was not significantly related to the length of time the partners had been together, but was strongly related to the amount of time spent on sex for both women with women and women with men ($p < 0.001$). We found that the typical sex acts associated with orgasm for women (regardless of gender of partner) were kissing ($p < 0.001$), non-genital touching ($p < 0.006$), receiving oral sex ($p < 0.001$), digital-vaginal stimulation ($p < 0.001$), and the use of sex toys ($p < 0.01$). Of these acts, kissing ($p < 0.001$), nongenital touching ($p < 0.01$), digital-vaginal stimulation ($p < 0.001$), and use of toys ($p < 0.001$) were more likely to be practiced by women with other women than by women with men.

Lesbian relationships revisited

If we incorporate new information about the lesbian community with the results of more recent research and theory about female sexuality, the picture is more complex than the old stereotype portrays. First, we see increased support for the idea that legal marriage is related to longevity of relationship, for better or worse. Second, while it may be true that women in lesbian relationships have somewhat less sex than their heterosexual counterparts, it is by no means true that the typical lesbian relationship becomes asexual. Women in relationships with other women are less likely to have sex because their partner wants it, which may account for part of the difference in sexual frequency. Furthermore, there is evidence to suggest that lesbian sexuality includes behaviors that are more associated with women's sexual satisfaction: it lasts longer, is more varied, includes more sex acts likely to lead to orgasm for women, and is in fact more correlated with orgasm. Indeed, if one measured sex not by frequency but, say, by Kinsey's original standard – sexual contact to the point of orgasm – women with women have more sex than women with men, and are more likely to have sex of their own volition. Assimilating this information can radically change the professional's paradigm of sexual relationship health. Perhaps we should stop asking so much about sexual frequency, and instead ask more about female orgasm and pleasure, about quality versus quantity.

Lesbian sexual dysfunction

There are few nonclinical data on the nature of lesbian sexual dysfunction compared with those of heterosexual women. Clinical data suggest that sexual desire discrepancy between partners and/or low sexual desire are the most common problems lesbians face, as with heterosexual women.[35,36] In the Internet study, participants were given a list of sexual problems (e.g., lack of lubrication, decreased sexual arousal, less desire than partner, more desire than partner, feeling guilty, feeling anxious). An analysis was conducted on self-identified lesbians versus heterosexuals, and a second analysis investigated women with women versus women with men. The results from both analyses showed that lesbians or women with women reported fewer sexual problems than heterosexuals or women with men ($p < 0.01$, $p < 0.001$, respectively).

Table 8.1.2 shows percentages of the overall sample of lesbians and heterosexual women as they reported sexual dysfunction, and for which problems there was a significant difference between the two groups. Table 8.1.3 presents the same data broken down for women with women versus women with men. Not surprisingly, lack of interest in sex and/or having

less desire than one's partner were the most frequently reported problems for all women, followed by problems with orgasm, problems experiencing more desire than one's partner, trouble lubricating, and anxiety about sex. Many of the differences between groups were significant, and only one problem – feeling more desire than one's partner – was reported more frequently for lesbians/women with women, although not at a statistically significant level.

If lesbians have fewer sexual problems than heterosexual women, and only slightly less sex, how can we account for clinical accounts of "lesbian bed death"? Several possibilities exist. First, it is possible that greater social acceptance of homosexuality over the last two decades has made lesbians feel less internalized shame and homophobia and therefore less self-imposed sexual repression – note that in the Internet sample fewer lesbians than heterosexual women felt guilty about sex. In other words, "lesbian bed death" may have been more common 20 years ago than it is now. Another explanation may lie in the high percentage of lesbians who participate in psychotherapy – clinicians may see a disproportionate number of lesbian couples with sex problems, and lack of interest in sex is by far the most common sexual complaint of all women.

Summary and conclusions

The sexual health professional who works with lesbian clients is rewarded with a broadened and enriched perspective on female sexuality in general. The provider must, as with all minority groups, be sensitive to and respect cultural differences in sexual expression. When one practices within the lesbian community, he or she must be comfortable with patients' sexual fluidity in both behavior and self-identification, as well as with a broader range of gender identity. Sexually transmitted infections are less common among lesbians, and sexual dysfunction may be less common as well, although lesbians are highly likely to seek counseling when they do have problems.

Table 8.1.2. Frequency of sexual problems in lesbian and heterosexual women

Type of sexual problem	Lesbian %"yes"	Hetero %"yes"	Total Sample %"yes"	Significance level $p <$
No interest in sex	40	45	42	
Difficulty/unable to reach orgasm	29	41	33	0.02
Pain with penetration	20	30	23	0.02
Unable to be penetrated	6	5	6	
Persistent, unwanted arousal	10	17	13	
Trouble lubricating	13	30	20	0.000
Sex possible, but not pleasurable	19	27	22	
Guilt about sex	16	24	19	
Anxiety about sex	29	32	30	
More desire than partner	36	28	33	
Less desire than partner	37	46	40	

Results based on the Institute for Personal Growth Internet Study; lesbian women $n = 231$; heterosexual women $n = 132$; bisexual women excluded.

Table 8.1.3. Frequency of sexual problems among women currently in relationships with women versus women in relationships with men

Type of sexual problem	Female–female %"yes"	Female–male %"yes"	Total Sample %"yes"	Significance level $p <$
No interest in sex	39	51	44	0.02
Difficulty/unable to reach orgasm	32	41	36	
Pain with penetration	22	34	28	0.02
Unable to be penetrated	6	4	5	
Persistent, unwanted arousal	11	17	14	0.02
Trouble lubricating	18	32	25	0.002
Sex possible, but not pleasurable	20	32	26	0.000
Guilt about sex	18	22	20	
Anxiety about sex	28	34	31	
More desire than partner	36	34	35	
Less desire than partner	39	52	45	0.008

Results based on the Personal Growth Internet Study; women in relationships with women (female–female) $n = 205$; women in relationship with men (female–male) $n = 179$.

Most importantly, the sexual behavior of women with other women is different from that of women with men, and probably more consonant with the attainment of female orgasm. Although lesbian couples appear to have sex less frequently than their heterosexual counterparts, they have sex because both partners want to, they spend more time on sex and include more nongenital, non-penis-oriented acts, and their sexual activity more frequently results in orgasm for both partners. Indeed, when questioning not only lesbians but heterosexual women about their sexual practices, it may be useful for the practitioner to focus more closely on female sexual pleasure and to consider quantity of sex less important than quality.

References

1. Laumann E, Gagnon J, Michael R et al. *The Social Organization of Sexuality: Sexual Practices in the United States.* Chicago: University of Chicago Press, 1994.

2. Diamond L. Was it a phase? Young women's relinquishment of lesbian/bisexual identities over a 5-year period. *J Pers Soc Psychol* 2003; 84: 352–64.

3. Ryan C, Bradford J. The National Lesbian Health Care Survey: an overview. In L Garrets, D Kimmel, eds. *Psychological Perspectives on Lesbian and Gay Male Experiences.* New York: Columbia University Press, 1993: 541–56.

4. Nichols M, Williamson D, Menahem S et al. First results of the IPG Internet study of female sexuality/lesbian sexuality. *Growing Diversity*. Available at: www.ipgcounseling.com/growing_diversity.html.

5. Conrad F. The Ladder 1959: DOB questionnaire reveals some facts about lesbians. *J Lesbian Stud* 2001; 5: 1–24.

6. Roberts S, Sorenson L, Patsdaughter C et al. Sexual behaviors and sexually transmitted diseases of lesbians: results of the Boston Lesbian Health Project. *J Lesbian Stud* 200; 4: 49–70.

7 Chivers M, Rieger G, Latty E et al. Men's sexual arousal is targeted; women's sexual arousal is bisexual. Paper presented at the annual meeting of the International Academy of Sex Research, Hamburg, Germany, 2002.

8. Peplau L. Human sexuality: how do men and women differ? *Curr Dir Psychol Sci* 2003; 12: 37–40.

9. Peplau L. Rethinking women's sexual orientation: an interdisciplinary approach. *Pers Relat* 2001; 8: 1–19.

10. Peplau L. A new paradigm for understanding women's sexuality and sexual orientation. *J Soc Issues* 2000; 56: 329–50.

11. Diamond L. What does sexual orientation orient? A biobehavioral model distinguishing romantic love and sexual desire. *Psychol Rev* 2003; 110: 173–92.

12. Weise E. *Closer to Home: Bisexuality and Feminism.* Seattle: Seal Press, 1992.

13. Nichols M. Therapy with bisexual women: working on the edge of emerging cultural and personal identities. In M Mirkin, ed. *Women in Context: Toward a Feminist Reconstruction of Psychotherapy.* New York: Guilford Press, 1994: 149–69.

14. Bernstein F. On campus, rethinking Biology 101. *New York Times*, 7 March 2004.

15. Levy A. Where the bois are. *New York Magazine*, 12 January 2004: 23–7.

16. Hines M, Brook C, Conway G. Androgen and psychosexual development: core gender identity, sexual orientation, and recalled childhood gender role behavior in women and men with congenital adrenal hyperplasia (CAH). *J Sex Res* 2004; 41: 75–81.

17. Singh D, Vidaurri, M, Zambarano R et al. Lesbian erotic role identification: behavioral, morphological, and hormonal correlates. *J Pers Soc Psychol* 1999; 76: 1035–49.

18. Blumstein P, Schwartz P. *American Couples: Money, Work, and Sex.* New York: Morrow, 1983.

19. Hall M. Lesbians, limerance, and long-term relationships. In J Loulan, *Lesbian Sex.* San Francisco: Spinsters Ink, 1984: 141–50.

20. Loulan J. *Lesbian Sex.* San Francisco: Spinsters Ink, 1984.

21. Nichols M. Lesbian sexuality: issues and developing theory. In Boston Lesbian Psychologies Collective, eds. *Lesbian Psychologies:*

Explorations and Challenges. Chicago: University of Illinois Press, 1987: 97–125.

22. Nichols M. Low sexual desire in lesbian couples. In S Leiblum, R Rosen R eds. *Sexual Desire Disorders.* New York: Guilford Press, 1988: 387–412.

23. Nichols M. Lesbian relationships: implications for the study of sexuality and gender. In D McWhirter, S Sanders, J Reinisch, eds. *Homosexuality/Heterosexuality: Concepts of Sexual Orientation.* London: Oxford University Press, 1990: 351–63.

24. Kaschak E, Tiefer L. *A New View of Women's Sexual Problems.* New York: Haworth, 2001.

25. Kleinplatz P. *New Directions in Sex Therapy: Innovations and Alternatives.* Philadelphia: Brunner Routledge, 2001.

26. Rothblum E, Brehony K. *Boston Marriages: Romantic but Asexual Relationships Among Contemporary Lesbians.* Amherst: University of Massachusetts Press, 1993.

27. Iasenza S. Beyond 'lesbian bed death': the passion and play in lesbian relationships. *J Lesbian Stud* 2002; 6: 111–20.

28. Cole E. Is sex a natural function: implications for sex therapy. In E Rothblum, K Brehony, eds. *Boston Marriages: Romantic but Asexual Relationships Among Contemporary Lesbians.* Amherst: University of Massachusetts Press, 1993: 188–93.

29. Schwartz P. *Love Between Equals.* New York: Simon & Schuster, 1994.

30. Matthews A, Tartaro J, Hughes T. A comparative study of lesbian and heterosexual women in committed relationships. *J Lesbian Stud* 1994; 7: 101–14.

31. Iazenza S. The relations among selected aspects of sexual orientation and sexual functioning in females. *Dissertation Abstracts International.* Ann Arbor: University Microfilms International, 1991.

32. Nichols M. Sex therapy with sexual minorities. In S Leiblum, R Rosen, eds. *Principles and Practice of Sex Therapy,* 3rd edn. New York: Guilford Press, 2002: 335–67.

33. Bolonik K. Girls gone wild. *New York Magazine,* 12 January 2004: 18–23.

34. Munson M, Stelboum J. The lesbian polyamory reader: open relationships, non-monogamy, and casual sex. *J Lesbian Stud* 1999; 3: 1–7.

35. Loulan J. *Lesbian Passion.* San Francisco: Spinsters Ink, 1997.

36. Nichols M. Sexual desire disorder in a lesbian couple: the intersection of therapy and politics. In R Rosen, S Leiblum, eds. *Case Studies in Sex Therapy.* New York: Guilford Press, 1995: 161–75.

8.2 Sexual function in women with men: partners with sexual dysfunction

Michael Sand, William A Fisher, Raymond C Rosen, Irwin Goldstein

Introduction

Couples share their sexual dysfunctions. In this chapter, the issue of female sexual dysfunction that is associated with male sexual dysfunctions will be reviewed.

Studies such as that by Riley et al. in 2002 have noted a high prevalence of sexual problems in women whose men also had sexual problems. In this specific investigation, Riley et al. found, regarding men with erectile dysfunction, that women had frequent sexual concerns about their own function. The problem included relationship dissatisfaction, fear of intimacy, diminished sexual desire, and dyspareunia.[1] Is the association between female sexual dysfunction and male sexual dysfunction related to aging factors within each member of the couple? Can a woman who is otherwise sexually functional and healthy develop a sexual dysfunction because her male partner has a sexual dysfunction?

There are limited data on the topic. This chapter will review the evidence supporting the potentially strong association between female sexual dysfunction and sexual dysfunction in the male partner.

Women with men who have erectile dysfunction

Introduction

Women with men who have erectile dysfunction may have their own sexual function adversely affected. In particular, a woman's sexual attitudes, sexual beliefs, sexual experiences, sexual function (desire, arousal, and orgasm) and sexual quality of life may be impaired by her partner's erectile dysfunction. Furthermore, among women with male partners, it is not known whether the woman's sexual function and sexual quality of life are altered when her partner is successfully treated for erectile dysfunction with safe and effective agents such as selective phosphodiesterase type 5 inhibitors.

While substantial investigation has taken place on the effects of selective phosphodiesterase type 5 inhibitors on men with erectile dysfunction, little attention has been given to the sexual responses of their female partners. A typical inclusion criterion in the selective phosphodiesterase type 5 inhibitor trial on such couples was the existence of a stable heterosexual relationship. Participation of the woman was voluntary and limited to assessments of treatment satisfaction. The female partners of men with erectile dysfunction were thought to support unconditionally their partners' sexual treatment. The perspective of the woman, her well-being, quality of life, sexual function, and sexual satisfaction, either in relation to existing erectile dysfunction or successfully treated erectile dysfunction, were not taken into consideration.

Data

What are the scientific data available concerning changes in the woman's sexual function among women whose partners have erectile dysfunction? Clinically, it has been frequently anecdotally observed that women have discontinued their sexual activity if their male partners develop erectile dysfunction. Unfortunately, there are limited investigations on the subject. In one study, Blumel et al. examined a sample of 534 otherwise healthy women who had ceased sexual activity with their male partners.[2] It was noted that, among the cohort under age 45, erectile dysfunction was the most frequently cited reason for cessation of the woman's sexual activity.

There have recently been a series of studies investigating the effects of a woman's sexual function when her male partner has erectile dysfunction. Initial studies were, however, obtained with data from the man's perspective. Past research in this area involved inquiries of the men with erectile dysfunction about the effect their sexual problem had on their women partners. For example, in 2001, Paige et al. hypothesized that since erectile dysfunction could have a significant influence on the lives of the couple, the restoration of erectile function should then be associated with an enhancement of health-related quality of life in the couple.[3] Focusing on the relationship involving women whose men had erectile dysfunction, this study showed that significant improvement in the marital interaction score was noted when men with erectile dysfunction used a selective phosphodiesterase type 5 inhibitor. Moreover, when the men were asked whether using the selective phosphodiesterase type 5 inhibitor improved the relationships with their women partners, 29% indicated that it definitely had.[3]

Contemporary research has finally begun to address the issue from the woman's perspective. Current investigations have begun to shed light on the previously poorly explored effects of erectile dysfunction and its treatment among women whose partners experience this sexual dysfunction.

In the following five investigations, data are derived from the woman herself, as her own study subject. In the first study, Cayan et al. recently reported on a prospective study assessing the sexual function of women with men who had erectile dysfunction.[4] All women in the trial completed a Female Sexual Function Index score. The study involved 38 women whose men had erectile dysfunction and 49 women whose men did not have erectile dysfunction. Women's sexual function, including sexual arousal, lubrication, orgasm, satisfaction, pain, and total score, was significantly diminished among women with men who had erectile dysfunction in comparison with women in the control group. Among those women whose male partners received treatment (penile prosthesis insertion, oral phosphodiesterase type 5 inhibitor treatment) for their erectile dysfunction, significant improvements in sexual arousal, lubrication, orgasm and satisfaction in the women were identified.[4]

In the second study, Ichikawa et al. evaluated the sexual function and satisfaction of women with men who received treatment (phosphodiesterase type 5 inhibitor) for erectile dysfunction.[5] Of the 98 women who were invited to participate, only 30 (31%) accepted. Of these, most women (90%) reported that the treatment was effective, and a majority of women (60%) reported improvement in their quality of life. Interestingly, 20% of women whose men's erectile dysfunction

was treated with phosphodiesterase type 5 inhibitors were concerned about adverse events. A significant number of women disappointed with the erectile dysfunction treatment had female sexual dysfunction.[5]

In the third study, Montorsi et al. investigated thoughts, views, and intercourse satisfaction in 930 women whose male partners were taking a selective phosphodiesterase type 5 inhibitor to manage erectile dysfunction.[6] Women with men using a selective phosphodiesterase type 5 inhibitor had significantly higher intercourse satisfaction than women whose men used a placebo.[6]

In the fourth study, Chevret et al. developed and validated the Index of Sexual Life to measure women's sexual function in relationships with men who had erectile dysfunction.[7] Women partnered with men with erectile dysfunction were found to have significantly diminished sexual drive and sexual satisfaction compared with women whose male partners did not have erectile dysfunction.[7]

In the fifth study, Oberg et al. examined data from a nationally representative cross-sectional population investigation of sexual life, attitudes, and behavior in Sweden.[8] A total of 926 women, aged 18–65 years, were sexually active in a steady, heterosexual relationship during the 12 months prior to the investigation. Data from women who claimed personally distressing sexual dysfunctions quite often, nearly all the time, or all the time were compared with data from women that had no distressing sexual dysfunction. Women distressed by low sexual interest or orgasmic dysfunction were very likely to have a partner with an erectile dysfunction (odds ratios 47.6 and 20.0, respectively).[8]

There are two additional data sets that have been utilized to investigate the sexual function of women whose male partners have erectile dysfunction. One new source of scientific data has been obtained from a large observational study, the Female Experience of Men's Attitudes to Life Events and Sexuality study.[9–11] In this investigation, data were analyzed from 283 women in eight countries whose male partners had erectile dysfunction. Women with men who had erectile dysfunction were asked multiple questions comparing their sexual activity, sexual function, and beliefs about sexuality before and since their partners experienced difficulty with their erections. Data from the women were stratified by the man's self-reported degree (mild, moderate, or severe) of erectile dysfunction.[9] In the Female Experience of Men's Attitudes to Life Events and Sexuality study, women whose partners had erectile dysfunction reported a lower frequency of sexual activity currently compared with before their partner developed erectile difficulties.[9,10] Significantly fewer women reported that they experienced sexual desire, sexual arousal, orgasm, or sexual satisfaction ("almost always" or "most times") currently compared with before their partners developed erectile difficulties. There was a significant correlation between the reduction in frequency of the woman's orgasm, the reduction in her sexual satisfaction, and the degree of her partner's self-reported erectile dysfunction (mild, moderate, severe).

Women had the lowest frequency of orgasm and the lowest satisfaction with the sexual experience when their partners had severe erectile dysfunction.

The diminished sexual response in these women was analyzed by current-use versus nonuse of phosphodiesterase type 5 inhibitors by the male partner.[10] Women whose partners were current users of phosphodiesterase type 5 therapy reported significantly greater frequency of desire (54% vs 43%), arousal (56% vs 40%), and orgasm (46% vs 30%) than did women whose partners were not current phosphodiesterase inhibitor type 5 users.

This study showed that a woman partnered with a man who had erectile dysfunction had significant negative sexual experiences compared with before her partner developed erectile dysfunction, and that the woman's loss of orgasm and satisfaction with the sexual experience correlated with the man's perception of the severity of his erectile dysfunction.[10]

The second source of scientific data has been obtained from a double-blind, multicenter, 3-month, randomized trial involving men with erectile dysfunction in heterosexual couples who were in a stable relationship for at least 6 months.[11] In this trial, women whose male partners had erectile dysfunction were asked at initial screening to complete the validated Female Sexual Function Index. Couples in which the female partner did *not* have sexual dysfunction, based on their baseline responses, were enrolled in the trial. Male partners with erectile dysfunction received placebo or selective phosphodiesterase type 5 inhibitor for 1 month, with an option to adjust the dose higher or lower based on erectile response after each of two consecutive, 1-month intervals. One outcome variable was the improvement of the woman's sexual quality of life. This was determined objectively by the woman's response to the quality of life domain of the modified Sexual Life Quality Questionnaire as well as other patient responses to that questionnaire.[11]

The selective phosphodiesterase type 5 inhibitor significantly improved the erectile quality of the men with erectile dysfunction compared to placebo. Compared with those men with erectile dysfunction treated with placebo, women whose partners were randomized to receiving active drug had significantly higher (1) sexual quality of life, (2) sexual confidence, (3) sexual pleasure, and (4) orgasm satisfaction.[11]

Summary

In summary, accumulating scientific evidence indicates that there are adverse effects on the sexual function of women whose male partners have erectile dysfunction. In addition, accumulating data support the hypothesis that there is an independent improvement in the sexual quality of life of women whose partners have erectile dysfunction and receive successful erectile dysfunction treatment. This supports the theory that that there is a close relationship between women's sexual response and the quality of the erectile responses of their male partners.

Women with men who have premature ejaculation

Introduction

Women with men who have premature ejaculation may have their own sexual function adversely affected. Since premature ejaculation is the most common male sexual dysfunction,[12] affecting approximately 25% of men, it is likely that many women experience a sexual relationship with a man with premature ejaculation. In addition, since only 5–10% of men receive treatment for premature ejaculation,[13] it is likely that women with men with premature ejaculation will have to deal with his sexual problem on a long-term basis. Premature ejaculation is objectively determined with a stopwatch to record intravaginal ejaculatory latency time defined as the time between vaginal intromission and intravaginal ejaculation. It has been suggested that an intravaginal ejaculatory latency time of 2 min or less may serve as a criterion for defining premature ejaculation.[14] Note that the diagnosis of premature ejaculation is somewhat controversial.[15]

Data

Women with men who have premature ejaculation may have significant distress, interpersonal difficulties, and dissatisfaction with sexual intercourse. The woman's distress is a common reason for the man to consult a clinician about premature ejaculation.

Byers et al. investigated the effect of premature ejaculation on 152 couples' sexual function.[16] Concerning the couple's perceptions of whether the premature ejaculation was a problem, reports of women and men were only moderately correlated. Women saw less of a problem for the men than the men reported for themselves. For both the women and the men, having more premature ejaculation characteristics was related to lower sexual satisfaction. The results suggest that, for most couples, the premature or early timing of ejaculation adversely affects sexual satisfaction.[16]

Patrick et al. carefully selected patients with and without premature ejaculation based on stopwatch testing.[15] The mean intravaginal ejaculatory latency time was 1.8 min in the 207 men with premature ejaculation. This was significantly lower than the time (7.3 min) in the 1380 men without premature ejaculation. Women whose men had premature ejaculation were found to differ significantly from women whose men did not have premature ejaculation in terms of decreased satisfaction with sexual intercourse and increased interpersonal difficulty and distress ($p < 0.0001$). More women partners of men with premature ejaculation than women whose partners did not have premature ejaculation claimed "poor" or "very poor" for satisfaction with sexual intercourse (28% vs 2%, respectively) and gave worse ratings ("quite a bit" or "extremely") for personal distress, couple relationship (44% vs

3%, respectively), and interpersonal difficulty (25% vs 2%, respectively) ($p < 0.0001$).[16]

Summary

Women whose partners experience premature ejaculation are adversely affected by the men's sexual dysfunction.

Conclusion

Both members of a couple experience aspects of the sexual dysfunction of the affected individual. Initial findings suggest that the woman whose male partner has erectile dysfunction or premature ejaculation often has concerns and distress about her own sexual function. It is important for clinicians to recognize that sexual dysfunction and its treatment are likely to have an effect on both members of the affected couple.

References

1. Riley A. The role of the partner in erectile dysfunction and its treatment. *Int J Impot Res* 2002; 14: S105–9.
2. Blumel JE, Castelo-Branco C, Cancelo MJ et al. Impairment of sexual activity in middle-aged women in Chile. *Menopause* 2004; 11: 78–81.
3. Paige NM, Hays RD, Litwin MS et al. Improvement in emotional well-being and relationships of users of sildenafil. *J Urol* 2001; 166: 1774–8.
4. Cayan S, Bozlu M, Canpolat B et al. The assessment of sexual functions in women with male partners complaining of erectile dysfunction: does treatment of male sexual dysfunction improve female partner's sexual functions? *J Sex Marital Ther* 2004; 30: 333–41.
5. Ichikawa T, Takao A, Manabe D et al. The female partner's satisfaction with sildenafil citrate treatment of erectile dysfunction. *Int J Urol* 2004; 11: 755–62.
6. Montorsi F, Althof SE. Partner responses to sildenafil citrate (Viagra) treatment of erectile dysfunction. *Urology* 2004; 63: 762–7.
7. Chevret M, Jaudinot E, Sullivan K et al. Quality of sexual life and satisfaction in female partners of men with ED: psychometric validation of the Index of Sexual Life (ISL) questionnaire. *J Sex Marital Ther* 2004; 30: 141–55.
8. Oberg K, Fugl-Meyer KS. On Swedish women's distressing sexual dysfunctions: some concomitant conditions and life satisfaction. *J Sex Med* 2005; 2: 169–80.
9. Fisher W, Rosen R, Sand M et al. Is there a correlation between ED severity and level of sexual concerns in the female partner? The FEMALES study. Abstract presented at 20th EAU Congress, Istanbul, Turkey, 2005.
10. Rosen R, Eardley I, Fisher W et al. *Effect on the Sexual Function of Female Partners of PDE5 use in Men with ED: The F.E.M.A.L.E.S. Study. J Sex Med* 2005; Suppl 1.
11. Fisher W, Rosen R, Brock G et al. Vardenafil improves treatment satisfaction and sexual pleasure in men with erectile dysfunction and their Partners. Abstract presented at 20th EAU Congress, Istanbul, Turkey, 2005.
12. Rowland DL, Perelman MA, Althof S et al. Self-reported premature ejaculation and aspects of sexual functioning and satisfaction. *J Sex Med* 2004; 1: 225–32.
13. Rosen R, Porst H, Montorsi F. The premature ejaculation prevalence and attitudes (PEPA) survey: a multi-national survey [abstract]. 11th World Congress of the International Society of Sexual and Impotence Research, 17–21 October 2004.
14. Rowland DL, Cooper SE, Schneider M. Defining premature ejaculation for experimental and clinical investigations. *Arch Sex Behav* 2001; 30: 235–53.
15. Patrick D, Althof S, Pryor JL et al. Premature ejaculation: an observational study of men and their partners. *J Sex Med* 2005; 2: 358–67.
16. Byers ES, Grenier G. Premature or rapid ejaculation: heterosexual couples' perceptions of men's ejaculatory behavior. *Arch Sex Behav* 2003; 32: 261–70.

Section 3

PSYCHOLOGIC AND BIOLOGIC MANAGEMENT

PATIENT HISTORY AND
PHYSICAL EXAMINATION

9.1 Classification and diagnosis of female sexual disorders

Sandra R Leiblum

The diagnosis of sexual behavior as either healthy or dysfunctional is mutable and subject to varying social and cultural expectations about sexual conduct, as well as being affected by greater sophistication of scientific knowledge, sexual psychophysiology, and current clinical practice. Consequently, it should come as no surprise that the classification of female sexual dysfunction is somewhat arbitrary, imprecise, and changeable.

In fact, the classification and diagnosis of sexual disorders are a challenging undertaking. Certain behaviors that were once considered aberrant are now widely accepted as normal (e.g., homosexual behavior), and what once was considered normal (e.g., lack of sexual enthusiasm or interest in women) has come to be considered dysfunctional. Women who displayed too much sexual interest were considered to be nymphomaniacs a century ago and were the object of medical attention and concern. Nowadays, hypoactive rather than hyperactive sexual desire is the most common female sexual dysfunction.[1,2]

Despite the fact that classification systems are changeable, they are necessary. They help order our knowledge and understanding of behavior. The classification of sexual disorders helps differentiate sexual complaints, that is, short-lived and transient disruptions or dissatisfactions with current sexual function, from sexual dysfunctions, persistent problems causing genuine personal distress (see Chapters 2.1–2.4 in this volume).

Thoughtful diagnoses help legitimatize sexual disorders as warranting attention and intervention from health professionals. A sound sexual nosology helps justify treatment reimbursement by insurance carriers and/or managed care providers. Identification of agreed-upon diagnostic entities serves as a stimulus for research and treatment. Well-defined diagnoses of sexual problems permit the development of assessment instruments and help with the identification of reasonable endpoints for treatment, whether pharmacologic or psychologic (see Chapter 16.1). A widely accepted diagnostic nomenclature provides a common language for communication between health-care professionals involved in the remediation of those disorders. Perhaps most important in recent years has been the recognition that accurate, reliable, and valid diagnoses are essential for determining inclusion or exclusion into research or clinical trials that investigate new pharmacotherapy, and hormonal or psychologic treatment interventions (see Chapter 11.2).

Historical overview

In reviewing how definitions of sexual dysfunction have evolved over the last 50 years, changes in the American Psychiatric Association's *Diagnostic and Statistical Manual of Mental Disorders* (DSM) provide a good starting point. In the first edition (DSM-I), which appeared in 1952,[3] there were no diagnostic terms for sexual dysfunction, although the manual did include a section on sexual deviations. The second edition (DSM-II) (1968) included two sets of diagnostic terms for sexual disorders, which appeared in the section entitled "Psychophysiologic disorders". These were described as physical symptoms caused by emotional factors involving a single organ system, as in relation to menstruation, micturition, and the two sexual disorders of dyspareunia (painful intercourse) and impotence (difficulties in obtaining or maintaining an erection). There was no identification of possible problems involving sexual drive, orgasm, or early or delayed ejaculation. The underlying hypothesis guiding these terms was the belief that the problems were basically psychophysiologic in nature, although both DSM-I and DSM-II were based on psychoanalytic theories. This approach to psychiatric diagnosis was abandoned by American psychiatry in 1980 with the publication of the third edition (DSM-III).

The nomenclature of female sexual dysfunction changed dramatically as a consequence of the publication of *Human Sexual Response* by Masters and Johnson in 1966[4] and their subsequent volume, *Human Sexual Inadequacy* (1970).[5] Masters and Johnson described a sexual response cycle which they considered characteristic of both men and women. It consisted of four phases: excitement, plateau, orgasm, and resolution. Shortly after their description of the sexual response cycle, Helen Singer Kaplan (1977)[6] amended it to include a salient missing phase, namely, that of sexual desire (see Chapter 1.1).

Sexual dysfunctions were then linked to each phase, and these became the foundation on which the psychosexual diagnoses described in the third edition of the DSM (DSM-III, 1980) were based. Inhibition of the appetitive or psychophysiologic changes that characterize the normal sexual response cycle was considered pathologic. However, the diagnosis of a psychosexual dysfunction was not made if the disorder was considered to be primarily due to organic factors such as a physical disease or condition, medication, or another Axis I disorder.

DSM-III included five terms for psychosexual disorders: inhibited sexual desire, inhibited sexual excitement (variously described as frigidity or impotence), inhibited female orgasm, inhibited male orgasm, premature ejaculation, functional dyspareunia, and functional vaginismus. In order to qualify for diagnosis, the disorder had to be due to something other than organic factors.

A notable change occurred in the revision of the third edition of the DSM (DSM-III-R), published in 1987. What had formerly been described as psychosexual dysfunction were now described as "sexual dysfunctions", but the essential feature of diagnosis remained the belief that the responsible agent underlying dysfunction was psychologic inhibition. Interestingly, DSM-III-R acknowledged that, while there was no empirical evidence of an association between personality traits and sexual dysfunction, it was clear that anxiety, high internal standards for sexual performance, and unusual sensitivity to real or imagined rejection by a sexual partner predisposed the individual to the development of sexual disorder.

DSM-III-R did include greater recognition of subjective experience as relevant to diagnosis. For instance, in the diagnosis of female arousal disorder, "persistent or recurrent lack of a subjective sense of sexual excitement and pleasure during sexual activity" was integral to diagnosis. However, the definition of orgasmic disorders retained the term "inhibited", suggesting an underlying psychologic etiology.

Things changed significantly with the publication of the fourth edition (1994) of the DSM (DSM-IV), which devoted an entire section to the diagnosis of sexual disorders. The belief that psychologic inhibition interfers with the ability to experience orgasm had not been supported by an evidence-based review of the literature; therefore, the diagnosis of orgasmic disorders was substantially changed. The idea that psychopathologic disorders are caused primarily by psychologic inhibition was abandoned. Psychosexual disorders were described as disturbances, in sexual desire and in the psychophysiologic changes that characterize the sexual response cycle, which cause marked distress and interpersonal difficulty.

There was no attempt to specify a specific frequency of sexual behavior or activity as normative or deviant. Rather, the determination of whether a condition warranted diagnosis was to be made by the clinician, taking into account such factors as the age and experience of the individual, the frequency and chronicity of symptoms, the degree of subjective distress, and the impact on other areas of function. In addition, the clinician was advised to consider the contributions of an individual's ethnic, cultural, religious, and social background which might influence sexual desire, expectations, and attitudes to sexual performance.

With the growing recognition that general medical conditions and substance use affect sexual function, DSM-IV includes diagnoses for sexual dysfunction caused by a medical condition and substance-induced sexual dysfunction. The essential feature of sexual dysfunction caused by a general medical condition was the assumption that the sexual dysfunction was a result of the direct physiologic effects of a generalized medical condition: "there must be evidence from the history, physical examination, or laboratory findings that the dysfunction is fully explained by the direct physiologic effects of a general medical condition".[3]

It is now widely acknowledged that it is nearly impossible to separate conditions that are primarily due to organic causes from those with psychologic etiologies, since the overlap is so considerable.[7] Indeed, in most instances, the exact pathogenesis of sexual dysfunction is uncertain, and multiple psychologic, interpersonal, and organic contributions are involved.

Female sexual dysfunction reconsidered: recent developments

Many clinicians and researchers were dissatisfied with the DSM-IV diagnoses of female sexual problems.[8,9] They objected to the heterosexist, phallocentric model of sexual behavior on which the diagnoses were based, with intercourse being considered the reference standard or referent for many of the diagnoses. They believed that it was inaccurate to present male and female disorders as parallel representations of the same phenomenon when, in fact, women's arousal and pain disorders were quite different from those experienced by men.

The diagnostic categories in DSM-IV were organized in such a way as to suggest that sexual response unfolded in a clear-cut linear sequence of desire, arousal, and orgasm, although there was evidence that a more circular and interactive model applied with arousal and desire influencing and stimulating each other. Moreover, research evidence indicated that diagnoses tended to co-occur, with desire and arousal being particularly difficult to separate.[10]

Of particular importance was the lack of recognition of the

emotional and interpersonal aspects of sexual exchange. There was little acknowledgment that sexual behavior usually occurs in an interpersonal context and that the adequacy and acceptability of past and current relationship, partner function/dysfunction, sexual incentives and motivation, adequacy of stimulation, and other environmental and contextual variables are crucial in assessing and evaluating sexual function or dysfunction.

Finally, the DSM-IV separation of disorders into those due primarily to either medical or psychologic factors was felt to be unjustified, since as noted above, the etiology of nearly all sexual dysfunctions tends to be a complicated admixture of organic, psychogenic, and interpersonal factors.

Consensus conferences to reconsider diagnosis of female sexual dysfunction

With these limitations in mind, a consensus conference was convened by the sexual function health council of the American Foundation for Urologic Disease in 1998 to review and update the classification of female sexual disorders.[11] A multidisciplinary group of European and North American academic and clinical experts in the field of women's sexuality reviewed the published evidence, debated and discussed the current nosology, and recommended modifications of the DSM-IV definitions of female sexual dysfunction.

Although the resulting document continued to rely on the traditional model of sexual response, small but important modifications were made to each definition. For example, the DSM-IV definition of hypoactive sexual desire was amended to emphasize the importance of receptive as well as intrinsic desire for women. In DSM-IV, hypoactive sexual desire disorder was defined as "persistently or recurrently deficient (or absent) sexual fantasies and desire for sexual activity". The consensus conference redefined the disorder as "persistent or recurrent deficiency (or absence) of sexual fantasies, and/or desire for, or receptivity to, sexual activity which causes personal distress".[11] This was based on research highlighting the finding that many women do not routinely experience spontaneous sexual desire but are receptive to, and interested in, sexual activity once underway and subjective sexual excitement is experienced.[12]

The revised definition of orgasmic disorder emphasized the importance of sufficient sexual stimulation and sexual arousal as intrinsic to the diagnosis of orgasmic disorder. If sexual arousal is insufficient or inadequate, the appropriate diagnosis would be arousal disorder.

The sexual pain disorders were extended to include a third category of pain, noncoital sexual pain, to acknowledge that pain may be experienced and reported by the woman during sexual activities other than intercourse.

Female sexual arousal disorder proved to be the sexual dysfunction most difficult to describe accurately, since, historically, it had rarely been diagnosed independently of desire or orgasm disorders. While the presence of lubrication was generally seen as the hallmark of sexual arousal, a sizeable body of psychophysiologic research highlighted the fact that the correlation between lubrication or vasocongestion and women's report of subjective arousal was rather inconsistent.[13-16] In order to acknowledge the importance of mental or subjective arousal as primary when making a diagnosis, the new definition of female sexual arousal disorder became "persistent or recurrent inability to attain or maintain sufficient sexual excitement causing personal distress. It may be expressed as a lack of subjective excitement or a lack of genital lubrication/swelling or other somatic response."[11]

Each specified disorder had to be accompanied by the women's report of personal distress about the complaint. This was emphasized in order to avoid pathologizing normative variations in female sexual response and to underline the fact that women experience alterations in their sexual life that are often not experienced as personally distressing even though they may be distressing to a partner (e.g., failure to attain an orgasm during intercourse).

Subtypes of disorders were to be specified as either lifelong or acquired, generalized or situational. In order to acknowledge that the causes of sexual dysfunction are often unknown, it was suggested that a new category be added to the list of etiologic determinants. Thus, the etiologic specifiers of a disorder became organic, psychogenic, mixed, or unknown. It was hoped that the addition of the "unknown" category would stimulate innovative research.

Problems with diagnoses remain

While these changes were valuable, there remained dissatisfaction with the revised diagnoses. In part, the problem stemmed from the continued reliance on what was seen to be an invalid model of women's sexual response cycle. The traditional model, namely, that described by Masters and Johnson in 1966,[4] seemed to fit men better than women with its inherent linearity and sequential stages of desire, arousal, and orgasm.[1] Basson[17] and others[18,19] challenged the assumption that desire invariably precedes arousal when, in fact, sexual arousal appears to trigger awareness and feelings of sexual desire for many women. Further, the lack of specificity regarding the various presentations of sexual arousal problems was viewed as problematic, since deficits in genital arousal are typically due to different causes and necessitate different interventions than deficits in subjective or mental arousal.

In light of these shortcomings, a second consensus conference was convened by the Sexual Health Council of the American Foundation of Urologic Diseases in 2003. The group was charged with undertaking a comprehensive review of the evidence supporting or refuting the existing definitions and was asked to offer recommendations for revision.

Latest recommendations proposed by the second consensus conference on female sexual nosology (2003)

As with the first consensus conference, an international and interdisciplinary group of clinical and research experts in female sexuality was recruited to revise and update the diagnoses. After a comprehensive, evidence-based review of published research, the following revisions in the diagnostic nomenclature of women's sexual dysfunctions were made (Table 9.1.1).[1]

Hypoactive sexual desire disorder was renamed "women's sexual interest/desire disorder" and was defined as follows: absent or diminished feelings of sexual interest or desire, absent sexual thoughts or fantasies, and lack of responsive desire. Motivation (here defined as reasons/incentives) to attempt to become sexually aroused is weak or absent. The lack of interest is considered to be beyond a normative lessening with life cycle and relationship duration.

The word "interest" was used along with the word "desire" in the new definition to reflect the fact that many women engage in sex for reasons other than intrinsic physical desire. In fact, a multiplicity of motives for initiating or engaging in sex exist apart from physical desire, including such incentives as wanting to please or placate a partner, wanting a "reward" from a partner, or, more negatively, wanting to forestall anticipated anger or punishment.[19–21]

The new definition acknowledges that there are fluctuations in desire that occur with age, life cycle, and relationship duration as well as with current contextual factors, and that lack of desire may be normative and even adaptive depending on the circumstances of a woman's life. Furthermore, the de-emphasis on sexual fantasies or thoughts as a hallmark of desire was deliberate, since many women report a total absence of sexual thoughts and/or fantasies despite good arousal and receptive desire.[22–24] What is considered crucial in the new definition is the persistent absence of receptive desire and motivation to be sexual along with personal distress about the condition.

Considerable changes were made in the diagnoses of sexual arousal (Table 9.1.2). In order to highlight the repeated observation that subjective arousal does not always strongly correlate with genital congestion,[13–16] the definition of female sexual arousal disorder was subdivided into three specific categories: subjective, genital, and combined. The new definitions are as follows:

● "subjective sexual arousal disorder": absence of or markedly diminished feelings of sexual arousal (sexual excitement and sexual pleasure) from any type of sexual stimulation. Vaginal lubrication or other signs of physical response still occur.
● "genital sexual arousal disorder": complaints of absent or impaired genital sexual arousal. Self-reports may include minimal vulval swelling or vaginal lubrication from any type of sexual stimulation and reduced sexual sensations from caressing genitalia. Subjective sexual excitement still occurs from nongenital sexual stimuli.

● "combined genital and subjective arousal disorder": absence of, or markedly diminished feelings of, sexual arousal (sexual excitement and sexual pleasure) from any type of sexual stimulation as well as complaints of absent or impaired genital sexual arousal (vulval swelling, lubrication).

While genital and combined arousal disorders reflect complaints that are quite common among certain populations of women (e.g., those who have undergone surgical menopause without hormonal replacement, who are receiving chemotherapy, or who have sustained autonomic nerve impairment), women who complain about lack of mental excitement or subjective arousal often report no problems with vaginal lubrication. In fact, they may have perfectly adequate vasocongestion but feel an absence of mental excitement or a feeling of being "turned on". Consequently, the treatment of women who lack mental excitement may be quite different from that of women who report lack of genital arousal. The former group of women may benefit from treatment that helps them better focus on their sexual arousal and overcome existing feelings of guilt, inhibition, or distraction due to their past history or present circumstance, whereas women with genital or combined arousal disorders may derive greater benefit from hormonal therapy or pharmacotherapy.[24]

The combined subjective/genital arousal disorder is the most common sexual arousal complaint and is usually comorbid with a lack of sexual desire/interest that must be treated along with (or instead of) the arousal complaint.

Finally, a new category of female arousal disorder was described and recommended for provisional inclusion in the revised diagnostic system, namely, persistent sexual arousal syndrome.[25,26] This syndrome was based on the reports of many clinicians who had seen (or were seeing) women who complained of excessive and persistent vaginal and clitoral sexual arousal in the absence of conscious feelings of sexual desire. The feelings of genital arousal were described as unwanted and intrusive and did not subside with one or more orgasms. A normal refractory or resolution period was missing, and the feelings of genital vasocongestion and tingling occurred without an identifiable stimulus or trigger.

"Persistent sexual arousal disorder" was defined as spontaneous, intrusive, and unwanted genital arousal (e.g., tingling, throbbing, pulsating) in the absence of sexual interest and desire. Any awareness of subjective arousal is typically but not invariably unpleasant. The arousal is unrelieved by one or more orgasms, and the feelings of arousal persist for hours or days.

It was hoped that by offering a provisional definition of this complaint, research in the etiology, epidemiology, and treatment of persistent arousal would be stimulated.

The definition of orgasmic disorder was clarified in order to emphasize that adequate sexual arousal must be present before making the diagnosis, since, in the past, the criterion of high or "adequate" arousal was often ignored.

The revised diagnosis of "women's orgasmic disorder"

(Table 9.1.3) now specifies that, despite the self-report of high sexual arousal/excitement, there is either lack of orgasm, markedly diminished intensity of orgasmic sensations, or marked delay of orgasm from any kind of stimulation.

The definitions of dyspareunia and vaginismus were updated and amended (Table 9.1.4).

"Dyspareunia" is defined as persistent or recurrent pain with attempted or complete vaginal entry and/or penile vaginal intercourse. This definition avoids the emphasis on pain during coitus as being essential to the diagnosis, since pain may be experienced with any attempt at vaginal insertion or even with only the anticipation of vaginal pain from past experiences.

The new definition of "vaginismus" is persistent difficulty in allowing vaginal entry of a penis, a finger, and/or any object, despite the woman's expressed wish to do so. There is variable involuntary pelvic muscle contraction, (phobic) avoidance, and anticipation/fear/experience of pain. Structural or other physical abnormalities must be ruled out/addressed. The new

Table 9.1.1. Changing definitions of women's sexual desire disorders

DSM-IV-TR[30] definition of hypoactive sexual desire disorder
Persistently or recurrently deficient (or absent) sexual fantasies and desire for sexual activity. The judgment of deficiency or absence is made by the clinician, taking into account factors that affect sexual functioning such as age and the context of the person's life. The disturbance causes marked distress or interpersonal difficulty. The sexual dysfunction is not better accounted for by another Axis I disorder (except another sexual dysfunction) and is not due exclusively to the direct physiologic effects of a substance (e.g., a drug of abuse, a medication) or a general medical condition.

Consensus Conference 2000 definition of hypoactive sexual desire disorder
The persistent or recurrent deficiency (or absence) of sexual fantasies/thoughts, and/or desire for or receptivity to sexual activity, which causes personal distress.

Consensus Conference 2003 definition of women's sexual interest/desire disorder
Absent or diminished feelings of sexual interest or desire, absent sexual thoughts or fantasies and a lack of responsive desire. Motivations (here defined as reasons/incentives), for attempting to become sexually aroused are scarce or absent. The lack of interest is considered to be beyond a normative lessening with life cycle and relationship duration.

DSM-IV-TR definition of sexual aversion disorder
Persistent or recurrent extreme aversion to, and avoidance of, all (or almost all) genital contact with a sexual partner. The disturbance causes marked distress or interpersonal difficulty. The sexual dysfunction is not better accounted for by another Axis I disorder (except another sexual dysfunction).

Consensus Conference 2000 definition of sexual aversion disorder
Persistent or recurrent phobic aversion to and avoidance of sexual contact with a sexual partner, which causes personal distress.

Consensus Conference 2003 definition of sexual aversion disorder
Extreme anxiety and/or disgust at the anticipation of/or attempt to have any sexual activity.

Table 9.1.2. Changing definitions of women's sexual arousal disorders

DSM-IV-TR[30] definition of female sexual arousal disorder
Persistent or recurrent inability to attain, or to maintain until completion of the sexual activity, an adequate lubrication–swelling response to sexual excitement. The disturbance causes marked distress or interpersonal difficulty. The sexual dysfunction is not better accounted for by another Axis I disorder (except another sexual dysfunction) and is not due exclusively to the direct physiologic effects of a substance (e.g., a drug of abuse, a medication) or a general medical condition.

Consensus Conference 2000 definition of female sexual arousal disorder
The persistent or recurrent inability to attain or maintain sufficient sexual excitement, causing personal distress, which may be expressed as a lack of subjective excitement, or genital (lubrication/swelling) or other somatic responses.

Consensus Conference 2003 definition of subjective sexual arousal disorder
Absence of or markedly diminished feelings of sexual arousal (sexual excitement and sexual pleasure) from any type of sexual stimulation. Vaginal lubrication or other signs of physical response still occur.

Consensus Conference 2003 definition of genital sexual arousal disorder
Absent or impaired genital sexual arousal. Self-report may include minimal vulval swelling or vaginal lubrication from any type of sexual stimulation and reduced sexual sensations from caressing genitalia. Subjective sexual excitement still occurs from nongenital sexual stimuli.

Consensus Conference 2003 definition of combined genital and subjective arousal disorder
Absence of or markedly diminished feelings of sexual arousal (sexual excitement and sexual pleasure) from any type of sexual stimulation as well as complaints of absent or impaired genital sexual arousal (vulval swelling, lubrication).

Consensus Conference 2003 definition of persistent sexual arousal disorder (provisional diagnosis)
Spontaneous, intrusive and unwanted genital arousal (e.g., tingling, throbbing, pulsating) in the absence of sexual interest and desire. Any awareness of subjective arousal is typically but not invariably unpleasant. The arousal is unrelieved by one or more orgasms, and the feelings of arousal persist for hours or days.

definition avoids the suggestion that a vaginal spasm is responsible for the inability to tolerate vaginal insertion, given the recent empirical finding that the vaginal muscle spasm is unreliable.[27] Rather, reflexive involuntary contraction of the pelvic muscles in addition to thigh adduction, contraction of the abdominal muscles, and the description of fear and/or anxiety are associated with attempts to insert any object, be it a penis, tampon, speculum, or finger, into the vaginal introitus. When accompanied by great discomfort and pain, vaginismus may be diagnosed even if vaginal insertion is possible.

Finally, sexual aversion disorder was retained as a sexual diagnosis, although some felt that it might be better seen as a phobia and treated as such. The decision to retain it as part of sexual nosology was based on the sexual context in which the symptoms occur, its typical etiology, and the reliance on sex therapy interventions for successful resolution.

Table 9.1.3. Changing definitions of female orgasmic disorder

DSM-IV-TR[30] Definition of female orgasmic disorder
Persistent or recurrent delay in, or absence of, orgasm following a normal sexual excitement phase. Women exhibit wide variability in the type or intensity of stimulation that triggers orgasm. The diagnosis of female orgasmic disorder should be based on the clinician's judgment that the woman's orgasmic capacity is less than would be reasonable for her age, sexual experience, and the adequacy of sexual stimulation she receives. The disturbance causes marked distress or interpersonal difficulty. The orgasmic dysfunction is not better accounted for by another Axis I disorder (except another sexual dysfunction) and is not due exclusively to the direct physiological effects of a substance (e.g., a drug of abuse, a medication) or a general medical condition.

Consensus Conference 2000 definition of female orgasmic disorder
Persistent or recurrent difficulty, delay in or absence of attaining orgasm following sufficient sexual stimulation and arousal, which causes personal distress.

Consensus Conference 2003 definition of women's orgasmic disorder
Despite the self-report of high sexual arousal/excitement, there is either lack of orgasm, markedly diminished intensity of orgasmic sensations, or marked delay of orgasm from any kind of stimulation.

Table 9.1.4. Changing definitions of women's sexual pain disorders

DSM-IV-TR[30] definitions of sexual pain disorders
Dyspareunia: recurrent or persistent genital pain associated with sexual intercourse. The disturbance causes marked distress or interpersonal difficulty. The disturbance is not caused exclusively by vaginismus or lack of lubrication, is not better accounted for by another Axis I disorder (except another sexual dysfunction), and is not due exclusively to the direct physiologic effects of a substance (e.g., a drug of abuse, a medication) or a general medical condition.
 Vaginismus: recurrent or persistent involuntary spasm of the musculature of the outer third of the vagina that interferes with sexual intercourse. The disturbance causes marked distress or interpersonal difficulty. The disturbance is not better accounted for by another Axis I disorder (e.g., somatization disorder) and is not due exclusively to the direct physiologic effects of a general medical condition.

Consensus Conference 2000 definitions of sexual pain disorders
Dyspareunia: recurrent or persistent genital pain associated with sexual intercourse.
 Vaginismus: recurrent or persistent involuntary spasm of the musculature of the outer third of the vagina that interferes with vaginal penetration, which causes personal distress.
 Noncoital pain disorder: recurrent or persistent genital pain induced by noncoital sexual stimulation.

Consensus Conference 2003 definitions of sexual pain disorders
Dyspareunia: persistent or recurrent pain with attempted or complete vaginal entry and/or penile vaginal intercourse.
 Vaginismus: persistent difficulties to allow vaginal entry of a penis, a finger, and/or any object, despite the woman's expressed wish to do so. There is variable involuntary pelvic muscle contraction, (phobic) avoidance, and anticipation/fear/ experience of pain. Structural or other physical abnormalities must be ruled out/addressed.

"Sexual aversion disorder" was defined as extreme anxiety and/or disgust at the anticipation of/or attempt to have any sexual activity.

Etiologic specifiers recommended

In addition to revising the existing definitions of female sexual dysfunction, the committee felt it was important to include some indication as to the possible etiologic or maintaining factors associated with the problem. It was believed that if the significant contextual and interpersonal contributions to the problem could be determined at the time of diagnosis, more relevant and sensible treatment interventions could be offered.

 It was recommended that the following three classes of specifiers or descriptors be included when making a diagnosis:

I. Negative upbringing/losses/trauma (physical, sexual, emotional), past interpersonal relationships, cultural/religious restrictions
II. Current interpersonal difficulties, partner sexual dysfunction, inadequate stimulation, and unsatisfactory sexual and emotional contexts
III. Medical conditions, psychiatric conditions, medications, substance abuse.

For many women, all three classes of factors are implicated in the development and maintenance of a problem: a developmental history marred by loss, trauma or inhibition, an unsatisfactory partner relationship characterized by conflict or partner sexual dysfunction, and medications which interfere with sexual desire or arousal. In these cases, all three descriptors should be given along with the diagnosis.

 As in the past, it was recommended that disorders be identified as either lifelong or acquired, generalized, or situational.

Assessment of distress

Finally, in light of the fact that women report varying levels of distress associated with sexual difficulties, it was recommended that an indication of relative distress be included as part of the diagnosis. Ratings of subjective distress may have important implications for treatment motivation and outcome. At the simplest level, it was recommended that a rating of none, mild, moderate, or severe distress might suffice, based on the women's self-report, although validated distress measures were seen as preferable, such as the Female Sexual Distress Scale[28] or the Sexual Satisfaction Scale for Women, which includes measures of personal and interpersonal distress.[29]

Conclusions

As is evident from this brief review of changes in the conceptualization and description of women's sexual response cycle and definition of female sexual disorders, reasonable and accurate diagnosis of sexual dysfunction in women is a challenging undertaking. As greater sophistication and understanding of the biologic, neurologic, psychologic, interpersonal, and cultural contributions to women's sexuality occur, there will be a need for still more diagnostic amendments.

The recently revised definitions of female sexual disorders are certainly an improvement over earlier definitions. They are based on a model of women's sexual response cycle that is a more accurate depiction of women's sexual reality, as well as being based more closely on evidence-based research. The revised definitions provide greater specificity in and refinement of the variety of sexual arousal disorders in women that should prove helpful in guiding both research and clinical intervention. Although the diagnoses are more specific and detailed than earlier iterations, they do reflect the complexity of women's sexuality and are currently guiding the development of standardized diagnostic interviews.

However, the revised diagnoses remain recommendations at this time. They have not yet been officially adopted by the DSM or the World Health Organization's *International Classification of Diseases*. At present, the most widely accepted nomenclature for the diagnosis of women's sexual disorders continues to be those found in the "Text Revision" of DSM-IV (DSM-IV-TR), published in 2000, or the first consensus conference.[11]

Finally, these definitions will undoubtedly continue to evolve with new research and clinical data illuminating the anatomic, neurologic, physiologic, psychologic, interpersonal, and cultural contributions to women's sexual function.

References

1. Lauman E, Paik A, Rosen R. Sexual dysfunction in the United States: prevalence and predictors. JAMA 1999; 281: 537–44.
2. Fugl-Meyer A, Fuel-Meyer S. Sexual disabilities, problems and satisfaction in 18 to 74 year old Swedes. Scand J Sexol 1999; 2: 79–105.
3. American Psychiatric Association. DSM-I: Diagnostic and Statistical Manual of Mental Disorders. Washington, DC: American Psychiatric Press, 1952.
4. Masters WH, Johnson VE. Human Sexual Response. Boston: Little, Brown, 1966.
5. Masters WH, Johnson VE. Human Sexual Inadequacy. Boston: Little, Brown, 1970.
6. Kaplan SH. Hypoactive sexual desire. J Sex Marital Ther 1977; 3: 3–9.
7. Basson R, Leiblum S, Brotto L et al. Definitions of women's sexual dysfunction reconsidered: advocating expansion and revision. J Psychosom Obstet Gynecol 2003; 24: 221–9.
8. Tiefer L. Historical, scientific, clinical and feminist criticisms of the "human sexual response cycle" model. Annu Rev Sex Res 1995; 6: 32–76.
9. Leiblum SR. Definition and classification of female sexual disorders. Int J Impot Res 1998; 10: S104–6.
10. Segraves KB, Segraves RT. Hypoactive sexual desire disorder: prevalence and comorbidity in 906 subjects. J Sex Marital Ther 1991; 17: 55–8.
11. Basson R, Berman J, Burnett A et al. Report of the international consensus development conference on female sexual dysfunction: definitions and classifications. J Urol 2000; 163: 888–93.
12. Lunde I, Larson GK, Fog E et al. Sexual desire, orgasm and sexual fantasies: a study of 625 Danish women born in 1910, 1936 and 1958. J Sex Educ Ther 1991; 17: 111–15.
13. Meston CM, Gorzalka BB. The effects of sympathetic activation on physiological and subjective arousal in women. Behav Res Ther 1995; 33: 651–64.
14. Meston CM, Gorzalka BB. The effects of immediate, delayed and residual sympathetic activation on physiological and subjective sexual arousal in women. Behav Res Ther 1996; 34: 143–8.
15. Laan E, Everaerd W. Determinants of female sexual arousal: psychophysiological theory and data. Annu Rev Sex Res 1995; 6: 32–76.
16. Brotto LA, Gorzalka B. Genital and subjective arousal in postmenopausal women: influence of laboratory induced hyperventilation. J Sex Marital Ther 2002; 28S: 39–53.
17. Basson RJ. Using a different model for female sexual response to address women's problematic low sexual desire. J Sex Marital Ther 2001; 27: 395–403.
18. Leiblum S. Sexual problems and dysfunction: epidemiology, classification and risk factors. J Gend Specific Med 1999; 2: 41–5.
19. Leiblum S. Redefining sexual response. Contemp Obstet Gynec 2000; 45: 120–6.
20. Basson R, Leiblum S, Brotto L et al. Definitions of women's sexual dysfunction reconsidered: advocating expansion and revision. J Psychosom Obstet Gynecol 2003; 24: 221–9.
21. Galyer K, Conaglen H, Hare A et al. The effect of gynecological surgery on sexual desire. J Sex Marital Ther 1999; 25: 81–8.
22. Hill CA, Preston LK. Individual differences in the experience of sexual motivation: theory and measurement of dispositional sexual motives. J Sex Res 1996; 33: 27–45.
23. Regan P, Berscheid E. Belief about the states, goals, and objects of sexual desire. J Sex Marital Ther 1996; 22: 110–20.
24. Leiblum S. Arousal disorders in women: complaints and complexities. Med J Aust 2003; 6: 638–40.
25. Leiblum S, Nathan S. Persistent sexual arousal in women: a not uncommon but little recognized complaint. Sex Relat Ther 2002; 17: 191–8.
26. Leiblum S, Grazziottin A. Il disturbo dell'eccitazione sessuale persistente nelle donne. Principi e practica di terapia sessuale. In S Leiblum, R Rosen, A Graziottin, eds. Roma: CIC Edizione Internazaionali, 2004: 239–47.
27. Reissing ED, Binik YM, Khalifé S et al. Vaginal spasm, pain, and behavior: an empirical investigation of the diagnosis of vaginismus. Arch Sex Behav 2004; 33: 5–17.
28. Derogatis L, Rosen R, Leiblum S et al. The female sexual distress scale (FSDS): initial validation of a standardized scale for the assessment of sexually related personal distress in women. J Sex Marital Ther 2002; 28: 317–30.

29. Meston CM, Trapnell PD. Development and validation of a five factor sexual satisfaction and distress scale: the Sexual Satisfaction Scale for Women (SSS-W). *J Sex Med* 2005; 2: 66–81.

9.2 Medical history, including gynecologic history

Kalli Varaklis

Introduction

The medical history represents a comprehensive overview of the patient's health, with detailed information regarding the specific issue that has caused the patient to seek medical attention. It is obtained primarily from the patient as well as available past medical records. The history is collected in a logical sequence, allowing the patient's issues to be organized for the practitioner and other health-care providers as needed. The general outline of the medical history includes the chief complaint, history of the present illness, gynecologic history, obstetric history, past medical and surgical history, medications, allergies, personal habits, social history, family history, and review of symptoms. Regarding the gynecologic history, areas to be included are menstrual history, sexual history, contraception, gynecologic infection, Pap smear history, gynecologic surgery history, urologic history, and gynecologic review of systems.

General guidelines for history taking

The patient interview should take place in a room that ensures complete privacy and has enough space for the patient to feel comfortable. The health-care professional should knock on the door first, and make eye contact with the patient when entering. The health-care professional should introduce themself to the patient and to any accompanying persons. The relationships of those persons to the patient should be ascertained at the beginning of the interview. The health-care professional should always be courteous and professional, and it is always appropriate to address the patient formally. Although this may be difficult at times, the health-care professional should try to be relaxed so that the patient does not feel rushed.

The interview should start with an exploratory approach, using open-ended questions to allow the patient to use her own words and express herself freely. This will allow the patient to bring up issues that are perceived as more interesting and more acute to her. This also affords the interviewer the opportunity to listen for verbal cues that are indications of any other issues that are important to the patient. Listening carefully and attentively will convey to the patient that the physician is interested and concerned about her issues.

As the interview continues, open-ended questions should probe the issue that brought the patient to the health-care provider. Then progress to more directed questions will allow development of a more precise and complete history of the present problem. However, one should try not to ask questions that require only a "yes" or "no" answer from the patient, and be wary of asking leading questions, which may elicit answers the patient thinks her physician wants to hear. If there is a language barrier, make every effort to have an independent, professional interpreter available. If the patient has brought an interpreter with her, be aware of the relationship to the patient and how that may influence the completeness of the history being given, particularly if there are sensitive issues to discuss. Note any additional barriers that may influence the medical history the patient is giving. Issues around substance use, domestic violence, and noncompliance can sometimes influence the accuracy and completeness of the history.

During the interview, try to maintain as much eye contact as possible and make notes sparingly. As many office practices are turning to computerized office note systems, it is imperative that the health-care provider not look at the computer monitor and type while the patient is speaking. Language that the patient will understand should be used, avoiding unnecessarily complex medical terminology. Choose words that are understandable to the patient, yet are not overly simple or demeaning. Avoid any terms of endearment, as they may be perceived as patronizing by the patient.

At the end of the history taking, the health-care professional should try to give a summary of what was understood, and offer the patient the opportunity to add anything she may have forgotten. "Is there anything else you think would be important for me to know?" Further signal the end of the interview segment of the visit by explaining to the patient what will happen during the physical examination, if that is to follow the history.

Taking a comprehensive patient history

Chief complaint

The chief complaint is the brief summary of why the patient is seeking medical attention, in the patient's own words. The health-care practitioner should ask an open-ended questions in order to elicit the main purpose of the visit: "What is the problem that has brought you in to the clinic today?", "What concerns do you have for today's visit?", "What brings you in today?" are examples of a good way to start a conversation that does not assume that there is a problem. The patient should be allowed to express herself without interruption. Other significant secondary issues may surface during this introduction and should be thoroughly explored.

History of present of illness

The history of present of illness describes the detailed information that is relevant to the chief complaint. It should answer when the problem started, the duration of the condition, the detailed symptoms and their development over time. Organizing this section chronologically is a very reasonable way to understand the nature of the problem. It is preferable to start this portion of the interview with open-ended questions and then utilize more directed questions to elicit specific information. The objective of this section is to generate a hypothesis about what could be causing the problem. During this section of the history, the physician can ask specific questions to test further the hypothesis being formulated.

Gynecologic history

Obtaining a thorough gynecologic history is imperative for the patient who presents for evaluation of female sexual dysfunction. For some patients, the gynecologic history is a sensitive subject that may elicit feelings of embarrassment or shame. The physician should be sensitive to any signs of discomfort. Asking questions in an objective, matter-of-fact way, using formal but understandable language, will help the patient to feel more comfortable discussing sensitive issues.

Menstrual history

The health-care professional should start by asking the date of the last menstrual period. Note the regularity of the menstrual cycle, and the duration of the bleeding, as well as the character of the blood loss. Inquire about the symptoms associated with menses. Does the patient have dysmenorrhea, and, if so, does she miss time from work or school because of her pain? Has she always had dysmenorrhea or has this developed recently? Does she have diarrhea, sweating, or migraine with her menses? What kind of sanitary protection does she use? Does the patient describe herself as suffering from premenstrual symptoms? If so, what are her symptoms? When do the premenstrual symptoms start in terms of her menstrual cycle, and are they relieved by the onset of menses? Note also the age of menarche. If there was any developmental delay, inquire about when secondary sexual characteristics appeared and whether any workup was initiated.

Sexual history

This section of the gynecologic history will be covered in great depth later in Chapter 9.4 of this volume.

Contraception

The patient should be asked whether she currently uses any form of contraception (see Chapter 7.6). If so, what kind of contraception does she use currently and what has she used in the past? Has she had any side effects or complications from any kind of contraception in the past? Does she use the contraception reliably? If she is not using any form of contraception currently, does she want to start some method of contraception? If not, is she taking prenatal vitamins?

Gynecologic infection history

A history of any previous vaginal infections should be obtained, as well as a detailed account of what treatments have been prescribed for these infections, and what medications and treatments the patient has used without a prescription (see Chapter 7.7). Predisposing conditions preceding the infections should be elicited, as well as whether these infections were related to sexual activity. A history of what kinds of soaps, detergents, and perfumes that the patient uses is often helpful. The patient should be asked whether she douches. She should be asked whether she has ever been diagnosed with any sexually transmitted diseases in the past, and, if so, what treatments were prescribed. Did she complete the entire course of treatment? Was her partner treated? Each patient should be asked whether she has been tested for human immunodeficiency virus (HIV) and offered testing again if appropriate.

Papanicolaou history

A thorough history of the patient's previous Papanicolaou history should be explored. If there is a history of abnormal Pap smears, detailed information regarding colposcopic examinations and any treatment should be recorded. The patient should be asked specifically about any history of genital warts.

Previous gynecologic surgical history

A gynecologic surgical history should be obtained (see Chapter 16.7). If the patient has had gynecologic surgery, detailed information about the indications for surgery, exact surgical procedure, and complications, if any, should be carefully recorded.

Urologic history

The urologic history should be thoroughly taken (see Chapter 17.4). Any history of incontinence, recurrent urinary tract infections, pyelonephritis, hematuria, or kidney stones should be developed in great detail. Any treatment that the patient has received should also be recorded, including detailed information about any surgical procedures.

Gynecologic review of symptoms

Obtaining the gynecologic review of systems at the end of the gynecologic history is a good way to elicit any additional gynecologic issues that would be significant in the patient with female sexual dysfunction. The patient should be asked about any pelvic pain and whether it is related to menses, urination, defecation, or intercourse. A history of abnormal uterine bleeding should be elicited, with careful attention to when the bleeding is happening with respect to the menstrual cycle or intercourse and the duration, frequency, and character of the bleeding. The patient should be asked whether she has any unusual vaginal discharge (see Chapter 9.5). A history of difficulty in getting pregnant should be explored. Patients, especially older and parous women, should be asked about symptoms of pelvic relaxation such as urinary and fecal incontinence, relaxed vaginal introitus, and difficulty in defecating.

Obstetric history

All previous pregnancies should be documented (see Chapter 7.5). Dates of all deliveries should be recorded, noting the gestational age at delivery, as well as mode of delivery, outcome, and complications. Indications for all operative deliveries should be recorded, including forceps and vacuum deliveries. If the patient has had a cesarean section, she should be asked whether it was emergent or elective, and uterine scar type should be ascertained. Although this usually requires obtaining the operative report from the previous surgery, many patients will be able to give some clue about incision site. "My last doctor told me that I would always need a C-section because of the way she needed to cut my womb" would suggest that the patient had required a vertical uterine incision.

The gestational age of all spontaneous abortions should be noted, as well as whether the patient had a dilation and evacuation after the event. If the patient has had multiple miscarriages, inquire about any workup she may have had for recurrent pregnancy loss. Any history of therapeutic abortions should be recorded, including the gestational age at time of termination, the date of the procedures, whether they had surgical or medical abortion, and whether there were any complications.

Medical and surgical history

This portion of the medical history is a summary of the overall assessment of the patient's health. It is of great value in assessing the current complaint and also provides a context for the condition that brought the patient to seek medical attention.

The medical history comprises the general state of health, past illnesses, and surgical history. Inquiring about the general state of health affords an opportunity for the patient to summarize her general health in one sentence, such as "I have excellent general health." Past illnesses should include all illnesses that occurred in adult life as well as significant childhood illnesses. Details of treatment for any illnesses should be carefully documented to the best of the patient's recollection. Any hospitalizations should be recorded, including hospitalizations for any psychiatric conditions. The past surgical history should include all surgeries, even dental procedures, documented with the date of the surgery as well as any complications, including any complications of anesthesia.

Medications, allergies, personal habits, social history

All current medications taken by the patient should be recorded, including dosage and actual use by the patient. In addition, nonprescription medications and home remedies should also be recorded. Having the patient bring in her medications can improve the accuracy of this history.

All allergies should be carefully recorded, as well as a detailed account of the reaction. The history should not be limited to allergies related to medications, but should also include food, and environmental agents.

An attempt should be made to elicit a history of childhood immunizations, although many patients will not remember specifics and only be able to state that they were immunized. Information about the last purified protein derivative antigen used to aid in the diagnosis of tuberculosis infection, tetanus, and hepatitis immunizations should also be obtained.

A social history including the personal status of the patient is important to obtain. This includes the patient's place of birth, current address, and with whom she lives. This is a wonderful opportunity to ask whether the patient feels safe at home from domestic violence, to ascertain whether the patient has a smoke detector at home, and to determine whether the patient has any religious proscriptions in her medical care.

It is important for the health-care professional to ascertain the patient's personal habits. If tobacco is being currently used, the type should be noted (smoking or chewing) and when the patient started using tobacco. The amount used per day should be documented as well. Be careful to elicit a history of previous tobacco use, even if the patient has ceased use. If the patient has quit, ask whether the patient used or is currently using any medical or pharmaceutic smoking cessation aids.

The US Preventive Services Task Force recommends screening to detect problem drinking for all adult and adolescent patients.[1,2] The patient should be asked whether she drinks alcohol, and, if so, how many drinks per week she consumes. A history of binge drinking should be elicited as well. Screening tests for alcohol-related problems, such as the CAGE questionnaire, can be incorporated into the social history. The acronym "CAGE" aids the health-care professional in remembering the questions on *c*utting down, *a*nnoyance by criticism, *g*uilty feeling, and *e*ye-openers. The CAGE questionnaire asks, "Have you ever felt the need to cut down on drinking?", "Have you ever felt annoyed by criticism of your drinking?", "Have you ever had guilty feelings about your drinking?", "Have you ever taken a morning eye-opener?" Appropriate referrals for alcohol-related problems should be made.

Additionally the patient should be asked about any use of illegal drugs, current or past. The type of drug used should be documented as well as the route of administration. Duration of use should be noted as well. The patient should also be asked about use or abuse of any prescription medications.

Each patient should be asked about the frequency and type of exercise done, if any. General questions about diet should be asked, as well as dietary restrictions, and the use of caffeine-containing beverages.

Included in this interview should be questions regarding the patient's occupational history. A record of where the patient currently works should be obtained, specifically trying to elicit a history of exposure to potential environmental substances that are known to cause illness. The patient should also be asked about stress at work, as well as stress as a result of not working.

Family history

It is important for the health-care professional to develop a brief history of each member of the immediate family, including the age and cause of death of any deceased family members. If there is a history of a hereditary disease, it is useful to extend the family history to grandparents, aunts, uncles, and cousins. In certain circumstances, it may be useful to document information in a pedigree diagram. Included in the family history should be a determination of the ethnicity of the patient, as some conditions are seen more often in distinct ethnic groups.

Review of systems

The review of systems should be organized in terms of body systems. The many symptoms that may pertain to the history of present illness and the past medical history will also be elicited in this section, although some health-care practitioners choose to record pertinent symptoms in the history of present illness section. In addition, thoroughly reviewing all the possible symptoms may uncover symptoms of an undiagnosed condition for which the patient is not specifically presenting. It is best to organize the questions in a systematic fashion. It is unlikely that all aspects of each system will be asked at each patient visit; however, the health-care professional should be able to ask some questions about each system. Depending on the history of

present illnesses, more detailed questions about an affected system may be asked. Some practices have considered an extensive questionnaire for the patient to complete prior to her visit as a way for thorough review of the extensive review of systems (Table 9.2.1).

Conclusions

In sexual medicine, in particular, obtaining a "good" history is critical to patient management. In general, history taking for women with sexual health concerns involves a detailed sexual, medical, and psychosocial history. This chapter reviewed the key aspects of the medical history; see Chapters 9.3 and 9.4 for detailed information on the psychosocial and sexual history.

Table 9.2.1. Common symptoms asked about in a comprehensive review of systems

General: weight changes, weakness, fatigue, unexplained fevers, chills, malaise

Skin: rashes, changes in mole pigmentation, lumps, bumps, hair loss, hirsutism

Head: headache, dizziness, lightheadedness

Eyes: Visual changes, change in prescription strength, double vision, blurred vision, glaucoma, cataracts

Ears: hearing loss, tinnitus, vertigo, pain

Nose: nasal stuffiness, discharge, polyps, epistaxis, loss of smell

Mouth and throat: mouth lesions, halitosis, sore throat, bleeding gums, petechiae, dental problems, decreased taste

Neck: lymphadenopathy, goiter

Breasts: soreness, lumps, adnexal masses, nipple discharge, asymmetry

Lungs: cough, dyspnea, hemoptysis, wheezing, sputum

Cardiac: angina, dyspnea, dyspnea on exertion, palpitations, orthopnea, paroxysmal nocturnal dyspnea, edema

Gastrointestinal: heartburn, stomach upset, excessive burping, bloating, nausea, vomiting, diarrhea, constipation, abdominal pain (note frequency and location) food intolerance, excessive flatus, jaundice, hemorrhoids, change in bowel habits

Urinary: incontinence, retention, hematuria, dysuria, polyuria, decrease in urinary stream, dribbling, dark, tarry stools, change in stool caliber

Musculoskeletal: joint pain, muscle weakness, leg cramps, varicose veins, history of blood clots, arthritis, gout, stiffness, backache

Neurologic: fainting, seizures, numbness, paralysis, tremors

Hematologic: anemia, easy bleeding or bruising, history of blood transfusions (with year and location of transfusion)

Endocrine: cold or heat intolerance, excessive sweating, thyroid history, polydypsia, polyuria, increased appetite, change in glove size, hirsutism

Psychiatric: depression, mood, anxiety, memory changes, difficulty in concentrating

References

1. US Preventive Services Task Force. *Guide to Clinical Preventive Services*, 2nd edn. Baltimore: Williams and Wilkins, 1996.
2. Cleary PD, Miller M, Bush BT et al. Prevalence and recognition of alcohol abuse in primary care population. *Am J Med* 1988; 85: 466.

Further reading

Barker LR, Burton JR, Zieve PD. *Principles of Ambulatory Medicine*, 4th edn. Baltimore: Williams & Wilkins, 1994: 30–41.

Bickley LS. *Bate's Guide to Physcial Examination and History Taking*, 7th edn. Philadelphia: Lippincot Williams & Wilkins, 1999: 2–38.

Droegmueller W, Herbst AL, Mishell DR et al. *Comprehensive Gynecology*. St Louis: Mosby, 1987: 131–5.

Jones III HW, Wentz AC, Burnett LS. *Novak's Textbook of Gynecology*, 11th edn. Baltimore: Williams & Wilkins, 1981: 3–26.

Sapira JD. *The Art and Science of Bedside Diagnosis*. Baltimore: Urban & Schwarzenburg, 1989: 33–45.

Seidel HM, Ball JW, Dains JE et al. *Mosby's Guide to Physical Examination*, 4th edn. St Louis: Mosby, 1999: 4–46.

Williams JL, Schneiderman HS, Algranati PS. *Physical Diagnosis – Bedside Evaluation of Diagnosis and Function*. Baltimore: Williams and Wilkins, 1994: 1–32.

9.3 Psychosocial history

Michael A Perelman

Introduction

The etiology of female sexual dysfunction is frequently multi-dimensional. Health-care professionals treating female sexual dysfunction must consider the psychologic, social, cultural, and behavioral aspects of their patient's diagnosis and management, as well as organic causes and risk factors. Our current paradigm recognizes the important role of both organic and psychosocial factors in predisposing, precipitating, maintaining, and reversing female sexual dysfunction. Despite the existence of organic pathogenesis, female sexual dysfunction has always had a psychogenic component – even if the female sexual dysfunction was initially the result of constitution, illness, or treatment (see Chapter 17.6 of this book). This chapter highlights a methodology for assessing the psychologic forces which affect a woman's sex life beyond organic illness and mere performance anxiety. The methodology, referred to as the "Cornell model", is adapted from the work of Helen S. Kaplan (see Chapter 1.1).[1,2] The psychosocial interview can be understood as an interview that provides a broad understanding of the current sexual experience within the context of the woman's life history. Establishing the "sex status" rapidly identifies the numerous common maintaining causes of sexual dysfunction (e.g., insufficient stimulation, depression) and points toward predisposing and precipitating factors (see Chapters 3.1–3.4 and 11.1–11.5).

The ideal history is an integrated, fluid assessment in which the patient's response is continually re-evaluated. Assessing response to the initial pharmaceutic and behavioral prescriptions, which functions as a therapeutic probe, is a critical component of the psychosocial evaluation process. The proper evaluation of female sexual dysfunction requires that medical and psychologic concepts and diagnostic procedures be integrated in a comprehensive manner.

The successful treatment of both male and female sexual dysfunctions requires a specific data set that provides answers to three key questions regarding diagnosis, etiology, and treatment:

1. Does the patient really have a sexual disorder and what is the differential diagnosis?
2. What are the underlying organic and/or psychosocial factors?
   a. What are the organic factors?
   b. What are the "immediate" maintaining psychosocial causes (e.g., current cognitions, emotions, and behaviors)?
   c. What are the potential "deeper" psychosocial causes (predisposing, precipitating)?
3. Should the patient be treated or not? Is the severity of the underlying organic and psychosocial factors enough to require direct treatment, or can treatment of these factors be bypassed or concurrent? These decisions are dynamic and should be consistently re-evaluated as treatment proceeds.

The methodology used to answer these questions is a focused history integrating psychosexual and medical factors. This method is a flexible one. For instance, it can be adapted by a primary care physician with only 7 min available or by a sex therapist with 45 min to interview the patient. Once this method is mastered, all necessary data can be captured, even if multiple consultations or a referral is required to facilitate this process. The health-care professionals should obtain the necessary information to answer the above three questions in a manner that does not sabotage the relationship with the patient. First, an attempt should be made to establish what medical, organic, or psychosocial factors require "pretreatment" prior to symptom reversal. Treatment for the female sexual dysfunction should be started as soon as possible, with continuing re-evaluation of the patient's responses as treatment proceeds. A fuller comprehension of psychosocial issues optimizes patient response and minimizes relapse potential. Since many different professions of origin are involved in the care of women with female sexual dysfunction, this chapter refers to health-care professionals as a generic term for these clinicians.

This history-taking model suggests a rapid assessment of the immediate and remote causes of sexual dysfunction, using a four-phase model of human sexual response (i.e., desire, excitement, orgasm, and resolution) while maintaining rapport with the patient. Keeping this model in mind becomes a useful heuristic device to guide assessment.[3–6] This model is not necessarily linear and causes could become effects. For example, anorgasmia might diminish desire. However, generally speaking, sexual dysfunctions are disruptions in any of these four phases and/or the sexual pain and muscular disorders. Furthermore, while these dysfunctions can occur independently of each other, they frequently cluster together.

The history is the most important tool to assess the woman's sexual function. The primary goal of the evaluation session is to obtain the necessary information to help assess the nature of the female sexual dysfunction and to begin developing a treatment plan. However, empathy and rapport with the patient must never be sacrificed in the service of obtaining the critical details. The creation/maintenance of a therapeutic alliance is uppermost. This alliance will be strengthened if the patient is asked direct questions in a comfortable, reassuring, empathic manner. Both patient and clinician will obtain an understanding of the problem and a mutually derived treatment plan. The therapeutic context works best when it is humanistic, emphasizing good communication and mutual respect.

Numerous Continuing Medical Education programs have addressed the problem of encouraging health-care professionals both to initiate and discuss sexual issues by emphasizing the importance of sexual dysfunction as a biologic marker of disease, among other reasons. Health-care professionals must use a direct approach with inquiry initiated in a neutral manner, using nonjudgmental screening questions. Yet, the quest for details must be balanced by a sensitivity to the patient's anxiety as the information is collected. Changes the patient has experienced in her sexual function and her beliefs as to what the causes of those changes are should be inquired about directly.[7,8] Her story should be allowed to unfold in the available time, yet she should be carefully guided with a predetermined list of questions. The health-care professional must be mindful not to interject in the middle of the woman's explanation of her chief complaint.

While most patients are eager to "tell their story" to an accessible, knowledgeable clinician, others may be ambivalent about discussing details. This anxiety must be appreciated even as the clinician gently proceeds. If needed, the health-care professional can reassure the patient, saying, "I appreciate that discussing these details may be uncomfortable, but understanding them is the way to help you. We can proceed as slowly as you wish." This usually relaxes the patient and encourages her to continue. Reciprocally, the interviewing must be conducted at the health-care professional's comfort level. While pursuing an analysis of sexual behavior, it is essential that health-care professionals monitor their own comfort in order to instill the greatest confidence and promote openness on the patient's part.

The format for both evaluation and treatment can vary, as patients may be single or coupled. Whether single or coupled, most patients visiting a health-care professional will be seen alone. When time permits, for women in a relationship, the health-care professional should encourage partner attendance. However, the issue should not be forced. Treatment format is a psychotherapeutic issue, and rapport should never be sabotaged. While conjoint consultation is a good policy, it is not always the right choice. Health-care professionals should remember that while important information can be obtained from the partner's perception of the problem, partner cooperation is more important than partner attendance in the evaluation and treatment of sexual dysfunction.[9] If the patient wants her "obnoxious, dominating partner" to be present, he should be welcomed, although an individual follow-up with her may be necessary. These are all strategic issues to manage in treatment, although the intricacies are beyond the scope of this chapter.

The psychosocial history captures a pyramid of important pieces of information, beginning with the chief complaint on top and expanding through a relevant developmental history-taking. To any extent possible, both the precipitating and predisposing psychosocial factors should be illuminated. While flushing out a deep understanding of the etiology of a woman's dysfunction is helpful, understanding the current picture (i.e., maintaining or immediate factors) should be the first priority.

The method

The diagnostic evaluation of female sexual dysfunction focuses on finding potential physical and specific psychosocial factors relating to the disorder. The sexual symptom, the history of the sexual symptom, and the sex status examination must be pursued in detail for all patients during the first meeting. All patients who are being evaluated for sexual difficulties should be briefly screened for psychopathology. However, this does not need to be pursued in depth unless there is evidence of a significant emotional disorder. Additionally, an assessment of the medical status must be conducted or arranged, depending on the health-care professional's training and competencies. Certain basic information must be obtained from the patient's history and physical examination, regardless of the specific female sexual dysfunction presented. This exploration will provide a clear understanding and will determine the treatment.

All health-care professionals should have a general understanding of the numerous physiologic and pharmaceutic risk factors that must be assessed when evaluating women complaining of female sexual dysfunction. For instance, they must familiarize themselves with commonly used medications that may cause a central and/or peripheral inhibition of sexual response. Assessment of the medical status must determine whether the patient has an illness or is taking a drug that could be causing the symptom. However, the current chapter presumes the necessary assessment steps and procedures, including the physical examination of the genital and reproductive organs, as well as laboratory tests, have been conducted (see Chapter 9.5). The current chapter will focus on the relevant psychosocial material. However, the health-care professional should not arbitrarily separate the psychosocial/sexual history from the medical history. An integrated medical and sexual history yields a significant amount of information regarding all aspects of a woman's sexual health and relationships. The health-care professional must identify which variables are most relevant to understanding the etiology of the chief complaint, and focus the interview accordingly.

Identifying the sexual complaint

The health-care professional should obtain a clear and detailed description of the patient's sexual symptoms, as well as information about the onset and progression of symptoms. The details of the physical and emotional circumstances surrounding the onset of a difficulty are important for the assessment of both physical and psychologic causes. The health-care professional must elicit these details, if not spontaneously offered. Diagnosis will be partially determined by the specific sexual complaint(s). Past and present modifiers should be incorporated, ascertained from key elements obtained from the sex status examination and from reviewing relevant psychosocial and developmental history.[9,10]

The sexual status examination is the next step in the assessment process. A detailed description of the patient's current sexual experience and an analysis of her sexual behavior and of the couple's erotic interaction help rule out organic causes and identify current operating psychosocial antecedents of the disorder. The sexual status examination is the single most important diagnostic tool at the health-care professional's disposal, and is most consistent with the "review of systems" common to all aspects of medicine.[2,9] The interview is rich in detail and clarifies many aspects of the individual's sexuality. A focused sex status critically assists in understanding and identifying the immediate cause of the sexual dysfunction (i.e., the actual behavior and/or cognition causing or contributing to the sexual disorder). Armed with this information, a diagnosis can be made and a treatment plan formulated. Significantly, the sexual information evoked in history taking will help anticipate non-compliance with medical and surgical interventions. Modifying immediate psychologic factors may result in less medication being needed, regardless of the specific female sexual dysfunction. In general, physicians will intervene with pharmacotherapy and brief sex coaching, which address immediate causes (e.g., insufficient stimulation) directly and intermediate issues (e.g., partner issues) indirectly, and will rarely focus on deeper issues (e.g., sex abuse) (see Chapter 3.4). In fact, when deeper psychosocial issues are the primary obstacles, it is usually time for referral.[11]

It is particularly useful for the health-care professional, when initiating the discussion of sex with the patient, to obtain a description of a recent experience that incorporates the sexual symptom. One question that will help pin down many of the immediate and remote causes is, "Tell me about your last sexual experience." Common immediate causes of female sexual dysfunction will be quickly evoked by the patient's response. There are several frequently identified contributors to female sexual dysfunction, including insufficient stimulation (e.g., lack of adequate friction), lack of subjective feelings of arousal, fatigue, and negative thinking.[12]

When possible, the health-care professional should ascertain the patient's thoughts during various types of sexual behavior. The following questions can be helpful: When does antisexual thinking emerge? Is the patient anxious about sexual failure early in the day before sex is even on the horizon? Does she worry that she "is taking too long" while her partner performs cunnilingus? What is the content of her negative thinking? Do her fantasies cause her distress? Is there a fear of negative behavioral consequences, such as urination or flatulence? Is she afraid of what her partner thinks and/or is she judging herself negatively? The mind is capable of derailing normal sexual arousal as well as interfering with the restorative benefit of current and future sexual pharmaceuticals. Understanding cognition can be key to facilitating sexual recovery and satisfaction. Why this person has intrusive thoughts that are of a frequency and intensity that interfere with her sexual function is an issue that generates focus for additional psychosexual history taking.

Which psychosocial factors are currently maintaining the psychic structure that results in the distracted thoughts and implicitly/explicitly reduces sexual arousal? It is interesting to understand what predisposed the patient to have that type of distressing thought and to know her full psychosocial history. However, it is critical to know and understand the current psychosocial obstacles that are maintaining the dysfunctional process.

Health-care professionals should follow up with focused, open-ended questions to obtain a clear picture (e.g., "What is your masturbation technique?"). Inquiries should be made about desire, fantasy, frequency of sex, and effects of drugs and alcohol. Idiosyncratic masturbation may be a hidden cause of female sexual dysfunction.[13] The role of masturbation in understanding the pathogenesis of orgasm disorders in particular has not been fully explored. Disparity between the woman's masturbatory sexual fantasy (whether unconventional or not) and the reality of sex with the partner should be explored. This disparity takes many forms (e.g., body type, orientation, sex activity performed). The health-care professional will become implicitly aware of the patient's sexual script and expectations, leading to more precise and improved recommendations and management of patient expectations.[9,12] For example, a health-care professional could improve outcome by briefly clarifying whether a patient was better off with practicing masturbating or with reintroducing sex with a partner.

Exploring other psychosocial issues

Primary versus secondary

It is not necessary to do an exhaustive sexual and family history for most evaluations. The investigation of these issues should be selective so that the interview does not become unnecessarily lengthy. The patient's description will probably indicate whether she experiences the difficulty at all times or only under certain circumstances. However, a fluctuating pattern does not necessarily discriminate between psychogenic and organic etiology. In cases of a secondary problem, the clinician will hear of an important change from function to dysfunction. Was the change preceded by or concurrent with major life stress (e.g., change in the structure of the family, loss of a job by herself or a partner)? The patient may guide the health-care professional to the specific cause, or the health-care professional may need to examine the time period of the sexual change for clues to causation. The health-care professional should examine any of the areas known to alter sexual function from the point of view of psychosocial stress, including, but not limited to, health, family, and work.

It is often less important to get a detailed history of earlier developmental issues in cases of secondary sexual dysfunction. Time is more valuably spent exploring the circumstances of life that changed concomitant with the change in sexual function. This hunt for the precipitating factors will likely reveal a pattern within the mindset or experience of the patient which would help explain the shift in sexual function. Sometimes the patient will tell the clinician the cause of change herself. For example, a 35-year-old mother of two might tell the health-care professional, "Sex was great, till I got a venereal disease from my husband's dalliance with a prostitute on his business trip. Things have never been the same. Every time I start to get excited, I can't get the image of him with her out of my mind." This is of course different from the 52-year-old recently menopausal woman who obsesses about lost youth when she notices her diminished lubrication. The guideline is frequently to "interview the crisis", meaning that the health-care professional should get not only a clear picture of the current situation, but also a full understanding of exactly what occurred and the patient's response to the change.

In long-standing cases of primary dysfunction, it is more important to look for precipitating causes with an emphasis on what is currently maintaining the dysfunction. For instance, if there was a traumatic or painful first sexual experience, is the woman still afraid that sex will hurt? Is fear causing painful muscular contractions during attempts at coitus? Coital pain for a virginal woman is not uncommon. However, the critical differentiator is the continuation of pain, fear, and their relation to the presenting dysfunction. Greater exploration is warranted, whereas, if later experiences were positive, it would not be necessary to explore "first sex" in great detail. In other words, the health-care professional should identify when the problem began and try to understand its source in a linear, relational manner, rather than assessing all aspects of a person's sexual history.

Sometimes the patient will provide too much detail on background information which is tangentially relevant, but not primary. In this situation, the health-care professional should gently interrupt, acknowledging the potential importance of the patient's statement, and move the interview forward. For example, the health-care professional could say, "That's very interesting, but I wonder if we might postpone those details. I'd like to come back to that, but today I need a broader understanding of your problem." Alternatively, "That's helpful, but what happened next?" The goal should be to establish and maintain rapport while gathering the relevant details.

Previous treatment approaches

Depending on the particular patient, the discussion of the last sexual experience and an elaboration of current function will inevitably also evoke information about what previous approaches the patient has attempted. Many women have attempted a variety of treatments for their conditions, including herbal therapies, folk therapies, and professional treatment. The effects of such treatments should be assessed. Additionally, past treatment for psychiatric issues (e.g., depression), early sexual experiences and developmental issues, substance use or abuse, and partner issues may be mentioned by the patient. The health-care professional should decide which material seems most important to understand the sexual disorder's etiology, following the pattern that emerges naturally from the patient's description. The following are some helpful ways to examine these other aspects of the psychosocial factors in greater detail, but only the screening elements are required during the first session.

Psychiatric considerations

The health-care professional should briefly screen all patients for obvious psychopathology that would significantly interfere with the initiation of treatment for the female sexual dysfunction. Yet, the health-care professional will also want to know whether psychiatric symptoms, if present, are the cause and/or the consequence of the sexual disorder. In addition, it is important for the health-care professional to know whether the patient is receiving appropriate treatment for any psychiatric disorder. The skillful and experienced health-care professional can make judgments about a patient's or a couple's psychiatric status by observations of, and interactions with them, by attending to their appearance, speech, and demeanor, by the way they relate to the health-care professional and to each other, and by the feelings they evoke. If any psychiatric issue is severe enough, the health-care professional may decide to refer the patient for psychiatric help prior to initiating treatment for the sexual disorder. Yet, even when a patient and/or her partner seem to be mentally healthy, answers to the following four questions should be obtained:

1. What is her experience with emotional or mental illness?
2. If the patient was in psychotherapy, why was treatment sought and what was learned?
3. Was she ever hospitalized for an emotional or mental disorder?
4. What psychoactive drugs has she taken?[2]

There is a statistically significant increase in depression for individuals with female sexual dysfunction. If the patient is depressed, the severity of her depression should be clarified. Furthermore, all patients who experience major depression should be queried about suicide risk. Treatment of female sexual dysfunction may improve mild reactive depression, while depressive symptoms might alter response to therapy for female sexual dysfunction.[14] A clinician's history taking must parse out the question of whether the sexual dysfunction is causing depression or whether the depression and its treatment (e.g., selective serotonin reuptake inhibitors) are causing the sexual dysfunction (see Chapters 16.2, 17.2, and 17.3). Besides depression, panic attacks are often associated with sexual complaints, so almost all patients should be asked whether they have any phobias and have ever experienced a panic attack.

A brief review of each partner's functioning in the work, social, and family areas will also help measure mental and emotional status. If the patient relates in a pleasant, sensitive manner, if her story makes sense, if she enjoys work, if she has friends, and if her answers to the questions about mental health are reassuring, then serious psychopathology can be ruled out. However, if the health-care professional senses that the patient may be suffering from an undiagnosed or unsuspected mental or emotional disorder, further assessment should be arranged.[2]

When a patient with a variety of psychopathologic states (e.g., stress, phobias, personality disorders) is evaluated for sexual complaints, the health-care professional must consider whether that patient's emotional conflicts are too severe for a focused treatment of the sexual problem, and whether such treatment should either be safely postponed for another time or occur concurrently with treatment for the emotional distress. In more severe situations, the modal choice is likely to be a simultanous initiation of the sexual dysfunction treatment and referral to a mental health practitioner to facilitate patient management. For example, actively psychotic patients are clearly not appropriate candidates for brief treatment, even when they have a real sexual problem. Yet, treatment for a sexual disorder is not contraindicated for many persons with a history of severe psychiatric disturbance who are in a compensated phase of a psychiatric illness. Many such individuals have been successfully treated with sex therapy and have benefited in terms of their overall psychologic well-being. The same will be true for today's women receiving sexual pharmaceuticals and/or sex therapy. More subtle personality factors, such as fragile self-esteem and fear of being negatively evaluated by others, are frequently prevalent in women with sexual concerns, especially those with low sexual desire. Yet, usually, this would not result in postponing treatment for the sex problem.[2]

Special populations

A person who is currently addicted to drugs and/or alcohol is not a suitable candidate for treatment until she has been detoxified and is off the drug. Many mentally retarded individuals, especially those with borderline to moderate impairment, are physically normal and have normal sexual urges. Sexual problems in the mentally retarded tend to involve inappropriate sexual expression and unwanted pregnancy, as well as problems associated with fear of sex and lack of information about sex.[2]

Family and early psychosexual history

A psychosexual and family history may provide insight into the deeper causes of the patient's problem and may reveal cultural and/or neurotic origins of the problem. Negative factors from the past might include losses, traumas, negative past sexual relationships, and negative past interpersonal relationships. They may also include cultural and religious restrictions. The health-care professional should obtain a brief sketch of family background and of sexual development landmarks. Sex pioneer Helen Kaplan asked every patient, "What sort of sexual message did you receive when you were growing up?"[2] Possible predisposing factors such as traumatic sexual experiences (e.g., sex abuse, rape) and body image and gender identification issues (initially assessed by asking about response to first menses) should be explicitly ruled out. These avenues should be pursued in depth only if warranted by the manifest emotions and content of the reply to inquiry. The health-care professional should tread doggedly but gingerly, with confidence that rapport will preserve another opportunity.

Partner/relationship issues

While sex therapists assess the pattern and quality of the woman's romantic relationships, health-care professionals typically obtain a brief status of the current relationship. For all women, health-care professionals should assess marital status as well as living and dating arrangements. Contextual factors, including difficulties with the current interpersonal relationship and whether the partner has a sexual dysfunction, should be clarified. The health-care professional may grasp the couple's interactions from the first interview's sex status. It remains to be determined whether deeper difficulties in the couple's relationship determine the patient's sexual problem.

Previous sexual scripts also need assessment.[15] Several questions should be asked, including whether sexual relations were ever good with the current partner, what changed, and what the patient's view of causation is. Numerous partner-related psychosexual issues may also adversely affect outcome. Reassurance and inquiry (e.g., "No one's relationship is perfect. What do you argue about?") can be helpful, as can an evaluation of the degree of acrimony when the patient describes her complaints (e.g., is the anger, resentment, hurt, or sadness a maintaining or precipitating factor, or are the emotions more mild manifestations of the frustrations of daily life?).

For all women, whether or not the problem is partner-specific needs to be determined. If the problem is partner-specific, the health-care professional must ascertain which of several categories are etiologically relevant (e.g., inadequate sexual technique, poor communication, incompatible sexual script or fantasies, no physical attraction). Power struggles, transferences, partner psychopathology, and commitment/intimacy issues are elusive and may have implications for the sexual problem. A woman will often "turn off" if the only time her husband is interested in her feelings is prior to intercourse. Women give multiple reasons for having and wanting sex, with lust being only one of numerous possible emotions present prior to the experience. This is especially important to assess in women with diminished desire. Initially, all that is required is to decide whether the degree of relationship strife is too severe to initiate the female sexual dysfunction treatment. Otherwise, concurrent relationship treatment is provided, or a referral is made and female sexual dysfunction treatment is postponed. However, it will be the bias of many to err on the side of giving the relationship and female sexual dysfunction treatment every possible chance (see Chapters 8.1 and 8.2).

Follow-up

Initial treatment failures should be examined at follow-up. Sometimes the most critical information is made evident by the patient's reaction to the health-care professional's first suggestions. The pharmaceutic or behavioral interventions can act as therapeutic probes, illuminating the cause of failure or nonresponse. Retaking a quick "sex status" provides a convenient model for managing follow-up.[11] It is also helpful to increase success by scheduling follow-up the first day either a pharmaceutic or behavioral intervention is prescribed. Follow-up is essential to ensuring optimal treatment. Components of follow-up include monitoring side effects, assessing success, and considering whether an alteration in dose or treatment is needed. A continuing dialog with patients is critical to facilitate success and prevent relapse. There are several psychologic issues to consider which evoke noncompliance, including fear of complications; reactions to changes associated with aging; reactions to chronic diseases or injury; changes associated with medications, alcohol, and smoking; and changes associated with life stressors. These are important issues in differentiating treatment nonresponders from "biochemical failures" in order to enhance success rates. Early failures can be reframed into learning experiences and eventual success.[9,12,16–18]

Partner cooperation must be anticipated before treatment, and follow-up provides opportunity to confirm whether or not such cooperation is present. If cooperation is not present, the recognition of a need for contact with the partner should increase. If the partner's support for successful resolution of the sexual dysfunction is not present, active steps must be taken to evoke it. Sometimes referral for adjunctive treatment to a sex therapist for the partner may be required.[9] It is likely that the more problematic the relationship, the less likely that patient–partner sex education can augment treatment in and of itself. Inevitably, a mental health referral would be required, albeit not necessarily accepted.

Referral

Identifying psychologic factors does not necessarily mean that the health-care professional must treat them. Health-care professionals are encouraged to practice at their own comfort level. If not inclined to counsel or if uncomfortable with counseling, the health-care professional may refer or work conjointly with a sex therapist. However, in more complex cases, significant intrapsychic and relationship problems must be investigated by someone.[12]

Health-care professionals may want to optimize the patient's response to treatment. In doing so, it is important that health-care professionals do not collude with the patient's unrealistic expectations. Health-care professionals should be mindful of a patient's potential idealized notion of her sexual capacity and/or idealization of the treating clinician's abilities. There are situations when it is appropriate either to make a referral or to decline to treat a patient. Significant, process-based, developmental predisposing factors usually indicate to the need for resolution of psychic wounds prior to the introduction of sexual pharmaceuticals. The more determinants of female sexual dysfunction are driven by developmental processes, the more likely the patient will benefit from sex therapy in addition to pharmacotherapy. There are situations when it is appropriate to postpone treating the patient for the female sexual dysfunction until psychotherapeutic consultation is able to assist the individual in developing a more reality-based view. While this can sometimes be done simultaneously, at other times treatment for female sexual dysfunction must be postponed.

The single patient

The single patient with a psychosexual dysfunction must be assessed in the same manner as if the patient was in a relationship. The patient's sexual symptom may or may not relate to difficulties in her relationships. Women seeking treatment for primary anorgasmia, and some cases of vaginismus, are suitable for initial intervention for the patient alone. The health-care professional's time constraints and competencies, along with patient predilections, will determine whether the patient's single status becomes a therapeutic focus. This issue must be managed with extreme emotional and political sensitivity. Needless to say, sexual orientation issues, for both single and coupled women, require the same if not even greater sensitivity on the health-care professional's part.

Questionnaires

Questionnaires can be used in both training and research. In training, questionnaires provide students with a range of potentially relevant material of interest in the diagnosis and treatment of female sexual dysfunction. In research, questionnaires both allow standardization of diagnostic data collection and provide recognized consistent endpoints. Therefore, the student of female sexual dysfunction treatment and research should have a passing familiarity with commonly used paper-and-pencil tests (for a complete review of this topic, see Chapter 11). Additionally, health-care professionals may choose to use current or future instruments to facilitate history taking. Such instruments must be incorporated in a manner which does not interfere with rapport.

Conclusion

Health-care professionals should make the patient a partner in her care and share conclusions with her. Patients are often anxious and eager to know what is wrong. Interim conclusions should be expressed throughout the interview, especially when they are encouraging. Health-care professionals should make recommendations and/or let the patient know when further evaluation is needed. However, the more complex the symptomology and etiology, the more likely additional time is required to make a diagnosis and develop a treatment plan.

Combination treatments for sexual dysfunction, where sex therapy strategies and treatment are integrated with sexual pharmaceuticals, may provide the best solution. There is a synergy to this approach that is not yet supported by empirical evidence, but that is rapidly gaining adherents, who eventually will document its successful benefits. Research on male sexual disorders in the last few years indicates that combination therapy will be the treatment of choice for all sexual dysfunction, as new pharmaceuticals are developed for desire, arousal, and orgasm problems in both men and women.[12,19,20] Sexuality is a complex interaction of biology, culture, developmental, and current intra- and inter-personal psychology. A biopsychosocial model of sexual dysfunction provides a compelling argument for integrating sex therapy and sexual pharmaceuticals. Restoration of lasting and satisfying sexual function requires a multidimensional understanding of all of the forces that created the problem, whether a solo physician or multidisciplinary team approach is used. Health-care professionals must carefully evaluate their own competence and interests when considering the treatment of female sexual dysfunction, so that, regardless of the modality used, the patient receives the best care. This sensibility should infuse the perspective on taking a psychosexual history from a woman suffering from female sexual dysfunction.

References

1. Perelman MA. Commentary: pharmacological agents for ED and the human sexual response cycle. *J Sex Marital Ther* 1998; 24: 309–12.

2. Kaplan H. *The Evaluation of Sexual Disorders: Psychologic and Medical Aspects.* New York: Brunner/Mazel, 1995.

3. Perelman MA. The urologist and cognitive behavioral sex therapy. *Contemp Urol* 1994; 6: 27–33.

4. Perelman M. Letter to the editor: regarding ejaculation: delayed and otherwise. *J Androl* 2003; 24: 496.

5. Masters WH, Johnson VE. *Human Sexual Inadequacy.* Boston: Little, Brown, 1970.

6. Kaplan HS, Perelman MA. The physician and the treatment of sexual dysfunction. In G Usdin, J Lewis, eds. *Psychiatry in General Medical Practice.* New York: McGraw-Hill, 1979.

7. Warnock JK. Assessing FSD: taking the history. *Prim Psychiatry* 2001; 8: 60–4.

8. Viera AJ. Managing hypoactive sexual desire in women. *Med Aspects Hum Sex* 2001; 1: 7–13.

9. Perelman MA. Sex coaching for physicians: combination treatment for patient and partner. *Int J Impot Res* 2003; 15(Suppl 5): S67–S74.

10. Basson R, Burnett A, Derogatis L et al. Report of the international consensus development conference on female sexual dysfunction: definitions and classifications. *J Urol* 2000; 163: 888–93.

11. Perelman, M. Combination therapy: integration of sex therapy and pharmacotherapy. In R Balon, R Seagraves, eds. *Handbook of Sexual Dysfunction.* New York: Marcel Dekker, 2005.

12. Perelman M. Sex and fatigue. *Contemp Urol* 1994; 6: 27–33.

13. Perelman M. Retarded ejaculation. In M O'Leary, ed. *Current Sexual Health Reports.* Philadelphia: Current Science, 2004.

14. Seidman SN, Roose SP, Menza MA et al. Treatment of erectile dysfunction in men with depressive symptoms: results of a placebo-controlled trial with sildenafil citrate. *Am J Psychiatry* 2001; 158: 1623–30.

15. Gagnon J, Rosen R, Leiblum S. Cognitive and social science aspects of sexual dysfunction: sexual scripts in therapy. *J Sex Marital Ther* 1982; 8: 44–56.

16. Althof, SE. New roles for mental health clinicians in the treatment of erectile dysfunction. *J Sex Educ Ther* 1998; 23: 229–31.

17. McCarthy BW. Integrating Viagra into cognitive-behavioral couple's sex therapy. *J Sex Educ Ther* 1998; 23: 302–8.

18. Barada, JA. Successful salvage of sildenafil (Viagra) failures: benefits of patient education and re-challenge with sildenafil. Presented at the 4th Congress of the European Society for Sexual and Impotence Research 2001, Rome, Italy.

19. Perelman MA. FSD partner issues: expanding sex therapy with sildenafil. *J Sex Marital Ther* 2002; 28: 195–204.

20. Lue TF, Basson R, Rosen R et al. *Sexual Medicine: Sexual Dysfunctions in Men and Women.* Paris: Health Publications, 2004.

9.4 Sexual history

Ulrike Brandenburg, Anneliese Schwenkhagen

The aim of this chapter is, first, to encourage health-care professionals to overcome the awkwardness or embarrassment they might feel in discussing sexual matters with their patients; second, to advocate the value of taking a detailed sexual history; and third, to make clear how taking such a history constitutes, in itself, the beginning of treatment. As a resource for practitioners, the chapter also incorporates a selection of analytic questions that can contribute to developing a thorough sexual history.

Sexual dysfunction is not absolute. It stands in opposition to sexual fulfillment, within the sexual norms of the culture. Sexual dysfunction differs from culture to culture, and from time to time. Similarly, each patient has her individual sexual norms that differ from one time of her life to another, as does her health-care professional. Consequently, any sexual dysfunction will, inevitably, present as an individually defined disturbance (see Chapters 3.1–3.4 of this book).

There is often considerable inhibition that must be overcome before the patient will bring up a sexual problem. The problem may, however, have been troubling her for a long time. Health-care practitioners who do not bring up the topic of sexual health, because of their own uneasiness, contribute to the patient's suffering.

The challenge of the sexual conversation

Speaking with a patient about sex is very different from speaking with her about high blood pressure, cardiac health or orthopedic problems. In these areas, there are clear definitions, clear questions to ask, and (relatively) clear answers. Physicians do not feel inhibited in bringing up these topics with a patient, quite in contrast to talking about sex. The health-care professional must examine his or her own comfort level in discussing sex, separating the professional side from personal emotions, and putting aside feelings of awkwardness, embarrassment, hesitation, or intimidation from the patient.

The discomfort of the health-care professional in talking about sexual health should help in empathizing with patients, giving some insight into how they are likely to feel when discussing their sexual life. Neither physicians nor patients have learned how to conduct such conversations, as they are not part of cultural training, and are rarely part of professional training.

Waiting for the physician to speak

While speaking with patients about sexual matters is a challenge for many, it is a topic patients are waiting for their health-care providers to broach. Considering the prevalence of sexual dysfunction among women young and old, the challenge needs to be met. Sexual dysfunction frequently leaves the patient feeling inadequate and deeply flawed as a person. It affects her self-image more deeply than most medical conditions. For the patient simply to discover she is not the only one with the problem can be a relief, in addition to knowing that there is someone who understands the condition. One woman said, "I was so happy when I finally got to learn that my illness had a name, a diagnosis."

Many patients have gone from one physician to another, from consultant to psychologist to psychotherapist, struggling to discuss the problem, only to feel frustrated by suggestions to relax, or drink a glass of water, or simply to wait for the right partner. The discomfort the practitioner feels in bringing up the topic of sexual behavior has condemned patients to a fruitless odyssey.

Avoiding the sexual conversation

Sexual problems exist, and they contribute to all manner of symptoms. If the patient is not engaged in the sexual conversation, the physician must be avoiding it. What strategies are used to avoid talking about sex with patients? One gynecologist related a conversation concerning the oral contraceptive pill. As she was leaving the room, the patient said, "Oh, by the way, I don't have an orgasm." After catching her breath, the physician responded by suggesting a physical examination. However, as she conducted the examination, the gynecologist felt sure that it was not the appropriate diagnostic intervention. After completing the examination, she told the patient everything was fine, and then found herself able to say, "It's good that you mentioned this problem. It is something we need to deal with," and made a further appointment with the woman.

As awkward as it may be to talk to patients about sex, and no matter how helpless or embarrassed it may make the physician feel, patients may be every bit as uncomfortable themselves. The responsibility to initiate the sexual conversation belongs to the professional.

Initiating the sexual conversation

The hardest part of the conversation about sexual health is often simply getting started. Although the patient may bring up a sexual problem, she is often waiting for the invitation from the health-care professional. Frequently, the woman is presenting for other complaints, anything from cardiac problems to chronic osteoporosis. In studies, patients clearly indicate that they would welcome their doctor saying something like, "By the way, I just wanted to mention that if you find yourself having any sexual problems at any point, that is something we should talk about." In contrast, there are ways to start the sexual conversation in a manner that immediately stops it in its tracks. The direct approach, such as asking, "What about your sex life?", tends to elicit the response that everything is fine even when that may not be true. Patients seem to experience the direct approach as an attack. They prefer a respectful, low-key invitation. To the earlier question, if they respond by saying, "Well, yes, I actually do have a problem," you might say, "Tell me about it." Many patients, particularly older ones, are embarrassed to talk about a sexual problem even though they want to, and therefore may recoil from the idea. But once it has been broached, they feel at liberty to discuss it again in future. It is helpful to be aware of the kind of conversation that will be of most use, both in terms of providing comfort to the patients and a detailed sexual history to the clinician.

Concrete sexual conversation

It is important to talk about sexual problems in a concrete manner. The patient must understand that the purpose of the conversation is to understand the problem, and what it means to the woman, so that the health-care provider can make an accurate diagnosis and recommend an effective course of treatment. When doctors are embarrassed to talk about sexual matters, they rarely take enough time to understand the problem. For instance, many patients present with the complaint that they are unable to achieve orgasm, appearing to have general orgasmic dysfunction. However, when pursuing the matter further, it may turn out that the woman does not have experience in trying to have an orgasm, or has attempted it incorrectly, thus showing a lack of experience rather than a dysfunction.

It may take a lot of courage for an older woman even to mention her orgasm problem. She needs to be encouraged to

tell exactly what she has done to attempt to achieve orgasm. Concrete questions may help, such as the following. Have you ever examined your vagina? Have you looked at your labia? Have you seen your clitoris? Have you ever touched these areas? Have you ever caressed them? Have you ever put some saliva on your fingers and tried to arouse yourself? It often turns out that a nonorgasmic woman has done little of the above. She may have tried only coitus.

A similar situation pertains to cases of female sexual desire disorder. Typically, when a patient says she has no desire, she answers no to the query, "Have you had any sexual thoughts or fantasies recently?" But when asked, "Please take a moment more to think carefully. Have you had any sexual thoughts at all in recent weeks?", she will reply that indeed she did. When asked about masturbation, the answer was also yes. However, when asked, "Have you been attracted recently to any man or woman?", the response was, "No, of course not." Obviously, this response is consistent with how the patient presented her problem. While patients express how things are in general, their focus is on the problem that is in the forefront of their minds and they fail to notice the exceptions to the rule. It is often necessary to say, "Please think again, just to make sure you are being completely accurate." In this case, that question elicited the response, "Oh, yes, there was a man at a party." Without careful questioning, the patient would not have brought him to mind. She felt guilty in thinking of him, almost denying to herself the attraction she felt toward him. The attraction may have been slight, but the health-care provider's proceeding in this manner shows the situation to be less black-and-white than when first presented. As a result, the monumental quality of the problem may be undermined and its dependence on technique and situational factors revealed, with the consequence that it becomes more manageable.

Often in cases of lack of desire, when questioned appropriately, the woman remembers a recent instance when she felt some sexual attraction toward her partner, although it does not come readily to mind. Careful questioning can reveal that many women supposedly suffering from hypoactive sexual desire disorder do have sexual fantasies and masturbate from time to time. In such cases, it would be inappropriate to treat them with medication.

Meaningful sexual conversation

Obtaining concrete details concerning the patient's sexual problem is only half of the problem. There is also the question of what those facts mean to the patient. Physicians tend to be trained to focus on facts; however, these cannot be isolated from their meaning, whether that results in pleasure or discomfort.

It is not the symptoms that cause problems to patients but their significance which determines how they are viewed. Indeed, the doctor may discover a problem that does not distress the patient, who is unlikely to do anything about it. For that reason, a full sexual history needs to incorporate the meaning and significance of any symptom under discussion, and these may not be at all what the practitioner expected. Thus, questions about the significance of symptoms need to be as thorough as the factual questions about the details themselves.

Questions for a detailed sexual history

The diagnostic dimension of a sexual history involves interplay between the facts and their significance. Listed here are a number of suggested questions to address separately sexual function and the meaning of sexual dysfunction. The questions, therefore, comprise three elements: the functional aspect, the meaning of these functional problems for the patient, and the past sexual experiences of the patient and their significance. The questions do not need to be asked in order but should be asked in a comfortable sequence.

Function

- What is the problem?
- When did it begin?
- How often does it (the symptom) happen?
- When it happens, how much or how often does it happen?
- In which situation does it (the symptom) appear?
- In which situation does it not appear?
- From which activities/technique does it appear?
- From which activities/techniques does it not appear?
- In which kind of relationship does it appear?
- In which kind of relationship does it not appear?
- How often do you have sexual desire? arousal? orgasm? satisfaction?
- Do you sometimes masturbate?
- How often?
- What works well for you?

Significance

- What does it (the symptom) mean to you?
- Does it lead you to any feelings of shame or frustration?
- Are you anxious about not satisfying your own expectations?
- Do you feel your own sexual potency to be in some way lacking?
- What would it mean to you if it (the symptom) disappeared? What would be different?

Interpersonal

- What does (the symptom) mean to your partner?
- Who suffers from what?
- Who do you feel suffers more?
- Do you talk about sex with your partner?

- As a result of it (the symptom), is there any withdrawal from the relationship? On your part or that of your partner? Emotionally, sexually, or both?
- Does your partner feel responsible or guilty in some way because of your having it (the symptom)?
- Do you think your partner has anxieties about not satisfying your expectations?
- What would it mean for your relationship if it (the symptom) disappeared?
- Sometimes it (the symptom) can protect a couple from having to deal with some other issue; if that were the case, what do you imagine it could be for the two of you?

Past sexual experience

- What were your first experiences with sexuality?
- What were your parents' attitudes toward sexuality?
- What do you remember of your first experiences with masturbation?
- How did you experience puberty and adolescence?
- When did you have your first sexual experiences with a partner?
- Did you ever have any issues regarding whether you were more attracted to men or women?
- When did you have your first experience with sexual intercourse?
- What were the early experiences like for you?
- Have you had children?
- Did you ever want to have children?
- Have you been pregnant?
- Have you had an abortion?
- How have you practiced contraception?
- Have you had any unconventional sexual experiences (ones other people might think unusual or odd)? Have you ever wished to have any such experiences?
- Have you ever experienced sexual violence or sexual misconduct?

Talking tips

While knowing the kind of questions to ask is of considerable help in feeling comfortable and able to start a conversation on sexual matters, the practitioner may be more at ease by recognizing the following:

- Don't be too focused on finding a solution. Sexual problems can be complex. For instance, there may be relationship issues involved, but simply airing the problem will be bringing some measure of relief to the patient.
- Don't think that talking about sexual health problems has to take more time than talking about others sorts of health problems.
- Don't put yourself under time pressure. When a patient finally discusses her sexual problem, the pressure she feels

may project onto the practitioner. It is important to remember that sexual problems are usually long-standing, not acute. If time runs out the patient can always return for another office visit.

Talking as a treatment

While such concrete questions have clear value for diagnostic purposes, they can also be of benefit to the patient. Patients have the opportunity to ask questions as diverse as, "Am I disturbed because I don't feel any desire for sex?", "Do I have the right kind of orgasms?", and "Is it okay for me to still be wanting sex when I am seventy-two?" Such questions may have been weighing on the patient's mind for a long time; the issue can be cleared up quite simply in such a conversation.

Additionally, referring back to the anorgasmic older women who had simply not been using an effective technique, it may not be the so-called problem that requires treatment, and recognizing this may be the end of the matter. Once again, it is a matter of delicate questioning. The patient might be asked, "Now you know that, is it okay for you, or do you want to change anything?" Patients are often satisfied with that new knowledge and do not want to do anything further. Others may prefer to be coached on how to achieve orgasm.

The therapeutic value of the diagnostic conversation is that it often reveals a completely new perspective for the patient. For this reason, it is important to include the partner in the conversation. A more comprehensive understanding of the sexual problem is likely to emerge. However, in general, it is better to have the initial talk with the woman alone to allow her the

opportunity to speak about those things she might be reluctant to bring up in front of her partner, such as past sexual abuse or other partners. In a conversation with the couple, the woman's lack of desire, which may have been viewed as her problem, might be revealed as being much more of an interaction or communication problem between the two people.

Taking a sexual history is usually seen as part of the first diagnostic step on the road toward a solution to the sexual problem. It can be much more than that. The conversation about the patient's sexual history is actually the beginning of treatment. Feedback from patients often reveals that if they had realized the intimate questions they were going to be asked they would never have had the courage to come. But they also say, "I am so happy we had this talk." When they come again, it is discovered they have taken the talk as a model of what is possible, that conversation about sexual health is possible, and that they have taken the first step in getting past their paralysis. Many patients use their conversation with their physician as a model to strike up a conversation with their partner, their close friend, or their sister, and report this on their return visit. This is the start of treatment.

Conclusion

The benefit of taking the kind of precise and detailed sexual history advocated here is that it provides a clear basis for any necessary next steps for treatment. For the health-care professional, this provides a very thorough understanding of the situation, rather than wasting time waiting for the information to emerge over time.

9.5 Physical examination in female sexual dysfunction

Elizabeth Gunther Stewart

Introduction

When a woman has found the courage to speak up about sexual dysfunction, the problem is unlikely to be a new one. Women vainly await spontaneous regression, and try available modalities to achieve resolution. Reassurance for them at this point will come only from adequate history and examination. Scheduling time for thorough investigation or referring to an experienced colleague will address their concern. The physical examination is key in identifying physical abnormality underlying female sexual dysfunction.

History factors that influence physical examination

General influences on the physical examination

The physical examination should be tailored to the chief complaint, to rule out a physical reason for dysfunction in desire, arousal, and/or orgasm, and to search for a physical cause of irritative symptoms or pain. The examination should focus on specific areas elucidated in the history of the present illness, such as meticulous evaluation of the skin if pruritus interferes with sexual function, or careful examination of the abdominal wall and bimanual evaluation of pelvic organs if deep dyspareunia is the complaint. By the end of a patient's history, the clinician should have a reasonable idea of what the diagnosis may be. Hence, time spent taking a careful history (see Chapters 9.2 and 9.4 of this book) is invaluable.

The physical examination addresses problems in communication. Unable to use the proper anatomic descriptor, a patient needs to point out the location of the problem. When she has difficulty communicating what "inside" means to her, the examination distinguishes the vulvar vestibule from an endovaginal or endopelvic locus. Table 9.5.1 covers history information that will help direct the physical examination when pain is the source of the dysfunction.

Specific history influencing the examination

In women under the age of 50 years, vestibulodynia is the leading cause of superficial dyspareunia.[1] A total of 56% of women over the age of 50 years experience dyspareunia as a result of atrophy,[2] whereas premature ovarian failure can occur at any age from the teens to age 40.

It is important to note the duration of dyspareunia. If painful intercourse has persisted since sexual activity commenced, the physician must consider the possibility of a congenital anomaly, female circumcision, or vestibulodynia, in addition to any psychosexual issues. Acquired dyspareunia has multiple etiologies.

Cyclical discomfort can suggest *Candida* or endometriosis. Seminal plasma allergy can manifest as itching and burning immediately on penetration or with ejaculation. Discomfort with certain partners suggests a possible problem with the relationship, although this does not rule out a physical etiology. These differences in presentation require that the clinician be attentive to the timing of the dyspareunia.

The discomfort may be located superficially or deep. Superficial pain suggests dermatitis or dermatosis, vaginal infection, or vulvodynia. Deep dyspareunia may represent a painful focus in the abdominal wall, pelvic pathology, or impaction against the cervix.

Table 9.5.1. History questions that direct the physical examination when pain causes dysfunction[3]

Question to patient	Information obtained	Physical diagnosis to consider
When do you feel the pain?	Timing of dyspareunia	
	Arousal: pain with increased blood flow	Vestibulitis, clitorodynia, vulvodynia
	Foreplay: pain with touching	Vestibulitis, vulvodynia, *Candida. albicans*
	Penetration: pain on entry	Vestibulitis, lichen planus, lichen sclerosus
	Throughout: pain from start to finish	Vulvovaginal diseases, mixed pain of vestibulitis and vulvodynia
	Postcoital: itching, burning, stinging, soreness, and edema develop after sex	*C. albicans*, contactant (lubricant, latex, spermicide), seminal plasma allergy, dermatitis, vestibulitis, vulvodynia
Where do you feel the pain? (probably need to have patient point during examination)	Location of the discomfort	Pelvic dyspareunia versus lower genital dyspareunia
	Abdominal wall	Trigger point from intra-abdominal disease, abdominal wall muscle
	Uterus, adnexal	Pelvic: endometritis, adenomyosis, large posterior fibroid, pelvic inflammatory disease, endometriosis, adnexal pathology
	Clitoris, labia, perineum	Lower genital: clitorodynia or clitoral lesion, dermatitis, dermatosis, vulvodynia
	Vestibule	Lower genital: vestibulitis, dermatitis, lichen sclerosus, lichen planus, lesion, Bartholin pathology, atrophy
	Vagina	Lower genital: vaginitis, lichen planus, lesion, levator hypertonicity, vulvodynia, atrophy
What is the discomfort like?	Itching	Seminal plasma allergy with penetration or postcoital latex allergy if condom used, *C. albicans*, LSC
	Resistance, "hitting something"	Rectocele with stool, pelvic floor muscle hypertonicity, cervical contact
	Sharp pain, ripping	Vestibulitis, synechiae of LS, LP, fissuring
Does discomfort occur at other times?	Pain only with sex	Vestibulitis
	Symptoms at other times	Vulvar disease, vaginitis, vulvodynia
What have you tried for help?	Successful aids give clues to pathology	Estrogen relieves atrophy
		Topical steroids treat dermatitis, dermatosis
		Fungal suppression controls recurrent or cyclical candidiasis

LSC = lichen simplex chronicus; LS = lichen sclerosus; LP = lichen planus.

Planning tactics before the pelvic portion of the physical examination

If this is the first pelvic examination for a young woman, the value of adequate education beforehand by the health-care professional or one of the staff must not be forgotten. Some women have had negative experiences with pelvic examinations or may not be able to tolerate a pelvic examination because of psychosexual issues. Asking about previous experience with this examination and taking measures to reduce anxiety and discomfort give the patient control over the experience. Use of premedication or the presence of a support person may be helpful. Other considerations may be a contract with the patient to stop the examination if requested, or the use of a pediatric speculum. This may allow full cooperation with a complete evaluation. Occasionally, the pelvic examination may need to be scheduled for performance under anesthesia or deferred until desensitization with a sexual therapist has been achieved.

The physical examination should be scheduled carefully. It is ideal to avoid menses. If physical symptoms are part of the problem, it is helpful to see a patient when it is flaring up. If there is dysfunction that occurs at a specific time, such as midcycle dyspareunia, the examination should be scheduled at that time. Patients with postcoital complaints may need instructions to have intercourse just before the examination. Otherwise, patients should be instructed not to have intercourse or douche for 24 h before the examination, and to discontinue 2 weeks before it all topical preparations applied to the vulva and all oral and topical antifungal medications.

Such scheduling can be challenging and may require two visits: one to start on the history and examination, and another during the worst symptoms while medication free.

The physical examination

Purpose of the examination

The goals of the examination for a woman with sexual dysfunction are to detect pathology, educate the woman about normal anatomy and physiology, and, if pain is a feature, reproduce and localize the pain.

The examination consists of the general examination with focus on the specific points listed below, the abdominal examination, the detailed pelvic examination including a rectovaginal examination, and any indicated diagnostic studies.

Step-by-step discipline is important, since omission of steps or a change in the order can lead to a missed diagnosis or obscured clues. The progression of steps also reserves the least comfortable parts of the evaluation for the end of the examination.

Step one: general examination

The practitioner should look for physical signs of diseases that may lead to sexual dysfunction. The following systems should be examined for each new patient.

Constitutional

Weight loss or gain from diabetes: with vascular disorder or chronic candidiasis (failure to arouse, anorgasmia, or dyspareunia), depression (low desire, libido-reducing drugs), anorexia (amenorrhea, low estrogen), or thyroid disorder (low desire).

Oral cavity

- lacy white reticules, cherry red gingival erosions from: lichen planus (dyspareunia)
- aphthae (also found on the vulva)
- cold sores (herpes simplex virus 1, HSV-1, can be transferred to vulva).

Integumentary

- acne, rosacea: treated with antibiotics leading to candidiasis (dyspareunia)
- psoriasis on extremities: often accompanied by vulvar lesions
- purple polygonal plaques: lichen planus may accompany the vulvovaginal gingival variant of lichen planus (dyspareunia)
- white patches: lichen sclerosus
- scaling patches: eczema (common on vulva)
- spiders, palmar erythema: alcoholism (low desire, anorgasmia).

Cardiovascular

Hypertension, output failure: cardiovascular disease (medications altering sexual function).

Pulmonary

Wheezing, diminished breath sounds: asthma, frequent antibiotics or steroids that cause candidiasis (dyspareunia); chronic obstructive pulmonary disease: fatigue (low desire).

Hepatic

Spiders, palmar erythema, hepatomegaly: alcoholic cirrhosis (low desire).

Breast

Lumpectomy or mastectomy: breast cancer, altered body image, chemotherapy with ovarian failure, low estrogen (low desire, dyspareunia). Tamoxifen can estrogenize the vagina and lead to chronic candidiasis (dyspareunia).

Kidney

Renal failure, dialysis (low desire).

Endocrine

- vascular abnormality, painful neuropathy: diabetes (candidiasis, anorgasmia, dyspareunia)
- goiter: hypothyroidism (low desire, orgasm)
- tachycardia, exophthalmos: hyperthyroidism: (low desire)
- pigment changes: Addison's disease (orgasm)
- trunkal obesity, buffalo hump, striae: Cushing's disease (orgasm, dyspareunia)
- short stature, webbed neck, ovarian failure: Turner's syndrome (orgasm, dyspareunia)
- amenorrhea, atrophy: premature ovarian failure, hypoestrogenism (low desire, dyspareunia)
- galactorrhea: hyperprolactinemia: (low desire).

Neurologic

- seizures: epilepsy (medications inhibit desire)
- paraplegia, hemiplegia, painful spasticity: cerebrovascular accident (mechanical difficulty with intercourse)
- weakness, paralysis: multiple sclerosis (possible association with vulvodynia).

Connective tissue

- joint inflammation: arthritis (pain restricting movement)
- dry eye, mouth: Sjögren's syndrome (vaginal dryness)
- skin, muscle, joint abnormality: lupus (vulvar lesions, steroids promoting candidiasis).

Step two: abdominal examination

The physician should palpate the abdominal wall with attention to any tender area the patient points out. Such painful spots can represent myofascial injury, or trigger points for pain referred from intraperitoneal disease within the abdomen or pelvis. If these areas are still tender to palpation as the patient flexes her abdominal wall muscles (by raising her shoulders off the table), the source is probably the muscle itself.

To identify deep tenderness, mass, or bladder tenderness, deep palpation of the lower quadrants should be performed.

Step three: the pelvic examination

The pelvic examination involves systematic evaluation from the external to the internal genitalia. There are six sequential steps to the pelvic examination. First the physician should inspect and palpate the mons, labia majora, and perineum, progressing to the labia minora, prepuce, and clitoris, and then the urethra, vestibule, and introitus. Table 9.5.2 lists the physical causes of dyspareunia, the location affected, and the specific condition and associated history.

Next, the health-care professional should perform the Q-tip test, as illustrated in Fig. 9.5.1. This should be followed by a single-digit examination. Then the physician should do a speculum examination of the vagina and collect specimens. A bimanual examination should be performed, followed by a rectovaginal examination.

Vulvar inspection

Anatomy
Vulvar anatomy, especially the prepuce and labia minora, can be silently or symptomatically altered by disease. Only careful inspection will reveal synechiae of the labia minora anteriorly and/or posteriorly, which can narrow the introitus to cause painful intromission. Fusion of the prepuce buries the glans clitoris, sometimes reducing sexual response, although this occurs often without symptoms.

During this portion of the examination, it is ideal to use a large mirror to inform the woman about normal anatomy or abnormal findings.

The physician should use gentle palpation to confirm the presence of the elastic retractable clitoral hood or prepuce. Scarring of the hood to the glans clitoris or fusion of the hood over the glans (phimosis) is a classic symptom of lichen sclerosus or lichen planus (in rare cases, pemphigus) and should prompt a search for other lesions posteriorly on the vulva. The skin on or near the prepuce should be examined for subtle white reticules of lichen planus (see Fig. 12.2.11, Chapter 12.2).

The glans clitoris should be checked to confirm that it is normal. With the prepuce gently retracted, the glans clitoris should be inspected for masses or lesions of lichen sclerosus or lichen planus under the hood. The physician should palpate the glans through the prepuce for a mass. The area should be examined for periclitoral fissures or small erosions. Vulvodynia can cause clitoral or periclitoral pain without any physical findings. Hypertrophy of the glans (>1 cm) should prompt a workup for excess androgens, but is not usually a cause of pain.

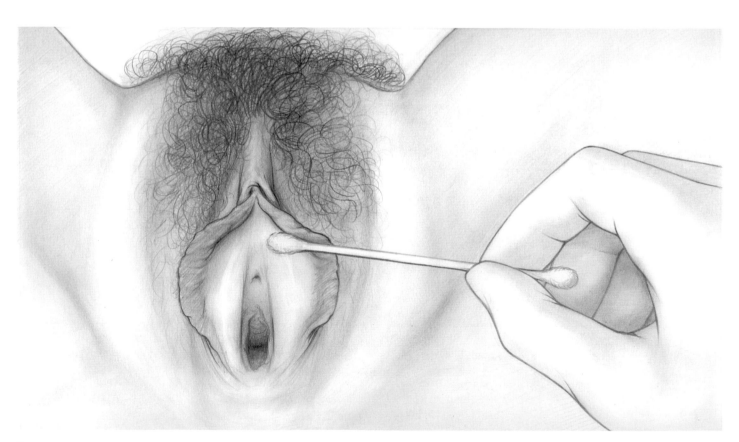

Figure 9.5.1. The Q-tip test.[4] Original drawing courtesy of Dawn Danby and Paul Waggoner.

Table 9.5.2. Differential diagnoses for physical causes of dyspareunia[5]

Location affected	Specific condition	Important history	Source of dyspareunia	Comments and caveats
Vulva and vestibule	Dermatitis (eczema)	Atopic history, other eczema	Erythema, scaling, fissuring	Look for *Candida* also
	Dermatosis: lichen sclerosus	Itching, recent or lifelong, soreness, possibly no symptoms	Fissures, ulceration, scarring	Look for *Candida* also
	Dermatosis: lichen planus	Itching, irritation, burning	Erosions, ulcers, scarring	Many drugs exacerbate
	Ulcerative disease: herpes simplex or zoster, chancroid, GI, aphthae, Behçet's disease	Episodic outbreaks	Ulceration varying in size, tenderness	Behçet's disease very rare, involves oral ulcers, uveitis, other systems
	Labial hypertrophy	Irritation with physical activity	Elongation of labia	Look for vestibulitis
	Female circumcision	Ethnicity and country of origin	Absence of clitoris and prepuce, labial fusion	
	Generalized dyesthesia (Vulvodynia)	Episodic or virtually constant burning, stinging, soreness irritation, rawness	Often no findings; or erythema and edema, areas of hyper- or hypo-esthesia	Long history of unsuccessful UTI, yeast, BV treatments
	Radiation	History of gynecologic or urinary tumor	Pallor, alopecia, loss of elasticity	
Urethra and bladder	Urinary tract infection	Dysuria, frequency, urgency	Tenderness over bladder	Sx with negative cultures suggests vulvodynia
	Urethral diverticulum	Dysuria, dribbling, pain with penetration	Urethral tenderness, mass	
	Interstitial cystitis	Pelvic pain, dysuria, urgency, frequency, nocturia	Tenderness over bladder, along anterior vaginal wall	Look for vestibulitis
Vestibule and vagina	Atrophy: low or absent estrogen	Dryness, irritation, hx breast feeding, oligo/amenorrhea, low estrogen/high androgenic OCP, depo-Provera, anorexia, exercise, chemotherapy, radiation, BSO, premenopausal tamoxifen, aromatase inhibitors	Reduction in labial size, mucosal color and textural change, fissures; elevated vaginal pH, atrophic wet preparation	Can occur at *any* age
	Vulvovaginitis: *Candida albicans*	Antibiotics, steroids, estrogen, immunosuppression	Itching, erythema, edema, discharge, fissures; or few sx	Look for superimposed vestibulitis
	Desquamative inflammatory	Irritative sx, profuse discharge	Erythema, sheets of wbc, parabasals, no lactobacilli	Atypical Pap. Look for vestibulitis
	Vulvovaginitis: *Trichomonas*	Itching, discharge, or few sx	Mobile trichomonads; plus culture	
	Bartholin cyst or abscess	Swelling and pain	Cystic mass at base of vestibule	
	Seminal plasma allergy	Itching on entry or ejaculation	Edema and erythema after coitus	Trial of condom helps
	Dermatosis: lichen sclerosus	Itching or no symptoms	Fissures, scaring around introitus	*Candida*, vulvodynia
	Dermatosis: lichen planus	Itching, burning, discharge	Erosions, ulceration, scarring	As above, atypical Pap
	Inadequate lubrication, dryness	Poor sexual technique, sexual dysfunction, Sjögren's syndrome, OCP, medications, vestibulitis	Dryness, tenderness	No good test for lubrication; hard to judge on examination; history important

Table 9.5.2. (Continued)

Location affected	Specific condition	Important history	Source of dyspareunia	Comments and caveats
	Radiation	History of gynecologic or urinary tumor	Pallor, loss of elasticity, scarring	
Vestibule only	Vestibulitis	Pain mainly with penetration, tampon or speculum	Tenderness on touch or pressure, erythema	Easily missed without Q-tip testing
Perineum and anus	Episiotomy	Vaginal delivery with episiotomy	Nonhealing, tenderness	
	Dermatitis (eczema)	Itching, irritation	Erythema, edema, fissuring	Look for *Candida*
	Inflammatory bowel: Crohn's disease	Diarrhea, bleeding, pain	Edema, tags, fissures, sinuses	May precede bowel sx
Rectum	Rectocele	Sensation of vaginal obstruction	Protrusion of stool-filled rectum	
Vagina	Pelvic floor hypertonus	Aching pain, vaginismus	Levator spasm on palpation	
	Congenital anomaly: vaginal agenesis, imperforate hymen	Inability to be penetrated	Absent vagina, absent hymen	
Pelvis	Retroverted or prolapsed uterus	Pain with thrusting	Uterine retroversion or descent	
	Leiomyomata	Pain with thrusting	Tender uterine masses	Uncommon cause of pain
	Endometriosis, adenomyosis	Cramping, deep dyspareunia; history of menorrhagia, dysmenorrhea	Tender uterus, fixed uterus, nodules cul de sac rv septum, adnexal tenderness or masses	
	Adnexal pathology	Deep dyspareunia, cyclical	Tenderness in adnexa	
	Pelvic inflammatory disease	Chronic pelvic pain, deep dyspareunia	CMT, uterine, adnexal tenderness	
	Abdominal wall trigger points	Abdominal wall injury or intra-abdominal disease	Myofascial injury or intra-abdominal pathology	Tender point on flexion of abdominal wall muscle suggests pain from muscle itself
	Irritable bowel syndrome	Deep dyspareunia	None; or pelvic tenderness	

GI = gastrointestinal; UTI = urinary tract infections; BV = bacterial vaginosis; sx = symptoms; wbc = white blood cell; BSO = bilateral salpingoophorectomy; OCP = oral contraceptive pill; rv = rectovaginal; CMT = cervical motion tenderness.

The presence of the labia minora must be confirmed bilaterally. Flattening, resorption, and loss of a portion of labia minora posteriorly suggest the existence of lichen sclerosus or lichen planus (see Fig. 12.2.12, Chapter 12.2). Hypertrophy of the labia minora (>5 cm in width) can be a mechanical cause of dyspareunia.

The health-care professional should confim that the introitus is patent in order to rule out a thickened, inelastic hymen or the rare congenital absence of the vagina. In addition to narrowing the opening of the synechiae of the labia minora anteriorly or posteriorly, lichen planus or sclerosus can cause pain on downward retraction or painful fissuring with intromission.

Female circumcision, depending on the type, will significantly alter the genital anatomy. Atrophy associated with normal menopause or premature ovarian failure that may occur at any age may cause flattened labia, thin, dry tissue, and infantile anatomy.

Skin color

The skin should be examined for color and quality. It should be pink, supple, and elastic. Thin, dry tissue is characteristic of atrophy or Sjögren's syndrome. Epidermal whitening and thickened, lichenified tissue is seen with lichen simplex chronicus, hypertrophic lichen planus, or lichen sclerosus. Whitening and thin inelastic tissue is also characteristic of radiation change. Erythema is a nonspecific finding, but subtle erythema is often seen under the hymenal remnants in cases of vestibulodynia.

Accurate testing for moisture and lubrication does not exist. Careful examination can give clues for atrophy, but only careful history gives information about lubrication.

Epithelial integrity

The skin should be intact. Fissures on any surface or along anatomic margins suggest *Candida* (see Fig. 12.2.5, Chapter 12.2), herpes, dermatitis (eczema), or dermatosis (lichen planus, lichen sclerosus, or lichen simplex chronicus) (see Fig. 12.2.17, Chapter 12.2). Flaking of the skin characteristic of eczema is often not seen on the moist vulva, but may be seen on the labia majora. Papules, pustules, and vesicles may represent a variety of disorders. Erosions classic for lichen planus are seen in the vestibule with glassy erythema and denudation of the surface (see Fig. 12.2.12, Chapter 12.2); often these have a white linear or lacy, reticulate border (Wickham's striae) (see Fig. 12.2.11, Chapter 12.2). *Candida* and herpes (see Fig. 12.2.2, Chapter 12.2) are leading causes of small ulcerations; aphthous ulcers can also be found (see Fig. 12.2.19, Chapter 12.2). These, like the ulcers of Epstein–Barr infection (see Fig. 12.2.10, Chapter 12.2), can be confused with the ulcers of Behçet's disease, which are rare and always associated with other lesions, often oral or occular.

It is important to recognize that vulvodynia frequently gives no physical findings.

Vulvar palpation

Palpation should be over the vulva, in the clitoral area, and on the perineum. The physician should take a moistened Q-tip and gently touch over the external vulvar surfaces to rule out a focus of tenderness (Fig. 9.5.1). Women with vulvodynia will often describe such activity as unpleasant (raw, abrasive, like sandpaper), but not painful. Using the fingertips, the practitioner should gently palpate in the clitoral area to rule out painful focus or mass. The hood should be checked again for retraction. Painful scarring at an episiotomy site is a possible cause of dyspareunia. It should be palpated carefully. Women often indicate that the perineum is the source of pain, but it is actually coming from the vestibule.

If the physician does not evaluate the vestibule but moves immediately to examination by speculum, it is easy to miss any tenderness in the vulvar vestibule. To evaluate vestibular pain, the labia minora should be gently separated and palpated with a moistened Q-tip starting at 12 o'clock and progressing around the vestibular "clock face" within Hart's line, posterior to hymenal remnants. Tenderness may be diffuse or isolated. The sites of Bartholin ducts and the epithelium at 6 o'clock in the vestibule are often the most tender foci. While atrophy is a frequent cause of dyspareunia, a urethral caruncle is an unusual cause.

Palpation: single digit

The discomfort of the speculum examination and bimanual evaluation may cause enough pain to terminate the examination prematurely, or prevent satisfactory evaluation because the pain caused may render a woman unable to localize her symptoms. For this reason, it is important to perform the single-digit palpation before the speculum examination.

This part of the examination searches for primary or secondary vaginismus. Primary vaginismus from a psychosexual source may manifest as extreme anxiety about the examination, difficulty in assuming and maintaining the lithotomy position, or inability to cooperate, leading to termination of the evaluation. While secondary vaginismus from the repeated pain of vestibulodynia may also manifest as above, it often generates milder anxiety and tensing, with ability to complete the examination, identifying the painful tightness and muscle spasm.

To perform the single-digit palpation, the physician must gently slide a single finger into the vaginal opening and depress the bulbocavernosus muscle, looking for tightness (spasm) and pain. This should be done in the midline, then to the left and to the right. To avoid stimulating the pain of vestibulodynia, the vestibule should be avoided by gentle and slow insertion of the digit in the exact center of the vaginal orifice. Then, to do the evaluation, the finger should be crooked so that only the tip touches the muscle.

Speculum examination with pH determination and sample collection
For the patient's comfort, a warm, well-lubricated speculum should be used. If the woman has pain, a narrow or pediatric speculum may be necessary.

With the speculum opened, apply the pH paper to the upper third of the vaginal wall, just inside the speculum. A normal pH (< 4.5) rules out infection other than by *Candida*. An elevated pH (> 4.5) is nonspecific and can reflect infection, atrophy, recent intercourse, or bleeding.

The vagina should be evaluated for adequate estrogenization, inflammation, fissures, erosion, ulcer, and masses. Atrophy manifests first as erythema, and then pallor with flattening of rugae and sometimes petechiae. Lichen planus (and rarely pemphigus) can cause scarring of the vagina, leading to telescoping posteriorly, and eventually causing foreshortening and obliteration.

The discharge should be examined for location, amount, color, and consistency. The appearance of the discharge should not form the basis for diagnosis as this indicator is extremely unreliable.[6] Measuring the pH and performing microscopy and other diagnostic studies are essential.

The health-care professional should collect samples of vaginal secretions for wet mount and yeast culture in Sabouraud's medium; cervical swabs may be sent for gonorrhea, chlamydia, and herpes. Vaginal bacterial culture grows normal commensals, is nonspecific, and therefore is not recommended. A normal pH and wet mount, with lactobacillus dominating the flora, rule out infection.

Before removing the speculum, the physician should rotate it gently to obtain visualization of all portions of the vagina and hymenal ring. Subtle, painful fissures of the ring may be seen only in this fashion.

Palpation: bimanual and evaluation of pelvic floor

Evaluation of the pelvic floor for trigger point tenderness is essential for the evaluation of dyspareunia, but this is not a skill familiar to many physicians. A physical therapist skilled in such assessment can be an invaluable part of the diagnostic team (see Chapter 4.4 on pelvic floor anatomy, and Chapter 12.3 on physical therapy).

The bulbospongiosis and levator vaginae portions of the levator ani that enclose the introitus need to be evaluated. These muscles are readily identified by having the patient squeeze the examining fingers inserted at the orifice. The muscles can then be examined for trigger points by gentle pincer palpation around the opening. Trigger points manifest as tender, taut bands that refer the ache to the vagina and perineum, reproducing the patient's pain complaint.[7]

The ischiocavernosus muscle is evaluated by pressing directly laterally from within the distal vagina against the edge of the pubic arch. A trigger point will refer pain to the perineal region.

A simple assessment of the levators and the underlying obturator internus may be achieved if the examiner places two fingers against the lateral wall of the pelvis just beyond the inside margin of the pubic arch over the obturator membrane. The upper finger overlies the anterior portion of the obturator internus while the lower finger palpates the levator ani and the underlying posterior portion of the obturator. Palpate the muscle fiber for tenderness or taut bands indicative of trigger points. Trigger points in both the levator ani and the obturator internus can cause vaginal pain.[7]

The lower examining hand should then evaluate the fornices and vaginal sidewalls for mass, nodularity, or tenderness. Bladder tenderness is assessed by upward palpation through the vaginal wall and downward pressure over the pubis. A tender mass along the urethra representing a diverticulum may be palpated through the anterior vaginal wall. The uterus and adnexa are then evaluated for masses, tenderness, and mobility.

Rectovaginal examination

Next, the physician should evaluate the anal sphincter tone and rectovaginal septum. Sphincter spasm may be associated with pelvic floor dysfunction; nodularity of the septum is associated with endometriosis. A rectocele filled with stool can interfere with penetration.

Step four: diagnostic studies

Wet mount

For a wet mount, the health-care professional must first mix vaginal secretions with a few drops of saline, cover this with a cover slip, and examine the slide under the microscope. The examiner needs to look for four features, epithelial cells, background flora, pathogens, and white blood cells.

Epithelial cells are large rectolinear, clean-bordered, superficial cells with small nuclei. Smaller oval cells with larger nuclei suggest parabasal cells representing atrophy or inflammation. Borders that are ragged occur with clue cells of bacterial vaginosis.

Background flora should consist mainly of long and short, motile rods representing the lactobacillus. Lack of lactobacilli is not a feature of candidal infection.

Presence or absence of pathogens should be noted. The wet mount is not highly specific; both *Candida albicans* and *Trichomonas* may be present in the vagina but are not seen on wet mount. Trichomonads must be motile. Addition of potassium hydroxide (KOH) to the secretions eliminates cells and allows better evaluation for *Candida*. Hyphae of *C. albicans* have smooth, parallel borders. They are opalescent, and spores can be seen within the hyphus, budding off the sides or ends, or adjacent and free. If yeast or trichomonads are not seen, only specific cultures rule out these infections. A negative KOH does not rule out *Candida*.

Multiple white blood cells are present when there is more than one white blood cell per epithelial cell. The finding is non-specific and can represent vaginal infection with yeast or *Trichomonas*, inflammatory vaginitis, or lichen planus, cervicitis, gonorrhea, herpes, chlamydia, fistula, or upper tract disease, and possibly allergy.

Cultures

Material for cultures must be obtained at the time of speculum examination.

Biopsy

A biopsy can be an important diagnostic test to rule out dermatitis, dermatosis, intraepithelial neoplasia, or neoplasia. Index of clinical suspicion is also important. A review by a dermatopathologist may prove to be invaluable. If a biopsy is negative in a woman with whitening and/or scarring and loss of architecture, lichen sclerosus or lichen planus is likely and needs follow-up and treatment.

Serology

Since hormonal abnormalities are a common cause of sexual dysfunction, a panel of blood tests is indicated in the workup. Basic tests would include glucose and HbA1c, and the appropriate serology to test for any hormone-related condition in question (see Chapter 14.7). Herpes serology is invaluable to rule out the virus as a source of irritative symptoms. Other specialized testing may be indicated.

Special studies

Referral for other testing is dictated by history and clinical findings. Helpful testing may include pelvic ultrasound, magnetic resonance imaging of the pelvis or spine, duplex Doppler ultrasound, biothesiometry, vaginal photoplethysmography, thermal testing, and diagnostic nerve blocks.

Conclusion

With the completion of the workup of history, physical examination, and associated testing, the clinician will have the necessary components to assess the role of a physical problem underlying female sexual dysfunction. Figure 9.5.2 gives a helpful algorithm for the diagnosis of vulvar pain.

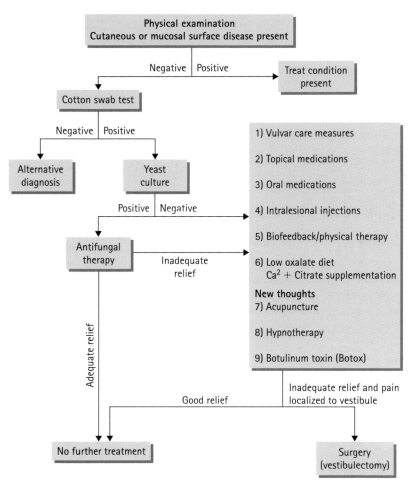

Figure 9.5.2. Algorithm for vulvar pain.[5]

References

1. Meana M, Binik YM, Khalife S et al. Biopsychosocial profile of women with dyspareunia. *Obstet Gynecol* 1997; 90: 583–9.

2. Jalbuena JR. Atrophic vaginitis in Filipino women. *Climacteric* 2001; 87: 55–8.

3. Stewart EG. Approach to the woman with dyspareunia. In BD Rose, ed. *Up To Date*. Wellesley: 2003.

4. Stewart EG, Spencer P. *The V Book*. New York: Bantam Books, 2002.

5. Haefner HK, Collins ME, Davis GD et al. The vulvodynia guideline. *J Low Genit Tract Dis* 2005; 9: 40–51.

6. Sobel JD. Overview of vaginitis. In BD Rose, ed. *Up to Date*. Wellesley: 2003.

7. Simons DG, Travell JG. *Myofascial Pain and Dysfunction: The Trigger Point Manual*, vol 2. *The Lower Extremities*. Philadelphia: Lippincott, Williams & Wilkins, 1993: 121–7.

SPECIALIZED LABORATORY TESTING

10.1 Blood flow: vaginal photoplethysmography

Nicole Prause, Erick Janssen

The most widely used method for assessing vaginal blood flow (see Chapters 4.1–4.3 and 5.4–5.6 of this book) is vaginal photoplethysmography. The vaginal photoplethysmograph, introduced by Palti and Bercovici[1] and refined by Sintchak and Geer,[2] is made of clear, acrylic plastic and is shaped like a menstrual tampon. Embedded in the device is an incandescent light that projects toward the vaginal wall. Some of the light is reflected back to a photosensitive cell within the body of the probe, while the rest of the light, presumably, is dispersed through the vaginal tissue (for tissue absorption estimates, see Niklas et al.[3]). Researchers generally assume that more light will return to the photosensitive cell as the amount of blood in the vaginal blood vessels increases. The change is represented as a change in mV from a basal value. In later years, an infrared light-emitting diode was introduced as an alternative to incandescent light,[4] a phototransistor replaced the photocell,[4] and a stabilizing, acrylic plate was developed that can be attached to the external cord of the device.[5] These innovations are thought to reduce potential signal drift (possibly produced by warming of the incandescent light), minimize probe movement, and allow for standardization of probe position. The vaginal photoplethysmograph can be easily placed by the participant herself and usually is cleaned with glutaraldehyde-based antiseptics (e.g., Cidex Plus, Cidex PA, or Metricide).

The photometer output typically is filtered to yield two signals. One signal is the direct current signal, also referred to as the vaginal blood volume, which is thought to provide an index of the total blood volume change in the vaginal wall.[6] The other signal is the alternating current signal, or vaginal pulse amplitude, which is thought to reflect pressure changes within the blood vessels of the vagina's vascular walls.[7] Signal cleaning usually includes reducing high-frequency noise and manually deleting artifacts. Next, response levels are computed for the time periods of interest. The length of the time period can vary from 5- or 10-s intervals over a condition to the entire condition. Within the selected period(s), signal values (in mV) are either averaged or the maximum value is taken. Response for the vaginal blood volume is represented by the actual value of

the signal, whereas response for the vaginal pulse amplitude is represented by the amplitude of each complete cycle in the signal. Typically, researchers use a baseline period to calculate difference scores for use in analyses.

The sensitivity and specificity of the vaginal photoplethysmograph for assessing sexual arousal, as opposed to general arousal, has been supported by several studies (e.g., Henson et al.[8] or Zingheim and Sandman[9]). Available data strongly suggest that vaginal blood volume is the less sensitive measure,[5,10,11] so vaginal blood volume will not be discussed further. The influence of anxiety-inducing, sexually threatening, or neutral film excerpts on vaginal pulse amplitude responses is specific, increasing only to film excerpts with sexual content.[5,12] Mirroring participants' self-reported sexual arousal, genital response increased significantly from baseline during the presentation of a sexually threatening film, but increased further during a nonthreatening sexual film.[5,12] In general, these findings demonstrate response specificity of vaginal pulse amplitude to sexual stimuli.

Alternative measures of genital response

Over the years, several instruments have been developed to assess physiologic sexual arousal in women (see Chapters 10.2–10.4). For example, thermography is a method for detecting and measuring heat from various regions of the body, including the genital area, which can be recorded photographically.[13] This approach, however, lacks convincing validity data, having been tested in only one male and one female. Devices also have been designed to measure vaginal pH.[14,15] On average, vaginal pH increases with increasing sexual arousal. Measurement of vaginal pH, however, requires potentially disruptive experimenter involvement, and pH seems to vary nonsystematically across different areas of the vagina.[16] A heated electrode to measure oxygen pressure and heat dissipation also has informed researchers about vaginal changes that accompany sexual arousal, and is minimally affected by artifacts.[17,18] However, this instrument must be placed directly by an experimenter, and the heating element and suction cup to attach it could cause tissue damage if left in place too long. Finally, some researchers have used Doppler ultrasonography to record clitoral vascular changes by quantifying changes in blood velocity.[19] However, this method currently requires a technician to hold the probe in place over the clitoris.[20]

Several studies have been reported on the relationship between labial temperature and the vaginal photoplethysmograph. Henson and coworkers[21] examined the reliability of the two instruments across two sessions. Although both the general response pattern and response amplitude proved fairly reliable for both instruments, labial temperature was the most consistent on both parameters. In a second study, Henson and coworkers[8] found high correlations between subjective sexual arousal and both vaginal pulse amplitude and labial temperature changes. Although the labial temperature clip currently is used in few laboratories, it offers several advantages over vaginal photoplethysmograph. The labial temperature clip offers an absolute scale of measurement, is less sensitive to movement artifacts than the vaginal photoplethysmograph (as discussed in a later section), and may be more easily be used during menses. Some have criticized the labial clip because it requires the control of ambient temperature and does not consistently return to baseline levels.[22,23] However, the vaginal photoplethysmograph also does not consistently return to baseline levels (e.g., Graham et al.[24]). The slow return to baseline genital response levels may not be a problem with the vaginal photoplethysmograph *per se*, especially considering that the labial thermistor also rarely returns to baseline levels, and it may reflect an actual, slow physiologic process in females.

Another new approach, the labial photoplethysmograph, relies on measurements of genital responses that are similar to the vaginal photoplethysmograph. The labial photoplethysmograph is a small, plastic clip, originally designed to measure blood flow in the ear lobe (BIOPAC Systems, Model TSD100). It can be attached to the labium minorum. In a small study (n = 10), the labial photoplethysmograph was compared simultaneously with the vaginal photoplethysmograph while participants viewed neutral, sexual, sexually threatening, and threatening film clips.[12] Both instruments were specific to sexual content and correlated strongly with participants' own ratings of their sexual arousal. Although participants reported that the labial photoplethysmograph was somewhat more difficult to place and less comfortable, the labial device exhibited fewer movement artifacts than the vaginal photoplethysmograph. Given the potentially large impact that movement artifacts may be having on the analysis of vaginal photoplethysmograph data,[25] the labial photoplethysmograph warrants further development.

In summary, several promising alternatives to the vaginal photoplethysmograph exist. In particular, it is unclear why the labial thermistor is not more widely used. The thermistor has

particularly strong advantages over the vaginal photoplethysmograph, including an absolute scale of measurement and resistance to movement artifacts.

Interpreting vaginal pulse amplitude

Despite the title of this chapter, the vaginal photoplethysmograph does not necessarily measure vaginal blood flow. The vagina consists of a layered, scaly cell epithelium with numerous folds (but without sweat or hair glands), surrounded by sheaths of smooth muscle.[76,77] Although the vascular vaginal walls are supplied by an extensive anastomotic network of blood vessels, the vagina itself is almost anaerobic. The amount of blood in the vaginal walls increases with sexual arousal, although the mechanism causing the increase has recently become a topic of debate. Historically, researchers described the increased blood flow as a process of vasocongestion, a gradual increase in capillary blood flow. Levin and Goddard[28] have suggested that vasomotion, the oscillation of vascular tone in capillaries,[29] may better characterize changes in vaginal pulse amplitude. As support for this idea, they cite a pattern of large and small amplitude peaks in vaginal pulse amplitude that change in proportion with increasing sexual arousal. Vasomotion refers to the phenomenon that capillaries are, essentially, open or closed, and different capillaries are recruited at different levels of sexual arousal (cf. motor unit recruitment). Increased blood volume in the vaginal walls increases the force in the vaginal walls, which drives transudation of $NaCl^+$-rich plasma through the vaginal epithelium, coalescing into the slippery film of vaginal lubrication and neutralizing the vagina's usually acidic state (see Chapters 4.1–4.3 and 5.4–5.6).[16,30] Given the many and complex changes that occur in vaginal physiology during sexual arousal, it is too early to assume that vaginal pulse amplitude indexes changes in blood flow alone, if at all. More comprehensive models of vaginal physiology and its relationship to other (central and peripheral) systems are yet to be developed.

Levin[31] stated that one of the basic assumptions underlying the use of the vaginal photoplethysmograph is that changes in vaginal pulse amplitude reflect vascular events only in the genitalia. He further suggests that vaginal pulse amplitude reflects rather complex interactions between sympathetic and parasympathetic regulatory processes and between circulatory and vaginal blood pressure. Vaginal blood flow changes could partly reflect increases in general circulatory blood pressure that occur with sexual, as well as general, arousal.[32] However, some preliminary data argue against that idea.[12]

Part of the difficulty in deciphering what vaginal pulse amplitude represents lies in its lack of an absolute scale. Since the scale is relative and no published calibration method exists, the use of vaginal pulse amplitude in between-subjects designs requires caution when drawing conclusions. Vaginal pulse amplitude has not been shown to represent any specific physiologic process or event, and may, in fact, reflect multiple physiologic processes or events. Disentangling which components of vaginal pulse amplitude indicate which physiologic phenomena would allow researchers to select filters more accurately, based on the specific phenomenon they wish to investigate.

Artifacts

Artifacts in vaginal pulse amplitude are common and variable in appearance. The detection of artifacts is not standardized, and the procedures used often are not described in research publications. Movement artifacts are inferred when the signal has sudden, strong fluctuations in amplitude. Not only distinct body movements (such as sitting back in a chair), though, but also less conspicuous behaviors (such as tensing one's abdominal or pelvic muscles, or crossing one's ankles) can affect the vaginal photoplethysmograph's output,[33,34] and these artifacts are not always as easy to detect. They may increase or decrease the amplitude, cause a basal shift, or obliterate the signal for a period of time. Moreover, some circumvaginal muscular contractions during sexual arousal are normal.[35–37] As a result, artifacts threaten the validity of vaginal pulse amplitude data, and ignoring their presence or editing them in inconsistent or ill-defined ways could render vaginal pulse amplitude findings unreliable.

Two potential strategies exist for managing artifacts. The most apparent strategy is to prevent them. For instance, providing a reclining chair or an examination table and instructing participants to try not to move or tense their muscles, especially during stimulus presentations, may help considerably to reduce the number of movement artifacts. More realistically, researchers may manage artifacts after data collection is complete. Usually, each individual artifact is edited out of a signal after visual inspection by a researcher. The potentially low reliability of single raters begs for better standardization. Standardization is achieved in other fields by signal processing algorithms,[38–40] which could benefit sexual psychophysiologists who use the vaginal photoplethysmograph as well. Owing to high intra- and inter-participant artifact variability, however, developing algorithms for the editing of vaginal pulse amplitude signals is a challenge. Standardization would minimize processing time, and encourage the operationalization of artifacts. If laboratories cannot develop artifact processing algorithms, they should, at a minimum, articulate what methods were used to identify and edit signal artifacts in publications.

Menstruation

Several psychophysiologic studies in women have found that levels of subjective sexual arousal in response to sexual stimuli tend to remain stable across phases of the menstrual cycle. However, a more complex picture emerges for genital sexual response. Some studies have found stable response patterns across menstrual phases.[41,42] Others have found higher response levels during the premenstrual as compared to the periovulatory

phase.[43,44] Still others have reported complex interactions between menstrual phases and the order in which the phases were tested.[24,45] Among the factors that may have contributed to this lack of consistency are differences in the method used for determining cycle phase, experimental design, and participant characteristics.[46] Although there is no consensus about the possible effects of menstrual cycle phase on sexual arousal, it is important to control for, or, at the very least, assess participants' menstrual phase.

Relationship of physiologic and subjective sexual arousal

As in other psychophysiologic research areas, physiologic and subjective indices of sexual arousal do not correlate perfectly (cf. Lang and Cuthbert[47]). Correlations between vaginal pulse amplitude and subjective sexual arousal vary widely, whether subjective arousal is measured discretely[48] or continuously.[49] Women typically are reported to exhibit lower concordance between physiologic and subjective sexual arousal than men,[50–53] although men with and without sexual dysfunction also frequently exhibit discordance between their erection level and subjective reports of sexual arousal.[10,54–56] Since sexual arousal is a construct that may not be captured best by vaginal pulse amplitude,[22,57] it is inappropriate to characterize correlations in women as "poor". Variations in concordance may occur for many different reasons which, upon further investigation, might contribute to our understanding of vaginal pulse amplitude.

One reason for the variability in concordance could be that components of sexual arousal are under the control of multiple mechanisms.[58] Janssen et al.[59] presented a model that highlights the interaction between automatic (unconscious) and controlled (conscious) cognitive processes, and proposed that different levels of processing may differentially affect subjective and physiologic sexual arousal. The model states that unconscious processes help explain the automaticity of the genital response, whereas subjective feelings of sexual arousal are under the control of higher-level, conscious, cognitive processing. Several studies suggest that preconscious, automatic activation of sexual cognitive networks are possible in both men and women, and that subsequent conscious evaluations of sexual stimuli do not always match subjectively reported sexual arousal or sexual attraction.[60–63]

The variability in concordance could also be due to different women attending to different cues, or even different cues at different points of their sexual response. Laan et al.[64] found that women's subjective and physiologic indices of sexual arousal were more strongly correlated at later moments of sexual stimulation (presumably at greater levels of sexual arousal). Physical cues may become more salient at higher levels of sexual arousal when, for instance, vaginal lubrication increases and is more easily detected.

Finally, the variability in women's concordance may appear

low because of the way that they are asked to report their level of sexual arousal. Research suggests that if women are asked to report on their genital changes, rather than on their sexual arousal, the agreement between their genital and subjective measures will be stronger.[65,66] This supports the contention of researchers who have suggested that women attend to many factors in addition to their genital response when reporting their level of sexual desire or arousal (e.g., Basson[67]). If the latter is true, and if men tend to focus more on physiologic cues in estimating their sexual arousal, then a lower correlation between genital blood flow and reported sexual arousal in women than men is to be expected. Low correlations are not, de facto, problematic. Discerning what factors alter the relationship between subjective and physiologic components of sexual arousal in women could inform better models of female sexual function. In view of the variability in physiologic and subjective response patterns, it is arbitrary to promote either response as the gold standard. Sexual arousal is, at this time, best approached as a construct with multiple (affective, physiologic, and behavioral) indicators.[68]

Clinical application

Clinical diagnoses, in general, are based on the presence of stable tendencies that are designated as dysfunctional and present in some individuals, but not in others. Since the vaginal photoplethysmograph cannot reliably be used in between-subject designs, vaginal pulse amplitude response alone is an inadequate basis for diagnosing sexual dysfunction. On the other hand, psychophysiologic measures are used to compare diagnostic groups in other research areas even though they also lack an absolute scale and are not associated with a single physiologic process (e.g., electroencephalography[69]). Certainly, less is understood about vaginal pulse amplitude than many of these other measures, and vaginal pulse amplitude appears more variable between individuals. In summary, researchers should use a within-participants design whenever possible with vaginal pulse amplitude. Should they use a between-participants design, attempts should be made to recruit large samples, and between-participant differences in vaginal pulse amplitude should be interpreted with caution.

One way that vaginal pulse amplitude may be useful for diagnostic purposes is through the identification of patterns of dysfunctional sexual response. For instance, Wouda et al.[70] found that the vaginal response of women with dyspareunia decreased during the portion of an erotic video portraying penetrative sex, compared with portions portraying oral sex or petting, although genital response to the penetrative sex portion increased further in women without dyspareunia. Moreover, Tuiten et al.[71] demonstrated that women with hypothalamic amenorrhea exhibited a smaller vaginal pulse amplitude increase from baseline to fantasy than controls, but that they exhibited increases to sexual films similar to nonamenorrheic women; the decreased response to fantasy in the patient group was eliminated with testosterone

administration. While not diagnostic ipso facto, this may prove a useful addition to diagnostic approaches if future research confirms its incremental validity.[72]

Vaginal pulse amplitude has also been used to assess treatment effects. For example, Morokoff and Heiman[73] compared a group of women entering sex therapy for treatment of low arousal with a control group of sexually functional women across two sessions. In addition to the problems associated with the use of between-subject designs when measuring vaginal pulse amplitude, the comparison of women's responses over two sessions introduces new complications. This approach requires that women reinsert the vaginal photoplethysmograph, which is not likely to result in exactly the same positioning. As a result, the vaginal photoplethysmograph may record from different tissue(s) leading to potentially substantial differences in observed baseline and response levels.

Even measuring vaginal pulse amplitude within participants during a single session (for example, to assess the effects of a drug) can be problematic. One problem is that vaginal pulse amplitude baselines within a single, brief session often cannot be re-established (e.g., Graham et al.[24]). If physiologic arousal truly dissipates so slowly, studies testing drugs with a long time-to-efficacy or a slow clearance rate, as is typical of many selective phosphodiesterase type-5 inhibitors, require careful interpretation of vaginal pulse amplitude when using a single-session, within-participants design. In those cases, unless extensive return-to-baseline periods are used, counterbalancing conditions will more likely than not reveal order effects. Moreover, whether or not this failure of vaginal pulse amplitude to return to baseline levels reflects a true physiologic process (possibly representing the presence of a sustained genital response), the relative scaling means that an increase of 10 mV over baseline in one condition is not necessarily equivalent to an increase of 10 mV over a second baseline in a later condition.

Signal acquisition and processing

Hardware and software

Laboratory equipment for the measurement of vaginal pulse amplitude is available from various manufacturers. No hardware brand is necessarily better than another for recording vaginal pulse amplitude, although selecting hardware that is already made to work with the vaginal photoplethysmograph may simplify laboratory setup. The more significant components to consider during hardware selection are amplifiers and any external filters. Many hardware components offer the option to adjust manually amplification and filter settings. In fact, some vaginal photoplethysmograph users adjust amplification for individual participants to equate better (visually, at least) the highly variable vaginal photoplethysmograph output between participants. Modern signal-processing software and greater data storage capacity make this practice outdated. The vaginal pulse amplitude signal is fairly easy to detect and requires little amplification. In the past, experimenters amplified the vaginal pulse amplitude signal as much as 100 mV/cm,[8] but amplification settings of 1 mV/cm are now common.[74] Researchers now also often oversample vaginal pulse amplitude purposefully and make filtering decisions post-acquisition.

Many laboratories currently use Biopac Systems' MP100 or MP150 hardware and its accompanying software package, AcqKnowledge. AcqKnowledge has the advantage of a point-and-click environment and requires relatively little startup knowledge. The trade-off is that its analytic capabilities are limited, and the description of its existing functions sometimes lacks an appropriate level of detail. In contrast, a software program such as MatLab[75] has different strengths and weaknesses. Compared with AcqKnowledge, MatLab requires extensive startup knowledge and is more often used for data analysis than for data collection. Conversely, MatLab has a highly accessible, freely available, flexible code, offers extensive help, and can perform more advanced data manipulation and statistical analyses than AcqKnowledge.

Sampling

Sampling rates for the vaginal photoplethysmograph vary widely. Researchers often fail to report sampling rates, but published reports vary from 511 to 200 Hz.[65] Two factors determine the acceptable range of sampling rates for signal collection. First, the Nyquist frequency indicates the lowest sampling rate that will still capture the signal of interest. Second, available data storage capacity may suggest a reasonable upper sampling range.

The Nyquist theorem states that only the frequencies in the waveform below half of the sampling frequency are recorded in a digitized signal. The Nyquist frequency is therefore the highest frequency that can be represented in a digital signal of a specified sampling frequency, and it will determine the lowest reasonable sampling rate. Vaginal pulse amplitude is unlikely to exceed 3 Hz (180 bpm); thus, sampling at 6 Hz should capture the signal of interest. However, the inter-beat-interval of vaginal pulse amplitude does vary, and artifacts can also make the signal irregular, so recording at only 6 Hz, where artifacts may be less identifiable, is not recommended. The highest recommended sampling rate is truly limited only by the size of files for which storage is available. Often researchers will sample beyond the Nyquist frequency of their signal, which conservatively avoids aliasing and seems reasonable given the increased capacity of modern computers and storage devices.

Filtering and smoothing

The alternating current signal is usually band-pass filtered (0.5–30 Hz). The basis for the selection of these specific settings is unclear, aside from convention and avoiding 60 Hz light cycles. The sawtooth-shaped vaginal pulse amplitude signal generally peaks once for each heart beat. Heart rate variability during sexual arousal, then, could inform researchers which

frequency spectrum of the vaginal pulse amplitude signal would be most appropriate for analysis.

Resting heart rate is approximately 60 beats per minute (bpm) or about 1 cycle per second (Hz). Masters and Johnson[14] reported increases in heart rate up to 175 bpm (during the "plateau" phase) and a slightly greater heart rate with orgasm. Laboratory studies typically record much lower heart rate levels, even to erotic films (e.g., maximum = 80 bpm),[48] with often only a few bpm increase to erotic films over resting heart rate.[5] This suggests that the frequencies of the vaginal pulse amplitude that are of greatest interest to researchers might fall between 1 (60 bpm) and 2 (120 bpm) Hz. Indeed, using Fast Fourier Transform to extract the 1–2 Hz spectrum of interest from vaginal pulse amplitude yields very similar results to peak amplitude analyses.[25] Polan et al.[76] found similar results with a 0.7–1.2 Hz spectrum, which varied slightly between participants. Since the 0.7–1.2 Hz band varied by individuals based on a visual judgment of the Fast Fourier Transform power peak, this data-driven spectral band selection will require better standardization and replication before its value is understood.

Signals rarely contain only the frequency of interest. In addition to previously discussed movement artifacts, the vaginal pulse amplitude signal may also contain high- and low-frequency noise. High-frequency noise includes waves that occur above the frequency of interest. Visually, these are seen as small "jitter" on top of the 1–2 Hz vaginal pulse amplitude signal. High-frequency noise can be minimized during data acquisition by altering the alternating current band pass filter and selecting a lower high-band limit (e.g., 20 instead of 30 Hz). Alternatively, the signal can be smoothed or low-pass filtered after data collection. Smoothing and low-pass filtering can have the same effect, but are usually differentiated in software programs. The extensive literature on filters cannot be thoroughly reviewed here (for an introduction, see Cunningham[77]). The main point is that selecting filter parameters always involves a tradeoff between cutting undesired noise and biasing the signal of interest (e.g., vaginal pulse amplitude peaks decrease as one increases the filter window).

Low-frequency noise may also be decreased by increasing the low end of the band pass filter (e.g., from 0.05 to 0.08 Hz). High-pass filters also are useful. Researchers have speculated that low-frequency noise is related to breathing.[1] This proposition, however, lacks empirical support, and the slow waves' unpredictable appearance in parts of some signals suggests a different physiologic process. A gradual, steady rise in the signal suggests that the vaginal blood volume frequency band was not sufficiently filtered out, and detrending could be used to remove linear drift and improve the quality of the data.

Amplitude calculation

In the past, researchers calculated vaginal pulse amplitude peak amplitude by hand with a ruler (e.g., Wincze et al.[78]). While this method encourages thorough screening of raw data, the reliability of this procedure is unknown. Computerized algorithms to remove artifacts and detect peaks standardize measurement and significantly reduce processing time. However, computerization is hampered by the high between-subject signal variability of the vaginal pulse amplitude, particularly with regard to artifacts and low-frequency noise. Wavelets may overcome this variability (for a relevant example of this method, see Browne and Cutmore[79]). Researchers are encouraged to develop an algorithm to promote standardization across laboratories, but at the same time to evaluate critically the assumptions underlying the peak-detection algorithms used in their software packages (e.g., Prause and Janssen[80]).

Binning

Most researchers report using relatively large (e.g., 30-s) intervals, or bins.[23] Averaging across (or using the maximum of) entire conditions is problematic because it prohibits the exploration of changes over time. When presenting participants with a composite stimulus, such as a video clip containing different sexual behaviors (e.g., 1 min of petting, 1 min of oral sex, and 1 min of sexual intercourse), stimulus intensity could be used as a within-participants factor when conducting statistical analyses. For the assessment of concordance between physiologic and subjective sexual arousal at a within-participants level, even smaller windows would be preferable (e.g., 10-s intervals). Smaller bins also permit examination of time-lagged correlations (cross-correlations). Large bins may obscure patterns over time. They also can make the identification of outliers more difficult and, even when they are identified, could cause additional data loss.

Analysis of vaginal pulse amplitude

While a few researchers use raw vaginal pulse amplitude data, the data are usually transformed before analysis. Transformations could include z-scores, percentage of "full" response, or difference scores. z-Score transformations may decrease between-subject variability, possibly by correcting for anatomic differences or variations in probe placement, but, currently, little empirical support exists for its assumed increased validity. Percentage scores are quite problematic because participants have to reach their maximum sexual response in the laboratory. Not only might this procedure increase volunteer bias and session time, but the likely variability in participants' subjective identification of a "maximum" response is problematic.

In repeated-measures designs, difference scores are most commonly used, but calculating these scores becomes problematic because participants' vaginal pulse amplitude often does not return to initial baseline levels. Using distraction tasks (e.g., counting backward from 1000) and lengthening the time between testing conditions may increase the likelihood of vaginal pulse amplitude returning to initial baseline levels; alas, our limited knowledge of vaginal physiology makes it difficult to say whether it is reasonable to expect a return even to initial

baseline level. At the very least, few criteria exist for deciding when return-to-baseline levels are "close enough" to the initial baseline. Usually, the initial baseline is used for calculation of difference scores unless the vaginal pulse amplitude does not decrease to initial baseline levels between subsequent testing conditions. In that case, researchers could calculate difference scores, using the baseline immediately preceding each testing condition, or use those baselines as covariates for the test condition following each.[7]

A repeated-measures analysis of (Co)variance (AN(C)OVA) or multivariate analysis of (Co)variance (MAN(C)OVA) is often used to test hypotheses statistically. Within participants designs are standard given the relative nature of the vaginal pulse amplitude. An additional within-participants factor of bin (or interval) is sometimes added to examine patterns of change over time and to increase statistical power.

Conclusion

The vaginal photoplethysmograph has proven to be a useful instrument in psychophysiologic sex research, but its considerable limitations are not always taken into account. Perhaps the most pressing problem is that researchers know relatively little about precisely what physiologic processes the vaginal photoplethysmograph detects. This lack of knowledge means that vaginal pulse amplitude provides only a relative scale, which limits the conclusions that researchers can draw when comparing participants. Without a better theoretic understanding of vaginal physiology, the clinical utility of the vaginal photoplethysmograph will remain limited.

In addition to our limited understanding of what the vaginal photoplethysmograph measures, large differences in signal-processing procedures across laboratories are problematic as well. High interlaboratory variability in data processing hardly is unique to sexual psychophysiology (cf. Jennings et al.[81]), but methods for vaginal pulse amplitude processing are far less standardized than for signals in many other research areas. In particular, managing movement artifacts is potentially a significant source of variability in vaginal pulse amplitude processing. Publishing detailed descriptions of signal-processing procedures (e.g., the proportion of data deleted for artifacts) could increase standardization, and thereby comparability, of study findings.

The construct of sexual arousal is also still poorly understood and defined. This leaves researchers with limited understanding of the causes or determinants of concordance between physiologic and psychologic response components, as well as with problems in selecting the most appropriate measures of sexual arousal in both basic and clinical research.

Finally, potentially useful signal-processing and analysis advances (e.g., time series) are not well utilized. Fourier decomposition, lagged correlations, and wavelet-based signal-cleaning algorithms are all promising candidate techniques and warrant exploration in the analysis of vaginal pulse amplitude. New techniques may increase not only its reliability but also our understanding of what the signal represents.

References

1. Palti Y, Bercovici B. Photoplethysmographic study of the vaginal blood pulse. *Am J Obstet Gynecol* 1967; 97: 143–53.
2. Sintchak G, Geer JH. A vaginal plethysmograph system. *Psychophysiology* 1975; 12: 113–15.
3. Niklas M, Moser U, Buehrer A et al. Attenuation of the near-infrared and red photoplethysmographic signal by different depth of tissues. *Eur J Med Res* 1998; 3: 241–8.
4. Hoon PW, Wincze JP, Hoon EF. Physiological assessment of sexual arousal in women. *Psychophysiology* 1976; 13: 196–204.
5. Laan E, Everaerd W, Evers A. Assessment of female sexual arousal: response specificity and construct validity. *Psychophysiology* 1995; 32: 476–85.
6. Hatch JP. Vaginal photoplethysmography: methodological considerations. *Arch Sex Behav* 1979; 8: 357–74.
7. Janssen E. Psychophysiological measurement of sexual arousal. In MW Wiederman MW, BE Whitley Jr, eds. *Handbook for Conducting Research on Human Sexuality*. Mahwah: Lawrence Erlbaum Associates, 2002: 139–71.
8. Henson C, Rubin HB, Henson DE. Women's sexual arousal concurrently assessed by three genital measures. *Arch Sex Behav* 1979; 8: 459–69.
9. Zingheim PK, Sandman CA. Discriminative control of the vaginal vasomotor response. *Biofeedback Self Regul* 1978; 3: 29–41.
10. Heiman JR. A psychophysiological exploration of sexual arousal patterns in females and males. *Psychophysiology* 1977; 14: 266–74.
11. Meston CM, Gorzalka BB. The effects of sympathetic activation on physiological and subjective sexual arousal in women. *Behav Res Ther* 1995; 33: 651–64.
12. Prause N, Cerny J, Janssen E. The labial photoplethysmograph: a new instrument for assessing genital hemodynamic changes in women. *J Sex Med* 2005; 2: 58–65.
13. Seeley TT, Abramson PR, Perry LB et al. Thermographic measurement of sexual arousal: a methodological note. *Arch Sex Behav* 1980; 9: 77–85.
14. Masters WJ, Johnson VE. *Human Sexual Response*. Boston: Little, Brown, 1966.
15. Shapiro A, Cohen HD, DiBianco P et al. Vaginal blood flow changes during sleep and sexual arousal. *Psychophysiology* 1968; 4: 394.
16. Wagner G, Levin RJ. Human vaginal fluid, pH, urea, potassium and potential difference during sexual excitement. In R Gemme, CC Wheeler, eds. *Progress in Sexology: Selected Proceedings of the 1976 International Congress of Sexology*. New York: Plenum Press, 1976: 335–44.
17. Levin R, Wagner G. Human vaginal blood flow – absolute assessment by a new, quantitative heat wash-out method. *J Physiol* 1997; 504: 188–9.
18. Laan E, Everaerd W. Physiological measures of vaginal vasocongestion. *Int J Impot Res* 1998; 10(S107–10): 124–5.
19. Lavoisier P, Aloui R, Schmidt MH et al. Clitoral blood flow increases following vaginal pressure stimulation. *Arch Sex Behav* 1995; 24: 37–45.
20. Berman JR. Vaginometry, vaginal pH, duplex ultrasonography, vaginal resistance. Paper presented at New Perspectives in the Management of Female Sexual Dysfunction, Burlington, VT, 1998.
21. Henson DE, Rubin HB, Henson C. Analysis of the consistency of objective measures of sexual arousal in women. *J Appl Behav Anal* 1979; 12: 701–11.
22. Rosen RC, Beck JG. *Patterns of Sexual Arousal: Psychophysiological Processes and Clinical Applications*. New York: Guilford Press, 1988.
23. Meston CM. The psychophysiological assessment of female sexual function. *J Sex Educ Ther* 2000; 25: 6–16.
24. Graham CA, Janssen E, Sanders SA. Effects of fragrance on female sexual arousal and mood across the menstrual cycle. *Psychophysiology* 2000; 37: 76–84.
25. Prause N, Janssen E. Four approaches to the processing of vaginal pulse amplitude (VPA) signals. Paper presented at International Academy of Sex Research, Helsinki, Finland, 2004.
26. Krantz KE. Anatomy of the urethra and anterior vaginal wall. Paper presented at 61st Annual Meeting of the American Association of Obstetricians, Gynecologists, and Abdominal Surgeons, Hot Springs, VA, 1950.
27. Sefton A, Richters J. Understanding the vagina: structure and function. *Healthright* 1986; 5: 13–16.
28. Levin R, Goddard A. Photoplethysmographic evidence for vasomotion in the vaginal circulation – drug-induced vasodilation changes both the vaginal pulse amplitude and the ratio of low to high pulses recorded in the basal trace. Paper presented at International Academy of Sex Research, Helsinki, Finland, 2004.
29. Nilsson H, Aalkjær C. Vasomotion: mechanisms and physiological importance. *Mol Interv* 2003; 3: 79–89.
30. Levin RJ. A journey through two lumens! *Int J Impot Res* 2003; 15: 2 9.
31. Levin RJ. Assessing human female sexual arousal by vaginal photoplethysmography – a critical examination. *Sexologies* 1998; 6: 26–31.
32. Levin RJ. The mechanisms of human female sexual arousal. *Annu Rev Sex Res* 1992; 3: 1–48.
33. Carpenter D. Vaginal photoplethysmography artifacts: a pilot study. Unpublished manuscript, 1999.
34. Rogers GS, Van de Castle RL, Evans WS et al. Vaginal pulse amplitude response patterns during erotic conditions and sleep. *Arch Sex Behav* 1985; 14: 327–42.
35. Bohlen JG, Held JP, Sanderson MO. Response of the circumvaginal musculature during masturbation. In B Graber, ed. *Circumvaginal Musculature and Sexual Function*. New York: Karger, 1982: 43–60.
36. Bardwick JM, Behrman SJ. Investigation into the effects of anxiety, sexual arousal, and menstrual cycle phase on uterine contractions. *Psychosom Med* 1967; 29: 468–82.
37. van der Velde J, Everaerd W. The relationship between involuntary pelvic floor muscle activity, muscle awareness and experienced threat in women with and without vaginismus. *Behav Res Ther* 2001; 39: 395–408.

38. Gratton G, Coles MG, Donchin E. A new method for off-line removal of ocular artifact. *Electroencephalogr Clin Neurophysiol* 1983; 55: 468–84.

39. Relente A, Sison LG. Comparison of LMS and RLS in adaptive filtering of motion artifacts in photoplethysmograms. Paper presented at ECE Conference, Quezon City, Philippines, 2002.

40. Kaiser W, Findeis M. Artifact processing during exercise testing. *J Electrocardiol* 1999; 32: 212–19.

41. Slob AK, Koster J, Radder JK et al. Sexuality and psychophysiological functioning in women with diabetes mellitus. *J Sex Marital Ther* 1990; 16: 59–69.

42. Hoon PW, Bruce KE, Kinchloe B. Does the menstrual cycle play a role in sexual arousal? *Psychophysiology* 1982; 19: 21–7.

43. Schreiner-Engel P, Schiavi RC, Smith H et al. Sexual arousability and the menstrual cycle. *Psychosom Med* 1981; 43: 199–214.

44. Meuwissen I, Over R. Female sexual arousal and the law of initial value: assessment at several phases of the menstrual cycle. *Arch Sex Behav* 1993; 22: 403–13.

45. Slob AK, Ernste M, Van der Werff ten Bosch JJ. Menstrual cycle phase and sexual arousability in women. *Arch Sex Behav* 1991; 20: 567–77.

46. Hedricks CA. Female sexual activity across the human menstrual cycle. *Annu Rev Sex Res* 1994; 5: 122–72.

47. Lang PJ, Cuthbert BN. Affective information processing and the assessment of anxiety. *J Behav Assess* 1984; 6: 369–95.

48. Heiman JR, Rowland DL. Affective and physiological sexual response patterns: the effects of instructions on sexually functional and dysfunctional men. *J Psychosom Res* 1983; 27: 105–16.

49. Wincze J, Hoon P, Hoon E. Sexual arousal in women: a comparison of cognitive and physiological responses by continuous measurement. *Arch Sex Behav* 1977; 6: 121–32.

50. Schreiner Engel P, Schiavi RC, Smith H. Female sexual arousal: relation between cognitive and genital assessments. *J Sex Marital Ther* 1981; 7: 256–67.

51. Speiss WF. The psychophysiology of premature ejaculation: some factors related to ejaculatory latency. *Diss Abstr Int* 1977; 38B: 1424.

52. Laan E, Everaerd W, van Bellen G et al. Women's sexual and emotional responses to male- and female-produced erotica. *Arch Sex Behav* 1994; 23: 153–69.

53. Laan E, Everaerd W, Van Aanhold M-T et al. Performance demand and sexual arousal in women. *Behav Res Ther* 1993; 31: 25–35.

54. Janssen E, Everaerd W. Determinants of male sexual arousal. *Annu Rev Sex Res* 1993; 4: 211–45.

55. Mavissakalian M, Blanchard EB, Abel GC et al. Responses to complex erotic stimuli in homosexual and heterosexual males. *Br J Psychiatry* 1975; 126: 252–7.

56. Kockott G, Feil W, Ferstl R et al. Psychophysiological aspects of male sexual inadequacy: results of an experimental study. *Arch Sex Behav* 1980; 9: 477–93.

57. Laan E, Everaerd W. Determinants of female sexual arousal: psychophysiological theory and data. *Annu Rev Sex Res* 1995; 6: 32–76.

58. Bancroft J. *Human Sexuality and Its Problems*, 2nd edn. Edinburgh: Churchill Livingstone, 1989.

59. Janssen E, Everaerd W, Spiering M et al. Automatic processes and the appraisal of sexual stimuli: toward an information processing model of sexual arousal. *J Sex Res* 2000; 37: 8–23.

60. Howard R, Longmore F, Mason P. Contingent negative variation as an indicator of sexual object preference: revisited. *Int J Psychophysiol* 1992; 13: 185–8.

61. Spiering M, Everaerd W, Laan E. Conscious processing of sexual information: mechanisms of appraisal. *Arch Sex Behav* 2004; 33: 369–80.

62. Spiering M, Everaerd W, Elzinga B. Conscious processing of sexual information: interference caused by sexual primes. *Arch Sex Behav* 2002; 31: 159–64.

63. Bradley MM, Codispoti M, Cuthbert BN et al. Emotion and motivation. I. Defensive and appetitive reactions in picture processing. *Emotion* 2001; 1: 276–98.

64. Laan E, Everaerd W, van der Velde J et al. Determinants of subjective experience of sexual arousal in women: feedback from genital arousal and erotic stimulus content. *Psychophysiology* 1995; 32: 444–51.

65. Brotto LA, Gorzalka BB. Genital and subjective sexual arousal in postmenopausal women: influence of laboratory-induced hyperventilation. *J Sex Marital Ther* 2002; 28: 39–53.

66. Prause N, Graham CA, Janssen E. Effects of different instructions on within- and between-subject correlations of physiological and subjective sexual arousal in women. Paper presented at Annual Meeting of the International Academy of Sex Research, Montreal, Canada, 2001.

67. Basson R. The female sexual response: a different model. *J Sex Marital Ther* 2000; 26: 51–65.

68. Conte HR. Multivariate assessment of sexual dysfunction. *J Consult Clin Psychol* 1986; 54: 149–57.

69. Costa L, Bauer L. Quantitative electroencephalographic differences associated with alcohol, cocaine, heroin and dual-substance dependence. *Drug Alcohol Depend* 1997; 46: 87–93.

70. Wouda JC, Hartmen PM, Bakker RM et al. Vaginal plethysmography in women with dyspareunia. *J Sex Res* 1998; 35: 141–7.

71. Tuiten A, Laan E, Panhuysen G et al. Discrepancies between genital responses and subjective sexual function during testosterone substitution in women with hypothalamic amenorrhea. *Psychosom Med* 1996; 58: 234–41.

72. Sechrest L. Incremental validity: a recommendation. *Educ Psychol Meas* 1963; 23: 153–8.

73. Morokoff PJ, Heiman JR. Effects of erotic stimuli on sexually functional and dysfunctional women: multiple measures before and after sex therapy. *Behav Res Ther* 1980; 18: 127–37.

74. Meston CM, Gorzalka BB. Differential effects of sympathetic activation on sexual arousal in sexually dysfunctional and functional women. *J Abnorm Psychol* 1996; 105: 582–91.

75. MatLab [computer software program]. Version 7; 2004.

76. Polan ML, Desmond JE, Banner LL et al. Female sexual arousal: a behavioral analysis. *Fertil Steril* 2003; 80: 1480–7.

77. Cunningham EP. *Digital Filtering: An Introduction*. Boston: Houghton Mifflin, 1992.

78. Wincze JP, Albert A, Bansal S. Sexual arousal in diabetic females: physiological and self-report measures. *Arch Sex Behav* 1993; 22: 587–601.

79. Browne M, Cutmore TRH. Low-probability event-detection and separation via statistical wavelet thresholding: an application to psychophysiological denoising. *Clin Neurophysiol* 2002; 113: 1403–11.

80. Prause N, Janssen E. *New VPA Peak Picking Procedure.* Unpublished manuscript, 2004.

81. Jennings JR, Berg KW, Hutcheson JS et al. Publication guidelines for heart rate studies in man. *Psychophysiology* 1981; 18: 226–31.

10.2 Blood flow: magnetic resonance imaging and brain imaging for evaluating sexual arousal in women

Kenneth R Maravilla

Introduction

It is a fundamental concept that increased blood flow to the genital structures and pelvic tissues is closely associated with and is a major contributor to the sexual arousal response (see Chapters 6.1–5.6 of this book). While this is true for both men and women, it has been particularly difficult to observe the blood flow changes in women in a nonintrusive manner (see Chapters 10.1, 10.3, and 10.4). It is even more problematic to attempt to quantify these changes. Magnetic resonance imaging has been applied in recent years as a new method to evaluate changes in tissue signal intensity that are associated with sexual arousal in women.[1,2] These signal intensity changes are a direct result of increases in local blood flow and in regional blood volume.

In the past few years, magnetic resonance techniques have been applied to observation and analysis of two aspects of the female sexual arousal response that are located in two widely separate and functionally diverse anatomic locations: the pelvic genital area and the brain. This chapter describes the basic principles of using magnetic resonance for monitoring the female sexual arousal response, describes the basic methodologies used, and outlines some initial research results using these new techniques. The first section describes changes in genital engorgement observable with magnetic resonance imaging that document and quantify the physical arousal response in women.

Since the cerebral response to a sexual stimulus is tightly coupled with genital sexual arousal, the second section addresses functional magnetic resonance imaging of the brain as a tool to monitor regions of brain activation that occur during arousal, as well as highlighting the initial experience with this exciting area of research.

Magnetic resonance imaging

Magnetic resonance imaging is a revolutionary medical imaging technique that was introduced into clinical use approximately 20 years ago. It has rapidly gained widespread acceptance because it offers several advantages over traditional medical imaging techniques such as radiography, computed tomography, ultrasound, and radioisotope scanning. For example, magnetic resonance is exquisitely sensitive to subtle changes in tissue composition, is noninvasive, and uses no ionizing radiation. It can provide dynamic assessment of tissue changes over time, and also quantitative physiologic information on areas such as three-dimensional volumes of anatomic structures, regional blood flow changes, and regional metabolite composition (magnetic resonance spectroscopy). In recent years, a few research centers worldwide, including ours at the University of Washington, have begun to explore the application of magnetic resonance techniques to improve knowledge and understanding of female sexual arousal response. Different types of magnetic resonance techniques were devised to evaluate female sexual arousal response in two separate areas of the body: the pelvic genital region and the brain. Assessments in both of these anatomic areas have their fundamental basis in observational measurements in changes of regional blood flow and regional blood volume.

Historical perspective

Until now, it has been very difficult to observe and monitor female sexual arousal response in an objective, reliable, and nonintrusive manner. Methods used in the past, such as temperature probes,[3,4] vaginal photoplethysmography,[5–7] and ultrasound monitoring of intravascular flow in pelvic blood vessels,[8–10] provide limited information, are difficult to reproduce, and, in some cases, such as vaginal photoplethysmography (which requires vaginal insertion of a measurement probe), may confound or interfere with the physiologic response one is trying to measure. Dynamic magnetic resonance evaluation, on the other hand, can provide quantifiable information that is reproducible and may be used to compare dynamic changes that occur within subjects at different time points.[1,2,11–14]

Initial attempts to employ magnetic resonance to observe arousal changes in pelvic genital structures in women utilized a gadolinium-based blood pool contrast agent.[1,11] Since blood flow changes and engorgement are a major factor in physical sexual arousal, it was hypothesized that the best chance of observing such changes on the magnetic resonance scan would occur if a marker of blood pool volume in arteries, veins, capillaries, and cavernous structures was enhanced with a contrast agent. A new investigational contrast agent, MS-325 (EPIX Medical, Waltham, MA, USA), was used. This magnetic resonance contrast agent remains in the vascular system with a long half-life compared with conventional, extracellular, gadolinium contrast agents that rapidly "leak" from the vascular system into the interstitial tissues of the body.[15] The contrast agent MS-325 also reversibly binds to serum albumin that serves both to retain the contrast agent in the vascular system and to increase significantly the enhancement effect provided by the contrast agent.[15–17] These properties enabled excellent enhancement of the genital tissues that lasted for up to several hours of observation and imaging. In particular, the erectile tissue within the clitoris and vestibular bulb was especially well enhanced. Imaging of the target structures, both before and after intravenous contrast injection, also enabled quantitative calculation of relative regional blood volume changes that occurred during arousal.[1] The major disadvantage of this technique is that it is not totally noninvasive, since it requires injection of a magnetic resonance contrast agent with the attendant risk, albeit small, of an adverse reaction.

Therefore, alternative methods for observing female sexual arousal response were explored with magnetic resonance techniques that did not require intravenous contrast media injection. It was found that T_2-weighted images with fat suppression could also provide precise anatomic detail of the genital structures.[2,12] In addition, changes related to engorgement with arousal that are similar in appearance to those shown to occur with contrast-enhanced images of the clitoris could also be observed by noncontrast, T_2-weighted techniques.[12] Magnetic resonance imaging is exquisitely sensitive to even small changes in water content, and this is probably the reason that engorgement can be visualized on noncontrast magnetic resonance. As blood and serum are mostly water, an increase in regional blood volume that accompanies arousal and engorgement results in increased regional water content and thus an increase in T_2 signal intensity along with an observable change in anatomic volume. The change in clitoral volume can be measured and provides a quantifiable means by which it is possible to compare the arousal response at different time points or across different subjects, as with the types of clitoral volume measurements done with the investigational contrast agent MS-325.[2,11,12] Thus, this method provides a totally noninvasive technique to observe physical genital arousal in women. One limitation of the noncontrast magnetic resonance technique is that it is no longer possible to obtain quantitative regional blood volume measurements. However, since this has already proved to be less robust than three-dimensional, anatomic clitoral volume measurements,[1] it is not felt to be a significant limitation.

Principles for evaluating the pelvic genitalia with dynamic magnetic resonance imaging

The magnetic resonance technique currently used for genital evaluation consists of obtaining high-resolution, three-dimensional, T_2-weighted images of the pelvic genital area. A technique is used that suppresses signal from subcutaneous and interstitial fat in this region to provide better visualization of the clitoris and adjacent genital structures. The suppression of magnetic resonance signal from fat also facilitates better visualization of signal changes within the genital structures themselves. Sequential, serial, three-dimensional images of the genital region are obtained at approximately 3-min intervals while the patient views an audiovisual presentation comprising first a 15-min neutral documentary video and then a 15-min segment of sexually stimulating content. Audiovisual stimulus is delivered to the patient in the magnet by a magnetic resonance-compatible, fiber-optic video display and headphones (Fig. 10.2.1). Changes in size and signal intensity of key genital structures caused by an increase in regional blood volume with tissue engorgement are readily observed. Images are analyzed, and quantitative, volumetric measurement of the clitoris in mm^3 at each time-point in the magnetic resonance imaging series is performed.

Although several analysis techniques were explored, our early research studies showed measurement of total clitoral volume to be the most robust measure. Attempts at measuring changes in regional blood volume were also shown to be quite

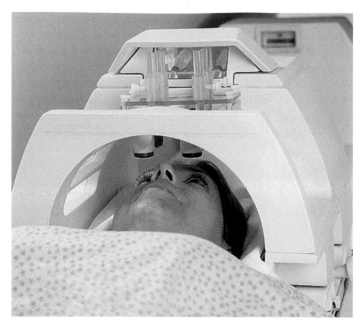

Figure 10.2.1. Subject lying in the magnetic resonance magnet with head in head-imaging coil. Fiber-optically coupled goggles allow subject easily to view the video presentation while the head is being imaged.

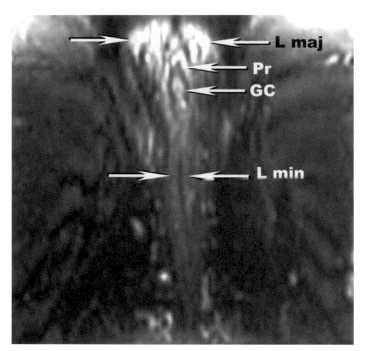

Figure 10.2.2. All cross-sectional images in this chapter are oriented identically; the anterior portion of the subject's anatomy is at the top, and the right side of the subject's anatomy is at the reader's left. Image through the superficial portion of the introitus shows the major (L maj; labia majorus) and minor labia (L min; labia minora). Note the tip of the glans clitoris (GC), and the prepuce (Pr) or hood is also visible at this level.

good but were not as robust as the clitoral volume measurements. Measurements of other structures, including analysis of vaginal mucosa, vaginal wall thickness, changes in the labia, or vestibular bulb changes, all proved either unsuccessful or far less reproducible than the clitoral volume measurements.[1] High-detail (high-resolution and high signal-to-noise ratio) magnetic resonance imaging techniques are needed, since the clitoral volume is very small. In our studies, the clitoris ranged in volume from approximately 1.5 ml to 5.5 ml in the nonaroused state, increasing significantly in size with sexual arousal to a maximum of approximately 10 ml among our subject population. Thus, lower resolution imaging, employing a relatively large picture element volume (pixel) size, would result in unacceptably large standard deviations for measurements of this small structure.

Anatomy

Magnetic resonance imaging can define the normal anatomic relationships of the female genital structures *in vivo*. This provides a more accurate picture and a better understanding of the functional anatomy of women than cadaver dissection studies. Our studies focused mainly in the area of the introitus. Three-dimensional images are acquired and displayed mainly in the axial (horizontal) plane.[18] Beginning most superficially (inferior or caudally), one can define the major and minor labia along with the tip of the glans clitoris (Fig. 10.2.2). As we image slightly deeper (superiorly or rostrally), we begin to see the glans clitoris along with the frenulum, which forms the junction of the minor labia and can be seen just posterior to the base of the glans clitoris and just superficial to the body of the clitoris (Fig. 10.2.3). Just

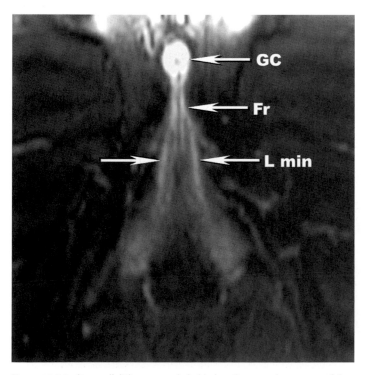

Figure 10.2.3. Image slightly more cephelad in location now shows some of the structures slightly deeper in the introitus. The base of the glans clitoris (GC) is now visible along with the labia minora (L min), which come together at the frenulum (Fr).

deep to the glans clitoris is the body of the clitoris, which is only seen in the magnetic resonance imaging and is not visible upon direct visual examination of the introitus. The clitoral body is seen as a paired structure that gives rise to the two crura of the clitoris, which are also hidden from direct visual examination (Fig. 10.2.4). Beginning at about the level of the body of the clitoris are the vestibular bulbs, which are oblong-shaped structures on either side of the vaginal opening in the midline. They form a slight concavity in the center and track alongside the clitoral crura, forming an inverted V-shaped configuration (Fig. 10.2.5). O'Connell et al.,[19] who has done extensive gross and microscopic studies of the female genitalia, believes that the vestibular bulbs should be considered part of the clitoris. The histologic appearance is similar and there are many vascular spaces, although fewer sensory nerve endings than in the clitoris itself. Our magnetic resonance studies support this concept, since the signal intensity changes in the bulbs roughly parallel those of the clitoris, and there is a similar, although lesser, increase in volume with arousal. The clitoris itself is a complex, wishbone-shaped structure (Fig. 10.2.6). The glans clitoris forms the head of the wishbone, followed by the body and then the two crura that diverge posteriorly on either side of the vaginal canal. The two elongated crura track along the inner and inferior surface of the ischial rami. Just posterior to the point where the two crura join to form the body of the clitoris and also where the two vestibular bulbs join are the urethra and periurethral tissues (Fig. 10.2.7).

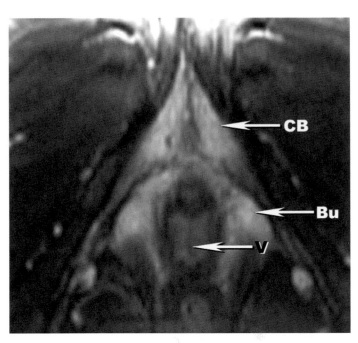

Figure 10.2.5. Anatomic section at this level shows the upper part of the clitoral body (CB) as it widens to form the base of the crura. The upper part of the vestibular bulbs (Bu) is well demonstrated at this level along with the vaginal opening (V).

The bulbourethral glands, also known as Bartholin's glands, are also well visualized at this level; they are pea-shaped structures embedded in the posterolateral introitus near the posterior aspect of the vestibular bulbs. The periurethral tissues do not appear to change in signal intensity or size with arousal, so our studies do not confirm this area as the "G-spot"[20–22] that some investigators believe to be associated with the sexual response of women.

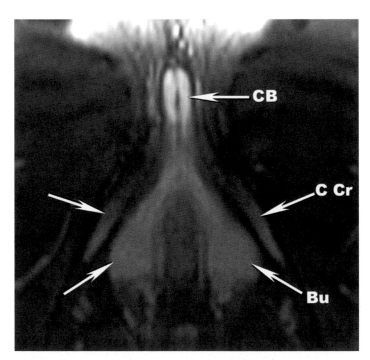

Figure 10.2.4. Image at this level shows the paired structures that form the body of the clitoris (CB) along with the inferior-most aspects of the crura of the clitoris (CCr). Note also that the paired vestibular bulbs (Bu) that lie on either side of the vaginal opening are also visible at this level. All of these structures lie deep to the superficial tissues of the introitus and are not visible upon direct visual examination of the subject.

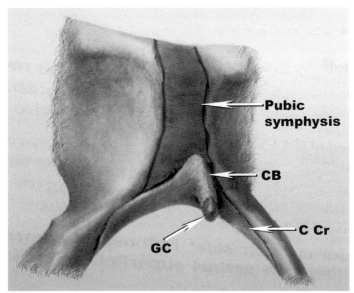

Figure 10.2.6. Anatomic drawing shows the complex, three-dimensional structure of the clitoris forming a wishbone-shaped structure that lies close to and parallels the inferior surface of the pubic symphysis and the ischial rami. CB = clitoral body, CCr = clitoral crura, GC = glans clitoris.

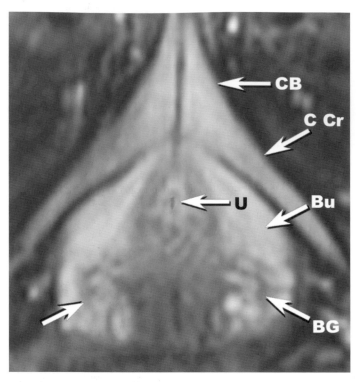

Figure 10.2.7. At this level, one can see a good demonstration of the clitoral body (CB) and the clitoral crura (CCr) on either side. They surround vestibular bulbs (Bu) and the bulbourethral glands (BG), which are very well shown at this level. Note the position of the urethra (U) and periurethral tissues. The vaginal opening lies just posterior to this.

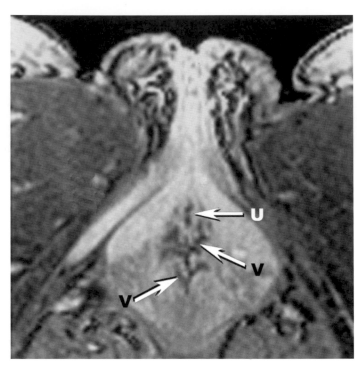

Figure 10.2.8. Image of a premenopausal woman at the level of the vaginal canal (V). Note the irregular contours of the mucosal surface, which form an irregular rugal pattern that is characteristic of the premenopausal vaginal canal. U = Urethra and periurethral tissue.

The vaginal mucosa appears as an H-shaped, irregular rugal pattern in most premenopausal women (Fig. 10.2.8). In the postmenopausal state, however, the vaginal mucosa shows a smoother appearance to the lining of the vaginal canal, presumably due to atrophy of the mucosa in the postmenopausal state (Fig. 10.2.9).

Magnetic resonance images show characteristic changes in key anatomic structures with engorgement during arousal. These changes are most evident in the clitoris, especially in the crura and body of the clitoris. During arousal, these structures demonstrate a very prominent increase in size and signal intensity that is easily discernible upon visual inspection of the images (Fig. 10.2.10). In addition, there are similar, although less robust, changes present within the vestibular bulbs. Obvious changes to visual observation are not present in the major and minor labia, the vaginal wall, or the vaginal mucosa, although careful anatomic measurements of the images do show a slight increase in size of the major and minor labia.[23] The vaginal mucosa does not show any increase in size and signal intensity, most probably because it is only a few cell layers thick and is below the limit of resolution of the magnetic resonance imaging technique. Thus, the vaginal mucosa is not resolvable separate from the muscular wall of the vagina itself.

Initially, it was postulated that one might be able to see changes within the vaginal canal due to the watery secretions

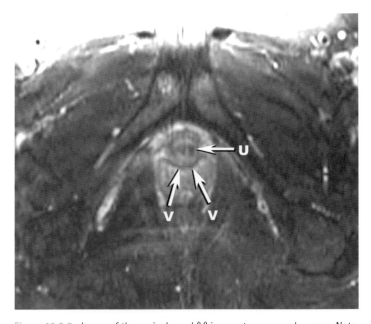

Figure 10.2.9. Image of the vaginal canal (V) in a postmenopausal woman. Note the smooth, regular configuration of the vaginal canal in the postmenopausal state. The irregular rugal pattern has now atrophied due to the hormonal changes that occur with menopause. This smooth appearance of the vaginal opening is characteristic of the postmenopausal state in contrast to the irregular rugal pattern shown in Fig. 10.2.8. U = Urethra and periurethral tissue.

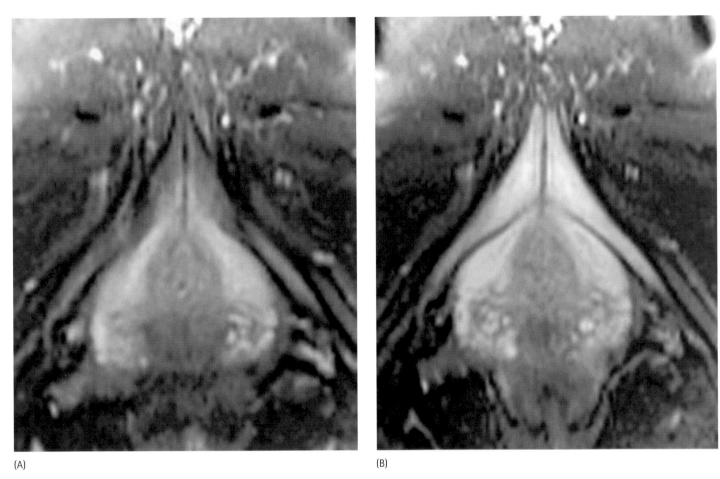

(A)   (B)

Figure 10.2.10. Images of the same subject taken at the same anatomic position illustrating the prearousal or neutral state (A) and the postarousal or stimulated state (B) after viewing of audiovisual sexual stimulus. Note the prominent change in both the size as well as the increased signal intensity of the clitoral body and crura. There is also a slight increase in signal intensity within the vestibular bulbs on either side, although the size of the vestibular bulbs is not significantly changed.

that form lubrication during arousal. However, such changes are not visible on the magnetic resonance images; this is probably due to the small amount of lubrication fluid that forms a thin film over the surface of the vaginal canal, and this thin film is also below the limit of resolution of magnetic resonance imaging.

Quantitative analysis

As already stated, quantitative analysis of a number of genital structures was attempted, including measurements of the major and minor labia, vaginal wall thickness, and vestibular bulb changes. Of all the measurements attempted, the two that were found to be most robust were anatomic clitoral volume measurements and relative regional blood volume measurements. The latter set of measurements could be performed only on contrast-enhanced magnetic resonance scans, and these measurements were less reproducible than anatomic clitoral volume measurements. Thus, the primary measurement used in our studies has been comparison of changes in anatomic clitoral volume before, during, and after sexual arousal by an audiovisual sexual stimulus.

After acquisition of the magnetic resonance image series as previously described, quantitative measurements of the anatomic clitoral volume are obtained by the planometric technique to outline clitoral structures on each individual image at each time point. The various slices that contain portions of the clitoral anatomy are then summed, and a total volume of the clitoris at each imaging time point is determined. A curve of anatomic clitoral volume versus time is plotted, as illustrated in Fig. 10.2.11. An average value of all neutral time points is then compared with the average clitoral volume obtained during all stimulus time points, and a measure of percent change in clitoral volume is calculated. This provides a quantitative measure of arousal by which one can compare results within subjects as well as across different subjects and different subject populations. Results of these comparisons are presented in Table 10.2.1.

As can be seen, there is an excellent correlation within subject comparisons at two different imaging time points, with an r value equal to 0.95 (Fig. 10.2.12), and there is more variability across subjects than within subjects. The average increase in clitoral volume measured approximately 90% when

MRI Time Response Curve During Video Viewing

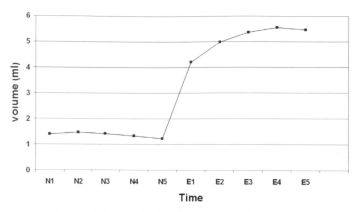

Figure 10.2.11. Plot of anatomic clitoral volume versus time shows the time response curve of a typical, normal subject during the neutral video phase (time points labeled N) with the rapid increase in clitoral volume during the sexual stimulus portion of the video (time points marked E).

Clitoral MRI Correlation Between 2 Imaging Sessions: All subjects (n = 7)

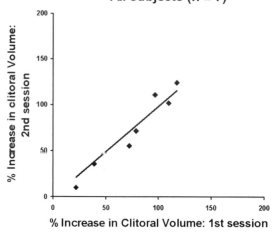

Figure 10.2.12. Correlation curve plotted from the data in Table 10.2.1 shows the high correlation coefficient of 0.95 obtained when comparing the anatomic clitoral volume change obtained with arousal at two different time points within each subject.

compared with a baseline average for all subjects. Furthermore, in our various studies, there was also good correlation between clitoral volume changes observed at two different time-points within each subject in a premenopausal group compared with that seen in a postmenopausal group. The numbers of subjects in each group, however, are very small at this point in time, so these early results should be interpreted with caution.

The level of sexual arousal achieved in each subject was documented by a validated sexual arousal score questionnaire.[13,14] This questionnaire used a seven-point scale scoring system and presented queries that probed for overall feelings of sexual arousal, mental sexual arousal, and feelings of physical sexual arousal. Scores from the various questions were totaled, and an average arousal score between 1 (no feelings of sexual arousal) and 7 (most intense feelings of arousal) was calculated. Results from one group of subjects are shown in Table 10.2.1. While subjective, these scores provided a reasonable level of documentation regarding subject arousal status. These scores were also correlated with the measurement of percent change in

clitoral volume, where it was found that there was a reasonably good correlation, with an r score greater than 0.7 (Fig. 10.2.13).

To date, all of our published data have involved evaluation of healthy, volunteer, pre- and post-menopausal women without reported sexual difficulties. We have initiated studies utilizing these magnetic resonance techniques to evaluate women with selected types of sexual arousal disorder, and these studies are underway. We are exploring the possibility that differences in the pattern and quantitative measurements of the arousal response and/or the degree of reproducibility within subjects may provide valuable information that would help to clarify the underlying dysfunctional physiology, and eventually may help to design and validate better treatment methods. These techniques also provide a possible basis for monitoring response to therapy. This should also prove useful in testing new drugs or other therapies to treat patients with sexual arousal disorders and to determine the effectiveness of proposed new therapies.

Table 10.2.1. Comparison of clitoral volume and arousal score data obtained at two time points for a normal volunteer group of women (n = 7)

Subject Number	Session 1			Session 2		
	CV (ml) Neutral/Erotic	% CV Increase	Arousal Score	CV (ml) Neutral/Erotic	% CV Increase	Arousal Score
1	2.0/4.4	128	6	1.7/3.6	115	4.7
2	5.6/10.4	84	4.3	5.6/9.5	70	3.7
3	1.9/3.2	71	3.3	1.8/3.1	74	2.7
4	1.8/3.9	115	5	1.8/4.0	117	5.7
5	1.3/2.1	64	3.7	1.4/2.2	58	2
6	2.9/5.7	95	4	3.5/5.7	62	3.7
7	1.7/3.1	85	5	1.8/3.2	75	6

CV = clitoral volume.

SEQ Score vs. Clitoral Volume Change

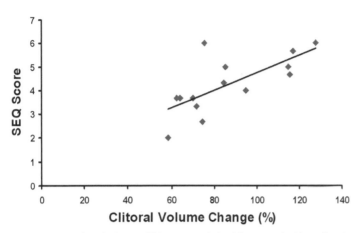

Figure 10.2.13. Correlation coefficient curve derived for a set of subjects listed in Table 10.2.1 shows a correlation between the average clitoral change in volume and the subjective arousal score. There was moderately good correlation with an *r* value of approximately 0.70.

Functional brain imaging during sexual arousal

Definition

In its most basic definition, functional brain imaging is the use of rapid, dynamic magnetic resonance imaging to observe anatomic sites of brain activation in response to a specific task performed by a subject. This technique is often referred to as "functional magnetic resonance imaging", and in the few short years since its introduction, it has gained widespread acceptance in clinical and experimental brain imaging research. First applied as a method to define eloquent areas of the brain, such as activation of motor or visual cortex, the technique has been refined and become more sensitive and is now being applied to define brain activation that occurs in association with subtle, cognitive tasks. Thus, this technique is an ideal tool for exploring brain function associated with emotional attraction, feelings of pleasure, and even sites of activation associated with sexual arousal.

Theory of method and techniques

Functional brain imaging is most easily understood by illustrating what happens when a subject performs a simple motor task. If a subject taps the fingers of one hand and functional magnetic resonance imaging images are obtained during that task, these images can be analyzed to demonstrate the area of brain activation in the contralateral motor cortex that is responsible for performance of this motor task (Fig. 10.2.14). However, if one looks at a single echo planar functional magnetic resonance image, the change in the magnetic resonance

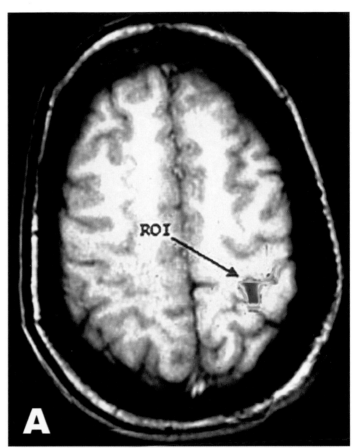

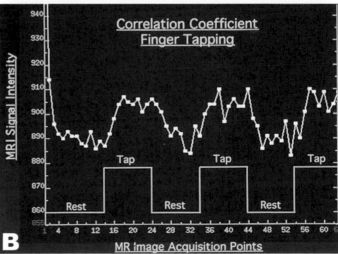

Figure 10.2.14. Functional magnetic resonance imaging (fMRI) (A) and time response signal intensity curve (B) illustrating the fMRI activation seen in association with tapping of the right fingers. (A) Axial image through the upper portion of the brain shows the area of activation in the left motor cortex highlighted in red. (B) Signal intensity time response curve shows the changes in signal intensity (irregular white line) and their correlation with the activation of rest versus finger tapping of the right hand (solid blue line). Note that the change in signal intensity correlates very nicely with the period of time that the subject is tapping the fingers of the right hand. Note also that the amount of signal change is very slight and measures only approximately 2% of the total signal intensity. This small amount of signal intensity change is not visible on visual inspection of the images but can only be discerned on accurate statistical analysis of the images.

image is very slight, and there is no visual indication of this activation (Fig. 10.2.15). So how does one identify the area(s) of motor activation, and why does this work?

There are several key points to be aware of regarding functional magnetic resonance imaging. The first is that functional magnetic resonance imaging is based on changes in regional cerebral blood flow that occur when focal areas of the brain are activated. The second is that with changes in brain activity there are also local blood flow changes within the same region of the brain. These local blood flow changes result in a slight change in magnetic resonance signal intensity that is very subtle and is not discernible by eye on visual inspection of a single image. Third, the areas that are activated are identified by statistical analysis of a series of images that are rapidly acquired during rest and during performance of a task. By statistical comparison of the magnetic resonance signal pattern in a set of dynamic images acquired during a resting state with those acquired during performance of a task (finger tapping), the area of activation in the motor cortex can be identified.

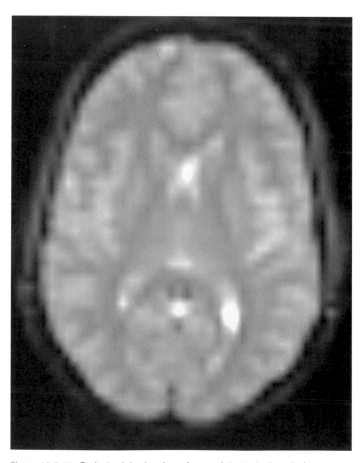

Figure 10.2.15. Typical axial echo planar image of the brain done during performance of a functional activation task does not show any obvious areas of signal intensity change. As already stated, only detailed statistical analysis of an entire sequence of dynamic images can show the subtle changes that occur with brain activation.

Theory of activation

The functional magnetic resonance imaging technique is based upon changes that occur with blood flow due to changes that occur in the level of blood oxygenation. These changes in signal intensity that occur with changes in oxygen level are referred to as blood oxygen level-dependent tissue contrast. These changes were first defined by Ogawa,[24] who demonstrated differences between images of oxyhemoglobin and deoxyhemoglobin. Blood containing oxyhemoglobin, that is, hemoglobin that is fully oxygenated, is diamagnetic and has a neutral effect on the magnetic resonance signal derived from oxygenated blood when compared with surrounding tissues. Deoxyhemoglobin, which represents the state of hemoglobin when oxygen has been extracted, is a paramagnetic substance and has a high magnetic susceptibility relative to surrounding tissues, leading to loss of signal intensity on T_2-weighted (susceptibility-weighted) magnetic resonance imaging sequences. Thus, in the normal resting state, oxygenated blood entering the brain has a slightly higher baseline signal intensity, while blood in the venous system of the brain, because it has had much of the oxygen extracted as it passed through the capillary bed, has a subtly lower signal intensity.

Let us now consider what happens in the motor cortex when a subject begins to tap fingers. In this case, the neurons in the cortex become activated and begin to fire rapidly in order to produce motion in the fingers. With activation of the neurons, there is an increased oxygen demand in order to supply energy to the neurons. This increased oxygen demand is met by a signal from the brain to increase blood flow to that local area of the cortex with the neurons that have become active. This increased flow brings increased oxyhemoglobin. However, the mechanism described many years ago by Fox et al.,[25] termed "decoupling", results in an excess of blood flow to the area of neuronal or brain activation. That is, the amount of increased blood going to the tissues is greater than what is needed to supply the increased oxygen requirements of the active neurons and, thus, an excess of oxyhemoglobin is delivered. The venous blood draining from the area of activation then carries both the deoxygenated hemoglobin that has supplied oxygen to the neurons and the excess oxyhemoglobin that was not needed by the tissues. This results in a local decrease in the concentration of deoxyhemoglobin during the activation state when compared with the resting state. Since deoxyhemoglobin normally causes a mild decrease in signal intensity on susceptibility-weighted (T_2) images, the decreased concentration in deoxyhemoglobin results in a slight increase in signal intensity on these activated images compared with the resting (baseline) state. The magnitude of this signal increase is very small, but it is reproducible and generally measures 1–5% of baseline signal intensity. Thus, such a small change in intensity is not detectable by merely looking at the magnetic resonance images.

However, if one were to subtract an image acquired during the resting state with the subject lying quietly with both hands by their sides from an image acquired during the activation state when the subject was tapping their fingers, we would be able to see a very slight signal increase in the motor cortex of the opposite hemisphere responsible for the finger tapping. In practice, however, rather than doing a simple image subtraction, a rapid series of images is acquired over a few minutes and then statistically analyzed to show this subtle change in signal that occurs over time.

Each magnetic resonance image is a digital image that is composed of a number of picture elements, or pixels. A pixel is a single, digitized "dot" that has a measurable gray level, that is, a certain level of whiteness or blackness that contributes to the picture. Pictures are made up of a matrix of pixels that is defined by the number of pixels on the longitudinal axis versus the number of pixels on the vertical axis. Thus, a 256×256 image is composed of 256 pixel rows in the vertical direction and 256 pixel columns in the longitudinal or horizontal direction. The larger the number of pixels in the matrix, the higher the resolution of the image and the more detail it can provide (Fig. 10.2.16). Unlike a digital picture taken with a camera, which is a two-dimensional representation of the surfaces that reflect light, in magnetic resonance each image of the brain is a "slice" though the brain of a certain thickness – generally 5–10 mm. Because of this slice thickness or depth of the tissue, each picture element is more often referred to as a "voxel" (the three-dimensional equivalent of a pixel).

Rapid dynamic images called echoplanar images are acquired of the entire brain and then repeated every 2 or 3 s for the time required to perform a repetitive task (such as finger tapping) that is alternated with a control time interval (rest) – usually about 2–5 min. During these few minutes of echoplanar image acquisition, the subject alternately lies still and performs the finger-tapping task at specified intervals in response to a verbal or visual signal. Each voxel in each image of this series of images is then statistically analyzed to determine voxels that change in signal intensity over time. In comparing voxels that change signal intensity with the periods of finger tapping and rest, only those voxels that show a pattern of signal change that matches or correlates with the times of task performance are selected or highlighted (Fig. 10.2.16B). This statistical image-analysis technique is referred to as a correlation coefficient, and is far more powerful than a simple subtraction of two images, since it averages signal intensity from a large number of images to reduce interference from the random signal fluctuation due to background noise that normally occurs with all magnetic resonance images.

Once the voxels responsible for finger tapping are statistically identified, they can be highlighted in color and their location superimposed (or mapped) over a detailed anatomic magnetic resonance image of the brain acquired at the same magnetic resonance session with the subject's head in the same position (Fig. 10.2.16A). This allows the specific anatomic areas associated with the activation task (finger tapping) to be visually displayed, and produces the resulting functional magnetic resonance imaging image.

These same principles can be applied to cognitive tasks.

However, in general, the amount of associated signal change is greater for motor tasks than for cognitive tasks. In addition, while eloquent areas of brain associated with motor function, vision, or speech production are well defined and well localized, most cognitive functions are widely dispersed across multiple areas of the brain that act in association with each other in complex, and often incompletely understood, patterns to produce the cognitive task. Thus, the combination of very low signal change and widely distributed areas of activation makes it difficult to analyze and interpret functional magnetic resonance imaging scans done for complex cognitive tasks. Nevertheless, through a painstaking and methodical series of research experiments, scientists are slowly unraveling some of the mysteries of the brain that are associated with learning, problem solving, and emotional responses.

There are several limitations to functional brain imaging that the reader should be aware of. The most problematic of these are artifacts caused by head motion. Since each voxel in a series of images is compared over time, even small amounts of head motion in the range of 1–2 mm during the functional magnetic resonance imaging acquisition session can result in severe artifacts or completely uninterpretable results. In addition, air has a very high magnetic susceptibility difference from brain tissue. Thus, artifacts from local areas of magnet field disturbance at the skull base caused by air in the adjacent paranasal sinuses may also produce uninterpretable results due to local areas of signal void on the image (Fig. 10.2.17). Air, like deoxyhemoglobin, has high magnetic susceptibility differences from adjacent tissues, leading to this loss in signal. Fortunately, most of the brain is well away from the areas affected by this magnetic field disturbance. However, tasks related to the inferior frontal lobes of the brain adjacent to large frontal and ethmoid sinuses or the inferior portions of the posterior temporal lobes in subjects with large mastoid sinuses can be affected. Disturbances in magnetic field leading to image distortion and/or signal loss can also be caused by small amounts of metal in the skin, hair, or teeth. Past traumatic injuries occasionally result in small fragments of embedded metal, or a subject may forget to remove a hair ornament or earring. While most dental fillings do not interfere with magnetic resonance, there are a few – especially certain types of root canal device or bridge work – that can interfere with the images.

Finally, paradigm design is a major consideration that must be carefully formulated in order to produce the intended result. The brain is a very complex organ and responds in multiple different ways. Trying to isolate a specific function without interference from other tasks that may be performed simultaneously by the brain is a difficult undertaking.

Results from functional magnetic resonance imaging studies

There have been a number of studies applying functional magnetic resonance imaging techniques to the evaluation of sexual

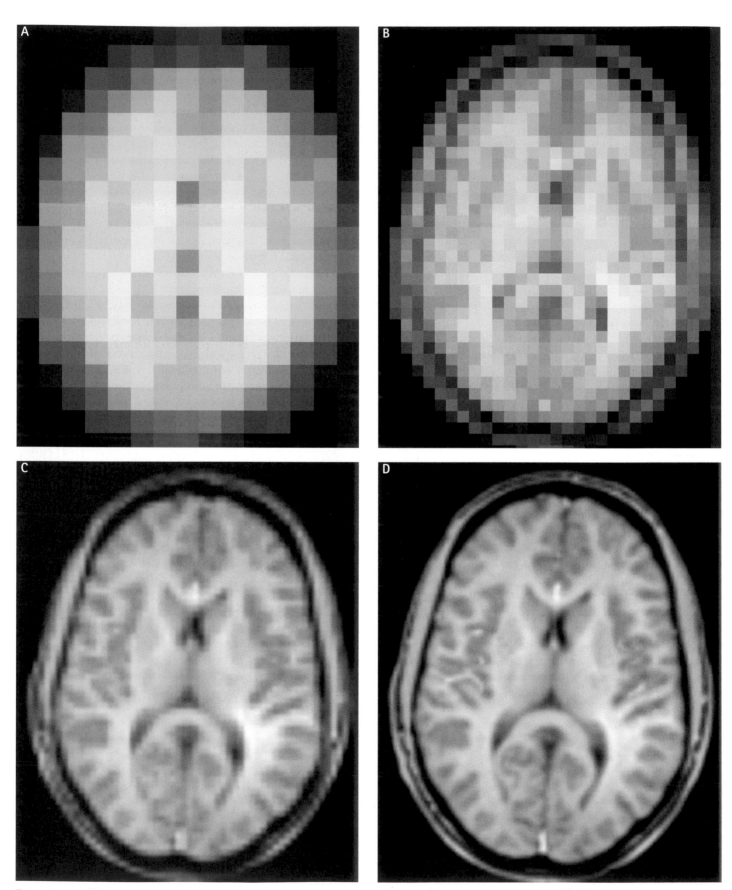

Figure 10.2.16. Illustration showing changes in resolution that occur with increasing matrix size (decreasing size of imaging pixels): (A) 16 × 16, (B) 32 × 32, (C) 64 × 64, (D) 128 × 128 (continued overleaf)

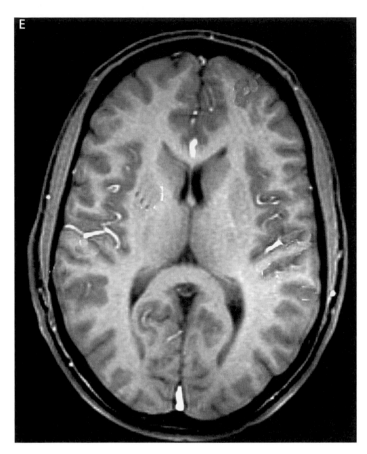

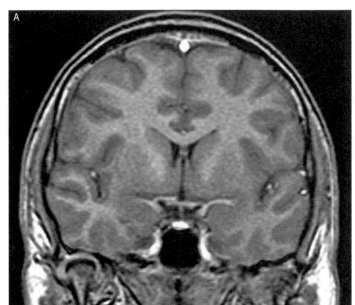

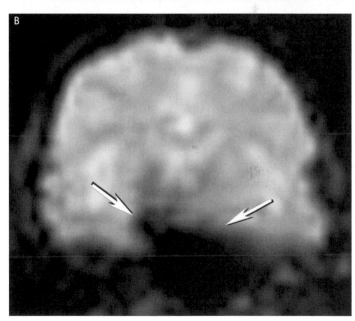

Figure 10.2.16. (continued) (E) 256 × 256 matrix sizes, respectively. Note that there is no usable anatomic information at matrix sizes of 16 or 32. Limited resolution is obtained at matrix sizes 32 and 64 and improves at levels of 128, but is best shown on a 256 × 256 matrix.

Figure 10.2.17. Coronal image of the brain at the level of the sphenoid sinus. (A) Anatomic image (B) echoplanar image obtained for fMRI study. Note the prominent loss of signal at the base of the brain surrounding the area of the sphenoid sinus (arrows) in image (B). This is due to the high susceptibility difference of air in the sphenoid sinus compared with the surrounding brain tissue as described in the text.

arousal or emotional response in both men and women. Initial imaging studies analyzing the functional neuroanatomic correlates of visually evoked sexual arousal in human males were performed by positron emission tomography scanning, and results from these studies were first reported by Stoleru et al.[26] In these studies, the brain activation response in eight male subjects to sexually explicit video clips was compared with emotionally neutral control film clips and humorous control film clips. The researchers found visually evoked areas of cerebral activation that correlated with the sexual arousal response in the posterior temporal-occipital cortices (a visual association area); the right insula and right inferior frontal cortex (paralimbic areas related to processing of sensory information with motivational states); and the left anterior cingulate cortex, another paralimbic area known to control autonomic and neuroendocrine functions. Thus, this study identified for the first time the ability to define brain regions whose activation was associated with visually evoked sexual arousal in men.

Park et al.,[27] using blood oxygen level-dependent functional magnetic resonance imaging techniques, such as those

described above, published the first study evaluating regions of cerebral activation associated with the female sexual arousal response. This group studied six healthy, premenopausal women volunteers with a mean age of 33. Using a real-time video presentation with alternatively presented erotic and nonerotic film clips, they were able to identify several brain regions activated in association with the sexual arousal response. These areas included the inferior frontal lobes, anterior cingulate gyrus, insula, corpus callosum, thalamus, caudate nucleus, globus pallidus, and inferior temporal lobes. Thus, they were able to demonstrate that functional magnetic resonance imaging can also show sexual arousal response within the brain in women undergoing visual sexual stimulus.

A group from Stanford University led by Arnow[28] used a novel paradigm and analysis method to define areas of brain activation associated with sexual arousal in healthy, heterosexual males. Rather than correlating the brain response associated with sexual arousal simply with the time of presentation of neutral versus erotic film clips, these researchers used a novel technique to correlate also the cerebral arousal response with erection. To do this, they constructed a device that measured the presence and degree of penile turgidity while the subject was in the magnetic resonance machine during presentation of the video material (alternating arousing and nonarousing video clips) while collecting functional magnetic resonance imaging data. They subsequently analyzed the data by two statistical methods: the traditional cross-correlation analysis already described that uses the time of presentation of the neutral versus arousing video clips, and a second cross-correlation using penile turgidity measures as the covariant. The team found a stronger activation response with the penile turgidity method than with the timing of the film clips, probably because penile turgidity correlated more precisely with the actual onset of arousal. Nevertheless, they defined areas of activation that were similar to several previous studies that included the right insular region, claustrum, left caudate, right middle occipital and middle temporal gyri, and bilateral cingulate gyri.

Another interesting study was reported by Karama et al.[29] These authors compared the responses of men and women during viewing of erotic video film clips. This study is unique in that it used identical techniques and the same team of researchers to study groups of 20 male and 20 female subjects. This provided direct comparison of the cerebral responses in men and women. Their results demonstrated that the observed levels of cerebral activation that correlated with sexual arousal, as measured by the blood oxygen level-dependent functional magnetic resonance imaging technique, was significantly higher in the male group of subjects than the female group of subjects. They also found that there were many similar areas of brain activation between both genders, including the anterior cingulate, prefrontal, orbital frontal, insular, and occipitotemporal cortices, as well as the amygdala and the ventral striatum in both groups. They did find, however, that activation of the thalamus and hypothalamus was significantly greater in male subjects. Furthermore, the greater levels of arousal observed in male subjects were also correlated with greater levels of sexual arousal among the male subjects as reported by subjective questionnaire.

Our group also studied a group of 10 healthy, premenopausal women without reported sexual difficulties. Analysis was done of the blood oxygen level-dependent functional magnetic resonance imaging studies, and two types of analyses were performed. The first analysis was the conventional blood oxygen level-dependent activation analysis to define areas of positive (increased) activation associated with the sexual arousal response. A second analysis was done to assess areas of the brain that showed decreased activation during sexual arousal. It was found that positive activation occurred in association with sexual arousal in many brain areas previously reported by several other groups. These areas include the orbital frontal region, the amygdala, the right caudate, the anterior cingulate, and the posterior temporal-occipital cortex on both sides (Fig. 10.2.18). Analysis of areas showing decreased activation revealed that there were localized areas of decreased regional cerebral blood flow during sexual arousal in both temporal lobes, predominately in the superior and middle temporal gyri. Additionally, the areas of decreased activation on the right were significantly greater than those observed on the left (Fig. 10.2.19). Interpretation of these data supports the hypothesis that the temporal lobe areas represent areas of normally active inhibition that underwent a decrease in their level of activation during the sexual arousal response. In support of this theory, similar anatomic sites in the superior and middle temporal gyri on the right side have been associated with moral judgment in previous cognitive functional magnetic resonance imaging studies.[30-32]

While the preceding studies demonstrate that the functional magnetic resonance imaging, blood oxygen level-dependent technique can define areas of activation associated with the sexual arousal response, this suggests that application of this technique could answer several questions about the cerebral component of the sexual arousal response. By defining normal areas of activation, one can begin to define the multiple associated cerebral components of the sexual arousal response. Through comparison of these arousal-related regions with other functional magnetic resonance imaging studies of the brain, we can begin to construct a model of the normal cerebral sexual arousal response and the various components that are associated with it. One can also begin to see the similarities and differences between male and female brain responses. It is interesting, although not unexpected, that early studies suggest that the

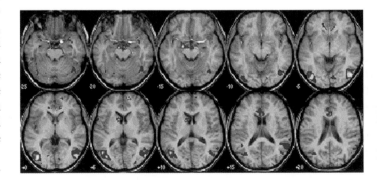

Figure 10.2.18. Axial functional magnetic resonance imaging of brain showing results of a group analysis of 10 normal subjects that demonstrate areas of activation. Specific areas of activation are highlighted in red and their anatomic location is discussed in the text.

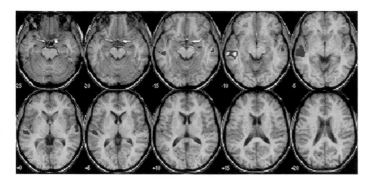

Figure 10.2.19. Functional magnetic resonance imaging study showing results of a group analysis of areas of decreased levels of activation during sexual arousal response. Note the dominant areas of decreased activation present in both temporal lobes. The decreased level of activation on the right is significantly greater than that seen on the left.

major regions of activation are similar for both men and women, although there is a greater magnitude of response in males. Thus, these techniques show promise of eventually providing a better understanding of previously elusive information regarding the brain components related to sexuality.

Of even greater importance, however, is the fact that these techniques may prove useful to analyze possible new methods of treatment, whether they are pharmacologic treatments or new approaches to psychotherapy. For example, a study done by Montorsi et al.[33] analyzed brain activation patterns in men during video sexual stimulation both before and after administration of apomorphine, a known stimulator of the erectile process. The role of apomorphine in initiating the erectile process has been defined in animal models, though there has not been any direct data confirming its effectiveness in humans. The study by Montorsi utilized sublingual apomorphine versus a placebo control agent to study 10 male patients with psychogenic arousal (erectile) dysfunction. Their response was assessed by functional magnetic resonance imaging of the brain during visual stimulation by a video of alternating neutral and erotic content. Six volunteers with no history of erectile dysfunction were used as controls. In the patients with psychogenic erectile dysfunction, the sublingual apomorphine produced an increase in extent of the activated networks of the brain plus additional activation in deep structures, including the nucleus accumbens, hypothalamus, and mesencephalon, that was greater than in the placebo control group of patients. In addition, the pattern of increased responses among the apomorphine group of patients more closely resembled the functional magnetic resonance imaging response pattern seen in control subjects without erectile dysfunction. This study demonstrates the potential utility of functional magnetic resonance imaging techniques to help confirm the positive response to a pharmacologic therapy as well as to define possible anatomic sites within the brain at which the pharmacologic therapy acts to produce its effect.

Finally, another area of functional magnetic resonance imaging activity that is helping to define normal and abnormal

brain responses to sexual arousal has been explored by Komisaruk et al.[34] This group studied the brain response to vaginal-cervical self-stimulation in women with complete spinal cord injury. These researchers were able to define the ability of women with a complete spinal cord injury to achieve orgasm by self-stimulation. They found that cervical self-stimulation increased activity in the region of the nucleus of the solitary tract, which is the brainstem nucleus to which the vagus nerves project. Their findings suggest that the vagus nerve can convey genital sensory input directly to the brain in women with spinal cord injury, thus completely bypassing the spinal cord injury.

Conclusion

Magnetic resonance imaging both in the genitalia and in the brain is a powerful tool that can provide unique information unobtainable by any other method. Its exquisite sensitivity and total noninvasiveness allow us to apply this technique in large numbers of subjects and even to perform repetitive serial studies without difficulty. Our understanding of the pelvic genital responses and the ability to quantify certain measures related to engorgement in women may eventually lead to a better understanding of the genital physiology during sexual arousal. This, in turn, may enable discoveries for new avenues of research into treatment of sexual dysfunction and to evaluate the effect of new therapies to improve genital sexual response in women.

Understanding of brain function associated with sexual arousal and response represents a truly unique and exciting area of application of functional magnetic resonance imaging. This previously mysterious and inaccessible region is now open to research and analysis by large numbers of cognitive brain scientists and human sexuality researchers. No doubt these and similar techniques will be applied in as yet unimagined ways to answer questions about normal human sexuality and dysfunction. The hope is that such increased understanding will inevitably lead to better methods of treatment. Thus, these exciting technologies promise to improve the quality of life for many in the coming years.

References

1. Deliganis AV, Maravilla KR, Heiman JR et al. Female genitalia: dynamic MR imaging with use of MS-325 initial experiences evaluating female sexual response. *Radiology* 2002; 225: 791–9.
2. Maravilla KR, Heiman JR, Garland PA et al. Dynamic MR imaging of the sexual arousal response in women. *J Sex Marital Ther* 2003; 29(Suppl 1): 71.
3. Levin RJ, Wagner G. Orgasm in women in the laboratory – quantitative studies on duration, intensity, latency, and vaginal blood flow. *Arch Sex Behav* 1985; 14: 439–49.
4. Wagner G, Levin RJ. Effect of atropine and methylatropine on human vaginal blood flow, sexual arousal and climax. *Acta Pharmacol Toxicol (Copenh)* 1980; 46: 321–5.

5. Beck JG, Barlow DH, Sakheim DK. Operating characteristics of the vaginal photoplethysmograph. *Arch Sex Behav* 1984; 13: 595–6.

6. Henson DE, Rubin HB, Henson C. Labial and vaginal blood volume responses to visual and tactile stimuli. *Arch Sex Behav* 1982; 11: 23–31.

7. Laan E, Everaerd W. Physiological measures of vaginal vasocongestion. *Int J Impot Res* 1998; 10(Suppl 2): S107.

8. Farquhar CM, Rae T, Thomas DC et al. Doppler ultrasound in the nonpregnant pelvis. *J Ultrasound Med* 1989; 8: 451–7.

9. Lavoisier P, Aloui R, Schmidt MH et al. Clitoral blood flow increases following vaginal pressure stimulation. *Arch Sex Behav* 1995; 24: 37–45.

10. Taylor KJ, Burns PN, Woodcock JP et al. Blood flow in deep abdominal and pelvic vessels: ultrasonic pulsed-Doppler analysis. *Radiology* 1985; 154: 487–93.

11. Maravilla KR, Cao Y, Heiman JR et al. Serial MR imaging with MS-325 for evaluating female sexual arousal response: determination of intrasubject reproducibility. *J Magn Reson Imaging* 2003; 18: 216–24.

12. Maravilla K, Cao Y, Heiman J et al. Noncontrast dynamic magnetic resonance imaging for quantitative assessment of female sexual arousal. *J Urol* 2005; 173: 162–6.

13. Meston CM, Heiman JR. Ephedrine-activated physiological sexual arousal in women. *Arch Gen Psychiatry* 1998; 55: 652–6.

14. Heiman JR. A psychophysiological exploration of sexual arousal patterns in females and males. *Psychophysiology* 1977; 14: 266–74.

15. Grist TM, Korosec FR, Peters DC et al. Steady-state and dynamic MR angiography with MS-325: initial experience in humans. *Radiology* 1998; 207: 539–44.

16. Lauffer RB, Parmelee DJ, Ouellet HS et al. MS-325: a small-molecule vascular imaging agent for magnetic resonance imaging. *Acad Radiol* 1996; 3(Suppl 2): S356.

17. Prasad PV, Cannillo J, Chavez DR et al. Contrast-enhanced MR angiography and first-pass renal perfusion imaging using MS-325, an intravascular contrast agent. *Acad Radiol* 1998; 5(Suppl 1): S219.

18. Suh DD, Yang CC, Cao Y et al. Magnetic resonance imaging anatomy of the female genitalia in premenopausal and postmenopausal women. *J Urol* 2003; 170: 138–44.

19. O'Connell HE, Hutson JM, Anderson CR et al. Anatomical relationship between urethra and clitoris. *J Urol* 1998; 159: 1892–7.

20. Grafenberg E. The role of the urethra in female orgasm. *Int J Sexol* 1950; 3: 145–8.

21. Goldberg DC, Whipple B, Fishkin RE et al. The Grafenberg spot and female ejaculation: a review of initial hypotheses. *J Sex Marital Ther* 1983; 9: 27–37.

22. Whipple B, Perry JD. The G-spot: a modern gynecologic myth. *Am J Obstet Gynecol* 2002; 187: 519; reply, 520.

23. Suh DD, Yang CC, Cao Y et al. MRI of female genital and pelvic organs during sexual arousal. *J Psychosom Obstet Gynecol* 2004; 25: 153–62.

24. Ogawa N. [Central acetylcholinergic systems in the normal aged and in the patient with Alzheimer-type dementia (ATD)]. *Rinsho Shinkeigaku* 1989; 29: 1529–31.

25. Fox PT, Mintun MA, Raichle ME et al. A noninvasive approach to quantitative functional brain mapping with H2 (15)O and positron emission tomography. *J Cereb Blood Flow Metab* 1984; 4: 329–33.

26. Stoleru S, Gregoire MC, Gerard D et al. Neuroanatomical correlates of visually evoked sexual arousal in human males. *Arch Sex Behav* 1999; 28: 1–21.

27. Park K, Kang HK, Seo JJ et al. Blood-oxygenation-level-dependent functional magnetic resonance imaging for evaluating cerebral regions of female sexual arousal response. *Urology* 2001; 57: 1189–94.

28. Arnow BA, Desmond JE, Banner LL et al. Brain activation and sexual arousal in healthy, heterosexual males. *Brain* 2002; 125: 1014–23.

29. Karama S, Lecours AR, Leroux JM et al. Areas of brain activation in males and females during viewing of erotic film excerpts. *Hum Brain Mapp* 2002; 16: 1–13.

30. Greene JD, Nystrom LE, Engell AD et al. The neural bases of cognitive conflict and control in moral judgment. *Neuron* 2004; 44: 389–400.

31. Heekeren HR, Wartenburger I, Schmidt H et al. An fMRI study of simple ethical decision-making. *Neuroreport* 2003; 14: 1215–19.

32. Moll J, de Oliveira-Souza R, Bramati IE et al. Functional networks in emotional moral and nonmoral social judgments. *Neuroimage* 2002; 16: 696–703.

33. Montorsi F, Perani D, Anchisi D et al. Brain activation patterns during video sexual stimulation following the administration of apomorphine: results of a placebo-controlled study. *Eur Urol* 2003; 43: 405–11.

34. Komisaruk BR, Whipple B, Crawford A et al. Brain activation during vaginocervical self-stimulation and orgasm in women with complete spinal cord injury: fMRI evidence of mediation by the vagus nerves. *Brain Res* 2004; 1024: 77–88.

10.3 Blood flow: duplex Doppler ultrasound

Sandra Garcia Nader, Scott R Maitland, Ricardo Munarriz, Irwin Goldstein

Introduction

The biologic evaluation of women with sexual health problems involves an assessment of the integrity of multiple systems contributing to physiologic sexual function, including endocrinologic, neurologic, and vascular factors[1] (see Chapters 10.1, 10.2, and 10.4–10.7 of this book). Concerning genital hemodynamic physiology in women, sexual arousal is dependent on the structural and functional integrity of tissue, primarily of vascular and nonvascular smooth muscle as well as arterioles, and involves complex neurovascular processes modulated by various local neurotransmitters, vasoactive agents, sex steroid hormones, and growth factors[2] (see Chapters 5.1–5.6). The increased pelvic blood flow through the ilio-hypogastric-pudendal arterial bed leads to increased perfusion of the sexual organs, specifically the vagina, clitoris, and labia (see Chapters 4.1–4.3). The resultant increase in blood flow leads to increased engorgement of the clitoral, labial, and vaginal erectile tissues; increased diameter of the clitoral corpora cavernosa and the labial corpora spongiosa (vestibular bulb erectile tissue); and increased diameter and length of the vagina.[2,3]

Vasculogenic female sexual dysfunction

Animal model data indicate that arterial occlusive pathology in the ilio-hypogastric-pudendal arterial bed is associated with impaired sexual (pelvic nerve stimulation) arousal response.[3–7] The altered sexual response includes diminished arterial inflow, diminished lubrication, decreased vaginal wall pressures, decreased vaginal length and width changes, and increased intraluminal pressures compared to control animals. Park et al. reported in the animal model that atherosclerosis of the hypogastric-vaginal-clitoral arterial bed was associated with

marked impairment in pelvic nerve-mediated changes in genital blood flow.[6] These findings were associated with cavernosal artery atherosclerotic changes, loss of corporal smooth muscle, and increase in corporal connective tissue in atherosclerotic compared with control animals. It was concluded that vaginal and clitoral engorgement depend on increased blood inflow and that atherosclerosis is associated with vaginal and clitoral engorgement insufficiency. This and other studies have suggested that at least some cases of female sexual arousal dysfunction might be associated with arterial vascular insufficiency[3–7] (see Chapter 5.6).

Selective internal iliac arteriography of women with peripheral vascular disease and claudication reveals that there is significant arterial occlusive disease in the pudendal and cavernosal arteries. An unpublished pilot study at our center reviewed pelvic arteriographic studies performed in women who presented with claudication and peripheral vascular disease symptoms. Twenty-seven per cent of the women had severe or completely occluded internal pudendal arteries, 23% had severe or complete occlusion of the hypogastric arteries, and 9% had severe or complete occlusion of the common iliacs. It was concluded that women with peripheral vascular disease had pelvic atherosclerotic arterial occlusive disease.

The clinical relevance of hemodynamic investigations has not yet been established in women with sexual dysfunction. It is likely that there are sexual arousal problems and tissue integrity changes in women that are associated with ilio-hypogastric-pudendal arterial occlusive disease.[8] Vascular assessment by duplex Doppler ultrasound may be important in the evaluation of women with sexual dysfunction, particularly in women with arousal disorders.[9–11] Women in the menopause and women associated with vascular risk factor exposure may be candidates for duplex Doppler ultrasonography.[12] Nevertheless, it must be emphasized that the presence of arterial pathology is not always indicative of organic sexual dysfunction. Further research is needed to clarify the relationship between the hemodynamic integrity of the hypogastric-pudendal arterial bed and peripheral genital arousal responses.

Nonultrasound genital blood flow measures in women

Physiologic measures to assess genital blood flow during arousal in women have been used for psychophysiologic research since the 1970s. The first physiologic method involved vaginal photoplethysmography[13–15] (see Chapter 10.1). Vaginal photoplethysmography consists of a tampon-sized device containing a light source (infrared) to illuminate the capillary plexus in the lamina propria under the vaginal epithelium, and a phototransistor as a light detector that senses the backscattered light from the vaginal epithelium. With alternating current coupling, the phasic changes in vaginal engorgement with each heartbeat are measured by "vaginal pulse amplitude". The higher the vaginal pulse amplitude, the greater the vaginal tissue blood content. Although the vaginal photoplethysmograph can be inserted by the subject and is well tolerated, it is not reliable during movement such as masturbation, clitoral vibration, and orgasm.[16,17]

The other physiologic method involves an oxygen-temperature measuring system and was developed in 1977 by Levin and Wagner[18] (see Chapter 10.4). The oxygen-temperature measuring system consists of an oxygen electrode heated by an electric current to a set temperature, and joined to the vagina via a suction cup. During an increase in vaginal blood perfusion, the electrode records increased heat loss. A greater power output is needed to maintain the electrode at the set temperature. The electrode also measures the amount of oxygen, reflecting transient changes in blood flow, diffusing across the vaginal epithelium. Although the oxygenation-temperature measure does not seem to be impaired by movement such as masturbation, clitoral vibration, and orgasm, the electrode needs to be attached by the experimenter (not the subject) and cannot be applied for long periods.

Ultrasound genital blood flow measures in women

Despite the recognition that medical factors are associated with sexual dysfunction, there have been limited medically focused diagnostic evaluations in women with sexual dysfunction. Duplex ultrasonography can be adapted for measuring vaginal, clitoral, and labial blood flow during arousal. Lavoisier et al. first reported on the use of Doppler ultrasonography to measure blood velocity in the clitoral cavernosal artery and to record changes in flow associated with intravaginal pressure changes.[19] Sarrel utilized laser Doppler velocimetry to measure vaginal blood flow in postmenopausal women receiving estrogen alone versus estrogen and androgen.[20] While such studies suggest that

genital blood flow can be objectively measured by ultrasound technology, there have been few publications concerning duplex ultrasonographic findings in women with sexual dysfunction.[9–11]

Duplex Doppler ultrasonography with a high-frequency (12.5 MHz) external probe can be used to provide continuous, real-time imaging of arterial and erectile tissue components recorded at baseline and after sexual stimulation with an erotic video on a surround sound headset and a vibrator. Only visual stimulation is maintained during the actual ultrasound examination.[9–11]

Duplex Doppler ultrasonography can assess the changes in peak systolic velocity in centimeters per second that occur in the right and left clitoral cavernosal and labial artery during sexual arousal[9–11] or after intracavernosal clitoral injection.[21] Genital tumescence is visually demonstrated on ultrasound, anatomically by increased venous pooling, and physiologically by increased end-diastolic velocities in the genital arteries. Duplex Doppler ultrasonography can also be used to assess the changes in clitoral and labial diameter associated with sexual stimulation. A transvaginal probe may be used to measure right and left vaginal, iliac, and uterine arterial peak systolic velocity changes.

Duplex Doppler ultrasonography is useful as a measure of genital blood flow before and during arousal in women who present for sexual dysfunction evaluation. Of great concern is the paucity of "control" duplex Doppler ultrasound data in women without sexual dysfunction. Prior to consideration of the use of duplex Doppler ultrasonography in the evaluation paradigm, women seeking treatment should undergo psychologic interview and history and physical examination.[1] If indicated, consideration should be given for blood testing for steroid hormones and laboratory tests such as duplex Doppler ultrasonography.[1]

Clinical experience with duplex Doppler ultrasound in a women's sexual health clinic

The following issues need to be addressed before duplex Doppler ultrasound becomes a robust component of the diagnostic evaluation of women with sexual dysfunction. Data are needed regarding normal values of volumetric/morphologic and hemodynamic data in women without sexual dysfunction. Technical issues such as probe size and ultrasound frequency need further development. The equipment utilized in duplex Doppler ultrasonography is summarized in Table 10.3.1.

A critical consideration is that the audiovisual–mechanical sexual stimulation in the office setting may result in incomplete genital smooth muscle relaxation yielding suboptimal vascular responses. Vasoactive pharmacologic strategies with or without sexual stimulation should be employed to maximize smooth muscle relaxation and vascular responses.

Table 10.3.1. Equipment utilized for duplex Doppler ultrasound

Videos
Visual stimulation with 3-D surround sound headset
Vibrator
Ultrasound duplex Doppler with high-frequency (11–12.5 MHz)
    small-parts probe
Ultrasound suite with quiet, relaxing, secure room for patient privacy
    containing an electronic communicating system enabling the patient
    to inform staff when she feels arousal has maximized.

The induction of an arousal response in an office setting is not always well accepted by patients, and there is concern for lack of privacy; both factors may lead to suboptimal vascular responses. Both to improve patient acceptance and achieve more reliable hemodynamic data, Becher et al. reported on duplex Doppler assessment of clitoral vascular changes with topical prostaglandin E_1 administration.[22] Becher et al. documented that prostaglandin E_1 gel application modified the vascular response of the clitoral artery, suggesting that vasoactive drugs might improve sexual response in patients with sexual dysfunction. In addition, Becher reported that the use of topical prostaglandin E_1 administration during duplex Doppler assessment of clitoral vascular changes resulted in better patient acceptance and more reliable hemodynamic data.[22]

In women with sexual health concerns, duplex Doppler ultrasonography has been used to assess genital morphologic, volumetric, and hemodynamic changes during sexual arousal.[9–11,19–22] Diagnostic ultrasonography is routinely performed in gray scale and duplex modes. The gray-scale ultrasound technique provides relevant clinical information on: (1) the integrity of clitoral and corpora spongiosa erectile tissue and tunica albuginea and (2) the clitoral and corpora spongiosa diameter. Classic duplex Doppler ultrasonography provides quantitative clitoral and spongiosal hemodynamic-focused data.

There have been few publications concerning duplex ultrasonographic findings in women with sexual dysfunction.[9–11,19–22] One aim of this chapter is to report gray-scale, volumetric, and duplex hemodynamic ultrasound data before and after sexual stimulation in a large population of women with sexual dysfunction.

This retrospective study of 142 (mean age 38.2 ± 9.7 years) women who underwent duplex Doppler ultrasound (GE Logic 400) arousal testing for sexual dysfunction in an outpatient clinic over 12 months was Institutional Review Board approved. For consistency, the same ultrasound technologist performed all studies. The angle of the clitoral shaft formed by the suspensory ligament was the sonographic landmark used for volumetric measurement.

Technique

To simplify volumetric/morphologic data collection and to minimize the duration of the vascular evaluation, only clitoral shaft diameter data were measured. The high-frequency (MHz)

small-parts probe was placed on one side of the clitoris, and clitoral diameter was measured from the medial tunica albuginea of the ipsilateral corporal body across the septum to the tunical albuginea of the contralateral corporal body at the level of the midshaft (Fig. 10.3.1). Gray-scale scanning of the tunica and corporal erectile tissue was performed. Hemodynamic clitoral data were recorded (Fig. 10.3.1C and D). While this sonographic landmark was maintained, the small parts probe was then swept laterally to evaluate the hypoechoic, ill-defined, carrot-shaped ipsilateral corpus spongiosum, which possesses a thin, occasionally visualized tunica. The width of the corpus spongiosum was obtained from the lateral to the medial aspect of the hypoechoic region at the predetermined sonographic landmark (Fig. 10.3.1B and E). Hemodynamic data from the ipsilateral corpus spongiosum artery was measured (Fig. 10.3.1E).

In summary, after audiovisual-sexual stimulation with or without vasoactive agents, diagnostic duplex Doppler ultrasonography was performed in gray-scale and duplex modes. Gray-scale ultrasound technique provides relevant clinical information on the integrity of clitoral and corpora spongiosa erectile tissue and tunica albuginea, and the clitoral and corpora spongiosa diameter before and after sexual stimulation. Classic duplex Doppler ultrasonography provides both quantitative clitoral and spongiosal hemodynamic-focused data.

The nursing staff carefully instructed patients and were available for assistance. Patient privacy was maximized. An electronic communication system was used to inform staff when the patient felt that arousal was maximized. Sexual stimulation was achieved and maintained with a 15-min standardized erotic video (Sinclair Institute; Femme Productions) on a 3-D surround sound headset (I.O. Display Systems LLC) and a vibrator (Ferticare, ILTS, Inc.) (frequency: 100 Hz; amplitude: 2.5 mm). After arousal, gray-scale, hemodynamic, and volumetric measurements were repeated by similar sonographic techniques (Fig. 10.3.1).

Gray-scale scanning of the clitoris revealed that 138 women had homogeneous erectile tissue throughout, with a smooth, continuous tunica albuginea (thickness ≤ 2 mm). The labial corpora spongiosa erectile tissue was uniformly hypoechoic with a thin or absent tunica albuginea in 139 women. Volumetric and hemodynamic data in the subject population are summarized in Table 10.3.2. We found that the increase in pre- and postarousal clitoral and corpus spongiosum diameter directly correlated ($p < 0.05$) with an increase in both the pre- and postarousal clitoral and corpus spongiosum end-diastolic velocity values. All data were analyzed by paired t-test. Differences between paired comparisons were considered statistically significant when p values were less than 0.05. Duplex Doppler ultrasound data (peak systolic velocity, end-diastolic velocity, resistive index) were expressed as the mean ± standard error of the mean.

Duplex Doppler ultrasound studies in women with sexual dysfunction were useful in a diagnostic and therapeutic context. A woman with persistent sexual arousal syndrome was found to have

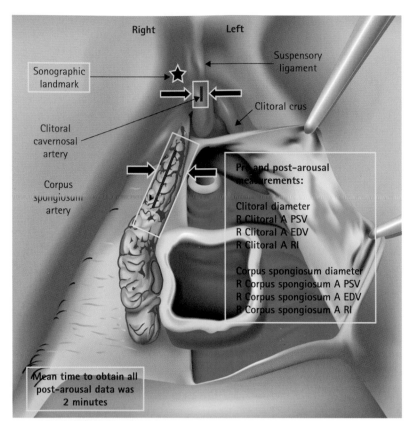

A

Figure 10.3.1. (A) Schematic illustration of the sonographic landmark for transducer probe placement. (B) Gray-scale ultrasound provides clinical information on the diameter of the clitoral corpora cavernosa and corpus spongiosum. (C) Gray-scale ultrasound provides diameter of the clitoral corpora cavernosa before and after sexual stimulation. Classic duplex Doppler ultrasonography provides quantitative, hemodynamically focused data, including clitoral peak systolic velocity values and clitoral end-diastolic velocity values. (D) A patient undergoing gray-scale ultrasound diameter determination of the clitoral corpora cavernosa. Duplex Doppler ultrasound revealed quantitative, hemodynamically focused data, including clitoral peak systolic velocity values and clitoral end-diastolic velocity values. (E) A patient undergoing gray-scale ultrasound diameter determination of the corpus spongiosum. Duplex Doppler ultrasound revealed quantitative, hemodynamically focused data, including corpus spongiosum peak systolic velocity values and end-diastolic velocity values.

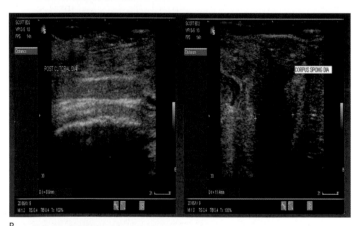

B

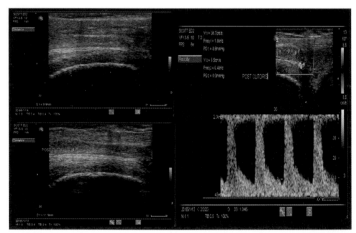

C

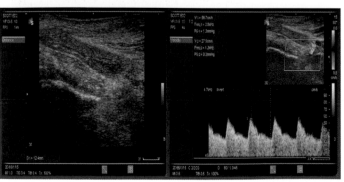

D

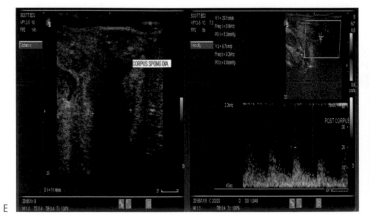

E

Table 10.3.2. Clitoral and corpus spongiosal hemodynamic and volumetric data before and after audiovisual-mechanical sexual stimulation

	Baseline	Postarousal	*p* values
Clitoral diameter	0.9 ± 0.33	1.2 ± 0.48	< 0.001
Clitoral peak systolic velocity	12.2 ± 3.8	21.6 ± 7.4	< 0.001
Clitoral end-diastolic velocity	2.9 ± 1.9	6.7 ± 3.7	< 0.01
Clitoral resistance index	0.57 ± 0.11	0.69 ± 0.09	0.10
Corpus spongiosum diameter	1.2 ± 0.7	1.8 ± 0.9	0.05
Corpus spongiosum peak systolic velocity	10.8 ± 4.6	19.4 ± 9.4	< 0.05
Corpus spongiosum end-diastolic velocity	4.0 ± 3.2	7.8 ± 3.0	0.05
Corpus spongiosum resistance index	0.45 ± 0.59	0.64 ± 0.08	0.40

elevated peak systolic velocity values in the clitoral cavernosal artery (Fig. 10.3.2A) and the corpus spongiosum artery (Fig. 10.3.2B), and a pelvic arteriovenous malformation was noted during vaginal ultrasound (Fig. 10.3.2C). Another patient with persistent sexual arousal syndrome had elevated peak systolic velocity values in the clitoral cavernosal artery (Fig. 10.3.3A) and the corpus spongiosum artery (Fig. 10.3.3B), but no abnormal arteriovenous malformation was noted during vaginal ultrasound. Another patient with persistent sexual arousal syndrome had significant prolapse of urethral mucosa and elevated peak systolic velocity values in the urethral artery. No abnormal arteriovenous vessels were noted during vaginal ultrasound (Fig. 10.3.4A and B). Another patient had pudendal nerve entrapment after childbirth with prolonged forceps use. We perform interval vaginal ultrasound-directed pudendal nerve blocks, administering the steroid–lidocaine mixture just lateral to the pudendal artery, as visualized easily on ultrasound (Fig. 10.3.5). Another patient fell onto a bicycle bar as a child. Ultrasound revealed a hyperechoic lesion just above the tunica consistent with thickening of the tunica (Peyronie's disease) (Fig. 10.3.6).

Conclusion

Female sexual dysfunction is a highly prevalent disorder that has underlying psychologic, physiologic, and interpersonal

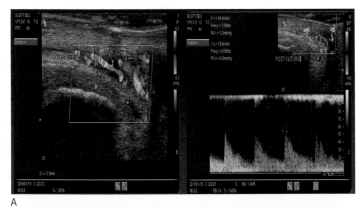

A

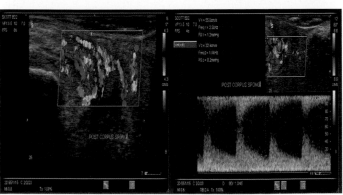

B

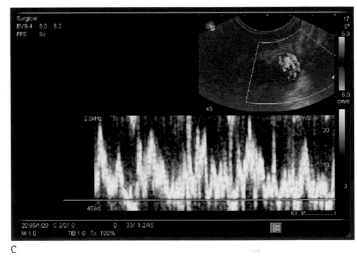

C

Figure 10.3.2. A woman with persistent sexual arousal syndrome was found to have elevated peak systolic velocity values in the clitoral cavernosal artery (A) and the corpus spongiosum artery (B), and a pelvic arteriovenous malformation was noted during vaginal ultrasound (C).

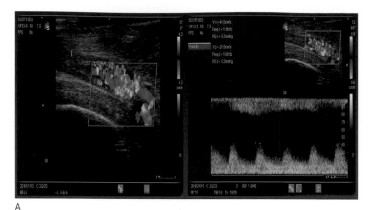

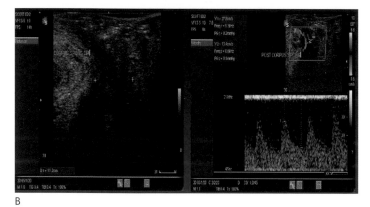

Figure 10.3.3. A patient with persistent sexual arousal syndrome had elevated peak systolic velocity values in the clitoral cavernosal artery (A) and the corpus spongiosum artery (B), but no abnormal arteriovenous malformation was noted during vaginal ultrasound.

relationship factors. Recognized biologic pathophysiologies include: (1) hormonal insufficiency states associated with menopause and androgen insufficiency; (2) neurologic disorders, such as spinal cord injury and multiple sclerosis; and (3) arterial occlusive disease in the ilio-hypogastric-pudendal arterial bed in association with cardiovascular risk factor exposure, as in aging, hypertension, diabetes, high cholesterol, and heart disease.[1,2,12] In general, there has been limited investigation of the mechanisms whereby biologic factors adversely affect sexual function in women, partly because of the lack of validated and standardized clinical diagnostic instruments and methodologies. In particular, there has been a paucity of research on vascular factors in female sexual function and dysfunction.

The study reported in this chapter revealed that duplex Doppler ultrasonography can record significant volumetric (clitoral and corpora spongiosa diameters) and hemodynamic (peak systolic and end diastolic) changes in women with sexual dysfunction before and after sexual stimulation. These changes were greater in the clitoris than in the corpus spongiosum, probably due to differences in the size of the vascular lumina and the characteristics of the erectile tissues.

Resistive index measurements, which are indicative of veno-occlusive function, did not significantly change before

and after arousal in either the clitoris or corpora spongiosa. This implies that genital arousal in women is associated with a volumetric increase not accompanied by significant veno-occlusion. In fact, it was found that the increases in pre- and post-arousal clitoral and corpus spongiosum diameters correlated with an increase in both the pre- and post-arousal clitoral and corpus spongiosum end-diastolic velocity values. This implies that genital engorgement in women is better assessed by the determination of end-diastolic velocity values.

Gray-scale imaging revealed tunical thickening and/or plaque of the clitoris in several patients. In addition, we found microcalcifications within the erectile tissue of the clitoris and/or corpora spongiosa (Fig. 10.3.6). All of these patients with abnormal gray-scale findings recalled a specific episode of blunt perineal trauma such as falling onto a bicycle crossbar.

While this duplex Doppler ultrasound study in 142 women with sexual dysfunction showed that ultrasound may by utilized in women with sexual dysfunction, there remain many issues

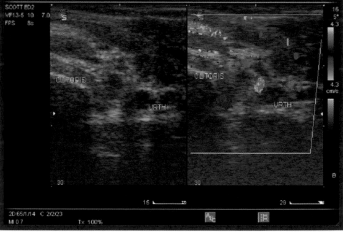

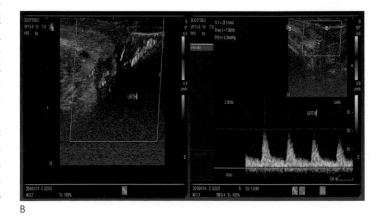

Figure 10.3.4. A patient with persistent sexual arousal syndrome had a significant prolapse of her urethral mucosa and had elevated peak systolic velocity values in the urethral artery. No abnormal arteriovenous vessels were noted during vaginal ultrasound.

may result in incomplete genital smooth muscle relaxation, yielding suboptimal vascular responses. Third, vasoactive pharmacologic strategies with or without sexual stimulation need to be employed to maximize smooth muscle relaxation and vascular responses. Fourth, there are technical issues, such as probe size and ultrasound frequency, which need further delineation.

References

1. Basson R, Althof S, Davis S et al. Summary of the recommendations on sexual dysfunctions in women. *J Sex Med* 2004; 1: 24–34.
2. Giraldi A, Marson L, Nappi R et al. Physiology of female sexual function: animal models. *J Sex Med* 2004; 1: 237–53.
3. Giuliano F, Allard J, Compagnie S et al. Vaginal physiological changes in a model of sexual arousal in anesthetized rats. *Am J Physiol Regul Integr Comp Physiol* 2001; 281: R140–9.
4. Traish AM, Kim NN, Munarriz R et al. Biochemical and physiological mechanisms of female genital sexual arousal. *Arch Sex Behav* 2002; 31: 393–400.
5. Munarriz R, Kim NN, Goldstein I et al. Biology of female sexual function. *Urol Clin North Am* 2002; 29: 685–93.
6. Park K, Goldstein I, Andry C et al. Vasculogenic female sexual dysfunction: the hemodynamic basis for vaginal engorgement insufficiency and clitoral erectile insufficiency. *Int J Impot Res* 1997; 9: 27–37.
7. Park K, Tarcan T, Goldstein I et al. Atherosclerosis-induced chronic arterial insufficiency causes clitoral cavernosal fibrosis in the rabbit. *Int J Impot Res* 2000; 12: 111–16.
8. Tarcan T, Park K, Goldstein I et al. Histomorphometric analysis of age-related structural changes in human clitoral cavernosal tissue. *J Urol* 1999; 161: 940–4.
9. Munarriz R, Maitland S, Garcia SP et al. A prospective duplex Doppler ultrasonographic study in women with sexual arousal disorder to objectively assess genital engorgement induced by EROS therapy. *J Sex Marital Ther* 2003; 29(Suppl 1): 85–94.
10. Bechara A, Bertolino MV, Casabe A et al. Duplex Doppler ultrasound assessment of clitoral hemodynamics after topical administration of alprostadil in women with arousal and orgasmic disorders. *J Sex Marital Ther* 2003; 29(Suppl 1): 1–10.
11. Khalife S, Binik YM, Cohen DR et al. Evaluation of clitoral blood flow by color Doppler ultrasonography. *J Sex Marital Ther* 2000; 26: 187–9.
12. Lewis RW, Fugl-Meyer KS, Bosch R et al. Epidemiology/risk factors of sexual dysfunction. *J Sex Med* 2004; 1: 35–9.
13. Geer JH, Morokoff P, Greenwood P. Sexual arousal in women: the development of a measurement device for vaginal blood volume. *Arch Sex Behav* 1974; 3: 559–64.
14. Sintchak G, Geer JH. A vaginal photoplethysmograph system. *Psychophysiology* 1975; 12: 113–15.
15. Korff J, Geer JH. The relationship between sexual arousal experience and genital response. *Psychophysiology* 1983; 20:121–7.
16. Levin RJ. Assessing human female sexual arousal by vaginal photoplethysmography: a critical examination. *Sexologies* 1997; 6: 25–31.

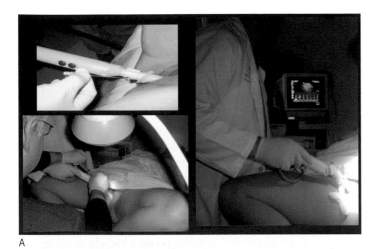
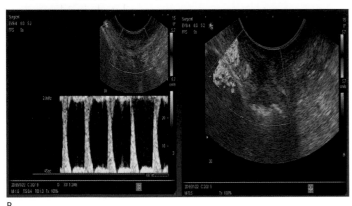

Figure 10.3.5. A patient had pudendal nerve entrapment after childbirth with prolonged forceps use. We perform interval vaginal ultrasound-directed pudendal nerve blocks (A), administering the steroid–lidocaine mixture just lateral to the pudendal artery, as visualized easily by ultrasound (B).

that need to be addressed before this diagnostic modality becomes a standard part of the evaluation. First, there are insufficient data regarding normal values of volumetric and hemodynamic data in women without sexual dysfunction. Second, audiovisual–mechanical sexual stimulation in the office setting

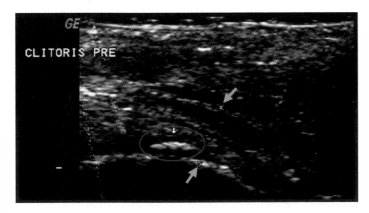

Figure 10.3.6. Ultrasound revealed a hyperechoic lesion just above the tunica consistent with thickening of the tunica (Peyronie's disease).

17. Laan E, Everaerd W, Evers A. Assessment of female sexual arousal: response specificity and construct validity. *Psychophysiology* 1995; 32: 476–85.

18. Levin RJ, Wagner G. Haemodynamic changes of the human vagina during sexual arousal assessed by a heated oxygen electrode. *J Physiol* 1977; 75: 23P–4P.

19. Lavoisier P, Aloui R, Schmidt MH et al. Clitoral blood flow increases following vaginal pressure stimulation. *Arch Sex Behav* 1995; 24: 37–45.

20. Sarrel PM. Ovarian hormones and vaginal blood flow: using laser Doppler velocimetry to measure effects in a clinical trial of postmenopausal women. *Int J Impot Res* 1998; 10(Suppl 2): S91–3.

21. Akkus E, Carrier S, Turzan C et al. Duplex ultrasonography after prostaglandin E1 injection of the clitoris in a case of hyperreactio luteinalis. *J Urol* 1995; 153: 1237–8.

22. Becher EF, Bechara A, Casabe A. Clitoral hemodynamic changes after a topical application of alprostadil. *J Sex Marital Ther* 2001; 27: 405–10.

10.4 Blood flow: heated electrodes

Roy J Levin

Introduction: measuring vaginal blood flow with heated electrodes

Vaginal blood flow assessed by the heated oxygen electrode

The heated oxygen electrode employed was a commercial electrode (E5250) and oxygen monitor (TCM1) manufactured by Radiometer (Copenhagen, Denmark) for use in intensive care units to measure the arterial partial pressure of oxygen (P_{O2}) transcutaneously.* In essence, it is a Clarke-type oxygen electrode fitted with a temperature-measuring device and an electrical heater that could be set to heat up the skin to a depth of about 3 mm.[1] The electrode is normally applied to the skin surface by a special adhesive holder. The temperature of the electrode can be set to temperatures above that of blood so that the tissue underneath becomes maximally vasodilated, allowing the fast-flowing capillary blood to be similar to that of arterial blood, and the oxygen that diffuses out of the blood onto the surrounding tissues closely mirrors that of the arterial partial pressure of oxygen. While this itself is a useful measure of the blood perfusion of the tissue, the real bonus of the electrode is that it can be set to operate at a particular temperature above that of blood (say, 41°C), and the electronic circuit of the device gives a readout of the electrical power (in milliwatts) needed to maintain the device at that set temperature. This power is a measure of the heat loss of the electrode, representing both (1) the heat loss by conduction into the tissue beneath the electrode, influenced mainly by the blood flow and (2) heat losses from the housing of the electrode to the environment by convection, conduction, and radiation. If the heat loss by conduction to the skin because of the blood flow is very much greater than the heat loss due to the other nonspecific process, then the actual power consumption of the electrode will be a reasonable indirect measure of the blood flow underneath the heated electrode. The attachment of the electrode to the relatively dry skin is by a special holder with an adhesive surface. This cannot be used in the vagina, as the walls of the organ are usually coated with a slippery, basal fluid secretion. Wagner and Levin[2] designed a holder the electrode can be placed in that is then held onto the vaginal wall by a grooved suction rim (Fig. 10.4.1). The grooved rim is connected to a vacuum pump and the device is held onto the vaginal wall by the suction, which is sufficient to hold the electrode in contact against the vaginal epithelium even during the vaginal contractions of an orgasm. It is thus possible to follow the changing power consumption throughout sexual stimulation, including an orgasm.

The graphs in Fig. 10.4.2 show the changes in blood flow of the vaginal walls during arousal to orgasm (and after) by clitoral stimulation in three subjects. Two separate heated oxygen electrodes were employed attached to the lateral walls on either side of the vagina. The practically identical changes measured by both electrodes in all the subjects show that the increases in blood flow induced by the clitoral stimulation is not discrete but involves the whole vagina.

Obviously, to give the best index of the blood flow, the heat losses by the non-blood-flow processes need to be kept to the minimum. The ideal correction for these heat losses would be to attach the electrode to the vaginal wall and stop all blood flow; the heat lost (power consumption) would then be only that from non-blood-flow processes. Of course, while this can be achieved in an animal vagina by clamping of the arterial blood supply, it cannot be accomplished in the human vagina *in situ*. In humans, the best correction that can be made, if high accuracy is demanded and it is felt essential, is to attach the electrode to the volar surface of the subject's arm and measure the power needed to keep the electrode at its vaginal fixed temperature with normal skin blood flow and after the inflation of a

---

* The original Radiometer heated oxygen electrode has now been replaced by a solid-state electrode, but the specifications are the same as the E5250. The present model, TCM4 monitor, still allows the power measure to be obtained, with the added advantage that the trend curve can be shown and printed out. Radiometer's website is www.tc-monitoring.com.

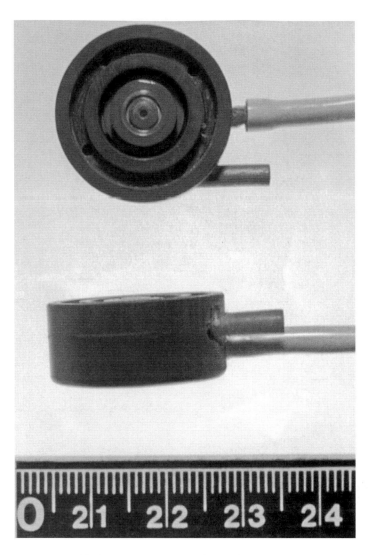

Figure 10.4.1. The heated oxygen electrode (model E5250, Radiometer, Copenhagen) mounted inside the suction capsule for attachment to the vaginal wall. The short tube opens into the groove around capsule's rim and is where the suction is applied. The scale beneath is in centimeters (reproduced with permission from Wagner and Levin[2]).

blood pressure cuff to approximately 200 mmHg to stop arterial inflow to the arm (Fig. 10.4.3). The amount of power used when the arterial blood flow to the arm is blocked off can be used as a correction for the non-blood-flow heat losses. It can be subtracted from the original readings of the power consumption ("calculated blood flow index" in Fig. 10.4.3). After the correction, the shape of the blood flow curve is identical to that previously obtained; the only difference is that the actual power consumption figures are now obviously much smaller and mirror more accurately the blood flow.

Another simple experiment confirms that the electrode loses heat to the vaginal wall and external milieu even if there is no blood flow underneath the electrode. An electrode was attached to the vaginal wall, and a subepithelial injection of adrenaline was given immediately underneath the electrode. This causes the contraction of the peripheral blood vessels underneath the electrode, as indicated by the sharp drop to zero of the surface partial pressure of oxygen (Fig. 10.4.4). There is still, however, a significant loss of heat by the electrode to the environment and to the underlying tissue by conduction.

For many practical purposes, the direct reading of the electrode's power consumption without correction gives a reasonable index of the vaginal blood flow and congestion (pooling). As heat loss is proportional to the difference in temperature between the electrode's surface and the tissue it is resting on, if there is blood pooling as well as blood flow, the loss of heat will be affected by the volume of fluid that the heat is being lost to, because a large volume of fluid can absorb a greater amount of heat for a smaller increase in its temperature. Thus, heat loss from any heat electrode attached to the vaginal wall will be influenced both by tissue blood flow and by blood pooling.

The heat electrode technique has been used in a number of laboratory studies. It was first employed in the vagina to measure the changes in oxygen tension of its epithelial surface,[2] and in later work on vaginal wall blood flow during arousal to orgasm.[3,3a] In other studies, it was used: to ascertain which hemodynamic measure gives the best assessment of sexual arousal;[4] to investigate the effect of atropine on vaginal blood flow, sexual arousal, and climax;[5] to monitor simultaneously the vaginal hemodynamics by three independent methods during sexual arousal;[6] to record the vaginal blood flow and the duration, intensity, and latency of orgasm in women in the laboratory;[3] to evaluate the action of thyrotropin-releasing hormone on vaginal blood flow in conscious humans and anesthetized sheep;[7] and to monitor the veracity of claimed subjective sexual arousal in a subject in the laboratory.[8] Since its introduction, the heated oxygen electrode has been used by a number of other workers in a variety of studies on vaginal blood flow (see review by Levin[9] for references). One group, overlooking the initial employment and subsequent early studies by Wagner and Levin, claimed, in 2001, that it was a new technique for assessing female arousal (see comment by Levin and Wagner[10]).

Advantages of the heat electrode

The advantages of using the heated oxygen electrode as a device to monitor vaginal blood flow are: (1) it can be employed throughout all phase of sexual arousal, even when orgasm is induced, as it is not affected by movement; (2) the data it produces are transferable; (3) the basis of its measurement (that is, heat loss to the tissue) is reasonably well understood; (4) although it is intrusive (residing in a body cavity), it is not invasive (does not go beneath the skin layer); (5) it is relatively safe; (6) it is commercially available and relatively cheap; (7) repeated measures can be obtained in the same subject by heating and allowing the electrode to cool and then reheating; (8) it can even be used during menstruation if the surface of the vagina is first wiped free of any blood (the photoplethysmograph cannot be used if there is free blood in the vagina) (see Chapters 10.1–10.3).

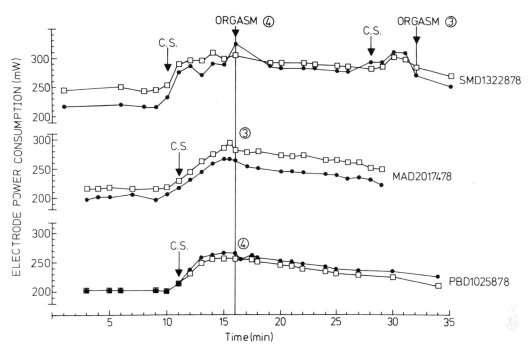

Figure 10.4.2. Power consumptions of two heated oxygen electrodes attached to the right and left hand sides of the vaginal walls in three subjects during sexual arousal by clitoral stimulation (C.S.) to orgasm (self-graded in the encircled number on a scale 1 = poor to 5 = excellent). In all the records, the decrease in electrode power consumption after orgasm is not very marked, and it slowly returns to the prearousal levels, suggesting that a single orgasm does not dissipate rapidly the vaginal blood flow/congestion. The first subject (SMD 1322878) induced a second orgasm 16 min after the first; note the very obvious decreased power response to the second arousal and orgasm compared with the first (Levin and Wagner, unpublished data), with the moderate decrease in subjective assessment of the second orgasm (from 4 to 3).

Disadvantages of heat electrode

Its main disadvantages are: (1) it needs to be applied to the vaginal surface by the experimenter, and this appears to be a drawback in some cultures, although having a female laboratory assistant or nurse do the application satisfies most ethical committees; (2) it should not be left stuck onto the vaginal wall for periods greater than 2–3 h; (3) its unit of measurement (milliwatts) is indirect rather than in direct terms of flow (ml/100 g tissue/min).

The clearance concept and the heat electrode

Measuring the blood flow in human organs *in situ* has always been a challenge, as it is usually impossible to measure the arterial inflow or to cannulate the venous drainage and directly collect all the flow coming from the organ. Because of this difficulty, various indirect methods of measuring blood flow have been developed, many using the concept of "clearance". In essence, a substance is injected into the organ or applied to a tissue surface and the rate of its local disappearance monitored; this local rate is the clearance of the substance from the site, and it is practically exclusively removed by the blood.

Substances employed for the clearance have to be nontoxic and not metabolized, must equilibrate rapidly between tissue and blood, and must be easily and accurately estimated. Examples are radioactive sodium (Kety[11]) and xenon-133

(Lassen et al.[12]). Wagner and Ottesen[13] were the first to employ the clearance of xenon-133 to estimate the vaginal blood flow in the quiescent, nonsexually aroused state (median 10, range 6–20 ml/100 g tissue per min, n = 7) and its increase during sexual arousal (median 29, range 22–45 ml/100 g tissue per min). However, because the technique is invasive (it uses an intraepithelial needle injection of the xenon-133 in saline) and uses a radioactive gas, it has remained a research technique and has not been employed by others for routine clinical studies on the vaginal blood flow.

Changes in the extraction of heat from a variety of probes has often been used to monitor tissue blood flow indirectly, but because heat fits all of the requirements for an ideal washout "substance", it can be used to calculate the tissue's blood flow in real terms of ml/100 g tissue per min as if it were an actual "substance".

The heated oxygen electrode used for "heat washout" experiments

At the Panum Institute in Copenhagen, Middttun et al.[14] developed a simple technique to measure the blood flow of the human skin with a modified Radiometer transcutaneous partial pressure of oxygen electrode. The disk electrode was attached to the skin and the initial skin temperature (T_b) measured. The electrode was heated until the underlying tissues reached the

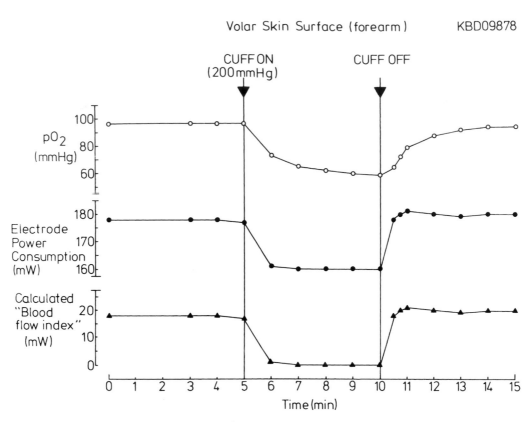

Figure 10.4.3. Electrode power consumption of a heated oxygen electrode (model E5250, Radiometer, Copenhagen) mounted on the volar skin surface of a female subject's forearm. On application of the pressure to 200 mmHg in the arterial pressure cuff around the arm (CUFF ON) for 5 min, there is a fall in pO_2 on the skin surface of approximately 50% and a decrease in the power consumption of approximately 15 mW. Subtracting the power consumption that remains after the pressure is applied yields the curve of calculated "blood flow" index, which is of identical shape to uncorrected values (Levin and Wagner, unpublished data).

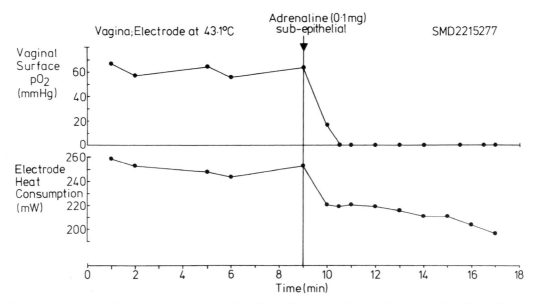

Figure 10.4.4. Vaginal surface pO_2 and electrode heat power consumption (in milliwatts) before and after subepithelial injection of adrenaline under the electrode. Note that the surface pO_2 falls within 1 min to zero, but that the power consumption initially falls in 1 min by approximately 30 mW and then slowly decreases to a 50-mW fall (Levin and Wagner, unpublished data).

selected steady-state temperature (usually 37–45°C). The heat was then switched off, and the temperature, T, was recorded every 10 s until a stable baseline temperature, T_b, similar to that obtained before the heating, was obtained. On the forearm, this took 5–10 min, but on the pulp of the thumb (with a much higher blood flow), this could take as little as 1.5–3 min. When plotted semilogarithmically against time in seconds, the differential rate of cooling of the electrode ($T = T - T_b$), after the first few curvilinear readings presumably caused by heat equilibration between probe and tissue, yields a straight line, indicating an exponential heat washout. The blood flow (in ml/100 g tissue per min) was calculated by Kety's[11] formula, in which λ, the tissue-to-blood partition coefficient for heat, was assumed, for simplification, to be 1 ml/g (its actual value is 0.954 ml/g) (Perl and Cucinell[15]), and the slope of the straight line graph k equal to $\log_e 2$ divided by the half-time of the change in T.

Levin and Wagner[16] adapted the technique to measure human vaginal blood flow. The Radiometer heated oxygen

electrode was held against the vaginal surface by the same suction holder as that previously employed for oxygen measurements. The unheated, steady-state temperature of the vaginal surface was recorded. The electrode was usually heated to 41–43°C and then switched off. The cooling curve of the electrode's temperature was followed every 5–10 s until the temperature reached the previously recorded unheated state. This usually took 2–3 min. The initial basal temperature was subtracted from each of the cooling temperatures and plotted semilogarithmically to obtain the slope of the linear portion of the cooling curve. An example of the results obtained is shown in Fig. 10.4.5, where the subject had her basal vaginal blood flow recorded initially, and then the flow was measured when she actively sexually fantasized. The much steeper slope of the latter graph shows the greater heat clearance induced by the mental sexual arousal. A feature of the technique that at first seems remarkable is that whatever temperature the electrode is initially set at (within the limits of 37–43°C) to obtain the

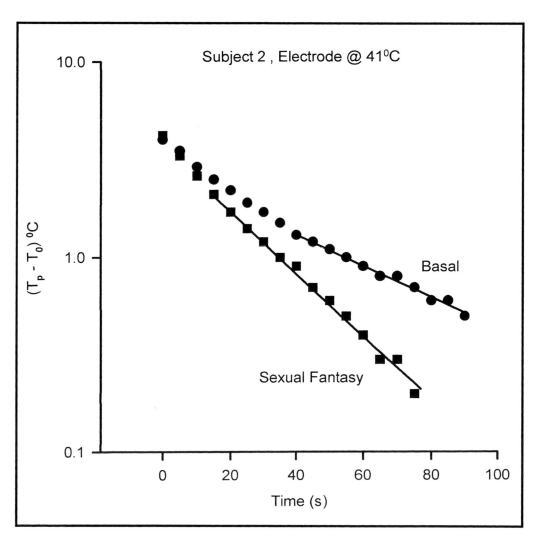

Figure 10.4.5. Heat washout responses of the heated oxygen electrode mounted on the vaginal wall of a subject in a basal, nonstimulated condition and when sexually aroused by fantasy. In the basal condition, her vaginal flow was 44 ml/100 g tissue per min, which increased to 173 ml/100 g per min by sexual fantasy (reproduced with permission from Levin and Wagner[16]).

blood flow by heat clearance, the same calculated flow is obtained.[14] In one subject, for example, with the electrode set at 39°C, 41°C, and 43°C, the calculated vaginal blood flows in three separate serial measurements were approximately 80, 70, and 70 ml/100 g per min, respectively.

One weakness of the method using the unmodified Radiometer electrode is the significant heat loss from the electrode that is not related to blood flow but is due to heat losses, especially to the surrounding environment from the back of the electrode. In order to reduce these losses as much as possible, a simplified Sheffield heat electrode was designed, developed, and manufactured at the Department of Biomedical Science, University of Sheffield, UK, by Tony Carter, one of the department's electronic technicians, and myself (Fig. 10.4.6).

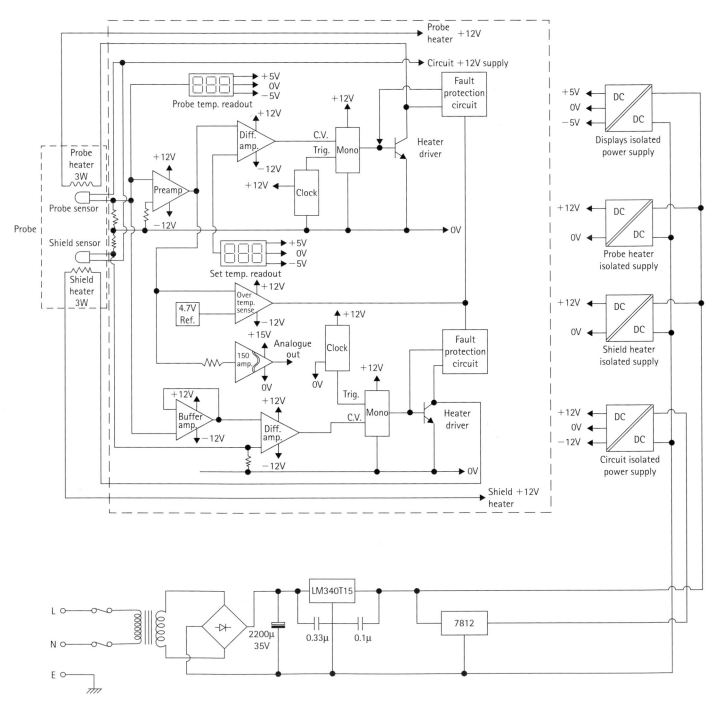

Figure 10.4.6. A diagrammatic representation of the electrical circuitry used in the Sheffield heat electrode (probe). See text for details (copyright RJ Levin & T Carter).

The simplified Sheffield heat electrode used for heat "washout"

The Sheffield heat electrode dispensed with the oxygen-measuring device and was simply a gold disk (diameter approximately 18 mm) heated electrically by a surface-mounted, 47 Ω, 3-W ceramic resistor from a 12-V, subject-isolated power supply with an analog output circuit to record its temperature. The disk, heater, and temperature sensor were housed in a ceramic (Makor) holder (diameter 25 mm, height 14 mm) that also had a second "shield" heater circuit behind the disk that was driven to the same temperature as that of the disk. This reduced heat losses from the back of the housing to the environment. The electrode could be used with the shield heater circuit switched on or off. The disk was held in contact against the vaginal wall by suction through a 1–2-mm-wide and -deep groove cut around the periphery of the front face of the holder connected to a portable clinical vacuum pump (Fig. 10.4.7).

The whole unit needed to be sealed very carefully to make it waterproof so that it could be routinely chemically sterilized. Good sealing is essential because the fluids used for sterilizing the electrode between subjects have searching qualities and can find the smallest of entry points into the electrode's inner compartment and destroy the electrical circuits. A number of early prototype models were damaged beyond repair because of this problem. All electrodes were calibrated against an accurate glass thermometer and could read temperatures to 0.1°C.

The control unit consists of a heater digital display so that the temperature that the heating current creates in the disk can be set while a second digital display gives the actual temperature of the disk when the heater is switched off. Other switches control the shield heater, and one turns the whole unit off. A fail-safe circuit was built in so that the temperature of the gold disk can never rise beyond 47°C. Three electrodes were constructed and calibrated; each one loses a different amount of heat to the environment, so that when corrections are made for this heat loss, the actual electrode used must be known. The corrections for each electrode's heat loss were obtained by applying the electrode to the volar surface of the subject's arm and measuring the cooling of the electrode (initially run at the temperature used in the vagina) on the arm with an arterial cuff at 200 mmHg. The calculated "blood flow" from this cooling curve can then be subtracted from that obtained in the vagina, yielding a lower corrected vaginal blood flow.

Repeated measures of vaginal blood flow in the same subject can be obtained simply by allowing the electrode to cool down to the original vaginal temperature and then heating it again, switching it off, and repeating the cooling process. It is thus possible to measure vaginal blood flow many times in an hour in the same organ, a highly desirable feature if one wants to follow the action of a drug, hormone, or specific condition.

Final words

The control unit and the Sheffield electrodes have now been in service for approximately 6 years, and many measurements have been made in both the basal and sexually aroused conditions. We have recently finished a study, undertaken at the Sexual Physiology Laboratory at the Porterbrook Clinic, Sheffield, to compare, in a number of subjects, the vaginal flow measured by the Sheffield heat electrode in both basal and sexually aroused states simultaneously with photoplethysmographic recording of vaginal pulse amplitude. On the basis of this study, a large drug firm is manufacturing a number of the Sheffield electrodes for research.

The simultaneous technique (heat and vaginal pulse amplitude recording) allows one to calibrate the nontransportable vaginal pulse amplitude data (normally measured in arbitrary units) for each subject, and convert the beat-by-beat vaginal pulse amplitude signal into quantitative, transportable beat-by-beat data as ml/100 g tissue per min flow.

Because it needs some 3–5 min of temperature cooling recorded data, it is obvious that the heat electrode technique cannot follow rapid changes in vaginal blood flow, so it should not be used during an orgasm. However, if the double recording method as explained previously is used, it may be possible to use the vaginal pulse amplitude record obtained during orgasm to monitor the flow quantitatively. The great advantage of the electrode, however, is that it generates a quantitative measure of vaginal blood flow that is in ml/100 g tissue per min, and these data are completely transferable, unlike the vaginal pulse amplitude from the photoplethysmograph. The vaginal blood flows of different women, at different times of the month (menstrual cycle) or year, with different drugs and doses, can all be directly and quantitatively compared with one another. This method has yet to invade the clinical arena, but this is mainly because

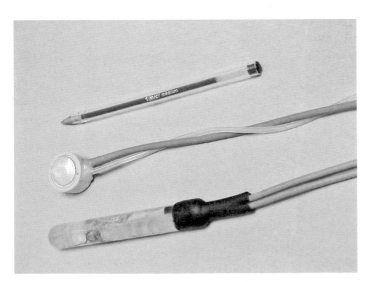

Figure 10.4.7. The Sheffield heat electrode and the photoplethysmograph used in the study combining simultaneous photoplethysmography and heat electrode recordings. The two attachments to the heated electrode are the translucent suction tubing and the cabling for the electronics. The ballpoint pen is 140 mm long and 7 mm wide. See text for details.

hardly any measurements of blood flow are undertaken by any method on women (or for that matter any other genital function) to characterize female sexual dysfunction, as opposed to the many that are in use for male genital dysfunction.[17]

Acknowledgments

Grateful acknowledgment is made to Tony Carter, who converted my simple thoughts and sketches by his expertise and skill into the working reality of the Sheffield heat electrode, and to Gorm Wagner and his Sexual Physiology Laboratory at Copenhagen, where the Sheffield electrode first came into contact with a human vagina.

References

1. Jaszczak P, Baumbach P. A combined tc-PO2 and skin blood flow sensor. *Acta Anaesthesiol Scand* 1985; 29: 623–8.

2. Wagner G, Levin RJ. Oxygen tension of the vaginal surface during sexual stimulation in the human. *Fertil Steril* 1978; 30: 50–3.

3. Levin RJ, Wagner G. Orgasm in women in the laboratory – quantitative studies on the duration, intensity, latency and vaginal blood flow. *Arch Sex Behav* 1985; 14: 439–49.

3a. Levin RJ, Wagner G. Haemodynamic changes of the human vagina during sexual arousal assessed by a heated oxygen electrode. *J Physiol* 1978; 275: 23P.

4. Levin RJ, Wagner G. Sexual arousal in women – which haemodynamic measure gives the best assessment? *J Physiol* 1980; 392: 22–3P.

5. Wagner G, Levin RJ. Effect of atropine and methyl atropine on human vaginal blood flow, sexual arousal and climax. *Acta Pharmacol Toxicol* 1980; 46: 321–5.

6. Levin RJ, Wagner G, Ottesen B. Simultaneous monitoring of human vaginal haemodynamics by three independent methods during sexual arousal. *Sexology* 1981; 114–20.

7. Levin RJ, Wagner G. TRH and vaginal blood flow – effects in conscious women and anaesthetized sheep. *J Physiol* 1986; 378: 83P.

8. Levin RJ, Wagner G. Self-reported central sexual arousal without vaginal arousal- duplicity or veracity revealed by objective measurement. *J Sex Res* 1987; 23: 540–4.

9. Levin RJ. The mechanisms of human sexual arousal. *Annu Rev Sex Res* 1992; 3: 1–48.

10. Levin RJ, Wagner G. Re-measurement of vaginal and minor labial oxygen tension for the evaluation of female sexual function. *J Urol* 2001; 166: 2324–5.

11. Kety SS. Measurement of regional circulation by the local clearance of radioactive sodium. *Am Heart J* 1949; 38: 321–8.

12. Lassen NA, Lindbjerg IF, Munck O. Measurement of blood flow through skeletal muscle by intra-muscular injection of xenon-133. *Lancet* 1964; ii: 686.

13. Wagner G, Ottesen B. Vaginal blood flow during sexual stimulation. *Obstet Gynaecol* 1980; 56: 621–3.

14. Midttun M, Sejrsen P, Colding-Jørgensen M. Heat-washout: a new method for measuring cutaneous blood flow rate in areas with and without arteriovenous anastomoses. *Clin Physiol* 1996; 16: 259–74.

15. Perl W, Cucinell SA. Local blood flow in human leg muscle measured by a transient response thermoelectric method. *Biophys J* 1965; 5: 211–30.

16. Levin RJ, Wagner G. Human vaginal blood flow – absolute assessment by a new, quantitative heat wash-out method. *J Physiol* 1997; 504P: 88P–9P.

17. Levin RJ. Measuring female genital functions – a research essential but still a clinical luxury? *Sex Relatsh Ther* 2004; 19: 191–200.

10.5 Neurologic testing: quantified sensory testing

Yoram Vardi, Uri Gedalia, Ilan Gruenwald

Introduction

Neurologic disorders, such as multiple sclerosis, peripheral neuropathy, and lumbar radiculopathy, are major and frequent potential etiologies of female sexual dysfunction (see Chapters 16.5 and 16.6 of this book). Nevertheless, female sexual dysfunction due to neurologic causes has been poorly explored. Clearly, the integrity of the genital innervations plays a significant role in the sexual cycle, and any damage to the somatic or autonomic neural system may affect the normal sexual response (see Chapters 4.1–4.4 and 5.3). In the female, even more than the male counterpart, intact genital sensation is a major component in this process.

Therefore, the need for quantitative measurement of the neural function of the female genitalia, specifically sensory function, has become obvious (see Chapter 10.6). In suspected neurologic disorders, vibratory, thermal, or painful stimuli are often used for quantification of sensation because they provide information on the neuroanatomic pathways with their discrete fiber types.[1] We have implemented this neurophysiologic technique, using quantitative sensory testing (QST) to study sensation in the female genital organs, and have established a set of age-corrected normal threshold values of vibratory and thermal sensations. Moreover, we were able to show that in neuropathic female patients, quantitative sensory testing could identify abnormal sensory states with high specificity, and could aid in diagnosis of neurogenic female sexual dysfunction.[2]

In this chapter, we will describe this diagnostic test and its role in the evaluation armamentarium for women's sexual disorders.

Fibers innervating the genitalia

It is assumed that any neural lesion, central or peripheral, that causes female sexual dysfunction should have sensory deficit as its mainstay. The important role of the sensory neural pathways is anatomically expressed by the rich innervation of the external genitalia, mainly at the clitoral level.

These afferents include three principal fiber subtypes, the first of which is *the large* (and fastest conducting), peripheral A-*beta myelinated fibers*, responsible for conveying sensations of touch, mild pressure, and vibration. These fibers most probably have a major role in normal sexual function, since vibratory stimuli are known to evoke an intense sexual excitatory response. Their dysfunction could potentially affect some of the sensory input, and could hinder the natural progression of the sexual cycle. On the other hand, *the small-fiber system* mediates modalities of temperature and pain. This fiber system is composed of *small, A-delta myelinated* fibers that mediate cold sensation and initial pain, and of *smaller, C-unmyelinated* fibers (slowest) that mediate warm and major pain sensation. In sexual dysfunction, these sensations probably are of secondary importance. However, the true value of performing a test to evaluate these small fibers in the female genitalia lies in their structural and functional similarity to the autonomic nerve fibers (which are also small C-nerve fibers). Therefore, pathologic results in thermal testing may indirectly suggest dysfunction of the autonomic fibers. As a result, quantitative sensory testing may help to detect autonomic nerve fiber damage in neurologic disorders such as diabetic neuropathy[3] or multiple sclerosis.[4,5] These data are crucial, as, until now, there was no direct test that could provide such quantitative information on autonomic nerve function, rendering this test the closest one available to autonomic evaluation.

Quantitative sensory testing

Quantitative sensory testing is a common test used in neurophysiologic laboratories to assess sensory function in neurologic disorders (as in pain disorders, peripheral neuropathies, toxic neuropathies, uremic neuropathy, and legal proceedings).[1] Only during the last few years was it adapted and applied to the evaluation of sensory function in the female genitalia. This test, in essence, is based on the administration of quantified stimuli (such as temperature or vibration) in a controlled manner. The subject determines the sensation threshold either verbally or by electronic means (i.e., pressing a button). The collected data are compared with a normal set of threshold values to determine whether sensory hyper- or hypo-sensitivity is present.

Methodology

Apparatus

The only apparatus available today that has specially designed probes for the quantitative measurement of sensation of the female genitalia is the Thermal/Vibratory Sensory Analyzer system (TSA-3000 and VSA-3000; Medoc, Israel) for the vaginal and clitoral region. The apparatus includes an adjustable arm with appropriate probe holders, in order to ensure steady and constant contact with the stimulated region. The adjustable probe-holder provides user-defined control of the pressure applied (Fig. 10.5.1). There are two special probes; each is anatomically designed for use at the vagina and clitoris, one for vibratory and the other for thermal stimulation. Both share the same basic cylindric design; the large part of the probe is for the vaginal region, whereas the distal end is used for the clitoris and is shaped like a thick button. This design reduces the need for multiple repositioning of the probes and is thus beneficial for the patient, avoiding unnecessary discomfort.

The thermal probe (Fig. 10.5.2)

The vaginal part of the probe has its metal contact element on the outside, cylindric surface, and is 28 mm in diameter and 125 mm in length. The thermal element has an active cooling/heating area of 16×32 mm. The distal clitoral part ("button") is smaller, measuring 25-mm diameter with a thermal contact element on the outer end.

This probe has a working temperature range of 0–50°C at both thermal surfaces.

The vibration probe (Fig. 10.5.3)

The vaginal part of the probe is 24 mm in diameter and 100 mm in length. The distal clitoral part is 10 mm in diameter and 5 mm in length. The vibratory probe is smaller in order to compensate for the vibration amplitude. Both parts vibrate throughout and do not have a particular point for surface contact. For both vaginal and clitoral components, the vibration frequency is fixed at 100 Hz, with an amplitude range of 0–130 μm.

Technique

Because this test is of subjective nature, the patient needs to be acquainted with the procedure. For this purpose, it is important to instruct the patient properly, and to familiarize her with the

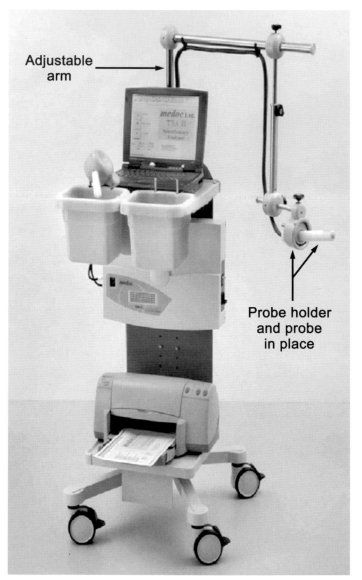

Adjustable arm

Probe holder and probe in place

Figure 10.5.1. Thermal/Vibratory Sensory Analyzer system (courtesy of Medoc Ltd, Israel).

type of stimuli administered. This is achieved by first applying the stimuli to the patient's hand.

The test starts with the subject lying down comfortably in the supine position. Either thermal or vibratory stimuli may be administered first; the order is of no particular importance. The thermal probe is inserted to the point where the thermode makes contact with one of the distal vaginal walls. The test can be performed on either anterior or posterior, or both vaginal walls.[6] Thermal stimulus is increased/decreased gradually (for warm and cold, respectively). This is repeated four times; each time the subject indicates the onset of the perceived sensation by pressing a button. By doing so, the individual's threshold limit to the specific sensory stimulus is defined and automatically recorded (method of limits). An average of the four recorded measurements is calculated in order to establish the mean threshold.

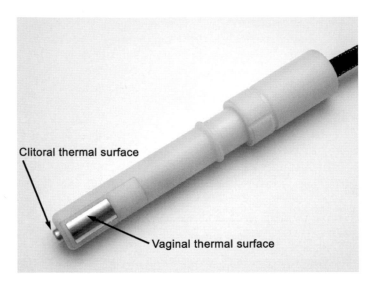

Clitoral thermal surface

Vaginal thermal surface

Figure 10.5.2. The thermal probe.

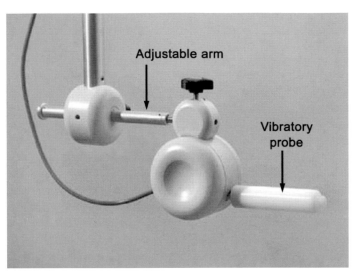

Adjustable arm

Vibratory probe

Figure 10.5.3. The vibration probe.

When the vaginal vibration probe is used, it is inserted to its full length into the vagina, without pressure on the vaginal walls. The patient is requested to report when she is comfortable with the probe in place. The adjustable holder is then locked and the probe remains set in place. Stimulation and measurements take place at this stage. The same stimuli are then given to the clitoral region by the designed probes. In general, positioning of the clitoral probe is trickier and requires a certain amount of experience.

Like any other sensory measuring test, the quantitative sensory testing is not fully objective, as it is dependent on the patients' subjective feeling and individual reaction time until pressing the button.[6-8] Although this method is often criticized, results are consistently repeatable and therefore can be used as a valid tool to evaluate the sensory state of the genital area in the female.[9,10]

Interpreting the test results

After the average threshold of each stimulus is obtained, it is plotted on the available normogram. Figure 10.5.4 depicts the age-corrected normograms for vibratory and thermal sensory thresholds at the clitoral and vaginal levels, for the upper, lower, and normal thresholds.[6] As evident in this figure, the validity of the quantitative sensory testing is further strengthened by the fact that the age dependency of the genital vibratory threshold is very similar to its age dependency for the skin in the limbs.[7] The smaller age effect found in the clitoris may be due to the relatively rich innervation of this organ. The normograms were constructed taking into account (log) coefficients of repeatability (r) as part of the analysis in order to minimize the unavoidable inaccuracies.

Vibration thresholds detected with quantitative sensory

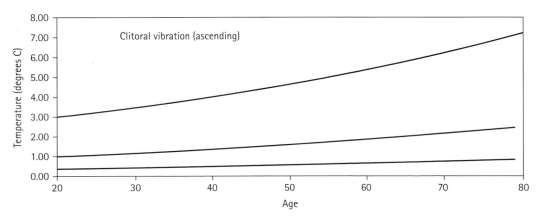

Figure 10.5.4. Age-corrected nomograms for vibratory and thermal sensory thresholds at the clitoral and vaginal levels, showing upper, lower and normal thresholds.

testing represent the function of the large, myelinated A-beta sensory fibers and their central connections. These thresholds have a better repeatability profile than the other modalities, indicating higher sensitivity and specificity in diagnosing dysfunction. In fact, preliminary data showed that vibratory threshold is the most sensitive parameter in identifying neurologic deficit in patients with female sexual dysfunction caused by peripheral neuropathies or radiculopathies.[6]

The role of sensory testing in the evaluation of a suspected neurologic etiology in women with sexual dysfunction

We suggest that genital sensory testing should be included in the evaluation of the female patient whenever a neurologic etiology is suspected (see diagnostic algorithm in Fig. 10.5.5). This should be based mainly on the patient's history and physical examination. Quantitative sensory testing may also be of value in cases where the basic neurologic assessment is inconclusive, insufficient, or contradictory; whenever vascular or endocrine evaluations are unconvincing, there is need for more objective, quantitative data on the sensory status of the external genital region. The neurogenic origin should always be sought, as it may point to disorders that could be treated and cured (surgery for lumbosacral disk herniation, surgical release of pudendal nerve entrapment, etc.) (see Chapters 10.6, 16.5, and 16.6).

Apart from its use in the etiologic evaluation, quantitative sensory testing may have other applications for female sexual disorder. In medicolegal cases, this method can be used as part of the total assessment of patients suffering from sexual dysfunction after an accident/trauma, or from iatrogenic causes. This tool can be used to assess the initial damage caused, and can also be used to monitor recovery or deterioration. Munarriz et al. published a study on 13 women with a history of blunt perineal trauma and associated sexual dysfunction (mainly orgasmic disorders and clitoral pain). This study had also shown abnormal genital sensory testing in all subjects,[11] suggesting a neurogenic etiology of sexual dysfunction.

Another potential and important clinical role for quantitative sensory testing is objective patient follow-up. Specifically, it could be used in the quantitative evaluation of pain in females with vestibulitis. Baseline pain could be quantified and progress of treatment could be monitored.[12]

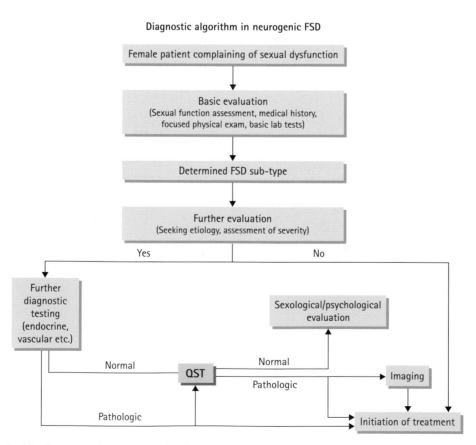

Figure 10.5.5. Diagnostic algorithm for suspected neurologic etiology in women with sexual dysfunction. QST = quantitative sensory testing; FSD = female sexual dysfunction.

In research, quantitative sensory testing can be used to assess pre- and post-surgical genital sensory status in patients undergoing surgery, mainly pelvic procedures (i.e. hysterectomy) and vaginal deliveries. Our group has also found significant abnormal genital quantitative sensory testing findings in 41 females 3 months after undergoing hysterectomy.[13]

We finally have a reliable research tool that can be used to assess possible side effects of new future medications suspected of influencing the sensation of the external genitalia. For pharmaceutics, there is no doubt that this test will be of importance in assessing the efficacy of new drugs and other therapeutic options for female sexual dysfunction as they emerge. The feasibility, efficiency, and cost-effectiveness of the potential applications are yet to be demonstrated, and more studies are needed to provide sufficient data on the maximal role of quantitative sensory testing in the clinical set-up and in research of female sexual dysfunction.

Summary

The plethora of scientific studies and research in the field of female sexual dysfunction in recent years has already provided substantial theoretic and clinical knowledge. Nevertheless, our knowledge remains very limited, as this field is only in its infancy. We have yet to reach the point where the treatment solution for sexual dysfunction in women is as effective as it is for men. To achieve this goal, we need effective, validated diagnostic tools for evaluating female patients, such as quantitative sensory testing. Clinically, genital sensation deficits are probably responsible for a considerable number of the female sexual dysfunction cases. Since female sexual dysfunction with neurogenic etiology is probably more common in women than in men, and probably more significant, quantitative sensory testing can be an effective way of assessing neural deficit and the extent of the disease process. Only in the years to come will we be able to appreciate fully the contribution of this and other solid and reliable diagnostic tools to the scientific advancement of this field.

References

1. Shy ME, Frohman EM, So YT et al. Report of the Therapeutics and Technology Assessment Subcommittee of the American Academy of Neurology. *Neurology* 2003; 60: 898–904.
2. Gruenwald I. Female sexual dysfunction in multiple sclerosis. *Neurology (submitted for publication)*.
3. Berman JR, Berman LA, Lin H et al. Female sexual function: new perspectives on anatomy, physiology, evaluation, and treatment. *AUA Update Series* 2000; 34: 266–76.
4. Zaslansky R, Yarnitsky D. Clinical applications of quantitative sensory testing. *J Neurol Sci* 1998; 153: 215–38.
5. Yang CC, Bowen JR, Kraft GH et al. Cortical evoked potentials of the dorsal nerve of the clitoris and female sexual dysfunction in multiple sclerosis. *J Urol* 2000; 164: 2010–13.
6. Vardi Y, Gruenwald I, Sprecher E et al. Normative values for female genital sensation. *Urology* 2000; 56: 1035–40.
7. Dyck PJ, Karnes J, O'Brien P et al. Detection thresholds of cutaneous sensation in humans. In PJ Dyck, PK Thomas, JW Griffin et al., eds. *Peripheral Neuropathy*. Philadelphia: WB Saunders, 1993: 706–28.
8. Yarnitsky D, Ochoa JL. Studies of heat pain sensation in man: perception thresholds, rate of stimulus rise and reaction time. *Pain* 1990; 40: 85–91.
9. Yarnitsky D, Ochoa JL. Warm and cold specific somato-sensory systems. Psychophysical thresholds, reaction times and peripheral conduction velocities. *Brain* 1991; 114: 1819–26.
10. Yarnitsky D, Sprecher E. Thermal testing: normative data and repeatability for various test algorithms. *J Neurol Sci* 1995; 125: 39–45.
11. Munarriz R, Talakoub L, Somekh N et al. Characteristics of female patients with sexual dysfunction who also had a history of blunt perineal trauma. *Sex Marital Ther* 2002; 28(Suppl 1): 175–9.
12. Lowenstein L, Vardi Y, Deutsch M et al. Vulvar vestibulitis severity-assessment by sensory and pain testing modalities. *Pain* 2004; 107: 47–53.
13. Gruenwald I, Deutsch M, Gertman I et al. Does hysterectomy affect genital sensation? *Int J Impot Res* 2003; 15(Suppl 6): S40.

10.6 Neurophysiologic evaluation of female genital innervation

Ugur Yilmaz, Claire C Yang

Introduction

Neurophysiologic testing of female genital innervation is an extension of the genital physical examination, and is used to search for evidence of motor and sensory nerve disruption. The nervous system is intricately involved with female sexual function, but how the central nervous system and peripheral nerves mediate the sexual response is still largely unknown (see Chapters 4.1–4.4, 5.3, 10.5, 16.5, and 16.6 of this book). Existing electrodiagnostic methods for evaluating the integrity of the components of the nervous system, such as nerve conduction studies, somatosensory evoked potentials, and electromyography, can be used in clinical and research settings not only to define genital neuropathology, but also to clarify the physiology of the sexual response.

In this chapter, we describe (a) basic principles used in electrodiagnostic tests, (b) anatomic correlates of the procedures, (c) extant genital neurophysiologic tests, and (d) future applications in clinical female sexual function research.

Basic technical principles in clinical neurophysiology

Equipment

Most clinical neurophysiology tests require sophisticated electronic instruments that include computer-based software programs. A standard electromyography/evoked potential unit comprises amplifiers, display, loudspeaker, and data storage device, and can deliver stimuli and record specific signals through electrodes. The electrodes, surface/cutaneous, needle, or affixed to probes, can be used for both neural stimulation and recording of bioelectric signals in accordance with the specific testing procedure. Surface electrodes are usually square or round metal plates made of platinum or silver, applied to the skin with adhesive plates or fixed with tape and conducting jelly. A surface electrode records signals from a wider region (recording radius of 20 mm), whereas a needle electrode is useful to select signals from a smaller area (recording radius of 0.5 mm).[1] Needle electrodes, such as concentric (coaxial), monopolar, bipolar, or single-fiber needles, vary according to procedure.

Recording procedures

Electrical activity is recorded through electrodes, and the bioelectrical potentials are amplified and displayed for visual analysis. Bioelectrical potentials can be "evoked", or generated in response to a stimulus (e.g., nerve conduction studies or somatosensory evoked potential tests). Potentials can also be measured in muscle during rest or during contraction, as in electromyography.

The recording settings of the instrument vary with the parameters of the bioelectrical signal, and they should have appropriate gain, sweep (time-base), and frequency filters. For instance, a slow-frequency signal, such as a sympathetic skin response, can be recorded with a longer duration of sweep (1 s/div) and a narrower frequency window (0.1–100 Hz) than a somatosensory evoked potential test, which involves a shorter sweep (100 ms/div) and wider frequency limits (10–3000 Hz). For responses with small amplitudes (e.g., somatosensory evoked potential recordings), the evoked potentials must be averaged to obtain a better signal-to-noise ratio. Typically, at least 200 stimuli are delivered and the corresponding époques are averaged. In tests of sympathetic activation, the response amplitudes are usually large and subject to habituation (fading); therefore, averaging is not employed. In most situations, tests should be repeated at least twice to demonstrate the reproducibility of the response.

Responses are characterized by the shape of waveforms, latency, and amplitude measurements. Response latencies are measured either from the onset of response (e.g., sacral reflex tests) or from the individual peaks of the potentials (e.g., somatosensory evoked potentials). Amplitudes are measured relative to the baseline or "peak to peak" (Fig. 10.6.1).

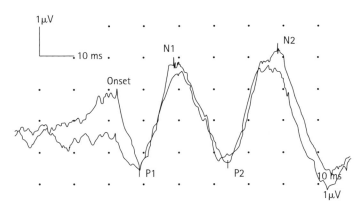

Figure 10.6.1. The waveform of a pudendal somatosensory evoked potential (SEP) test. After the onset, the response follows a downward deflection (P1: first positive peak) and an upward deflection (N1: first negative peak). The second positive (P2) and negative (N2) peaks follow. The latency of the responses is usually measured at P1 response. The amplitude of the response is measured between the first peak-to-peak distance (P1–N1).

Stimulus delivery

Stimulation of a nerve should evoke a recordable, reproducible, and defined response. Several different types of stimuli, such as electrical, mechanical, or magnetic, can be delivered to depolarize a nerve. In clinical neurophysiology applications, electrical stimulus is the most commonly applied stimulus type, and it is defined by several parameters characterizing its duration, intensity, and pattern of delivery. In somatosensory evoked potential tests, an electrical stimulus with a rectangular pulse, 0.1-ms duration, two to three times of sensory threshold intensity, and recurrent pattern is typically employed. An example of stimulus parameters for the sympathetic skin response is a rectangular pulse of 0.2-ms duration, 10–15-mA intensity, and nonrecurrent pattern.[2]

Female genital neuroanatomic correlates of neurophysiologic tests

The female genitalia are innervated by both somatic and autonomic nerve fibers (Fig. 10.6.2). Somatic nerves are myelinated, and thus of large diameter, and conduct neural impulses

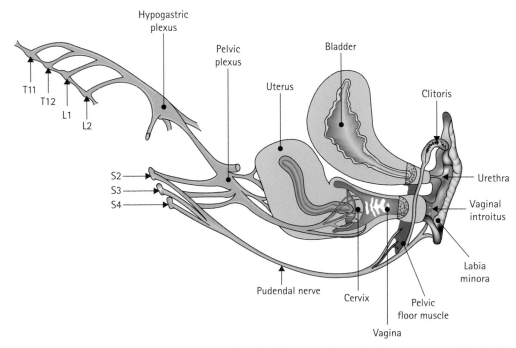

Figure 10.6.2. Innervation of female genitalia. Thoracolumbar sympathetic fibers (T_{11}–L_2), coursing through the hypogastric nerve, join with the sacral parasympathetic fibers (S_2–S_4) to form the pelvic plexus on either side of the bladder. The pelvic plexus supplies the autonomic innervation of genital organs, including the uterus, cervix, proximal vagina, clitoris, bulbs, and bladder. Somatic sensory branches innervating the distal vagina, clitoris, and perineum join to form the pudendal nerve (S_2–S_4), the motor branches of which innervate the pelvic floor and perineal muscles.

relatively rapidly. Somatic motor fibers mediate impulses to skeletal muscles (under *voluntary* control), and somatic sensory fibers mediate information from the skin, skeletal muscles, and joints. Autonomic fibers are of small diameter, and poorly myelinated or nonmyelinated, and conduct neural impulses relatively slowly. Their motor impulses mediate *involuntary* responses such as sweat gland release, blood flow, and gut peristalsis. Autonomic sensory fibers are known as visceral afferents, and conduct sensory information from the viscera and blood vessels (see Chapter 4.2).

Somatic innervation

The somatic sensory and motor innervation of female genitalia is carried via branches of the pudendal nerve. The pudendal nerve arises from sacral spinal segments 2–4 (S_2–S_4). The nerve enters the perineum after traveling through Alcock's canal.[3] There are three branches of the pudendal nerve (dorsal clitoral, perineal, and inferior rectal), each carrying sensory input to the S_2–S_4 spinal levels from the genital structures, which is relayed through the central nervous system via ascending spinal tracts.[4,5] The skeletal pelvic floor muscles receive somatic innervation mainly from the motor branches of the pudendal nerve (perineal nerve, inferior rectal nerve).[6,7]

The exact pathways of the genital autonomic fibers within the human have not been documented, but they generally follow the major arteries of the abdomen and pelvis. The pelvic plexus is the main crossroad for autonomic nerves, consisting of parasympathetic fibers from the sacral nerve roots (S_2–S_4) and sympathetic nerve fibers from the thoracolumbar sympathetic nerve roots (T_{11}–L_2). The plexus lies on either side of the bladder and rectum, and supplies all the pelvic viscera, including the bladder and urethral sphincter, the uterus and upper vagina, and the female genital tissue.[8] These autonomic fibers are especially important since they regulate the blood flow to the vagina, clitoris, and bulbs.[9–11]

Neural testing of somatic nerves

This section will briefly review the neurophysiologic testing applicable to the somatic innervation of the female genitalia. Neurophysiologic testing involves the assessment of both the afferent (sensory) and efferent (motor) nerves. Sensory innervation is usually tested by stimulating the sensory branch and recording either from the somatosensory cortex (e.g., somatosensory evoked potentials) or from the distal end of the sensory nerve, as in nerve conduction studies. The motor component is evaluated with electrodes from the innervated muscle or muscle groups, with or without nerve stimulation.

Somatic sensory tests

Somatosensory tests are evaluations of nerve conduction, which primarily evaluate large myelinated nerve fibers, without regard to the smaller fibers. The genital somatosensory pathway can be

evaluated along the whole neuraxis with pudendal somatosensory evoked potentials and, in theory, on certain segments of the nerve pathway with lumbar evoked potentials to localize a neural lesion.

Somatic sensory nerve pathways can also be assessed by quantitative sensory tests, which are based on subjective reports of sensory experience (see Chapter 10.5). Although it is possible to evaluate small-diameter, unmyelinated nerve fibers by quantitative sensory testing, this method depends on the psychophysical/cognitive factors of the subject tested and therefore lacks the objectivity of nerve conduction studies. Quantitative sensory testing measures the integrity of the entire sensory pathway without the capacity to localize abnormal findings.[12]

Pudendal somatosensory evoked potentials

The technique of pudendal somatosensory evoked potentials involves stimulation of a pudendal nerve branch, such as the dorsal clitoral nerve or perineal nerve, with recurrent electrical square wave stimuli, and recording multiple responses with averaging techniques in order to increase the signal-to-noise ratio. The recording is done with scalp electrodes placed over the somatosensory cortex where genital sensation is mapped. At this point, the highest amplitude response can be obtained (Cz –2 cm: Fz of the International 10–20 electroencephalogram System).[4]

The primary method to perform pudendal somatosensory evoked potential testing is to depolarize the dorsal clitoral nerve. It can be stimulated with self-adhesive surface electrodes placed bilaterally on each side of the clitoral body, allowing assessment of each clitoral nerve branch separately.[13] The stimulus intensity is usually two to four times the sensory threshold. A vaginal probe mounted with electrodes can depolarize the perineal nerve in the distal vagina and labia minora to elicit somatosensory evoked potentials similar to those obtained with depolarization of the dorsal clitoral nerve (Fig. 10.6.3).[14]

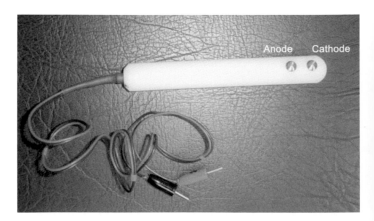

Figure 10.6.3. Vaginal probe used to depolarize the perineal nerve in female subjects. The cathode electrode (distal) is positioned to the introitus, and the anode (1 cm proximal) is in contact with the labia minora.

The response in healthy women is a W-shaped potential, and the latency is measured at the first positive (downward) peak, called P1. The P1 response occurs at approximately 40 ms. This first response is followed by an upward deflection of the waveform, defined as the first negative peak at about 55 ms (N1 response). The amplitude of the response is measured between the onset and first positive peak or between the first positive and negative peaks[4,15,16] (Figs 10.6.1 and 10.6.4).

The amplitude of an evoked potential is a reflection of the axon density of the nerve population, while the latency is a reflection of the myelin content and number of synapses through the afferent pathway. However, in most neurophysiology laboratories, somatosensory evoked potential latency measurements are regarded as more informative and reliable than the amplitude measurements, which are highly variable and are dependent on the intensity of stimuli delivered.[17]

The clinical utility of the pudendal somatosensory evoked potential test is that it is an assessment of the genital somatic innervation. Genital somatic sensation is crucial to the generation and maintenance of male sexual reflexes,[18,19] and this paradigm, although not yet demonstrated, is also presumed to apply to women. The only study correlating neurophysiologic

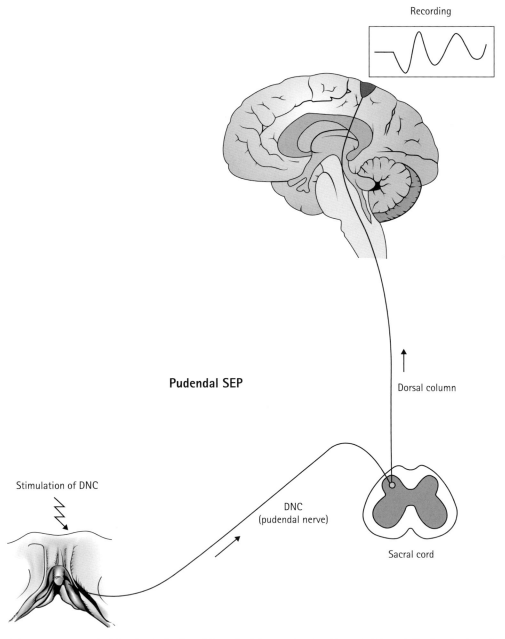

Figure 10.6.4. The pudendal somatosensory axis. After depolarization of the pudendal nerve, the signal is carried through the dorsal column in the spinal cord to the somatosensory cortex. The recording is usually made with surface electrodes placed on the scalp. A normal pudendal somatosensory evoked potential test demonstrates the integrity of the sensory axis from the dorsal clitoral nerve to the sensory cortex (DNC dorsal clitoral nerve; SEP sensory evoked potential).

findings with sexual function in women was by Yang et al., evaluating women with multiple sclerosis.[13] They found that women with abnormal dorsal clitoral nerve somatosensory evoked potentials had a very high incidence of orgasmic dysfunction. These abnormal somatosensory evoked potentials also were associated with subjective loss of genital sensation.

Perineal nerve somatosensory potentials evoked with a vaginal probe were less consistently obtained than the dorsal clitoral nerve somatosensory evoked potentials (69% vs 90%), probably because of a decreased axon density of the perineal nerve at the level of the introitus.[14] Therefore, the presence of a normal perineal somatosensory evoked potential can confirm the integrity of perineal innervation, but an absent response is not necessarily an indication of neuropathology.

Lumbar evoked potentials

Several authors have attempted to record evoked potentials from the spinal level by the stimulation of the dorsal clitoral/penile nerve.[4,20] In theory, knowing the latencies of lumbar evoked potentials and somatosensory evoked potentials can help to identify a neuroanatomic lesion along the sensory neuroaxis (Fig. 10.6.5). However, the amplitudes of the potentials are small with low signal-to-noise ratio, and it is difficult to record lumbar evoked potentials in women and in healthy, obese men. Therefore, the technique is not feasible for routine clinical application. A combination of sacral reflex latency measurements (see below) and pudendal somatosensory evoked potentials gives ample information about the integrity of afferent pudendal pathways.

Somatic motor tests

The pelvic floor skeletal muscles are important in the female sexual response. Inability to contract the pelvic muscles during

arousal and orgasm appears to affect a woman's sexual responsivity.[21] Thus, methods to evaluate the nerves to the pelvic muscles and their function may be helpful in the diagnosis of certain sexual dysfunctions.

Genital somatic motor pathways can be tested by (a) sacral reflex measurements, (b) directly stimulating motor nerves (e.g., pudendal terminal motor latency measurement), (c) anterior sacral root stimulation, (d) stimulation of the motor cortex with a transcranial cortical stimulator, or, (e) electromyography.

Sacral reflex measurements

The integrity of the sacral reflex arc is assessed by sacral reflex latency measurement, which typically involves stimulating the sensory branches of the pudendal nerve and recording the reflex response from the bulbocavernosus (*bulbocavernous reflex*) or external anal sphincter muscles (*pudendal-anal reflex*), both of which are innervated by branches of the pudendal nerve[22–24] (Fig. 10.6.6). Motor potentials from the external anal sphincter can be recorded with a concentric needle electrode, anal plug electrode, or surface electrodes on the perineal skin.[17]

There are several different applications of sacral reflexes, and each gives information about the reflex pathway tested. Several types of stimuli such as electrical, mechanical, or magnetic stimulation can be used to elicit sacral reflexes.[25] Electrical stimulation can be applied at the dorsal clitoral nerve,[26] the perineum,[27] and the vesicourethral junction,[28] and to bladder mucosa with a catheter-mounted ring electrode.[29] If the vesicourethral junction or bladder mucosa is stimulated and the reflex is recorded from the bulbocavernosus muscle, the reflex arc involves a *viscerosomatic pathway*, meaning that the afferents are visceral and the efferents are somatic nerve pathways. If the dorsal clitoral nerve is stimulated and the response is recorded from the bulbocavernosus muscle or external anal sphincter – the most commonly applied technique – the reflex arc is a *somatosomatic pathway*.

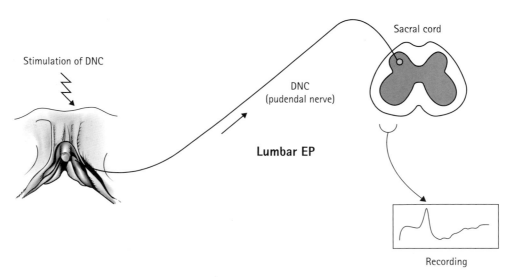

Figure 10.6.5. Pudendal lumbar evoked potentials. Although it is theoretically possible to assess the sensory branches distal to the spinal cord with this technique, the low-amplitude responses in female subjects are difficult to record (DNC dorsal clitoral nerve).

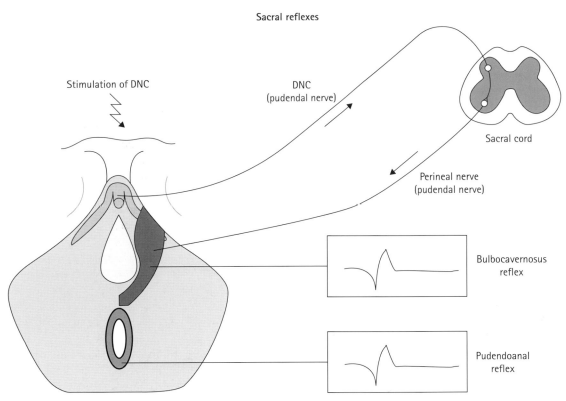

Figure 10.6.6. Sacral reflex arc. After depolarization of the dorsal clitoral nerve (DNC), the sacral reflexes are carried through the perineal branch of the pudendal nerve to the bulbocavernosus and external anal sphincter muscles, where the recording can be made.

The latency of sacral reflexes after stimulation of the dorsal clitoral nerve is consistently obtained at 31–38.5 ms.[17,22,30–33] The latency of the viscerosomatic reflex pathway is longer (50–65 ms) than the somatosomatic reflex pathway, and this is probably due to the differences in myelin content of the afferent branches and the number of spinal synapses involved in the reflex arc.[28,34]

Most studies of electrophysiologic sacral reflex latency measurements in women were in the context of voiding function, not sexual function.[22,35,36] Even though the importance of sacral reflexes is well understood in the evaluation of male sexual dysfunction,[23] there is no neurophysiologic study in women for the evaluation of sacral reflexes in the context of sexual function. One study involving a clinical (physical examination only) assessment of the bulbocavernosus reflex in men and women found deficiency of a clinically obtained bulbocavernosus reflex in a substantial proportion of cases of primary anorgasmia in both sexes.[37] However, no reliable conclusion can be drawn from that study, since electrophysiologic bulbocavernosus reflex testing is more sensitive to the clinically assessed bulbocavernosus reflex response.[38] Sacral reflex latency measurements can potentially be used in the evaluation of deficient orgasmic pelvic contractions.

Sacral reflex measurements, as with other tests of nerve conduction, are not sensitive to partial axonal lesions. In a neurophysiologic evaluation protocol, the combination of sacral reflex latency measurements with pudendal somatosensory evoked potentials gives more reliable information about the somatic innervation of the pelvic floor and external genitalia than either test alone. However, subtle, partial lesions are not always detectable.

Pudendal terminal motor latency

Pudendal nerve terminal motor latency measurement assesses the distal motor branches of the pudendal nerve, similar to the technique routinely used in the evaluation of limb motor nerves: a motor nerve is stimulated proximally, and a compound motor action potential is measured in the appropriate muscle or muscle groups.[39] The technique can be employed by recording with a concentric needle electrode from the bulbocavernosus, the external anal sphincter, or the urethral sphincter muscles in response to bipolar surface stimulation in the perianal/perineal region. It is easier, however, to use a special surface electrode assembly fixed on a gloved index finger, known as the St Mark's electrode, consisting of a bipolar stimulating electrode on the tip of the gloved finger and a recording electrode pair placed 8 cm proximally on the base of the finger.[40] The pudendal nerve can be accessed through the rectum or vagina with the tip of the finger placed close to the ischial spine. With the St Mark's electrode, the distal motor latency for the anal sphincter is approximately 2 ms.[41,42]

Most of the studies involving pudendal nerve terminal motor latency measurements were directed to assess the urinary and fecal continence functions after delivery, but the value of the test in clinical practice is still controversial.[43] There is no study explaining the role of pudendal nerve terminal motor latency in female sexual dysfunction. Theoretically, such a study may provide information on pelvic floor dysfunction and how it relates to the female sexual response.

Other somatic motor nerve tests

Transcutaneous stimulation of the anterior sacral nerve roots can be performed, with responses recorded in the muscles of the pelvic floor.[27] Transcortical stimulation of the motor cortex also results in recordable responses in the pelvic floor muscula-ture.[25,44,45] Both these tests are difficult to perform, and their clin-ical utility in sexual function evaluations has not been determined.

Pelvic floor electromyography

Pelvic floor electromyography can evaluate the integrity of muscle innervation, as well as identify primary muscle patho-logy. The primary means of evaluation is the recording of motor unit potentials through needle electrodes. A motor unit is represented by a single motor neuron and the muscle fibers innervated by its branches.

The motor unit potentials are analyzed for their amplitude and duration (Fig. 10.6.7). The innervation status of a skeletal muscle can be assessed by motor unit potential characteristics. After complete denervation, no motor unit potentials can be recorded for several days. With time, reinnervation occurs, and is reflected as abnormal motor unit potentials. Needle electro-myography has frequently been used to assess peripheral nerve injury, multiple system atrophy, neuropathic conditions involv-ing spinal segments, and cauda equina lesions.[46] Even though pelvic floor electromyography has been classically directed to the assessment of voiding function, it may have value in the evaluation of female sexual disorders involving the pelvic floor. In one study involving women with vaginismus and healthy control subjects, pelvic floor electromyography activity was

increased both at rest and on induction of pelvic floor spasm in women with vaginismus.[47] Hypertonicity of the pelvic floor muscles is one of the recognized pathophysiologic processes in genital pain disorders; therefore, needle electromyography may be a valuable diagnostic tool before the initiation of pelvic floor training programs. Electromyographic monitoring with surface electrodes for biofeedback training could be useful in women with genital pain disorders.[48,49]

Neural testing of autonomic nerves

The autonomic nervous system plays an important role in the female sexual response. Sacral parasympathetic (S_2–S_4) and thoracolumbar sympathetic (T_{11}–L_2) spinal segments represent the autonomic pathways to female genital tissue, as shown in animal studies with retrograde labeling techniques.[50] The similarity of autonomic nervous system responses between males and females has also been demonstrated with animal studies.[10,11,51] Autonomic neuropathy, such as occurs in dia-betes, can result in sexual dysfunction in both genders.[52,53] Therefore, the assessment of afferent and efferent autonomic pathways has critical importance in the evaluation of sexual dysfunction. Autonomic nerve assessments differ in technique from somatic nerve electrodiagnostic tests, although the neurophysiologic principles are essentially the same as for somatic innervation.

Autonomic (visceral) afferent pathway assessment

Since the sensory innervation of the proximal urethra, bladder neck, and bladder wall is mediated by visceral afferent fibers sharing the same derivation as those fibers innervating the genital tissue, cerebral evoked potentials after stimulation of these areas theoretically gives direct information about the vis-ceral afferent pathways to the genitalia[28,54–56] (Fig. 10.6.8). The recording technique is similar to the pudendal somatosensory evoked potentials tests except for the use of a transurethral catheter for stimulation. There has been no study demonstrat-ing the utility of visceral somatosensory evoked potentials in the evaluation of female sexual function.

Autonomic efferent pathway assessment

Female genital tissue receives both parasympathetic and sym-pathetic innervation. This is homologous to the innervation of the male corpus cavernosum and corpus spongiosum by the cavernous nerves,[57] although the patterns of innervation are not well defined in the human female. The sexual arousal response with pelvic organ engorgement is similarly mediated by the autonomic component of the cavernous and pelvic nerves.[9–11] In males, corpus cavernosum electromyography and evoked cavernous activity have been proposed for the assessment of

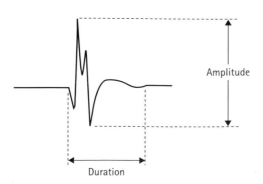

Figure 10.6.7. A normal motor unit potential (MUP). The amplitude of the MUP is measured from peak to peak, and the duration is measured from the first deflection to the return to baseline.

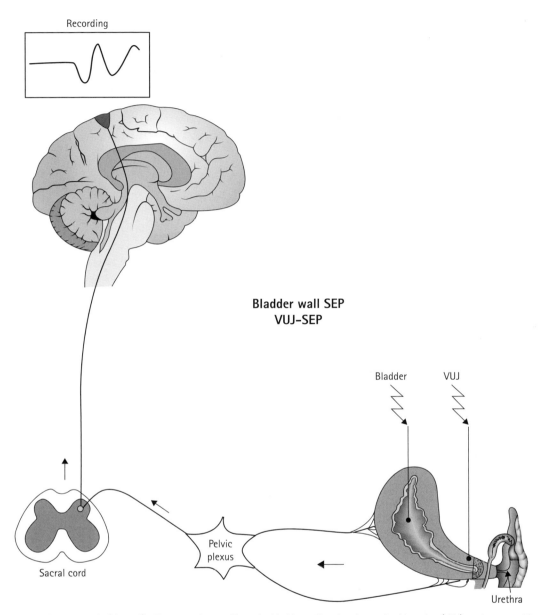

Figure 10.6.8. Evaluation of the autonomic (visceral) afferent pathways. Since the bladder wall and vesicourethral junction (VUJ) are innervated by the autonomic fibers, evoked potentials by the stimulation of these areas can give information about the integrity of pelvic visceral afferent pathways. The depolarization is carried via the pelvic plexus to the sacral spinal cord, and recording can be made from the somatosensory cortex (SEP sensory evoked potential).

genital autonomic innervation.[58,59] These tests presumably assess the sympathetic autonomic pathways to the corpus cavernosum. In men with erectile dysfunction, corpus cavernosum electromyography has been found to have deteriorated.

Currently, information on female autonomic genital innervation can be obtained by *indirect* clinical assessment tools, such as vaginal blood flow or vaginal pulse amplitude measurements, which are end-organ response autonomic impulses.[60–62] However, work is being done with neurophysiologic techniques, such as clitoral electromyography and evoked bulbar/clitoral activity, for *direct* assessment of autonomic innervation. We developed a technique similar to the male autonomic neurophysiologic methods to record both spontaneous and evoked

electrical activity from the clitoris.[63] In a subsequent study, we also showed that electrical activity could be obtained from the bulbs, which are large erectile structures on either side of the urethra.[64] The bulbar evoked activity is more robust and easier to elicit than clitoral evoked activity. Spontaneous electrical activity recordings of both structures are highly variable and subject to artifacts, and thus are not as reliable as evoked recordings (Fig. 10.6.9).

Briefly, the technique involves placement of concentric needle electrodes in the clitoral body and bulb. The median nerve is electrically stimulated to evoke a generalized sympathetic discharge, as in the procedure applied in sympathetic skin response testing. The frequency filters for recording are set

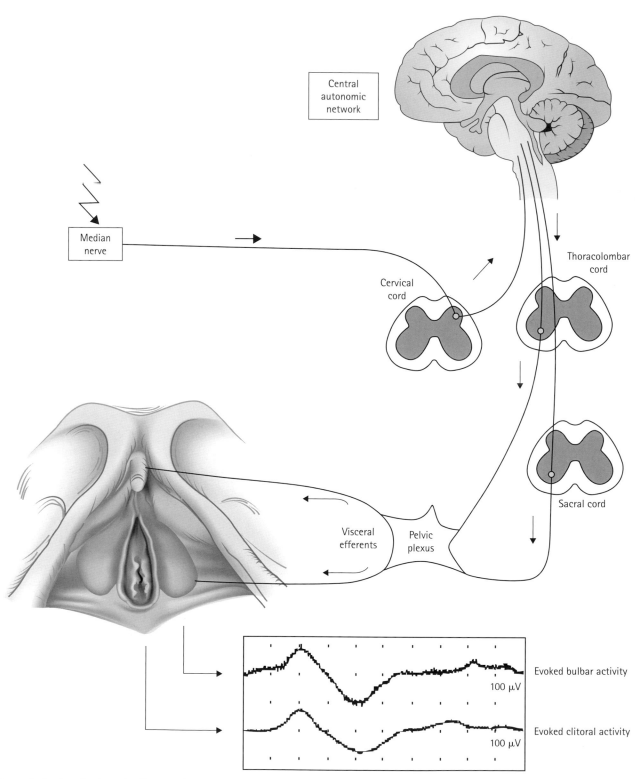

Figure 10.6.9. Evaluation of autonomic efferent pathways. A startling electrical stimulus to the median nerve activates the sympathetic nervous system, resulting in evoked electrical activity in the clitoris and bulbs, similar to sympathetic skin responses. The activities can be recorded with concentric needle electrodes with a sweep of 1 s/div.

within 0.2 and 100 Hz. The recorded responses are much slower than the evoked potential and sacral reflex tests, with an onset latency of 410–3080 ms, requiring a long sweep of 1 s/div. The test appears promising in the assessment of female genital autonomic innervation.

Sympathetic skin response

Sympathetic skin response tests are one of the most commonly employed autonomic neurophysiologic assessments of sweat gland activity, which is mediated by the sympathetic nervous system. Sympathetic skin response tests have been applied to evaluate the autonomic innervation of the genital skin. Changes in sweat gland activity are recordable as spontaneous oscillating waveforms with surface electrodes placed on the palmar, plantar, and dorsal sides of the hands and feet. Noxious stimulation, such as a sudden noise or an electrical impulse, creates a potential shift in the sweat gland activity, and the recorded response is known as the sympathetic skin response of the corresponding area. Sympathetic skin response tests are useful in the assessment of small-fiber neuropathy.[2] The reflex arc involves a myelinated somatosensory nerve, the central autonomic network, and a sympathetic efferent limb with postganglionic, nonmyelinated C fibers.

Sympathetic skin responses are recordable from the perineum and the penis, and abnormal responses are associated with male erectile dysfunction.[65–68] A few studies assessed the value of the test in autonomic neuropathy and voiding dysfunction.[69–71] Shorter latency and higher amplitude measurements of genital sympathetic skin response have been found in women with vaginismus than in healthy individuals. This finding suggests that there is increased sympathetic activity within the pelvis (unpublished data). Further work is needed to substantiate the value of female genital sympathetic skin responses in sexual pain disorders.

General comments and the future

Neural testing in the clinical assessment of female sexual function is still in its infancy. Very few tests are indicated on a routine basis, and those that are, are typically indicated for those with a neurologic disease or injury. Furthermore, the number of persons trained (and willing) to perform such tests is limited. This is not to say that these methods have no place in the study of female sexual function. Neural testing is limited only because of our finite knowledge of the role of the central and peripheral nervous system in female sexual function. The integrity of the nervous system is critical for healthy sexual function, but the details of sexual reflex arcs and central nervous system integration still need to be unraveled. To this end, the role of neural testing as a research entity has much promise: it is one of the means by which these problems can be solved. Neurophysiologic examinations can help to determine which neural pathways are involved with the female sexual response,

and, once this is determined, whether that pathway is intact. As with all human conditions, only a better understanding of the physiology can lead us to better diagnosis and treatment of female sexual dysfunction.

References

1. Barkhaus PE, Nandedkar SD. Recording characteristics of the surface EMG electrodes. *Muscle Nerve* 1994; 17: 1317–23.
2. Shahani BT, Halperin JJ, Boulu P et al. Sympathetic skin response – a method of assessing unmyelinated axon dysfunction in peripheral neuropathies. *J Neurol Neurosurg Psychiatry* 1984; 47: 536–42.
3. Barber MD, Bremer RE, Thor KB et al. Innervation of the female levator ani muscles. *Am J Obstet Gynecol* 2002; 187: 64–71.
4. Haldeman S, Bradley WE, Bhatia NN et al. Pudendal evoked responses. *Arch Neurol* 1982; 39: 280–3.
5. Guerit JM, Opsomer RJ. Bit-mapped imaging of somatosensory evoked potentials after stimulation of the posterior tibial nerves and dorsal nerve of the penis/clitoris. *Electroencephalogr Clin Neurophysiol* 1991; 80: 228–37.
6. Nakanishi T. Studies on the pudendal nerve. I. Macroscopic observation on the pudendal nerve in humans. *Kaibogaku Zasshi* 1967; 42: 223–39.
7. Shafik A, Doss S. Surgical anatomy of the somatic terminal innervation to the anal and urethral sphincters: role in anal and urethral surgery. *J Urol* 1999; 161: 85–9.
8. Butler-Manuel SA, Buttery LD, A'Hern RP et al. Pelvic nerve plexus trauma at radical and simple hysterectomy: a quantitative study of nerve types in the uterine supporting ligaments. *J Soc Gynecol Investig* 2002; 9: 47–56.
9. Giuliano F, Rampin O, Allard J. Neurophysiology and pharmacology of female genital sexual response. *J Sex Marital Ther* 2002; 28(Suppl 1): 101–21.
10. Giuliano F, Allard J, Compagnie S et al. Vaginal physiological changes in a model of sexual arousal in anesthetized rats. *Am J Physiol Regul Integr Comp Physiol* 2001; 281: R140–9.
11. Vachon P, Simmerman N, Zahran AR et al. Increases in clitoral and vaginal blood flow following clitoral and pelvic plexus nerve stimulations in the female rat. *Int J Impot Res* 2000; 12: 53–7.
12. Chong PS, Cros DP. Technology literature review: quantitative sensory testing. *Muscle Nerve* 2004; 29: 734–47.
13. Yang CC, Bowen JR, Kraft GH et al. Cortical evoked potentials of the dorsal nerve of the clitoris and female sexual dysfunction in multiple sclerosis. *J Urol* 2000; 164: 2010–13.
14. Yang CC, Kromm BG. New techniques in female pudendal somatosensory evoked potential testing. *Somatosens Mot Res* 2004; 21: 9–14.
15. Haldeman S, Bradley WE, Bhatia NN et al. Cortical evoked potentials on stimulation of pudendal nerve in women. *Urology* 1983; 21: 590–3.
16. Opsomer RJ, Guerit JM, Wese FX et al. Pudendal cortical somatosensory evoked potentials. *J Urol* 1986; 135: 1216–18.
17. Vodusek DB. Pudendal SEP and bulbocavernosus reflex in women. *Electroencephalogr Clin Neurophysiol* 1990; 77: 134–6.

18. Seftel AD, Resnick MI, Boswell MV. Dorsal nerve block for management of intraoperative penile erection. *J Urol* 1994; 151: 394–5.

19. Dick HC, Bradley WE, Scott FB et al. Pudendal sexual reflexes. Electrophysiologic investigations. *Urology* 1974; 3: 376–9.

20. Opsomer RJ, Caramia MD, Zarola F et al. Neurophysiological evaluation of central-peripheral sensory and motor pudendal fibres. *Electroencephalogr Clin Neurophysiol* 1989; 74: 260–70.

21. Graber B, Kline-Graber G. Female orgasm: role of pubococcygeus muscle. *J Clin Psychiatry* 1979; 40: 348–51.

22. Dilkey WJ, Awad FA, Smith AD. Clinical application of sacral reflex latency. *J Urol* 1983; 129: 1187–9.

23. Krane RJ, Siroky MB. Studies on sacral-evoked potentials. *J Urol* 1980; 124: 872–6.

24. Rodi Z, Vodusek DB. Intraoperative monitoring of the bulbo-cavernosus reflex: the method and its problems. *Clin Neurophysiol* 2001; 112: 879–83.

25. Loening-Baucke V, Read NW, Yamada T et al. Evaluation of the motor and sensory components of the pudendal nerve. *Electroencephalogr Clin Neurophysiol* 1994; 93: 35–41.

26. Opsomer RJ, Guerit JM, Van Cangh PJ et al. Electrophysiological assessment of somatic nerves controlling the genital and urinary functions. *Electroencephalogr Clin Neurophysiol Suppl* 1990; 41: 298–305.

27. Ghezzi A, Callea L, Zaffaroni M et al. Perineal motor potentials to magnetic stimulation, pudendal evoked potentials and perineal reflex in women. *Neurophysiol Clin* 1992; 22: 321–6.

28. Nordling J, Andersen JT, Walter S et al. Evoked response of the bulbocavernosus reflex. *Eur Urol* 1979; 5: 36–8.

29. Badr GG, Fall M, Carlsson CA et al. Cortical evoked potentials obtained after stimulation of the lower urinary tract. *J Urol* 1984; 131: 306–9.

30. Rushworth G. Diagnostic value of the electromyographic study of reflex activity in man. *Electroencephalogr Clin Neurophysiol* 1967; (Suppl 25): 65–73.

31. Vereecken RL, De Meirsman J, Puers B et al. Electrophysiological exploration of the sacral conus. *J Neurol* 1982; 227: 135–44.

32. Varma JS, Smith AN, McInnes A. Electrophysiological observations on the human pudendo-anal reflex. *J Neurol Neurosurg Psychiatry* 1986; 49: 1411–16.

33. Bartolo DC, Jarratt JA, Read NW. The cutaneo-anal reflex: a useful index of neuropathy? *Br J Surg* 1983; 70: 660–3.

34. Sarica Y, Karacan I. Bulbocavernosus reflex to somatic and visceral nerve stimulation in normal subjects and in diabetics with erectile impotence. *J Urol* 1987; 138: 55–8.

35. Blaivas JG, Zayed AA, Labib KB. The bulbocavernosus reflex in urology: a prospective study of 299 patients. *J Urol* 1981; 126: 197–9.

36. Koldewijn EL, Van Kerrebroeck PE, Bemelmans BL et al. Use of sacral reflex latency measurements in the evaluation of neural function of spinal cord injury patients: a comparison of neuro-urophysiological testing and urodynamic investigations. *J Urol* 1994; 152(2 Pt 1): 463–7.

37. Brindley GS, Gillan P. Men and women who do not have orgasms. *Br J Psychiatry* 1982; 140: 351–6.

38. Blaivas JG, Sinha HP, Zayed AA et al. Detrusor-external sphincter dyssynergia. *J Urol* 1981; 125: 542–4.

39. Amarenco G, Kerdraon J. Pudendal nerve terminal sensitive latency: technique and normal values. *J Urol* 1999; 161: 103–6.

40. Kiff ES, Swash M. Slowed conduction in the pudendal nerves in idiopathic (neurogenic) faecal incontinence. *Br J Surg* 1984; 71: 614–16.

41. Rogers J, Laurberg S, Misiewicz JJ et al. Anorectal physiology validated: a repeatability study of the motor and sensory tests of anorectal function. *Br J Surg* 1989; 76: 607–9.

42. Pedersen E, Klemar B, Schroder HD et al. Anal sphincter responses after perianal electrical stimulation. *J Neurol Neurosurg Psychiatry* 1982; 45: 770–3.

43. Barnett JL, Hasler WL, Camilleri M. American Gastro-enterological Association medical position statement on ano-rectal testing techniques. American Gastroenterological Association. *Gastroenterology* 1999; 116: 732–60.

44. Ghezzi A, Callea L, Zaffaroni M et al. Motor potentials of bulbo-cavernosus muscle after transcranial and lumbar magnetic stimulation: comparative study with bulbocavernosus reflex and pudendal evoked potentials. *J Neurol Neurosurg Psychiatry* 1991; 54: 524–6.

45. Brostrom S, Jennum P, Lose G. Motor evoked potentials from the striated urethral sphincter and puborectal muscle: reproducibility of latencies. *Clin Neurophysiol* 2003; 114: 1891–5.

46. Vodusek DB, Fowler CJ. Clinical neurophysiology. In Fowler CJ, ed. *Neurology of Bladder, Bowel, and Sexual Dysfunction*. Boston: Butterworth-Heinemann, 1999: 109–43.

47. Shafik A, El-Sibai O. Study of the pelvic floor muscles in vaginismus: a concept of pathogenesis. *Eur J Obstet Gynecol Reprod Biol* 2002; 105: 67–70.

48. Bergeron S, Binik YM, Khalife S et al. A randomized comparison of group cognitive–behavioral therapy, surface electromyographic biofeedback, and vestibulectomy in the treatment of dyspareunia resulting from vulvar vestibulitis. *Pain* 2001; 91: 297–306.

49. Glazer HI, Rodke G, Swencionis C et al. Treatment of vulvar vestibulitis syndrome with electromyographic biofeedback of pelvic floor musculature. *J Reprod Med* 1995; 40: 283–90.

50. Nadelhaft I, Booth AM. The location and morphology of pregan-glionic neurons and the distribution of visceral afferents from the rat pelvic nerve: a horseradish peroxidase study. *J Comp Neurol* 1984; 226: 238–45.

51. McKenna KE, Chung SK, McVary KT. A model for the study of sexual function in anesthetized male and female rats. *Am J Physiol* 1991; 261(5 Pt 2): R1276–85.

52. Blanco R, Saenz de Tejada I, Goldstein I et al. Dysfunctional penile cholinergic nerves in diabetic impotent men. *J Urol* 1990; 144(2 Pt 1): 278–80.

53. Enzlin P, Mathieu C, Vanderschueren D, *et al.* Diabetes mellitus and female sexuality: a review of 25 years' research. *Diabet Med* 1998; 15: 809–15.

54. Ganzer H, Madersbacher H, Rumpl E. Cortical evoked potentials by stimulation of the vesicourethral junction: clinical value and neurophysiological considerations. *J Urol* 1991; 146: 118–23.

55. Schmid DM, Reitz A, Curt A et al. Urethral evoked sympathetic

skin responses and viscerosensory evoked potentials as diagnostic tools to evaluate urogenital autonomic afferent innervation in spinal cord injured patients. *J Urol* 2004; 171: 1156–60.

56. Hansen MV, Ertekin C, Larsson LE. Cerebral evoked potentials after stimulation of the posterior urethra in man. *Electroencephalogr Clin Neurophysiol* 1990; 77: 52–8.

57. Paick JS, Donatucci CF, Lue TF. Anatomy of cavernous nerves distal to prostate: microdissection study in adult male cadavers. *Urology* 1993; 42: 145–9.

58. Stief CG, Kellner B, Hartung C et al. Computer-assisted evaluation of the smooth-muscle electromyogram of the corpora cavernosa by fast Fourier transformation. *Eur Urol* 1997; 31: 329–34.

59. Sasso F, Stief CG, Gulino G et al. Progress in corpus cavernosum electromyography (CC-EMG) – third international workshop on corpus cavernosum electromyography (CC-EMG). *Int J Impot Res* 1997; 9: 43–5.

60. Heiman JR. Female sexual response patterns. Interactions of physiological, affective, and contextual cues. *Arch Gen Psychiatry* 1980; 37: 1311–16.

61. Rogers GS, Van de Castle RL, Evans WS et al. Vaginal pulse amplitude response patterns during erotic conditions and sleep. *Arch Sex Behav* 1985; 14: 327–42.

62. Polan ML, Desmond JE, Banner LL et al. Female sexual arousal: a behavioral analysis. *Fertil Steril* 2003; 80: 1480–7.

63. Yilmaz U, Soylu A, Ozcan C et al. Clitoral electromyography. *J Urol* 2002; 167(2 Pt 1): 616–20.

64. Yilmaz U, Kromm BG, Yang CC. Evaluation of autonomic innervation of the clitoris and bulb. *J Urol* 2004; 172: 1930–4.

65. Ertekin C, Almis S, Ertekin N. Sympathetic skin potentials and bulbocavernosus reflex in patients with chronic alcoholism and impotence. *Eur Neurol* 1990; 30: 334–7.

66. Ertekin C, Ertekin N, Mutlu S et al. Skin potentials (SP) recorded from the extremities and genital regions in normal and impotent subjects. *Acta Neurol Scand* 1987; 76: 28–36.

67. Daffertshofer M, Linden D, Syren M et al. Assessment of local sympathetic function in patients with erectile dysfunction. *Int J Impot Res* 1994; 6: 213–25.

68. Opsomer RJ, Boccasena P, Traversa R et al. Sympathetic skin responses from the limbs and the genitalia: normative study and contribution to the evaluation of neurourological disorders. *Electroencephalogr Clin Neurophysiol* 1996; 101: 25–31.

69. Ueda T, Yoshimura N, Yoshida O. Diabetic cystopathy: relationship to autonomic neuropathy detected by sympathetic skin response. *J Urol* 1997; 157: 580–4.

70. Schurch B, Curt A, Rossier AB. The value of sympathetic skin response recordings in the assessment of the vesicourethral autonomic nervous dysfunction in spinal cord injured patients. *J Urol* 1997; 157: 2230–3.

71. Rodic B, Curt A, Dietz V et al. Bladder neck incompetence in patients with spinal cord injury: significance of sympathetic skin response. *J Urol* 2000; 163: 1223–7.

10.7 Measurement of circulating levels of total and free testosterone

Frank Z Stanczyk

One of the key androgens in sexual dysfunction in women is testosterone (see Chapters 5.5, 6.1–6.3, and 13.1–13.3 of this book). In blood, testosterone is found predominantly in a protein-bound form. It is bound with high affinity but limited capacity to sex hormone-binding globulin, and with lower affinity but higher capacity to albumin; only about 1–2% is non-protein-bound (free).[1] However, it is the free testosterone fraction that has physiologic importance, since it is available for androgen action or metabolism and subsequent clearance. Both total and free testosterone are measured in serum for diagnostic purposes. Total testosterone is measured routinely in diagnostic testing laboratories by immunoassay methods. Reliable measurement of free testosterone requires a more specialized assay that is carried out in relatively few laboratories.

The purpose of this chapter is to discuss the different assay methods that are used to quantify total and free testosterone levels. I will begin with a summary of the development and validation of the first steroid immunoassays, specifically, radioimmunoassays with preceding purification steps. This will be followed by a discussion of direct steroid immunoassays, which were developed to avoid the purification steps in the initial radioimmunoassay methods. After that, the current status of mass spectrometry assays to measure testosterone will be addressed. The final part of the chapter will deal with the different methods used to measure free testosterone. A particular emphasis in this chapter will be the advantages and limitations of the different assay methods used to quantify total and free testosterone (see Chapter 6.3).

Measurement of total testosterone

Historical aspects

In 1959, Yalow and Berson[2] described an assay method that eventually revolutionized the entire field of endocrinology. This assay method arose from studies on the effects of ^{131}I-labeled proteins in vivo, in which it was demonstrated that insulin-requiring diabetics usually have a circulating insulin-binding protein.[3] The same study showed that ^{131}I-insulin could be displaced from the insulin-binding protein by excess of unlabeled insulin. It also showed that the binding of ^{131}I-insulin was quantitatively related to the total amount of insulin present. These observations formed the basis for the first radioimmunoassay. Subsequently, specific antisera to human insulin were prepared in guinea pigs and resulted in the first radioimmunoassay with sufficient sensitivity to detect endogenous insulin in human blood.[4]

In 1963, Greenwood et al.[5] developed a method of coupling iodine to growth hormone that was far superior to any previous method. The coupling was accomplished by using a mild oxidizing agent, chloramine-T. This method made it possible to bind all proteins with radioactive iodine, with minimal damage to the protein. Along with the improvement in protein iodination, antibody production methods were also improved, yielding good titers. Subsequently, a new era in reproductive endocrinology was launched in 1967 when Odell et al.[6] developed the radioimmunoassay for luteinizing hormone and in 1969 Abraham[7] did the same for estradiol. The success of the radioimmunoassay method can be attributed to the fact that it offers a general system for measurement of an immensely wide range of compounds of clinical and biologic importance.

First steroid radioimmunoassay

The estradiol assay method first reported by Abraham[7,8] consisted of purification of estradiol in serum or plasma samples by organic solvent extraction and column chromatography prior to its quantification by radioimmunoassay. The rationale for the purification steps in the estradiol radioimmunoassay method was to separate estradiol from interfering metabolites. Table 10.7.1 shows numerous unconjugated metabolites of estradiol present in blood. Whenever a steroid molecule contains a hydroxyl group, it may be conjugated to form a sulfated or glucuronidated derivative. Thus, many of the metabolites shown in Table 10.7.1 are also found in a conjugated form in serum or plasma. The unconjugated and conjugated estradiol metabolites may interfere with the specificity of the estradiol radioimmunoassay if they are not separated from estradiol. In contrast to steroid hormones, protein hormones such as luteinizing hormone and follicle-stimulating hormone are transformed only to a relatively minor extent. Therefore, luteinizing hormone and follicle-stimulating hormone immunoassays do not require purification of the analytes.

In the estradiol radioimmunoassay method reported by Abraham,[7,8] purification of estradiol in serum or plasma was carried out as follows. First, after taking an aliquot of each sample, a very small amount of tritiated estradiol, approximately 1000 disintegrations per minute (d.p.m.), with high specific activity to minimize the mass, was added to the aliquots. The tritiated estradiol served as the internal standard for monitoring losses during extraction procedures. Then, an organic solvent (diethyl ether) extraction was used to remove the conjugated steroids, which remain in the aqueous layer, and to dissociate the estradiol from sex hormone-binding globulin. This step was followed by LH-20 column chromatography to separate interfering unconjugated steroids from estradiol. After evaporating the organic solvent in which estradiol was eluted off the columns, the residues were reconstituted in assay buffer. Duplicate aliquots of each reconstituted residue were taken for radioimmunoassay, and a single aliquot was taken to determine procedural losses.

Radioimmunoassay of the purified estradiol in buffer was carried out, together with varying concentrations of authentic estradiol, also in assay buffer, and used to generate a standard curve. The procedure consisted of adding to each sample and standard a constant amount of tritiated estradiol (approximately 10,000 d.p.m.) and the appropriate dilution of antibody

Table 10.7.1. Unconjugated metabolites of estradiol

Position on carbon	Estrogen metabolite	Position on carbon	Estrogen metabolite
C-1	1-Hydroxyestrone	C-11	11β-Hydroxyestrone
			11-Ketoestrone
C-2	2-Hydroxyestrone		11β-Hydroxyestradiol
	2-Hydroxyestradiol		11-Ketoestradiol
	2-Hydroxyestriol		Δ(9,11)-Dehydro-17α-estradiol
			Δ(9,11)-Dehydroestrone
C-4	4-Hydroxyestrone		
	4-Hydroxyestradiol	C-14	14α-Hydroyestrone
	4-Hydroxyestriol		14α-Hydroxyestradiol
C-6	6α-Hydroxyestrone	C-15	15α-Hydroxyesterone
	6β-Hydroxyestrone		15β-Hydroxyestrone
	6-Ketoestrone		15α-Hydroxyestradiol
	6α-Hydroxyestradiol		15α-Hydroxyestriol (estetrol)
	6β-Hydroxyestradiol		
	6-Ketoestradiol	C-16	16α-Hydroxyestrone
	6α-Hydroxyestriol		16β-Hydroxyestrone
	6-Ketoestriol		16-Ketoestrone
C-7	7α-Hydroxyestrone		16α-Hydroxyestradiol (estriol)
	7β-Hydroxyestrone		16-Epiestriol
	7α-Hydroxyestradiol		16-Ketoestradiol
	7β-Hydroxyestradiol		16,17-Epiestriol
	7-Ketoestradiol	C-17	17α-Estradiol
	7α-Hydroxyestriol		17-Epiestriol
		C-18	18-Hydroxyestrone

raised in rabbits against estradiol. After overnight incubation, antibody-bound estradiol was separated from unbound estradiol with dextran-coated charcoal. After centrifugation, an aliquot of each supernatant was taken for counting in a liquid scintillation counter. The aliquots taken previously for determining procedural losses were also counted. After the estradiol standard curve was plotted, the concentration of estradiol in each sample was determined by extrapolation from the standard curve, using a programmed calculator, and each value was subsequently corrected to account for procedural losses.

The extraction/chromatography radioimmunoassay method described for estradiol soon started to be used to measure other steroid hormones by a growing number of investigators in a variety of studies. In the early 1970s, this methodology was used at our institution to measure sex hormones, including testosterone.[9,10] Our assay methodology for quantifying steroid hormones has remained essentially the same since that time. Some changes made include replacement of radioligands with iodinated steroid derivatives, resulting in more sensitive radioimmunoassays, and use of ethylacetate:hexane instead of diethyl ether for extraction to obtain a purer extract. Moreover, although steroid hormones can be measured in either serum or plasma, serum is the preferred matrix, because sometimes clotting occurs in plasma after repeated freezing, thawing, and refreezing cycles.

Reliability of extraction/chromatography radioimmunoassays

Ever since the first steroid radioimmunoassay was developed, determination of assay sensitivity, accuracy, precision, and specificity has been deemed critical for validity and reliability of immunoassay methods.[11] Each new immunoassay that is developed or an existing immunoassay that is being set up for the first time in a laboratory should be thoroughly validated before using it to measure an analyte in a sample.

Sensitivity

Assay sensitivity can be defined as the minimal detection limit of an assay. From the practical standpoint, assay sensitivity is the lowest concentration of a steroid standard in a sample, which can be distinguished from a sample without a standard. The sensitivity can be calculated by first determining the mean±standard deviation of the antibody-bound counts of replicates of the zero standard, and subtracting two standard deviations from the mean counts.[11] The difference in counts is then used to read the steroid concentration off the standard curve. The sensitivity of an immunoassay can be improved by making certain changes in the assay methodology, the most important of which are reducing the amount of antibody and increasing the time of incubation.

Precision

The precision of an assay refers to the variability in the concentration of a substance observed when multiple measurements are made on the same sample. In practice, the interassay preci-

sion and interassay precision are calculated as the per cent coefficient of variation of replicate measurements. Quality control samples containing low, medium, and high levels of the appropriate steroid hormone can be used in a single assay (intraassay) and in several assays to determine the coefficients of variation of the measurements. At least five replicates of each level of the steroid hormone in the quality control samples should be used for determination of assay precision.

Specificity

Assay specificity refers to the degree of interference or cross-reaction encountered from substances other than the one that is measured in the assay. Specificity can be divided into two types.[11] One type refers to interference by identifiable compounds that are physicochemically similar to the analyte being measured and may therefore possibly react directly with the antibody in the radioimmunoassay. This type of specificity may be assessed by determining the percentage crossreaction from the amount of material required to produce 50% inhibition of the antibody-bound tracer, after plotting curves of different concentrations of the relevant standard and the potential interfering compounds, such as relevant metabolites.[11] Cross-reactivity of the antiserum in an immunoassay may lead to overestimation of an analyte being measured in a sample.

The other type of specificity-related interference in an assay involves factors other than those that can be clearly identified by their physicochemical similarity to the ligand. A commonly used synonym for this type of nonspecificity is "matrix effect". It may lead to an underestimation or, more commonly, an overestimation of the amount of an analyte in a sample. A variety of materials can interfere with antibody–ligand reactions, and the effects can vary in different assay methods. High levels of serum lipids are particularly notorious for causing matrix effects. Other materials that may interfere include hemoglobin, heparin, salts, acids, alkalines, nucleic acids, and sodium azide.[11]

Accuracy

Assay accuracy can be defined as the extent to which a given measurement of a substance agrees with the actual value. Accuracy of an extraction/chromatographic radioimmunoassay method can be established by "spiking" known amounts of the appropriate steroid standard to serum and determining the amount of steroid recovered, after measuring the steroid by radioimmunoassay in the spiked and some unspiked samples. The expected recovery of the "spiked" steroid is generally ±10% for each of the amounts added. Moreover, regression analysis of the data should give a line that is parallel to that obtained with the standard curve.

Quality control of extraction/chromatographic steroid radioimmunoassays

Quality control parameters used to determine the reliability of each extraction/chromatographic radioimmunoassay include those related to the standard curve and the analyte being measured in samples. Parameters related to the standard curve include the following: total counts added to each radioimmunoassay tube, nonspecific binding, binding of the zero standard, slope, y-intercept, and doses of the standard at which per cent bound/maximum bound (B/B_o) is equal to 20, 50, and 80. Parameters related to the analyte include the results of quantifying the analyte in quality-control samples and the performance characteristics of pipettes and instruments. However, the single most important quality-control parameter includes the result of repeated measurements of the low, medium, and high levels of the analyte in samples prepared to monitor the reliability of each assay. These quality-control samples are analyzed in the same manner as serum samples containing unknown concentrations of the analyte. Typically, one set of low, medium, and high quality-control samples and a buffer blank that is used to monitor potential assay contaminants are placed at the beginning and end of the samples with unknown concentrations of the analyte. Assays are accepted or rejected on the basis of the limits of rejection for different quality-control parameters, which are set by the individual laboratory.

Advantages and disadvantages of extraction/chromatographic steroid radioimmunoassays

Extraction/chromatographic radioimmunoassays have advantages and disadvantages. The advantages include the following: (a) steroid-binding proteins are denatured by the organic solvent in the extraction step, resulting in release of steroid hormones such as testosterone from sex hormone-binding globulin; (b) both conjugated and unconjugated metabolites are separated from the analyte prior to its quantification; (c) relatively large serum aliquots can be used, allowing the analyte in a sample to be measured on an accurate part of the standard curve. High assay reliability is achieved when the assay method is properly validated.

Disadvantages of the extraction/chromatographic radioimmunoassay include potential errors from counting very small amounts of tritiated labeled internal standard, such as tritiated testosterone in the testosterone radioimmunoassay, to follow procedural losses, and from use of factors to account for dilutions used in assay procedures. In addition, the assay method is somewhat cumbersome, takes about 2 days for analysis of around 40 samples, and is relatively costly.

Direct steroid immunoassays

Because extraction/chromatographic radioimmunoassays for quantifying steroids were so time-consuming and laborious, the need for rapid, direct immunoassay methods, i.e., without purification steps, became obvious. In the late 1970s, such assays started to become available commercially, initially using commercial kits that contained reagents to perform assays manually.

An iodinated steroid derivative, instead of a tritiated radioligand, was used in the assay methodology to reduce the time of counting the radioactivity. Subsequently, the kits were used in an instrument so that the assay could be performed automatically.

Automated immunoassay methods employ a chemiluminescent, fluorescent, or enzyme tag, which avoids use of radioactivity and prolonged counting times, as well as the high cost of radioactive material. The money saved from decreased labor costs and not having to pay for radioactivity disposal offsets the initial cost of purchasing an automated instrument. Thus, direct steroid immunoassays are simple, convenient, rapid, and relatively inexpensive.

Unfortunately, direct steroid immunoassays can have disadvantages. First, steroids that bind with high affinity to the plasma binding proteins, such as testosterone to sex hormone-binding globulin and cortisol to corticosteroid-binding globulin (CBG), sometimes may not be released efficiently from the protein. Manufacturers of steroid immunoassay kits often use a low pH in one of the reagents in the kit, such as the radioligand solution, to release the steroid from sex hormone-binding globulin or corticosteroid-binding globulin. If the pH is not correct, testosterone will not be dissociated from sex hormone-binding globulin, and a patient can be considered to be hypogonadal on the basis of a subnormal testosterone measurement.

A second deficiency of direct steroid immunoassay involves differences between the matrix containing the analyte being measured and the matrix containing the different concentrations of standard. The matrix often used by kit manufacturers for the different concentrations of steroid standard is defibrinated, delipidated, charcoal-stripped plasma, which is a clear, buffer-like solution. In contrast, serum samples often contain interfering materials that may cause a "matrix effect" and consequently an overestimation or underestimation of an analyte in a sample, as pointed out earlier. Serum samples that are hemolyzed should not be used in a direct assay.

A third deficiency of direct steroid immunoassays arises from the fact that there are several hundred different steroids, in an unconjugated or conjugated form, present in serum. Some of these steroids are closely related in chemical structure to the analyte being measured, and may therefore be recognized by the antiserum used in the assay. It is rare that an antiserum against a certain steroid is so highly specific that it measures solely the analyte that it is intended to measure. Due to the presence of crossreacting compounds, measures of analytes are often overestimated in direct immunoassays.

Evidence showing that direct steroid immunoassays carried out with reagents in commercial kits are not reliable can be found in several studies. In our study,[12] we evaluated four different commercially available direct testosterone immunoassay kits and used our extraction/chromatographic testosterone radioimmunoassay as a standard for comparison. Our results show that the assays using the kits performed generally well for male serum samples, but gave poor intraclass correlations and/or failed validity for both premenopausal and postmenopausal serum samples. (The validity of an assay reflects its accuracy.) Our findings are consistent with those reported by Taieb et al.,[13] who measured serum testosterone levels in women, men, and children by use of 10 different direct testosterone immunoassay kits and by isotope dilution gas chromatography-mass spectrometry. On the basis of their results, they concluded that the direct assays were acceptable for measuring testosterone in male samples, but not in samples from women or children. In an accompanying editorial[14] on the article by Taieb et al.,[13] the editors concluded that "guessing appears to be nearly as good as most commercially available immunoassays and clearly superior to some".

Mass spectrometry assay methods

Gas chromatography–mass spectrometry and liquid chromatography–mass spectrometry are powerful analytic techniques that combine the resolving power of gas chromatography or liquid chromatography with the high sensitivity and specificity of the mass spectrometer. Separation of steroids by gas chromatography requires that they be first derivatized to increase their volatility, selectivity, and detectability. It is not necessary to derivatize steroids for separation by liquid chromatography, but derivatization is sometimes used to improve the ionization efficiency of steroids, a step which increases mass spectrometry assay sensitivity.

The mass spectrometer functions as a unique detector that provides structural information on individual solutes as they elute from the gas chromatography or liquid chromatography column. Addition of the appropriate internal standard to the sample enables accurate quantification in conjunction with a standard curve of known concentrations of the standard.

The mass spectrometry technique first involves ionization of the target compound at the ionization source. This is followed by separation and detection of the ions in the mass analyzer. A mass spectrum is produced, in which the relative abundance of a particular ion is plotted as a function of the mass-to-charge ratio.

Although a variety of gas chromatography–mass spectrometry and liquid chromatography–mass spectrometry assay methods exist, one of the most highly efficient of these methods is liquid chromatography combined with tandem mass spectrometry (liquid chromatography/tandem mass spectrometry). This technique involves use of a collision cell in which the ion of interest (precursor ion) undergoes collision-induced fragmentation into product ions. The mass of the product ion is then determined at the detector. Tandem mass spectrometry has the capability to achieve not only high sensitivity and specificity, but also high throughput. It is projected to become the reference standard for steroid hormone measurements. However, at present, measurement of testosterone by liquid chromatography/tandem mass spectrometry for diagnostic testing is restricted to only a few laboratories. This is due to the high cost of the mass spectrometry instrument (nearly US$500,000), the requirement for a highly trained technician to operate the instrument, and

the time required to develop the assay for quantifying a wide range of testosterone levels. Nevertheless, at least one laboratory (Quest Diagnostic Nichols Institute, San Juan Capistrano, CA, USA) is using liquid chromatography/tandem mass spectrometry to measure testosterone levels in women, children, and men for diagnostic testing. The initial high cost of the liquid chromatography/tandem mass spectrometry instrumentation and assay development is offset by the relatively rapid turnaround time of accurate testosterone results compared with the costly, cumbersome and time-consuming extraction/chromatography testosterone radioimmunoassay methodology.

Free and bioavailable testosterone

As mentioned earlier, testosterone is present in blood predominantly in a protein-bound form and only a very small portion is free. In premenopausal women, approximately 66% and 30% of total testosterone are bound to sex hormone-binding globulin and albumin, respectively, and the free fraction generally comprises under 2% of the total.[1] Testosterone is bound with high affinity ($K_a = 1.7 \times 10^9\,\mathrm{M^{-1}}$) and low capacity to sex hormone-binding globulin, and it is bound with low affinity ($K_a = 1 \times 10^4$ $\mathrm{M^{-1}}$ to $1 \times 10^5\,\mathrm{M^{-1}}$) but high capacity to albumin.[1,15]

For many years, it was accepted that only the free fraction of testosterone in the circulation can be taken up by tissues and that the protein-bound testosterone complex is inactive. However, some investigators observed that the fraction of testosterone bound to albumin dissociates rapidly and is taken up by tissues in a manner similar to that of the free steroid.[16–18] Testosterone bound to the large pool of albumin, together with the small amount of the free steroid, probably forms the circulating pool of bioavailable (non-sex hormone-binding globulin-bound) testosterone. The bioavailable fraction of testosterone enters cells where it may undergo metabolism or binds to the androgen receptor and exerts biologic activity.

Commonly used methods for measuring free testosterone involve the addition of a small amount of ³H-testosterone to serum or plasma and, after a suitable incubation period, separation of the protein (sex hormone-binding globulin and albumin)-bound fractions from the free fraction of testosterone by means of a membrane (e.g., equilibrium dialysis) or filter (e.g., centrifugal ultrafiltration). These barriers retain the protein-bound fractions but allow free testosterone to pass through. The percentage of tritiated free testosterone is then calculated on the basis of the total tritiated testosterone added. Recovery of free components through a barrier is sometimes monitored with a small labeled molecule such as ¹⁴C-glucose.

Several technical limitations exist in the assays used to measure free testosterone. The equilibrium dialysis method is influenced by dilution of the serum sample. The centrifugal ultrafiltration method is complex and subject to adsorption of testosterone to the membrane. Both the dialysis and ultrafiltration methods can be affected by impurities of tritiated testosterone not bound by sex hormone-binding globulin or albumin;

these impurities may increase the percentage of free testosterone. Moreover, the use of too large an amount of tritiated testosterone in the assays may increase the concentration of total testosterone and possibly disturb the equilibrium of endogenous testosterone.

Two methods used to determine the percentage of bioavailable testosterone in serum include centrifugal ultrafiltration with heat-treated serum and ammonium sulfate precipitation. In the centrifugal ultrafiltration method, the percentage of albumin-bound testosterone is determined after sex hormone-binding globulin is inactivated by heating the serum sample to 60°C for 1 h. After the temperature of the sample returns to 37°C, the testosterone dissociated from sex hormone-binding globulin is re-equilibrated in the serum, and the testosterone fraction bound to albumin can be determined by ultrafiltration. The fraction of testosterone bound to albumin along with the free testosterone fraction determined before heating the sample comprises the total bioavailable testosterone fraction. A much simpler method to determine bioavailable testosterone involves addition of a small amount of tritiated testosterone to serum and, after a suitable incubation period, precipitation of the globulins (including the sex hormone-binding globulin testosterone complex) with saturated ammonium sulfate, centrifugation, counting the tritium in the supernatant, and calculating the percentage of the total ^{3}H-testosterone that is not sex hormone-binding globulin bound.

Certain technical difficulties are also encountered in the measurement of bioavailable testosterone. When this fraction is measured by the barrier method after inactivation of sex hormone-binding globulin, the same technical problems exist as described for the measurement of free testosterone. The most frequently encountered sources of error in the ammonium sulfate precipitation assay are use of impure tritiated testosterone, insufficient counting time of the small amount of radiolabeled testosterone, and incomplete precipitation of globulins. The deficiencies in both assays are often the cause of poor intra-assay and interassay reproducibility.

By the methods described above, the concentration of free or bioavailable testosterone is usually calculated from the percentage of free or bioavailable testosterone multiplied by the total testosterone concentration, which is quantified separately by immunoassay. Free testosterone concentrations are sometimes measured directly in the dialysate after equilibrium dialysis. However, highly sensitive extraction/chromatography radioimmunoassays are required to measure the very low testosterone levels.

Because the assays described above for quantifying free or bioavailable testosterone are time-consuming and expensive, they are available in a limited number of reference laboratories. The most widely used assays for measurement of free testosterone in clinical laboratories are direct radioimmunoassays. In general, these assays use a ^{125}I-labeled testosterone analog that has very low affinity for sex hormone-binding globulin and albumin, and competes with free testosterone for binding sites on an immobilized specific testosterone antibody. Although this approach provides a simple and rapid test for quantifying free testosterone, it has been pointed out that the assay method has several deficiencies: these include low antibody affinity, major biasing effects due to dilution of serum samples, significant binding of the analog to serum proteins, and lack of parallelism between measurements of serially diluted serum samples and free testosterone.[19] For these reasons, the reliability of the analog-based free testosterone radioimmunoassay kit has been questioned.[20,21] One study[22] showed that plasma free testosterone levels in samples from normal women and patients with polycystic ovary syndrome were approximately three to four times higher when measured by a commercial analog-based radioimmunoassay kit than when measured by the equilibrium dialysis method. The results obtained with the latter method were comparable to published data. Nevertheless, good correlations were obtained between the results of the two methods. The investigators concluded that the free testosterone values measured by use of the kit had a mean bias of −76%, thereby making comparison with published data difficult. The higher levels of free testosterone measured by direct radioimmunoassay may result from the fact that the antibody in the radioimmunoassay system has a greater affinity for testosterone weakly bound to albumin than albumin does. This may allow the antibody to strip some of the testosterone that is bound to albumin. A subsequent study[23] showed that the direct testosterone radioimmunoassay had unacceptably high systematic bias and random variability, and did not correlate well with equilibrium dialysis. A letter to the editor by Rosner[24] about the direct free testosterone analog radioimmunoassay concluded, "the literature of science ought not to use a method so grossly inaccurate when better ones exist." In addition, Rosner[24] suggested, "The journal might choose to return manuscripts that use it without further evaluation to discourage its use."

Some laboratories and investigators that have measured total testosterone and sex hormone-binding globulin have used the ratio of testosterone/sex hormone-binding globulin, referred to as the free androgen index, as an estimate of free testosterone. The validity of the free androgen index as an accurate reflection of free testosterone has been questioned. One small study[20] showed the free androgen index to be unreliable, on the basis of its comparison with free testosterone quantified by equilibrium dialysis; the ratio of free androgen index to free testosterone determined by dialysis was 0.12–0.26. Another small study[25] found a high correlation coefficient (0.858) between the free androgen index and free testosterone levels determined by centrifugal ultrafiltration in serum samples from women, whereas in male samples the correlation was only 0.435. A more recent study[23] in women found a good correlation between free androgen index and equilibrium dialysis. However, the authors of that study pointed out that the free androgen index can be altered by changes in either testosterone or sex hormone-binding globulin, and that using this quotient alone can be misleading. Therefore, use of the free androgen index is limited.

Both free and bioavailable testosterone can also be calculated by an algorithm which requires the concentrations of total testosterone, sex hormone-binding globulin, and albumin, as well as the binding constants of testosterone to sex hormone-binding globulin and albumin obtained from published equations.[20] Calculated free testosterone levels in men and women were found to be nearly identical to corresponding values measured by equilibrium dialysis.[23,26,27]

It is important to realize that when indirect methods, such as equilibrium dialysis or centrifugal ultrafiltration, are used to determine free testosterone concentrations, the accuracy of the total testosterone concentration is very important. This is because those methods determine the percentage of total testosterone that is free, and the percentage is multiplied by the total testosterone concentration to obtain the free testosterone concentration. Thus, direct immunoassay methods should not be used for quantifying total testosterone levels in female samples; radioimmunoassays with preceding organic solvent extraction and chromatography steps will provide reliable values. Similarly, if the free androgen index or algorithm is used to calculate free testosterone, the accuracy of both total testosterone and sex hormone-binding globulin values is essential. Although the concentration of albumin is also required in the algorithm method, an average normal albumin value can be used without any significant change in the calculated free testosterone concentration.

Differences in sex hormone-binding globulin concentrations obtained with different commercially available sex hormone-binding globulin kits have been reported.[28] In one study,[23] an approximately twofold greater absolute value was found with an immunoradiometric assay than a radioimmunoassay, and better accuracy was found with the former assay. The immunoradiometric method was calibrated against a dihydrotestosterone-binding capacity assay, which is considered to provide sex hormone-binding globulin values that reflect more physiologically relevant sex hormone-binding globulin concentrations in blood. Thus, it seems reasonable to use sex hormone-binding globulin assay methods that correlate well with assay methods based on testosterone- or dihydrotestosterone-binding capacity.

Normal ranges of total and free testosterone

Once an immunoassay for a hormone in serum is developed and validated in a laboratory, normal ranges for females and/or males should be established. Serum samples must be obtained from normal, healthy subjects who are not on any treatment that may affect the normal range. It is also important to establish normal ranges in a large number of individuals; this number should be over 100. In addition, blood samples for normal ranges should be obtained at the same time of day, such as 08:00–10:00. This is essential for those hormones that undergo diurnal variation.

An example of female and male normal ranges for total testosterone quantified by extraction/chromatography radioimmunoassay and free testosterone determined by equilibrium dialysis is shown in Table 10.7.2. The values were obtained from Quest Diagnostics Nichols Institute.

Table 10.7.2. Normal ranges of total and free testosterone in women and men

Gender	Total testosterone (ng/dl)	Free testosterone (pg/ml)
Female		
Premenopausal	15–70	1–21
Postmenopausal	5–51	1–21
Male	260–1000	34–194

Conclusions

From the information presented in this chapter, the following conclusions can be made. (a) Extraction/chromatography radioimmunoassay methods for quantifying testosterone are highly reliable when thoroughly validated with respect to sensitivity, accuracy, precision, and specificity, and when the quality control of the assay is properly monitored. (b) It is essential that users of commercial direct immunoassay kits for measurement of any steroid hormone validate the assay methods thoroughly in their own laboratory; they should not merely accept the kit manufacturer's validation. It is especially important that steroid hormone values measured in a direct assay be compared with corresponding values determined by a well-established assay, i.e., either extraction/chromatography radioimmunoassay, or a gas chromatography–mass spectrometry or liquid chromatography–mass spectrometry assay. (c) Tandem mass spectrometry is projected to become the reference standard for steroid hormone measurements. However, interlaboratory comparisons using tandem mass spectrometry to quantify steroid levels are essential before any measurement is accepted as the reference standard. (d) Measurement of free testosterone concentrations by the analog-based free testosterone radioimmunoassay is highly unreliable and should never be used. (e) When free testosterone concentrations are quantified experimentally, the first step is to determine the percentage of free testosterone by methods such as equilibrium dialysis or ultrafiltration. Because this percentage is then multiplied by the total testosterone concentration to obtain the free testosterone concentration, a highly reliable immunoassay, such as the extraction/chromatography radioimmunoassay, must be used to measure total testosterone. (f) Use of the calculated method to determine the free testosterone concentration gives values that are similar to the equilibrium dialysis method, which is considered the reference standard for determination of free testosterone concentrations. The calculated method requires accurate measurement of not only total testosterone but also sex hormone-binding globulin.

A recent editorial by Matsumoto and Bremner[29] stated: "What is needed now is refocusing of attention to more rigorous validation and standardization of accuracy and normal ranges for these assays to alleviate the confusion that has arisen in the clinical and research community as a result of the variability and discrepancies in testosterone assays. We hope that assay vendors, endocrinologists, clinical chemists, and regulatory agencies can act together to achieve better standardization of hormone measurements, including testosterone assays."

References

1   Westphal U. *Steroid–Protein Interactions*. Berlin: Springer-Verlag, 1986.

2.   Yalow RS, Berson SA. Assay of plasma insulin in human subjects by immunological methods. *Nature* 1959; 184: 1648–9.

3.   Berson SA, Yalow R, Bauman A et al. Insulin-I-131 metabolism in human subjects: demonstration of insulin binding globulin in the circulation of insulin treated subjects. *J Clin Invest* 1956; 35: 170–90.

4.   Yalow RS, Berson SA. Immunoassay of endogenous plasma insulin in man. *J Clin Invest* 1960; 38: 1157–75.

5.   Greenwood FC, Hunter WM, Grove JS. The preparation of ^{125}I-labelled human growth hormone high specific radioactivity. *Biochem J* 1963; 89: 114.

6.   Odell WD, Ross GT, Rayford RL. RIA of luteinizing hormone in human plasma or serum: physiological studies. *J Clin Invest* 1967; 46: 248.

7.   Abraham GE. Solid-phase radioimmunoassay of estradiol-17β. *J Clin Endocrinol Metab* 1969; 29: 866–70.

8.   Abraham GE, Odell WD. Solid-phase radioimmunoassay of serum estradiol-17β: a semi-automated approach. In FG Peron, BV Caldwell, eds. *Immunologic Methods in Steroid Determination*. New York: Appleton-Century-Crofts, 1970: 87–112.

9.   Thorneycroft IH, Sribyatta B, Tom WK et al. Measurement of serum LH, FSH, progesterone, 17-hydroxyprogesterone, and estradiol-17β levels at 4-hour intervals during the periovulatory phase of the menstrual cycle. *J Clin Endocrinol Metab* 1974; 39: 754–8.

10. Goebelsmann U, Arce JJ, Thorneycroft IH et al. Serum testosterone concentrations in women throughout the menstrual cycle and following hCG administration. *Am J Obstet Gynecol* 1974; 119: 445–52.

11. Chard T. An introduction to radioimmunoassay and related technique. In PC Van der Vliet, ed. *Laboratory Techniques in Biochemistry and Molecular Biology*. Amsterdam: Elsevier, 1995.

12. Stanczyk FZ, Cho MM, Endres DB et al. Limitations of direct estradiol and testosterone immunoassay kits. *Steroids* 2003; 68: 1173–8.

13. Taieb J, Mathian B, Millot F et al. Testosterone measured by 10 immunoassays and by isotope-dilution gas chromatography – mass spectrometry in sera from 116 men, women, and children. *Clin Chem* 2003; 49: 1381–95.

14. Fitzgerald RL, Herold DA. Ciba Corning ACS: 180 direct total testosterone assay can be used on female sera. *Clin Chem* 1997; 43: 1466–7.

15. Westphal U. *Steroid–Protein Interactions*. Berlin: Springer-Verlag, 1971.

16. Manni A, Pardrige WM, Cefalus W et al. Bioavailability of albumin-bound testosterone. *J Clin Endocrinol Metab* 1985; 61: 705–10.

17. Pardridge W, Landaw EM. Tracer kinetics model of blood–brain barrier transport of plasma protein-bound ligands: empiric testing of free hormone hypothesis. *J Clin Invest* 1984; 74: 745–52.

18. Pardridge WM. Transport of protein bound hormones into tissues in vivo. *Endocr Rev* 1981; 2: 103–23.

19. Ekins R. Hirsutism: free and bound testosterone. *Ann Clin Biochem* 1990; 27: 91–4.

20. Vermeulen A, Verdonck L, Kaufman JM. A critical evaluation of simple methods for the estimation of free testosterone in serum. *J Clin Endocrinol Metab* 1999; 84: 3666–72.

21. Winters SJ, Kelley DE, Goodpaster B. The analog free testosterone assay: are the results in man clinically useful? *Clin Chem* 1998; 44: 2178–82 [Erratum 1999; 45: 444].

22. Cheng RN, Reed MJ, James VHT. Plasma free testosterone: equilibrium dialysis vs direct radioimmunoassay. *Clin Chem* 1986; 32: 1411.

23. Miller KK, Rosner W, Lee H et al. Measurement of free testosterone in normal women and women with androgen deficiency: comparison of methods. *J Clin Endocrinol Metab* 2004; 89: 525–33.

24. Rosner W. An extraordinary inaccurate assay for free testosterone is still with us [Letter]. *J Clin Endocrinol Metab* 2001; 86: 2903.

25. Kapoor P, Luttrell B, Williams D. The free androgen index is not valid for adult males. *J Steroid Biochem Mol Biol* 1993; 45: 325–6.

26. Morley JE, Patrick P, Perry HM III. Evaluation of assays available to measure free testosterone. *Metabolism* 2002; 51: 554–9.

27. Emadi-Konjin P, Bain J, Bromberg IL. Evaluation of an algorithm for calculation of serum "bioavailable" testosterone (BAT). *Clin Biochem* 2003; 36: 591–6.

28. Bukowski C, Grigg MA, Longcope C. Sex-hormone-binding globulin concentrations: differences among commercially available methods. *Clin Chem* 2000; 46: 1415–16.

29. Matsumoto AM, Bremner WJ. Editorial: serum testosterone assays – accuracy matters. *J Clin Endocrinol Metab* 2004; 89: 520–4.

PSYCHOLOGIC TREATMENT OF FEMALE SEXUAL DYSFUNCTION

History of psychologic treatments

Harold I Lief, Richard C Friedman

Introduction

Although psychologic treatment might be seen to include counseling and education as well as psychotherapy, for the purposes of the chapter on the history of psychologic treatments (see Chapter 1.1 of this book), we are restricting our overview to psychotherapy. The history of the typology of female sexual dysfunction is confusing, and the nosology remains unsettled and controversial (see Chapter 9.1). Before turning to the diagnostic labeling of female sexual dysfunctions and the psychotherapeutic methods and approaches that have evolved over the past century, we need to examine how society and the helping professions have perceived female sexuality.

Views of female sexuality

Throughout history, women have been viewed through male eyes. Men have defined the roles of women and, for the most part, have succeeded in characterizing female sexuality in terms of procreation and parenting.[1] With few exceptions, usually those of queens, empresses, and concubines, women were socially and politically powerless. In what today would be called the Third World, they were savagely persecuted by men. For example, the practice of female circumcision, in which the clitoris and labia minora are excised and frequently much of the vagina is sutured closed, began before the birth of Christ in what are now Islamic countries and has continued to be practiced upon millions of women for hundreds of years since. This assault upon female sexuality is outlawed in many countries today but is widely practiced nonetheless. A common notion during various phases of Western European history was that women who were openly erotically expressive were instruments

of the devil, whose purpose was to acquire power over the otherwise rational minds of men.

The minimizing of women's sexual function persisted until the twentieth century, when the rise of feminism, in conjunction with a quasi-sexual revolution, made it appropriate for women to enjoy sex and to be assertive in seeking sexual gratification. However, conflicts between motherhood and occupational and sexual roles persist today, and are mirrored in societal confusion about what are appropriate roles for women.

Severe suppression of female sexuality continued into the nineteenth century, as women were moving from farms to factories during the Industrial Revolution and as class differences were accentuated. Women of the rising middle class, emulating upper-class society, became "ladies" for whom modesty was the most important virtue. Sexual desire, sexual drive, and female orgasm were taboo subjects for conversation as well as for study and research. As Bullough et al.[1] put it, "The world came to be made up of good girls and bad girls. The bad girls represented sexuality, the good girls purity of mind and spirit, unclouded by the shadow of any gross or vulgar thought".

Although there was a widespread trend toward this repressive view of female sexuality, there had been more enlightened views as well. For example, physicians of the seventeenth and eighteenth centuries equated female desire and receptivity with those of the male and made a sharp distinction between desire and coital response. Ellis stated that "all the old medical authors carefully distinguished between the heat of sexual desire and the actual presence of pleasure in coitus".[2] He regarded sexual impulse as a combination of interest (i.e., drive, desire) and responsivity (i.e., arousal, orgasm), and stated, in summary, "Such facts and considerations as these tend to show that the sexual impulse is by no means so weak in women as many would lead us to think".

Around 1900, when Freud was developing his psychoanalytic theories, the professional view of female sexuality approximated the views of society, namely, that women's sexual desire and responsivity were pale imitations of the more robust sexual drive in men. Modern clinicians sometimes forget that Freud's famous phallocentrism and sexism placed him in the mainstream of nineteenth- and early twentieth-century European thought. When Freud began publishing his work, women throughout the then modern world still could not vote. In some countries, women could not inherit property. It was in this climate that Freud developed his ideas about human sexual development and functioning out of his self-analysis, carried out in 1897. Observations he made about himself were hypothesized to have universal validity. As numerous psychoanalytic critics have skeptically observed, the first psychoanalysis involved the male as a subject and an object, indicating that Freud's ideas about the way a woman's mind works were flawed. One such idea was that the clitoris was a tiny and inadequate penis. With this premise, Freud developed the vaginal transfer theory that clitoral responsivity has to be superseded in a *mature woman* by coital (i.e., vaginal) orgasm. The idea of "penis envy", in which the inadequate female develops envy and possibly angry feelings toward the male, was another conclusion based on the false premise of clitoral insufficiency.

Freud believed that the young child's reaction to the difference between male and female genitalia and her or his concerns about possible genital damage (e.g., castration anxiety) were of universal importance in sexual development. Vicissitudes in the way children respond to the genital difference were responsible for much sexual pathology. One of his more provocative observations about female psychosexuality was in a discussion of the anatomic differences between the sexes:

> The feminist demand for equal rights for the sexes does not take us far, for the morphological distinction [e.g., in their genitalia] is bound to find expression in differences of psychical development. "Anatomy is destiny," to vary a saying of Napoleon. The little girl's clitoris behaves just like a penis to begin with; but when she makes a comparison with a playfellow of the other sex she perceives that she has "come off badly" and she feels this as a wrong done to her and as a ground for inferiority. The essential difference thus comes about that the girl accepts castration as an accomplished fact, whereas the boy fears the possibility of its occurrence.[3]

Freud suggested that women start life with a genital defect, awareness of which emerges by toddlerhood. The notion of universal penis envy in women was thought by Freud to be part of the biologic "bedrock"; an innate, inherent influence not only on sexual development, but also on the development of the total personality of all women. This idea is, of course, now discredited – as are many of Freud's other ideas about sexual development. These include the theory that all little girls take their mothers as their first sexual/romantic love objects and that this fundamentally erotic relationship stimulates their (clitoral)

masturbatory fantasies. As they grow older, however, "mature development" dictates that they relinquish this sexual fantasy tie in favor of an imagined coital relationship with their fathers. The wish to be sexually stimulated by mother is (hypothetically) replaced by the wish to have father's baby. This latter wish is the "Oedipus complex" in girls – only to be repressed and replaced by a period of latency (e.g., latent quiescent sexual desire). Freud hypothesized that boys as well as girls experience Oedipal desires and castration fears and that this "complex", normally repressed, can continue to exert pathologic effects throughout life if development is derailed. In fact, he attributed virtually all psychopathology to abnormal processing of Oedipal conflicts. For reasons that we cannot discuss here, Freud also thought that the complex sexual developmental pathway of girls is responsible for the fact that their conscience structure is not as fully developed as boys.[4]

Freud put forth his theories prior to the cascade of knowledge about child development that led to modern gender psychology. Virtually all of his speculations about female sexual development have been abandoned by modern clinicians. Freud was sufficiently grounded in reality and imaginative enough to recognize that new biologic findings might destroy his hypotheses. His bold prediction was, "On the other hand it should be made clear that the uncertainty of our speculation has been greatly increased by the necessity for borrowing from the science of biology. Biology is truly a land of unlimited possibilities. We may expect it to give us the most surprising information and we cannot guess what answers it will return in a few dozen years to the questions that we have put to it. They may be of a kind which will blow away the whole of our artificial structure of hypotheses."[5]

Freud's prediction came true. In 1953, the embryologist and endocrinologist Jost discovered that the "constitutional sex in mammalian fetal development is female" and that "a functioning ovary is not required for the female phenotype, whereas a testes is mandatory for male development".[6] Much research has demonstrated that the presence or absence of fetal testosterone organizes the fetal brain for later prototypically masculine or feminine behavior. Studies of females with congenital adrenal hyperplasia, of males with androgen insensitivity syndrome, and of patients with a variety of intersex disorders have been of particular value in this regard. Sex stereotypic behavior begins to be expressed during childhood well before puberty and at a time when no differences in sex steroid hormones are found between females and males.

In 1951, Ford and Beach[7] expressed the view that the clitoris plays a primary role, if not the only role, in the female orgastic response, and Kinsey and his colleagues[8] stated their belief that the vaginal orgasm is a biologic impossibility. In 1954, Judd Marmor[9] criticized Freud's theory of the nature of female orgasm, but it took the groundbreaking physiologic studies of Masters and Johnson in the early 1960s to produce more of the biologic facts that undermined the transfer theory. In 1961, Therese Benedek and Helene Deutsch attacked the transfer theory. For example, Benedek[10] stated, "the expectation that clitoral sensation should be transferred to the vagina is inconsistent with the distribution of the sensory cells responsible for the perception of orgasm"; according to Benedek, Deutsch held that the clitoris is the primary sexual organ. Their ideas were simply not acceptable to the majority of psychoanalysts, who still believed the original Freudian theory.

The new findings did not penetrate the psychoanalytic community. For example, the vaginal transfer theory remained the hypothesis for psychoanalytic treatment of women for decades after the biologic facts began to emerge. Perhaps a historical vignette will illustrate the nature of this travesty. In 1947, the senior author was a student of A.A. Brill, one of the first American psychoanalysts and the translator of many of Freud's early works. A small group of us assembled in Brill's office one day to discuss a patient who had come to him with deep depression. She had been in treatment for this with another psychoanalyst. During the course of that analysis, the other analyst discovered that his patient could not have an orgasm with intercourse. It is uncertain how the analyst phrased it, but he made it clear to his patient that it was her immaturity that was keeping her from having a vaginal orgasm. She had had no trouble having an orgasm with clitoral stimulation, but had not been able to reach orgasm during coitus. The analyst's words were such a blow to her self-esteem that her depression deepened. She had the good sense to leave this analyst and seek the help of Brill, who told her that the vaginal transfer theory was rubbish. At that point, no analyst had criticized the theory, at least in print, and it would be 6 or 7 years before a paper by Judd Marmor would be the initial critique. After the class was over, I lingered behind, thinking that Brill's conclusions were so important that they should be in the literature, so I asked why he did not develop and write up his observations. Brill looked stunned and flushed, almost as if I had struck him across the face, and it became apparent to me that writing something in direct opposition to Freud, the "Master", was unthinkable – this was 8 years after Freud had died. It was clear that the institution of psychoanalysis had the trappings of a church with doctrinal absolutism and demand for unquestioned fidelity to its belief system.

Psychoanalytic therapy based on psychoanalytic theory

For many years, psychoanalysts were less interested in the woman's sexual function than in object choice (mainly sexual orientation) and personality development. Convinced of the universality of the libido theory and the Oedipus complex, analysts looked for their manifestations in every case. Case histories mainly concerned inappropriate partner choices, personality development, and masochistic relationships. In turn, the consequence of erotic feelings toward father substitutes was the guilty fear that ensued. Limited attention was paid to the inhibition of sexuality, usually played out against the theoretic superstructure

described earlier. Some cases do make the psychoanalytic approach useful, however. A patient that the senior author saw at the Psychoanalytic Clinic of Columbia University is illustrative. A woman in her late twenties had married her lover, with whom she had had a very satisfactory sex life prior to marriage, including orgasm. On her wedding night, she found herself completely unresponsive. This lack of responsivity, of almost of any hint of arousal, continued for 10 months until she and her husband decided that there was no way that they could live together with this degree of sexual dissatisfaction. On the night that they separated, having had otherwise a satisfying relationship, they had sex and she was orgastic once again. As one might imagine, she had had a close, somewhat too dependent relationship with her father. (The dynamics in this case are much more common in men, creating what Freud termed the Madonna prostitute complex.) The guilty fear over her unconscious fixation on her father transferring to her husband by virtue of the symbolism of marriage is an example of unconscious mental processes, arguably the most important of Freud's contributions.

In the treatment of sexual dysfunctions, the primary emphasis for many years was on the woman's failure to have an orgasm during coitus. It was not until midcentury that doubts were expressed about the vaginal transfer theory. It takes a long time for criticisms to change belief systems. If only the analysts had been able to follow the dictum of Sandor Rado, who told his students, "Don't marry a theory in a state that does not recognize divorce."

Cognitive-behavioral therapy

The field of sex therapy was radically changed by the innovative research and clinical work of Masters and Johnson (see Chapters 17.2 and 17.3). Their ideas were presented in two books, *Human Sexual Response* (1966)[11] and *Human Sexual Inadequacy* (1970).[12] Until then, the only form of therapy was psychoanalytic or psychodynamic psychotherapy based on psychoanalytic theory and observations. With the results of Masters and Johnson's treatment protocol, cognitive-behavioral therapy of sexual dysfunctions was widely accepted and practiced.

For the clinician, the most important findings of Masters and Johnson were as follows:

1. There is no separate vaginal orgasm; indeed, there is no such thing as a vaginal orgasm, although orgasm may occur during coitus.
2. The human female has the capacity to have intense and multiple orgasms without a refractory period. After males experience orgasm, there is a variable period of time when they are "refractory" to sexual stimulation and arousal. This is not true of females.
3. There are four stages of the human sexual response: excitement, plateau, orgasmic phase, and the resolution phase.
4. There is a need to treat the couple rather than an individual.

Masters and Johnson's studies also indicated that there is great variability between women in their sexual response profiles, whereas men seem to follow a linear progression from excitement to plateau to orgasm, to resolution, to refractory period. Different women seem to follow different pathways. Responses may include a single orgasm, multiple orgasms, extreme sexual excitement/arousal without an apparent orgasm, or even orgasm without awareness of arousal, yet fall within a range experienced as being normal by a particular woman or couple. The four points described above became the bedrock of sexual therapy carried out by sexologists over the last quarter of a century. Later, the desire phase was added to the four phases described by Masters and Johnson, to make a five-phase approach.

Some early efforts at behavioral therapy preceded the work of Masters and Johnson. For example, in 1963, Arnold Lazarus[13] treated "frigidity" with systematic desensitization. Early behavioral therapists proceeded on the assumption that behavioral changes would create changes in attitude. In order to avoid cognitive dissonance, it was assumed that the patient would change her attitudes so that they would be congruent with her changed behavior. This was just the opposite of the thinking of psychoanalysts, who had always assumed that it was necessary to change attitudes before there would be behavioral changes.

The principles of behavioral therapy as reported by Bancroft in 1977[14] still remain the key elements of this type of therapy. Those principles are (1) systematic desensitization, (2) shaping of fantasies, (3) operant methods, and (4) role rehearsal. There is an overlap between the operant methods of appraisal and systematic desensitization. In this approach, actual behaviors are described in detail in a hierarchal positioning from the least to the most troublesome. With systematic desensitization, these behaviors from the least to the most anxiety-provoking are faced in fantasy and then in reality. This includes homework assignments from session to session. In each session, the difficulties encountered in carrying out the assignments or the negative affects evoked are discussed. Rewarding positive reinforcers and eliminating negative ones are key concepts. As Bancroft states, "The patient is always given something to do between sessions, and not only does this represent behavioral progress during treatment, but it is a remarkably powerful method for revealing the underlying problems and the attitudes that block change". He made this statement at a time before cognitive therapy had begun to dominate the thinking of therapists and before the integration of cognitive and behavioral therapy. It is therefore of interest to see the comment, "It is in the modification of such attitudes that the behavioral approach is less clearly defined and it is here that the main source of variance between therapists, and overlap with other psychotherapeutic approaches occurs". The early behavioral therapists, while generally subscribing to the dictum that "behavioral changes precede attitudinal changes", began to recognize that change would not take place simply by changing behavior; attitudes had to change as well. In some cases, attitudes were changed by behavioral changes, but in others they were not. Therefore, attention had to be paid directly to attitude change. In was in this setting that cognitive therapy arose. Attitudes could be changed by changes in cognitions or beliefs. Getting at thoughts, often preconscious, that triggered maladaptive behaviors was the key to cognitive therapy. It was in this way that behavioral therapy metamorphosed into cognitive-behavioral therapy.

It should be noted that the history of psychologic treatments is a history of steps in integrative psychotherapy. We have already seen one such step, namely, the integration of behavioral and cognitive therapies. Another step was the integration of individual and couple therapy. A third step was the integration of cognitive-behavioral therapy with psychodynamic or interpersonal therapies. At about the time (c.1970) that Masters and Johnson published their first report of their treatment methods, cognitive-behavioral therapy was just getting started, and psychologic therapy for women's sexual dysfunction, psychoanalytic or briefer forms of psychodynamic psychotherapy, was still dominant.

In reviewing Masters and Johnson's methods, it is clear that they used the principles of behavior therapy. Emphasizing sensual rather than erotic pleasure, and only gradually approaching vaginal penetration, is a form of systematic desensitization. Giving homework assignments between sessions, monitoring the couple's responses, using positive reinforcers, and eliminating negative reinforcers is a form of operant conditioning. Role behavior, including role rehearsal, is an additional attribute of the method of Masters and Johnson. While exploration of fantasies does not seem to play an important role, Masters and Johnson's methods certainly led to the unearthing of beliefs and attitudes, allowing the negative ones to be constantly challenged. Cognition was hardly neglected. A major emphasis was on effective communication. In this way it can be said that their methods were not behavioral alone; they were cognitive-behavioral therapy. Perhaps, in the long run, the major contribution of Masters and Johnson will turn out to be their insistence on couple therapy and their de-emphasis of therapy aimed at the individual.

Couple sex therapy

Couple sex therapy was given an enormous boost by the methods of Masters and Johnson. In the treatment of individual patients there had always been two key issues: (1) how nonsexual problems in a relationship affected the sexual function of the patient and (2) how changes in therapy would play out in the relationship. Masters and Johnson dealt with this head-on. They insisted on seeing only couples in a committed relationship and treating both at the same time. In at least half their cases, both partners had significant sexual problems and, even if that was not the case, relationship factors played an integral role in the development of symptoms of sexual dysfunction and in the process of therapy. By handing out homework assignments (as in behavioral therapy), they were able to elicit nonsexual problems, such as those dealing with power, intimacy, communication, respect, and role conflict, and discover the negative reinforcers used by the couple. By using systematic desensitization surrounding sensate focus, they enabled the couple to overcome negative affects, such as shame, anxiety, and anger. They also rewarded positive responses to increasing sensual and erotic pleasure through words of encouragement, thus changing the couple's attitudes. The use of conjoint therapists reinforced the notion that sexual problems existed in the context of a relationship.

Despite the therapy research of Masters and Johnson demonstrating the effectiveness of couple therapy for sexual dysfunctions, couple therapy expanded slowly. Perhaps this was due to a need for a therapist to learn two methods of approach; relationship therapy as well as sex therapy. Most training programs emphasized only one approach or the other. McCarthy et al.,[15] in a chapter on the integration of sex and couple therapy citing Basson, noted that sexual responsivity in women is usually limited to "an opportunity to be sexual, an awareness of the potential benefits to her and the relationship". Facilitating that responsivity occurs when the woman learns to develop her "sexual voice" so that "she can request the type and sequence of touching and erotic scenarios that promote her sexual receptivity and responsivity." They define the woman's sexual voice as her sexual and erotic feelings and needs. Recognizing these, she can proceed at her own pace rather than be driven by the man's erection and his needs. Another guiding principle is that a woman's orgasm is much more varied than a man's. There are a variety of normal sexual response patterns; certainly, the inability to have an orgasm during vaginal penetration is not a sexual dysfunction. Included in couple therapy is the enhancement of bridges to sexual desire, the essence of which is positive anticipation and the woman's feeling that she deserves sexual pleasure.

The integration of cognitive-behavioral therapy and dynamic psychotherapy

We have discussed how behavior therapy became integrated with the field of cognitive psychology leading to cognitive-behavioral therapy. As Goldfried[16] puts it, "Although desensitization was found to be very effective clinically, there were instances where one could readily observe that cognitively mediated anxiety undermined its effectiveness". What drew psychodynamic therapists to cognitive-behavioral therapy was the recognition that the notion of "schema" could be a useful bridge between the two modalities. Cognitive-behavioral therapy was heavily reliant on the "here and now" appraisal of a patient's problems, whereas psychodynamic therapies made extensive use of past experiences, including past relationships. Schema refers to a cognitive representation of one's past experiences in situations or with people. It organizes one's perceptions based on these past experiences and serves as a filter through

which a person perceives current events in his or her life. It is selective in that it takes in those perceptions that fit the schema and excludes perceptions that do not seem to fit. In this way it is self-reinforcing. Briefly, it is the way we organize our perceptions based on past experience. It also serves to integrate perceptions and emotional reactions which tend to occur automatically in similar situations. In some ways this resembles Freud's "repetition compulsion" and is manifest in transference phenomena. The analysis of schemas allows the therapist to understand the beliefs, attitudes, and accompanying emotions that may enhance, but too often undermine, sexual satisfaction.

The commonalities between cognitive-behavioral therapy and psychodynamic psychotherapy are far greater than the differences. The goal of reducing the anxiety that leads to the inhibition of pleasure-seeking behavior or of pleasure itself and the goal of reducing or eliminating maladaptive behaviors that decrease the chances of intimacy are the same for both modalities. Therapy techniques used to seek or reach these goals are also similar. These include increasing the woman's capacity to identify her thoughts and feelings, her bodily sensations, and eventually her schemas and scripts. This helps the woman feel safe and secure in situations that provoke anxiety by providing her with corrective emotional experiences[17] brought about by desensitization, role rehearsal, repetition of positive behaviors, recognition of positive responses in her partner, and changes in her own feelings and sensations. As a woman's fearful expectations and negative responses are replaced by pleasurable anticipation, she begins to sense her own potential for growth and the new possibilities in her relationship with her partner.

The linkage between cognitive-behavioral therapy and psychodynamic psychotherapy is provided by the analysis of schemas and scripts. The perceptual mindsets and the consequent rules for sex-oriented behaviors become the centerpiece of therapy. If it tilts to the behavioral end of the spectrum, less attention is paid to schemas (they may never be identified to the patient), and attention is moved to the changed behaviors themselves. The more psychodynamic, the greater the attention to the less-than-conscious aspects of the schema.

The exploration of dreams and fantasies may be very helpful in uncovering psychic material that the patient may resist becoming conscious of. If dream metaphors are analyzed in terms of themes and are connected to the emotional events in the day or two preceding the dream, the underlying schema through which the patient views herself in the world may come into focus. The therapist must avoid using dreams as a way of uncovering childhood trauma. That path is treacherous, as "recovered memory" therapists have discovered. If sexual abuse in childhood has been corroborated, the connection between trauma, dreams, and fantasies may be useful.

Impetus to the integration of psychodynamic therapy with cognitive-behavioral therapy came from the clinical studies of Helen Kaplan. In *The New Sex Therapy*, published in 1974, Kaplan[18] stated, "When sexual exercises are combined with psychotherapy conducted with skill and sensitivity, psychotherapy becomes immensely important, and in fact, is indispensable to the success of the new sex therapy" (p 221). Kaplan, probably projecting herself as the ideal therapist, set out requirements for sex therapy that few could claim. She said, "A sex therapist should have extensive knowledge of the theory and practice of psychoanalysis, marital therapy, and behavior therapy, and know how and when to apply these theoretic and therapeutic concepts to the couple's specific sexual problems" (p 222).

Kaplan used her knowledge of psychoanalysis and psychotherapy and of sex therapy in a very specific and limited way. She suggested that dynamic therapy be used to overcome the blocks or impediments to more effective sexual function. In this way, she hoped to keep sex therapy a short-term therapy of a few weeks to a few months, and to avoid the lengthy treatment usually associated with psychoanalysis. It is not at all clear how many sex therapists have been able to carry out this type of integrative model of sex therapy. We suspect that it remains more of an ideal than a realized model.

In the 1970s, sexual desire was added to the four parts of the response cycle set forth by Masters and Johnson. Although Lief[19] was the first clinician in the modern era to describe inhibited sexual desire as a serious clinical problem, Kaplan[20] developed the concept in detail. This led to a change in the classification of women's sexual dysfunction to include problems of desire along with problems of arousal and orgasm.

Nosology

There used to be a single category for women's sexual problems termed "frigidity". The historical development of the classification of women's sexual dysfunction can be traced in the successive editions of the *Diagnostic and Statistical Manual of Mental Disorders* (DSM) described elsewhere in this book. The sexual experiences of women are so much more varied than those of men that the classification of women's sexual dysfunction has become a battleground for people of diverse and intense beliefs.[21] The main objections to the current DSM (fourth edition; DSM-IV) classification are as follows:

1. The medical model of women's sexual function is male-based and orgasm-centered.
2. The biopsychosocial model is discarded in favor of a biologic model.
3. The standard for sexual function in the female is based on the human sexual response cycle as defined by Masters and Johnson and modified by Kaplan. Selection bias is a problem in their research. In other words, the volunteer subjects in Masters and Johnson's studies were nonrepresentative, as they were orgastic, came from a particular social class, and were enthusiasts about becoming good sexual "performers". It is questionable whether the "cycle" discussed by Masters and Johnson should be considered a norm.
4. The DSM-IV classification is based on symptom description rather than etiology, and presumes that etiologies, including

social, personal, relational, or medical ones, should be the basis of classification.
5. Satisfaction in sexual experiences may involve intimacy, comfort, safety, self-validation, power-sharing, or other experiences not entirely or even specifically erotic.
6. Sexual desire is multifaceted and therefore must always be viewed with a biopsychosocial perspective.
7. The desynchronization of psychologic sexual arousal and physiologic excitement (i.e., vasocongestion/lubrication) is so frequent that a "normal" sexual response is impossible to identify and label.
8. Sexual satisfaction is dependent on factors other than orgastic capacity, which may play no role or a limited role.

It is for all these reasons that female sexual response is so varied and so resistant to arbitrary classification.

Conclusions

If we compare 1900 with 2000, it is clear that enormous strides have been made in understanding woman's sexual function and in the sophistication of psychologic methods of treatment of dysfunction. Sexual responses in females are much more varied than in males, and sexual dysfunctions are more difficult to diagnose. Treatment has to be based on a biopsychosocial perspective (see Chapter 17.6), has to be multifaceted, has to be oriented toward the woman's relationships, and, wherever possible, has to involve the partner in couple therapy. Sexual problems provide an excellent opportunity for the integration of a number of therapeutic modalities, including cognitive-behavioral and psychodynamic, individual and couple, and biologic and psychologic.

References

1. Bullough VL, Shelton B, Slavin S. *The Subordinated Sex: A History of Attitudes Toward Women*. Athens: University of Georgia Press, 1988.
2. Ellis H. The sexual impulse in women. In *Studies in the Psychology of Sex*, vol 3. New York: Random House, 1905 (1942 edn): 189–256.
3. Freud S. The dissolution of the Oedipus complex [1924]. In *The Standard Edition of the Works of Freud*, vol 19. London: Hogarth Press, 1953–66: 172–9.
4. Friedman RC, Downey JI. *Sexual Orientation and Psychoanalysis*. New York: Columbia University Press, 2002.
5. Freud S. *Beyond the Pleasure Principle* [1920]. In *The Standard Edition of the Works of Freud*, vol 18 (1955). London: Hogarth Press, 1953–66: 3–64; cited in Sherfey MJ. *The Nature and Evaluation of Female Sexuality*. New York: Random House, 1972.
6. Hughes IA. Fetal development – all by default? *N Engl J Med* 2004; 351: 748–50.

7. Ford CS, Beach FA. *Patterns of Sexual Behavior.* New York: Harper, 1951.

8. Kinsey A, Pomeroy WB, Martin CE et al. *Sexual Behavior in the Human Female.* Philadelphia: WB Saunders, 1953.

9. Marmor J. Some considerations concerning orgasm in the female. *Psychosom Med* 1954; 16: 240–5.

10. Benedek T. On orgasm and frigidity in women. *J Am Psychoanal Assoc* 1961; 571–84.

11. Masters WH, Johnson VE. *Human Sexual Response.* Boston: Little, Brown, 1966.

12. Masters WH, Johnson VE. *Human Sexual Inadequacy.* Boston: Little, Brown, 1970.

13. Lazarus AA. The treatment of chronic frigidity by systematic desensitization. *J Nerv Ment Dis* 1963; 136: 272–8.

14. Bancroft J. The behavioral approach to treatment. In J Money, J Musaph, eds. *Handbook of Sexology.* Amsterdam: Excerpta Medica, 1977: 1197–1225.

15. McCarthy BW, Bodnar LE, Handal M. Integrating sex therapy and couple therapy. In JH Harvey, A Wenzel, S Sprecher, eds. *The Handbook of Sexuality in Close Relationships.* London: Erlbaum Associates, 2004: 573–93.

16. Goldfried MR. *From Cognitive Behavior Therapy to Psychotherapy Integration.* New York: Springer, 1955.

17. Alexander F. The dynamics of psychotherapy in light of learning theory. *Am J Psychiatry* 1963; 120: 440–8.

18. Kaplan HS. *The New Sex Therapy. Active Treatment of Sexual Dysfunctions.* New York: Brunner/Mazel, 1974.

19. Lief HI. What's new in sex research? Inhibited sexual desire. *Med Aspects Hum Sex* 1977; 11: 94–5.

20. Kaplan HS. *Disorders of Sexual Desire.* New York: Brunner/Mazel, 1979.

21. Kaschak E, Tiefer L. *A New View of Women's Sexual Problems.* New York: Haworth Press, 2001.

11.2 Psychologic assessment and self-report questionnaires in women: subjective measures of female sexual dysfunction

Raymond C Rosen, Jennifer L Barsky

Introduction and overview

Despite the prevalence (see Chapters 2.1–2.3 of this book) and frequent distress (see Chapter 2.4) associated with sexual dysfunction in women, there are few standardized or evidence-based methods available to assess women's sexual function (see Chapters 9.1–9.5). This is a significant concern for researchers and clinicians alike, for whom the lack of available measures has served as a significant barrier to clinical research and treatment of sexual problems in women. In contrast, sexual problems in men, such as erectile dysfunction, are routinely diagnosed and assessed by means of either physiologic methods (e.g., Rigiscan) or standardized and widely used self-report instruments (e.g., International Index of Erectile Function).[1,2] Currently available techniques for measuring physiologic arousal in women, such as vaginal photoplethysmography or pelvic magnetic resonance imaging, have not proven to be sufficiently sensitive or reliable for diagnosis or assessment of clinical outcomes associated with treatment.[3] Although vaginal photoplethysmography (see Chapter 10.1) and other laboratory methods (see Chapters 10.2–10.7) have provided valuable insights into the interplay of physiologic and psychologic processes in women's sexual arousal, the clinical utility or "real-world" application of these methods is extremely limited. Instead, assessment of sexual function and dysfunction in women is based almost exclusively on self-report measures, including structured interviews, diary or event log measures, or, most commonly, self-report questionnaires. These latter measures are reviewed in detail in this chapter.

Prior to considering the psychometric properties and application of these measures, some key theoretic and conceptual points are worth noting. First, the definitions and classification of sexual dysfunction in women are undergoing rapid change and evolution.[4,5] Major changes have been proposed in the categories of desire and arousal disorders in particular, which may necessitate development of new foci and methods of assessment (e.g., subjective sexual arousal) (see Chapter 9.1). Second, the linear sexual response cycle model, first proposed by Masters and Johnson[6] and modified subsequently by Kaplan,[7] has been strongly criticized in recent years for failing to emphasize the psychologic complexities of sexual desire in women, and the importance of subjective aspects of female sexual response. It is uncertain what effect these new models of sexual response will have on self-report measures in women. Third, the sensitivity of current self-report measures to treatment response has been difficult to assess in the absence of well-defined and effective treatments for women's sexual dysfunction. Thus, while there is evidence for discriminant and convergent validity of various self-report measures,[8] the paucity of data supporting their sensitivity to treatment effects is a major omission to be addressed in future clinical trials.

Models of sexual response in women: the interplay of subjective and physiologic factors

The sexual response cycle model, developed originally by Masters and Johnson[6] and modified subsequently by Kaplan[7] and others, consists of a linear progression of sexual desire, arousal, and orgasm in both men and women. This influential model forms the basis of both the diagnostic classification system for sexual dysfunction in both genders, and the corresponding self-report measures used to assess disturbances in each phase of the sexual response cycle. Despite its widespread adoption, criticism has been directed at the conceptual and clinical foundations of the traditional sexual response cycle model. Alternative formulations have recently been proposed, most notably the cyclical or interactive sexual response cycle model of Basson,[9] in which sexual desire and arousal are conceptualized as interactive and mutually reinforcing aspects of sexual response. Sexual and emotional satisfaction are viewed as integral components of the process of sexual response in women. According to this model, the physiologic and subjective aspects of sexual response are described as separate, albeit integral components of sexual response. A new classification schema for sexual dysfunction in women has recently been proposed, in which separate categories of genital and subjective arousal disorder are described in detail.[5] An obvious consequence of the revised sexual response cycle model and diagnostic classification schema has been to focus increasing attention on assessing subjective aspects of sexual response in women.

Assessment methods

Self-administered questionnaires

Although subjective sexual function can be assessed in several ways, the preferred and most widely used method is the self-administered questionnaire. Self-administered questionnaires have the advantages of assessing multiple components of sexual response, ease of administration and scoring, and ability to be translated and adapted for use in multinational settings. The principal limitation of self-administered questionnaires is that they do not directly assess physiologic aspects of sexual response; consequently, information about the genital aspects of sexual response is necessarily indirect and possibly less reliable

than other responses. This may be especially true in women, as past research has frequently shown a marked discordance between subjective and physiologic aspects of female sexual response.[10,11]

At present, several self-administered questionnaires are in widespread use, including the Brief Index of Sexual Functioning for Women,[12,13] the Female Sexual Function Index,[14] and the Sexual Function Questionnaire.[15] These self-administered questionnaires typically assess sexual functioning across a number of domains (e.g., sexual desire, arousal, orgasm, satisfaction) and measure average responses over a specified time period (e.g., 4 weeks). Scoring algorithms are provided for each of the sexual functioning domains and the entire questionnaire.

In selecting a self-administered questionnaire measure for use in a clinical trial, several criteria should be considered. Overall, self-administered questionnaires have been much more widely used in outpatient (at-home) treatment studies in both men and women. These measures are also most suitable when used in a prospective study design, in which each patient is assessed before and after a treatment intervention in order to assess changes associated with treatment.

Event logs and daily diaries

A variety of event logs and daily diaries have been used in clinical trials of male and female sexual dysfunction. Diaries or event logs are designed to be completed after each episode of sexual activity and assess sexual functioning and satisfaction during each sexual episode. There are currently no standardized or validated sexual event logs for women, although several instruments have been proposed or are currently in development. Results from the sexual event log are typically regarded as primary or secondary endpoints from a regulatory perspective. According to the US Food and Drug Administration Guidance Document of Female Sexual Dysfunction, event log measures of satisfying sexual events should be used as primary endpoints in clinical trials of female sexual dysfunction.

Structured interviews

Assessments that are directly administered by the researcher, such as the Derogatis Interview for Sexual Functioning,[16] can provide more detailed and specific information about sexual functioning. Although the breadth of information that can be obtained from an interview is potentially valuable, structured interviews are more time-consuming to administer than self-administered questionnaires and are potentially more burden-some for both patients and investigators. To date, this assessment strategy has seldom been used in clinical trials.

Criteria for assessment instruments

The two most fundamental and desirable characteristics for measures of sexual function in women are reliability and validity. Reliability refers to the consistency or replicability of results, with reliability coefficients serving as quantitative indicators of measurement consistency. Validity reflects the degree to which an instrument measures what it purports to measure. Unlike reliability, which is established through a specific, rigorously prescribed series of statistical exercises, the validation of a measuring instrument is ongoing and iterative in nature.

The two essential indicators of validity for measures of sexual function are discriminant validity and sensitivity to therapeutically induced change. The former refers to an instrument's capacity to discriminate sexually dysfunctional individuals from persons without sexual problems (sensitivity and specificity in epidemiologic terms, or discriminant validity in psychometric terms), while the latter criterion refers to an instrument's sensitivity to clinical change associated with treatment (longitudinal validity in psychometric terms). These are both essential criteria of measures designed to serve as diagnostic and/or treatment efficacy measures in either clinical or research settings. The reliability and validity of the most widely used self-administered questionnaire measures for female sexual function are described below.

Specific self-administered questionnaires for assessment of female sexual function

Self-report measures, such as questionnaires and daily diaries, are greatly preferred to other assessment methods for large-scale, multicenter trials. Simple self-report scales, such as the International Index of Erectile Function, have been shown to be highly sensitive and reliable indicators of treatment efficacy in men,[1,2] and efforts have been made to achieve a similar degree of precision and reliability with self-administered questionnaires for female sexual function.

Brief Index of Sexual Functioning for Women

Description

This is a 22-item, multidimensional, self-report measure for women that assesses sexual function in seven dimensions: sexual thoughts/desires, arousal, frequency of activity, receptivity/initiation, pleasure/orgasm, relationship satisfaction, and sexual problems.[12] In addition to these domain scores, this measure yields an overall composite score. It takes about 15–20 min to complete and is intended for use among both clinical and nonclinical samples of heterosexual and homosexual women.

Psychometric evaluation

The Brief Index of Sexual Functioning for Women was validated in a normative sample of 225 healthy women aged 22–55 years, 187 of whom had sexual partners, and in a clinical sample of 104 surgically menopausal women of the same age with impaired sexual function.[13] This measure was able to discriminate between normal women with and without sexual partners

and between the normative and clinical sample groups on six out of seven dimensions and overall composite scores. In particular, the surgically menopausal women scored the lowest on the domains pertaining to sexual desire, arousal, and frequency of activity. The internal consistency of this measure ranged from 0.39 for the arousal domain to 0.72 for the dimensions of sexual desire and orgasm. Test–retest reliability of the original three-factor scores ranged from 0.68 to 0.78 at baseline and a 1-month interval. A high concurrent validity was found through comparison with relevant scales of the Derogatis Interview for Sexual Function.[16] Recently, this measure was found to be sensitive to effects of testosterone therapy in a sample of women with bilateral oophoectomy.[17]

Comments

The Brief Index of Sexual Functioning for Women was one of the first self-administered questionnaires of female sexual function and satisfaction to provide a detailed assessment of broad areas of function. One of the weaknesses of this measure is a relatively low internal consistency for three of the seven domains. Some of these inconsistencies may result from the fact that the design of this measure was based largely on the male version, the Brief Sexual Function Questionnaire. Thus, some of the items in this measure may not be as specific to female sexual function as more recently developed instruments.

Sexual Function Questionnaire (SFQ)

Description

The Sexual Function Questionnaire is a brief, multidimensional, patient-centered measure of women's sexual functioning that was developed for use in clinical trials.[15] Items were generated through semistructured interviews with 82 women aged 19–65 years old from seven countries (UK, USA, Australia, the Netherlands, Denmark, France, and Italy) and included women with and without female sexual dysfunction. Phrases used by these women to describe experiences of female sexual dysfunction were incorporated into the measure. Through factor analysis, seven domains of women's sexual functioning were identified: desire, physical arousal-sensation, physical arousal-lubrication, enjoyment, orgasm, pain, and partner relationship. The Sexual Function Questionnaire can be used in three forms: a 34-item version that consists of the seven domains mentioned plus additional items and the arousal-cognitive domain, a 26-item version that consists of seven domains, and a short-item version (Abbreviated Sexual Function Questionnaire) that includes four of the seven domains (desire, arousal-sensation, arousal-lubrication, and orgasm). This measure takes 10–15 min to complete and is intended for women in a sexual relationship or who have participated in sexual activity within the previous month.

Psychometric evaluation

This measure was initially validated in a sample of 982 women aged 19–65 years. The sample included women both with and without a clinical diagnosis of female sexual dysfunction.[15]

Internal consistency of the domains was reasonably high, with Cronbach's alphas ranging from 0.65 to 0.91. Test–retest reliability was conducted over a 4-week period, and coefficients ranged from 0.42 to 0.78 for individual items. Discriminant validity for this measure was high; women with sexual dysfunction scored significantly lower than women without dysfunction on all seven domains at baseline. In addition, all seven domains of the Sexual Function Questionnaire were able to discriminate between women who reported improvement in their sexual functioning at the end of the study (responders) and those who reported no improvement (nonresponders). Construct validity was found to be acceptable through correlations between the Sexual Function Questionnaire domains and relevant domains of the Derogatis Interview for Sexual Functioning,[16] the Fugl-Meyer Life Satisfaction Checklist,[18] and the Hospital Anxiety and Depression Scale.[19]

Female Sexual Function Index (FSFI)

Description

The Female Sexual Function Index is a 19-item, multidimensional, self-report instrument used to assess key domains of female sexual function.[14] This measure was initially designed to assess female sexual arousal disorder. Responses are based on sexual activity within the past 4 weeks. Six domains were identified through a factor analysis: desire, subjective arousal, lubrication, orgasm, satisfaction, and pain. A full-scale score that represents overall sexual function may be calculated from the domain scores. This measure takes about 15 min to complete and is intended for use in clinical trial and community populations and among both heterosexual and homosexual women.

Psychometric evaluation

This measure was initially validated in a sample of 128 heterosexual women with female sexual arousal disorder and 131 age-matched heterosexual healthy women aged 21–69 years.[14] Internal consistency was high, as all domains had Cronbach's alphas above 0.82. Test–retest reliability was high over a 2–4-week period, ranging from 0.79 to 0.86 for the domains, and 0.88 for the full-scale score. Significantly lower scores were reported by women with female sexual arousal disorder in all domains and overall, demonstrating discriminant validity. The largest differences between the groups were in the domains of lubrication and arousal. A second study showed the Female Sexual Function Index subscales and full-scale score to discriminate reliably between women without sexual dysfunction and women with female orgasmic disorder.[20] Recently, discriminant validity was further established in samples of women with hypoactive sexual desire disorder, sexual pain disorders, and multiple sexual dysfunctions.[21]

Divergent validity was established through comparison with the Locke–Wallace Marital Adjustment Test.[22] In the first study, correlations between the relevant domains on these scales were of modest size, ranging from 0.19 for the desire subscale, to 0.57 for the satisfaction with partner subscale, in the full sample of both female sexual arousal disorder patients and controls. The full-scale score yielded a correlation of 0.41 with the Locke–Wallace Marital Adjustment Test.[14] These expected levels of association between the theoretically related constructs of sexual function and marital adjustment support the construct validity of the Female Sexual Function Index. The second validation supported these findings regarding the divergent validity of the Female Sexual Function Index with the same comparison scale.

Comments

The Female Sexual Function Index is easy to administer and score, and is currently being used in a number of clinical trials. This measure has been extensively studied and has generally been shown to perform extremely well in psychometric analyses. However, this scale has not yet been evaluated for its specificity to treatment-related change.

Menopausal Sexual Interest Questionnaire (MSIQ)

Description

This measure is a very brief (10-item), unidimensional instrument that measures sexual function in postmenopausal women.[23] Although the Menopausal Sexual Interest Questionnaire includes some items addressing other aspects of sexual response, this measure primarily focuses on sexual desire, given the prevalence of hypoactive sexual desire disorder in postmenopausal women. Initial item selection was performed by a panel of experts in the field of sexual dysfunction, and pilot testing was then conducted with women attending menopause management groups at 18 sites across the USA. Three domains were identified through factor analysis: desire, responsiveness, and satisfaction; however, the constructs assessed by these domains seem to overlap considerably. A full-scale score is also available. This measure takes approximately 5 min to complete and is intended for use by postmenopausal women.

Psychometric evaluation

This measure was validated in a sample of 111 postmenopausal women without hypoactive sexual desire disorder and an age-matched sample of 221 women with a clinical diagnosis of hypoactive sexual desire disorder who were participating in a treatment trial.[23] Internal consistency of the three domains was very high. Cronbach's alphas for the items within each domain were 0.87 and higher. One-month test–retest reliability was acceptable, with Pearson coefficients ranging from 0.52 to 0.76 for individual items and 0.79 for the overall scale. Each Menopausal Sexual Interest Questionnaire domain and the full score were able to discriminate between women with and without hypoactive sexual desire disorder. Convergent validity was established through comparison with the thought/desire domain of the Brief Index of Sexual Functioning for Women (BISF-W)[12] and found to be high, yielding a correlation coefficient of 0.82

for the desire domain of the Menopausal Sexual Interest Questionnaire, and 0.81 for the full-scale score. Divergent validity was established by comparing the full-scale score of the Menopausal Sexual Interest Questionnaire with the anxiety and depression domains of the Kellner Symptom Questionnaire (KSQ)[24] and the sexual domain of the Menopause Specific Quality of Life Questionnaire (MENQOL).[25] The correlations were −0.002, −0.14, and −0.42, respectively. These findings support the construct validity of the Menopausal Sexual Interest Questionnaire. The Menopausal Sexual Interest Questionnaire also demonstrated sensitivity to therapeutic effects in a clinical trial, showing increases in scores pre- to post-treatment among self-identified responders, but not in nonresponders.[23]

Profile of Female Sexual Function (PFSF)

Description

The Profile of Female Sexual Function is a somewhat lengthy (37-item), patient-centered, multidimensional measure that targets the assessment of low sexual desire and associated symptoms in postmenopausal women suffering from hypoactive sexual desire disorder.[26] This measure was developed and tested for language coherence through interviews with surgically and naturally menopausal women from the USA, Germany, the UK, Italy, France, the Netherlands, Canada, and Australia. This scale consists of six domains: sexual pleasure, sexual desire, responsiveness, arousal, orgasm, sexual self-image, and sexual concerns. This measure is intended for use in clinical trial populations.

Psychometric evaluation

This scale was validated in a sample of 325 oophorectomized women with hypoactive sexual desire disorder and an age-matched sample of 255 premenopausal control women in the USA, Canada, Europe, and Australia.[26] Cronbach's alpha coefficients, assessing internal consistency within each of the domains, ranged from 0.79 to 0.96 in the low-libido group and 0.50 to 0.96 in the control group. Intraclass correlation coefficients reflecting 2-week test–retest reliability ranged from 0.52 to 0.90 in the low-libido group and from 0.66 to 0.92 in the control group. A second validation study including naturally menopausal women[27] found similar results to support the internal consistency (Cronbach's alpha = 0.74–0.95), and 4-week test-retest reliability (intraclass correlation coefficients = 0.57–0.91) of the six domains. Domain intercorrelations ranged from 0.18 to 0.66, with a median of 0.50, indicating relatively little redundancy. The Profile of Female Sexual Function and its individual domains discriminated between oophorectomized women with low libido and age-matched controls across geographic regions.[26] Discriminant validity was further supported in samples of both surgically and naturally menopausal women with hypoactive sexual desire disorder.[27] The sensitivity, specificity, and positive predictive value of this measure were calculated according to each domain, and ranged from 0.67 to 0.94, 0.86 to 0.95, and 0.86 to 0.94, respectively. Convergent validity was established through statistically significant correlations with relevant domains of the Derogatis Sexual Functioning Inventory (DSFI-SR).

Comments

The Profile of Female Sexual Function has demonstrated excellent psychometric properties and is notable for its international patient-based development and validation. However, the Profile of Female Sexual Function is not yet readily available for general use in clinical trials.

Female Sexual Distress Scale (FSDS)

Description

This is a 12-item, unidimensional scale measuring sexual distress in women.[28] The Female Sexual Distress Scale was developed to reflect recent classifications of female sexual dysfunction that take into account sexually related personal distress as an important factor in the diagnosis of female sexual dysfunction.[4] Prior to this measure, no methods of evaluating sexually related personal distress were available. This measure takes about 5 min to complete and is intended for use with women presenting for an evaluation concerning sexual dysfunction.

Psychometric evaluation

The reliability of the Female Sexual Distress Scale was established over the course of three separate clinical trials, consisting of a control group and several groups of women with various sexual dysfunctions.[28] Through a principal components analysis, items that did not load substantially on a principal component of the original 20 items were eliminated, leaving a 12-item version. Internal consistency of the items in this measure was very high, with Cronbach's alphas ranging from 0.86 to 0.97. Test–retest reliability coefficients ranged from 0.80 to 0.92. Discriminant validity was established through comparisons between both naturally and surgically menopausal women and healthy age-matched controls. In this trial, the Female Sexual Distress Scale demonstrated both sensitivity and specificity of 0.93, and a positive predictive value of approximately 0.90. These measures were highest when using a cutoff score of ⩾ 15 on this scale. Findings indicated that this measure was also highly sensitive to treatment-induced change from baseline to termination of treatment. Construct validity was established through comparisons between the Female Sexual Distress Scale and other measures of psychologic distress, which yielded correlations of moderate magnitude in the expected direction.

Comments

The Female Sexual Distress Scale offers potential for specifically targeting women's sexually related personal distress, a relatively new concept and a key component in the diagnosis of female sexual dysfunction. The Female Sexual Distress Scale is recommended as an instrument to complement, rather than replace, other multidimensional measures in the evaluation of female sexual dysfunction.

Golombok Rust Inventory of Sexual Satisfaction

Description

The Golombok Rust Inventory of Sexual Satisfaction is a 56-item (28 items for women and 28 items for men), self-report measure designed to assess the presence and severity of sexual problems among sexually active individuals and heterosexual couples.[29] Originally developed for use with sex therapy clients, it is intended to be used to assess each partner's individual sexual functioning as well as that of the overall relationship. When assessing individuals, the men's and women's items may be presented as two separate forms. This measure consists of 12 four-item domain scores: five for women, five for men, and two scores in common for both. Men's domains consist of the following: premature ejaculation, impotence, avoidance, nonsensuality, and dissatisfaction. The equivalent domains for women are anorgasmia, vaginismus, avoidance, nonsensuality, and dissatisfaction. The two domains in common to both men and women are frequency of sexual contact and noncommunication. An overall composite score is calculated to summarize the quality of sexual and relationship functioning in the couple. This measure takes approximately 15 min to administer and is targeted for use with heterosexual sex therapy clients.

Psychometric evaluation

The Golombok Rust Inventory of Sexual Satisfaction was originally developed with a standardized sample of 44 heterosexual couples (88 individuals) seeking marital or sex therapy.[29,30] The split half reliability was 0.94 and 0.87 for the main female and male scales, respectively. Internal consistencies for the domain subscales ranged from 0.61 to 0.83, with an average of 0.74. Test–retest reliability coefficients, assessed using pre- and post-treatment scores, were 0.76 and 0.65 for the male and female overall scores, respectively, and ranged from 0.47 to 0.84 for the domain subscales. However, because of improvements due to therapy, these reliability coefficients are likely to be underestimates.

The overall female and male scores were able to discriminate subjects with a clinical diagnosis of a sexual problem from a control group consisting of general medical patients. In addition, specific dysfunctional groups differed from the control subjects on the relevant subscales. Therapists' ratings of problem severity correlated with both the female and male scale scores (correlations of 0.56 and 0.53, respectively). Therapists' ratings of improvement after five sex therapy sessions also correlated with change scores in the female and male scale score (correlations of 0.54 and 0.43, respectively).[30]

More recently, the Golombok Rust Inventory of Sexual Satisfaction has been translated into Dutch and tested for its psychometric properties in a Dutch population.[31,32] In the first study, this measure was tested in 305 heterosexual couples with a sexual problem and 68 student couples.[31] This study provided further support for the 12-factor structure of the Golombok Rust Inventory of Sexual Satisfaction, and lent additional support for the reliability and validity of the measure. Internal consistencies, as assessed by Cronbach's alpha, ranged from 0.55 to 0.85 for the domain subscales, and 0.87 for the overall scale. A high degree of intercorrelation was found among the subscales, suggesting that the measure might assess overlapping constructs. Test–retest reliability coefficients in the nonclinical couples ranged from 0.63 to 0.94 over a 2-week period. The Golombok Rust Inventory of Sexual Satisfaction was found to predict the presence of sexual dysfunction in individual men in a urologic clinic.[32]

Discussion and conclusion

Although physiologic measures such as vaginal photoplethysmography have contributed to our understanding of basic mechanisms in female sexual response, these are of limited benefit in diagnostic assessment or clinical studies of female sexual dysfunction. To provide a multidimensional assessment of sexual function, a number of self-administered questionnaires have been developed in recent years. Several of these measures have demonstrated adequate psychometric properties, including test–retest reliability, internal consistency, and discriminant validity. Self-administered questionnaires are widely used at present to assess sexual function in women.

Daily diary and sexual event log measures have also been developed for use in clinical trials of female sexual dysfunction. These are typically used in conjunction with self-administered questionnaires measures, and have been recommended for use as endpoints in clinical trials by the US Food and Drug Administration. However, daily diary measures have not been adequately validated and lack the potential for multidimensional assessment.

Although self-administered questionnaires offer a valid and user-friendly means of assessing sexual function, several limitations should be noted. First, these measures provide information only on current level of sexual function and cannot substitute for a detailed sexual, psychologic, or medical history. Furthermore, the current questionnaires do not provide information on specific background or etiology, or the role of comorbid medical or psychiatric conditions. Additionally, some patients may experience discomfort or embarrassment while completing questionnaires or symptom scales, or may have difficulty with comprehension. Steps should always be taken to ensure privacy and confidentiality and to assist the patient with comprehension when indicated. Finally, questionnaires or symptom scales should not be used as an alternative to or substitute for direct inquiry or face-to-face clinical interaction with the clinician.

References

1. Rosen R, Riley A, Wagner G et al. The International Index of Erectile Function (IIEF): a multi-dimensional scale for assessment of male erectile dysfunction (MED). Urology 1997; 49: 822–30.

2. Rosen R, Cappelleri J, Gendrano N. The International Index of Erectile Function (IIEF): a state-of-the-science review. *Int J Impot Res* 2002; 4: 1–17.

3. Rosen R. Measurement of male and female sexual dysfunction. *Curr Psychiatry Rep* 2001; 3: 182–7.

4. Basson R, Berman J, Burnett A et al. Report of the international consensus development conference on female sexual dysfunction: definitions and classifications. *J Urol* 2000; 163: 888–93.

5. Basson R, Leiblum S, Brotto L et al. Defintions of women's sexual function reconsidered: advocating expansion and revision. *J Psychosom Obstet Gynaecol* 2004; 24: 221–9.

6. Masters WH, Johnson VE. *Human Sexual Inadequacy.* Boston: Little, Brown, 1970.

7. Kaplan HS. *The New Sex Therapy.* New York: Brunner Mazel, 1974.

8. Rosen RC. Assessment of female sexual dysfunction: review of validated methods. *Fertil Steril* 2002; 77: S89–93.

9. Basson R. The female sexual response: a different model. *J Sex Marital Ther* 2000; 26: 51–65.

10. Rosen RC, Beck JG. *Patterns of Sexual Arousal: Psychophysiological Processes and Clinical Applications.* New York: Guilford Press, 1988.

11. Laan E, Everaerd W, van der Velde J et al. Determinants of subjective experience of sexual arousal in women: feedback from genital arousal and erotic stimulus content. *Psychophysiology* 1995; 32: 444–51.

12. Taylor JF, Rosen RC, Leiblum SR. Self-report assessment of female sexual function: psychometric evaluation of the Brief Index of Sexual Function for Women. *Arch Sex Behav* 1994; 23: 627–43.

13. Mazer NA, Leiblum SR, Rosen RC. The Brief Index of Sexual Functioning for Women (BISF-W): a new scoring algorithm and comparison of normative and surgically menopausal populations. *Menopause* 2000; 7: 350–63.

14. Rosen R, Brown C, Heiman J et al. The Female Sexual Function Index (FSFI): a multidimensional self-report instrument for the assessment of female sexual function. *J Sex Marital Ther* 2000; 26: 191–208.

15. Quirk FH, Heiman JR, Rosen RC et al. Development of a sexual function questionnaire for clinical trials of female sexual dysfunction. *J Womens Health Gend Based Med* 2002; 11: 277–89.

16. Derogatis LR. The Derogatis Interview for Sexual Functioning (DISF/DISF-SR): an introductory report. *J Sex Marital Ther* 1997; 23: 291–304.

17. Shifren JL, Braunstein GD, Simon JA et al. Transdermal testosterone treatment in women with impaired sexual function after oophorectomy. *N Engl J Med*, 2000; 343: 682–8.

18. Fugl-Meyer AR, Lodnert G, Branholm IB et al. On life satisfaction in male erectile dysfunction. *Int J Impot Res* 1997; 9: 141–8.

19. Zigmond, AS, Snaith RP. The Hospital Anxiety and Depression Scale. *Acta Psychiatr Scand* 1983; 67: 361–70.

20. Meston CM. Validation of the Female Sexual Function Index (FSFI) in women with female orgasmic disorder and in women with hypoactive sexual desire disorder. *J Sex Marital Ther* 2003; 29: 39–46.

21. Wiegel M, Meston C, Rosen RC. The Female Sexual Function Index (FSFI): cross-validation and development of clinical cutoff scores. *J Sex Marital Ther* 2005; 31: 1–20.

22. Locke H, Wallace K. Short marital adjustment and prediction tests: their reliability and validity. *Marriage Fam Living* 1959; 2: 251–5.

23. Rosen RC, Lobo RA, Block BA et al. Menopausal Sexual Interest Questionnaire (MSIQ): a unidimensional scale for the assessment of sexual interest in postmenopausal women. *J Sex Marital Ther* 2004; 30: 235–50.

24. Kellner R, Sheffield BF. A self-rating scale of distress. *Psychol Med* 1973; 3: 88–100.

25. Hilditch JR, Lewis J, Peter A et al. A menopause–specific quality of life questionnaire: development and psychometric properties. *Maturitas* 1996; 24: 161–75.

26. McHorney CA, Rust J, Golombok S et al. Profile of Female Sexual Function: a patient-based, international, psychometric instrument for the assessment of hypoactive sexual desire in oophorectomized women. *Menopause* 2004; 11: 474–83.

27. Derogatis L, Rust J, Golombok S et al. Validation of the Profile of Female Sexual Function (PFSF) in surgically and naturally menopausal women. *J Sex Marital Ther* 2004; 30: 25–36.

28. Derogatis LR, Rosen R, Leiblum S et al. The Female Sexual Distress Scale (FSDS): initial validation of a standardized scale for assessment of sexually related personal distress in women. *J Sex Marital Ther* 2002; 28: 317–30.

29. Rust J, Golombok S. The Golombok Rust Inventory of Sexual Satisfaction. *Br J Clin Psychol* 1985; 24: 63–4.

30. Rust J, Golombok S. The GRISS: a psychometric instrument for the assessment of sexual dysfunction. *Arch Sex Behav* 1986; 15: 157–65.

31. Ter Kuile MM, van Lankveld JJDM, Kalkhoven P et al. The Golombok Rust Inventory of Sexual Satisfaction (GRISS): psychometric properties within a Dutch population. *J Sex Marital Ther* 1999; 25: 59–71.

32. Van Lankveld JJDM, van Koeveringe GA. Predictive validity of the Golombok Rust Inventory of Sexual Satisfaction (GRISS) for the presence of sexual dysfunctions within a Dutch urological population. *Int J Impot Res* 2003; 15: 110–16.

11.3 Psychologic-based desire and arousal disorders: treatment strategies and outcome results

Lori A Brotto

Introduction

Since the US Food and Drug Administration approval of selective phosphodiesterase type 5 inhibitors for erectile dysfunction, there has been a search for a panacea for women's sexual difficulties. In the past 6 years, there have been at least two dozen placebo-controlled studies exploring the efficacy of various pharmacologic preparations for hypoactive sexual desire disorder and female sexual arousal disorder. This enthusiastic effort has renewed interest in female sexual dysfunction and its treatment, with more research centers in diverse disciplines turning their attention to women's sexuality. Unfortunately, the research exploring psychologic treatments for female sexual dysfunction has not been as proliferative, and the field has not advanced significantly beyond the treatments that were developed three decades ago (see Chapter 11.1 of this book).

This chapter focuses on the evidence-based literature for treatments of desire and arousal disorders in women. This chapter does not represent an exhaustive overview of all treatments, as hormonal approaches to management are the focus of Chapters 13.1–13.3. The available data to date on psychologic as well as nonhormonal pharmacologic treatments for hypoactive sexual desire disorder and female sexual arousal disorder will be reviewed. This chapter will center on hypoactive sexual desire disorder and female sexual arousal disorder that are "psychologic-based", defined here as having a presumed etiology that is largely psychologic, and not organic (although this is a false dichotomy with limited utility, and management of sexual complaints is best when treatment providers adopt a biopsychosocial approach) (see Chapter 17.6). As the reader will note, the evaluation of treatment efficacy rarely relies upon presumed psychologic versus organic etiology as inclusion and exclusion criteria when selecting participants – except in some cases where pharmacologic antidotes to antidepressant-induced sexual dysfunction are being investigated (see Chapter 11.2). There is a discrepancy between empirical investigations and management in the real clinical setting, the latter situation consisting of treatment regimens that follow logically from a well-conceptualized case formulation that takes etiology into consideration. With the increasing sophistication of instruments to explore the physiologic components of the sexual response (e.g., laser Doppler, functional magnetic resonance imaging) (see Chapters 10.1–10.7), we may be in a better position in the future to infer when a sexual difficulty has more of a physiologic than psychologic basis.

Much of the published outcome literature on psychologic interventions involves participants who met criteria for one of the conventional diagnoses according to the recent versions of the *Diagnostic and Statistical Manual of Mental Disorders*, fourth edition, text revised (DSM-IV-TR),[1] or the *International Statistical Classification of Diseases and Related Health Problems*, 10th revision.[2] However, the clinical picture is typically more complex with a high degree of comorbidity between sexual difficulties. Moreover, rather than unambiguous symptoms, complaints of dissatisfaction and distress[3] often do not fit neatly into discrete diagnostic categories. A later chapter in this text will illustrate such complexity through a series of case vignettes.

Brief history of sex therapy approaches, beginning with Masters and Johnson

Masters and Johnson's extensive research program can be credited for bringing research on sex therapy to the forefront (see Chapter 1.1). Their book *Human Sexual Inadequacy*,[4] published in 1970, presents data on 790 men and women treated in their St Louis clinic along with 5-year follow-up data on a smaller subsample. The treatment consisted of education in sexual responsivity, sensate focus, and encouragement of verbal communication (for all subtypes of sexual dysfunction), followed by specific techniques tailored to the particular sexual concern. Treatment was administered daily over 2 weeks by a male–female therapist team, and outcome was assessed with one clinician-determined item based on perceived success or failure. They reported astounding success rates of 72–98% for women and only a 5% relapse rate after 5 years. Attempts to replicate these findings have been unsuccessful, and many critics attribute this to the entirely subjective endpoint used, the expensive, intensive, and unfeasible delivery of their sex therapy, and the highly selective sample of participants on which their data were based (e.g., patients had to be willing to "isolate themselves from the social or professional concerns of the moment" (p 20)).[4] Their findings did, however, prompt interest in research on the efficacy of sex therapy over the next several years that aimed at determining which components of Masters and Johnson's intensive program were most efficacious.

In a modified Masters and Johnson sex therapy approach that involved weekly sessions by one therapist (versus daily therapy with a male–female therapist team), Hawton et al.[5] found that only 61% of the 140 couples completed treatment. By the end of treatment, 26% of couples had their sexual problem completely resolved with at least partial remission in another 50%. The authors do not provide recurrence rates for each sexual dysfunction separately, though they note that results for vaginismus were "excellent, so that total resolution of this problem can be expected in most couples"; however, results for inhibited female desire were not as positive. Seventy-six per cent were available for follow-up, which took place, on average, 3 years after treatment. Interestingly, whereas 75% of couples had either recurrence or continuing difficulties at follow-up, only 34% were concerned about this. Another, more recent, large-scale study involved 365 married couples presenting to a sex therapy clinic with heterogeneous sexual complaints.[6] Treatment was behavioral and occurred weekly over 7 weeks, and outcome was defined dichotomously as success or failure.

Sixty-five per cent of all couples responded favorably to behavior therapy, equal numbers of men and women showing improvement. Less than 50% of those who benefited from treatment returned at the 3-month follow-up. Of those, 74% reported having maintained treatment gains.

Overall, the data from the outcome research of Masters and Johnson and other large-scale studies that followed suggest that psychologic treatment of sexual dysfunction appears to be beneficial with good maintenance effects. Approximately 65–98% of participants reported at least moderate improvement by the end of treatment, and 5–34% experienced relapse, depending on the type of therapy employed and the degree of sexual difficulty (Table 11.3.1). However, methodological limitations prevent one from drawing any firm conclusions about the effects of therapy on specific sexual dysfunctions. Specifically, these limitations include the lack of comparison control groups that account for nonspecific factors, and highly subjective endpoint measures.

Psychologic treatment approaches for desire disorder

Low sexual desire in women represents the most frequent complaint (approximately 30–34%) among women in recent large-scale nationally representative samples in the USA[7] and Sweden.[8] Interestingly, female low desire and erectile difficulty appear to be related, as recent data show that 60% of female partners of men with erectile dysfunction meet criteria for hypoactive sexual desire disorder.[9] There have been a number of studies (Table 11.3.2) evaluating the efficacy of Masters and Johnson's treatment or other treatments derived from it, specifically for hypoactive sexual desire disorder, which DSM-IV-TR defines as "persistent or recurrent deficiency or absence of sexual thoughts, fantasies, desire for, or receptivity to sexual activity which causes personal distress".[1] Schover and LoPiccolo[10] assessed the efficacy of 15–20 weekly behavior therapy sessions on couples in which either partner experienced low desire. The dropout rate was negligible at 2–3%. They found significant improvements in initiation of sexual activity, sexual satisfaction, and frequency of sexual activity, but only a minor improvement in marital satisfaction, with relatively stable maintenance after 1 year. In the UK,[11] a modified Masters and Johnson approach applied over 12 sessions for couples in which women experienced low desire, found significant improvement for 57% of the couples. Improvement was defined as intercourse either with no difficulties or minor difficulties. However, unlike the prior study, there was a significant attrition rate of 37% that was found to be largely dependent upon the male partner's level of motivation before treatment. One significant limitation of this study was the sole reliance on clinician-determined perceived intercourse ability as the primary outcome variable. Theorizing that treatment of orgasmic difficulties may lead to improvements in sexual desire, Hurlbert[12] compared the effects of

Table 11.3.1. Published studies that have evaluated Masters and Johnson's sex therapy, or one of its modified versions, on heterogeneous sexual complaints in couples

Publication	Participants	Therapy details	Efficacy rates	Misc.
Masters and Johnson 1970[4]	790 men and women	Daily therapy for 2–3 weeks by male–female team; 5-year follow-up data available	72–98% for women with only 5% relapse rate after 5 years	Efficacy determined by one clinician-determined item of success vs failure
Hawton et al. 1986[5]	140 couples	Modified Masters and Johnson treatment with 15 weekly sessions; 3-year follow-up data available	26% had complete resolution of problem with at least partial remission in another 50%; 75% had either recurrence or continuing difficulties at follow-up	Despite recurrence, the majority were not bothered by their symptoms
Sarwer and Durlak 1997[6]	365 couples	Behavioral sex therapy with 7 weekly sessions (4-hour group sessions); 3-month follow-up data available for < 50% of couples	64% of women and men showed significant improvement. 70% reported maintained treatment gains at follow-up. Treatment success for HSDD, impaired orgasm, and dyspareunia were 65%, 65%, and 58%, respectively	Limitation: treatment outcome defined dichotomously as "successful" or "unsuccessful"

HSDD = hypoactive sexual desire disorder.

marital sex therapy with and without orgasm consistency training in women with hypoactive sexual desire disorder. Treatment was a primarily cognitive-behavioral approach that incorporated elements of directed masturbation, sensate focus, and the coital alignment technique. Whereas all women improved on measures of sexual desire and arousal, those who also received orgasm consistency training had even greater levels of sexual arousal and assertiveness, and these group differences were maintained at the 6-month follow-up assessment.

Cognitive-behavioral therapy for low desire has also been investigated (see Chapter 11.1). In one uncontrolled study, cognitive-behavioral therapy was helpful for approximately 50% of women that met criteria for various sexual complaints, including low desire.[13] In a recent controlled study, Trudel and colleagues[14] compared the effects of cognitive-behavioral therapy with wait-list control in 74 couples in which women met criteria for hypoactive sexual desire disorder. Treatment consisted of 12 weekly, 2-h group-therapy sessions that included homework exercises and reading assignments. The treatment included psychoeducation, couple exercises, sensate focus, communication training, emotional communication training, mutual reinforcement training, cognitive challenging, and sexual fantasy training. Seventy-four per cent of women no longer met diagnostic criteria for hypoactive sexual desire

Table 11.3.2. Support for psychologic interventions for hypoactive sexual desire disorder (HSDD) in women

Mode of treatment	Empirical support	Level of efficacy
Modified Masters and Johnson treatment	Hawton et al. 1991[11]	Significant improvements in 57% of sample
Behavioral sex therapy	Schover and LoPiccolo 1982[10]	Significant improvements in marital adjustment, sexual satisfaction, sexual frequency, initiating of sexual activity, sexual responsivity, and masturbation
Marital sex therapy plus orgasm consistency training	Hurlbert 1993[12]	Significant improvements in sexual arousal and sexual assertiveness with sex therapy plus orgasm consistency training vs sex therapy alone
Cognitive-behavioral therapy	McCabe 2001[13] Trudel et al. 2001[14]	< 50% improved 74% no longer met diagnostic criteria; significant improvements in quality of marital life, individual sexual and cognitive functioning, sexual arousal, satisfaction
Systemic and multielement treatments	No empirical data	Clinical reports of treatment utility in treating low desire in a couple

disorder by the end of the treatment, and this stabilized to 64% at 1-year follow-up.[14] Nearly all other measures of individual and interpersonal dimensions improved with treatment, including quality of marital life, and individual, sexual, and cognitive functioning. Notably, the perception of sexual arousal also increased in this group of women with hypoactive sexual desire disorder. At the end of treatment, women reported a high level of satisfaction with treatment, and added that they would recommend the treatment to others. There have been other investigations of psychologic treatments for women's low desire; however, failure to present data for specific sexual complaints limits our ability to drawn conclusions from them.[15,16]

To date, there are no published empirical studies on the efficacy of treatments for low desire despite the rich clinical literature supporting these treatments among individuals and couples.[17,18] This is probably due to the difficulty in manualizing treatment protocols for psychodynamic and systemic treatments. Multielement treatments that incorporate cognitive and behavioral ingredients with systemic approaches have also been described, and appear especially useful for the difficult-to-treat couple.[19] The treatments require rigorous scientific testing before any definitive conclusions can be drawn as to their efficacy.

Recent efforts to redefine hypoactive sexual desire disorder[20] to make it more consistent with the evidence-based literature[3] and the clinical presentations of women[21,22] has called into question the utility of the traditional four-stage Masters and Johnson human sexual response cycle as a way of understanding women's sexuality. It has also been argued that previous reports of the prevalence of hypoactive sexual desire disorder are markedly inflated, given that survey questions did not simultaneously assess levels of distress.[3] Instead, newer models[22] focus on the normalization of age- and relationship duration-related declines in spontaneous sexual desire, and encourage couples to focus treatment on aspects of the interpersonal relationship or context that may not promote responsive sexual desire. Also central to this reconceptualization is the notion of sexual arousability, or the ease with which women become sexually aroused when the context and stimuli that promote sexual response are adequate. What makes newer models unique and especially relevant for women in long-term relationships is the focus on sexual motivation that is intimacy-based.[23] Efforts to incorporate this new model in the treatment of couples where low desire is the primary complaint have been promising;[24,25] however, future studies that assess the model's efficacy in the context of controlled clinical trials are needed. Another notable attempt to provide a more useful classification of women's sexual problems is the "new view of women's sexual problems",[26] which has replaced diagnostic labels such as "hypoactive sexual desire disorder" with descriptions that relate to a number of sociocultural, interpersonal, psychologic, and medical factors. To date, there are no published data on treatment efficacy in women who are diagnosed according to the "new view".

Sexual aversion disorder is included in the sexual desire disorders section of the DSM-IV-TR,[1] but it has received considerably less attention than hypoactive sexual desire disorder. Moreover, because of the avoidance component, the precise prevalence for this distressing condition is unknown. In general, it has been found that sexual aversion disorder is less responsive to behavioral treatment than is hypoactive sexual desire disorder.[10] However, systematic desensitization in the context of behavior therapy (akin to the approaches used in the treatment of anxiety disorders) has been described as very effective in two published case studies.[27,28]

Psychologic treatment approaches for arousal disorder

Epidemiologic data suggest that the prevalence of problematic sexual arousal, according to the DSM-IV-TR definition of female sexual arousal disorder as "persistent or recurrent inability to attain, or to maintain until completion of the sexual activity an adequate lubrication, swelling response of sexual excitement", is approximately 12–21%.[7,8] In the clinical setting, however, arousal complaints that are independent of desire and/or orgasm complaints are rarely seen. This has led some to dispute the validity of female sexual arousal disorder as a discrete clinical entity.[29] Others have suggested that there may be a subgroup of women with genital vascular insufficiency that interferes specifically with vaginal engorgement and clitoral erectile capacity while desire remains unaffected.[30] Certainly, the literature on treatment for female sexual arousal disorder reflects this lack of consensus, as there are no published trials of a psychologic intervention for female sexual arousal disorder. Instead, owing to the success of vasoactive agents in the treatment of male erectile dysfunction, various pharmaceutic companies have initiated an eager search for a comparable medication in the treatment of women's impaired arousal.

Factors associated with favorable outcome in sex therapy

Before we review the literature on pharmacologic approaches to desire and arousal disorders, the variables that have been linked to a positive treatment outcome in psychologic outcome studies will first be addressed. Although very little has been published on this topic recently, the work of Hawton and colleagues[5,11,31,32] has been helpful in identifying important prognostic variables. Better long-term treatment outcome was associated with couples who reported being able to communicate about anger[5] and the general functioning of the relationship[5,33] (with ratings by women being more strongly predictive than those of men).[31] Compliance with homework early on,[31] as well as in the final sessions of treatment,[6] was found to be highly predictive of outcome success. Pretreatment motivation by both partners, but especially of the male,[34] was a strong positive predictor of a favorable outcome,[31,33] as well as of which couples would complete treatment.[11] Looking specifically at treatment outcome for hypoactive sexual desire disorder, Hawton[32] found that degree of physical attraction between partners and interpersonal communication were important positive predictors. Others have shown that attention to systemic issues in the relationship is also positively related to outcome.[35,36]

Factors that predict a poorer outcome have also been identified. These include having a history of psychiatric disorder, and marital separation in the past.[5,31] Variables not found to predict significantly outcome success have included age or social class of the couples,[31] whether one or both partners experienced a sexual problem, presence of prior treatment (although this has been found to be a predictor in one study[11]), perception of the sexual problem, how well the partners were informed about sexuality, number of children, duration of the relationship, and strength of religious beliefs.[31]

Investigational, nonhormonal, pharmacologic treatments for hypoactive sexual desire disorder and female sexual arousal disorder

At the time of writing (July 2004), there are no approved nonhormonal pharmacologic treatments for either hypoactive sexual desire disorder or female sexual arousal disorder. The androgens, estrogen, and progestins have been the topic of a number of investigations, but their potential role in women's sexual complaints is the focus of Chapters 13.1–13.3, and therefore they are not covered here. The place for pharmacologic treatment of desire and arousal complaints in women is still unclear (see Chapters 14.1 and 14.2). As knowledge about the precise etiologies of sexual dysfunction continues to advance, we may be in a position in the future to determine which pharmacologic agent might be useful for which specific aspect of impaired sexual response.

Numerous studies on nonhormonal agents have been conducted or are underway, and the limited published data available from those placebo-controlled investigations will be briefly reviewed. In general, the nonhormonal investigational agents for desire and arousal fall into the following categories:[37] (1) dopaminergic agonists, (2) melanocortin-stimulating hormone and its agonists, (3) adrenoceptor antagonists, (4) prostaglandins, and (5) nitric oxide system agents (see Chapters 14.1 and 14.2).

Among the dopaminergic agonists, bupropion has been the subject of a few investigations based on the assumption that dopaminergic dysregulation may underlie some forms of hypoactive sexual desire disorder. A single-blind study of bupropion HCl (150 mg twice daily) in nondepressed women with hypoactive sexual desire disorder was found to have a 29% response rate.[38] In a more recent, double-blind, placebo-controlled investigation in women with hypoactive sexual

desire disorder,[39] buproprion sustained release (300 mg) had no effect on the traditional markers of desire as defined by the DSM (e.g., spontaneous sexual thoughts or fantasies). On the other hand, the drug significantly improved sexual arousability – or the ease with which women become sexually aroused when the context and stimuli that promote sexual response are adequate. The lack of effect on spontaneous desire coupled with the recent reconceptualization of hypoactive sexual desire disorder that focuses on responsive desire[20] has implications for future pharmacologic agents that might help women with low desire. It is possible that as clinical trial endpoints begin to shift focus away from spontaneous desire or fantasies and toward more relevant aspects of responsive desire and sexual arousability, beneficial drug effects, if any, may become more apparent. The dopaminergic agonist, sublingual apomorphine, was also investigated in a study of 55 premenopausal women with comorbid hypoactive sexual desire disorder and female sexual arousal disorder.[40] There was no significant drug effect when apomorphine (2 or 3 mg) was taken "as needed", but there were significant improvements in desire, arousal, orgasm, enjoyment, satisfaction with sexual frequency, and overall intercourse frequency when sublingual apomorphine was taken daily.

Another agent with potential utility for the treatment of low desire in women is the melanocortin agonist, PT-141, which selectively binds to central melanocortin receptors. When solicitation behavior in the female rodent was taken as an analog of human female desire, PT-141 was found to facilitate significantly and selectively this aspect of appetitive sexual behavior.[41] Although these findings are promising, until safety and efficacy data are available in women, any speculation about the role of melanocortin agonists in women's desire is highly tentative.

Phentolamine mesylate acts as an antagonist via the alpha-1 and alpha-2 receptors and has been used for decades in the treatment of erectile dysfunction through intracavernosal injections. In a single-blind, placebo-controlled pilot study of six postmenopausal women,[42] 40 mg of the drug was found to improve self-reported lubrication and tingling sensations significantly, with no effect on physiologic sexual arousal, subjective pleasure, or arousal. In a double-blind replication with 41 postmenopausal women by Rubio-Aurioles et al.,[43] vaginally applied, but not oral, phentolamine, resulted in a statistically significant increase in physiologic arousal in women receiving hormone therapy. Moreover, only among women receiving hormone therapy did both vaginally applied and oral phentolamine significantly improve subjective measures of arousal, lubrication, tingling, and warmth with no effect on pleasure. To my knowledge, there have been no other published reports of phentolamine since Rubio-Aurioles et al. published this paper in 2002.

Prostaglandins have a long history in the successful treatment of erectile dysfunction, and few studies have examined their potential efficacy for female sexual dysfunction. Prostaglandin E_1 was the focus of a randomized, double-blind, placebo-controlled investigation in 94 premenopausal women with female sexual arousal disorder.[44] There were no significant effects of prostaglandin E_1 (500, 1000, or 1500 µg) over placebo on the mean arousal success rate, Female Sexual Function Index total score, or sexual distress, and only a marginal trend toward increased satisfaction with arousal. Prostaglandin E_1-based formulations are currently being studied in a number of investigations.

Selective phosphodiesterase type 5 inhibitors have been the subject of a handful of conflicting investigations. Although the large-scale studies failed to find benefit of selective phosphodiesterase type 5 inhibitors for women with mixed sexual dysfunction that included arousal complaints,[45,46] findings are more promising in more diagnostically homogeneous groups of women. For example, selective phosphodiesterase type 5 inhibitors were found to improve arousal and orgasm significantly in 53 premenopausal women with female sexual arousal disorder limited to genital arousal complaints.[47] In postmenopausal women with adequate estrogen repletion, selective phosphodiesterase type 5 inhibitors (adjustable to 25 or 100 mg) were found to improve significantly genital sensation/feeling and satisfaction with intercourse/foreplay only in women who did not experience comorbid desire complaints, and whose plasma free testosterone was within a narrow range.[48] Another investigation found that the vaginal photoplethysmograph was useful in identifying this small subsample of women with genital arousal complaints (and no comorbid problematic desire) who might respond positively to a selective phosphodiesterase type 5 inhibitor.[49] Given these findings, it is likely that a beneficial effect, if any, of selective phosphodiesterase type 5 inhibitors in women might be detected only among specific subsamples of women (e.g., spinal cord injury[50]).

The nitric oxide precursor, L-arginine, has been the focus of a double-blind, placebo-controlled investigation combined with yohimbine, an adrenergic antagonist, in women with female sexual arousal disorder.[51] The combination significantly facilitated physiologic arousal (measured by a vaginal photoplethysmograph) but had no effect on subjective measures of arousal or affect.

At present, there is one product approved by the US Food and Drug Administration for the treatment of female sexual arousal disorder. The EROS clitoral therapy device (CTD; Urometrics, St Paul, MN, USA) is a small, hand-held, battery-operated device that is placed over the clitoris and increases vasocongestion through a gentle suction. In a noncontrolled design, this device was found to improve significantly all measures of sexual response and satisfaction in women with female sexual arousal disorder.[52] However, because this device has not been subject to placebo-controlled designs, the specific effects of the gentle vacuum above and beyond nonspecific attentional effects are unknown.

Future directions

Based on the findings from both psychologic and pharmacologic trials, we might conclude that specific prognostic variables will guide future studies to target their interventions to specific subsamples of women. The data on sildenafil suggest that female sexual arousal disorder itself may be a heterogeneous diagnostic entity comprised of different subtypes that may differentially respond to vasoactive agents. The published recommendations for revising the female sexual dysfunctions[20] (see Chapter 9.1) include the division and expansion of female sexual arousal disorder into "genital sexual arousal disorder", "subjective sexual arousal disorder", and "combined genital and subjective sexual arousal disorder". Because women with subjective sexual arousal complaints have adequate genital vasocongestive responses, it is highly unlikely that a pharmaceutic agent designed to promote blood flow will be useful in ameliorating the sexual concerns in this group of women.[53] Instead, it is in this group that psychologic interventions designed to target lack of sexual excitement and pleasure, and promote the seeking of adequate sexual stimuli and context, may prove most useful. It is anticipated that in addition to continued investigation into compounds similar to those described earlier, we may see an increasing number of investigations using herbal remedies or other natural products.[54]

There is an urgent need for more empirical investigations into psychologic treatments of female sexual arousal disorder and hypoactive sexual desire disorder. Methodological strictness must be integrated in order for new conclusions about efficacy to be reached. For example, accurate documentation of sexual difficulty in addition to distress are necessary, and endpoints that reflect the important aspects of sexuality for women must be addressed (e.g., pleasure, enjoyment, satisfaction, or passion)[3] instead of intercourse frequency as the reference standard. Both participant- and investigator-derived definitions of success should be outlined, given that these can often be discordant. The differentiation between statistical and clinical significance is also essential. An extensive review of the literature in 1997[55] recommended that better descriptions of therapeutic technique, larger sample sizes, adequate control groups, group randomization, and inclusion of long-term follow-up data will help to build our evidence-based repertoire of treatments. Again, identification of prognostic variables will allow researchers to tailor both psychologic and pharmacologic treatments to samples of women. We hope that by the next edition of this textbook on female sexual dysfunction, more data on psychologic as well as combined psychologic-pharmacologic treatments will be available.

References

1. American Psychiatric Association. *Diagnostic and Statistical Manual of Mental Disorders*, 4th edn, text revised (DSM-IV-TR). Washington, DC: American Psychiatric Press, 2000.
2. World Health Organization. *International Statistical Classification of Diseases and Related Health Problems* (ICD-10). Geneva: WHO, 1992.
3. Bancroft J, Loftus J, Long JS. Distress about sex: a national survey of women in heterosexual relationships. *Arch Sex Behav* 2003; 32: 193–208.

4. Masters WH, Johnson VE. *Human Sexual Inadequacy*. Boston: Little, Brown, 1970.

5. Hawton K, Catalan J, Martin P et al. Long-term outcome of sex therapy. *Behav Res Ther* 1986; 24: 665–75.

6. Sarwer DB, Durlak JA. A field trial of the effectiveness of behavioral treatment for sexual dysfunctions. *J Sex Marital Ther* 1997; 23: 87–97.

7. Laumann EO, Paik A, Rosen RC. Sexual dysfunction in the United States: prevalence and predictors. *JAMA* 1999; 281: 537–44.

8. Fugl-Meyer AR, Sjogren Fugl-Meyer K. Sexual disabilities, problems and satisfaction in 18–74 year old Swedes. *Scand J Sexol* 1999; 2: 79–105.

9. Sjogren Fugl-Meyer K, Fugl-Meyer AR. Sexual disabilities are not singularities. *Int J Impot Res* 2002; 14: 487–93.

10. Schover LR, LoPiccolo J. Treatment effectiveness for dysfunctions of sexual desire. *J Sex Marital Ther* 1982; 8: 179–97.

11. Hawton K, Catalan J, Fagg J. Low sexual desire: sex therapy results and prognostic factors. *Behav Res Ther* 1991; 29: 217–24.

12. Hurlbert DF. A comparative study using orgasm consistency training in the treatment of women reporting hypoactive sexual desire. *J Sex Marital Ther* 1993; 19: 41–55.

13. McCabe MP. Evaluation of a cognitive behavior therapy program for people with sexual dysfunction. *J Sex Marital Ther* 2001; 27: 259–71.

14. Trudel G, Marchand A, Ravart M et al. The effect of a cognitive-behavioral group treatment program on hypoactive sexual desire in women. *Sex Relatsh Ther* 2001; 16: 145–64.

15. Crowe MJ, Gillan P, Golombok S. Form and content in the conjoint treatment of sexual dysfunction: a controlled study. *Behav Res Ther* 1981; 19: 47–54.

16. Zimmer D. Does marital therapy enhance the effectiveness of treatment for sexual dysfunction? *J Sex Marital Ther* 1987; 13: 193–209.

17. Schnarch D. Desire problems: a systemic perspective. In SR Leiblum, RC Rosen, eds. *Principles and Practice of Sex Therapy*. New York: Guilford Press, 2000: 17–56.

18. Verhulst J, Heiman JR. A systems perspective on sexual desire. In SR Leiblum, RC Rosen, eds. *Sexual Desire Disorders*. New York: Guilford Press, 1988: 243–67.

19. Pridal CG, LoPiccolo J. Multielement treatment of desire disorders. In SR Leiblum, RC Rosen, eds. *Principles and Practice of Sex Therapy*. New York: Guilford Press, 2000: 57–81.

20. Basson R, Leiblum S, Brotto L et al. Definitions of women's sexual dysfunction reconsidered: advocating expansion and revision. *J Psychosom Obstet Gynaecol* 2003; 24: 221–9.

21. Basson R. Human sex-response cycles. *J Sex Marital Ther* 2001; 27: 33–43.

22. Basson R. Rethinking low sexual desire in women. *Br J Obstet Gynaecol* 2002; 109: 357–63.

23. Basson R. Biopsychosocial models of women's sexual response: applications to management of "desire disorders". *Sex Relat Ther* 2003; 18: 107–15.

24. Basson R. Using a different model for female sexual response to address women's problematic low sexual desire. *J Sex Marital Ther* 2001; 27: 395–403.

25. Gehring D. Couple therapy for low sexual desire: a systemic approach. *J Sex Marital Ther* 2003; 29: 25–38.

26. Tiefer L. Beyond dysfunction: a new view of women's sexual problems. *J Sex Marital Ther* 2002; 28(Suppl 1): 225–32.

27. Finch S. Sexual aversion disorder treated with behavioural desensitization. *Can J Psychiatry* 2001; 46: 563–4.

28. Kingsberg SA, Janata, JW. The sexual aversions. In SB Levine, CB Risen, SE Althof, eds. *Handbook of Clinical Sexuality for Mental Health Professionals*. New York: Brunner-Routledge, 2003: 153–65.

29. Segraves KB, Segraves RT. Hypoactive sexual desire disorder: prevalence and comorbidity in 906 subjects. *J Sex Marital Ther* 1991; 17: 55–8.

30. Goldstein I, Berman JR. Vasculogenic female sexual dysfunction: vaginal engorgement and clitoral erectile insufficiency syndromes. *Int J Impot Res* 1998; 10(Suppl 2): S84–90.

31. Hawton K, Catalan J. Prognostic factors in sex therapy. *Behav Res Ther* 1986; 24: 377–85.

32. Hawton, K. Treatment of sexual dysfunctions by sex therapy and other approaches. *Br J Psychiatry* 1995; 167: 307–14.

33. Whitehead A, Mathews A. Factors related to successful outcome in the treatment of sexually unresponsive women. *Psychol Med* 1986; 16: 373–8.

34. Hirst JF, Watson JP. Therapy for sexual and relationship problems: the effects on outcome of attending as an individual or as a couple. *Sex Marital Ther* 1997; 12: 321–37.

35. Besharat MA. Management strategies of sexual dysfunctions. *J Contemp Psychother* 2001; 31: 161–80.

36. Milan RJ Jr, Kilmann PR, Boland JP. Treatment outcome of secondary orgasmic dysfunction: a two- to six-year follow-up. *Arch Sex Behav* 1988; 17: 463–80.

37. Fourcroy JL. Female sexual dysfunction: potential for pharmacotherapy. *Drugs* 2003; 63: 1445–57.

38. Segraves RT, Croft H, Kavoussi R et al. Bupropion sustained release (SR) for the treatment of hypoactive sexual desire disorder (hypoactive sexual desire disorder) in nondepressed women. *J Sex Marital Ther* 2001; 27: 303–16.

39. Segraves RT, Clayton A, Croft H et al. Bupropion sustained release for the treatment of hypoactive sexual desire disorder in premenopausal women. *J Clin Psychopharmacol* 2004; 24: 339–42.

40. Caruso S, Agnello C, Intelisano G et al. Placebo-controlled study on efficacy and safety of daily apomorphine SL intake in premenopausal women affected by hypoactive sexual desire disorder and sexual arousal disorder. *Urology* 2004: 63: 955–9.

41. Pfaus JG, Shadiack A, Van Soest T et al. Selective facilitation of sexual solicitation in the female rat by a melanocortin receptor agonist. *Proc Natl Acad Sci USA* 2004; 101: 10201–4.

42. Rosen RC, Phillips NA, Gendrano NC 3rd et al. Oral phentolamine and female sexual arousal disorder: a pilot study. *J Sex Marital Ther* 1999; 25: 137–44.

43. Rubio-Aurioles E, Lopez M, Lipezker M et al. Phentolamine mesylate in postmenopausal women with female sexual arousal disorder: a psychophysiological study. *J Sex Marital Ther* 2002; 28(Suppl 1): 205–15.

44. Padma-Nathan H, Brown C, Fendl J et al. Efficacy and safety of topical alprostadil cream for the treatment of female sexual arousal

disorder (FSAD): a double-blind, multicenter, randomized, and placebo-controlled clinical trial. *J Sex Marital Ther* 2003; 29: 329–44.

45. Basson R, McInnes R, Smith MD et al. Efficacy and safety of sildenafil citrate in women with sexual dysfunction associated with female sexual arousal disorder. *J Womens Health Gend Based Med* 2002; 11: 367–77.

46. Kaplan SA, Reis RB, Kohn IJ et al. Safety and efficacy of sildenafil in postmenopausal women with sexual dysfunction. *Urology* 1999; 53: 481–6.

47. Caruso S, Intelisano G, Lupo L et al. Premenopausal women affected by sexual arousal disorder treated with sildenafil: a double-blind, cross-over, placebo-controlled study. *Br J Obstet Gynaecol* 2001, 108. 623–8.

48. Berman JR, Berman LA, Toler SM et al. Safety and efficacy of sildenafil citrate for the treatment of female sexual arousal disorder: a double-blind, placebo controlled study. *J Urol* 2003; 170: 2333–8.

49. Basson R, Brotto LA. Sexual psychophysiology and effects of sildenafil citrate in oestrogenised women with acquired genital arousal disorder and impaired orgasm: a randomised controlled trial. *Br J Obstet Gynaecol* 2003; 110: 1014–24.

50. Sipski ML, Rosen RC, Alexander CJ et al. Sildenafil effects on sexual and cardiovascular responses in women with spinal cord injury. *Urology* 2000; 55: 812–15.

51. Meston CM, Worcel M. The effects of yohimbine plus L-arginine glutamate on sexual arousal in postmenopausal women with sexual arousal disorder. *Arch Sex Behav* 2002; 31: 323–32.

52. Billups KL, Berman L, Berman J et al. A new non-pharmacological vacuum therapy for female sexual dysfunction. *J Sex Marital Ther* 2001; 27: 435–41.

53. Basson R. Pharmacotherapy for sexual dysfunction in women. *Expert Opin Pharmacother* 2004; 5: 1045–59.

54. Ferguson DM, Steidle CP, Singh GS et al. Randomized, placebo controlled, double blind, crossover design trial of the efficacy and safety of Zestra for women with and without female sexual arousal disorder. *J Sex Marital Ther* 2003; 29(Suppl 1): 33–44.

55. Heiman JR, Meston CM. Empirically validated treatments for sexual dysfunction. *Annu Rev Sex Res* 1997; 8: 148–94.

11.4 Female orgasmic disorder: treatment strategies and outcome results

Cindy M Meston

The definition of orgasmic problems in women

The *Diagnostic and Statistical Manual of Mental Disorders*, fourth edition, text revision (DSM-IV-TR),[1] defines "female orgasmic disorder" as a persistent or recurrent delay in, or absence of, orgasm after a normal sexual excitement phase. The inability to obtain orgasm does not always lead to sexual distress or dissatisfaction in women,[2] and if the disorder does not cause the woman marked distress or interpersonal difficulty, a diagnosis of female orgasmic disorder should not be made. The diagnosis of this disorder should be based on the clinician's judgment that the woman's orgasmic capacity is less than would be reasonable for her age, sexual experience, and the adequacy of sexual stimulation she receives. Indeed, Laumann et al.[3] found that the youngest group of women (18–24 years) showed rates of orgasm lower than the older groups for both orgasm with a partner and orgasm during masturbation. This is likely to be attributable to age differences in sexual experience (see Chapter 6.4 of this book).

In diagnosis of female orgasmic disorder, it is particularly important to keep in mind that women exhibit wide variability in the type or intensity of stimulation required to attain orgasm. Research indicates that orgasm in women can be induced via erotic stimulation of a number of genital sites, including the clitoris and vagina (the most usual sites), periurethral glans,[4] breast/nipple, or mons[5] (see Chapters 4.1–4.3). Nongenital forms of stimulation reported to induce orgasm include mental imagery or fantasy[6] and hypnosis.[7] There have also been a few isolated cases of "spontaneous orgasm" described in the psychiatric literature in which no obvious sexual stimulus could be ascertained.[8]

The DSM-IV-TR uses the terms "lifelong" versus "acquired" and "generalized" versus "situational" to further describe female orgasmic disorder. However, most studies examining orgasmic dysfunction in women refer to orgasm problems as either "primary orgasmic dysfunction" or "secondary orgasmic dysfunction". These different diagnostic labels lead to some confusion when interpreting the literature on women's orgasm. In general, the term "primary orgasmic dysfunction" is used to describe women who report never having experienced orgasm under any circumstances, including masturbation. According to the DSM-IV-TR, this would refer to those women who meet criteria for lifelong and generalized female orgasmic disorder. "Secondary orgasmic dysfunction" relates to women who meet criteria for situational and/or acquired lack of orgasm. By definition, this encompasses a heterogeneous group of women with orgasm difficulties. For example, it could include women who were once orgasmic but are now so only infrequently, as well as women who are able to obtain orgasm only in certain contexts, with certain types of sexual activity, or with certain partners. The DSM-IV-TR does not directly address the issue of women who can obtain orgasm during intercourse with manual stimulation but not intercourse alone. However, the generally accepted clinical consensus is that she would not meet criteria for clinical diagnosis if she is able to obtain orgasm during masturbation unless she is distressed by the frequency of her sexual response.

Studies of women diagnosed with DSM-IV-TR female

orgasmic disorder report that a high percentage of these women also meet DSM-IV-TR criteria for female sexual arousal disorder.[9–11] This suggests that, although the DSM-IV-TR explicitly states that the absence or delay in orgasm is to follow "a normal sexual excitement stage", this criterion is often ignored. In light of this and other shortcomings of the traditional nosology of women's sexual disorders, an international multidisciplinary group recently proposed changes to the existing diagnostic system.[12] In hopes of highlighting the fact that a DSM-IV-TR diagnosis of female orgasmic disorder precludes one of arousal disorder, the committee proposed the following criteria for diagnosing women's orgasmic disorder: "Despite the self-report of high sexual arousal/excitement, there is either lack of orgasm, markedly diminished intensity of orgasmic sensations or marked delay of orgasm from any kind of stimulation."

The prevalence of orgasmic problems in women

Based on findings from the National Health and Social Life Survey,[13] orgasmic problems are the second most frequently reported sexual problem in American women (see Chapters 2.1–2.4). Results from this random sample of 1749 women (ages 18–59) indicated that 24% reported a lack of orgasm in the past year for at least several months or more. This survey also suggested that unmarried women and women who have not graduated from college are at greater risk of developing orgasm problems.

This percentage is comparable to clinic-based data. Orgasmic problems were noted by 29% of 329 healthy women (aged 18–73 years) who attended an outpatient gynecologic clinic[11] and by 23% of 104 women (aged 18–65+ years) attending a UK general practice clinic.[14] Similarly, absence of orgasm was reported in 28% of 67 women (aged 34–75 years) with chronic hypertension.[15] Although vascular abnormalities are a hallmark of this condition, it is interesting to note that the prevalence of orgasm dysfunction in this population is comparable to that of the general population.

The treatment of female orgasmic disorder (see Chapters 11.1 and 11.3)

Female orgasmic disorder has been treated from psychoanalytic, cognitive-behavioral, pharmacologic, and systems theory perspectives.[16] Substantial empirical outcome research is available only for cognitive-behavioral and pharmacologic approaches; hence, this review will focus specifically on these two methods of treatment (Table 11.4.1). Regardless of the treatment approach used, one needs to keep in mind that relationship factors such as marital satisfaction, marital adjustment, happiness, and stability have been linked to orgasm consistency, quality, and satisfaction in women.[17] A relation between

childhood sexual abuse (see Chapter 3.4) and various sexual difficulties has also been reported.[18] Although they are correlational in nature, these findings highlight the need for clinicians carefully to consider contextual factors such as a woman's sexual and relational history when designing a treatment approach.

Cognitive-behavioral approaches (see Chapters 11.1 and 11.3)

Cognitive-behavioral therapy for female orgasmic disorder focuses on promoting changes in attitudes and sexually relevant thoughts, decreasing anxiety, increasing the link between positive emotions and sexual behavior, and increasing orgasmic ability and satisfaction. As described below, the behavioral exercises used to induce these changes traditionally include directed masturbation, sensate focus, and systematic desensitization. Sex education, communication skills training, and Kegel exercises are also often included in cognitive-behavioral treatment programs for anorgasmia.

Directed masturbation (see Chapter 11.1)

Directed masturbation is most frequently prescribed for women with primary anorgasmia. LoPiccolo and Lobitz[19] were the first to detail a program of directed masturbation, and since then, several other researchers have provided variations.[20,21] The successive stages of directed masturbation train a woman to locate and manually stimulate genital areas that bring her sexual pleasure. The process begins with a visual exploration of the body, using a mirror and educational material depicting female genital anatomy. After visual and manual identification of the sensitive genital areas that elicit pleasure, a woman is instructed to apply targeted manual stimulation to these regions. Training on self-stimulation is directed toward the woman's achieving orgasm alone. Once she has accomplished this, her partner is incorporated into the directed masturbation sessions. The reasons for partner inclusion are twofold: first, the partner's presence serves as desensitization. As the woman learns to experience sexual arousal and orgasm openly in the company of her partner, anxiety accompanying sexual encounters lessens. Second, the partner observes how to stimulate the woman effectively.

To the extent that focusing on nonsexual cues can impede sexual performance,[22] masturbation exercises can help a woman to direct her attention to sexually pleasurable physical sensations. Because masturbation can be performed alone, any anxiety that may be associated with partner evaluation is necessarily eliminated. Moreover, because the amount and intensity of sexual stimulation is directly under the woman's control, she is not reliant upon her partner's knowledge or her ability and/or comfort with communicating her needs to her partner. Empirical support for this treatment approach is provided by research that shows a relation between masturbation and orgasmic ability. Kinsey et al.[23] reported that the average woman reached orgasm 95% of the time she engaged in masturbation compared with 73% during intercourse. More recently, Laumann et al.[3] reported a strong relation between frequency of masturbation and orgasmic ability during masturbation. Sixty-seven per cent of women who masturbated one to six times a year reported orgasm during masturbation compared with 81% of women who masturbated once a week or more.

Women with female orgasmic disorder have been treated successfully by directed masturbation in a myriad of therapy settings, such as group, individual, couples therapy, and bibliotherapy. A number of outcome studies and case series report directed masturbation is highly successful for treating primary anorgasmia. In an uncontrolled outcome study, Barbach[24] reported that 92% of 83 women with primary anorgasmia became orgasmic during masturbation after 10 sessions of group directed masturbation. In a wait-list controlled study, Delehanty[25] reported an 82% success rate in 28 women with primary anorgasmia who were treated with directed masturbation and assertiveness training in a 10-week group cotherapy format. Heinrich[26] reported that at 2-month follow-up, 100% of women with primary anorgasmia were able to attain orgasm during masturbation, and 47% were able to attain orgasm during intercourse after 10 sessions of therapist-directed group masturbation training. Among the women treated by self-directed masturbation training (bibliotherapy), 47% reported becoming orgasmic during masturbation and 13% during intercourse. In comparison, among the women who were assigned to wait-list control, only 21% were able to attain orgasm during masturbation, and none were able to attain orgasm during intercourse. McMullen and Rosen[27] compared the effectiveness of directed masturbation using bibliotherapy versus directed masturbation using instructional videotape versus wait-list control in 60 women with primary anorgasmia. They reported 65% of women who used a text and 55% of women who used videotapes had experienced orgasm during masturbation. Fifty per cent and 30%, respectively, were orgasmic during intercourse after 6 weeks. None of the wait-list control women had attained orgasm.

Few controlled studies have examined the exclusive effects of directed masturbation for treating secondary anorgasmia. Fitchen et al.[28] compared minimal therapist contact bibliotherapy with a variety of techniques, including directed masturbation, relaxation exercises, Kegel exercises, sensate focus, and sexual communication training, and found no change in orgasmic ability among 23 women with secondary anorgasmia. Hurlbert and Apt[29] recently compared the effectiveness of directed masturbation with coital alignment technique in 36 women with secondary anorgasmia. Coital alignment is a technique in which the woman assumes the supine position and the man positions himself up and forward on the woman. Thirty-seven per cent of the women receiving instructions on coital alignment technique versus 18% of those receiving directed masturbation reported substantial improvements (> 50% increase) in orgasmic ability during intercourse after four 30-min sessions. The benefits of this technique result from the fact that clitoral contact and possibly paraurethral stimulation are maximized.

Anxiety reduction techniques

Anxiety could potentially impair orgasmic function in women by disrupting the processing of erotic cues and causing the woman to focus instead on performance-related concerns, embarrassment, and/or guilt. This, in turn, could lead the woman to engage in self-monitoring during sexual activity, an experience Masters and Johnson[30] referred to as "spectatoring". Barlow[22] proposed that deficits in sexual function due to inhibited excitement are largely caused by disruptions in the processing of erotic cues necessary for arousal. These disruptions occur when sexual performance cues (i.e., those which occur during spectatoring) activate performance anxiety. This, in turn, leads to a shift in attention from reward-motivated focus on arousal cues to threat-motivated focus on sexual failure. Negative affect may perpetuate this cycle of dysfunctional sexual responding by contributing to an avoidance of erotic cues and consequent focus on nonerotic cues.[22] Indeed, a number of laboratory studies have demonstrated that cognitive distraction can impair sexual arousal in women.[31,32] Anxiety reduction techniques could be beneficial for helping women attain orgasm by enabling them to focus on pleasurable sexual thoughts and sensations that enhance arousal.

Systematic desensitization, first described by Wolpe,[33] and sensate focus, originally conceived by Masters and Johnson,[30] are the two most commonly used anxiety reduction techniques for treating female orgasmic disorder. Deep relaxation exercises in systematic desensitization enable the woman to replace fear responses with relaxation responses. A succession of anxiety-provoking stimuli is developed by the woman and the therapist to represent increasingly threatening sexual situations. The woman's task is to experience fearful and relaxed responses alternately, resulting in a net decrease of anxiety. After the woman can successfully imagine her hierarchy of anxiety-provoking situations without anxiety, she engages in the hierarchy of actual activities. Sensate focus is primarily a couple's skills-learning approach designed to increase communication and awareness of sexually sensitive areas between partners. Couples practicing sensate focus are instructed first to explore their partner's nonsexual body regions without the potential for sexual activity. The couple increasingly practice sexual touching without the pressure of sexual intercourse. The sexual touching allows a woman eventually to guide genital manual and penile stimulation to enhance her arousal. Conceptually, the removal of goal-focused orgasm, which can cause performance concerns; the hierarchic nature of the touching exercises; and the instruction not to advance to the next phase before feeling relaxed about the current one, suggest that sensate focus is also largely an anxiety reduction technique and could be considered a modified form of in vivo desensitization.

The success of using anxiety reduction techniques to treat female orgasmic disorder is difficult to assess because most studies have used some combination of anxiety reduction, sexual techniques training (e.g., directed masturbation), sex education, communication training, bibliotherapy, Kegel exercises, and/or pharmacologic agents, and have not systematically evaluated the

Table 11.4.1. Controlled outcome studies for the psychologic treatment of orgasm dysfunction

Reference	n	Subject characteristics	Definition of anorgasmia	Treatment	Outcome
Directed masturbation					
Heinrich[26]	44	M age = 25; 20 married, 24 with regular partner	Primary anorgasmia	DM (G) vs DM bibliotherapy (I) vs WL; DM: 10 sessions/5 weeks; DM bibliotherapy: 1 session	2 months: DM: 100% orgasmic with masturbation (om), 47% coitally orgasmic (co); DM bibliotherapy: 47% om, 13% co; WL: 21% om, 0% co
Munjack et al.[41]	22	12 prim, 10 sec	Primary and secondary anorgasmia	SD, DM, assertiveness training, modeling, sexual edu (I/C) vs WL; 22 weekly sessions	Tx > WL orgasmic ability; no difference between prim and sec
Riley and Riley[42]	SF (n = 15) DM + SF (n = 20)	M age = 26; married	Primary anorgasmia, defined as orgasmic inability regardless of type of sexual stimulation	DM and SF (C) vs SF (C); 6 weekly and 6 bimonthly sessions	DM and SF: 18/20 orgasmic; SF: 8/15 orgasmic; 1-year follow-up: gains maintained
McMullen and Rosen[27]	DM Bibliotherapy (n = 20) DM Instructional (n = 20) WL (n = 20)	M age = 29; 30 married, 30 single	Primary anorgasmia, defined as orgasmic inability through any sexual stimulation; assessed via clinician interview, self-report, and Sexual Behavior Inventory	DM Bibliotherapy (I) vs DM Instructional videotape (I) vs WL; 6 sessions/6 weeks	Bibliotherapy: 65% orgasm with masturbation (om), 50% coitally orgasmic (co); Instructional: 55% om, 30% co; WL: 0% om 0% co; 1-year follow-up: gains maintained/improved
Reisinger[43]	3	M age = 33; married 8–15 years	Secondary anorgasmia, coitally and by masturbation	DM with erotic video 8–13 sessions; stimulation by partner w/o training 2–6 sessions; stimulation by partner w/training 6–10 sessions; solitary stimulation w/o erotic aids 2–3 sessions; stimulation w/partner 4–7 sessions	DM: 3/3 orgasmic ability through masturbation; limited orgasmic success w/o partner training; 67% orgasmic ability with partner training; 2, 6-month follow-ups: 80% orgasmic ability with and without partner stimulation
Andersen[44]	30	M age = 25; 25 married, all with regular partners; some sexual aversion	Self-reported primary anorgasmia, also assessed via Sexual Interaction Inventory	SD (G) vs DM (G) vs WL; 10 sessions/5 weeks	DM > SD, WL on orgasmic response; 6-week follow-up: DM > SD on orgasmic response
Delehanty[25]	28	M age = 30	Preorgasmic: no history of orgasm within previous 5 years or primary anorgasmia; assessed via self-report and orgasm checklist	DM and assertiveness training in group cotherapy format for 10 weeks vs WL	82% orgasmic success with tx
Heiman and LoPiccolo[45]	41	M age = 30; 25 prim, 16 sec, absence of severe marital distress	Primary and secondary anorgasmia	CBT, communication training, DM, SF, systems conceptualization (C) vs WL; 15/1-h sessions	Prim and sec: increased duration foreplay and si; Prim: increased frequency si, increased orgasmic response during masturbation and si; sec: increased orgasmic response during si, increased initiation of sexual activity

Table 11.4.1. (Continued)

Reference	n	Subject characteristics	Definition of anorgasmia	Treatment	Outcome
Bogat et al.[46]	11	N/A	Self-reported preorgasmic (less than 10% of time) with desire to improve ability, also assessed with Women's Orgasmic Efficacy and Comfort Scale	DM vs no treatment (C); 10 sessions	80% Improvement in orgasmic success in tx vs controls
Eichel et al.[47]	CAT (n = 22) Control (n = 43 men and women)	CAT: M age = 40; Control: M age = 39; interest in sexual enhancement	Orgasmic function assessed via Orgasmic Attainment Criteria Scale	Coital alignment technique (C) vs no treatment (C)	CAT group: improvement in frequency of orgasm, simultaneous orgasm, and orgasm satisfaction compared to controls; use of CAT by both groups correlated with improved frequency of all orgasm variables
Hurlbert and Apt[29]	CAT (n = 19) DM (n = 17)	M age = 28; 36 sec; M years married = 5	Secondary anorgasmia, assessed via self-report and sex diary	Coital alignment technique (I) vs DM (I); 4 sessions of assertiveness training, communication, and SF	CAT: 37% substantially improved, 58% moderately improved orgasmic ability during si; DM: 18% substantially improved, 35% moderately improved orgasmic ability during si
Systematic desensitization					
Husted[48,49]	30	Mixed sexual dysfunction; all with partners; sexual anxiety	N/A	SD: imaginal (I) vs (C); vs in vivo (I) vs. (C) vs No-treatment control; Imaginal M = 8 sessions, in vivo M = 13 sessions	SD: decreased anxiety, increased coital frequency and orgasmic ability with masturbation; no difference (I) vs (C) or imaginal vs in vivo
Obler[50]	37	Mixed sexual dysfunction; marital status matched across groups	N/A	SD with videotapes (I) vs psychoanalytic tx with videotapes (G) vs WL; SD: 15 45-min sessions; Psychoanalytic: 10 75-min sessions	SD: 85% orgasmic; psychoanalytic: 36% orgasmic WL: 23% orgasmic SD > psychoanalytic, WL on decreased anxiety
Mathews et al.[51]	18	M age = 28; 13 prim, 5 sec; 17/18 low sexual desire/arousal	Primary and secondary anorgasmia	SD, sexual tx (C) vs SF, sexual tx (C) vs SF, bibliotherapy (C); 10 sessions; 3 sessions and 10-week mailing for SF, bibliotherapy	2/18 Increased orgasmic ability; no difference between groups; 4-month follow-up: no difference between groups
Wincze and Caird[52]	21	18–38 years old; 16 prim, 5 sec; 19/21 married; sexual anxiety	Frigidity, including "essential" sexual dysfunction	SD Imaginal (I) vs SD video (I) vs WL; M = 10 sessions/ 2–7 weeks	SD: 40% orgasmic; no difference between imaginal/video groups; 1–3-month follow-up: 25% orgasmic ability
Nemetz et al.[53]	SD (I) (n = 8) SD (G) (n = 8) Control (n = 6)	21–39 years old; 7 prim, 15 sec; sexual anxiety; all with regular partners	Primary and secondary anorgasmia	SD (I) vs SD (G) vs Control; 5 sessions/3 weeks	No difference between groups in orgasm; 3 weeks, 1yr follow-up: gains maintained

Table 11.4.1. (Continued)

Reference	n	Subject characteristics	Definition of anorgasmia	Treatment	Outcome
O'Gorman[54]	40	M age = 36; low sexual desire/arousal, some dysparuenia/vaginismus	Frigidity, including orgasm dysfunction	SD, sex edu (G), partner-only discussion groups vs SD, intravenous methoxitone sodium to induce relaxation (I with partner participation); SD (G) 20 1-hr sessions; SD (I) 15 10-min sessions/10 wk	SD, sex edu (G): 63% successful; SD, methoxitone sodium (I): 37% successful
Andersen[44]	30	M age = 25; 25 married, all with regular partners; some sexual aversion	Self-reported primary anorgasmia, also assessed via Sexual Interaction Inventory	SD (G) vs DM (G) vs WL; 10 sessions/5 weeks	DM > SD, WL on orgasmic response; 6-week follow-up: DM > SD on orgasmic response
Obler[55]	Integrated (n = 8) Couples (n = 8) No treatment (n = 10)	18–36 years old; married or cohabiting for over 2 years; no previous psychotherapy	N/A	42 weeks of Integrated hypnoanalytic/behavioral group vs 16 weeks of cotherapist/couples vs No tx; 1 year	Integrated: 7/8 self-reported orgasmic ability over 60% of time; cotherapist/Couples: 2/8 self-reported orgasmic ability over 60% of time; no tx: no self-reported orgasmic ability
Sensate focus/other					
Carney et al.[56]	Testosterone (n = 16) Diazepam (n = 16)	M age = 29; sexual anxiety; vaginismus or orgasm dysfunction as primary complaint excluded	Secondary anorgasmia assessed via self-report, clinician rating and independent assessor rating	SF weekly: testosterone, 10 mg daily (T) vs diazepam, 10 mg daily (C) vs. SF monthly: T vs diazepam (C); SF weekly: 16 sessions, SF monthly: 5 sessions	No difference in orgasm between weekly vs monthly T > diazepam frequency of orgasm; 6-month follow-up (after drug discontinuation): gains maintained
Roughan and Kunst[57]	PC group (n = 14) Relax (n = 12) Control (n = 14)	M age = 32; 14 with orgasmic dysfunction	Primary anorgasmia or secondary anorgasmia lasting over 2 years	PC (G): PC exercises, 5 times daily for 12 weeks vs relaxation (G): exercises for 12 weeks vs no tx	No relationship between PC muscle tone and orgasmic ability in any group
Fichten et al.[28]	23	M age = 33; M years married = 10	Secondary anorgasmia	Sexual information, relaxation, Kegel ex, DM, SF, sexual communication training, ban on si: (C) vs. (G) with minimal contact bibliotherapy; 14 weeks	SF: no change in orgasm; increase in enjoyment of noncoital sexual caressing and si
Chambless et al.[58]	16 (group n's not specified)	M age = 27	< 30% orgasm with coitus; assessed with Women's Sexuality Questionnaire	Kegel ex vs Attn. placebo (nonsexual imagery) vs. WL; 6 weeks	No differences in coital orgasmic frequency despite improvement in each group; no change in perceived vaginal stimulation during orgasm in any group
LoPiccolo et al.[59]	31	M age = 35; 12 prim, 19 sec; M years married = 13	Primary and secondary anorgasmia	CBT sexual therapy (LoPiccolo and Hogan, 1979) vs WL (C), both for 15 1-h sessions	Prim and sec: Increase in orgasm with masturbation; 3-month follow-up: gains maintained/improved
Kilmann et al.[38]	55	M age = 33; 51 married; all with partners; no dyspareunia or vaginismus, no premature ejaculation	Secondary anorgasmia for 5 months through si or clitoral stimulation and dissatisfied with coital orgasmic ability; assessed via clinician interview	2 2-h sessions sex education followed by communication skills (C/G) vs sexual skills (C/G) vs WL vs Attn-placebo	Communication and sexual skills > controls in coital orgasm ability; no difference between groups; 6-month follow-up: gains decreased, no difference between groups

Table 11.4.1. (Continued)

Reference	n	Subject characteristics	Definition of anorgasmia	Treatment	Outcome
Morokoff and LoPiccolo[60]	43	M age = 30; prim; M years married = 9; no male sexual dysfunction, no psychosis or depression	Primary anorgasmia, assessed via Sexual History Form	DM and bibliotherapy in either minimal therapist contact for 4 sessions (MTC; n = 14) vs full therapist contact for 15 sessions (FTC; n = 29)	Increased orgasmic ability with masturbation and si; MTC > FTC on increased frequency orgasm with masturbation
Kilmann et al.[61]	11	M age = 30; 10 married; no premature ejaculation in partners	Secondary anorgasmia, defined as 50% coital orgasm or less over 5 months and dissatisfaction with orgasmic frequency; assessed via structured interviews, Sexual Interaction Inventory and Sexual Behavior and Attitudes Questionnaire	2 2-h sessions sex education followed by communication and sexual skills vs WL vs Attn-placebo	Tx > WL, Attn-placebo: increase in orgasmic ability with tx
Milan et al.[62]	38	M age = 33; sec; M years relationship = 10; regular sexual partners with no dysfunction; 9% orgasmic frequency	Secondary anorgasmia, assessed via scale adapted from the Sexual Behavior and Attitudes Questionnaire	10 2-h sessions/5 weeks of sex education and either: communication skills vs sexual skills vs brief sex and communication skills vs didactic lecture vs WL 2-6 years:	No difference between tx groups, WL on sexual or relationship functioning
Van Lankveld et al.[63]	Bibliotherapy (n = 9) WL control (n = 9)	M age = 37; M sexual dysfunction duration = 8 years; hyposexual desire disorder; vaginismus; dyspareunia	DSM-IV diagnosis of orgasmic dysfunction via structured interview, with no distinction between primary and secondary anorgasmia; assessed via self-report and Golombok Rust Inventory of Sexual Satisfaction	Bibliotherapy (including communication skills, sexual education, and SF) and CBT with telephone support vs WL; 10 weeks	No improvement in orgasm in tx vs controls

SD = systematic desensitization, DM = directed masturbation, SF = sensate focus, CBT = cognitive-behavioral therapy, WL = wait-list, (I) = individual therapy, (C) = couples therapy, (G) = group therapy, (GI) = group/individual therapy, (GC) = group/couples therapy, prim = primary orgasmic dysfunction, sec = secondary orgasmic dysfunction, si = sexual intercourse, M = mean, tx = treatment.

independent contributions to treatment outcome. In addition, even within specific treatment modalities, considerable variation between studies exists. For instance, systematic desensitization has been conducted both imaginally and *in vivo*, has used mainly progressive muscle relaxation but also drugs[34] and hypnotic techniques[35] to induce relaxation, and has varied somewhat in the hierarchic construction of events. Variations in population demographics, sexual dysfunction severity, diagnoses, primary versus secondary anorgasmia, therapist characteristics, treatment settings, type of treatment, and duration of treatment further complicate systematic examination of anxiety reduction techniques for orgasmic function. With these limitations in mind, across controlled studies, women have reported decreases in anxiety and increases in the frequency of sexual intercourse and sexual satisfaction with systematic desensitization, but substantial improvements in orgasmic ability have not been noted (for review, see Meston et al.[36]). Similarly, of the few controlled studies that have included sensate focus as a treatment component, none have reported notable increases in orgasmic ability (for review, see Meston et al.[36]).

Other behavioral techniques

As discussed, female orgasmic disorder treatment outcome studies often contain a variety of treatments. To date, studies have not teased apart the independent contributions of each treatment component to account for improvement in orgasmic ability. However, these treatments have received wide support from the literature and thus warrant mention. Sex education has been a hallmark of sex therapy since the days of Masters and Johnson.[30] Education about female genital anatomy may help acquaint a woman with her body's pleasure-producing regions and consequently help alleviate orgasm difficulties. As demonstrated by Jankovich and Miller's study of women with primary anorgasmia,[37] seven out of 17 women experienced increased orgasmic capability after audiovisual sexual education sessions. In a comparison of the effectiveness of various sequences of sex education and communication skills training versus wait-list control, Kilmann and associates[38] found sex education to be beneficial for enhancing orgasmic ability in women with secondary anorgasmia at post-test but not at 6-month follow-up. Everaerd and Dekker[39] found sex therapy and communication skills training to be equally effective in improving orgasmic ability. Kegel[40] proposed that conducting exercises that strengthen the pubococcygeous muscle could facilitate orgasm by increasing vascularity to the genitals. Treatment comparison studies have generally found no differences in orgasmic ability between women whose therapy included using Kegel exercises and those whose therapy did not. However, to the extent that Kegel exercises may enhance arousal and/or help the woman become more aware and comfortable with her genitals, these exercises may enhance orgasm ability.

Pharmacologic approaches

Few placebo-controlled studies have examined the effectiveness of pharmacologic agents for treating female orgasmic disorder

(Table 11.4.2). Sustained release bupropion failed to improve orgasm in nondepressed women ($n = 20$) with orgasm dysfunction as compared to placebo. However, up to 20% of the sample experienced facilitated and/or more intense orgasms during bupropion treatment. These same individuals did not report comparable sexual effects with placebo.[64] Ito and colleagues[65] examined the effects of the female sexual health nutritional supplement ArginMax, a blend of ginseng, *Ginkgo biloba*, damiana leaf, and vitamins. After 4 weeks of using the supplement, approximately 47% of women treated with ArginMax reported an increase in the frequency of orgasm compared with approximately 30% of women treated with placebo – a marginally significant group difference. Baseline levels of sexual function were not established among participants, and thus it cannot be determined how many women would have met a clinical diagnosis of anorgasmia. Zajecka and associates[66] reported improvement in orgasm compared with baseline after 12 weeks of treatment with nefazodone, psychotherapy, or combined psychotherapy and nefazodone. The sample comprised depressed women who reported sexual dysfunction including orgasm difficulties. To date, there has been only one published placebo-controlled study of sildenafil for female anorgasmia.[67] In this study, 50 sexually healthy women (aged 19–38 years) were randomized to receive either 4 weeks' treatment with a selective phosphodiesterase type 5 inhibitor followed by a 2-week washout period and 4 weeks placebo, or the reverse sequence. The selective phosphodiesterase type 5 inhibitor significantly increased orgasmic function compared to both baseline and placebo.[67] Further placebo-controlled studies are needed to examine whether selective phosphodiesterase type 5 inhibitors facilitate orgasmic function in women diagnosed with female orgasmic disorder.

A number of studies have examined the effects of pharmacologic agents in treating antidepressant-induced anorgasmia. Because sexual dysfunction is itself associated with depression, a major weakness of research on antidepressant-induced sexual dysfunction is the inability to distinguish between dysfunction secondary to the depression or to the medications used to treat the depression. Furthermore, it is not known whether these agents would have the same treatment outcome effect on non-drug-induced versus drug-induced anorgasmia. These drugs include antiserotonergic agents, such as cyproheptadine, buspirone, mirtazapine, and granisetron; dopaminergic agents, such as amantadine, dextroamphetamine, bupropion, methylphenidate, and pemoline; adrenergic agents, such as yohimbine and ephedrine; cholinergic agents, such as bethanechol; and the selective phosphodiesterase type 5 inhibitor (see Chapters 14.1–14.2).[36] Numerous case reports and open-label studies report success in alleviating selective serotonin reuptake inhibitor-induced anorgasmia with some of these agents. Findings from the few placebo-controlled studies published are less optimistic.

In a 12-week study (4-week assessment period; 8-week treatment) conducted on premenopausal women with fluoxetine-induced sexual dysfunction, Michelson et al. compared the

Table 11.4.2. Controlled outcome studies for pharmacologic treatment of orgasm dysfunction

Reference	n	Subject characteristics	Antidepressant	Definition of anorgasmia	Treatment	Outcome
ArginMax						
Ito et al.[65]	77	M age = 43; 6 subjects with previous sexual dysfunction	N/A	Orgasm function assessed with Female Sexual Functioning Index	ArginMax herbal supplement for 4 weeks vs placebo	47% of ArginMax tx improved orgasm function at 4 weeks vs 30% in placebo
Bupropion						
Masand et al.[73]	Bupropion (n = 15) Placebo (n = 15)	Impairment of sex drive, arousal and/or vaginal lubrication	N/A	Impairment in orgasm and orgasm satisfaction assessed via Arizona Sexual Experiences Scale	Sustained release (SR) bupropion (150 mg) daily for 3 weeks vs placebo daily for 3 weeks	No difference bupropion vs placebo
Modell et al.[64]	20	21–54 years old; healthy	N/A	Self-reported secondary anorgasmia: inhibited or delayed orgasm	3 weeks placebo dose, 3 weeks SR bupropion (150 mg) once daily plus placebo dose, 3 weeks SR bupropion (150 mg) twice daily	No improvement in orgasm, satisfaction, or intensity beyond placebo with either 150– or 300-mg doses
Buspirone						
Landen et al.[69]	Buspirone (n = 16) Placebo (n = 11)	Major depressive disorder; decreased libido; orgasmic dysfunction (n = 19)	Citalopram (min 40 mg/day) or paroxetine (min 30 mg/day)	Orgasm dysfunction assessed in interview via Udvalg for Kliniske Undersøgelser Scale	Buspirone (20–60 mg/day) for 4 weeks vs placebo; SSRI continued during tx	8/15 showed remittance of sexual dysfunction at 4 weeks (change in orgasm function not specified)
Buspirone, Amantadine						
Michelson et al.[68]	Buspirone (n = 19) Amantadine (n = 18) Placebo (n = 20)	Depression; anxiety; obsessive compulsive disorder; PMS; decreased arousal and pleasure; premenopausal or estrogen therapy	Fluoxetine dosage by group: B (31.4 mg/day), A (28.4 mg/day), and P (25.7 mg/day)	Impaired orgasm, assessed by clinician, self-report, daily diary, and Interview Rating of Sexual Function Scale	Baseline and 4-week dose, respectively: amantadine (50, 100 mg/day) buspirone (20,30 mg/day) vs placebo; fluoxetine continued during tx	Improved orgasm with tx and placebo; no difference tx vs placebo
Ephedrine						
Meston[72]	19	Female sexual arousal disorder with complaints of decreased orgasm	Fluoxetine, sertraline, or paroxetine; min. 10 weekd	Orgasmic ability, intensity/ pleasure assessed via self-report	Two wk baseline, 8-week crossover design placebo vs 50 mg ephedrine 1 h prior to sexual activity	Improved orgasm intensity/pleasure with ephedrine tx and placebo; no difference in orgasm tx vs placebo
Ginkgo biloba						
Kang et al.[71]	G. biloba (n = 4) Placebo (n = 6)	G. biloba group: M age = 47; placebo group: M age = 46; depressive or anxiety disorders	Fluoxetine (20 mg/day), paroxetine (20–40 mg/day), or nortriptyline (30 mg/day)	DSM-IV diagnosis of sexual dysfunction; orgasm satisfaction and frequency via self-report and clinical interview	G. biloba at 120 mg/day for 2 weeks, 160 mg/day for following 2 weeks, 240 mg/day for final 4 weeks vs placebo doses on same schedule	No improvement in orgasm frequency or satisfaction with ginkgo vs placebo; 8 weeks: orgasm satisfaction improved with placebo

Table 11.4.2. (Continued)

Reference	n	Subject characteristics	Antidepressant	Definition of anorgasmia	Treatment	Outcome
Mirtazepine, Yohimbine, and Olanzapine						
Michelson et al.[70]	Mirtazepine (n = 36) Yohimbine (n = 35) Olanzapine (n = 38) Placebo (n = 39)	M age = 36; depression; decreased vaginal lubrication	Fluoxetine (20 mg/day or greater)	Self-reported orgasmic inhibition, at least moderate in severity	Random assignment to mirtazapine (15–30 mg/day), yohimbine (5.4–10.8 mg/day), olanzapine (2.5–5 mg/day), or placebo, taken 1–2 h before sex	No differences drug vs placebo in diary or self-report ratings of orgasm function
Sildenafil						
Caruso et al.[67]	n = 50	M age = 27; sexually healthy	N/A	Orgasm function assessed using Personal Experiences Questionnaire	Randomized, crossover study of 4 weeks placebo, 2-week washout, 4 weeks sildenafil (50 mg or reverse sequence	Significant improvement in orgasm with sildenafil vs placebo

effects of buspirone (20 mg/day; n = 19), amantadine (50 mg/day; n = 18), and placebo (n = 20) on sexual excitement, arousal, and orgasm.[68] Sexual function was evaluated before, during, and after treatment with daily sexual diaries, self-report measures, and clinical interviews. Women in the buspirone, amantadine, and placebo groups all showed improvements in orgasmic ability, and there were no statistically significant differences in improvement between groups. At higher dose levels (mean dose = 47 mg/day), 4-week treatment with buspirone relieved sexual dysfunction in 53% (8/15) of women with sexual dysfunction secondary to citalopram or paroxetine treatment. By comparison, improvements were noted in 18% (2/11) of the women who received placebo.[69] Unfortunately, the specific impact on orgasmic ability was not reported.

In a well-controlled study by Michelson and colleagues,[70] premenopausal women with either anorgasmia or impaired vaginal lubrication secondary to fluoxetine treatment were randomized to 6-week treatment with either placebo (n = 39), mirtazapine (30 mg/day; n = 36), yohimbine (10.8 mg/day; n = 35), or olanzapine (5 mg/day; n = 38). Results indicated no significant differences between groups on measures of orgasmic ability. Findings from an 8-week study evaluating the impact of *Ginkgo biloba* versus placebo on antidepressant-induced sexual dysfunction in depressed and anxious women (n = 10) revealed no significant difference between groups on measures of sexual dysfunction.[71] Most recently, the impact of 50 mg ephedrine on sexual function was examined in a randomized, double-blind, crossover study in women (n = 19) with sexual dysfunction secondary to fluoxetine, sertraline, or paroxetine treatment.[72] Ephedrine showed no significant effect on orgasmic ability beyond placebo.

Conclusions

In summary, directed masturbation has been shown to be an empirically valid, efficacious treatment for women diagnosed with primary anorgasmia, and may be beneficial for women with secondary anorgasmia who are uncomfortable touching their genitals. If the woman is able to attain orgasm alone by masturbation, but not with her partner, it may prove more beneficial to address issues relating to communication and trust, as well as to ensure that the woman is receiving adequate stimulation either via direct manual stimulation or intercourse positions designed to maximize clitoral stimulation (i.e., coital alignment technique). Anxiety does not appear to play a causal role in female orgasmic disorder; thus, anxiety reduction techniques are best suited for anorgasmic women only when anxiety is coexistent. Sex education, communication skills training, and Kegel exercises may serve as beneficial adjuncts to therapy. Used alone, they do not appear highly effective for treating either primary or secondary anorgasmia. To date, no pharmacologic agents have proven to be beneficial beyond placebo in enhancing orgasmic function in women with diagnosed female orgasmic disorder. Placebo-controlled research is needed to examine the effective-

ness of agents with demonstrated success in open-label trials or among sexually healthy women (i.e., bupropion, granisetron, and sildenafil) on orgasmic function in women with female orgasmic disorder.

References

1. American Psychiatric Association. *Diagnostic and Statistical Manual of Mental Disorders*, 4th edn, text revision (DSM-IV-TR). Washington, DC: 1994.
2. Frank E, Anderson A, Rubinstein D. Frequency of sexual dysfunction in "normal" couples. *N Engl J Med* 1978; 299: 111–15.
3. Laumann EO, Gagnon JH, Michael RT et al. *The Social Organization of Sexuality: Sexual Practices in the United States*. Chicago: University of Chicago Press, 1994.
4. Levin RJ. Sexual desire and the deconstruction and reconstruction of the human female sexual response model of Masters and Johnson. In W Everaerd, E Laan, S Both, eds. *Sexual Appetite, Desire and Motivation: Energetics of the Sexual System*. Amsterdam: Royal Netherlands Academy of Arts and Sciences, 2001: 63–93.
5. Masters WH, Johnson V. *Human Sexual Response*. Boston: Little, Brown, 1966.
6. Whipple B, Ogden G, Komisaruk BR. Physiological correlates of imagery-induced orgasm in women. *Archiv Sex Behav* 1992; 21: 121–33.
7. Levin RJ. The mechanisms of human female sexual arousal. *Annu Rev Sex Res* 1992; 3: 1–48.
8. Polatin P, Douglas DE. Spontaneous orgasm in a case of schizophrenia. *Psychoanal Rev* 1953; 40: 17–26.
9. Derogatis LR, Schmidt CW, Fagan PJ et al. Subtypes of anorgasmia via mathematical taxonomy. *Psychosomatics* 1989; 30: 166–73.
10. Meston CM. Validation of the Female Sexual Function Index (FSFI) in women with female orgasmic disorder and in women with hypoactive sexual desire disorder. *J Sex Marital Ther* 2003; 29: 39–46.
11. Rosen RT, Taylor JF, Leiblum SR. Prevalence of sexual dysfunction in women: results of a survey study of 329 women in an outpatient gynecological clinic. *J Sex Marital Ther* 1993; 19: 171–88.
12. Basson R, Leiblum S, Brotto L et al. Definitions of women's sexual dysfunction reconsidered: advocating expansion and revision. *J Psychosom Obstet Gynecol* 2003; 24: 221–9.
13. Laumann EO, Paik A, Rosen RC. Sexual dysfunction in the United States: prevalence and predictors. *JAMA* 1999; 281: 537–44.
14. Read S, King M, Watson J. Sexual dysfunction in primary medical care: prevalence, characteristics and detection by the general practitioner. *J Public Health Med* 1997; 19: 387–91.
15. Burchardt M, Burchardt T, Anastasiadis AG et al. Sexual dysfunction is common and overlooked in female patients with hypertension. *J Sex Marital Ther* 2002; 28: 17–26.
16. Heiman JR. Orgasmic disorders in women. In SR Leiblum, RC Rosen, eds. *Principles and Practice of Sex Therapy*, 3rd edn. New York: Guildford Press, 2000.

17. Mah K, Binik YM. The nature of human orgasm: a critical review of major trends. *Clin Psychol Rev* 2001; 21: 823–56.

18. Meston CM, Heiman JR, Trapnell PD. The relation between early abuse and adult sexuality. *J Sex Res* 1999; 36: 385–95.

19. LoPiccolo J, Lobitz WC. The role of masturbation in the treatment of orgasmic dysfunction. *Archiv Sex Behav* 1972; 2: 163–71.

20. Annon JS. The therapeutic use of masturbation in the treatment of sexual disorders. In RD Rubin, JP Brady, JD Henderson, eds. *Advances in Behavior Therapy*, vol. 4. New York: Academic Press, 1973.

21. Heiman JR, LoPiccolo L, LoPiccolo J. *Becoming Orgasmic: A Sexual Growth Program for Women*. Englewood Cliffs: Prentice-Hall, 1976.

22. Barlow DH. Causes of sexual dysfunction: the role of anxiety and cognitive interference. *J Consult Clin Psychol* 1986; 54: 140–8.

23. Kinsey AC, Pomeroy WD, Martin CE et al. *Sexual Behaviour in the Human Female*. Philadelphia: WB Saunders, 1953: 628.

24. Barbach LG. Group treatment of preorgasmic women. *J Sex Marital Ther* 1974; 1: 139–45.

25. Delehanty R. Changes in assertiveness and changes in orgasmic response occurring with sexual therapy for preorgasmic women. *J Sex Marital Ther* 1982; 8: 198–208.

26. Heinrich AG. The effect of group and self-directed behavioral-educational treatment of primary orgasmic dysfunction in females treated without their partners. Doctoral dissertation, University of Colorado, Boulder, CO, 1976.

27. McMullen S, Rosen RC. Self-administered masturbation training in the treatment of primary orgasmic dysfunction. *J Consult Clin Psychol* 1979; 47: 912–18.

28. Fitchen CS, Libman E, Brender W. Methodological issues in the study of sex therapy: effective components in the treatment of secondary orgasmic dysfunction. *J Sex Marital Ther* 1983; 9: 191–202.

29. Hurlbert DF, Apt C. Coital alignment technique and directed masturbation: a comparative study on female orgasm. *J Sex Marital Ther* 1995; 21: 21–9.

30. Masters WH, Johnson VE. *Human Sexual Inadequacy*. London: Churchill, 1970.

31. Dove NL, Wiederman MW. Cognitive distraction and women's sexual functioning. *J Sex Marital Ther* 2000; 26: 67–78.

32. Elliott AN, O'Donohue WT. The effects of anxiety and distraction on sexual arousal in a nonclinical sample of heterosexual women. *Arch Sex Behav* 1997; 26: 607–24.

33. Wolpe J. *Psychotherapy by Reciprocal Inhibition*. Stanford: Stanford University Press, 1958.

34. Brady JP. Brevital-relaxation treatment of frigidity. *Behav Res Ther* 1966; 4: 71–7.

35. Kraft T, Al-Issa I. Behavior therapy and the treatment of frigidity. *Am J Psychol* 1967; 21: 116–20.

36. Meston CM, Hull E, Levin RJ et al. Women's orgasm. In *Sexual Medicine*. Plymouth: Plymbridge Distributors, 2004.

37. Jankovich R, Miller PR. Response of women with primary orgasmic dysfunction to audiovisual education. *J Sex Marital Ther* 1978; 4: 16–19.

38. Kilmann PR, Mills KH, Caid C et al. Treatment of secondary orgasmic dysfunction: an outcome study. *Archiv Sex Behav* 1986; 15: 211–29.

39. Everaerd W, Dekker J. Treatment of secondary orgasmic dysfunction: a comparison of systematic desensitization and sex therapy. *Behav Res Ther* 1982; 20: 269–74.

40. Kegel AH. Sexual functions of the pubococcygeus muscle. *West J Surg Obstet Gynecol* 1952; 60: 521–4.

41. Munjack D, Cristol A, Goldstein A et al. Behavioral treatment of orgasmic dysfunction: a controlled study. *Br J Psychiatry* 1976; 129: 497–502.

42. Riley AJ, Riley EJ. A controlled study to evaluate directed masturbation in the management of primary orgasmic failure in women. *Br J Psychiatry* 1978; 133: 404–9.

43. Reisinger JJ. Generalization of treatment effects following masturbatory training with erotic stimuli. *J Behav Ther Exp Psychiatry* 1979; 10: 247–50.

44. Andersen BL. A comparison of systematic desensitization and directed masturbation in the treatment of primary orgasmic dysfunction in females. *J Consult Clin Psychol* 1981; 49: 568–70.

45. Heiman JR, LoPiccolo J. Clinical outcome of sex therapy. *Arch Gen Psychiatry* 1983; 40: 443–9.

46. Bogat GA, Hamernik K, Brooks LA. The influence of self-efficacy expectations on the treatment of preorgasmic women. *J Sex Marital Ther* 1987; 13: 128–36.

47. Eichel EW, Eichel JD, Kule S. The technique of coital alignment and its relation to female orgasmic response and simultaneous orgasm. *J Sex Marital Ther* 1988; 14: 129–41.

48. Husted JR. The effect of method of systematic desensitization and presence of sexual communication in the treatment of female sexual anxiety by counterconditioning. Doctoral dissertation, University of California at Los Angeles, CA, 1972.

49. Husted JR. Desensitization procedures in dealing with female sexual dysfunction. *Couns Psychol* 1975; 5: 30–7.

50. Obler M. Systematic desensitization in sexual disorders. *J Behav Ther Exp Psychiatry* 1973; 4: 93–101.

51. Mathews A, Bancroft J, Whitehead A et al. The behavioral treatment of sexual inadequacy: a comparative study. *Behav Res Ther* 1976; 14: 427–36.

52. Wincze JP, Caird WK. The effects of systematic desensitization in the treatment of essential sexual dysfunction in women. *Behav Ther* 1976; 7: 335–42.

53. Nemetz GH, Craig KD, Reith G. Treatment of female sexual dysfunction through symbolic modeling. *J Consult Clin Psychol* 1978; 46: 62–73.

54. O'Gorman EC. The treatment of frigidity: a comparative study of group and individual desensitization. *Br J Psychiatry* 1978; 132: 580–4.

55. Obler M. A comparison of a hypnoanalytic/behavior modification technique and a cotherapist-type treatment with primary orgasmic dysfunctional females: some preliminary results. *J Sex Res* 1982; 18: 331–45.

56. Carney A, Bancroft J, Mathews A. Combination of hormonal and psychological treatment for female sexual unresponsiveness: a comparative study. *Br J Psychiatry* 1978; 132: 339–46.

57. Roughan PA, Kunst L. Do pelvic floor exercises really improve orgasmic potential? *J Sex Marital Ther* 1981; 7: 223–9.

58. Chambless DL, Sultan FE, Stern TE et al. Effect of pubococcygeal

exercise on coital orgasm in women. *J Consult Clin Psychol* 1984; 52: 114–18.

59. LoPiccolo J, Heiman JR, Hogan DR et al. Effectiveness of single therapist versus cotherapy teams in sex therapy. *J Consult Clin Psychol* 1985; 53: 287–94.

60. Morokoff PJ, LoPiccolo J. A comparative evaluation of minimal therapist contact and 15–session treatment for female orgasmic dysfunction. *J Consult Clin Psychol* 1986; 54: 294–300.

61. Kilmann PR, Milan RJ, Boland JP et al. The treatment of secondary orgasmic dysfunction. *J Sex Marital Ther* 1987; 13: 93–105.

62. Milan RJ, Kilmann PR, Boland JP. Treatment outcome of secondary orgasmic dysfunction: a two- to six-year follow-up. *Arch Sex Behav* 1988; 17: 463–80.

63. Van Lankveld JJDM, Everaerd W, Grotjohann Y. Cognitive-behavioral bibliotherapy for sexual dysfunctions in heterosexual couples: a randomized waiting-list controlled clinical trial in the Netherlands. *J Sex Res* 2001; 38: 51–67.

64. Modell JG, May RS, Katholi CR. Effect of bupropion-SR on orgasmic dysfunction in nondepressed subjects: a pilot study. *J Sex Marital Ther* 2000; 26: 231–40.

65. Ito TY, Trant AS, Polan ML. A double-blind placebo-controlled study of ArginMax, a nutritional supplement for enhancement of female sexual function. *J Sex Marital Ther* 2001; 27: 541–9.

66. Zajecka J, Dunner DL, Gelenberg AJ et al. Sexual function and satisfaction in the treatment of chronic major depression with nefazodone, psychotherapy, and their combination. *J Clin Psychiatry* 2002; 63: 709–16.

67. Caruso S, Intelisano G, Farina M et al. The function of sildenafil on female sexual pathways: a double blind, cross-over, placebo-controlled study. *Eur J Obstet Gynecol* 2003; 110: 201–6.

68. Michelson D, Bancroft J, Targum S et al. Female sexual dysfunction associated with antidepressant administration: a randomized, placebo-controlled study of pharmacologic intervention. *Am J Psychiatry* 2000; 157: 239–43.

69. Landen M, Eriksson E, Agren H et al. Effect of buspirone on sexual dysfunction in depressed patients treated with selective serotonin reuptake inhibitors. *J Clin Psychopharmacol* 1999; 19: 268–71.

70. Michelson D, Kociban K, Tamura R et al. Mirtazapine, yohimbine, or olanzapine augmentation therapy for serotonin reuptake-associated female sexual dysfunction: a randomized, placebo controlled trial. *J Psychiatr Res* 2002; 36: 147–52.

71. Kang B, Lee S, Kim M et al. A placebo-controlled, double-blind trial of *Ginkgo biloba* for antidepressant-induced sexual dysfunction. *Hum Psychopharmacol* 2002; 17: 279–84.

72. Meston CM. A randomized, placebo-controlled, crossover study of ephedrine for SSRI-induced female sexual dysfunction. *J Sex Marital Ther* 2004; 30: 57–8.

73. Masand PS, Ashton AK, Gupta S et al. Sustained-release bupropion for selective serotonin reuptake inhibitor-induced sexual dysfunction: a randomized, double-blind, placebo-controlled, parallel-group study. *Am J Psychiatry* 2001; 158: 805–7.

11.5 Difficult cases: psychologic treatment of desire, arousal and orgasm disorders

Stanley E Althof, Linda Banner

Introduction

What do mental health clinicians mean when they say they are working with a difficult case? Are they suggesting that the symptom is especially severe, or the duration of the problem is lifelong, or that the patient is resistant to treatment? Before embarking on this chapter, it may be worthwhile to consider what experienced clinicians mean when they use the word "difficult". Levine[1] suggests there are four situations that define the difficult therapy patient: (1) the woman insists that her problem is entirely medical and is not open to any other interpretation; (2) the sexual problem is embedded in the interpersonal context and the partner is unwilling to participate, or support, the treatment; (3) the sexual symptom is comorbid with severe personality problems and/or addiction; and (4) the women's sexual problem is complicated by her menopausal status. Segraves and Segraves[2] define "difficult" in terms of mysterious, as when neither the therapist nor patient can reasonably explain the symptom in terms of any predisposing, precipitating, maintaining, or contextual factors. Finally, perhaps "difficult" refers to a case that is multidetermined with biologic, relational, cultural, religious, and psychologic overlays which all contribute to the onset and maintenance of the symptom.

Whatever one's definition of "difficult" might be, therapists have had their share of such difficult patients. Some are frustrating, others challenging, some even impossible. Hopefully, no matter how difficult the case may be, we all learn something from working with these patients. With this in mind, we present a series of difficult cases of women with psychologically based hypoactive sexual desire and female sexual arousal disorders.[3] A wide array of integrative techniques will be presented, including traditional psychodynamic/individual therapy, cognitive-behavioral interventions, behavioral prescriptions, hypnosis, and biblio-/videotherapy. We hope these case vignettes pique interest and stimulate readers to consider what they might have done in these situations.

While the nomenclature suggests that hypoactive sexual desire disorder and female sexual arousal disorder are discrete and separate disorders, women are seen typically in clinical practice with combined dysfunctions. Because the *Diagnostic and Statistical Manual of Mental Disorders*, fourth edition, text revision (DSM-IV-TR),[4] and the World Health Organization's *International Classification of Diseases* (ICD-10)[5] nosology was not in keeping with what was seen clinically, a consensus panel of experts met to revise the definitions of women's sexual dysfunction.[6] The panel recognized the saliency of contextual factors and differentiated between the subjective and physiologic aspects of female sexual arousal disorder. The panel recommended that female sexual arousal disorder be divided into three distinct subcategories: (1) physiologic sexual arousal disorder; (2) subjective sexual arousal disorder; (3) mixed physiologic and subjective arousal.

We use the following metaphor with patients to sort through the multiple etiologic considerations for hypoactive sexual desire disorder and female sexual arousal disorder. For some, hypoactive sexual desire disorder is like not being able to find the ignition to start the engine of a car (i.e., sexual response cycle). This could be due to a low battery (i.e., hormones), low fuel (i.e., tired and other psychologic distractions), or starter problems (i.e., knowing it will not be satisfactory – no orgasm or pain – so why start the process?). Female sexual arousal disorder is like not being able to get the fuel to the engine and allow it to warm up and ignite.

It is always challenging to present clinical case material. For purposes of confidentiality and to protect the patients' right to privacy, the material has been disguised and altered. The essential clinical problem and interventions, however, remain unaltered and described through the eyes of the therapist.

Case 1 – Sam and Sara

This was one of the most interesting and challenging cases because so much was going on to disrupt the couple's relationship, let alone the wife's libido. Sam, a 45-year-old businessman, had started and built up a successful construction company without support from anyone other than Sara, his 44-year-old wife of 27 years. They had been high-school sweethearts, had married when Sara left high school, and had quickly begun a family. Their older son had not gone to college because he struggled with substance abuse, while the younger attended college and was working with Sam.

Sara sought treatment for her low libido. Her childhood history revealed that she had been molested by several of her mother's boyfriends from about 9 to 12 years of age. Her mother neither believed nor protected her when she was told about the incidents. Consequently, Sara learned to use sex to get attention in high school and learned that it was not something special to be enjoyed. Sex was something she did to "get and keep a guy".

When she and Sam started dating in high school, she did not want to have sex on the first or second date because she wanted it to be "special with him". However, he had been accustomed to demanding and receiving sex, so he threatened to end the relationship after a couple of weeks unless "she put out". Ultimately, she complied. Sara was 14 at the time of her first sexual experience and she admitted that she never enjoyed it or experienced an orgasm. Due to Sara's sexual abuse history, she learned not to trust primary caregivers and to use sex in an unhealthy way. In their early years of marriage, Sam had numerous affairs and prodded Sara to join him in "swinging" parties. With great reluctance, she complied for a period of years.

Two years before beginning treatment, she had an affair with a family friend and considered divorce. However, she did not want to end up like her mother, with many men, so she chose to disclose the information to her husband, precipitating their beginning couples therapy.

Multiple predisposing, precipitating, maintaining, and contextual events helped explain Sara's hypoactive sexual desire disorder, including her history of sexual abuse and feeling that "women were not safe or valuable sexually"; feeling a lack of trust and respect from her husband's many affairs; and guilt from her affair and comparing her husband to the other man sexually. Sara also had perimenopausal symptoms of mood swings,

depression, and low libido. She had a hypercritical mother and absent father, and her older son's substance abuse problem was a significant distraction. Sara was the primary office person for her husband's business.

Sara's initial visits were individual, with attempts to quell her anxieties through guided relaxation tapes. Then, Sam and Sara began couples therapy. Sam was able to be consistently empathic to and supportive of Sara, and this helped her build trust and respect. She was reminded that the relationship she and Sam were creating was unlike anything either of them had experienced previously.

They were asked to make a list of positives about their partner and themselves and share it in the therapy room. They described their ideal relationship and steps to enable them to achieve mutual relationship satisfaction. They were instructed to take turns planning a relaxing and romantic evening for each other without the endpoint of erections, intercourse, or orgasm. The endpoints were relaxation, romance, sensuality, and pleasure. In addition they were to make a past, present, and future affection list and plan a surprise from these lists for each other. They watched educational videos and talked about sex openly with the emphasis on intimacy instead of performance. Sara reported that she had always experienced performance anxiety, so that was part of the reason for having her do the relaxation tapes. Additionally, Sara began a regimen of hormone therapy to help stabilize her moods.

The couple began to focus on fun and making time to get away from the household stressors. They also developed a mutually agreed upon plan for dealing with the oldest son's substance abuse. By working holistically and understanding the presenting problem from broad perspective, they were able to make the necessary changes to promote interpersonal growth and increased intimacy. Sara admitted she now actually felt closer to Sam than ever before – both emotionally and physically.

Case 2 – John and Jane

What made this next case difficult was that both partners were resistant to changing and "giving in" to the other partner. John, a 55-year-old computer consultant, and his wife of 32 years, Jane, a 55-year-old marketing manager, presented for treatment of low sexual desire. This couple had two children in their twenties attending college. A medical evaluation to assess hormonal status indicated that Jane was perimenopausal, with no significant alterations in hormone levels. During Jane's sex history taken separately from John,[2] she reported being aware of "using sex as her power within the marriage". She was the oldest of three children and as a child felt like she was "closer to her father than her mother". Jane was always the "responsible and good girl" and had been with a couple of partners during the "swinging '70s" but had been monogamous since marriage. When stressed, she became private and enjoyed being alone.

John had normal sexual function and a very high libido. He was the youngest of three children and had two older sisters. He was also quite responsible and yet learned to quiet his anxiety with "connecting". They were the classic isolator/fuser combination.[7]

Each partner tended to keep score of what the other did. Jane used sex as her power within the relationship. She felt she had to use this power because it was "what her husband wanted and she had control over it". When the children were growing up, she could stay busy being "supermom" and avoided sex by the excuse, "the children might hear us". However, when the children left home for college, John began requesting more sex. His desire for physical intimacy was about once or twice a week, after it had fallen to once a month during child-rearing years.

Both were committed to the marriage and had previously been to three other marriage counselors. This was their first experience with a sex therapist. In addition to hormonal assessment, Jane was evaluated for depression and anxiety. The psychiatrist prescribed a variety of psychotropic medications to treat her depression.

The treatment regimen for this couple included traditional cognitive-behavioral sex therapy, relationship counseling, communication and negotiation skills, and recorded hypnosis for Jane. Traditional cognitive-behavioral sex therapy included focusing on the "goods" about themselves and their partner; defining their relationship and sex therapy goals; identifying the "hot buttons" from their families of origin that would create barriers to intimacy; and taking turns with a special romantic, relaxation, and pleasure-focused evening where the endpoint was not intercourse. They were instructed to take turns with blindfolds and hand restraints during the sensate focus massage sessions to focus on increasing sensual awareness. Hence, the sexual responsiveness in the areas of visual and tactile hand responses was minimized, while that of the olfactory, skin, taste, and hearing were increased. This process has a double benefit of increasing intimacy and trust within the relationship and increasing anticipatory arousal.

When this couple watched an educational video series, they enjoyed being able to observe it in the comfort of their home, so that they could stop and start it as they desired. Many couples report stopping the video and trying some of the exercises presented and then continuing the video on another day. Again, the goal is not the endpoint of intercourse and orgasm, but rather of romance, relaxation, and pleasure (i.e., connection, communication, and intimacy).

In the case of John and Jane, real progress in their treatment plan was made once Jane felt heard by John due to their enhanced communication and negotiation skills. John was able to pull back on his sexual demands and empathize with Jane's depression. It is a fine line between "identified patient" and whole and healthy partner when doing couples counseling and cognitive-behavioral sex therapy. The therapist must be ever mindful of not getting into the middle of the couple's power struggle, and triangulating with the couple. Another difficult topic to address and be aware of is the potential for secondary gain for maintaining the problem. Jane knew that withholding sex was her only power in the relationship, so her motivation to

"fix" the problem was much lower than John's. This potential of secondary gain is what made this a difficult case to treat. It was further complicated by the long-term symptoms of depression, and her peri-menopausal symptoms of decreased libido and vaginal dryness.[8]

The good news was that once the integrative treatment began, and the couple worked collaboratively, progress was made in decreasing the sexual power struggle. Unfortunately, this couple faced many other stressors and distractions during the treatment process. Each spouse lost a parent and each lost their job at one time or another during our treatment process. Because of their commitment to therapy and their marriage, they persevered until their relationship moved to a place that allowed for the trust and safety that fostered relaxed physical intimacy together. The treatment process ended 2 years ago, although they still come back from time to time for tuneups and to refresh their intimacy skills.

Case 3 – James and Joan

This couple had been married 15 years but had never had intercourse or consummated their marriage. Joan was defensive in therapy and presented for treatment of pelvic pain and low sexual desire because of threats of divorce from James. Her motivation to fix the problem was more extrinsic than intrinsic. The case demonstrates the comorbidities associated with, and the complexity of, female sexual dysfunction. That they could remain married and friendly for that length of time without intercourse is remarkable, and underscores their commitment to the relationship. However, the chronicity of their asexual relationship suggested that this behavior was entrenched and would be difficult to change. James was a 43-year-old computer engineer, and Joan was a 44-year-old interior designer. She had been to other physicians and psychotherapists without success for treatment of low sexual desire and pelvic pain disorder. She had tried hormones and exercise, but was resistant to other medications.

The author[2] focused on helping her find her voice in the relationship and at work. As she developed feelings of safety and trust within her marriage, she also increased her self-confidence about her sexuality, and this allowed for more frequent physical intimacy.

In addition to the psychotherapy that included guided relaxation and recorded hypnosis to help quiet her anxieties around work and sexuality, Joan also worked with a physical therapist to treat her pelvic pain. She was advised to watch a video on physical intimacy in the context of emotional connection. It seemed that by using this collaborative and broad treatment protocol, this couple were able to overcome patterns of sexual inhibition that had plagued them for their entire married life. At the completion of treatment, the wife admitted looking forward to daily physical connection with her husband, whether it included intercourse or not. As her self-confidence and relationship satisfaction increased, the pelvic pain dissipated, as did the hypoactive sexual desire disorder.

Case 4 – Robert and Lana

Initially, Robert and Lana seemed like a straightforward case of combined desire/arousal disorder. What made this case difficult was that it seemed the explanation for Lana's problems had clear recent precipitants that could easily be turned around. This bright, insightful, couple in their early thirties were highly motivated to overcome their sexual dilemma. Additionally, the author felt good about this couple, liking them and enjoying the therapeutic work. There was only one catch; no matter what was done, her sexual symptoms never improved. Both grew as individuals but ultimately grew apart as a couple.

This case seemed simple because there were three clearly precipitating/contextual factors. First, the couple had purchased a "fixer-upper house" where anything that could go wrong did. After 2 years, they were still living between sheets of plastic to keep the drywall dust off their bed, the bathroom was barely useable, and progress on the home was agonizingly slow. Second, Lana's mother had unexpectedly passed away. Third, Robert's appetite for sex seemed insatiable.

Prior to their marriage of 2 years, the couple reported a frequent and satisfying sexual life. As the marriage approached, however, Lana noticed that she was losing interest in being sexual. She was no longer able to get aroused or easily achieve satisfying orgasms.

Lana's physical examination by her gynecologist was unremarkable – she took no medications and had no illness, her periods were regular, and she was athletic and fit. The gynecologist referred her for psychologic intervention, believing that the new sexual symptoms were the result of the stressful precipitating and contextual factors.

Weekly meetings were agreed upon to focus on the precipitating/contextual issues. Focus was on their feelings concerning the unfinished house. Robert felt he was to blame for them "living in a dump". He felt incompetent and overwhelmed by the complexity of the necessary repairs. Lana had grown weary of his "fumbling". Early in treatment, they decided to give up on their dream of building a "love nest" and hired a contractor, who quickly finished the job. Lana was also aided in the grieving process over her mother's death. As expected, Robert held ambivalent feelings toward her mother.

We also began to examine Robert's sexual insatiability. Two factors seemed responsible; as Lana withdrew sexually, he became increasingly anxious and calmed himself by being sexual (of course this pushed Lana to withdraw further). Second, the hypersexuality served as a compensatory mechanism for his wounded masculinity. He felt incompetent and inadequate because he could not successfully complete the home repairs. He agreed to initiate sexual interactions with Lana for the moment. These changes took place over the course of several months, and the couple seemed to be doing better; yet, surprisingly, Lana's symptoms persisted.

At this point, the author rethought the initial hypothesis, that the precipitating and contextual factors were responsible for Lana's sexual dysfunction. A new history was taken with an emphasis on finding predisposing factors that could help explain the impasse. Two facts emerged: at age 18, Lana had become pregnant and chose to have an abortion; and she recalled being molested as an 8-year-old by a baby sitter. At this point in her life, she no longer felt conflicted about the abortion and did not think it was related to her symptoms. She did, however, wonder about the impact of sexual abuse. It was still a mystery why she could have had 2 years of good premarital sex and then become symptomatic just prior to marriage.

Because the therapeutic work was now more focused on Lana's past life, she began to be seen individually. While treatment appeared to help Lana work through the complicated feelings of being sexually victimized, her sexual symptoms did not improve. While Lana was being seen individually, Robert disclosed that he had fallen in love with another woman and wanted to leave the marriage. He did, and the next 6 months was spent on helping Lana deal with his betrayal and abandonment. Obviously, the sexual symptoms took a back seat to helping maintain her mental health through the divorce process. Two years later, when she was feeling better, we agreed to end therapy. This case was difficult because no matter what the focus, predisposing, precipitating, or contextual factors, Lana's sexual symptoms never got much better.

A year after therapy ended, around Christmas, Lana sent a letter, stating, "First of all I owe you another big thank you. Shortly after we ended therapy, I felt something I didn't expect. It was a wonderful feeling directly related to the finality of treatment. I felt like you had given me permission to go on with my life. By ending therapy you indicated that I had grown up, that I could take care of myself and that you trusted me to do just that. What a wonderful feeling that was. And, so very different from my mother who never acknowledged me as an adult."

Five years later Lana telephoned, saying she had remarried. She talked about her new life and that she no longer had sexual problems. Perhaps the explanation had more to do with the relationship with Robert than originally thought. Or, perhaps the material discussed concerning her childhood allowed her to feel more adult and sexually comfortable in the new relationship.

Case 5 – Dan and Dawn

This next case is presented because it highlights several therapeutic difficulties, including the unwillingness of one partner to participate in treatment, childhood issues of mistrust and lack of respect from each partner's family of origin,[7] and the couple's resistance to allowing themselves to be helped by someone outside their relationship. This case was further complicated by their internal conflicts between professing openness and willingness to change, and their deep personal pain relating to their inherent mistrust in primary relationships from their unhealthy families of origin, which caused them to be very resistant to change and psychotherapy.

Dan and Dawn were both 35-year-old elementary schoolteachers who had been married for 10 years. Dawn presented with low libido after their second daughter had been born, 5 years previously. Both of them thought that, since they were teachers, they could learn skills to overcome this problem on their own. They had tried vacations without the children, weekend getaways without children, and date nights. None of these solutions had worked. Instead, a cycle evolved where intimacy was avoided, and each became angry and aggressive with the other. From Dawn's perspective, Dan would take his sexual frustrations out on her, and she would get defensive and resentful, further widening the wedge between them.

During the first meeting with Dawn, she said that because it was her problem, Dan was not interested in coming for sex therapy. However, he would participate in the homework that was sent home with her. The author began by taking a sex and family history from Dawn and establishing what their sex life was like before children, when things changed, and what solutions they had previously attempted. The family history revealed that Dawn had a history of always trying to please her parents but never succeeding. It was not surprising that she chose a husband who was also critical of her, whether it concerned her body image, sexuality, professional skills, parenting skills, or the way she combed her hair. She learned to develop better boundaries, and not react to Dan's critical nature that had caused her to feel defensive and angry.

Clearly, the defensiveness and anger within the relationship made it difficult for Dawn to allow herself to relax enough to become aroused, let alone want to initiate physical intimacy. Dan, like many men, wanted to do "makeup sex" after a confrontation; Dawn felt like it would be like "sleeping with the enemy" without resolving the source of the conflict. The couple became mired in the negative feedback loop of attack and defend, and did not make progress until Dawn began responding instead of reacting to Dan.

As Dawn's self-confidence increased and she learned not to personalize or react to Dan's critical nature, she was able to stay more balanced and, ultimately, loving and available to him. She was taught effective communication and negotiation skills so that the confrontations were minimal and there was more positive energy for the relationship. Dawn practiced with guided relaxation tapes to help quiet her anxiety so that she did not amplify Dan's inherent anxiety. She taught Dan breathing and connecting exercises so that they could both respond without reacting together. Dawn listed her past, present, and future ways of showing and sharing affection with Dan, and he made a similar list with her when she got home. They took turns planning a surprise from this list for each other each week. When treatment was finished, Dawn reported that she not only enjoyed the more frequent lovemaking with her husband, but she was also able episodically to initiate it. And, the more satisfied she was with their physical intimacy, the less anxious and angry Dan was with her. The negative feedback loop was converted to a positive feedback loop for this couple by giving them better physical intimacy skills in the context of the whole relationship.

Case 6 – Norm and Nancy

Norm and Nancy, a 30-year-old Asian couple, sought treatment because of her lack of desire, difficulty with lubrication, and total anorgasmia. What made this case difficult was her multiple sexual dysfunctions, the fact that they had not consummated their marriage, and Norm's family demanding grandchildren.

Theirs had been an arranged marriage. They had been married for 10 years and were desperate to have children. This added an additional layer of complexity to the case. This was their first foray into treatment because they had been focused on Nancy's establishing a professional career and gaining comfort living in America.

Another therapeutic hurdle involved cultural messages that directed her to keep personal problems within the family, especially sexual difficulties.

Treatment began with the usual family and sex history, with Norm doing most of the talking because Nancy's English was not as good as she would have liked it to be. After the histories, they were instructed about general sexual function and mechanics. Then, their enormous performance anxiety was addressed by giving them homework consisting of having them take turns doing a "special evening" with the emphasis on relaxation, romance, and pleasure and avoiding the goals of erection, intercourse, and orgasm. Norm prepared a special dinner for Nancy, dried her back when she got out of the bath, and did the "clean breast inspection". This is a playful activity that takes the performance anxiety away by having the man kiss the woman's breasts to make sure they are clean when she gets out of the bath. Then, Norm proceeded to give her a sensual massage while Nancy offered feedback about what ways and places he touched gave her pleasure. This was a good ice-breaker for this couple because it allowed them to get to know each other's bodies and their own ability to give and receive pleasure without the expectations that it lead to traditional sex.

They discussed what previous methods they employed to demonstrate affection, what they were doing presently, and what they would like in the future. Then, they planned a surprise for each other from this assignment. Nancy decided to buy some silk boxers for Norm and reported "getting aroused" while wrapping them in anticipation of his opening them and wearing them. It worked! When Norm put on the boxers she was excited and began rubbing her body against his on the living-room floor, and he proceeded to try to penetrate her. Unfortunately, he was not able to because her hymen was still intact.

They were referred to a gynecologist who specialized in infertility. She worked on helping to perforate her hymen, used dilators to prepare for penetration, and then verify that she was fully capable of becoming pregnant. Recorded relaxation tapes were prepared for Nancy to use prior to inserting the dilators. She would listen to the tapes, take a relaxing bath, practice with the dilators, and then begin placing her finger into her vagina. In small increments she progressed from inserting the dilators in the tub, to inserting them outside the tub with lubricant, to touching herself sensually and finally achieving orgasm.

Then, Nancy was instructed to masturbate in Norm's presence. He was encouraged to help Nancy relax by setting the mood with candles, stroking and kissing her body, and talking about how much he enjoyed touching her. She was eventually able to guide his hand to where she liked to be genitally touched. Norm responded with an erection when she did that with him. Next, Norm rubbed his erect penis on her leg as she was fingering herself. He then was able to put his finger into her vagina as well. He noticed that her natural lubrication seemed to be flowing, and sensed they might be ready for penetration. Because they trusted in their therapist's leadership, they were able to decrease performance anxiety and follow the treatment plan to achieve their ultimate goal of pregnancy. They sent a picture of their lovely new daughter some months later.

Conclusion

The goal in presenting these challenging cases was to share the treatment process and to demonstrate multiple sex therapy interventions used by the authors. There is no one right way to treat any of these cases and in different hands they might have received alternative treatment interventions. Psychotherapy remains part art and part science.

Psychotherapy seeks to restore women's desire and arousal to the optimal level possible, given the limits of physical well-being and life circumstances. Treatment attempts to overcome the psychologic barriers that preclude mutual sexual satisfaction. It is not about frequency of intercourse, intensity of arousal, or counting orgasms. Success is defined in terms of greater sexual satisfaction, enhanced intimacy, passion, and relational pleasure.

References

1. Levine S. Personal communication, 2004.
2. Segraves T, Segraves K. Personal communication, 2004.
3. Leiblum S, Rosen R. *Principles and Practice of Sex Therapy*, 3rd edn. New York: Guilford Press, 2000.
4. American Psychiatric Association. *Diagnostic and Statistical Manual of Mental Disorders*, 4th edn, text revised (DSM-IV-TR). Washington, DC: American Psychiatric Press, 2000.
5. World Health Organization. *International Classification of Diseases*, 10th Revision. Geneva: World Health Organization, 1989.
6. Basson R, Leiblum S, Brotto L et al. Definitions of women's sexual dysfunction reconsidered: advocating expansion and revision. *J Psychosom Obstet Gynaecol* 2003; 24: 221–9.
7. Hendrix H. *Getting the Love You Want*. New York: HarperCollins, 1988.
8. Barbach L. *The Pause*. New York: Penguin Putnam, 1993.

SEXUAL PAIN DISORDERS

12.1 Assessment, treatment strategies and outcome results: perspective of pain specialists

Kimberley A Payne, Sophie Bergeron, Samir Khalifé, Yitzchak M Binik

Introduction

Obtaining a proper diagnosis and treatment is a major obstacle for women suffering from sexual pain disorders. In a recent epidemiologic investigation,[1] only 54% of women surveyed sought treatment for their chronic vulvar pain, and of those, 60% saw three or more clinicians while only 61% obtained a diagnosis. These statistics are particularly alarming, given that prevalence estimates for dyspareunia and vaginismus range from 12% to 21%[1-4] (see Chapters 2.1–2.4 of this book).

Why so few women consult for dyspareunia or vaginismus remains uncertain, but this may be due to discomfort in discussing such issues with their doctor. One likely solution is to make a sexual pain assessment part of the routine gynecologic examination (see Chapters 9.1–9.5). However, prevalence data also suggest that health-care physicians lack expertise in diagnosing sexual pain disorders.[1] This possibly reflects an oversight in medical training, but also probably stems from confusion arising from current classification systems and nomenclature. Within the literature, various diagnostic labels are used to refer to dyspareunia, including vulvodynia, generalized and localized vulvar dysesthesia, dysesthetic vulvodynia, vestibulodynia, and vulvar vestibulitis syndrome. And while there appears to be some consensus regarding the use of the term "vaginismus",

criteria for this diagnosis remain controversial and are inconsistently applied.[5] Most notably, terminology within the sexual pain literature is not used consistently and at times fails to discriminate among conditions with different symptomatology. As a result, authors and clinicians alike commonly use the same labels to refer to different kinds of genital pain.

Classification

The five major classification systems with respect to sexual pain are as follows: that of the *Diagnostic and Statistical Manual of Mental Disorders* (DSM),[6] that of the *International Statistical Classification of Diseases and Related Health Problems* (ICD-10),[7] the International Association for the Study of Pain's *Classification of Chronic Pain*[8], and *ad hoc* classifications proposed by the American College of Obstetrics and Gynecology,[9] and the International Society for the Study of Vulvovaginal Disease.[10] These systems differ on the range of problems covered, diagnostic criteria for these problems, and underlying theoretic approach.

The revised third edition of the DSM (DSM-III-R) introduced the term "sexual pain disorder" to classify dyspareunia and vaginismus under the category of sexual dysfunctions.[11]

Today, the revised fourth edition of the DSM (DSM-IV-TR) has preserved this category, making dyspareunia and vaginismus the only pain conditions to be classified outside the category of pain or somatoform disorders.[6] Diagnostic criteria require that the sexual pain be specified as resulting from organic, psychologic, or mixed factors, lifelong or acquired, and global or situational. Ultimately very little discriminative diagnostic information is provided to make these distinctions. For example, what constitutes organic as opposed to psychologic causation is not specified, neither is any detail regarding the location, temporal duration, or quality of the pain. In addition, a woman who experiences a deep throbbing pain upon penile thrusting would obtain the same diagnosis as a woman who experiences a superficial burning sensation during vaginal insertion. Strictly speaking, according to the DSM-IV-TR, women who are not sexually active but experience pain during other activities involving vestibular pressure or vaginal insertion would not receive this diagnosis, as the pain is not interfering with sexual intercourse.

Interference with intercourse is also a central diagnostic feature for vaginismus in the DSM-IV-TR. Defined as an involuntary vaginal spasm that interferes with intercourse, pain is not required for the diagnosis of vaginismus. The ICD-10 and the American College of Obstetricians and Gynecologists[9] recommendations also identify vaginal spasm as the central criterion for a diagnosis of vaginismus. To date, however, very little empirical evidence exists for the validity of this diagnostic feature. Studies have failed to differentiate women with vaginismus from those with dyspareunia[5] or even healthy controls[12–14] by the presence of such a spasm. One study did find that women with vaginismus demonstrated increased pelvic muscle tonicity compared with women suffering from dyspareunia and healthy controls, and displayed more defensive and avoidance behaviors during pelvic examination.[5] The question of whether vaginismus constitutes a different clinical entity from other forms of dyspareunia or simply represents the extreme of a continuum remains unanswered.

Despite the limitations of the DSM-IV-TR system of classification in guiding the assessment and diagnosis of sexual pain disorders, this system is strikingly consistent with that of the ICD-10, which also classifies psychogenic dyspareunia and vaginismus as sexual dysfunctions,[7] while organic dyspareunia and vaginismus are classified as pain disorders. The implication is that if no physical findings can be found during medical examination, the disorder is necessarily of a sexual nature. The result is that too often women suffering from these conditions are similarly dismissed from the gynecologist's office with a referral to a sex therapist. While such a referral appropriately addresses the issue of sexuality in women suffering from pain during intercourse, the primary presenting symptom of pain is not being equally treated.

The International Association for the Study of Pain developed the Classification of Chronic Pain, which has inspired a new approach to the assessment and study of urogenital pain.[8] Within this classification system, pain is described according to the following five dimensions: location, system involved, temporal pattern, self-reported intensity and duration, and etiology. Considerable empirical research now exists for all five of these dimensions, particularly with reference to vulvar vestibulitis syndrome. This condition is believed to be the most common form of dyspareunia among premenopausal women[2,15,16] and is characterized by severe pain upon vestibular touch or attempted vaginal entry,[17] as opposed to idiopathic vulvodynia, in which the pain is unprovoked. The majority of women with vulvar vestibulitis syndrome report the onset of pain with penetration,[16] exhibit increases in pain after successive clockwise cotton-swab palpations of the vestibule,[18] and show habituation to suprathreshold pain.[19] Self-reported pain intensities in women with vulvar vestibulitis syndrome are normally distributed, representing a continuum of pain rather than an all-or-none phenomenon.[18] Moreover, in comparing thresholds for touch and pain, pain thresholds in women with vulvar vestibulitis syndrome match touch thresholds in pain-free controls.[19] An assessment according to the Classification of Chronic Pain provides a wealth of clinically relevant information, even in the absence of obvious disorder. A consideration of these pain dimensions should be included as part of any thorough urogenital pain assessment. Although not included in the formal axes, the International Association for the Study of Pain also places great value on self-reported pain quality, with the underlying assumption that similar pains may share similar etiology. In contrast, the DSM-IV-TR criteria for dyspareunia refer to a multitude of different pains, while, paradoxically, the category of vaginismus has little discriminative value.

The American College of Obstetrics and Gynecology and the International Society for the Study of Vulvovaginal Disease have attempted a more thorough classification of conditions causing urogenital pain. In 1997, the American College of Obstetrics and Gynecology released an educational bulletin[20] classifying vulvovaginal disorders according to the following four categories: lichen sclerosus, squamous cell hyperplasia, other dermatoses (including lichen simplex chronicus and lichen planus), and nonneoplastic epithelial disorders confined to the vulvar vestibule (including vulvar vestibulitis syndrome, vestibular papillomatosis, and idiopathic vulvodynia). This system of classification distinguishes vulvovaginal disease according to physical findings and also provides guidelines for the diagnosis and treatment of each, although any reference to vaginismus is lacking. Concerning the diagnosis of vulvar vestibulitis syndrome, the American College of Obstetrics and Gynecology suggests that evidence of inflammation and tenderness in response to pressure in inflamed areas, along with a clinical history, is sufficient for the diagnosis. However, the diagnostic criterion of erythema has received very little empirical support,[18] and the issue of inflammation remains a controversial one. Controlled histopathologic studies have revealed inflammatory infiltrates to be a relatively common finding in vestibular tissue,[21–23] while genetic evidence points to a dysfunctional inflammatory response in the pathogenesis of vulvar vestibulitis syndrome.[24–26] This condition therefore remains a diagnosis of exclusion when all other disorders have been ruled out, including idiopathic vulvodynia, although specific discriminative criteria are not provided for the latter.

In a newsletter,[10] the International Society for the Study of Vulvovaginal Disease recently circulated its newly formulated classification system for vulvar pain. In a dualistic approach similar to the DSM-IV-TR, vulvar pain is classified as due either to a specific disorder or to vulvodynia. The first category is further subdivided according to etiology as follows: (1) infectious; (2) inflammatory; (3) neoplastic; and (4) neurologic. Vulvodynia is categorized according to whether the pain is localized or not, and also whether the pain is provoked, unprovoked, or mixed. Under this newly proposed system, vestibulodynia, clitirodynia, and hemivulvodynia are provided as examples of localized pain, but no examples or official nomenclature are provided for the other criteria. It appears that in the absence of obvious disorder, vulvar pain is classified according to descriptive pain characteristics, similar to the International Association for the Study of Pain system. This represents a significant departure from the DSM-IV-TR, which would simply classify urogenital pain as psychogenic in the absence of obvious physical disorder. Although this approach does not make any specific mention of vaginismus, it encourages the careful assessment and diagnosis of pain regardless of physical findings.

Assessment

As with any sexual dysfunction or pain disorder, a multidisciplinary approach to the assessment of dyspareunia and vaginismus is encouraged to allow for a more comprehensive evaluation. This requires a clinical interview by a mental health professional in addition to a thorough physical examination by a gynecologist and pelvic floor physiotherapist. Although this may not be possible in every health-care setting, a multidisciplinary approach is encouraged to validate the patient's experience of the pain and its interference with sexual and couple functioning, rule out and/or treat identifiable physical pathology, and identify possible exacerbating/ attenuating factors and avenues for intervention. A multidisciplinary approach further allows the specialists to contribute their unique expertise to the understanding and evaluation of the problem in a complementary way.

The clinical interview

The clinical interview is essential when assessing any pain condition and should include questions on the history, onset, intensity, location, quality, and duration of the pain. If the pain is provoked, it is also important to assess which activities are likely to trigger it. Women with pain during intercourse in particular may have difficulty in identifying the location of the pain. In this instance, diagrams of both external and internal reproductive organs can be quite helpful. As pain is defined as

both a sensory and affective experience,[8] it is also important to assess both pain intensity and distress separately during the gynecologic examination and via retrospective reports. Some women may find even small amounts of pain distressing while others may report intense pain but not find it particularly upsetting. This information will help assess how the woman experiences and copes with her pain. Pain sensory and distress ratings should be assessed on a visual analog scale, which typically consists of a 10-cm line with verbal anchors labeling the ends from *no pain* at the left, to *unbearable pain* at the far right.[27] It is a well-established and validated pain measurement tool that has shown some advantages over simple verbal ratings, including sensitivity to changes in pain intensity and ratio scale properties.[28] Original formulations of the visual analog scale include simple paper-and-pencil administration; however, advances in technology have led to the development of an electronic version whereby pain ratings can be entered on hand-held computers.[29]

To obtain additional information regarding fluctuations in pain, a pain diary is a useful diagnostic and therapeutic tool (see Appendix).[30] This allows both patient and practitioner to track the fluctuations in pain with associated clinical phenomena, in addition to identifying potential antecedents to the pain and the success of current coping strategies. Like the visual analog scale, electronic diaries can facilitate the collection of clinical data.[31] Asking about past treatments, previous diagnoses, and remedies that helped or worsened the pain can also be informative.

Most importantly, when assessing patients with dyspareunia or vaginismus, it is crucial to determine the general impact of the pain on the patients' overall level of function. Is the pain threatening their sexual and relationship satisfaction? How has this affected their lives emotionally? Not surprisingly, women with dyspareunia report lower frequencies of intercourse and self-stimulation; lower levels of sexual desire, arousal, and pleasure; less success at achieving orgasm; and more negative attitudes toward sexuality than nonaffected women.[32-34] Unlike other nongenital pains, the inability to experience painless vaginal penetration may represent a threat to sexual and relationship satisfaction. Similarly, affected women report more catastrophizing with relation to coital pain than other noncoital pains,[19] in addition to difficulties with relationship adjustment and psychologic distress, including depression and anxiety.[32] Activities outside the realm of sexuality and intimate relationships may also be affected, such as gynecologic examinations, bicycle riding, tampon use, or even sitting for long periods of time.[18,32] Given the significant negative impact sexual pain disorders can have on multiple aspects of life, it is crucial to assess these in order to design an effective and targeted treatment plan.

The physical examination
(see Chapters 6.5, 9.5, and 12.2)

Before proceeding with a physical examination, physicians should assess the intensity of the pain and explain to the patient that, in order to obtain a diagnosis, an attempt will be made to replicate this pain. Empirical research has shown the pain of dyspareunia to be similar in intensity to that of chronic back or cancer pain;[17] therefore, both patient and physician should be aware that the experience is likely to be quite painful and potentially upsetting. Though the busy rush of patients through a general or gynecologic practice often precludes spending much time with each patient, extra care should be taken in assessing a woman in pain to explain each procedure before it is conducted and to assess how she is managing throughout the examination. Medical practitioners must be mindful of how vulnerable the patient could feel, and allow her to control the pace. Failure to do so may further worsen the situation or, in some cases of vaginismus, be traumatic. Women with dyspareunia and vaginismus in particular may have been avoiding regular gynecologic examinations because of the pain, and thus may not know what to expect.

The physical examination should include a cotton-swab palpation of the vulva and a pelvic examination in an effort to replicate the pain. It is important to ask the patient to distinguish between pain and discomfort. If pain is felt during the examination, the physician should assess whether this is the same pain the patient is consulting for, and if not, how does it differ? A careful examination of the vulvar vestibule with vaginal cultures and/or biopsy, where warranted, is required to rule out infection and/or dermatosis.[35,36] When assessing vulvar disease, Foster has developed a characterization of lesion type: macular (e.g., vulvar dermatosis); ulcer (e.g., vulvar neoplasia or herpes simplex); papule, nodule, cysts, or tumor (e.g., condyloma acuminata); pustule (Bartholin gland abscess); traumatic/anatomic (e.g., as a result of vaginal delivery); or neoplastic (e.g., vulvar intraepithelial neoplasia or melanoma).[37] Other conditions causing dyspareunia also need to be ruled out, including hypoestrogenism, endometriosis, ovaries in the cul-de-sac, fibroids, and pelvic infection.[38] Symptoms consistent with idiopathic, dysesthetic, or essential vulvodynia may also be caused by conditions such as pruritus vulvae or pudendal neuralgiae.[39] In assessing postmenopausal women with dyspareunia, it is important to assess carefully vulvovaginal atrophy and other anatomic changes experienced by aging women.[40,41] Dyspareunia may also result from pelvic or cervical surgery, radiotherapy, and pharmacotherapy;[42] therefore, a thorough medical history should be taken. In addition to the gynecologic examination, physiotherapists should assess the elasticity of the vaginal opening, pelvic floor muscle tonicity, and the patient's ability to isolate and voluntarily contract and release relevant muscle groups. Gynecologists and physiotherapists also have the unique ability to assess avoidance and fear behaviors during their examinations, such as vocalizations, crying, closing legs and knee withdrawal in an effort to avoid the examination.

Treatment and outcome

The treatment of sexual pain is largely hindered by the relative scarcity of randomized and controlled treatment outcome trials.

Without these, health professionals lack the information they need to treat their patients effectively and safely. Guided by dualistic diagnostic systems, clinicians have historically adopted treatment approaches starting with medical interventions, progressing to mental health ones when these fail, and finally surgery as a last resort. Medical interventions lie on a continuum from relatively minor to invasive methods, operating largely on a trial and error basis. Just about anything that can be applied to the vulva has been, in an effort to help patients suffering from various forms of dyspareunia (e.g. vulvar vestibulitis syndrome and idiopathic vulvodynia) and vaginismus. In most instances, there is no indication that these interventions are more effective than placebo, and some suspect that they could be iatrogenic.[43] Furthermore, many of these treatments are guided by etiologic theories of coital pain that have yet to be empirically validated.

In its 1997 educational bulletin, the American College of Obstetrics and Gynecology provided treatment recommendations for both vulvar vestibulitis syndrome and idiopathic vulvodynia (i.e. chronic vulvar pain).[20] Treatment recommendations for vulvar vestibulitis syndrome begin with local topical treatments (such as sitz baths), progressing to topical medical treatment involving corticosteroid, estrogen, or lidocaine cream, to oral medications such as calcium citrate, corticosteroids, or fluconazole. Should these interventions fail, progressively more invasive approaches are recommended, such as interferon injections, neurophysiologic treatments, and finally surgical excision via vestibuloplasty, or partial to total vestibulectomy. In patients with idiopathic vulvodynia, vestibulectomy is discouraged because it has been suggested to be less successful in this group of women.[44] Instead, the American College of Obstetrics and Gynecology recommends that these patients be treated with low-dose tricyclic antidepressants such as amitriptyline. Although the American College of Obstetrics and Gynecology recommendations accurately represent the hotchpotch of medical interventions that have been tried to treat dyspareunia and vaginismus, few of these approaches, with the exception of vestibulectomy, have received empirical support.

When medical interventions fail, women may be referred to a mental health professional such as a sex therapist. Sex therapy approaches range from psychoanalytic to the more commonly practiced cognitive-behavioral techniques. These often focus on impairment with intercourse and often assume poor adjustment and/or sexual knowledge on the part of the couple or elements of low sexual desire on the part of the patient. Others suggest impairment in sexual arousal leading to poor vaginal lubrication that causes pain, and likewise focus on improving sexual arousal. Behavioral strategies for dyspareunia and vaginismus also typically include some form of graded desensitization in combination with vaginal dilation with a heavy emphasis on relaxation training and anxiety reduction. More recent empirically proven behavioral strategies integrate a pain management component and focus on helping patients reconceptualize their dyspareunia or vaginismus as a pain problem influenced by behavioral, affective, cognitive, and relationship factors.[45] The partner is also encouraged to participate in these treatment efforts, as there is evidence that specific characteristics of romantic relationships are associated with pain and pain-related disability.[46]

Topical creams

Topical creams represent the standard first-line approach to the most common forms of dyspareunia involving vestibular pain. Topical anesthetics applied prior to intercourse are believed to relieve discomfort enough temporarily to make intercourse possible. However, many patients have difficulty in applying the cream in the correct area, and some report a burning sensation upon application. If applied too close to intercourse, the cream may also have a numbing effect on the partner. Finally, should the cream provide the desired anesthetic relief during coitus, the woman may be inclined to engage in vigorous thrusting, which may result in exacerbated pain after the cream has worn off. Other topical treatments such as antifungal, antibiotic, antiviral, and corticosteroid creams are generally believed to be ineffective, although few clinical trials exist. In addition to nightly applications of anesthetic cream,[47] other topical preparations have been investigated, including nitroglycerine,[48] glyceryl trinitrate,[49] capsaicin,[50] and estrogen-based creams.[51] However, evidence from randomized, placebo-controlled trials is lacking. The importance of placebo-controlled outcome trials was illustrated in one double-blind, randomized, placebo-controlled study comparing the effectiveness of 4% cromolyn cream with placebo cream.[52] Both groups improved significantly with no differences in the degree of improvement between groups. In addition, 46% of patients in the placebo condition felt they had a 50% or greater reduction in symptoms.

Oral medications

It has been suggested that excess oxalate in the urine irritates the vulvar epithelium, causing severe burning that can be relieved with calcium citrate tablets.[53] This theory, however, has never been supported by more than case reports. Acyclovir, an antiviral agent used in the treatment of genital herpes, has shown some promise in the treatment of idiopathic vulvodynia,[50] although it is rarely recommended to patients with sexual pain. This may be due to the fact that initial retrospective study results have not been replicated in a randomized, placebo-controlled treatment outcome trial.

Low-dose tricyclic antidepressants have been used widely in pain management. While some believe the use of amitriptyline is generally ineffective for women suffering from idiopathic vulvodynia, others have attempted to characterize the patients most likely to respond to this medication,[54] while yet another case study reported complete pain relief with nortriptyline.[55] Gabapentin, an anticonvulsant, has also been investigated in a small, uncontrolled treatment trial for idiopathic vulvodynia with promising results[56] that have yet to be replicated.

Injections

Interferon injections have been attempted to treat dyspareunia. Administered either intramuscularly, intralesionally, or intradermally, interferon is generally injected into the affected area several times a week for approximately 4 weeks.[57] Success rates from nonrandomized trials varied from 16% to 88%.[58] Interferon is rarely used today and is not recommended for the treatment of dyspareunia in the absence of suspected human papilloma virus infection. The efficacy of submucous infiltrations of methylprednisolone and lidocaine,[59] and betamethasone and lidocaine for dyspareunia,[60] and botulinum toxin for vaginismus[61] has also been investigated in small uncontrolled and case studies with some success. However, additional research is needed to establish the safety and efficacy of these treatments.

Surgical interventions

Vestibulectomy has been the most frequently investigated treatment for vulvar vestibulitis syndrome. This minor surgical procedure consists of the excision of the hymen and sensitive areas of the vestibule to a depth of approximately 2 mm, with some procedures involving the mobilization of the vaginal mucosa to cover the excised area.[17,62,63] Healing can take up to 8 weeks, after which women are instructed to resume intercourse gradually. To date, over 20 published studies exist reporting success rates ranging from 43% to 100%.[58] Most studies report success rates in excess of 60%, making vestibulectomy the treatment option with the best therapeutic outcome. Although many of these studies lack a control group, systematic pain measurement, or even an operational definition of therapeutic success, vestibulectomy has been validated in two randomized, controlled treatment outcome trials to date.[64,65] Recently, efforts have aimed at developing surgical techniques that are less invasive than total perineoplasty, with mixed results.[66–68]

CO_2 laser ablation of the vestibular area has also been investigated. This controversial modality, however, is believed to have potential aggravating effects, including delay in healing, chronic pain, scar tissue, and severe mucosal atrophy.[69] A flashlamp-excited dye laser believed, at the time, to have less negative consequences than the CO_2 technique has been used for selective photocoagulation of symptomatic vessels.[70] Although initial response rates seemed promising, this technique also resulted in negative effects; consequently, it is no longer used.

More recently, uterine suspension has been investigated in the treatment of dyspareunia and pelvic pain associated with uterine retroversion. This technique is motivated by the theory that deep dyspareunia may be the result of the penis colliding with the uterus and/or cervix. In a technique termed "UPLIFT" to denote uterine suspension and extraperitoneal ligament investment, fixation, and truncation, shortening of the ligaments that suspend the uterus results in a repositioning of the uterus in a slightly anteverted position.[71] This procedure takes approximately 12 min and is performed as same-day surgery. Although initial results seem promising for this and similar procedures, adverse effects have been reported.[72] Given the invasiveness of the procedure, more research is required to investigate the phenomena of "collision dyspareunia" and the effectiveness of uterine suspension as a safe and effective treatment option.

Cognitive-behavioral approaches

Cognitive-behavioral approaches have received some of the strongest empirical support to date, particularly in the treatment of vulvar vestibulitis syndrome. These include multidisciplinary treatment programs incorporating techniques from sex and pain management therapy, in addition to biofeedback and pelvic floor physiotherapy. These approaches are often guided by clear and empirically supported rationales.[73] Similar approaches for the treatment of vaginismus, however, have been somewhat empirically neglected.

Biofeedback training represents a treatment option that has been developed for the treatment of dyspareunia based on the finding that these women suffer from increased muscle tonicity potentially contributing to their pain.[5] Through biofeedback training, patients are provided with direct visual feedback on their level of muscle tension via a vaginal sensor connected to a display monitor. They receive pelvic floor muscle training with respect to contraction, relaxation, and the acquisition of voluntary control over these. In one uncontrolled study examining the efficacy of biofeedback in a mixed sample of women with vulvar pain, subjective pain reports decreased an average of 83% after 4 months of training.[74] Another study examined the effectiveness of biofeedback in the treatment of women with moderate to severe vulvar vestibulitis syndrome where 24 of the 29 participants reported negligible or mild pain after treatment.[75] Biofeedback also constitutes an important component of pelvic floor physiotherapy, in which the physiotherapist works directly with the patient to help relieve muscle tonicity. Results from one study revealed a significant improvement in over 70% of patients evaluated for the treatment of vulvar vestibulitis syndrome, after an average 16 months of treatment by this technique.[76]

Elements of pelvic floor physiotherapy and biofeedback have also been integrated into more comprehensive behavioral strategies. One such approach was compared with or without surgical intervention in the treatment of 48 women with vulvar vestibulitis syndrome.[64] In the first phase of the study, 14 patients were randomly assigned to either treatment condition. The behavioral approach included components of psychosexual education, pelvic floor muscle exercises aimed at reducing hypertonicity, small hygienic changes, and individual or couple sex therapy where deemed appropriate. Participants also randomized to surgery underwent modified perineoplasty. Follow-up data indicated that both treatments were equally effective, with all but two women reporting complete or partial improvement. Even for the two unimproved women, the pain was less of a problem. Similar results were obtained in a second nonrandomized phase of the study in which 34 women and their

partners were given the choice of treatment. Twenty-eight chose the behavioral intervention without surgery and showed similar improvements to those who chose surgery as well. The authors concluded that a behavioral approach should be the first-line treatment for vulvar vestibulitis syndrome, and that surgery should be used only as an adjunct in treatment-resistant patients.

In the only completely randomized, controlled treatment outcome trial for dyspareunia to date, group cognitive-behavioral pain management therapy was compared with vestibulectomy and biofeedback training in the treatment of vulvar vestibulitis syndrome.[65] In the behavioral treatment, patients were provided with psychoeducation on sexuality and pain, and with instruction on muscle relaxation, deep breathing, Kegel exercises and vaginal dilation, coping, communication, and cognitive restructuring, with the goal of increasing behaviors that decrease pain and facilitate sexual arousal and desire. A significant treatment effect was observed at post-treatment and 6-month follow-up in all three treatment groups; however, vestibulectomy resulted in approximately twice the pain reduction as the other two therapies. There was no treatment difference in overall sexual function and self-reported frequency of intercourse at the 6-month follow-up, and intercourse frequency for all groups remained below that for healthy women of similar age. All three groups continued to improve over time at a 2.5-year follow-up, and while vestibulectomy remained superior to the other two groups with respect to cotton-swab-induced vulvar pain in the gynecologist's office, women in the group therapy condition reported equal improvements in self-reported pain during intercourse.[77] These results suggest that the benefits of cognitive-behavioral group therapy may take longer to appear than surgery but can be just as great.

Similar randomized and controlled treatment outcome studies are lacking for vaginismus. A series of successful case studies has been published on behavioral approaches to the treatment of vaginismus; however, a review in 2004 of the literature found only two controlled studies.[78] One of the trials compared in vivo with in vitro forms of desensitization and found no difference in effectiveness between them,[79] while no data were supplied in the second publication, which allocated patients to waiting-list control, flooding, or systematic desensitization.[80] A third semicontrolled trial was also identified where patients were allocated to in vivo systematic desensitization ($n = 39$), in vitro desensitization ($n = 10$), or hypnotherapy ($n = 6$) on the basis of a neurosis scores.[81] Treatment success ranged from 100% in the hypnosis group and 94% in the in vivo group, to 70% in the in vitro group.

Other treatment options for dyspareunia and vaginismus include pain management techniques, such as acupuncture and hypnosis. Although few studies currently exist, there are promising data on the effect of acupuncture on pain reduction and overall quality of life in women with vulvar vestibulitis syndrome.[82] A case study has also been published whereby hypnosis reduced pain and helped re-establish sexual pleasure in yet another patient with vulvar vestibulitis syndrome.[83] As with most medical treatments, however, randomized, controlled trials are needed to establish the effectiveness of these newer modalities.

Summary

The multidisciplinary biopsychosocial approach to the assessment and treatment of dyspareunia and vaginismus has been the theme of this chapter. This model reflects the complexity of sexual pain. Even if the initiating pain could be reduced to an identifiable etiologic factor, it carries with it a snowball of physiologic, sexual, relationship, and cognitive-emotional sequelae that influence the maintenance of the sexual pain and significantly contribute to patient distress. Therefore, it is unlikely that any one "magic" pill, cream, or cognitive-behavioral technique will ever be found to cure all affected areas of function in women with sexual pain. The striking success of vestibulectomy does, however, contradicts this assertion. Although surgical removal of the affected area is effective in reducing pain, the question of what happens to the other psychosocial components of dyspareunia and vaginismus when the pain has been removed has yet to be fully investigated. Some evidence suggests that reducing the pain does not necessarily restore sexual function.[65] At this stage of knowledge, it is therefore crucial to address the *whole patient* and all the factors that affect quality of life.

References

1. Harlow BL, Wise LA, Stewart EG. Prevalence and predictors of chronic lower genital tract discomfort. *Am J Obstet Gynecol* 2001; 185: 545–50.

2. Harlow BL, Stewart EG. A population-based assessment of chronic unexplained vulvar pain: have we underestimated the prevalence of vulvodynia? *J Am Med Womens Assoc* 2003; 58: 82–8.

3. Laumann EO, Paik A, Rosen RC. Sexual dysfunction in the United States. *J Am Med Assoc* 1999; 281: 537–44.

4. Spector IP, Carey MP. Incidence and prevalence of the sexual dysfunctions: a critical review of the empirical literature. *Arch Sex Behav* 1990; 19: 389–408.

5. Reissing ED, Binik YM, Khalifé S et al. Vaginal spasm, pain, and behavior: an empirical investigation of the diagnosis of vaginismus. *Arch Sex Behav* 2004; 33: 5–17.

6. American Psychiatric Association. *Diagnostic and Statistical Manual of Mental Disorders*, 4th edn, text rev. (DSM-IV-TR). Washington, DC: 2000.

7. World Health Organization. *Manual of the International Statistical Classification of Diseases, Injuries, and Causes of* Death, 10th edn (ICD-10). Geneva: 1992.

8. Merskey H, Bogduk N. *Classification of Chronic Pain*, 2nd edn. Washington, DC: IASP Press, 1994.

9. American College of Obstetricians and Gynecologists. Vulvar nonneoplastic epithelial disorders. *Int J Gynecol Obstet* 1998; 60: 181–8.

10. International Society for the Study of Vulvovaginal Disease, Society Newsletter, 2004; 1: 1–3.

11. American Psychiatric Association. *Diagnostic and Statistical Manual of Mental Disorders*, 3rd edn rev. (DSM-III-R). Washington, DC: Author, 1987.

12. van der Velde J, Everaerd W. Voluntary control over pelvic floor muscles in women with and without vaginismic reactions. *Int Urogynecol J* 1999; 10: 230–6.

13. van der Velde J, Everaerd W. The relationship between involuntary pelvic floor muscle activity, muscle awareness and experienced threat in women with and without vaginismus. *Behav Res Ther* 2001; 39: 395–408.

14. van der Velde J, Everaerd W. Vaginismus, a component of a general defense mechanism: an investigation of pelvic floor muscle activity during exposure to emotion-inducing film excerpts in women with or without vaginismus. *Int Urogynecol J Pelvic Floor Dysfunct* 2001; 12: 328–31.

15. Harlow BL, Stewart EG. A population-based assessment of chronic unexplained vulvar pain: have we underestimated the prevalence of vulvodynia? *J Am Med Womens Assoc* 2003; 58: 82–8.

16. Meana M, Binik YM, Khalifé S et al. Dyspareunia: sexual dysfunction or pain syndrome? *J Nerv Ment Dis* 1997; 185: 561–9.

17. Friedrich EG. Vulvar vestibulitis syndrome. *J Reprod Med* 1987; 32: 110–14.

18. Bergeron S, Binik YM, Khalifé S et al. Vulvar vestibulitis syndrome: reliability of diagnosis and validity of current diagnostic criteria. *Obstet Gynecol* 2001; 98: 45–51.

19. Pukall CF, Binik YM, Khalifé S et al. Vestibular tactile and pain thresholds in women with vulvar vestibulitis syndrome. *Pain* 2002; 96: 163–75.

20. American College of Obstetrics and Gynecology. ACOG educational bulletin: vulvar nonneoplastic epithelial disorders. *Int J Gynecol Obstet* 1998; 60: 181–8.

21. Friedman M, Siegler E, Kerner H. Clinical and histopathological changes of the vulvar vestibulum in healthy subjects and in patients with vulvar vestibulitis. *XII International Congress of the International Society for the Study of Vulvar Disease*. Quebec City, Canada, 1993: Abstracts, p 21.

22. Lundqvist EN, Hofer PA, Olofsson JI et al. Is vulvar vestibulitis an inflammatory condition? A comparison of histological findings in affected and healthy women. *Acta Derm Venereol* 1997; 77: 319–22.

23. Slone S, Reynolds L, Gall S et al. Localization of chromogranin, synaptophysin, serotonin, and CXCR2 in neuroendocrine cells of the minor vestibular glands: an immunohistochemical study. *Int J Gynecol Pathol* 1999; 18: 360–5.

24. Gerber S, Bongiovanni AM, Ledger WJ et al. Interleukin-1? gene polymorphism in women with vulvar vestibulitis syndrome. *Obstet Gynecol* 2003; 107: 74–7.

25. Jeremias J, Ledger WJ, Witkin SS. Interleukin 1 receptor antagonist gene polymorphism in women with vulvar vestibulitis. *Am J Obstet Gynecol* 2002; 182: 283–5.

26. Witkin SS, Gerber S, Ledger WJ. Differential characterization of women with vulvar vestibulitis syndrome. *Am J Obstet Gynecol* 2002; 187: 589–94.

27. Ohnhaus EE, Adler R. Methodological problems in the measurement of pain: a comparison between the verbal rating scale and the visual analogue scale. *Pain* 1975; 1: 379–84.

28. Price DD, Bush FM, Long S et al. A comparison of pain measurement characteristics of mechanical visual analogue and simple numerical rating scales. *Pain* 1994; 56: 217–26.

29. Jamison RN, Gracely RH, Raymond SA et al. Comparative study of electronic vs. paper VAS ratings: a randomized, crossover trial using healthy volunteers. *Pain* 2002; 99: 341–7.

30. Bergeron S, Binik YM, Larouche J. Cognitive-behavioral pain relief therapy for vulvar vestibulitis syndrome. Université du Québec à Montréal, 2001, unpublished treatment manual.

31. Jamison RN, Raymond SA, Levine JG et al. Electronic diaries for monitoring chronic pain: one–year validation study. *Pain* 2001; 91: 277–85.

32. Meana M, Binik YM, Khalifé S et al. Biopsychosocial profile of women with dyspareunia. *Obstet Gynecol* 1997; 90: 583–9.

33. Reed BD, Advincula AP, Fonde KR et al. Sexual activities and attitudes of women with vulvar dysesthesia. *Obstet Gynecol* 2003; 102: 325–31.

34. Reissing ED, Binik YM, Khalifé S et al. Etiological correlates of vaginismus: sexual and physical abuse, sexual knowledge, sexual self-schema, and relationship adjustment. *J Sex Mar Ther* 2003; 29: 47–59.

35. Edwards L. New concepts in vulvodynia. *Am J Obstet Gynecol* 2003; 189: S24–30.

36. Foster D. Vulvar disease. *Obstet Gynecol* 2002; 100: 145–63.

37. Fischer G. Management of vulvar pain. *Dermatol Ther* 2004; 17: 134–49.

38. Steege JF, Ling FW. Dyspareunia: a special type of chronic pain. *Obstet Gynecol Clin North Am* 1993; 20: 779–93.

39. McKay M. Vulvodynia versus pruritus vulvae. *Clin Obstet Gynecol* 1985; 28: 123–33.

40. Hurd WW, Amesse LS, Randolph Jr JF. Menopause. In Berek JS, ed. *Novack's Gynecology*, 13th edn. Philadelphia: Lippincott Williams & Wilkins, 2002: 1109–42.

41. Willhite LA, O'Connel MB. Urogenital atrophy: prevention and treatment. *Pharmacotherapy* 2001; 21: 464–80.

42. Graziottin A. Etiology and diagnosis of coital pain. *J Endocrinol Invest* 2003: 26: 115–21.

43. Wesselmann U, Reich SG. The dynias. *Semin Neurol* 1996; 16: 63–74.

44. Bornstein J, Goldik Z, Stolar Z et al. Predicting the outcome of surgical treatment of vulvar vestibulitis. *Obstet Gynecol* 1997; 89: 695–8.

45. Pukall C, Payne KA, Kao A. Dyspareunia. In Balon R, Segraves RT, eds. *Handbook of Sexual Dysfunction.* New York: Marcel Dekker, *in press.*

46. Kiecolt-Glaser JK, Newton TL. Marriage and health: his or hers. *Psychol Bull* 2001; 127: 472–503.

47. Zolnoun DA, Hartmann KE, Steege JF. Overnight 5% lidocaine ointment for the treatment of vulvar vestibulitis. *Obstet Gynecol* 2003; 102: 84–7.

48. Walsh KE, Berman JR, Berman LA et al. Safety and efficacy of topical nitroglycerin for treatment of vulvar pain in women with vulvodynia: a pilot study. *J Gend Specif Med* 2002; 5: 21–7.

49. Peleg R, Press Y, Ben-Zion IZ. Glyceryl trinitrate ointment as a potential treatment for primary vaginismus. *Eur J Obstet Gynecol Reprod Biol* 2001; 96: 111–12.

50. Friedrich EG. Therapeutic studies on vulvar vestibulitis. *J Reprod Med* 1988; 33: 514–18.

51. Sarrel PM. Effects of hormone replacement therapy on sexual psychophysiology and behavior in postmenopause. *J Womens Health Gend Based Med* 2000; 9: S25–32.

52. Nyirjesy P, Sobel JD, Weitz MV et al. Cromolyn cream for recalcitrant idiopathic vulvar vestibulitis: results of a placebo controlled study. *Sex Transm Infect* 2001; 77: 53–7.

53. Solomons CC, Melmed MH, Heitler SM. Calcium citrate for vulvar vestibulitis: a case report. *J Reprod Med* 1991; 36: 879–82.

54. McKay M. Dysesthetic ("essential") vulvodynia. Treatment with amitriptyline. *J Reprod Med* 1993; 38: 9–13.

55. Stolar AG, Stewart JT. Nortriptyline for depression and vulvodynia. *Am J Psychiatry* 2002; 159: 316–17.

56. Ben-David B, Friedman M. Gabapentin therapy for vulvodynia. *Anesth Analg* 1999; 89: 1459–60.

57. Horowitz BJ. Interferon therapy for condylomatous vulvitis. *Obstet Gynecol* 1989; 73: 446–8.

58. Bergeron S, Binik YM, Khalifé S et al. Vulvar vestibulitis syndrome: a critical review. *Clin J Pain* 1997; 13: 27–42.

59. Murina F, Tassan P, Poberti P et al. Treatment of vulvar vestibulitis with submucous infiltrations of methylprednisolone and lidocaine. *J Reprod Med* 2001; 46: 713–16.

60. Segal D, Tifheret H, Lazer S. Submucous infiltration of betamethasone and lidocaine in the treatment of vulvar vestibulitis. *Eur J Obstet Gynecol Reprod Biol* 2003; 107: 105–6.

61. Brin MF, Vapnek JM. Treatment of vaginismus with botulinum toxin injections. *Lancet* 1997; 349: 252–3.

62. Marinoff SC, Turner MLC. Vulvar vestibulitis syndrome: an overview. *Am J Obstet Gynecol* 1991; 165: 1228–33.

63. Woodruff JD, Parmley TH. Infection of the minor vestibular gland. *Obstet Gynecol* 1983; 62: 609–12.

64. Weijmar Schultz WCM, Gianotten WL, van der Meijden WI et al. Behavioral approach with or without surgical intervention to the vulvar vestibulitis syndrome: a prospective randomized and non-randomized study. *J Psychosom Obstet Gynecol* 1996; 17: 143–8.

65. Bergeron S, Binik YM, Khalifé S et al. A randomized comparison of group cognitive-behavioral therapy, surface electromyographic biofeedback, and vestibulectomy in the treatment of dyspareunia resulting from vulvar vestibulitis. *Pain* 2001; 91: 297–306.

66. Bornstein J, Zarfati D, Goldik Z. Perineoplasty compared with vestibuloplasty for severe vulvar vestibulitis. *Br J Obstet Gynecol* 1995; 102: 652–5.

67. Bornstein J, Abramovici H. Combination of subtotal perineoplasty and interferon for the treatment of vulvar vestibulitis. *Gynecol Obstet Invest* 1997; 44: 53–6.

68. Kehoe S, Luesley D. Vulvar vestibulitis treated by modified vestibulectomy. *Int J Gynecol Obstet* 1999; 64: 147–52.

69. Tschanz C, Salomon D, Skaria A et al. Vulvodynia after CO_2 laser treatment of the female genital mucosa. *Dermatology* 2001; 202: 371–2.

70. Reid R, Omoto KH, Precop SL et al. Flashlamp-excited dye laser therapy of idiopathic vulvodynia is safe and efficacious. *Am J Obstet Gynecol* 1995; 172: 1684–96.

71. Carter JE. Carter–Thomason uterine suspension and positioning by ligament investment, fixation and truncation. *J Reprod Med* 2000; 1999: 417–22.

72. Batioglu S, Zeyneloglu HB. Laparoscopic placation and suspension of the round ligament for chronic pelvic pain and dyspareunia. *J Am Assoc Gynecol Laparosc* 2000; 7: 547–51.

73. Bergeron S, Lord M-J. The integration of pelvi-perineal re-education and cognitive-behavioral therapy in the multidisciplinary treatment of the sexual pain disorders. *Sex Relat Ther* 2003; 18: 135–41.

74. Glazer HI, Rodke G, Swencionis C. The treatment of vulvar vestibulitis syndrome by electromyographic biofeedback of pelvic floor musculature. *J Reprod Med* 1995; 40: 283–90.

75. McKay E, Kaufman RH, Doctor U et al. Treating vulvar vestibulitis with electromyographic biofeedback of pelvic floor musculature. *J Reprod Med* 2001; 46: 337–42.

76. Bergeron S, Brown C, Lord MJ et al. Physical therapy for vulvar vestibulitis syndrome: a retrospective study. *J Sex Marital Ther* 2002; 28: 183–92.

77. Bergeron S, Meana M, Binik Y et al. Painful genital sexual activity. In SB Levine, CB Risen, SE Althof, eds. *Handbook of Clinical Sexuality for Mental Health Professionals.* New York: Brunner-Routledge, 2003: 131–52.

78. McGuire H, Hawton K. Interventions for vaginismus. *Cochrane Database Syst Rev* 2004; 2.

79. Schnyder U, Schnyder-Luthi C, Ballinari P et al. Therapy for vaginismus: *in vivo* versus *in vitro* desensitization. *Can J Psychiatry* 1998; 43: 941–4.

80. Jarrousse N, Poudat F-X. Prise en charge thérapeutique: flooding ou désensibilisation systematique? [Vaginismus: therapeutic management: implosive therapy or systematic desensitization?] *Psychol Med (Paris)* 1986; 18: 771–2.

81. Lew-Starrowicz Z. Wyniki leczenia kobiet z roznaniem pochwicy [Results of treatment of women with diagnosed vaginismus]. *Ginekol Pol* 1982; 33: 691–4.

82. Danielsson I, Sjöberg I, Östman C. Acupuncture for the treatment of vulvar vestibulitis: a pilot study. *Acta Obstet Gynecol Scand* 2001; 80: 437–41.

83. Kandyba K, Binik YM. Hypnotherapy as a treatment for vulvar vestibulitis syndrome: a case report. *J Sex Marital Ther* 2003; 29: 237–42.

Appendix

Pain diary

To fill out after engaging in an activity that caused genital pain (e.g., intercourse, finger insertion, etc.). The items in italics (11, 12, 13, 14, and 15) refer only to pain experienced during sexual activities.

Name _____ Date _____

1. Day _____ 2. Time _____

3. Time of menstrual cycle _____ 4. Pain intensity (0 to 10) __

5. Cause of the pain _____ 6. Duration of the pain _____

7. Where were you? _____

8. What were you feeling and thinking just prior to the pain?___
_____

9. What were you feeling and thinking during the pain? _____
_____

10. What were you feeling and thinking after the pain? _____
_____

11. How much time did you spend on sex play? _____

12. How aroused were you (0 to 10)?_____

13. How lubricated were you (0 to 10)? _____

14. Up to what point were you in the mood for sex (0 to 10)? __

15. What was your partner's reaction to your pain? _____
_____

16. How relaxed did you feel (0 to 10)? _____

17. What did you do to try to reduce the pain? _____
_____

18. How effective was this? (circle the appropriate number).

0 = did not help at all   1 = helped very little

2 = helped somewhat   3 = helped a lot

4 = stopped the pain

<u>Additional comments:</u>
_____
_____
_____
_____

(Reproduced with permission from Bergeron et al.[30])

12.2 Overview of vulvar pain: pain related to a specific disorder and lesion-free pain

Lynette J Margesson, Elizabeth Gunther Stewart

Introduction

Vulvar pain and dyspareunia have been mysterious entities for many years, regarded until the mid-1980s as psychosexual in origin.[1] In 1983, the term "vulvodynia" was adopted by the International Society for the Study of Vulvovaginal Disease, sparking efforts to identify pathology. The US National Institutes of Health-sponsored conferences on vulvodynia in 1997 and in 2003 brought insights into the neurobiology of pain. Researchers at the Karolinska Institute in Sweden identified differences in the vestibule of women with pain compared with pain-free individuals. Drug companies have begun active efforts to develop medication that targets vulvodynia

Prevalence

Contrary to early suggestions that it is rare, chronic unexplained vulvar pain is a highly prevalent disorder. In a 2003 National Institutes of Health-sponsored study of 4915 women, 16% reported chronic burning, knifelike pain, or pain on vulvar contact that lasted for at least 3 months.[2] Similar findings have been reported on a Web-based survey.[3] In a 2002 survey of 1094 American women, 288 (27.9%) reported pain at the vulvar vestibule, 80 (7.8%) reporting pain within the past 6 months, 31 (3%) reporting pain that lasted 3 or more months, and 18 (1.7%) reporting vestibular pain lasting 3 or more months that occurred within the past 6 months.

Classification

The latest classification of vulvar pain agreed upon at the October 2003 Congress of the International Society for the Study of Vulvovaginal Disease[4] included two major headings: (1) vulvar pain related to a specific disorder and (2) vulvodynia. The first of these was subdivided as follows:

1. Infectious (candidiasis, herpes, etc.)
2. Inflammatory (erosive lichen planus, immunobullous disease, etc.)
3. Neoplastic (Paget's disease, squamous cell carcinoma, etc.)
4. Neurologic (herpes simplex and post-herpetic neuralgia, spinal nerve compression, etc.).

Vulvodynia was defined as "vulvar discomfort, most often described as burning pain, occurring in the absence of a relevant specific infectious, inflammatory, neoplastic, or neurologic disorder, either

1. Generalized, involving the whole vulva
   (a) provoked (sexual contact, nonsexual contact, or both),
   (b) unprovoke (spontaneous),
   (c) mixed (provoked and unprovoked), or
2. Localized, involving a portion or component of the vulva such as the vestibule, clitoris, hemivulva, or other specified site: vestibulodynia, clitorodynia, hemivulvodynia, etc.,
   (a) provoked (sexual contact, nonsexual contact, or both),
   (b) unprovoked (spontaneous),
   (c) mixed (provoked and unprovoked)."

Until the pathophysiology of pain is completely worked out, the definitions will continue to evolve. This chapter, fundamental to diagnosis of pain underlying female sexual dysfunction, covers essential material on common specific disorders as well as lesion-free causes of vulvar pain.

Vulvar pain related to a specific disorder

Infection

Herpes simplex virus infection

General description
Worldwide, herpes simplex virus is the commonest cause of vulvar ulceration and pain. Typically, it is characterized by recurrent painful outbreaks of grouped vesicles and erosions. The etiology is usually herpes simplex virus type II (80% of cases) and less commonly herpes simplex virus type I, although in some areas type I is becoming more prevalent. Primary herpes simplex virus infection is not commonly seen. Most patients have had unrecognized primary herpes simplex virus infection, and they present with nonprimary, recurrent disease.[5] Ninety per cent of herpes simplex virus II-positive women carriers are unaware of their infection. Up to 80% of women with herpes simplex virus II mistakenly think their symptoms are due to such things as vaginitis, soap allergy, poor lubrication, clothing irritation, urinary infection, or vaginitis. They are often shocked to find that their recurrent, variable, sore or painful vulvar problem is herpes simplex virus. The transmission usually is sexual, occurring during periods of asymptomatic viral shedding. Most affected individuals are unaware they are infectious.

Clinical features
Characteristic symptoms of primary disease are paresthesia, fever, malaise, headache, and myalgia. Pain varies from mild to deep, boring, and severe. Dysuria is common. Episodic itching, irritation, and burning signal recurrences. Women are often totally unaware of recurring herpes simplex virus.

In primary disease, there are often extensive groups of vesicles or pustules with surrounding redness and swelling (Fig. 12.2.1). These break, leaving tender erosions and ulcers that last 1–2 weeks. With primary herpes simplex virus, there can be large, impressive, painful ulcers (Fig. 12.2.2). Recurrent herpes simplex virus shows limited, scattered vesicles, pustules, and erosions that last 5–7 days (Figs 12.2.3 and 12.2.4). Less commonly, and often misdiagnosed, there are fissures or "pimples". Recurrent episodes of vulvar burning and itching with no skin signs can occur – herpes sine eruptione.[6,7]

Diagnosis
Herpes simplex virus culture is the reference standard if positive, but false negatives are common. Type-specific serology is

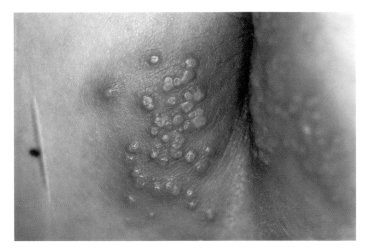

Figure 12.2.1. Primary herpes simplex in a baby, on labia majora with typical clusters of pustules.

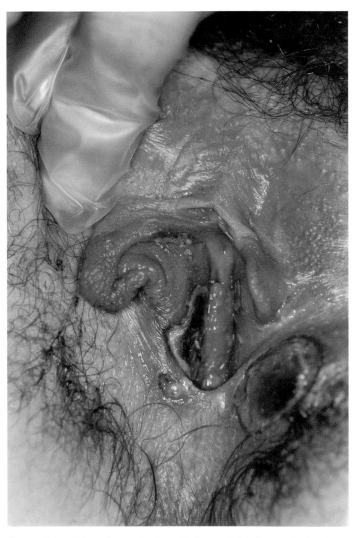

Figure 12.2.2. Primary herpes simplex with deep, painful ulcers at the introitus. Note classic clusters of pustules on the upper inner labia minora.

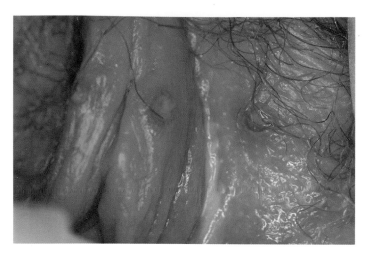

Figure 12.2.3. Typical recurrent herpes simplex with small painful erosions.

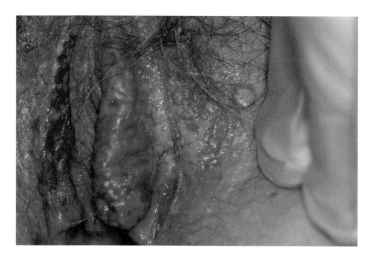

Figure 12.2.4. Severe, painful, recurrent herpes simplex showing swelling and erosion of the labia minora with pustules seen on left inner labium majus.

Candida

General description

Infection of the vulva and/or vagina by *Candida albicans* occurs once during their lives in 75% of women, 40–45% have more than one episode, and 5% have recurrent candidiasis, over four episodes yearly.[11] *Candida albicans* causes over 85% of cases.[12]

Candida pathogenesis involves colonization, and then transformation to symptomatic disease. Asymptomatic colonization does not require treatment. Major host factors facilitating transformation are antibiotic use, diabetes, sexual activity, and, possibly, dietary carbohydrate excess.[13] While the role of reproductive hormones remains unclear,[14] exogenous estrogens from oral contraceptive pills and hormone therapy, or local estrogen is believed to contribute.[15] Candidiasis often complicates dermatoses and topical steroid use.

Clinical description

Signs and symptoms of vulvovaginal candidiasis include a whitish, cheesy discharge with pruritus, irritation, soreness, dyspareunia, and dysuria. Erythema and fissuring may be seen (Figs 12.2.5 and 12.2.6). Burning is often a feature of pathogens other than *C. albicans*. No sign or symptom, individually or collectively, is pathognomonic.[16] Candidiasis can occur with low-grade symptoms and without discharge.

Diagnosis cannot be made by history and physical examination alone.[17] Microscopy and pH are essential, and since microscopy is only 40% specific, culture is imperative if yeast is not seen. Unfortunately, the diagnosis is made daily in thousands of women on the basis of a telephone conversation or noninclusive physical examination. Many other factors may account for identical signs and symptoms; hence, the need for laboratory confirmation is critical. Self-diagnosis is poor.[18] Other mimicking conditions include physiologic discharge, vestibulodynia, contact or irritant dermatitis, vulvovaginal atrophy, lichen sclerosus or lichen planus, and desquamative inflammatory vaginitis.

used to distinguish between herpes simplex virus I and herpes simplex virus II infection.[5,9]

Treatment[9,10]

One must first rule out other sexually transmitted diseases. For primary herpes simplex virus infections, local or oral analgesics and cool soaks can help. Specific oral antiviral treatment is indicated with valacyclovir 1 g twice a day for seven to ten days or famciclovir 250 mg three times a day for seven to ten days. For recurrent herpes simplex virus infection use valacyclovir 500 mg twice a day for three to five days or 1 g once daily for five days or famciclovir 125 mg twice a day for five days. To suppress herpes simplex virus infection use valacyclovir 1 g daily or famciclovir 250 mg twice a day. The length of suppressive therapy varies and needs to be evaluated yearly.

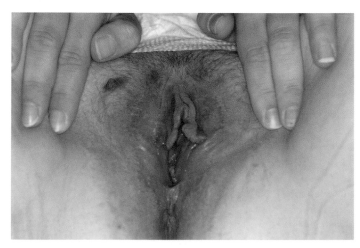

Figure 12.2.5. Vulvar candidiasis with diffuse erythema, swelling, and fissures.

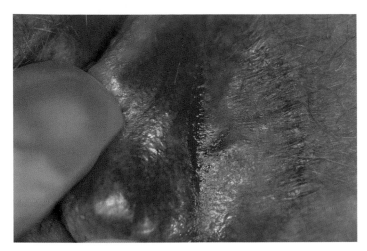

Figure 12.2.6. Close-up of the painful fissures in Fig. 12.2.5.

To facilitate treatment, candidiasis is classified.[17] Uncomplicated cases include mild to moderate severity, infrequent outbreaks, in a normal, nonpregnant host, showing pseudohyphae of *C. albicans* on microscopy. Complicated cases are moderate to severe, recur four or more times a year, can be non-*C. albicans*, and occur in an immunocompromised, diabetic, or pregnant host. Recurrence may also represent inadequately treated infection.[19] Ninety per cent of the patients who seek treatment for candidiasis have uncomplicated disease, treated with short-course therapy with a topical azole agent or a single 150-mg dose of fluconazole. Prolonged therapy necessary for complicated candidiasis includes two doses of 150-mg fluconazole 72 h apart, or 150 mg weekly for 6 months.[20]

Non-*C. albicans* yeasts, such as *C. glabrata*, respond poorly to azoles. They are treated with boric acid (600 mg) inserted vaginally nightly for 14 days.[21]

Trichomoniasis

General description
Vaginal infection with *Trichomonas vaginalis* is the most common sexually transmitted infection worldwide.[22] In the USA, trichomoniasis is second to chlamydia in estimated annual incidence. The protozoan is associated with sexual intercourse and is not generally spread by fomites. It frequently occurs with bacterial vaginosis and gonorrhea in women of all ages.

Trichomoniasis is no longer regarded as simply annoying, but may be associated with adverse pregnancy outcomes such as premature rupture of the membranes and preterm delivery.[23] It is also associated with increased human immunodeficiency virus (HIV) transmission.[13]

Clinical description
Trichomoniasis manifests as malodorous, profuse yellow-green discharge with vulvar pruritus and burning, but asymptomatic infection also can occur. If untreated, symptoms can persist for years.

Diagnosis
Trichomoniasis is diagnosed by microscopy of vaginal secretions with visualization of motile, ovoid, flagellated organisms. This method is 60–70% sensitive; backup culture is important if suspicion is high. Polymerase chain reaction testing has an 84% sensitivity[24] but is not approved by the US Food and Drug Administration.

Treatment of trichomoniasis with metronidazole 2 g orally as a single dose or 500 mg orally for 7 days has cure rates of 90–95%. Treating sex partners is encouraged. Vaginal gel is less efficacious; no other therapy is approved by the Food and Drug Administration. About 5% of cases are estimated to be resistant; most can be treated with increasing doses of metronidazole 500 mg b.i.d. for 7 days, or 2 g daily for 3–5 days.[25] Guidance from the Centers for Disease Control and Prevention is available for difficult cases.

Herpes zoster

General description
Herpes zoster (shingles) is an acute, painful blistering disease of the nerves of the skin and associated tissues. It usually affects one or two dermatomes and is caused by the varicella-zoster virus, another herpes virus. This virus lies latent in dorsal root ganglia after earlier varicella (chickenpox) infection. The virus is reactivated when immune surveillance is diminished by age, neoplasia, pharmacologic immunosuppression, or human immunodeficiency virus/acquired immunodeficiency syndrome.

Clinical features
With the onset of vulvar herpes zoster, pain and/or paresthesia are typically felt along the S3 dermatome. This occurs 1–5 days before the vesicular rash. Symptoms include a prodrome of headache, fever, and malaise. Before the eruption, there is usually pain, and as the pustules break, there is burning and dysuria. The involved skin is red and swollen with crops of grouped vesicles that become pustules and progress to crusted and/or open erosions (Figs 12.2.7–12.2.9). The pain can be severe. The course is 2–3 weeks. A debilitating postherpetic neuralgia, especially in the elderly, may follow, lasting months or years.[26–29]

Diagnosis
Usually the diagnosis is made clinically. Serologic testing or skin swab for direct immunofluorescence testing is available

Treatment
The treatment is valacyclovir 1 g t.i.d. for 7 days; famciclovir 500 mg t.i.d. for 7 days. Pain control is very important. For postherpetic neuralgia, treatment with tricyclic antidepressants, gabapentin, and oxycodone is effective. Start a tricyclic such as amitriptyline or nortriptyline in a low, gradually increasing dose (10 up to 50–75 mg) in older patients, as they are the ones at risk of postherpetic neuralgia. These drugs should be started immediately along with antiviral medications. Help from a pain clinic may be needed.[29–31]

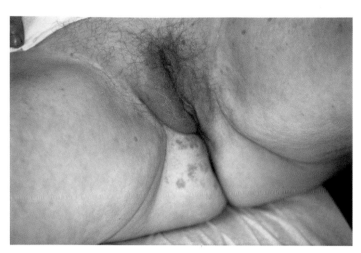

Figure 12.2.7. Vulvar herpes zoster with swelling of right labium majus and pustules on the buttock.

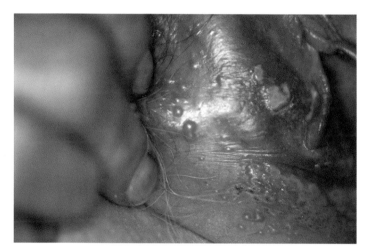

Figure 12.2.8. Close-up of Fig. 12.2.7 with painful vesicles and sheets of pustules on right medial labium majus.

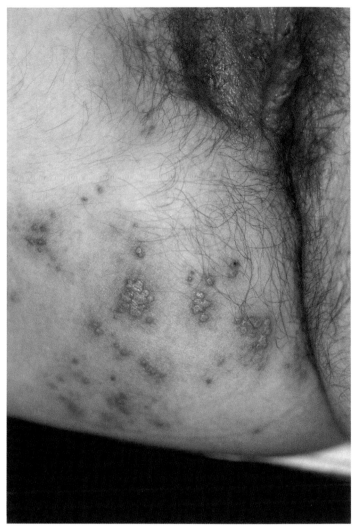

Figure 12.2.9. Typical herpetiform pustules of herpes zoster on buttock (from Figs 12.2.7 and 12.2.8).

Epstein–Barr virus

General description
Epstein–Barr virus is another herpes virus. Classically, it causes infectious mononucleosis. Occasionally, acute painful vulvar ulcers are seen in teenagers and young adults.

Clinical features
There may be a prodrome of fever, malaise, sore throat, mouth ulcers, and enlarged cervical glands. In the vulva, there is an acute onset of pain, burning, and dysuria with punched-out, red-rimmed, single or multiple, vulvar ulcers (Fig. 12.2.10). These last 1–2 weeks and resolve with no scarring. They are often mistaken for herpes simplex virus infection, but all tests for the latter are negative.

Diagnosis
The diagnosis of Epstein–Barr virus (EBV) is made with specific serology testing for the antibody to viral capsid antigen for EBV

on both acute and convalescent serum (the MonoSpot test may be negative).

Treatment:[7,32–35]
Only symptomatic treatment is needed.

Inflammatory disease

Lichen planus

General description
Lichen planus is a relatively common, lymphocyte-mediated, inflammatory, mucocutaneous dermatosis. Usually, it affects the oral cavity and skin, but it can involve the vulva and vagina in 5% of cases. This involvement is referred to as the vulvo-vaginal-gingival syndrome or erosive or ulcerative lichen planus. It can affect not only skin and mucous membranes but also ears, eyes, esophagus, bladder, and anus. The vulvovaginal disease may be in isolation or part of a more widespread

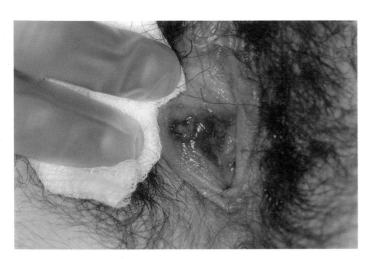

Figure 12.2.10. Severely painful ulcers right labium minus from Epstein–Barr virus infection.

eruption. It is of uncertain etiology but evidence supports an autoimmune, T-cell-mediated condition triggered by an exogenous antigenic stimulus. Erosive lichen planus can cause significant pain, dyspareunia, and apareunia. It may be self-limited, but the erosive form can be very chronic.

Clinical features

The typical patient is 30–60 years of age. There may be few to no symptoms, just variable itching and irritation. With the eroded and ulcerative form, symptoms are more severe with pain and dysfunction. Pain and burning are the main complaints and the physical findings often are missed, as they can be subtle or poorly recognized. With vaginal involvement, there can be complaints of dyspareunia, apareunia, and purulent, malodorous discharge. On physical examination, there may be a whitish, gray, lacy reticulated pattern on the vulvar mucous membranes (Fig. 12.2.11) with secondary excoriations or even

thickening due to scratching. In the painful erosive form, there is redness with partial or full-thickness erosions showing a gray or whitish edge (Fig. 12.2.12). The erosions are glossy red and classically present around the labia minora and vestibule. Normal architecture is lost, with destruction of labia minora and clitoris. Scarring causes synechiae on the vulva and in the vagina. The introitus may be stenosed. The vagina can become friable, atrophic, shortened, scarred, or even obliterated. Signs of lichen planus can be seen elsewhere, particularly the oral cavity, which may show the reticulated lacy pattern or even ulcers (Fig. 12.2.13). On the body is a purple to red, polygonal, itchy, papular, and sometimes scaling rash.

Diagnosis

Diagnosis can be made on the clinical pattern in the genital area, mouth, and skin. Biopsies should be examined with routine histopathology and direct immunofluorescence.

Treatment:[36–42]

Treatment is challenging. There is no single, universally effective treatment. All irritation to the area must stop. All infections (such as yeast) must be managed. Corticosteroids are the mainstay, being used as ointment, vaginal cream, or foam or systemically. Superpotent topical corticosteroid, halobetasol, or clobetasol 0.05% ointment, is usually chosen for primary treatment. Systemic steroids then may be required if there is no response.

Anecdotally reported treatments include hydroxychloroquine, cyclosporine, systemic retinoids, tetracyclines, dapsone, azathioprine, and methotrexate.

Surgery may be required for vaginal adhesions or in reconstruction of the vagina, although the success rate for these procedures is disappointing. There is a small risk of malignancy. These patients need long-term supervision with a lot of support, which is best done with a multidisciplinary team.

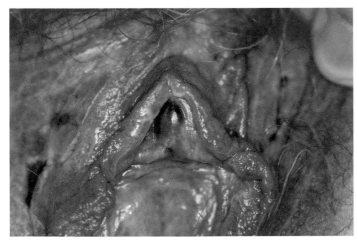

Figure 12.2.11. Painful, eroded vulvar lichen planus involving the clitoris and periclitoral areas. Note typical white, lacey pattern and scarring around the clitoris.

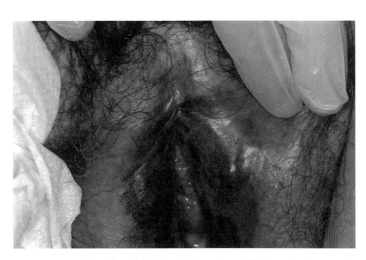

Figure 12.2.12. Severely painful vulvar lichen planus with glazed erythema and scarring plus loss of labia minora and most of clitoris.

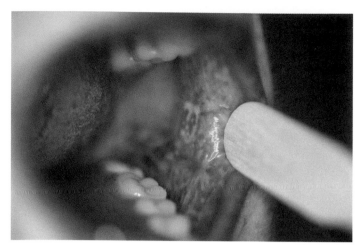

Figure 12.2.13. Typical lacey white pattern on the buccal mucosa in oral lichen planus.

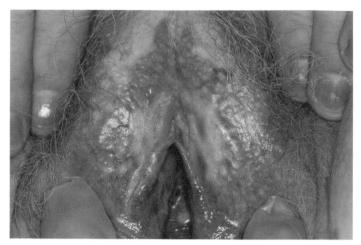

Figure 12.2.14. Shiny, white, patchy, cellophane-surfaced vulvar lichen sclerosus with periclitoral scarring.

Lichen sclerosus

General description

Lichen sclerosus is a common inflammatory mucocutaneous disorder of the vulva that presents with itching and/or irritation. Whiteness, thinning, and scarring changes are seen. Less commonly, there is pain, usually due to secondary factors. The definitive etiology is unknown, but most likely this is a multifactorial, autoimmune, familial condition. Family history is positive in 22% of patients, and up to 44% have various autoantibodies. The age of onset is 35–45 years of age, but children as young as 1½ years have been affected. Squamous cell carcinoma of the vulva develops in 3–4% of these patients.

Clinical features

The clinical picture is variable. Pruritus is the commonest complaint, usually with a mixture of itching, burning and dyspareunia. At times it is asymptomatic. Pain and burning may be the main, primary complaint. Usually pain is associated with open areas or fissures due to infection (bacteria and yeast), contactants (irritant or allergen), trauma (scratching or intercourse) or tumor (squamous cell carcinoma). Signs of lichen sclerosus range from the typical white, cellophane-surfaced (Fig. 12.2.14) shiny papules and scarred plaques to open erosions with secondary changes of purpura, ulcers, excoriation, lichenification, fissuring and crusting (Figs 12.2.15 and 12.2.16). There can be significant flattening of the normal vulvar architecture and scarring with loss of clitoris and labia minora and even introital stenosis. Involvement may form a figure of eight from the periclitoral area through the perineum to the perianal area.

Diagnosis

The diagnosis is made clinically and confirmed with biopsy.

Treatment[43–49]

The mainstay of treatment is topical superpotent corticosteroids, clobetasol, or halobetasol 0.05% ointment. These are

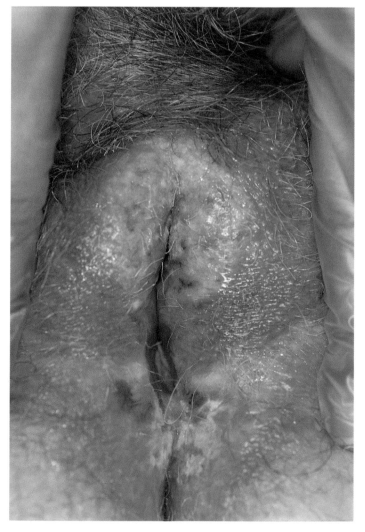

Figure 12.2.15. Shiny white plaques of vulvar lichen sclerosus showing scarring and loss of the clitoris and labia minora. Painful erosions are caused by scratching.

referred to as the "itch that rashes". This condition is defined by relentless pruritus but can be very painful when there are open eroded areas.

Clinical features

All patients present with a history of itching and scratching. Often they have had years of uncontrolled "chronic itch" that is worse with heat, stress, and menstruation. They have seen multiple practitioners and "nothing helps". At night, they wake up scratching. They try anything to get relief. The end result can be open, eroded areas with pain and chronic burning.

On examination, the vulvar skin is thickened with increased skin markings termed "lichenification". This thick, grayish skin develops due to chronic rubbing, like callused skin areas elsewhere. The involvement may be unilateral or bilateral with dyspigmentation (either hypo- or hyper-pigmentation or a combination), redness, excoriations, and variable serosanguineous crusts and fissures (Figs 12.2.17 and 12.2.18). Although this occurs anywhere in the perineum, the labia majora are most commonly involved. There may be hair loss from scratching. Lichen simplex chronicus can complicate other skin conditions. Look for psoriasis, candidiasis, lichen sclerosus, lichen planus, and contact dermatitis.

Secondary factors are often a problem and are the main cause of pain and burning. Infection from bacteria (usually streptococcus or staphylococcus) and/or yeast may develop. Irritant contact dermatitis is very common, as these patients resort to various caustic products to relieve itch. Allergic contact dermatitis may develop. The erosions, fissures, and ulcers associated with these infections and/or topical contactants can result in severe burning pain.

Diagnosis

This is a clinical diagnosis. Once the condition is quieter, a biopsy to look for underlying conditions can be helpful. A biopsy in the acute stage will show only secondary changes.

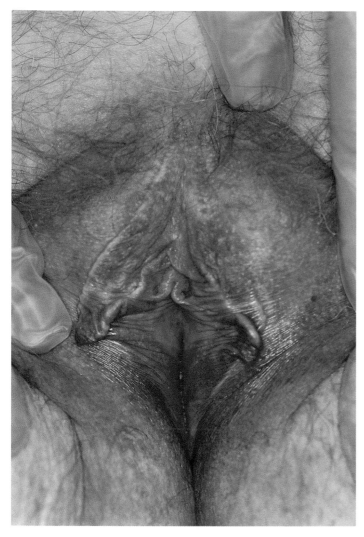

Figure 12.2.16. Scarring in the interlabial sulcus, clitoral area, and labia minora with painful erythema around the labium majus due to irritant contact dermatitis complicating vulvar lichen planus.

used for 3 months and then maintenance is one to three times a week. All irritating factors must be removed. This condition can be well controlled long-term but it is seldom "cured". Long-term follow-up is needed. Good patient education is imperative. Surgery may be necessary for dysfunctional scarring. Although the risk of malignancy is small, yearly follow-up is needed.

Lichen simplex chronicus

Synonyms

Lichen simplex chronicus is also called neurodermatitis, hyperplastic dystrophy, and squamous cell hyperplasia.

General description

Lichen simplex chronicus is the end stage of the itch–scratch–itch cycle. It is usually part of the atopic dermatitis spectrum. This is the chronic, localized, lichenified (thickened) form of atopic dermatitis. Less commonly, it is associated with secondarily scratched psoriasis or contact dermatitis. Sometimes it is

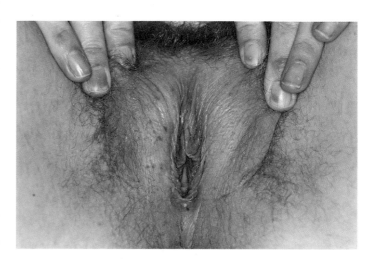

Figure 12.2.17. Thickened (lichenified) inner labia majora with excoriations and painful fissuring in vulvar lichen simplex chronicus.

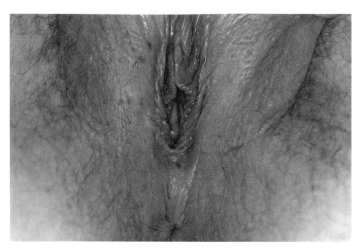

Figure 12.2.18. Close-up of Fig. 12.2.17 with tiny painful fissures at the base of the left labium majus and excoriations on the perineum.

Treatment[50–55]

Identify the underlying disease. Culture for yeast and bacteria. Stop all irritants and consider referral for patch testing to rule out an allergic contactant. Restore the skin barrier function with sitz baths and no cleansers. Follow this with an emollient such as plain petrolatum or vegetable oil to hold moisture in the skin. Reduce inflammation with superpotent steroids, halobetasol, or clobetasol 0.05% ointment b.i.d. for 2 weeks, once a day for 2 weeks, and then Monday–Wednesday–Friday for 2 weeks. Treat bacterial infections with 1 week of cephalosporin, and yeast infections with at least two doses a week of fluconazole 150 mg. Stop the itch–scratch–itch cycle with doxepin or hydroxyzine 25–100 mg at night, and in the morning add citalopram 20–40 mg or fluoxetine. Always look for multiple problems, such as contact dermatitis, lichen simplex chronicus, lichen sclerosus, and infection.

Aphthae

Synonym

Aphthae are also known as canker sores or complex aphthosis.

General description

Aphthous ulcers of the vulva are rare but very painful. Oral aphthae are common, with a lifetime incidence of 50%. Although these conditions do not occur concomitantly, they can be associated in the same individual and are referred to as complex aphthosis. Vulvar aphthae can be associated with inflammatory bowel disease such as Crohn's disease, or myeloproliferative diseases. They can be associated with cytotoxic drugs and some syndromes such as mouth and genital ulcers with inflamed cartilage and histiocytic necrotizing lymphadenitis.

Clinical features

Vulvar aphthous ulcers are painful, punched-out, round to irregularly outlined, red-based ulcers of sudden onset that may be single or multiple. They can occur anywhere on the vulva (Figs 12.2.19 and 12.2.20). They are often 1–2 cm in diameter and heal, perhaps with scarring, over 2–4 weeks. Dysuria is common. Recurrences are common at variable intervals. Systemic complaints are often minimal.

Diagnosis

This is a diagnosis of exclusion. Rule out, with appropriate serology, herpes simplex virus, Epstein–Barr virus, syphilis, and human immunodeficiency virus. Rule out chancroid with biopsy. Check on any possible precipitating drugs (particularly cytotoxic ones). Look for any association such as Behçet's disease, inflammatory bowel disease, and myeloproliferative disease or syndromes as above.

Treatment[56–61]

Corticosteroids are the first line of treatment. Topical superpotent halobetasol or clobetasol 0.05% ointment twice a day can be used. For resistant aphthae, intralesional triamcinolone acetonide 3.3 to 5 mg per mL can be injected with a 30 g needle into the base of the ulcer(s). For more difficult cases oral prednisone may be needed. For recurrent disease colchicine or avlosulfon are used. Colchicine 0.6 mg tablets, two to three daily is recommended or avlosulfon (Dapsone) 150–100 mg per day. Some cases require both these drugs together. For severe resistant disease, thalidomide may be needed.

Contact dermatitis

General description

Contact dermatitis is an inflammation of the skin from an external agent that acts either as an irritant or an allergen, producing a rash that can be acute, subacute, or chronic. It can be irritant or allergic. Primary irritant contact dermatitis is due to the caustic or irritating effects of a substance on the skin. It develops after prolonged or repeated exposure to substances

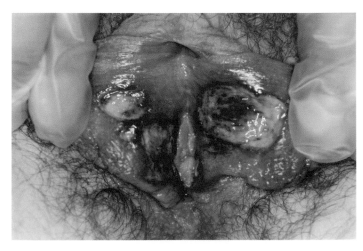

Figure 12.2.19. Deep, painful, punched-out vulvar aphthous ulcers in a teenager.

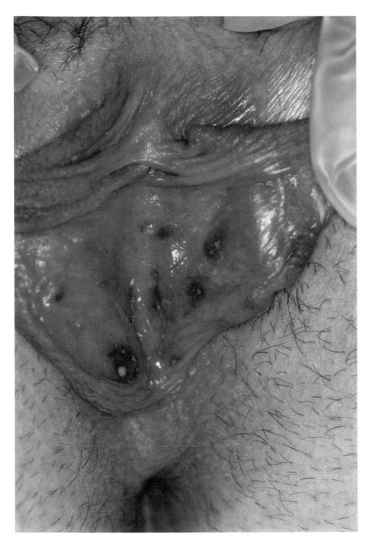

Figure 12.2.20. Same patient as in Fig. 12.2.19 with recurrent, but in this case less dramatically painful aphthous ulcers. All investigation, serology, and cultures repeatedly negative.

such as soap, urine, and feces – especially after over-zealous hygiene practices such as scrubbing. There is no immune reaction with this. Irritant contact dermatitis is more common on the vulva because vulvar skin is thin with a weaker barrier function. Patients with low estrogen, due to menopause, birth control pills, or giving birth have further thinning of the vulvar and vaginal tissue. Other risk factors include rashes such as lichen sclerosus or psoriasis. Incontinence of urine or feces (a very common problem in older women) and regular wearing of pads (that macerate and rub the skin) can cause further problems. To deal with their incontinence-related hygiene issues, some women compensate by washing and adding more topicals, compounding the burning and risking further incontinence-related sensitization.

Allergic contact dermatitis is caused by an allergy to a low dose of a chemical substance such as perfume, antibiotics (neomycin), or benzocaine, or poison ivy. This is a type IV, delayed-hypersensitivity reaction.

Clinical features

There are complaints of variable amounts of itching, burning, and irritation. Pain is not common unless there are open ulcers or erosions. The onset is slower for irritant contact dermatitis, as repeated exposure is necessary. Allergic contact dermatitis reactions are usually itchy with sudden onset with redness, swelling and, rarely in the vulva, vesiculation (Figs 12.2.21 and 12.2.22). More commonly, there is a chronic subacute pattern with dryness, scaling and redness (Fig. 12.2.23). Secondary changes such as scratching and thickening (lichenification) may be seen. Infection or a frank lichen simplex chronicus can occur. There may be a contact dermatitis superimposed on previous skin conditions such as psoriasis or lichen sclerosus.

Diagnosis

The diagnosis is usually clinical. A biopsy may be necessary. To find an allergic etiology, thorough patch testing by a dermatologist or allergist is needed.

Treatment[62-67]

Identify and stop all offending agents and practices. Patients should have lukewarm to cool soaks or sitz baths daily. Replace estrogen as indicated. Give topical corticosteroid, clobetasol, or halobetasol 0.05% ointment b.i.d. for 5–7 days, and then once a day for 5–7 days and a topical bland emollient such as petrolatum or vegetable oil. Night-time sedation with hydroxyzine or doxepin, as in lichen simplex chronicus, may be necessary. If the disease is severe, give oral prednisone tapering over 14 days or intramuscular triamcinolone 1 mg/kg. Treat secondary infection.

Squamous cell neoplasia

Squamous cell neoplasms of the vulva are classified by degree of invasiveness, either intraepithelial or invasive squamous cell carcinoma.

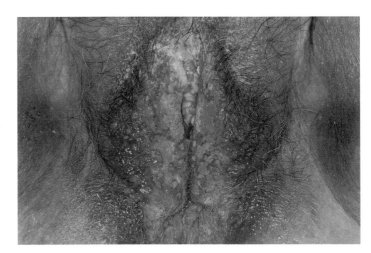

Figure 12.2.21. Severe painful swelling, erosions, and redness of the vulva due to contact dermatitis from benzocaine.

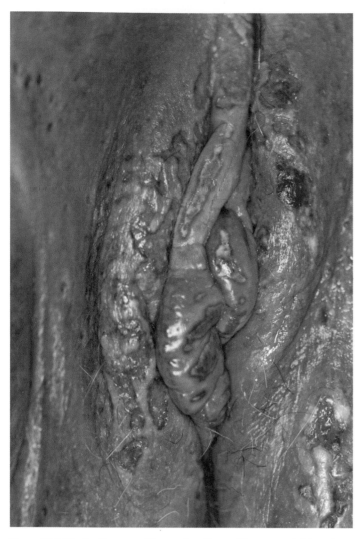

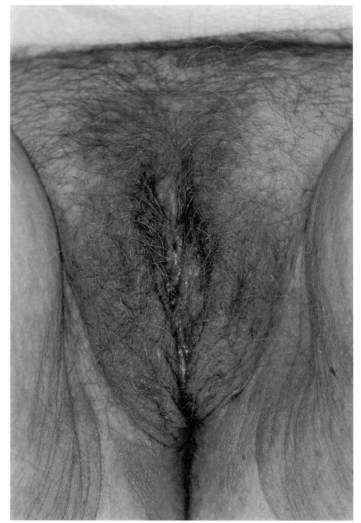

Figure 12.2.22. Another case of benzocaine allergy with severe painful erosions and swelling.

Figure 12.2.23. Swelling and redness due to contact dermatitis of the vulva from neomycin.

Vulvar intraepithelial neoplasia

General description
There are two different vulvar intraepithelial neoplasia patterns: (1) multifocal, human papilloma virus associated, occurring in women aged 20–50 years, and (2) the solitary lesions that occur in women aged 60–70 years.

Clinical description
Multifocal papules or small plaques are variably colored and may be isolated or involve the vulva extensively. The solitary lesion is a single, sharply marginated pink or reddish patch or plaque (Fig. 12.2.24). Lesions may be asymptomatic, or itchy and irritated. If fissuring occurs, the lesion becomes painful.

Diagnosis
This is a biopsy diagnosis. The disorganized histologic pattern of the epidermis in vulvar intraepithelial neoplasia shows variations in degree of dysplasia, cellular atypia, and mitotic activity. It is ranked from mild to severe.

Treatment
Depending on the location and extent of the lesions, treatment is by excision or destruction. Topical imiquimod (Aldara) cream 5% shows promise in the treatment of vulvar intraepithelial neoplasia.[68]

Invasive squamous cell carcinoma

General and clinical description
Invasive vulvar carcinoma occurs as a solitary lesion on the vulva in women older than 55 years. The lesion is usually asymptomatic but if exophytic, fissured, or ulcerated, it may bleed, or become pruritic, sore, or painful (Fig. 12.2.25). Squamous cell carcinoma may occur in the background of lichen planus; 4–96% of vulvar carcinomas are associated with

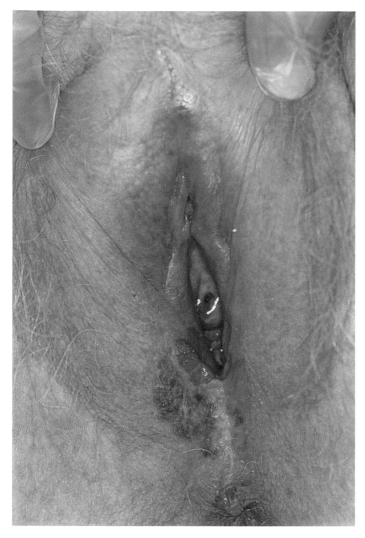

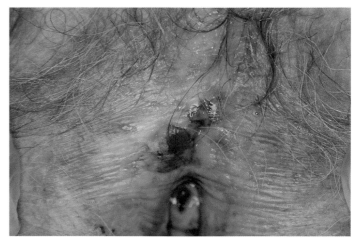

Figure 12.2.25. Painful ulcerated periclitoral squamous cell carcinoma in a case of vulvar lichen sclerosus.

Figure 12.2.24. Painful, superficial ulcer of right lower labium minus with hyperpigmented perineal plaque in vulvar intraepithelial neoplasia (VIN III). Note scarring of lichen sclerosus periclitorally.

surrounding lichen sclerosus, depending on the thoroughness of examination of the specimen.[69]

Diagnosis is by biopsy.
Treatment requires a gynecologic oncologist to stage and remove the tumor.

Neurologic conditions

Postherpetic neuralgia

Herpes zoster infection, or shingles, is caused by the clinical recurrence of varicella zoster virus that has been dormant in sensory ganglia. The infection causes postherpetic neuralgia in 10–34% of infected patients. Neuralgia is a debilitating neuropathic pain state that persists for 1–3 months after the resolution of the herpes zoster rash. Usually, the patients are older persons, and 70% are over 50 years of age. More than 50% of

patients over 60 years of age with herpes zoster develop postherpetic neuralgia due to an age-related decline in varicella zoster-specific T-cell-mediated immunity. It also occurs for the same reasons in the immunosuppressed, e.g. those with HIV infection, chemotherapeutic suppression, or cancer. Postherpetic neuralgia is more common in women (65%) than in men (35%). The lumbosacral nerves are affected in 15% of cases of herpes zoster. Vulvar shingles probably affects 1.5 million American women in their lifetime, and 150 000 have postherpetic neuralgia.[70–74]

After the initial outbreak of herpes zoster, there is a variable pattern of neuropathic pain. It may follow a continuum with the original acute pain or a relapsing and remitting pattern, or a pain-free period may occur after the infection, and then persistent pain.

The pain is described usually as severe, excruciating, debilitating, and incapacitating. There is constant aching and burning in the vulva and perineum with jabbing, lancinating, and shooting pain. The hallmarks of postherpetic neuralgia are allodynia (pain triggered by non-noxious stimuli, such as clothes and light touch) and hyperalgesia (exaggerated pain response to mild noxious stimuli). These occur in 70–90% of postherpetic neuralgia. Abnormal sensations of paresthesia ("pins and needles") and dysesthesia (other generally unpleasant abnormal sensations) also occur. Less commonly, there can be an incapacitating itch as the main feature – neuropathic pruritus. The discomfort may be continuous or intermittent day to day. Typically, it is worse with stress and fatigue – and fatigue worsens with continuing loss of sleep. It is very debilitating for elderly patients. The majority have resolution of pain in 12 months. Some patients are left with long-term, debilitating neuropathic pain.[70,73–77]

The most difficult patients are those who present generalized vulvodynia with all the hallmarks of allodynia, hyperalgesia, and dysesthesia, and no good history of antecedent infection. Their skin lesions may have been minor or there may have been no cutaneous findings.

Diagnosis is usually clinical with neuralgia as part of the original herpes zoster infection. Scraping of skin for direct immunofluorescence can be helpful with a turnaround time of 24 h. Viral serology may be necessary for diagnosis.

Treatment [73,78–80]

Vulvar herpes zoster in elderly women should be treated as an emergency with proper diagnosis and immediate treatment with antiviral and pain medication.

- For neuropathic pain, local anesthesia with 5% lidocaine gel is given.
- Tricyclic antidepressants, amitriptyline, or nortriptyline, provide 47–67% of patients with moderate to excellent response. It is recommended that these medications be started at the onset of the acute infection. The initial dose is 10 mg, slowly increased up to a maximum of 150 mg. Medication is given at night.
- Gabapentin is useful, starting at 100 mg and building up rapidly to three times a day and then to a total dose of 2600–3600 mg per day depending on the patient's age.
- Opiates such as morphine and oxycodone may be necessary.

Lesion-free causes of vulvar pain

Localized vulvodynia (vestibulodynia)

General description

Vestibulodynia is unprovoked pain in the vestibule; pain on touch at the vaginal vestibule with first tampon, pelvic examination, or intercourse (primary vestibulodynia), or after a period of comfort with these activities (secondary vestibulodynia). Vestibulodynia is recognized as the most common cause of dyspareunia in the woman under 50 years.[81] The dyspareunia of vestibulodynia can be psychosexually devastating.

The etiology of vestibulodynia is unknown. Theories proposed include abnormalities of embryologic development,[82] increased urinary oxalate excretion,[83] genetic/immune factors,[84] hormonal factors,[85] and *Candida*.[86] Human papilloma virus, long suspected, is not proven by recent studies.[87]

The role of inflammation in vestibulodynia is widely debated; currently, the term "vestibulitis" has been replaced by vestibulodynia in the International Society for the Study of Vulvovaginal Disease terminology, since some studies found a lack of association between excised tissue and inflammation. Nevertheless, the lack of a single common risk factor in vestibulodynia points to the common denominator of vulvar inflammation or trauma as the postulated initial event that releases a cascade of inflammatory cytokines.[88] This results in combined peripheral nerve sensitization and central sensitization, leading to the characteristic alterations in mechanical, thermal, and deep pressure pain threshold of vestibulodynia.[89] A genetic factor may operate susceptible individuals.[90]

Clinical description

Women are convinced that they have recurrent yeast infection, or that they are "too small" for comfortable sexual relations. Clinicians diagnose repeated infections, or dismiss the pain as psychologic. Women with vestibulodynia meet Friedrich's criteria, as follows:[91]

1. Severe pain on vestibular touch or attempted vaginal entry
2. Tenderness localized within the vestibule
3. Physical findings of erythema of various degrees.

Diagnosis is achieved by history and exclusion of vulvar pain related to a specific disorder. The distinct differences in pain response to light touch to the vestibule permit a clear, reliable diagnosis of vestibulodynia[92] by the Q-tip test. A moistened, cotton-tipped swab is used to touch around the vestibular "clock" (see Chapters 9.5 and 12.1); painful areas may be focal or diffuse.

A myriad of treatments are proposed (see Chapters 12.1 and 12.3–12.6); there is little evidence-based medicine for any of them. An accepted medical approach is to eliminate irritants, educate, and provide sexual counseling and support. Prescribe topical lidocaine to be applied several times a day to minimize afferent input to the dorsal horn, and an oral tricyclic starting at 10 mg q.h.s. and working up gradually to 100–150 mg q.h.s. Gabapentin in doses of 1000–3600 mg, in place of or in addition to the tricyclic, may be useful. Physical therapy to the pelvic floor with biofeedback complements this regimen.[93] If medical treatment fails, vestibulectomy with vaginal advancement has an 80% success rate,[94] reaching 95% in some studies.[95]

Generalized vulvodynia

General and clinical description

Burning, aching, stinging, and rawness are some of the descriptors for generalized vulvodynia and may involve all, half, or a focal point on the vulva. Symptoms may be constant or episodic, ranging from hours to days or weeks. Dyspareunia may or may not be a feature, although intercourse may trigger the pain. Other triggers include tight clothes and undergarments, prolonged sitting, standing, or walking. Urinary symptoms of burning are frequently reported.

The etiology of vulvodynia is unknown. The pain is likened to that of neuralgia, with hyperesthesia over the cutaneous distribution of the pudendal, iliohypogastric, ilioinguinal, or genitofemoral nerves from the mons to the anus. Nerve injury, compression, or entrapment is postulated.

Diagnosis is made by ruling out vulvar pain related to a specific disorder. As with other neurogenic pain, there are often no physical findings.

Treatment with tricyclic antidepressants in doses of 20–100 mg has been successful.[96] Gabapentin, effective for postherpetic neuralgia and diabetic neuropathy,[97,98] is also used, although it is unstudied for vulvodynia. If musculoskeletal causes are contributing to pain, physical therapy may be helpful. Surgery to release an entrapped pudendal nerve is being done in France and has just started to be performed in the USA.

Conclusion

The numerous etiologies for vulvar pain as a source of female sexual dysfunction mandate a careful history and physical examination to determine the source of pain and direct its treatment. An algorithm for vulvar pain is included in Chapter 9.5 (Fig. 9.5.2).

References

1. Steege JF, Ling FW. Dyspareunia. A special type of chronic pelvic pain. *Obstet Gynecol Clin North Am* 1983; 20: 779–93.
2. Harlow BL, Stewart EG. A population-based assessment of chronic unexplained vulvar pain: have we underestimated the prevalence of vulvodynia? *JAMA* 2003; 58: 82–8.
3. Reed BD, Crawford S, Couper M et al. Pain at the vulvar vestibule: a web-based survey. *J Lower Gen Tract Dis* 2004; 8: 48–57.
4. International Society for the Study of Vulvovaginal Disease, XVII World Congress, Jointly Sponsored by the American College of Obstetricians and Gynecologists, 12–16 October 2003, Salvador, Brazil.
5. Corey L, Handsfield HH. Genital herpes and public health: addressing a global problem. *JAMA* 2000; 283: 791–4.
6. Margesson LJ. Infectious diseases of the vulva. In BK Fisher, LJ Margesson, eds. *Genital Skin Disorders; Diagnosis and Treatment.* St Louis: Mosby, 1998: 131–3.
7. Oriel JD. Infective conditions of the vulva. In CM Ridley, SM Neill, eds. *The Vulva*, 2nd edn. London: Blackwell Science, 1999: 103–7.
8. Ashley RL, Wald A. Genital herpes: a review of the epidemic and potential use of type-specific serology. *Clin Microbiol Rev* 1999; 12: 1–8.
9. Yeung-Yue KA, Brentjens HM, Lee PC et al. Herpes simplex viruses 1 and 2. *Dermatol Clin* 2002; 20: 249–66.
10. Barton SE, Ebel CE, Kirchner JT et al. The clinical management of recurrent genital herpes: current issues and future prospects. *Herpes* 2002; 9: 15–20.
11. World Health Organization Department of HIV/AIDS. Global prevalence and incidence of selected curable sexually transmitted infection. 2001.
12. Laga M, Manoka A, Kivuvu M et al. Non-ulcerative sexually transmitted diseases as risk factors for HIV-1 transmission in women: results from a cohort study. *AIDS* 1993; 7: 95–102.
13. Donders GG, Prenen H, Verbeke G et al. Impaired tolerance for glucose in women with recurrent vaginal candidiasis. *Am J Obstet Gynecol* 2002; 187: 989–93.
14. Fidel PL, Cutright J, Steele C. Effects of reproductive hormones on experimental vaginal candidiasis. *Infect Immun* 2000; 68: 651–7.
15. Sobel JD. Management of patients with recurrent vulvovaginal candidiasis. *Drugs* 2003; 63: 1059–66.
16. Sobel JD, Faro S, Force RW et al. Vulvovaginal candidiasis: epidemiologic, diagnostic, and therapeutic considerations. *Am J Obstet Gynecol* 1998; 178: 203–11.
17. Schaaf VKM, Perex-Stable EJ, Borchardt K. The limited value of symptoms and signs in the diagnosis of vaginal infections. *Arch Intern Med* 1990; 150: 1929–33.
18. Ferris DG, Dekle C, Litaker MS. Women's use of over-the-counter antifungal pharmaceutical products for gynecologic symptoms. *J Fam Pract* 1996; 42: 595–600.
19. Horowitz BJ, Giaquinta D, Ito S. Evolving pathogens in vulvovaginal candidiasis: implications for patient care. *J Clin Pharmacol* 1992; 32: 248–55.
20. Sobel JD, Kapernick PS, Zervos M et al. Treatment of complicated *Candida* vaginitis: comparison of single and sequential doses of fluconazole. *Am J Obstet Gynecol* 2001; 185: 363–9.
21. Sobel JD, Chaim W, Nagappan V et al. Therapy of vaginitis due to *Candida glabrata*: use of topical boric acid and flucytosine. *Am J Obstet Gynecol* 2003; 189: 1297–1300.
22. World Health Organization, Department of HIV/AIDS. Global prevalence and incidence of selected curable sexually transmitted infections. 2001. Available at: www.who/int/docstore/hiv/GRSTI/006.htm.
23. Cotch MF, Pastorek JG, Nugent RP et al. *Trichomonas vaginalis* associated with low birth weight and pre-term delivery. The Vaginal Infections and Prematurity Study Group. *Sex Transm Dis* 1997; 24: 353–60.
24. Wendel KA, Erbelding EJ, Gaydos CA et al. *Trichomonas vaginalis* polymerase chain reaction compared with standard diagnostic and therapeutic protocols for detection and treatment of vaginal trichomoniasis. *Clin Infect Dis* 2002; 35: 576–80.
25. Centers for Disease Control and Prevention. Sexually transmitted diseases treatment guidelines. 2002. *MMWR Morb Mortal Wkly Rep* 2002; 51(RR-6): 44–5.
26. Margesson LJ. Infectious diseases of the vulva. In BK Fisher, LJ Margesson, eds. *Genital Skin Disorders; Diagnosis and Treatment.* St Louis: Mosby, 1998: 133–4.
27. Brown D. Herpes zoster of the vulva. *Clin Obstet Gynecol* 1972; 15: 1010–14.
28. Chen TM, George S, Woodruff CA et al. Clinical manifestations of varicella-zoster virus infection. *Dermatol Clin* 2002; 20: 267–82.
29. Gnann JW Jr, Whitley RJ. Clinical practice. Herpes zoster. *N Engl J Med* 2002; 347: 340–6.
30. Alder BS, Lewis PR. Treatment of postherpetic neuralgia: a systematic review of the literature. *J Fam Pract* 2002; 51: 121–8.
31. Johnson RW. Consequences and management of pain in herpes zoster. *J Infect Dis* 2002; 186(Suppl 1): S83–90.

32. Margesson LJ. Pediatric vulvar disorders. In M Black, M McKay. *Obstetric and Gynecologic Dermatology*, 2nd edn. London: Mosby, 2002: p 130.

33. Cheng SX, Chapman MS, Margesson LJ et al. Genital ulcers caused by Epstein–Barr virus. *J Am Acad Dermatol* 2004 (*in press*).

34. Sisson BA, Glick L. Genital ulceration as a presenting manifestation of infectious mononucleosis. *J Pediatr Adolesc Gynecol* 1998; 11: 185–7.

35. Hudson LB, Perlman SE. Necrotizing genital ulcerations in a premenarchal female with mononucleosis. *Obstet Gynecol* 1998; 92(4 pt2): 642–4.

36. Margesson LJ. Inflammatory Diseases of the Vulva. In Fisher DK, Margesson LJ, eds. *Genital Skin Disorders: Diagnosis and Treatment*. St. Louis: Mosby, 1998: 69–72.

37. Lynch PJ, Edwards L. Red plaques with papulosquamous features. In PJ Lynch, L Edwards, eds. *Genital Dermatology*. New York: Churchill Livingstone, 1994: 63–72.

38. Ridley CM, Neill SM. Non-infective cutaneous conditions of the vulva. In CM Ridley, SM Neill, eds. *The Vulva*, 2nd edn. London: Blackwell Science, 1999: 164–8.

39. Lewis FM, Shah M, Harrington CI. Vulval involvement in lichen planus: a study of 37 women. *Br J Dermatol* 1996; 135: 89–91.

40. Lewis FM. Vulval lichen planus. *Br J Dermatol* 1998; 138: 569–75.

41. Rogers RS III, Eisen D. Erosive oral lichen planus with genital lesions. The vulvovaginal-gingival syndrome and the peno-genital syndrome. *Dermatol Clin* 2003; 21: 91–8.

42. Ramer MA, Altchek A, Deligdisch L et al. Lichen planus and the vulvovaginal-gingival syndrome. *J Periodontol* 2003; 74: 1385–93.

43. Lynch PJ, Edwards L. White patches and plaques. In PJ Lynch, L Edwards, eds. *Genital Dermatology*. Baltimore: Churchill Livingstone, 1995: 149–58.

44. Ridley CM, Neill SM. Non-infective cutaneous conditions of the vulva. In CM Ridley, SM Neill, eds. *The Vulva*, 2nd edn. London: Blackwell Science, 1999: 154–64.

45. Margesson LJ. Inflammatory Diseases of the Vulva. In Fisher BK, Margesson LJ, eds. *Genital Skin Disorders: Diagnosis and Treatment*. St Louis: Mosby, 1998: 189–93.

46. Tasker GL, Wojnarwoska F. Lichen sclerosus. *Clin Exp Dermatol* 2003; 28: 128–33.

47. Neill SM, Tatnall FM, Cox NH. Guidelines for the management of lichen sclerosus. *Br J Dermatol* 2002; 147: 640–9.

48. Powell JJ, Wojnarowska F. Lichen sclerosus. *Lancet* 1999: 353: 1777–83.

49. Wakelin SH, Marren P. Lichen sclerosus in women. *Clin Dermatol* 1997; 15: 155–69.

50. Lynch PJ. Lichen simplex chronicus (atopic/neurodermatitis) of the anogenital region. *Dermatol Ther* 2004; 17: 8–19.

51. Lynch PJ, Edwards L. Red plaques with eczematous features. In PJ Lynch, L Edwards, eds. *Genital Dermatology*. New York: Churchill Livingstone, 1994: 27–34.

52. Ridley CM, Neill SM. Non-infective Cutaneous Conditions of the Vulva. In Ridley CM, Neill SM, eds. *The Vulva*, 2nd ed. London: Blackwell Science, 1999:151–2.

53. Ball SB, Wojnarowska F. Vulvar dermatoses: lichen sclerosus,

54. Virgili A, Bacilieri S, Corazza M. Evaluation of contact sensitization in vulvar lichen simplex. *J Reprod Med* 2003; 48: 33–6.

55. Virgili A, Bacilieri S, Corazza M. Managing vulvar lichen simplex chronicus. *J Reprod Med* 2001; 46: 343–6.

56. Rogers RS 3rd. Complex aphthosis. *Adv Exp Med Biol* 2003; 528: 311–16.

57. Rogers RS 3rd. Pseudo-Behcet's disease. *Dermatol Clin* 2003; 21: 49–61.

58. Rogers RS 3rd. Recurrent aphthous stomatitis in the diagnosis of Behcet's disease. *Yonsei Med J* 1997; 38: 370–9.

59. Rogers RS 3rd. Recurrent aphthous stomatitis: clinical characteristics and associated systemic disorders. *Semin Cutan Med Surg* 1997; 16: 278–83.

60. McCarthy MA, Garton RA, Jorizzo JL. Complex aphthosis and Behcet's disease. *Dermatol Clin* 2003; 21: 41–8.

61. Lynch PJ, Edwards L. Non-infectious primary ulcers. In PJ Lynch, L Edwards, eds. *Genital Dermatology*. New York: Churchill Livingstone, 1994: 213–16.

62. Margesson LJ. Contact dermatitis of the vulva. *Dermatol Ther* 2004; 17: 20–7.

63. Marren P, Wojnarowska F, Powell S. Allergic contact dermatoses and vulvar dermatoses. *Br J Dermatol* 1992; 126: 52–6.

64. Goldsmith PC, Rycroft RJ, White IR et al. Contact sensitivity in women with anogenital dermatoses. *Contact Dermatitis* 1997; 36: 174–5.

65. Kazaks EL, Lane AT. Diaper dermatitis. *Pediatr Clin North Am* 2000; 47: 909–19.

66. Lynch PJ, Edwards L. Red Plaques with Eczematous Features. In Lynch PJ, Edwards L, eds. *Genital Dermatology*. Edinburgh: Churchill Livingstone, 1994: 34–41.

67. Margesson LJ. Inflammatory Disorders of the Vulva. In Fisher BK, Margesson LJ, eds. *Genital Skin Disorders; Diagnosis and Treatment*. St. Louis: Mosby, 1998:155–7.

68. Van Seters M, van Beurden M, Burger MP et al. Preliminary results of a randomized controlled trial of imiquimod 5% cream in multifocal high grade vulvar intraepithelial neoplasia. International Society for the Study of Vulvovaginal Disease, XVII World Congress, 12–16 October, 2003, Salvador, Brazil.

69. Ridley CM, Neill SM. Non-infective cutaneous conditions of the vulva. In Ridley CM, Neill SM, eds. *The Vulva*. Oxford: Blackwell Science, 1999: 163.

70. Watson CPN. Post-herpetic neuralgia: clinical features and treatment. In HL Fields, ed. *Pain Syndromes in Neurology*. London: Butterworths, 1990: 223–38.

71. Ragozzino MW, Melton LJ III, Kurland LT et al. Population based study of herpes zoster and its sequelae. *Medicine (Baltimore)*. 1982; 61: 310–16.

72. Loeser JD. Herpes zoster and post-herpetic neuralgia. In JJ Bonica, ed. *The Management of Pain*, 2nd edn. Philadelphia: Lea and Febiger, 1990; 257–64.

73. Pappagallo M, Haldey EJ. Pharmacological management of post-herpetic neuralgia. *CNS Drugs* 2003; 17: 771–80.

74. Oaklander AL, Bowsher D, Galer B et al. Herpes zoster itch: preliminary epidemiological data. *J Pain* 2003; 4: 338–43.

75. Watson CP, Evans RJ, Watt VR et al. Post-herpetic neuralgia: 208 cases. *J Pain* 1988; 35: 289–97.

76. Brown D. Herpes zoster of the vulva. *Clin Obstet Gynecol* 1972; 15: 1010–14.

77. Nurmikko, T. Clinical features in pathophysiological mechanisms in post-herpetic pain neuralgia. *Neurology* 1995; 45(Suppl 8): S54–5.

78. Oaklander AL, Rissmiller JG. Post-herpetic neuralgia after shingles: an under-recognized cause of chronic vulvar pain. *Obstet Gynecol* 2002; 99: 625–8.

79. Rowbotham M, Harden N, Bernstein SB et al. Gabapentin for the treatment of post-herpetic neuralgia: a randomized control trial. *JAMA* 1998; 280: 1837–42.

80. Dworkin RH, Backonja M, Rowbotham M et al. Advances in neuropathic pain. Diagnosis, mechanisms and recommendations. *Arch Neurol* 2003; 60: 1524–34.

81. Meana M, Binik YM, Khalife S et al. Biopsychosocial profile of women with dyspareunia. *Obstet Gynecol* 1997; 90: 583–7.

82. Tarr G, Selo-Ojeme DO, Onwude JL. Coexistence of vulvar vestibulitis and interstitial cystitis. *Acta Obstet Gynecol Scand* 2003; 82: 969–71.

83. Solomons CC, Melmed MH, Heitler SM. Calcium citrate for vulvar vestibulitis. A case report. *J Reprod Med* 1991; 36: 879–82.

84. Witkin SS, Gerber S, Ledger WJ. Differential characterization of women with vulvar vestibulitis syndrome. *Am J Obstet Gynecol* 2002; 187: 589–94.

85. Bazin S, Bouchard C, Brisson J et al. Vulvar vestibulitis syndrome: an exploratory case-control study. *Obstet Gynecol* 1994; 83: 47–50.

86. Ashman RB, Ott AK. Autoimmunity as a factor in recurrent vaginal candidosis and the minor vestibular gland syndrome. *J Reprod Med* 1989; 34: 264–6.

87. Morin C, Bouchard C, Brisson J et al. Human papillomaviruses and vulvar vestibulitis. *Obstet Gynecol* 200; 95: 683–7.

88. Foster DC, Hasday JD. Elevated tissue levels of interleukin-1 beta and tumor necrosis factor-alpha in vulvar vestibulitis. *Obstet Gynecol* 1997; 89: 291–6.

89. Bohm-Starke N, Hilliges M, Brodda-Jansen G et al. Psychophysical evidence of nociceptor sensitization in vulvar vestibulitis syndrome. *J Pain* 2001; 94: 177–83.

90. Gerber S, Bongiouvanni AM, Ledger WJ et al. Defective regulation of the proinflammatory immune response in women with vulvar vestibulitis syndrome. *Am J Obstet Gynecol* 2002; 186: 696–700.

91. Friedrich EG. Vulvar vestibulitis syndrome. *J Reprod Med* 1987; 32: 110–14.

92. Bergeron S, Binik YM, Khalife S et al. Vulvar vestibulitis syndrome: reliability of diagnosis and evaluation of current diagnostic criteria. *Obstet Gynecol* 2001; 98: 45–51.

93. Glazer HI, Rodke G, Swencionis C et al. Treatment of vulvar vestibulitis syndrome with electromyographic biofeedback of pelvic floor musculature. *J Reprod Med* 1995; 40: 283–90.

94. Bergeron S, Binik YM, Khalife S et al. A randomized comparison of group cognitive-behavioral therapy, surface electromyographic biofeedback, and vestibulectomy in the treatment of dyspareunia resulting from vulvar vestibulitis. *J Pain* 2001; 91: 297–306.

95. Marinoff SC, Turner ML, Hirsch RP et al. Intralesional alpha-interferon: cost effective therapy for vulvar vestibulitis syndrome. *J Reprod Med* 1993; 38: 19–24.

96. McKay M. Dysesthetic ("essential") vulvodynia. Treatment with amitriptyline. *J Reprod Med* 1993; 38: 9–13.

97. Backonja M, Beydoun A, Edwards KR et al., for the Gabapentin Neuropathy Study Group. Gabapentin for the symptomatic treatment of painful neuropathy in patients with diabetes mellitus, a randomized controlled trial. *JAMA* 1998; 280: 1831–6.

98. Rowbotham M, Harden N, Stacey B et al., for the Gabapentin Neuralgia Study Group. Gabapentin for the treatment of post-herpetic neuralgia, a randomized controlled trial. *JAMA* 1998; 280: 1837–42.

12.3 Physical therapy for female sexual dysfunction

Hollis Herman

Introduction

Musculoskeletal dysfunctions are factors in the etiology and clinical manifestations of female sexual dysfunction. Gynecologists, urogynecologists, urologists, colorectal specialists, internists, family practice physicians, endocrinologists, sexual counselors, nurse practitioners, and physician assistants will benefit from consultation with practitioners skilled in examination and treatment of musculoskeletal dysfunction to decrease pain, increase muscle strength and improve function in their patients with female sexual dysfunction (see Chapters 4.4 and 6.5 of this book).

Complaints of sexual pain (see Chapters 12.1, 12.2, and 12.4–12.6) are common among women with thoracic, lumbar, pelvic, and lower extremity joint dysfunction.[1] Sexual pain is common in women with hypoactive and hyperactive pelvic floor disorders.[2-4] Low libido, vaginal dryness, dyspareunia and decreased sexual satisfaction are reported in women with urinary incontinence.[2] Inadequate lubrication, arousal, and orgasmic ability are present when there is pelvic floor muscle weakness.[5-7] Intolerance to introital penetration, pain during or after sex, fear of pain, and behavioral avoidance of intercourse occur when pelvic floor muscles are adaptively shortened, hypertonic, and weak,[8-11] pelvic nerves are inflamed, irritated, and injured or pelvic joints are hypomobile or hypermobile. White and Jantos[12] studied the changes in normal sexual behavior that accompany vulvar vestibulitis and found that subjects had no loss of sexual desire. Instead they experienced pain in the vulva tissues with contact, reducing their interest in intercourse and generating negative feelings toward it. In a study of vulvar vestibulitis patients, seven sessions of physical therapy for treatment of dyspareunia enabled participants to experience a significant decrease in pain during intercourse and gynecologic examinations. Up to 44 months later, levels of sexual desire and arousal and frequency of intercourse increased as a result of physical therapy intervention.[13]

This chapter addresses the musculoskeletal dysfunctions commonly associated with female sexual pain. It is written to help referring practitioners understand the role of musculoskeletal dysfunction in sexual pain and treatment options available.

The primary musculoskeletal findings in female sexual pain dysfunction are painful and restricted joints, hypertonic, short and weak pelvic floor muscles and irritated and inflamed nerves. Women complain of burning, stabbing, prickling, searing, knifelike pain in their vulva, clitoris, urethra, vagina, anus or rectum (see Chapters 9.2–9.5). They frequently suffer from constipation, urinary incontinence, or urinary frequency and urgency. They have histories of abdominal, perineal, or lumbar surgeries with scars that restrict tissue mobility or blood flow. They all have functional limitations in performing sexual intercourse and have pain during or after sexual activity.

The screening for musculoskeletal dysfunction involves many components listed in Table 12.3.1, including evaluation of the bony structure to assess static and dynamic alignment, symmetry, joint mobility, range of motion, and function. The evaluation proceeds to soft tissue assessment of sensation, muscle strength, length, recruitment, and function, which are often overlooked in the pelvic floor, leading to misdiagnoses of psychogenic pain.[14,15] Musculoskeletal structures of the abdomen, back, perineum, and lower extremities share segmental innervations with many urogenital structures. Referred pain from these musculoskeletal structures can mimic urogenital, gynecologic, and colorectal pain and interfere with the ability to participate in pain-free sexual activity (Table 12.3.2).

Table 12.3.1. Physical therapy components of evaluation and treatment for female sexual dysfunction

Evaluate and treat for postural changes in cervical, thoracic, lumbar, and pelvic regions

Evaluate and treat weakness, hypertonicity, and trigger points in the abdominal muscles

Evaluate and treat for diastasis recti

Evaluate and treat for weakness, hypertonicity, and trigger points in all muscles of the pelvic floor

Evaluate and treat for muscular restrictions to vaginal penetration

Evaluate and treat for vaginal canal movement restrictions

Evaluate for sensory disturbances of the perineum

Evaluate with surface electromyography for perineal muscle hyperactivity

Evaluate and treat for episiotomy and perineal laceration scar tissue restrictions

Evaluate and treat for psoas, iliacus, obturator internus, piriformis, adductor longus, adductor magnus, gluteal, abdominal, paraspinal, hamstring, and multifidus muscle weakness, strain, hypertonicity, and tender and trigger points

Evaluate and treat for pubic symphysis, coccyx, sacroiliac, lumbosacral, lumbar, thoracic, cervical , hip, knee, and ankle joint alignment dysfunctions

Evaluate and treat for pubic symphysis separation, upslip, downslip, anterior displacement, posterior displacement, coccyx hypermobility in flexion or extension, sacroiliac upslip, downslip, rotation, outflare, and inflare

Evaluate and treat muscles affected by spondylolythesis, spondylosis, sacralizations, and lumbarizations

Evaluate and treat for cesarean section scar tissue restrictions

Evaluate and treat for leg and vulvar varicosities with massage, compression, and exercise

Evaluate and treat for lumbar disk herniation, muscle strain, and supports

Evaluate and treat for functional impairment patterns, including poor trunk stability, increased spinal segmental flexibility, decreased proximal and distal limb joint flexibility, and inappropriate compensatory movements

Evaluate and treat for proper body mechanics during functional activities

Evaluate and treat for diminished thoracic and rib cage expansion

Evaluate and treat for first rib mobility restrictions

Evaluate and treat for musculoskeletal restrictions from ilioinguinal, iliohypogastric, genitofemoral, lateral femoral cutaneous, femoral, obturator, pudendal, and brachial plexus nerve entrapments

Evaluate and prescribe an individualized aerobic exercise program

Bony structure

Articulations of the lumbopelvic complex are the sacrum with the fifth lumbar vertebrae, two sacroiliac joints joining the ilium and the sacrum, the pubic symphysis joint, sacrococcygeal joints, intercoccygeal joints, and the femur with the innominate. All of these joints have established normal range of motion measured by goniometric devices, passive range of motion tests, and specific static and active mobility tests. Range of motion values less or significantly greater than expected during these passive and active motion tests are indicative of dysfunction predisposing the joint to abnormal biomechanics, which is a potential source of pain and functional limitation.

Observation of posture from front, back, and side views ideally aligns the joints to a plumb line. Palpation of bony landmarks for symmetry in standing, sitting, and supine, prone, and side lying provides information that alignment may be altered and a potential source of dysfunction. Passive joint testing for proper end feel and mobility can reproduce and isolate painful restrictions. Baker[16] lists a typical pattern of faulty posture in patients with musculoskeletal chronic pelvic pain, including anterior tilt of the pelvis with anterior rotation of the innominate and increased nutation of the sacrum, increased lumbar lordosis and hypomobility of the lumbar spine joints, hyperextension of the knees, anterior displacement of line of gravity in the pelvis and lower extremities, adaptive shortening and hypertonus of the iliopsoas and hip external rotators, lengthening of the iliofemoral ligament, loss of hip capsular extensibility, degenerative joint disease of the hips, loss of hip range of motion into internal rotation, weakness of the abdominal muscles, abdominal trigger points, hypermobility of the thoracolumbar facets, and degenerative joint disease of the thoracolumbar facets.

Soft tissue evaluation

The soft tissues of the lumbopelvic and abdominopelvic region are assessed by palpation for sensation, length, tension, strength, quality of contraction, and tender and trigger points. Muscles attaching to the pelvis are the pelvic floor muscles, including the levator ani (pelvic diaphragm), deep urogenital layer (perineal membrane), the superficial layer of muscles of the urogenital diaphragm, the abdominals, hip flexors, hip extensors, hip internal and external rotators, hip adductors and abductors and flexors and extensors of the spine (see Chapter 4.4).

Specific external assessment of the genitalia and superficial perineal structures begins with observation of skin integrity for redness, swelling, lesions, discoloration, hair loss, and discharge. Pelvic floor muscle contraction, relaxation, and lengthening are informative regarding the patient's awareness, voluntary control, and general resting state of her muscles. If the patient is unaware of the pelvic floor muscles, the excursion of the

Table 12.3.2. Referred pain sites

Structures	Innervation	Referred pain sites	Common disorders
Hip	T12–S1	Lower abdomen, anterior Medial thigh, knee	DJD, bursitis, inflammation, fracture
Lumbar facets, disks	T12–S1	Low back, lateral buttock posterior thigh	Instability, herniation capsular entrapment fracture
Sacroiliac joints	L4–S3	Posterior thigh, pelvic floor, buttock	Strain, laxity, malalignment
Symphysis pubis joint	L1–L5	Lower abdomen, anteromedial thigh, pelvic floor, hip	Strain, separation, laxity, fracture
Abdominal muscles	T5–L1	Abdomen, anteromedial thigh, pelvic floor	Weakness, strain, diastasis recti, TrP
Pelvic floor Muscles	S1–S4	Vagina, rectum, urethra coccyx, clitoris, labia	Adaptive shortening, TrP, protective guarding
Piriformis	L5–S3	Low back, buttock, pelvic	Adaptive shortening, TrP, protective guarding, weakness
Obturator Internus/externus	L3–S2	Pelvic floor, buttock, anterior thigh, clitoris, vagina, coccyx	Adaptive shortening, TrP, protective guarding

DJD: degenerative joint disease; TrP: trigger points.
Modified from Baker[16] and Travell and Simons.[18]

perineal body from the resting position to the shortened contracted position will be minimal, and lengthening of the tissues by gentle bulging will be absent. Often, patients who do not know how to lengthen the muscles suffer constipation or strain with defecation (see Chapters 9.5, 12.1, and 12.2).

External palpation of the pelvic floor muscles will reveal tender and trigger points, pain, and altered sensation and tone. A muscle trigger point will evoke a local twitch response in the taut muscle fibers upon palpation and produce specific referred autonomic phenomena in a pain reference zone. An active trigger point is always tender, prevents full lengthening of the muscle, weakens the muscle, and refers pain on direct compression.[17] Travell and Simons referenced pain zones in the coccyx, anus, rectum, buttock, and posterior thigh from trigger points in the levator ani, obturator internus, and gluteal, abdominal, lumbar, and lower extremity muscles.[18] Pelvic floor myofascial trigger points are a source of pain for voiding symptoms and a potential trigger for neurogenic bladder inflammation.[19] A muscle tender point produces a visible wince when palpated, and tenderness at the site of palpation. Figure 12.3.1 demonstrates a systematic method for documentation of tenderness, pain, and trigger points in the superficial transverse perineal, bulbocavernosus, ischiocavernosus, pubococcygeus, iliococcygeus, and ischiococcygeus muscles.

Midline episiotomies cause perineal trauma. There is a 50 times greater risk of grades three and four lacerations into the anal canal, more pain, more blood loss and slower healing than with spontaneous tears. Mediolateral episiotomies are associated with more pain and weaker pelvic floor muscles that provide less satisfactory cosmetic results and cause more painful intercourse than midline episiotomy or spontaneous tears.[20,21] Tissue restriction from the episiotomy scar may be a cause of pain during vaginal penetration. It may be a source of discomfort when sitting, painful defecation, urinary and fecal incontinence, constipation, altered sexual response and sensation, bleeding, and fissure. Tissue mobility of the episiotomy scar can be graded 1/3, 2/3, or 3/3 when palpated, depending on the amount of restriction present when compared with tissue mobility elsewhere in the body. Palpation of the scar may refer pain to the vaginal introitus, vaginal canal, rectum, and labia. Perineal massage (Table 12.3.3), heat, stretching with dilators or pediatric speculums, muscle re-education by surface electromyography biofeedback, and pelvic floor muscle exercises will increase tissue mobility, and decrease perineal pain and functional limitations. If not, surgical scar revision and reconstruction should be considered.

Muscle strength

Reissing et al.[8] reported higher vaginal and pelvic muscle tone and lower muscle strength in women with vaginismus and dyspareunia. Muscle testing for strength and endurance is performed manually according to established criteria and graded on the 0–5 Oxford scale. The muscles of the pelvic floor can be similarly tested by digital internal examination. The pelvic floor muscles: superficial, perineal membrane, and levator ani can be assessed independently to isolate muscle weakness at the different layers and the discrepancies between right and left sides that are common, particularly when there is concurrent sacroiliac,

1 = Ischiocavernosus
2 = Bulbocavernosus
3 = Superficial transverse perineal
4 = Levator ani
5 = Levator ani
6 = Perineal body
7 = Levator ani
8 = Levator ani
9 = Superficial transverse perineal
10 = Bulbocavernosus
11 = Ischiocavernosus
12 = Symphysis pubis

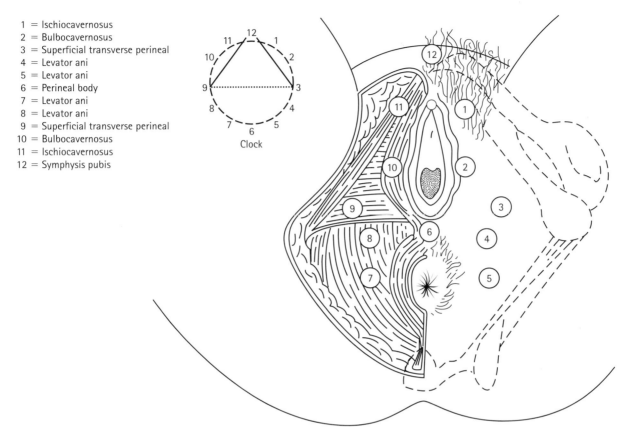

Figure 12.3.1. A systematic method for the documentation of tenderness, pain, and trigger points in the superficial transverse perineal, bulbocavernosus, ischiocavernosus, pubococcygeus, iliococcygeus and ischiococcygeus muscles.

pubic symphysis, hip, or lumbosacral joint dysfunction. In an attempt to standardize global pelvic floor muscle measurement, the International Continence Society Pelvic Floor Assessment Group has recommended a simpler grading system for the pelvic floor muscles of absent, weak, and strong.[22]

Treatment

Vaginismus is an involuntary vaginal muscle contraction making sexual intercourse difficult or impossible. Dyspareunia is defined as painful intercourse. Binik et al.[9] propose a reconceptualization of vaginismus and dyspareunia as sexual disorders characterized by pain, to pain disorders that interfere with sexuality. Physical therapy treatment coverage of dyspareunia may be denied under its primary *International Classification of Diseases*, ninth revision, code (625.9) if viewed as a psychiatric or sexual dysfunction rather than an anatomic or physiologic dysfunction. Graziottin[23] suggests that there are solid biologic factors causing vaginismus and dyspareunia, including muscular, neurologic, and vascular factors.

Possible musculoskeletal causes of dyspareunia are as follows: fissure, adhesion from prior surgery, endometriosis,[24] episiotomy, laceration, birthing trauma with forceps or vacuum extraction, vaginal infection, urinary tract infection, inflammation, skin irritation from chemicals, nerve irritation from entrapment, neurohormonal alteration (particularly estrogen deficiency),[25] instability of the pelvis,[26] prolapse, vasocongestion, and sexual trauma.

Marinoff and Turner[27] define three levels of dyspareunia. Level 1 refers to painful intercourse not severe enough to prevent the activity. Level 2 is painful intercourse that limits the frequency of the activity. Level 3 represents severe painful intercourse that causes abstinence.

Burning, stinging, irritation, rawness, tearing, and searing pain are the most common complaints reported during and after vaginal penetration. If these symptoms are felt at the vaginal introitus, superficial structures such as the vulva, perineal body, posterior fourchette, episiotomy site, and superficial muscle layer are implicated. If deeper vaginal pain occurs, restriction of the vaginal canal, levator ani, and obturator internus muscle trigger points, or sacroiliac, symphysis pubis, hip, or lumbosacral joint dysfunction may be implicated.

Once the musculoskeletal diagnosis for vaginismus and dyspareunia has been established, treatment should include the following steps:[28]

1. Correct any joint malalignment to promote pain-free joint mobility.
2. Teach the patient self-correction joint techniques.

Table 12.3.3. Perineal massage

Procedure 1

Practice lifting up and contracting the pelvic floor muscles, followed by relaxation

View in the mirror to see that the perineal body is pulled inward with the lift

While relaxed, slowly insert thumb fully into the vagina 1–1.5 inches (3–4 cm)

Pull down with the thumb

Stretch the bottom wall of the vagina toward the anus.

Hold steadily for 1–2 min

A feeling of burning in the stretched tissues usually subsides after 1–2 min

Pull the thumb down and to the right and stretch those tissues for 1–2 min

Pull the thumb down and to the left and stretch those tissues for 1–2 min

Combine stretching down and stretching to the sides in a sweeping motion

Slowly and gently massage back and forth over the lower half of the vagina, working the lubricant into the tissues for 3–5 min

Procedure 2

Insert your thumb partially into the vagina

Place your index finger outside the vagina on the perineal body

Roll the posterior wall of the vagina between the thumb and index finger

Roll the tissues for 3–5 min

Procedure 3

Place the index and middle finger on the perineal body without lubricant

Massage the tissues sideways back and forth to free up tissue mobility and scar adhesions

Massage for 3–5 min

For all procedures:

Trim fingernails

Wash hands

Semi-sitting with back supported against pillows

Knees bent up and open

Hold mirror for viewing

Cautions: Avoid the urinary opening to prevent urinary tract infections

Do not do this perineal massage if you have an active herpes lesion; it may spread the infection

Hints: Take a warm bath or place warm compresses on the perineum for 5–10 min before massage

Use K-Y jelly, Slippery Stuff, Astroglide, cocoa butter, vitamin E oil or pure vegetable oil, or none at all

Do this massage once a day

3. Inform about positions for sexual intimacy.
4. Eliminate tender and trigger points in all of the muscles.
5. Eliminate or reduce scar adhesions and tissue restrictions.
6. Teach pelvic floor muscle awareness with a biofeedback device.
7. Re-educate the pelvic floor muscles to be relaxed upon penetration.

8. Stretch the muscles surrounding the vagina by combining down-training with dilators.
9. Stretch the muscles surrounding the vagina by manual tissue techniques.
10. Correct muscle imbalances by down-training (relaxation) and up-training (strengthening).
11. Correct muscle imbalances by teaching correct muscle timing and recruitment.
12. Educate about lubricants.

Positions for sexual activity

Patients with orthopedic dysfunctions are often limited in the positions they can tolerate for intercourse, genital–manual manipulation, or genital–oral stimulation. A total of 46% of patients with chronic low back pain have reduced frequency of intercourse, marked discomfort during intercourse, and greater interference with all aspects of their sexual lives. Female patients with back pain prefer the supine to the prone position for intercourse,[29] although modifications may be required to place the lumbar spine in a neutral position for better comfort.

Dahm et al.[30] surveyed 254 members of the American Association of Hip and Knee Surgeons and found that 80% of surgeons do not discuss sexual positions with their hip arthoplasty patients. A total of 96% of surgeons who discussed postoperative sexual activity with patients spent 5 min or less on the topic. There are five positions for men and three positions for women that are considered acceptable by 90% of the surgeons to protect the hip replacement from dislocation. The most comfortable position reported by women is side-lying on the non-operative hip. Patients should be instructed in the use of wedges, cushions, and pillows to prevent the operated hip from falling into excessive adduction or flexion past 90°.

Hip dysplasia or symphysis pubis joint separation may limit comfortable lower extremity abduction, external rotation, and flexion. The typical missionary position will be too uncomfortable unless modifications are made by placing pillows and wedges lateral to the knees or placing the legs closer together to relax the hyperactive adductor longus and adductor magnus muscles and maintain joint alignment.

Patients with ilial rotation may prefer to straddle their supine partner or sit atop for intercourse. This musculoskeletal dysfunction is common in pregnant patients, early postpartum, and the luteal phase of the menstrual cycle.

Patients diagnosed with dyspareunia, vaginismus, vulvodynia, vestibulodynia, and pelvic floor muscle disorders need to find preferred sexual positions, because each position affords a different contact with the external vulva and internal pelvic organs.[31] Having tried one position unsuccessfully, patients and their partners will erroneously believe that all positions will hurt. Not all vaginal canals are at the same angle to the introitus. Patients and their partners benefit from instruction about female anatomy and how different positions may change the "fit" when attempting penetration. Depending on the shape and size of the pelvic outlet, penetration can be compromised. Patients are surprised to learn that limb and body positioning may increase or decrease the dimensions of the outlet. External perineal examination of the bony landmarks, muscle tone, and muscle tender and trigger point pain sites, and scar tissue mobility assessment offer specific information regarding factors that limit penetration and movement during intercourse. The external examination should be followed by an internal pelvic floor muscle examination without a speculum to determine which position is most suited for the patient and her partner. Digital examination inside the vaginal canal to determine elasticity of the tissues will contribute to an estimation of the circumferential dimensions the vagina can comfortably accommodate. Too often, patients are told, "just do it", or given a set of dilators without specific instruction about which one to start with and then how to progress through the sizes. Fear, pain, and lack of knowledge about how to use the dilators will prevent the patient from using these tools effectively. Simply suggesting that patients attempt vaginal penetration after orgasm by digital or oral stimulation may permit entry and a slower second time around.

In the missionary position, the erect penis reaches the anterior fornix and has contact with the anterior vaginal wall. The posterior bladder wall is pushed forward and upward, and the uterus pushed upward and backward. Patients with painful anterior wall tenderness, interstitial cystitis, painful bladder syndrome, endometriosis, or postsurgical tissue restrictions may find straddling their partner facing away, side lying, on hands and knees, or prone over a wedge more comfortable. In the rear entry position, the erect penis reaches the posterior fornix with contact of the posterior vaginal wall, and the bladder and uterus are pushed forward. Alternate positions are suggested in Table 12.3.4.

All patients should be instructed in self-correction of the lumbar vertebrae, symphysis pubis, hip, sacrum, and ilium by simple effective muscle energy techniques. After office treatment to correct the joint malalignment, the patient can continue with self-corrections at home, with the example of an anterior right ilial correction in Fig. 12.3.2.

Intravaginal manual therapy

Treating the myofascial trigger points in the pelvic floor, abdominal, gluteal, piriformis, and obturator internus muscles resolves or improves symptoms of chronic pelvic pain, sacroiliac joint dysfunction, interstitial cystitis, and irritative voiding.[32] Modified Thiele's massage, intravaginal manual therapy massage of the pelvic floor muscles, two times a week for 5 weeks, improved irritative bladder symptoms in patients with interstitial cystitis and decreased pelvic floor muscle tone.[33] In another study, similar intravaginal manual therapy massage to hypertonic pelvic floor muscles two times per week for 12 weeks effectively eliminated the symptoms of urinary urgency and frequency syndrome and interstitial cystitis.[17] To correct "short" painful pelvic floor muscles, Fitzgerald and Kotarinos[10,11] recommend external connective tissue massage to the lower extremities, abdomen, and pelvis, correction of the abdominal diastasis recti if present, muscle inhibition by proprioceptive neuromuscular facilitation antagonistic muscle patterns, and intravaginal manual therapy muscle massage and stretching. Treating the pelvic floor muscle trigger points by injections or dry needling in combination with intravaginal manual therapy massage techniques can be effective.[34]

Intrarectal manual therapy

Hypertonus in the pelvic floor muscles, poor intake of the correct fiber and fluid, and lack of activity may cause constipation.[35] This condition may contribute to pelvic and sexual pain through altered tone in the pelvic floor muscles. Relaxation of the pelvic floor muscles, specifically the puborectalis, during defecation is necessary to allow the canal to open and the anorectal angle to increase. Inability to relax the puborectalis muscle is termed a paradoxical contraction and necessitates straining during evacuation. Excessive straining can traction the pudendal nerve and alter perineal sensation. The electrical activity of the puborectalis muscle can be assessed by surface

Table 12.3.4. Positions for intercourse

Restrictions	Supine – supported knees	Supine – legs adducted	Prone – with pillow	All fours	Side–lying	Sitting	Straddling
Back pain	+	+	+	+	+	+	
Anterior ilium SIJ					+	+	+
Posterior ilium SIJ	+				+		
Herniated disk			+		+		+
Hip external rotation	+	+				+ facing away	
Neck pain					+	+	+
Prolapsed uterus	+ use a wedge	+ use a wedge		+	+		

SIJ = sacroiliac joint.

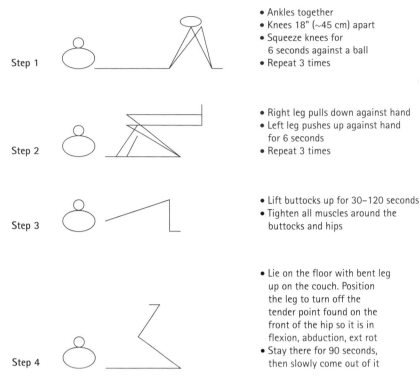

Step 1
- Ankles together
- Knees 18" (~45 cm) apart
- Squeeze knees for 6 seconds against a ball
- Repeat 3 times

Step 2
- Right leg pulls down against hand
- Left leg pushes up against hand for 6 seconds
- Repeat 3 times

Step 3
- Lift buttocks up for 30–120 seconds
- Tighten all muscles around the buttocks and hips

Step 4
- Lie on the floor with bent leg up on the couch. Position the leg to turn off the tender point found on the front of the hip so it is in flexion, abduction, ext rot
- Stay there for 90 seconds, then slowly come out of it

Figure 12.3.2. Anterior right ilial correction.

electromyography. In sitting, external surface sensors of one channel placed at the 3 and 9 o'clock positions around the anal rim, with the other channel monitoring the abdominal muscles, can demonstrate the patient's inability to relax the puborectalis muscle while teaching proper use of the abdominals. Re-education of both muscle groups is facilitated by surface electromyography, and proper muscle functioning reduces straining.

Thiele's massage Fig. 12.3.3 is a technique to address coccydynia directly by intrarectal manual therapy massage of the hypertonic piriformis, obturator internus, puborectalis, ischiococcygeus, and iliococcygeus muscles. Massage strokes are in the direction of the fibers or perpendicular to the muscle fibers. Intrarectal translation and traction mobilizations of the intracoccygeal and sacrococcygeal joints are effective 25% of the time to treat coccydynia. Intravaginal and intrarectal levator ani massage and muscle stretching were more effective in reducing pain than mobilization.[29]

External and internal soft tissue friction massage to a restricted anal fissure scar may reduce painful defecation or painful anal intercourse. Manual therapy techniques of sacral decompression, springing, rocking, strain–counterstrain, positional release, and myofascial release to the sacrum, ilium, connecting ligaments, and muscles will improve joint mechanics and reduce rectal pain.

Surface electromyography and pelvic floor muscle exercises

Surface electromyography was proposed[36] as an objective method of differential diagnosis between functional (musculoskeletal)

vulvovaginal pain syndromes and other sources of vulvovaginal pain such as infections. Battaglia et al.[37] proposed this as an effective therapeutic technique for patients with pelvic floor dyssynergia and slow-transit constipation. Bergeron et al.[38] compared the effects of cognitive-behavioral therapy, surface electromyography, and vestibulectomy in the treatment of dyspareunia and found all techniques significantly helped subjects in psychologic adjustment and sexual function from pretreatment to 6-month follow-up. Using surface electromyography with pelvic pain patients, Glazer et al.[36] demonstrated unstable and abnormally high resting baseline values. Unstable and weak amplitudes were recorded during phasic, tonic and endurance voluntary contractions. Shafik and El-Sibai[39] found that patients with vaginismus exhibited increased electromyography activity at rest and upon penetration when monitoring the levator ani, puborectalis and bulbocavernosus. Stabilizing muscle variability overall and predominantly at rest was a major factor in effective treatment rather than focus on increases in the contractile amplitude.

Glazer and MacConkey[40] proposed simultaneous use of different muscle combinations to enhance the pelvic floor muscles in order to "break" the resting tension level and reduce pain. The "Glazer protocol" (Table 12.3.5) consists of two 20-min exercise sessions per day. Each one is 60 repetitions of 10-s contractions alternating with 10-s relaxation phases. Patients are asked to contract the pelvic floor muscles maximally with all other surrounding muscles. They are required to use home surface electromyography training devices with intravaginal sensors. Gradually, the clinician may observe increased contractile amplitudes, decreased variability of the contraction and

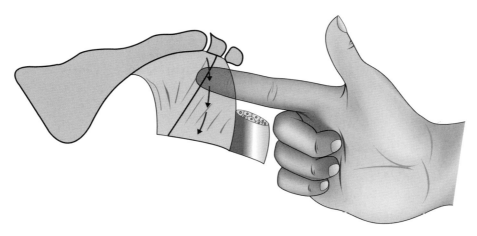

Figure 12.3.3. Theile's massage.

Table 12.3.5. Glazer's protocol and modified Glazer's protocol

Testing
1-min rest, pre-baseline
Five rapid contractions (flicks) with 10-s rest between each
Five 10-s contractions with 10-s rests between each
A single endurance contraction of 60 s
1-min rest post-baseline

Findings
The typical sEMG findings for pain patients are an elevated resting baseline, instability of the signal during resting measured by changes in standard deviation, and instability of the signal during the contraction

Home program
A home program is two 20-min exercise sessions per day
Patient is supine, semi-reclining, sitting, or standing
The patient contracts (shortens) the pelvic floor muscles up and in as hard as possible along with any other muscles
Hold the contraction for 10 s
Relax for 10 s
Repeat 60 times twice a day

Modifications
External surface sensors placed perianal (either side of the anal rim) rather than an internal surface sensor
Contractions can be performed by isolated pelvic floor muscles or in combination with accessory muscles
One session per day rather than two or two 15-min sessions

Daily
Use a one- or two-channel home rental sEMG unit for daily practice in varied positions of sitting, supine, and standing
Frequent self-monitoring of the pelvic floor muscles during daily activities is possible with focus concentration followed by pelvic floor muscle contractions
Gentle bulging to release and lengthen the pelvic floor muscles six times a day for 6 s
The goal is increased relaxation of the pelvic floor muscles most of the time when not activated for stability, posture, or activities

sEMG: surface electromyography.

relaxation amplitude, and faster rise and recovery times with subjective reports of less pain. According to Glazer, the surface electromyography changes demonstrate a reduction of the hypertonicity and instability associated with chronic uncoordinated discharge of fast twitch fibers seen in the resting surface electromyography of vulvovaginal pain patients. Variations on "Glazer's protocol" that have had equally significant treatment results are two 15- rather than 20-min sessions. Perianal external surface sensors can be used initially, progressing to a small intravaginal sensor the size of a tampon for those with Marinoff level 3 dyspareunia. McKay et al.[41] reported that 90% of patients with vulvar vestibulitis treated with home trainers, surface electromyography, and pelvic floor muscle exercises demonstrated decreased introital tenderness and the resumption of pain-free sexual activity within 6 months of the start of therapy. There are reasonably priced rental programs throughout the USA that offer month-long home use of a single-channel, surface electromyography unit, allowing most patients the opportunity to utilize this treatment. Tries[42] encourages standardization in protocols of biofeedback techniques using two or more channels of information to reinforce stable abdominal and bladder pressures concurrently with pelvic floor muscle contractions lasting up to 30 s. Patients should be instructed in at least four training sessions before home programs are used exclusively.

Fitzgerald and Kotarinos[10,11] suggest that hypertonic painful pelvic floor muscles are too short and need lengthening. They propose an alternative to the typical shortening contraction of pelvic floor muscles with pelvic floor muscles by "squat and drop" exercises to lengthen the muscles. Intravaginal manual therapy muscle stretching techniques are followed by active squatting coupled with gentle bulging and voluntary muscle relaxation.

After patients have learned to relax and lengthen the pelvic floor muscles, they can proceed with vaginal or rectal penetration, using progressively larger dilators and surface electromyography for muscle awareness and re-education. Step-by-step patient instructions are outlined in Table 12.3.6.

Table 12.3.6. Dilator instructions with sEMG

Now that you are able to contract and relax the muscles around the vagina and the rectum at will, it is time to use that knowledge to re-educate your muscles to stay relaxed while having penetration.

    The thought of having penetration (intercourse) can be enough to contract your muscles in anticipation of the pain. So, even before attempting penetration with the dilator, try these steps (also the idea of these exercises is to retrain your muscles to stay relaxed during penetration so that there is less discomfort). Under no circumstances should these exercises cause pain (some stretching feelings or slight tingling are acceptable), but not pain.

1. While connected to the sEMG machine, try to imagine the steps leading up to penetration (intercourse) and see if you can keep your muscles relaxed and the activity of your muscles quiet. Have 1 mv or less as your goal. If the muscles are more active, try squeezing them for 10 s and then relaxing for 10 s to get the baseline down.
2. Once you feel comfortable with that step, try bringing your hand down to your perineum and placing it on your labia. There may be a bit of movement in the graph or lights on the machine from the movement of your hand, but if the muscles are relaxed, the baseline should soon return to a low resting of 1 mv or less.
3. Then, try placing your hand on your labia and separating the labia. See if you can control the muscle activity to remain quiet.
4. You may find that having your legs in an open position is causing a strain on the inside (adductor) muscles and you may want to try positioning your knees on pillows so that they do not need to be held so far apart. Some women find that placing a pillow under the buttocks also can help the pelvic floor muscles relax.
5. Take the dilator, place water soluble lubricant on it, try a 10-s pelvic floor muscle squeeze, and then, while relaxing, slide the dilator into the vaginal canal for 2 inches. Remember, the canal usually angles down slightly toward the rectum, and for some women the canal can angle to the left or to the right. Try to relax with it in place for a few minutes (do not think you have to insert the dilator in all the way).
6. If the insertion of that dilator was comfortable and you wish to proceed with the next size, repeat step no. 5.
7. If that size was comfortable, try the next size until you feel that it is enough of a stretch.
8. Some women, try doing their Kegel exercises (pelvic floor muscle contractions) with the dilator in place inside the canal, but for some women it is too uncomfortable.
9. After removing the dilator, most women find that their resting baseline of muscle activity is practically zero because of the gentle stretching that occurred. Close your eyes and feel that muscle relaxation, for this is the muscle feeling you want to reproduce.
10. Take the dilator out of the vaginal canal, wash your perineum thoroughly with cold water, and wash the dilator with soap and water.
11. If you feel slight tingling or irritation around the opening of the vagina, rinse yourself with cold water, after urinating, for the next couple of hours, or place a bag of frozen peas to your perineum on the outside of your underwear to cool off the area.
12. Variations on this exercise using dilators can include placing the dilator into the vaginal canal when standing in the shower (like placing a tampon into the vagina), inserting the dilator while in the bathtub, having your partner carefully insert the dilator into your vagina with your instructions, moving the dilator in and out to mimic thrusting, pressing the tip of the dilator against a specific pain spot in the vagina and waiting for the muscle to relax, or using the dilator as an internal massage tool for a specific muscle trigger point.
13. Painfree insertion of the largest dilator is not an automatic indicator that penetration (intercourse) with your partner will be painfree and easy every time, but it helps to stretch out the tissues, re-educate the muscles to do what you want them to, break the anticipated pain response to penetration, and offer understanding and awareness as to what sexual positions might work best for you.

sEMG: surface electromyography.

Electrical stimulation

Patients experiencing dyspareunia and vaginismus benefited from electrical stimulation one time a week for 10 weeks by increasing their ability to contract the pelvic floor muscles. They had decreased pain measured on a visual analog scale and resumed sexual intercourse.[43] A 50-Hz setting utilizes the pudendal to pudendal nerve pathway to stimulate muscle contraction, and settings up to 250 Hz have been effective in reducing pelvic floor muscle pain.[44]

Ultrasound

A review of randomized, controlled studies on the application of ultrasound for perineal pain and dyspareunia is inconclusive based on minimal studies. Reduction of edema and inflammation through pulsed current, or increased tissue elasticity and mobility through continuous current have been documented. Standardization of settings for intensity and optimal duration have not been established.

Lubrication

Although aging results in changes in anatomy and physiology of the genitals, and many women have lubrication difficulty,[46,47] postmenopausal women preserve their genital responsivity when sufficiently sexually stimulated by viewing erotic imagery.[48] Vaginal dryness and dyspareunia experienced by some postmenopausal women may result from long-standing lack of arousal and diminished estrogen. The need for lubricant, the proper application of a lubricant, the benefits of a lubricant without propylene glycol if the vulva is hypersensitive, and the importance of foreplay to generate lubrication are topics to discuss with patients in preparation for pain-free penetration.

Transcutaneous electrical nerve stimulation

Transcutaneous electrical nerve stimulation is a noninvasive, affordable method for reducing perineal pain sensations. It has been used effectively to reduce pelvic pain during labor and delivery, and has been recommended for use in gynecologic pain conditions.[49] A two-channel unit costs under $60 to purchase, and transcutaneous electrical nerve stimulation can be self-administered with external electrodes placed over the L_4–L_5 and S_2–S_4 regions to address perineal pain.[50]

Nerve supply

The cutaneous nerve supply to the vulva includes the ilioinguinal nerve (L_1), the genital branch of the genitofemoral nerve (L_1–L_2), the perineal branch of the femoral cutaneous nerve (L_2–L_3), and the perineal nerve. The symphysis pubis is innervated by the iliohypogastric nerve (T_{12}) and branches of the genitofemoral nerve (L_1–L_2). Compression, traction, or entrapment of the nerves from abdominal surgeries, injury, or muscle hypertonus may contribute to sensory changes.[1] The perineum has sensory and motor innervation from the sacral plexus L_4–S_4 (Table 12.3.7). Patients with sexual pain often have histories of herniated or bulging lumbar disks

Table 12.3.7. Abdominal and pelvic neurophathies

Nerve	Symptoms–referred pain sites	Etiology
Ilioinguinal L1	Sensory–burning pain below inguinal ligament radiating to medial superior thigh and lateral scrotum or Labia majora Motor–weakness of transversus abdominus and internal oblique Bulging of anterior abdominal wall Ambulates with a flexed trunk	Blow to abdominal wall or incision (appendectomy, cesarean section, hysterectomy, inguinal hernia repair, sling suspension), trauma, pubis symphysis joint separation, ilial upslip
Iliohypogastric T12-L1	Sensory–iliac branch–posterior superior gluteals Hypogastric branch–anterior suprapubic Motor–weakness of transversus abdominus and internal oblique Bulging of anterior abdominal wall Ambulates with a flexed trunk	Blow to abdominal wall or incision (appendectomy, cesarean section, hysterectomy, inguinal hernia repair, sling suspension), trauma, pubic symphysis joint separation, ilial upslip
Genitofemoral L1-2	Sensory–femoral branch–proximal anterior thigh Genital branch- with round ligament to labia majora Motor–portion of the lateral bulbocavernous	Blow to abdominal wall or incision (appendectomy, cesarean section, hysterectomy, inguinal hernia repair, sling suspension), trauma, pubis symphysis joint separation, ilial upslip
Sciatic L4-S2	Sensory–radiating pain posterior thigh Paraesthesia posterior leg to foot Motor–weakness and atrophy of hamstring Gait instablity	Piriformis entrapment, disc injury Retroperitoneal or pelvic bleeding post-lower abdominal while on anticoagulant therapy, post hip surgery/trauma, lithotomy position
Femoral L2-4	Sensory–middle cutaneous-anterior thigh to above knee medial cutaneous – medial thigh, medial leg w/ saphenous nerve decreased patellar DTR Motor–weakness in quadriceps and iliacus and hip flexors	Lesions, tumors, trauma, childbirth lithotomy position, laceration or puncture at inguinal ligament retroperitoneal hematoma, pelvic surgery
Oburator T12-L1	Sensory–medial proximal thigh to inner knee often accompanied by femoral nerve deficit Motor–hip abductors and flexors Groin or medial thigh pain Wide based gait	Tumor, mass, lesion within pelvic girdle and psoas, childbirth, lower abdominal or gynecological surgery, trauma to pelvis, hip, ischial tuberosity, pelvic fracture, surgical positioning with prolonged hip flexion
Lateral femoral cutaneous L2-3	Sensory–lateral superior thigh with increased symptoms when standing, walking, – relieved when sitting	Injury to inguinal ligament (upper and lateral aspect), hernia repair, pregnancy
Posterior femoral cutaneous S2-3	Sensory–medial posterior buttock, posterior labia and posterior thigh	
Pudendal S2-4	Sensory–dermatomes S2-4, perineum, perianal Motor–anal sphincter, perineal muscles, periurethral skeletal muscles	Childbirth injury, entrapment, compression, traction injuries, pelvic fracture, joint malalignment

Modified from: Cindy Feldt PT-CSM Pelvic Girdle Preconference Course 2000. DTR = deep tendon reflex.

with or without laminectomy. Mobilizing the scar tissue or palpating lumbar or pelvic muscle trigger points will reproduce vulvar pain, vaginal pain, and coccyx, rectal, or even clitoral pain. Sensation of the perineum can be objectively assessed by Symmes–Weinstein monofilaments along established dermatomes.

The lesser sciatic foramen, the ischial spine, the sacrotuberous ligament, the ischial tuberosity, and Alcock's canal are potential sites for nerve entrapment or irritation. Physical or manual therapy techniques such as myofascial release, trigger point release, strain–counterstrain or positional release, ischemic pressure, friction massage, muscle energy techniques, and joint mobilization may alter tissue mobility or realign bony structures, thus reducing the pressure on the nerve and decreasing the symptoms. Addressing hypertonus in the levator ani, particularly the pubococcygeus and iliococcygeus,[51] iliopsoas,[27,52] piriformis, adductors,[19] quadratus lumborum, hamstrings, obturator internus, coccygeus, and gluteus medius[27] muscles is essential for complete treatment of this region.

Summary

The objective musculoskeletal findings in patients with sexual pain are: abnormal sensations and allodynia upon palpation of the vulva; burning, stinging, prickling, searing or pain in the clitoris, urethra, vagina, perineal body, anus, posterior thigh, and gluteal and abdominal areas;[19] lumbar, sacroiliac, coccyx, symphysis pubis, and hip joint restriction, and malalignment and instability of the pelvis;[27] functional impairment of sitting, walking, urination, defecation, sexual activity,[51] and household and community activities of daily living; high resting baseline on surface electromyography, excessive signal variability, and low net rise;[36] muscle hypertonus and trigger points external and internal to the urethral, vaginal, and rectal canals; and muscle weakness in the urogenital triangle muscles, levator ani, obturator internus, gluteals, iliopsoas, hip adductors, and internal and external hip rotator muscles. The commonality of all these findings results in restriction or inability to participate fully in pleasurable sexual activities.

Physical therapists specializing in women's health who have pelvic floor muscle training are skilled and knowledgeable in joint mechanics, muscle function, nerve innervation, tissue mobility, and functional application. They can assess and treat many of the mechanical joint, muscle, and nerve problems and train patients to work through the pain and fear and avoidance behaviors by demonstration of anatomy and functional anatomy, hands-on manual therapy techniques[53,54], biofeedback instruction, electrical modalities, and exercise prescriptions. They are vital participants in the interdisciplinary team to evaluate and treat female sexual dysfunction.

References

1. King P. Musculoskeletal origins of chronic pelvic pain: diagnosis and treatment. In Ling FW, ed. *Obstetrics and Gynecology Clinics of North America*, vol 20. Philadelphia: WB Saunders, 1993.

2. Handa VL, Harvey L, Cundiff GW et al. Sexual function among women with urinary incontinence and pelvic organ prolapse. *Am J Obstet Gynecol* 2004; 191: 751–6.

3. Liebling RE, Swingler R, Patel RR et al. Pelvic floor morbidity up to one year after difficult instrumental delivery and cesarean section in the second stage of labor: a cohort study. *Am J Obstet Gynecol* 2004; 191: 4–10.

4. Lewicky CE, Valentin C, Saclarides TJ. Sexual function following sphincteroplasty for women with third- and fourth-degree perineal tears. *Dis Colon Rectum* 2004; 47: 1650–4.

5. Marthol H, Hilz MJ. Female sexual dysfunction: a systematic overview of classification, pathophysiology, diagnosis and treatment. *Fortschr Neurol Psychiatr* 2004; 72: 121–35.

6. Berman JR, Berman LA, Werbin TJ et al. Clinical evaluation of female sexual function; effects of age and estrogen status on subjective and physiologic sexual responses. *Int J Impot Res* 1999; 11(Suppl 1): S31–8.

7. Graber B. *Circumvaginal Musculature and Sexual Function*. Omaha: Karger, 1982.

8. Reissing ED, Binik YM, Khalife S et al. Vaginal spasm, pain, and behavior: an empirical investigation of the diagnosis of vaginismus. *Arch Sex Behav* 2004; 33: 5–17.

9. Binik YM, Reissing E, Pukall C et al. The female sexual pain disorders; genital pain or sexual dysfunction? *Arch Sex Behav* 2002; 31: 425–9.

10. Fitzgerald MP, Kotarinos R. Rehabilitation of the short pelvic floor. I. Background and patient evaluation. *Int Urogynecol J* 2003; 14: 261–8.

11. Fitzgerald MP, Kotarinos R. Rehabilitation of the short pelvic floor. II. Treatment of the patient with a short pelvic floor. *Int Urogynecol J* 2003; 14: 269–75.

12. White G, Jantos M. Sexual behavior changes with vulvar vestibulitis syndrome. *J Reprod Med* 1988; 43: 783–9.

13. Bergeron S, Brown C, Lord MJ et al. Physical therapy for vulvar vestibulitis syndrome: a retrospective study. *Sex Marital Ther* 2002; 28: 183–92.

14. Graziottin A, Castoldi E, Montorsi F et al. Vulodynia: the challenge of "unexplained" genital pain. *J Sex Marital Ther* 2001; 27: 503–12.

15. Graziottin A Brotto LA. Vulvar vestibulitis syndrome: a clinical approach. *J Sex Marital Ther* 2004; 30: 125–39.

16. Baker PK. Musculoskeletal problems. In J Steege, D Metzger, B Levy, eds. *Chronic Pelvic Pain: An Integrated Approach*. Philadelphia: WB Saunders, 1998.

17. Costello K. Myofascial syndromes. In J Steege, D Metzger, B Levy, eds. *Chronic Pelvic Pain: An Integrated Approach*. Philadelphia: WB Saunders, 1998: 251–66.

18. Travell J, Simons D. *Myofascial Pain and Dysfunction: The Trigger Point Manual*. Vol 2, *The Lower Extremities*. Baltimore: Williams & Wilkins, 1992.

19. Weiss JM. Pelvic floor myofascial trigger points: manual therapy for interstitial cystitis and the urgency-frequency syndrome. *J Urol* 2001; 166: 2226–31.

20. Sartore A, De Seta F, Maso G et al. The effects of mediolateral episiotomy on pelvic floor function after vaginal delivery. *Obstet Gynecol* 2004; 103: 669–73.

21. Shiono P, Klebanoff M, Carey C. Midline episiotomies: more harm than good? *Obstet Gynecol* 1990; 75: 765–70.

22. International Continence Society. *Pelvic Floor Assessment Group Standarisation of Terminology March, 2003, www.icsoffice.org.*

23. Graziottin A. Etiology and diagnosis of coital pain. *J Endocrinol Invest* 2003; 26(Suppl 3): 115–21.

24. Blackwell R, Olive D. *Chronic Pelvic Pain: Evaluation and Management.* New York: Springer-Verlag, 1998.

25. Glazer HI, Romanzi L, Polanecsky M et al. Pelvic floor muscle surface electromyography. Reliability and clinical predictive validity. *J Reprod Med* 1999; 44: 779–82.

26. Lee D. *The Pelvic Girdle*, 3rd edn. London: Churchill Livingstone, 2004.

27. Marinoff S, Turner M. Vulvar vestibulitis syndrome. *Dermatol Clin* 1992; 10; 435–44.

28. McGuire H, Hawton K. Interventions for vaginismus. *Cochrane Database Syst Rev* 2003; 1: CD001760.

29. Maigne JY, Chatellier G. Assessment of sexual activity in patients with back pain compared with patients with neck pain. *Clin Orthop* 2001; 385: 82–7.

30. Dahm DI, Jacofsky D, Lewalen DG. Surgeons rarely discuss sexual activity with patients after THA: a survey of members of the American Association of Hip and Knee Surgeons. *Clin Orthop* 2004; 428: 237–40.

31. Fiax A, Lapray JF, Callede O et al. Magnetic resonance imaging (MRI) of sexual intercourse: second experience in missionary position and the initial experience in posterior position. *J Sex Marital Ther* 2002; 28(Suppl 1): 63–76.

32. Lukban J, Whimore K, Kellogg-Spadt S et al. The effect of manual physical therapy in patients diagnosed with interstitial cystitis, high-tone pelvic floor dysfunction, and sacroiliac dysfunction. *Urology* 2001; 57(Suppl 1): 121–2.

33. Oyama IA, Rejba A, Lukban JC et al. Modified Thiele massage as therapeutic intervention for female patients with interstitial cystitis and high-tone pelvic floor dysfunction. *Urology* 2004; 64: 862–5.

34. Doggweiler-Wiygul R, Wiygl JP. Interstitial cystitis, pelvic pain, and the relationship to myofascial pain and dysfunction: a report on four patients. *World J Urol* 2002; 20: 310–14 (Epub Oct 08).

35. Whitehead W. Gastrointestinal disorders. In J Steege, D Metzger, D Levy, eds. *Chronic Pelvic Pain: An Integrated Approach.* Philadelphia: WB Saunders, 1998: 205–24.

36. Glazer H, Rodke G, Swencionis C. Vulvar vestibulitis syndrome with electromyographic biofeedback of pelvic floor musculature. *J Reprod Med* 1995; 40: 283–90.

37. Battaglia E, Serrra AM, Buonafede G et al. Long-term study on the effects of visual biofeedback and muscle training as a therapeutic modality in pelvic floor dyssynergia and slow-transit constipation *Dis Colon Rectum* 2004; 47: 90–5 (Epub Jan 02).

38. Bergeron S, Binik YM, Khalife S et al. A randomized comparison of group cognitive-behavioral therapy, surface electromyographic biofeedback, and vestibulectomy in the treatment of dyspareunia resulting from vulvar vestibulitis. *Pain* 2001; 91: 297–306.

39. Shafik A, El-Sibai O. Study of the pelvic floor muscles in vaginismus: a concept of pathogenesis. *Eur J Obstet Gynecol Reprod Biol* 2002; 105: 67–70.

40. Glazer H, MacConkey D. Functional rehabilitation of pelvic floor muscles: a challenge to tradition. *Urol Nurs* 1996; 16: 68–9.

41. McKay E, Kaufman RH, Doctor U et al. Treating vulvar vestibulitis with electromyographic biofeedback of the pelvic floor musculature. *J Reprod Med* 2001; 46: 337–42.

42. Tries J. Protocol- and therapist-related variables affecting outcomes of behavioral interventions for urinary and fecal incontinence. *Gastroenterology* 2004; 126(Suppl 1): S152–8.

43. Nappi RE, Ferdeghini F, Abbiati I et al. Electrical stimulation (ES) in the management of sexual pain disorders. *J Sex Marital Ther* 2003; 29(Suppl 1):103–10.

44. Meadows E. Treatments for patients with pelvic pain. *Urol Nurs* 1999; 19: 33–5.

45. Hay-Smith EJ. Therapeutic ultrasound for postpartum perineal pain and dyspareunia. *Cochrane Database Syst Rev* 2000; 2: CD000495.

46. Laumann EO, Nicolosi A, Glasser DB et al. Sexual problems among women and men aged 40–80 y: prevalence and correlates identified in the global study of sexual attitudes and behaviors. *Int J Impot Res* 2005; 17: 39?57.

47. Nicolosi A, Laumann EO, Glasser DB et al. Sexual behavior and sexual dysfunctions after age 40: the global study of sexual attitudes and behaviors. *Urology* 2004; 64: 991–7.

48. Van Lunsen RH, Laan E. Genital vascular responsiveness and sexual feelings in midlife women; psychophysiologic, brain and genital imaging studies. *Menopause* 2004; 11: 741–8.

49. Kaplan B, Rabinerson D, Pardo J. Transcutaneous electrical nerve stimulation (TENS) as a pain-relief device in obstetrics and gynecology. *Clin Exp Obstet Gynecol* 1997; 24:123–6.

50. Van der Spank J, Cambier D, De Paepe H. Pain relief in labour by transcutaneous electrical nerve stimulation (TENS). *Arch Gynecol Obstet* 2000; 264: 131–6.

51. DeFranca G. *Pelvic Locomotor Dysfunction*. Maryland: Aspen, 1996.

52. Headley B. *When Movement Hurts*. Colorado: Innovative Systems of Rehabilitation, Inc., 1997.

53. Holland A. Physical therapy intervention for dyspareunia. *JSOWH* 2003; 27: 18–20.

54. Wurn &Wurn –2004 www.medscape.com/viewarticle/493989 Increasing Orgasm and Decreasing Dysareunia by a Manual Physical Therapy Technique

12.4 Medical management: perspective of the sexual medicine physician

Irwin Goldstein

Introduction

Sexual dysfunctions in women are recognized to be common health problems[1] (see Chapters 2.1–2.4 of this book). There has been limited clinical and basic science research investigation, and most of the investigatory focus has been on women who present with the most common of the sexual dysfunctions, that is, lack of interest, diminished orgasm, and/or decreased lubrication.[2] The sexual dysfunction that has received the least research and clinical attention is genital sexual pain (see Chapters 6.5, 12.1–12.3, 12. 5 and 12.6).

Genital sexual pain is considered a multifactorial syndrome of pain, sexual dysfunction, and psychologic disability. There are numerous mind, body, and relationship pathophysiologies linked to genital sexual pain.[3] Significant *psychologic* factors such as previous sexual trauma and abuse, sexual neuroses, sexual inhibitions or idiosyncracies, and/or interpersonal relationship issues may manifest as genital sexual pain disorders.[4] Significant *biologic* factors may occur in a multitude of peripheral genital organs and tissues secondary to such pertinent biologic factors as genital tissue infection, inflammation, abnormal immunologic conditions, abnormal hormonal states, tumors, mechanical compartment syndromes, blunt or penetrating traumatic injury, tissue weakness with organ prolapse, and others.[4]

Recent research in the psychophysics of pain and touch thresholds, as well as modern functional magnetic resonance imaging studies, robustly shows that genital sexual pain is not limited to the genitals and that genital sexual pain is similar in many ways to nongenital sexual pain. Furthermore, afflicted women with genital sexual pain demonstrate the intellectual survival strategies, such as hypervigilance and catastrophization, noted in women with nongenital sexual pain conditions. Contemporary researchers are emphasizing that genital sexual pain is a pain syndrome and that genital sexual pain research should consider the biopsychosocial mechanisms underlying chronic and recurrent pain.[5]

Ideal clinical management in women with genital pain disorders is *not* controversial. Preferably, women with genital pain should be diagnosed and treated by a multidisciplinary team, including biologic-focused health-care professionals trained to identify and manage specific biologic pathophysiologies, psychologic-focused health-care professionals trained to identify and manage specific psychologic pathophysiologies, physical therapists trained in women's sexual health disorders, and, if necessary, pain specialists trained in chronic and recurrent genital sexual pain problems and/or surgeons trained in genital sexual pain problems[2] (see Chapters 6.5, 12.1–12. 3, 12. 5 and 12.6).

While recognizing the need for multiple trained specialists in the overall management of women afflicted with genital sexual pain syndrome, this chapter aims to selectively provide the biologic-focused health-care professional relevant clinical information to help identify and treat specific biologic-based pathophysiologies. For the biologic-focused clinician, the general logic is that if the pathology or pathologies causing the peripheral genital sexual pain can be identified, management outcome may be successfully directed to the source pathophysiology.

Genital sexual pain disorders are associated with multiple

theories and anecdotes with little evidence-based medicine documentation. Unfortunately, randomized, controlled treatment-outcome studies in the management of women with genital sexual pain are limited. At the time of this writing, three treatments for genital sexual pain have been shown to be effective against placebo: cognitive-behavioral therapy, physical therapy/biofeedback, and surgery. No medications have yet been shown superior to placebo in randomized clinical trials for the management of women with genital sexual pain.[4,5]

The chapter will review the epidemiology, history, physical examination, laboratory testing, biologic pathophysiology, and medical treatment of many of the genital sexual pain disorders. The classification system for this chapter is an anatomic one that includes clitoral, urethral, vulvar, vestibular, vaginal, and pelvic floor disorders.

Anatomy/epidemiology

To understand genital sexual pain, it is important to appreciate relevant anatomy, especially the innervation of the various genital tissues such as the vagina, vestibule, and vulva (see Chapters 4.1–4.4).

Concerning vaginal innervation, many physicians concluded that, since biopsies of vaginal pathologic lesions can be performed without local anesthesia, the vagina is an organ devoid of sensory nerves. Contemporary research has shown that, based on immunohistochemical markers that stain axons and nerve terminals, all regions of the human vagina reveal profound innervation with multiple axons and nerve terminals.[6] Regional differences in nerve density are noted, such as the distal areas of the vagina having more fibers than proximal parts. The anterior vaginal wall is more densely innervated than the posterior vaginal wall, and there are free nerve endings only in the introital region.[6]

Concerning vulvar and vestibular innervation, there are four sensory and motor nerves which innervate the region. These include the iliohypogastric nerve (T-12, L-1, and L-2), the ilioinguinal nerve (L-1 and L-3), the genitofemoral nerve (L-1 and L-2), and the pudendal nerve (S-2-4). The pudendal nerve also includes the perineal nerve, the dorsal nerve of the clitoris, and the inferior hemorrhoidal nerve. The pelvic autonomic nerves to the genital organs pass through the hypogastric plexus. Parasympathetic input passes via the pelvic nerve, while sympathetic input travels via the hypogastric nerve.

There is an anatomic distinction between the vestibule and the vulva that is based, in part, on genital embryology and the keratin content of the skin epithelium. The vestibule is a rhomboidal area from the frenulum anteriorly to the mucocutaneous border of the perineum posteriorly. Laterally, the vestibule extends from the hymenal ring to Hart's line. The skin epithelium of the vulva is fully keratinized, while the epithelium overlying the vestibule has limited keratin content.

There are few epidemiologic studies on genital sexual pain. Contemporary epidemiologic studies show that genital sexual pain of varying degrees exists in approximately 10–20% of women. A recently published, population-based study of 8000 women, aged 18–64 years from seven ethnically and socioeconomically varied Boston-area communities, has shown that 16% of women have experienced vulvar pain lasting 3 months or longer. It is estimated that there are more than 15 million American women with genital sexual pain. Risk factors for genital sexual pain include being victimized as a child, lacking childhood family support, use of oral contraceptives in women reporting no pain at the time of first tampon use, and women first having intercourse before age 18 with a frequency of once per week or more.[3,7]

History of the patient with genital sexual pain

There are as yet limited consensed management paradigms for the diagnosis and treatment of women with genital sexual pain complaints. The cornerstone of diagnosis of women with sexual dysfunction, including those with genital sexual pain, is a detailed history and physical examination. Specifically, in women with sexual dysfunction, history taking is crucial. History taking establishes the diagnostic impressions and forms the basis of search on physical examination[2,4] (see Chapters 12.1 and 12.2).

For all clinical members of the multidisciplinary team, including biologic-focused health-care professionals, psychologic-focused health-care professionals, physical therapists, pain specialists, and surgeons, genital sexual pain problems in women are difficult, complex, and, unfortunately, not rare. Genital sexual pain disorders involve discomfort, throbbing, stinging, aching, soreness, burning, and/or tenderness. Genital sexual pain disorders usually interfere with satisfactory sexual function. Genital sexual pain disorders are often associated with a psychologic response, such as anxiety, depression, and/or an aversion response to sexual stimulation. Genital sexual pain disorders are often associated with a pelvic floor contraction and/or spasm response. There are multiple difficult interactive relationships that need to be addressed during history taking, in the overall assessment of women with genital sexual pain disorders.[2,4]

Genital sexual pain disorders are often so very distracting and disturbing that physiologic desire, arousal, and orgasm responses during sexual stimulation cannot manifest. In such cases, the patient with the genital sexual pain problem may erroneously consider the genital sexual pain a less relevant secondary sexual complaint. It is commonplace for women with significant, long-standing genital sexual pain history to present to the health-care provider mistakenly thinking that the primary sexual complaint is really a lack of interest, lubrication, or orgasm. A thorough and detailed sexual history will help elucidate the genuine primary sexual complaint of sexual pain, since defining the total sexual medical condition will be critical for successful clinical outcome.

For example, for women having sexual activity, inquiries should be made to assess whether the patient feels subjectively excited and feels her vagina become sufficiently moist during sexual stimulation. If the patient is engaging in intercourse, queries should be made concerning her thoughts and feelings prior, during, and after penetration. It is relevant to know whether the pain occurs with contact in the vulva or vestibule, with full entry, after thrusting, with her partner's ejaculation, after withdrawal, after urinary voiding, or days after sexual intercourse. If the pain is related exclusively to ejaculation, a rare seminal plasma allergy may exist. It is appropriate to question whether other forms of penetration hurt (tampons, fingers, sex toys). Is her body tensing or does she experience muscle spasms during penetration? Does touching her outside the genital area (nipples) also cause nongenital pain? It is important to know whether there is pain during nonsexual events such as riding a bicycle or when wearing tight clothes. What are the consequences of the genital sexual pain on her relationship? What is the personal distress or bother?[4]

Another important factor in history taking is the patient's age. Above age 50 years, it is likely that the cause is related to genital tissue atrophy and local estrogen deficiency. Below this age, the cause is probably related to vestibulodynia. The duration of the symptoms of the genital sexual pain is relevant. If the pain has always been a problem, even from the first sexual attempt, the cause is often related to vestibulodynia. The timing of the symptoms of the genital sexual pain is also of interest. A history of cyclical pain may indicate endometriosis. If the pain always occurs with certain partners, there may be an anatomic concern in the partner, such as Peyronie's disease or excessive phallic size, or a conflicting relationship issue. The location of the genital sexual pain may be pertinent. Patient-friendly anatomic diagrams of the female sexual and reproductive tract should be used, and the differences explained simply among the vulva, vestibule, vagina, cervix, uterus, and ovaries. Patients should localize pain sites from the anatomic drawing. If the patient describes on history taking that the pain is superficial and not deep, the cause may be more dermatologic, or consistent with vaginitis or vulvodynia. If the patient says that the pain is really deep inside her body, the pain may be more consistent with abdominal wall focus, pelvic pathology, or impaction against the cervix.[8–10]

Basic questions should be asked concerning tests done by other health-care providers, treatments already received by the patient, and the outcome of these various treatments.

Concerning the sexual history, it is appropriate for the clinician to use validated questionnaires to characterize the genital sexual pain. To help assess treatment outcome, questions are assessed at baseline and repeated at follow-up visits. The Female Sexual Function Inventory[11] utilizes three questions dedicated to the domain of genital sexual pain. The first question rates the patient's *experience* with discomfort or pain during vaginal penetration. The second rates how *often she experiences* discomfort or pain after vaginal penetration. Answers for the first two questions vary from not attempting intercourse (0

points), to almost always or always (1 point), to more than half the time (2 points), to about half the time (3 points), to less than half the time (4 points), and to almost never or never (5 points). The third question rates the patient's *level (degree) of discomfort or pain* during or after vaginal penetration. Answers vary from not attempting intercourse (0 points), to very high (1 point), to high (2 points), to moderate (3 points), to low (4 points), or to very low or none at all (5 points). The lower the score, the more the genital sexual pain complaints.

The McGill Pain Questionnaire[12] is more specific and extremely valuable in assessing women with genital sexual pain. The first series of 10 items helps in pain characterization. Is the genital sexual pain throbbing, shooting, stabbing, sharp, cramping, gnawing, hot-burning, aching, heavy, tender, and/or splitting? The second series of five items helps in understanding the patient's response to the pain. Is the genital sexual pain tiring-exhausting, sickening, fearful, and/or punishing-cruel? Answers are marked as none (0 points), mild (1 point), moderate (2 points), or severe (3 points). The worst score would be 45 points for the first two sets of queries. A Likert scale (10 cm) allows patients to rate the quality of the pain from no pain to worst pain (worst pain is 10 points). Finally, a series of descriptors is used to rate the overall intensity of the pain. Answers can range from no pain (0 points), to mild pain (1 point), discomforting pain (2 points), distressing pain (3 points), horrible pain (4 points), and excruciating pain (5 points). A patient with the worst genital sexual pain would score 60 points.

Physical examination of the patient with genital sexual pain

The peripheral genital examination is regularly a helpful and revealing clinical assessment, but its intimate character demands that a rational explanation exist for its inclusion in the diagnostic process. A focused peripheral genital examination is highly recommended in women with genital sexual pain disorder. It is particularly important that the patient with genital sexual pain have full communication with the health-care provider and final authority during the physical examination to terminate at any time, to ask questions, to have control over who is in attendance, and to understand the extent of the assessment. It is vital that the patient be aware of the purpose. Some of the goals of the physical examination are to confirm normal architecture; detect any existing lesions or abnormalities; and discover whether there are any tender areas of the vulva, vagina, or pelvis or whether there is any hypertonicity of the pelvic floor. Inclusion of the sexual partner, with permission of the patient, is advantageous and provides needed patient support. Allowing the patient (and the partner) to observe any pathology via mirrors or digital photography is often therapeutic, allowing, for the first time in many cases, an illustration and connection of a detected physical abnormality with the genital sexual pain problem. During the physical examination, the patient should point with her finger to the locations of the genital sexual pain.[2,4,8–10]

Whatever the gender of the examining health-care provider, it is strongly recommended that a *female chaperone health-care provider* be present in the examination room. The following equipment should be available: examination table, hospital gown, bedsheet, disposable absorbing chucks, patient covering sheet, surgical loupes or magnifying glass, examination light source, examination gloves, gauze, lubricant, Q-tip, speculum, pH paper, glass slide, saline, and microscope. The patient should wear a hospital gown and a sheet should cover her lower torso. The patient should be placed in the lithotomy position and the examining health-care provider, using magnified vision and a carefully focused light source, should be sitting comfortably.

The first part of the examination involves inspection. If appropriate, lubricant should be placed on the vulva. Gauzes can be grasped between thumb and index finger and used to retract the labia majora for a full inspection of the vestibular contents. Two gloved fingers are placed on either side of the clitoral shaft, and with an upward force in the cephalic direction, the prepuce is retracted to gain full exposure of the glans clitoris (usually more than 1 cm in diameter), corona, and right and left frenulum emanating at 5 o'clock and 7 o'clock off the posterior portion of the glans clitoris (Fig. 12.4.1). Using gauze to retract the labia minora, the labial-hymenal junction is identified. A Q-tip cotton-swab test is performed, gently applying pressure on Skene's glands and minor vestibular glands and documenting the quality of the discomfort or pain (Fig. 12.4.2). The Q-tip cotton swab may also be placed at multiple locations in the vulva and vestibule. Palpation is next performed by a single-digit examination. This procedure occurs before speculum insertion or bimanual searches for vaginismus. Single-digit palpation is achieved by sliding a finger into the vaginal opening and depressing the bulbocavernosus muscle. The test is positive if there is hypertonicity and pain.

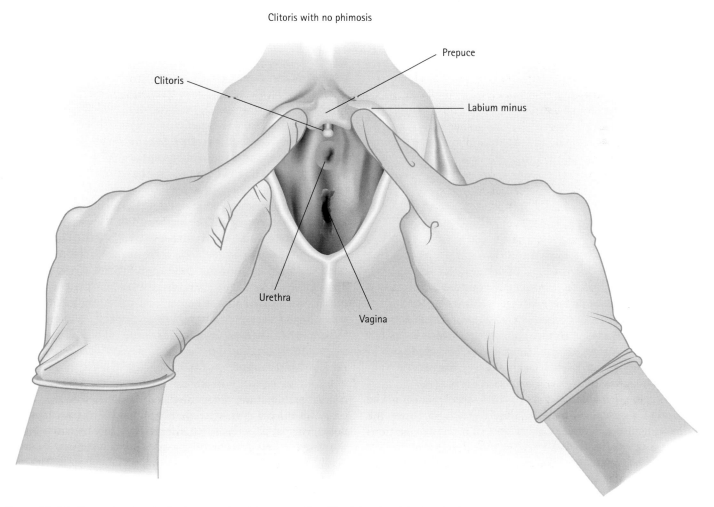

Clitoris with no phimosis

Prepuce

Clitoris

Labium minus

Urethra

Vagina

Figure 12.4.1. To examine the clitoris, place two gloved fingers on either side of the clitoral shaft, and, using an upward force in the cephalic direction, retract the prepuce to gain full exposure of the glans clitoris (usually more than 1 cm in diameter), corona, and right and left frenulum emanating at 5 o'clock and 7 o'clock off the posterior portion of the glans clitoris.

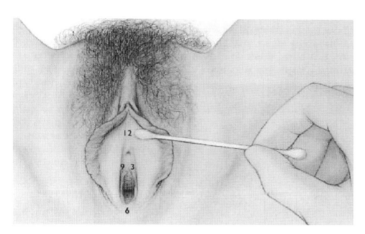

Figure 12.4.2. A Q-tip test is performed by gently applying pressure on the Skene's glands and minor vestibular glands and documenting the quality of the discomfort or pain. The Q-tip may also be placed at multiple locations in the vulva and vestibule.

A bimanual examination and evaluation of pelvic floor may be subsequently performed if indicated. Two fingers are placed against the lateral walls, and the levators and underlying obturator are assessed for tenderness or taut bands. In addition, a bimanual examination can evaluate the integrity of the fornices, bladder and urethral bases, and pelvic organs. A recto-vaginal examination and speculum examination can then be performed if indicated.

For the speculum examination, a warm, lubricated speculum is used. The vaginal wall is examined for estrogen milieu integrity, inflammation of the walls, and vaginal lesions.

Laboratory testing of the patient with genital sexual pain

Vaginal pH testing can be performed as indicated, especially if the physical examination identifies vaginal discharge or vaginal odor. The vaginal pH in a healthy vaginal milieu is approximately 3.5–4.5. An acid pH rules out bacterial vaginitis, but not candidiasis. For vaginal pH values more than 4.5, several conditions need to be considered, including vaginitis, vaginosis, and/or atrophic vaginitis[8] (see Chapters 9.5 and 12.2).

During the speculum examination, an evaluation should be performed for discharge. Samples should be collected for wet mount and culture. Normal vaginal secretions are odorless and are not associated with the clinical complaint of itching or irritation. On wet mount, one should note a heterogeneous suspension of desquamated vaginal epithelial cells with lactobacilli as the predominant microorganism. The wet prep[13,14] has four important elements: background flora, vaginal epithelial cells, pathogens, and white blood cells.

Concerning background flora, lactobacilli predominate in the healthy vagina. Lactobacilli may be best seen with the phase-contrast microscope. If lactobacilli are seen to dominate the background flora and the vaginal pH is acidic, it probably does not matter what vaginal culture grows. There is probably no bacterial infection, independent of any vaginal culture reports. If, however, there are absent lactobacilli in the background flora, there are several causes, including bacterial vaginosis, desquamative vaginitis, vaginal lichen planus, and the recent use of antibiotics. There is no evidence relating the presence of Candida albicans to lack of lactobacilli on a wet mount.[13,14]

Concerning vaginal epithelial cells, the frequency of noting parabasal cells on the wet mount can help the clinician assess the woman's estrogen status and/or presence or absence of inflammation. In normally estrogenized vaginal epithelium, the wet mount should reveal very few parabasal epithelial cells. If there is an ongoing inflammatory process in the vagina, the inflamed epithelium will shed, thereby increasing the occurrence of parabasal epithelial cells. In addition, the presence of so-called "clue cells" may be a sign of the existence of the condition of bacterial vaginosis.[13,14]

Vaginal pathogens may include Trichomonas and Candida (either C. albicans or non-C. albicans). It should be noted that Trichomonas and Candida may be identified on wet mount in approximately 60% of cases, and that in the remaining 40% of cases of true infection with these pathogens, wet mount will not disclose them. Vaginal cultures that show Escherichia coli, enterococcus, and/or group B streptococcus are normal vaginal organisms that have a commensal relationship, whereby one organism derives food or other benefits from the association while the other organism remains unharmed and unaffected. It should be noted that Gardnerella may be seen in the vaginal cultures of 50–70% of normal women.[13,14]

Concerning white blood cells on the wet mount, the observation of an increased white blood cell count is considered to be more than one white blood cell per epithelial cell. The observation of an increased white blood cell count on a wet mount may occur under the following conditions: vaginitis secondary to Trichomonas, yeast, and/or atrophy; cervicitis secondary to gonorrhea, chlamydia, and/or herpes; and upper genital/reproductive tract disease such as endometritis and/or pelvic inflammatory disease. An increased white blood cell count on a wet mount is not caused by bacterial vaginosis. One should consider a vaginal culture on Sabouraud's medium with the finding of an increased white blood cell count on a wet mount, especially if the vaginal pH is not acidic.[13,14]

Other laboratory testing procedures for assessment of genital sexual pain disorders include biopsy of a genital lesion; serology for lesions suggesting a sexually transmitted disorder; pelvic ultrasound of the ovaries, fallopian tubes, uterus, and cervix; magnetic resonance imaging of pelvis or spine; and sex steroid hormone blood testing. A genital biothesiometric examination and duplex Doppler ultrasound study before and during sexual stimulation may also help to assess underlying genital tissue function.

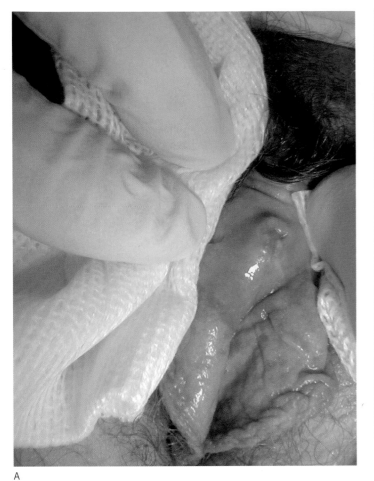

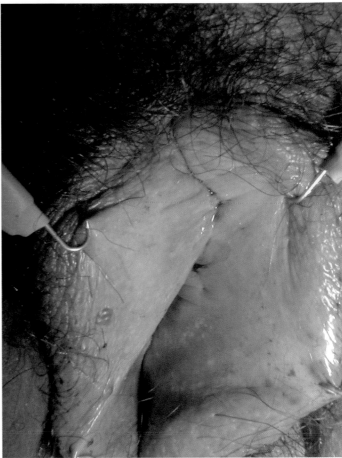

A

B

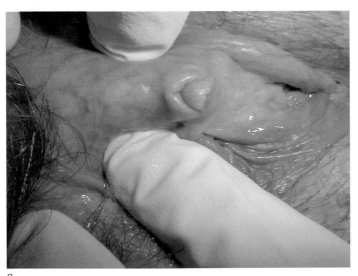

C

Figure 12.4.3. Phimosis which occurs in some female patients with sexual dysfunction, can be mild, moderate, or severe acording, in part, to the elasticity of the prepuce and its ability to retract on examination. Phimosis may create a closed compartment with an underlying balanitis disorder.

Biologic pathophysiologies and treatment strategies

Biologic pathophysiologies resulting in genital sexual pain may occur in the clitoris, urethra, vulva and vestibule, vagina, and pelvic floor muscles. In this chapter, the treatment strategies will be discussed within each anatomic region.

Clitoris, prepuce, and fenulae

Phimosis/balanitis

Careful inspection of the glans clitoris should be performed, especially in cases where the history suggests focused clitoral pain. Any smegma material can be removed by gentle manipulation with a Q-tip and/or with gauze. Failure to visualize the whole glans clitoris with the corona is consistent with some degree of prepucial phimosis.[15] Phimosis has been reported to occur in approximately one-quarter to one-third of all female patients with sexual dysfunction. There can be mild, moderate, or severe phimosis according to the elasticity of the prepuce and its ability to retract on examination (Fig. 12.4.3).

Phimosis *per se* does not imply clinically relevant disorder requiring intervention. Since phimosis may create a closed compartment, however, phimosis is often the underlying disorder in balanitis associated with the clinical symptoms of itching, burning, and recurrent fungal infections. Should clitoral glans balanitis be diagnosed, the physical examination usually reveals phimosis and the classic associated redness and tenderness of the visible glans clitoris. In cases of complete phimosis, the diagnosis cannot be made until surgical intervention. Initial treatment of clitoral glans balanitis should be conservative with topical estrogen and/or testosterone creams to see whether the prepuce can be made more elastic and retractile. Topical antifungal agents, such as nystatin, or oral antifungal agents, such as fluconazole, may be considered. Infections can also be related to herpes virus, and appropriate treatment, such as acyclovir, administered. If a chronic genital dermatitis condition, such as lichen sclerosus, involves the prepuce, phimosis and fusion of the prepuce are a likely sequela. An uncommon chronic genital dermatitis condition, lichen planus, may lead to hypertrophic, white scarring of the glans clitoris, prepuce, and frenulae. A useful treatment consideration for lichen sclerosus or lichen planus of the periglans clitoral tissue is clobetasol cream.

If appropriate conservative treatment is performed for any clitoral pain condition and the condition remains unchanged specifically due to the phimotic prepuce, surgical management by dorsal slit procedure should be considered so that medical management without the closed compartment can be re-initiated.

Prepucial infections

Severe swelling, pain, tenderness, fever, or purulent drainage may emanate from the prepuce. The most likely diagnosis is an

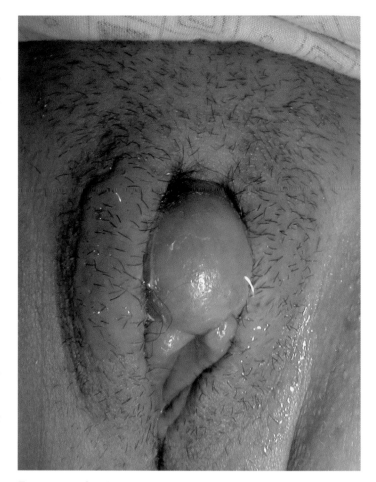

Figure 12.4.4. Swelling, pain, tenderness, fever, or purulent drainage may emanate from the prepuce or from vulvar tissue near the prepuce. The most likely diagnosis is infected sebaceous cyst with extension from surrounding vulvar or pubic skin into the prepuce.

infected sebaceous cyst with extension from surrounding vulvar or pubic skin into the prepuce (Fig. 12.4.4). Conservative treatments include antibiotics, soaking, and sitz baths. Often the situation is resolved only with incision and drainage.

Traumatic neuropathy

In some cases, women with genital sexual pain claim that symptoms started after traumatic injuries to regional or local nerves associated with childbirth, especially forceps delivery, regional anesthetic procedures, or postoperative injuries to the ileo-hypogastric or ileo-inguinal nerves, especially with wide lower abdominal Pfanenstiel incisions. Some women provide a history of sudden onset pain in the clitoris following a sharp blow to the perineum. This may result from bicycle-riding injuries, especially after a fall onto the nose of the saddle or the bar of the bicycle frame, or from other blunt perineal or pelvic trauma, as in a fall onto a tree branch or horn of a horse saddle, or after pelvic fracture as a result of a motor vehicle accident. In many such cases, the genital sexual pain is described as sharp, shooting, and burning, consistent with neuropathy and severe hypersensitivity. There is often diminished sensation of the clitoris and perineum on physical examination, including biothesiometric evaluation. On physical examination, Q-tip testing shows regions with no pain but highly specific localized regions with sharp pain, typically to the side of the clitoris.

Treatment should aim at correcting the primary disorder, but usually that is not possible. Psychotropic agents, such as amitriptyline or gabapentine, have become the mainstay of conservative therapy. Local genital pudendal neuromata can be identified after blunt perineal trauma, and these may be excised surgically in certain circumstances (Fig. 12.4.5). Unfortunately, there is a high recurrence rate after surgical excision of neuromata. Injection of the region with steroids may prevent recurrence of the neuromata after surgical excision.

Tumors

In women with a history of focused clitoral pain and increased sensitivity to touch, especially that which worsens with sexual contact, physical inspection of the clitoris may reveal a clitoral tumor. Occasionally, such women can feel a mass associated with and related to the clitoris during self-examination or self-stimulation. The most likely tumor of the clitoris is fibroepithelioma, a skin tumor composed of fibrous tissue intersected by thin, anastomosing bands of basal cells of the epidermis. Differential diagnosis would include condyloma, sebaceous cyst, or compound nevi. Careful surgical excision of the mass should be performed under local/general anesthesia with care to preserve as much as possible of the clitoral structure. It should be noted that fibroepitheliomas have a propensity to recur locally despite surgical excision. Fibroepitheliomas may also give rise to basal cell carcinoma of the nodular type (Fig. 12.4.6).

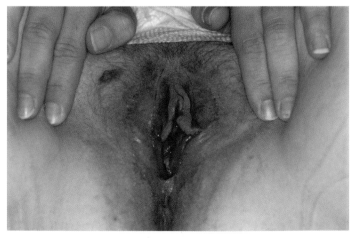

Figure 12.4.5. Local genital pudendal neuromata can be identified after blunt perineal trauma (in this case, a fall onto a bicycle bar). These may be excised surgically in certain circumstances.

Urethral meatus, urethra/bladder neck, Skene's glands

Gentle retraction of the labia minora should provide full view of the urethral meatus. This orifice is 1–2 cm posterior in the midline from the glans and frenula, and should be flush with the vestibule. The urethral meatus is 1–2 cm anterior to the 12 o'clock hymenal tissue at the vaginal introitus.

Urethral prolapse

Prolapse of the urethral mucosa out the urethral lumen is highly associated with estrogen-deficiency states such as after bilateral oophorectomy, natural menopause, or after chemotherapy for malignancy. Owing to breast cancer fears, many women with low estradiol values do not receive local or systemic estradiol treatment. It is not uncommon for such women with urethral prolapse to note urgency, frequency, and discomfort of urination and also observe spotting of blood on the toilet paper on wiping after voiding. The abnormal voiding history is often accompanied by a unique sexual history. Women with urethral prolapse often have the ability to have full sexual pleasure and satisfaction during self-stimulation of the clitoris; however, during sexual activity with the partner or with a mechanical device, they experience pain and/or urgency to urinate and/or inability to have orgasm secondary to distracting pain.

Physical examination of a urethral prolapse reveals a beefy, red, erythematous, protruding, inflamed, and edematous mucosa prolapsing from the meatus in different degrees. Conservative treatment options include topical or systemic estrogens. If necessary, surgical excision may be required (Fig. 12.4.7).

Skene's glands adenitis/urethral-vesical hyperreflexia

Skene's glands drain to the side of the meatus at various locations. It is at present unknown what the pathophysiology is of Skene's glands adenitis, but there appears to be a relation to abnormal immunologic and/or sex-steroid-deficiency states. The diagnosis is made by a history of significant, localized, urethral meatal discomfort and/or dysuria during penetrative sexual activity. Women able to have self-stimulation sexual activity that avoids contact with the urethral meatus can have excellent sexual satisfaction. The classic physical finding of Skene's glands adenitis is a swollen, edematous, protruding urethral meatus without mucosal prolapse. Conservative treatment is by topical and systemic sex steroid hormones, while in extreme cases surgical reconstruction of the meatus is required, with excision of the inflamed Skene's glands.

Urethral-vesical hyperreflexia is an unusual condition involving severe urgency and frequency during urethral meatal contact that is not associated with inflammation of Skene's glands. The pathophysiology is unknown and may be due to trauma to the perineum. The condition is diagnosed during physical examination. The urethral meatus appears otherwise normal except during Q-tip testing. Application of direct pressure by the Q-tip at the urethral meatus results in severe urgency. The diagnosis involves application of local lidocaine

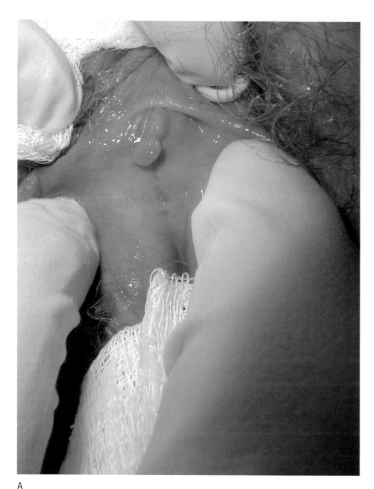

A

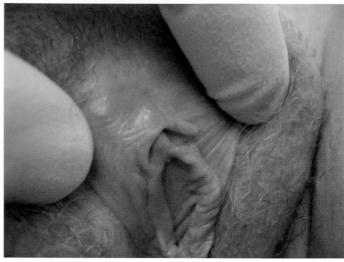

B

Figure 12.4.6. Occasionally, a women can feel a mass associated with and related to the clitoris during self-examination or self-stimulation. The most likely tumor of the clitoris is fibroepithelioma, a skin tumor composed of fibrous tissue intersected by thin anastomosing bands of basal cells of the epidermis. Differential diagnosis includes condyloma, sebaceous cyst, or compound nevi.

ointment at the meatus with immediate resolution of the irritative urethral symptoms. A long-term treatment plan may consist of local application of lidocaine prior to sexual activity. It is possible that recurrent kenalog steroid nerve blocks administered circumferentially around the meatus can help desensitize the hypersensitivity of the urethral meatus.

Urethra/bladder

Urethritis/recurrent urinary tract infections/interstitial cystitis

It is very common for women, especially during transition and in the menopause, to complain of irritative voiding symptoms, especially burning, frequency, urgency, and nocturia, which significantly interfere with sexual activity (see Chapter 17.4). In such women, the vulvovaginal and urinary irritative and burning symptoms are often poorly defined. The patient and physician confusion in this area occurs because the differential diagnosis of irritation and burning in the perineum, especially after coitus, involves multiple different urologic and gynecologic conditions. Urologic conditions that do not involve the urethral meatus include, for example, recurrent urethritis, recur-

rent urinary tract infections, urethral diverticulae, irritable bladder, cystocele, ureteral stones, and endometriosis of the ureter and/or bladder. Irritative symptoms during voiding, especially after coitus, may also be associated with inflammatory gynecologic conditions. In such situations, the contact of voided urine with the inflamed vestibular, vulvar, and/or vaginal tissues can result in significant perineal burning and stinging. Vaginal yeast infections, vulvar dermatitis conditions, and uterine prolapse with or without rectocele are common gynecologic pathophysiologies. In many cases, expert urologic and gynecologic consultations are required to confirm the various diagnoses involved in the individual patient so that varied specific focused treatments may be initiated.

A rare genital sexual pain condition that is confusing and ill-defined, interstitial cystitis, is associated with severe urogenital and pelvic pain, urgency, frequency, nocturia, and dyspareunia. Its pathophysiology is unknown, but it appears unrelated to any recognized bacterial pathophysiology. Interstitial cystitis symptoms, including dyspareunia, often increase with the menses, increase during bladder filling, and decrease with bladder emptying. There is no definitive diagnostic test for interstitial cystitis. History, physical examination,

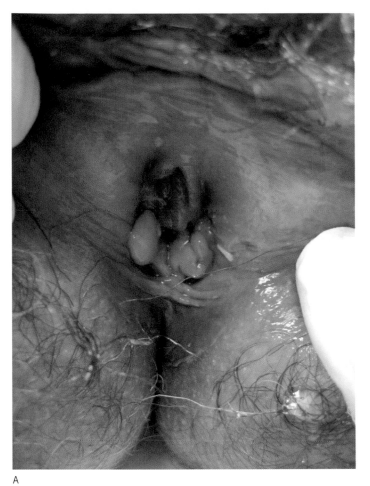

A

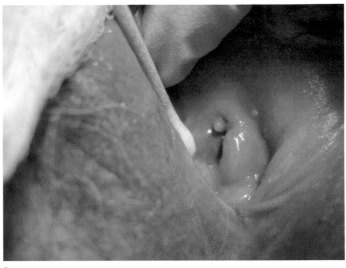

B

Figure 12.4.7. Urethral prolapse presents as a beefy, red, erythematous, protruding, inflamed, edematous mucosa, prolapsing from the meatus in different degrees. Conservative treatment options include topical or systemic estrogens. Surgical excision may be required.

urinalysis, urine culture, and maintenance of a voiding log are mandatory. Specific patient questionnaires are often useful. Other specific testing procedures include potassium sensitivity testing and cystoscopy with or without hydrodistention. As it relates to the dyspareunia and genital sexual pain component associated with interstitial cystitis, treatment of the underlying condition is important. Treatment of interstitial cystitis involves specific agents, such as oral pentosan polysulfate, and bladder instillations of dimethyl sulfoxide or heparin. Nonspecific agents include various antibiotics, anticholinergics, antihistamines, analgesics, and antidepressants.[16]

Vulva

Genital sexual pain in the vulva may be related to various specific disorders, such as infection secondary to *Candida*, herpes, etc. Another example may be inflammation resulting from lichen sclerosus or lichen planus. A neurologic etiology may derive from blunt perineal trauma, such as traumatic neuromata formation, or hyperpathia from postherpetic neuralgia.

Obstruction of the duct draining Bartholin's gland can lead to cyst formation, especially after sexual arousal. Another example is neoplasm from Paget's disease or squamous cell carcinoma.

Bartholin's cysts

Bartholin's (major vestibular) glands are located at 5 o'clock and 7 o'clock at the vaginal introitus, one on each side. During sexual stimulation, the function of Bartholin's glands is to secrete a lubricious fluid onto the mucosal surface of the labia. Bartholin's cyst develops when the exiting Bartholin's gland duct becomes obstructed. The fluid produced then accumulates, causing the gland to swell and form a cyst. Bartholin's cyst, typically in one of the two glands, results in discomfort and swelling of the labia near the entrance to the vagina, especially during sexual arousal. The labial physical examination may be normal in the baseline, nonsexually stimulated state. Ultrasound studies before and during sexual stimulation may be needed to make the diagnosis. Significant pain, swelling, and tenderness of a cyst that interfere with walking and sitting suggest that an abscess has developed, usually with such organisms as chlamydia or *E. coli*. Home treatment of Bartholin's cysts often involves sitz baths. Very large cysts or abscesses may require either incision and drainage or marsupialization, in which the lining of the cyst wall is sutured to the overlying skin in such a way as to create a permanent drain site. If needed, intraoperative ultrasound may help localize the cyst[17,18] (Fig. 12.4.8).

Lichen sclerosus/lichen planus

Lichen sclerosus is a chronic genital dermatitis condition that is associated with varying intensity of symptoms, including vulvar itch or burning and various degrees of vulvar scarring leading to narrowing of the introitus and dyspareunia. There is a wide variation in presentation symptoms. In some women, especially those not sexually active, there can be minimal symptoms, and the patient may be unaware of the condition of lichen sclerosus for years. Alternatively, the burning and itching symptoms can

be so intense as severely to interfere with sexual activity, day-to-day activities, and even sleep. If the scarring of lichen sclerosus involves the perianal area, the patient may also complain of perianal fissuring and painful defecation. The diagnosis of lichen sclerosus is suggested by physical examination showing white genital, vulvar, and vestibular tissue with paleness, loss of pigmentation, and characteristic "cigarette paper" wrinkling. Classically, the genital tissue changes do not involve the inside of the vagina, and if they involve the perianal area, there is a traditional figure of eight extension. The lichen sclerosus condition commonly involves the vestibule, with associated labia minora atrophy, and the vaginal introitus, with loss of elasticity and narrowing. The treatment of choice for lichen sclerosus is the ultrapotent fluorinated steroid, clobetasol. Safety and efficacy (especially for control of itching) studies for clobetasol treatment of vulvar lichen sclerosus have been reported for more than a decade[19,20] (Fig. 12.4.9).

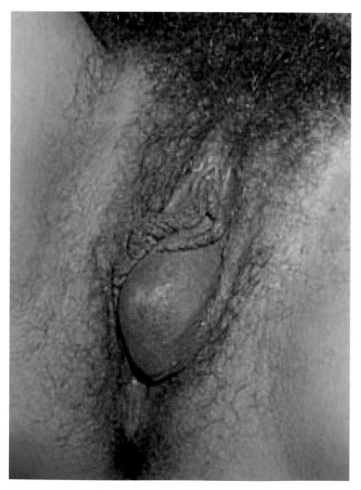

Figure 12.4.8. A Bartholin cyst, typically in one of the two glands, results in discomfort and swelling of the labia near the entrance to the vagina, especially during sexual arousal. The labial physical examination may be normal in the baseline, nonsexually stimulated state.

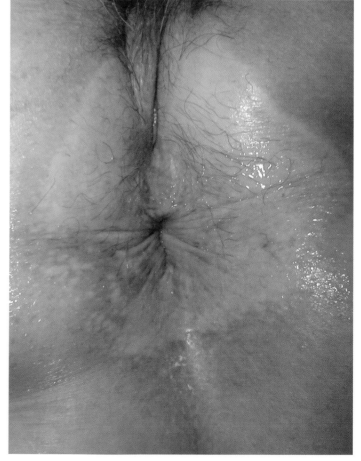

Figure 12.4.9. Lichen sclerosus is a chronic genital dermatitis condition associated with varying intensity of symptoms, including vulvar itch and/or burning and various degrees of vulvar scarring. If the scarring of lichen sclerosus involves the perianal area, the patient may also complain of perianal fissuring and painful defecation. The diagnosis of lichen sclerosus is suggested by physical examination showing white genital, vulvar and vestibular tissue with paleness, loss of pigmentation, and a characteristic "cigarette paper" wrinkling.

Lichen planus is another chronic genital dermatitis condition, probably pathophysiologically related to various altered immunologic disorders. The presenting symptoms vary widely in different patients, probably due to the varied pathophysiologies. Lichen planus may occur secondary to drugs, such as antihypertensives, diuretics, oral hypoglycemics, and nonsteroidal anti-inflammatory agents, that may rarely induce a lichen planus-like eruption. One type of lichen planus is primarily associated with itching and does not result in scarring. Another type of lichen planus is erosive and destructive. Overall, patient complaints may include severe vulvar itching, pain, burning, and irritation. Dyspareunia occurs in sexually active women secondary to vaginal introital scarring. Some types of lichen planus, unlike lichen sclerosus, may involve the vaginal mucosa. If there is vaginal involvement, a purulent malodorous discharge may be noted. Findings on physical examination of women with lichen planus vary widely. The pruritic type of lichen planus is associated with a purple color, and multiple papules and plaques on the vulva and vestibule. The erosive type is associated with vestibular ulcers, scarring, and clitoris and labia minora atrophy; occasionally, destruction of the vagina has been reported. A biopsy and dermatopathologic review may be needed to establish the diagnosis of lichen planus. Treatment of lichen planus involves use of ultrapotent topical steroids, such as clobetasol, topically and vaginally as indicated.[21,22]

Vestibule

Generalized vulvodynia

Generalized vulvodynia refers to a diffuse, constant, burning pain anywhere on the vulva, from mons to anus, which is hyperpathic and greatly out of proportion to the stimulus. Afflicted patients have a constant or sporadic awareness of the vulva with widespread "everything hurts", vulvar soreness, rawness, constant irritation, various paresthesias, aching, and/or stinging. Generalized vulvodynia may be considered as primary if it occurs with the first penetrative sexual encounter, or with a tampon or speculum examination. Generalized vulvodynia may be considered as secondary if it occurs after previous nonpainful vaginal penetrations. Although the pathophysiology of generalized vulvodynia is unknown, there are nociceptive and neuropathic theories.[23,24]

A nociceptive theory involves an initial "insult to genital tissues", not to genital peripheral nerve tissue. There have been multiple conditions proposed to induce the genital tissue insult and injury, including exposure to *C. albicans*, oxalate metabolite, chemotherapy, early and frequent intercourse at a young age, and inadequate estrogen milieu as with an oral contraceptive agent or menopause. Continuing genital tissue insult and damage lead to continual stimulation of nerve endings. This continuous stimulation leads to local sensitization of fibers and central sensitization potentiating chronic genital sexual pain. The chronic pain may exist to a degree that a nonnoxious stimulus, such as simple touch, produces pain or there is continuous pain appreciation.

A neuropathic theory also is proposed to explain generalized vulvodynia where there is "injury to the sensory nervous system" and the genital tissue is intact. In the neuropathic theory, transmission of pain signals occurs secondary to nerve. There are multiple possible etiologies, including injury to the pudendal nerve from childbirth, from vaginal surgeries such as transvaginal sacrospinous colpopexy surgery, or from disorder within the obturator internus. Other neuropathic etiologies of generalized vulvodynia include abnormalities of the sacroiliac joint, piriformis, or pubococcygeus; ruptured disk; scarring around nerve roots after disk surgery; or spinal stenosis.

The diagnosis of generalized vulvodynia is made by ruling out, on physical examination and laboratory testing, such diagnoses as *Candida* vaginitis and chronic genital dermatitis conditions, while Q-tip testing shows all vulvar areas positive for pain and/or tenderness. The treatment of any genital sexual pain disorder involves the multidisciplinary team approach. This is especially true for the disabling condition of generalized vulvodynia. Patient management includes education and support, especially regarding avoidance of contacts and practice of healthy vulvar hygiene; pelvic floor physical therapy treatment; management of concomitant depression; and management of any associated neurologic, dermatologic, gynecologic, orthopedic, or urologic conditions. Medical management includes amitriptyline and/or gabapentin.[23,24]

Vulvar vestibulitis syndrome/vestibular adenitis

Friedrich's criteria for vulvar vestibulitis syndrome are as follows. On history, there is severe pain on vestibular touch or attempted vaginal entry. On physical examination, there is erythema of various degrees within the vestibule. During Q-tip testing, there is tenderness to pressure "localized" within the vulvar vestibule. Often the tender localized region is along the labial hymen junction associated with the presence of minor vestibular glands.

Vulvar vestibulitis syndrome is one of the most likely causes of dyspareunia, especially in women less than 50 years old. Afflicted patients with vulvar vestibulitis syndrome complain of severe pain during sexual activity, often described as raw, red burning, and feeling like sandpaper or burnt tissue being rubbed. Most women experience the pain in the vulvar region with initial penetration. There is another group of women who do not experience pain during initial penetration, but experience severe pain upon deep penetration when the man's perineum comes into contact with the woman's perineum, resulting in the genital sexual pain. In the latter group of women, physicians are misguided to the cervix when the site of the pain trigger is really within the vulvar region. With vulvar vestibulitis syndrome, genital sexual pain may also be experienced with the use of ampons, during speculum examination, wearing tight pants, or straddling while cycling or horseback riding. Although there is no known pathophysiology, there are several possible pathophysiologic factors, including exposure to human papillomavirus, the irritant oxalate, abnormal immunologic conditions, psychopathology, and an abnormal sex steroid hormonal milieu.[25]

During physical examination, the diagnosis of vulvar vestibulitis syndrome is made by Q-tip testing. Q-tip point pressure mapping within the vestibule reveals localized areas without pain and localized areas with pain that can be graded on a 1–10 scale. Use of a spring-loaded Q-tip can result in a consistent pressure applied to the vestibule under all circumstances.[26] In many cases, the regions of pain are consistent with redness and tenderness in the ostea of the minor vestibular glands in the labial-hymenal junction. The diagnosis of vulvar vestibulitis syndrome can be further established with a lidocaine diagnostic nerve block test. This is performed with a few milliliters of 1% lidocaine administered by insulin syringe and 31-gauge needle in the region of positive Q-tip testing. In vulvar vestibulitis syndrome, unlike generalized vulvodynia, lidocaine administration results in virtual complete loss of pain (Fig. 12.4.10).

The treatment of vulvar vestibulitis syndrome includes conservative measures, including education, support, counseling, physical therapy, and/or biofeedback. The pain trigger should be eliminated. Topical estrogen and topical xylocaine creams and/or ointments should be considered. Systemic medications include tricyclic antidepressants or gabapentin. In women with vulvar vestibulitis syndrome, unlike generalized vulvodynia, if medical management fails, surgery, such as vestibulectomy, can be considered.[27–30]

Vagina

Atrophic vaginitis

Unfortunately, contemporary clinical research data show that the use of exogenous estrogen by women in menopause for control of menopausal symptoms, such as hot flashes and night sweats, and for maintenance of urogenital health is perplexing and controversial. What is not controversial, however, is the role of estradiol in the genital tissues. Estradiol is a sex steroid that is critical for the structure and function of multiple genital tissues, especially the vagina. All three layers of the vagina, the endothelium, lamina propria, and muscularis, require estradiol for their integrity. Persistently low estradiol levels in the vaginal tissues result in atrophic vaginitis, which is associated with low estradiol states, including natural menopause, bilateral oophorectomy, gonadotropin-releasing hormone agonist use, hypothalamic amenorrhea, radiation, and chemotherapy.

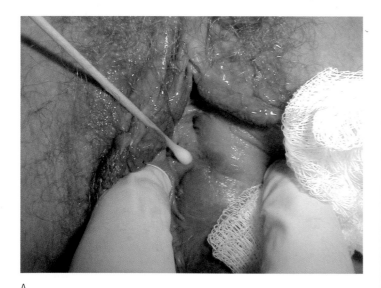

A

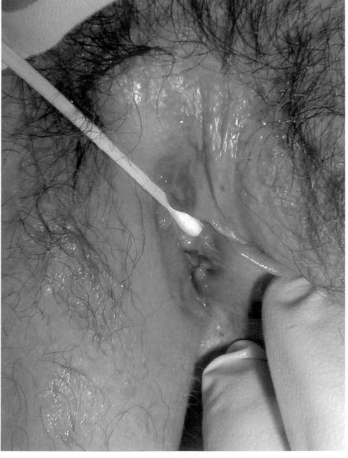

B

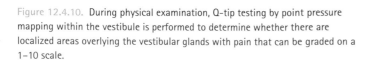

Figure 12.4.10. During physical examination, Q-tip testing by point pressure mapping within the vestibule is performed to determine whether there are localized areas overlying the vestibular glands with pain that can be graded on a 1–10 scale.

The symptoms of atrophic vaginitis include vaginal dryness, dyspareunia, stinging, bleeding, and dysuria. On physical examination, women with atrophic vaginitis reveal vaginal mucosal changes. The classic, healthy-appearing vagina has a pink hue with vaginal folds and rugae; when touched with a Q-tip, it reveals a shiny, lubricating substance and, when rubbed with a Q-tip, it does not bleed. In atrophic vaginitis, the vagina changes to an unhealthy pale complexion, with a lack of vaginal folds and

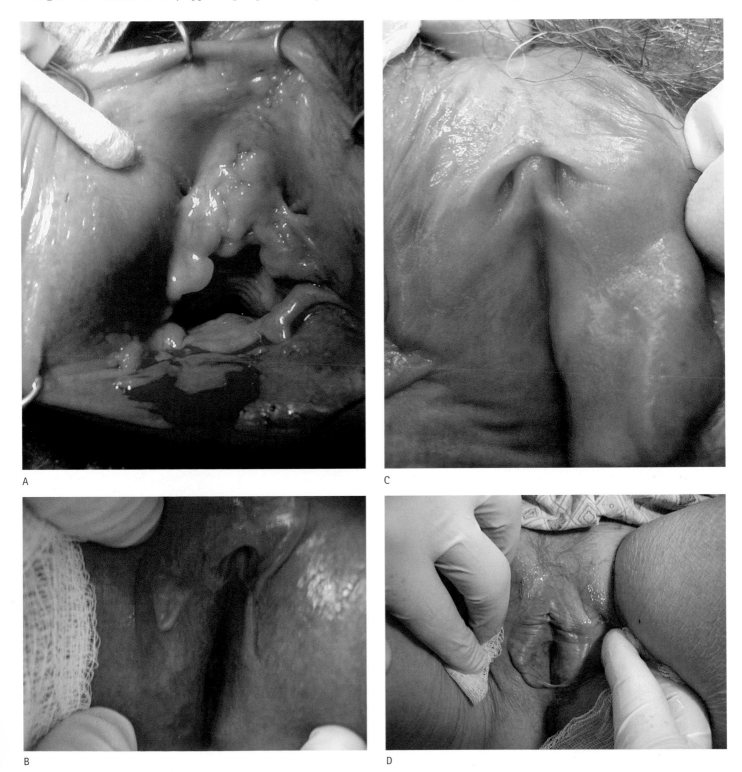

A

B

C

D

Figure 12.4.11. The classic, healthy-appearing vagina has a pink hue with vaginal folds and rugae; when touched with a Q-tip, it reveals a shiny, lubricating substance and, when rubbed with a Q-tip, does not bleed. In atrophic vaginitis, the vagina changes to an unhealthy pale complexion, with a lack of vaginal folds and rugae, and lubricating substance on the surface, and the tissue bleeds with minimal contact.

rugae, and a lack of lubricating substance on the surface, and the tissue bleeds with minimal contact (Fig. 12.4.11). On wet mount, the microscopic examination reveals parabasal cells, increased white blood cells, and absent background flora of lactobacilli. The vaginal pH is elevated to 6.0–7.0.

The conservative treatment involves the use of local topical vestibular and/or intravaginal estrogen. There are multiple products on the market, including intravaginal rings, and intravaginal pills and creams. In some rare patients, plasma estradiol levels may increase to values similar to those of systemic estrogen administration, so monitoring is required as indicated by the physician. Moreover, some patients are allergic to the various additives in the topical estradiol product. For example, some women react to the propylene glycol in several topical estrogen products. There are also multiple estrogen alternatives, such as soy, black cohosh, wild yam, chaste berry, angelica, damiana, nettle, red clover, and saw palmetto, although there are limited double-blind, placebo-controlled safety and efficacy trials with these products.[31,32]

Pelvic floor disorders (see Chapters 4.4 and 12.3)

In genital sexual pain disorders, spasms of the pelvic floor muscles may contribute to the overall pain and discomfort experienced by the patient. The spasms reflex to the spinal cord and back to the source of pain in a self-perpetuating circuit. Pain and spasm manifest as increased activity in the perineal muscles. Chronic spasm results in muscle anoxia responsible for deep, aching pain and additional genital sexual pain. Biofeedback utilizes an electromyographic transducer inserted into the vagina. The electromyographic output is connected to a computer for visual biofeedback. Physical therapists[33] organize a training process of contraction and relaxation of pelvic floor muscles similar to Kegel exercises.

Conclusions

Genital sexual pain problems are common and often disabling. Genital sexual pain disorders are multifactorial syndromes of pain, sexual dysfunction, and psychologic disability. Ideal patient management involves a multimodal approach, including psychologic support, sexual therapy, physical therapy, and medical management of the pain. The aim of this chapter was to provide the biologic-concentrated health-care professional with germane clinical data to aid in the management of specific biologic-based pathophysiologies of genital sexual pain.

The major lessons from this chapter are that there are multiple physiologic causes for genital sexual pain and that, as in other medical issues, accurate diagnosis is essential to appropriate treatment. The basis for diagnosis is history and physical examination with appropriate laboratory testing. Additional research is needed in this very significant aspect of women's sexual health.

References

1. Lewis RW, Fugl-Meyer, KS, Bosch R et al. Epidemiology/risk factors of sexual dysfunction. *J Sex Med* 2004; 1: 35–9.
2. Basson R, Althof S, Davis S et al. Summary of the recommendations on sexual dysfunctions in women. *J Sex Med* 2004; 1: 24–34.
3. Harlow BL, Wise LA, Stewart EG. Prevalence and predictors of chronic genital discomfort. *Am J Obstet Gynecol* 2001; 185: 545–50.
4. Basson R, Weijmar Shultz WCM, Binik YM et al. Women's sexual desire and arousal disorders and sexual pain. In Lue TF, Basson R, Rosen R et al., eds. *Sexual Medicine: Sexual Dysfunctions in Men and Women*. Paris: Health Publications, 2004: 851–974.
5. Binik YM. Sate of the art. IX. Genital sexual pain. *J Sex Med* 2004; 1: S7–S8.
6. Hilliges M, Falconer C, Ekman-Ordeberg G et al. Innervation of the human vaginal mucosa as revealed by PGP 9.5 immunohistochemistry. *Acta Anat (Basel)* 1995; 153: 119–26.
7. Harlow BL, Stewart EG. A population-based assessment of chronic unexplained vulvar pain: have we underestimated the prevalence of vulvodynia? *J Am Med Womens Assoc* 2003; 58: 82–8.
8. Stewart EG. Developments in vulvovaginal care. *Curr Opin Obstet Gynecol* 2002; 14: 483–8.
9. Harlow BL, Wise LA, Stewart EG. Prevalence and predictors of chronic lower genital tract discomfort. *Am J Obstet Gynecol* 2001; 185: 545–50.
10. Graziottin A, Castoldi E, Montorsi F et al. Vulvodynia: the challenge of "unexplained" genital pain. *J Sex Marital Ther* 2001; 27: 503–12.
11. Meston CM. Validation of the female sexual function index (FSFI) in women with female orgasmic disorder and in women with hypoactive sexual desire disorder. *J Sex Marital Ther* 2003; 29: 39–46.
12. Bergeron S, Binik YM, Khalife S et al. Vulvar vestibulitis syndrome: reliability of diagnosis and evaluation of current diagnostic criteria. *Obstet Gynecol* 2001; 98: 45–51.
13. Haefner HK. Current evaluation and management of vulvovaginitis. *Clin Obstet Gynecol* 1999; 42: 184–95.
14. Anderson MR, Klink K, Cohrssen A. Evaluation of vaginal complaints. *JAMA* 2004; 291: 1368–79.
15. Munarriz R, Talakoub L, Kuohung W et al. The prevalence of phimosis of the clitoris in women presenting to the sexual dysfunction clinic: lack of correlation to disorders of desire, arousal and orgasm. *J Sex Marital Ther* 2002; 28(Suppl 1): 181–5.
16. Stewart EG, Berger BM. Parallel pathologies? Vulvar vestibulitis and interstitial cystitis. *J Reprod Med* 1997; 42: 131–4.
17. Hill DA, Lense JJ. Office management of Bartholin gland cysts and abscesses. *Am Fam Physician* 1998; 57: 1611–16, 1619–20.
18. Downs MC, Randall HW Jr. The ambulatory surgical management of Bartholin duct cysts. *J Emerg Med* 1989; 7: 623–6.
19. Carlson JA, Lamb P, Malfetano J et al. Clinicopathologic comparison of vulvar and extragenital lichen sclerosus: histologic variants, evolving lesions, and etiology of 141 cases. *Mod Pathol* 1998; 11: 844–54.

20. Bracco GL, Carli P, Sonni L et al. Clinical and histologic effects of topical treatments of vulval lichen sclerosus. A critical evaluation. *J Reprod Med* 1993; 38: 37–40.

21. Lotery HE, Galask RP. Erosive lichen planus of the vulva and vagina. *Obstet Gynecol* 2003; 101(5 Pt 2): 1121–5.

22. O'Keefe RJ, Scurry JP, Dennerstein G et al. Audit of 114 nonneoplastic vulvar biopsies. *Br J Obstet Gynaecol* 1995; 102: 780–6.

23. Edwards L. Subsets of vulvodynia: overlapping characteristics. *J Reprod Med* 2004; 49: 883–7.

24. Lotery HE, McClure N, Galask RP. Vulvodynia. *Lancet* 2004; 363: 1058–60.

25. Graziottin A, Brotto LA. Vulvar vestibulitis syndrome: a clinical approach. *J Sex Marital Ther* 2004; 30: 125–39.

26. Pukall CF, Binik YM, Khalife S. A new instrument for pain assessment in vulvar vestibulitis syndrome. *J Sex Marital Ther* 2004; 30: 69–78.

27. Schover LR, Youngs DD, Cannata R. Psychosexual aspects of the evaluation and management of vulvar vestibulitis. *Am J Obstet Gynecol* 1992; 167: 630–6.

28. Reissing ED, Binik YM, Khalife S et al. Vaginal spasm, pain, and behavior: an empirical investigation of the diagnosis of vaginismus. *Arch Sex Behav* 2004; 33: 5–17.

29. Bergeron S, Brown C, Lord MJ et al. Physical therapy for vulvar vestibulitis syndrome: a retrospective study. *J Sex Marital Ther* 2002; 28: 183–92.

30. Bergeron S, Bouchard C, Fortier M et al. The surgical treatment of vulvar vestibulitis syndrome: a follow-up study. *J Sex Marital Ther* 1997; 23: 317–25.

31. Owen MK, Clenney TL. Management of vaginitis. *Am Fam Physician* 2004; 70: 2125–32.

32. Crandall C. Vaginal estrogen preparations: a review of safety and efficacy for vaginal atrophy. *J Womens Health (Larchmt)* 2002; 11: 857–77.

33. Kotarinos RK. Pelvic floor physical therapy in urogynecologic disorders. *Curr Womens Health Rep* 2003; 3: 334–9.

12.5 Management by anesthetic blocks

Ezio Vincenti, Alessandra Graziottin

Vulvar vestibulitis syndrome and vulvodynia, which clinically appear with symptoms typical of neuropathic pain, such as allodynia and hyperalgesia, represent the main cause of sexual pain disorders during the fertile age (see Chapters 12.1–12.4 and 12.6 of this book). Because of the severe vestibular pain when attempting vaginal entry, intercourse is increasingly avoided. When the disease is in an advanced state, pain is suffered spontaneously, almost while sitting or moving. In some chronic cases, pain/discomfort may radiate from the vulva to the perineum and into the groin and thigh.

If both current medical treatment and noninvasive anthalgic therapy fail to control pain, repeated anesthetic neural blockades may be the definitive solution. The rationale for this new approach is based on the results obtained in other chronic neuropathic pain diseases and from pathophysiologic data recently acquired in the specific vulvar field. In fact, recent histologic and biochemical findings from vestibular tissues of patients affected by vulvar vestibulitis syndrome or vulvodynia[1-3] have stimulated a new and more effective therapy for cases defined as intractable.

Anesthetic block of the impar ganglion (and specific somatic nerves) and ancillary anthalgic systemic supportive therapy have modified the general approach to the treatment of these patients, who previously were scheduled for ablative surgery of the vestibulus, i.e., vestibulectomy. Pathophysiologic considerations are necessary to elucidate the rational basis of this therapeutic approach.

Pathophysiologic scenario

Acute injury to the vulvar vestibule by bacterial, fungal, or viral infection, chemical irritants, or coital rubbing without lubrication and a defensively contracted elevator ani further reducing the vaginal entrance, as well as iatrogenic procedures, may cause acute pain triggered by the mucosal damage that lasts from several days to a few weeks. This causes an inflammatory response with a typical nociceptive pain, which may be resolved by the correct symptomatic and etiologic approach.[4] When the tissue damage is persistent because the predisposing and/or precipitating damaging factors remain undiagnosed and/or unaddressed, a chronic inflammation of variable intensity is maintained. The mast cells, key mediators of it, become upregulated. Their production of nerve growth factors promotes nerve pain fiber proliferation, which correlates with hyperalgesia, and superficially causes allodynia, the perceptive shift from tactile to burning pain.[1-4] This explains why pain may become persistent despite treatment. When nerves work in abnormally, signaling pain without apparent peripheral damage, the term "neuropathic pain" may be used. This pain also describes the process by which the neurons involved in pain transmission are converted from a state of normal sensitivity to one in which they are hypersensitive.

Initially, pain is due only to peripheral mechanisms, but later central mechanisms are progressively recruited. The pathophysiology of peripheral neuropathic pain is therefore based on both abnormal peripheral inputs and abnormal central processing.[1-5] Peripheral mechanisms include nociceptor sensitization, spontaneous activation of primary afferent fibers ectopically firing from the site of the lesion, and so-called neurogenic inflammation.

The last is characterized by the release of algogenic substances, which may move backward along the sensory nerves and/or be released by the upregulated mast cells through neurogenic activation of their degranulation. A close interaction between mast cells and pain nerve fibers, with reciprocal potentiation, seems to be a key feature of peripheral neuropathic pain. As far as the central mechanisms are concerned, a "wind-up" phenomenon occurs due to the progressive increase of cellular firing after repeated identical electrical stimuli.[6] Moreover, spinal and supraspinal propagation of abnormal local changes caused by peripheral nervous lesion is responsible for aberrant central elaboration. In the biochemical field, excitatory amino acids and N-methyl-D-aspartate receptors play a crucial role in the genesis of chronic neuropathic pain.[6]

The dorsal horn of the spinal cord seems to be extremely

important in the initiation and maintenance of neuropathic pain. Recently, Tsuda et al.[7] have demonstrated that activation of p38 mitogen-activated protein kinase in spinal hyperactive microglia of the dorsal horn contributes to pain hypersensitivity to innocuous stimuli (tactile allodynia) after peripheral nerve injury. In fact, intrathecal administration of a specific p38 mitogen-activated protein kinase inhibitor (SB203580) suppresses the development of the nerve injury-induced tactile allodynia. Other investigations[8] show that galectin-1 (one of the endogenous galactoside-binding lectins, involved in a variety of functions, such as neurite outgrowth, synaptic connectivity, cell proliferation, and apoptosis) increases in the dorsal horn at 1–2 weeks after axotomy. Furthermore, intrathecal administration of antirecombinant human galectin-1 antibody partially but significantly attenuates the upregulation of substance P receptor in the spinal dorsal horn and the mechanical hypersensitivity induced by the peripheral nerve injury. These data suggest that endogenous galectin-1 may support neuropathic pain after the peripheral nerve injury, at least partly, by increasing substance P receptor in the dorsal horn.

Tissue injury of almost any kind, but especially peripheral or central neural tissue injury, can lead to long-lasting spinal and supraspinal reorganization that includes the forebrain.[9] These forebrain changes may be adaptive and facilitate functional recovery, or they may be maladaptive, preventing or prolonging the painful condition.[9,10] In an experimental model of heat allodynia, functional brain imaging showed that: (a) the forebrain activity during heat allodynia is different from that during normal heat pain; (b) during heat allodynia, specific cortical areas, specifically the dorsolateral prefrontal cortex, can attenuate specific components of the pain experience, such as affect, by reducing the functional connectivity of subcortical pathways. The forebrain of patients with chronic neuropathic pain may undergo pathologically induced changes that can impair clinical response to all forms of treatment.

Therefore, both peripheral and central mechanisms are involved in maintaining intractable neuropathic pain arising from the vulvovaginal area. The new strategy of treatment is based on the destructuring of acquired anatomic and functional neuronal modifications during chronic pain, while respecting the anatomic integrity of the vestibular tissue. The ablative approach, which aims at removal of the inflamed vestibular mucosa, was proposed at a time when the pathophysiology of burning pain was not understood. Addressing the etiologic diversity of vulvar vestibulitis syndrome by multimodal treatment,[4] and specifically curing pain by appropriate anthalgic strategies, both peripheral and central, takes into account the current pathophysiologic understanding and the need for maintenance of anatomic integrity for a better sexual outcome.

Clinical aspects

The transition from nociceptive to neuropathic pain is key in vulvar vestibulitis syndrome/vulvodynia, as it underlies the shift from a sexual pain disorder, where intercourse elicits and provokes pain, to a progressively pure pain disorder that is spontaneously self-maintained despite the avoidance of any further coital intimacy. Some women with chronic vulvar vestibulitis syndrome/vulvodynia report distress from noncoital activity such as kissing or hugging their partner, dreaming, or watching an erotic movie, as even mild genital arousal (without direct contact) with the resultant vasocongestion immediately elicits a provocation of the genital pain.

From the nosologic point of view, neuropathic pain arising from vulvar vestibulitis syndrome and vulvodynia may be associated clinically with a complex regional pain syndrome[6] early recognized as reflex sympathetic dystrophy, an increasingly diagnosed entity. Spontaneous burning pain worsening over time, tenderness, and increasing psychologic involvement with a catastrophizing coping attitude are the main complaints of patients suffering from vulvar vestibulitis syndrome and vulvodynia. The pathophysiology of physical symptoms is related to the microscopic findings of proliferation of pain fibers, which are superficial within the vestibular tissue.

Persistent vulvar allodynia and hyperalgesia that cause dyspareunia lead to the avoidance of intercourse.[4] In the absence of appropriate treatment, pain tends to worsen and widen in the perineal and bladder area. Patients with vulvar vestibulitis syndrome have increased innervation and/or sensitization of thermoreceptors and nociceptors in their vestibular mucosa. In patients with vulvar vestibulitis syndrome, Bohm-Starke et al.[2] found the presence of allodynia to mechanical testing with von Frey filaments (14.3 ± 3.1 mN in the symptomatic posterior area compared with 158 ± 33.5 mN in healthy subjects), as well as to the pain threshold to heat ($38.6 \pm 0.6°C$ in patients and 43.8 ± 0.8 in controls). In addition, the pain threshold to cold was $21.6 \pm 1.2°C$ in patients, whereas cooling down to $6°C$ was usually not painful in controls.

The classic definition of vulvar vestibulitis syndrome by Friedrich[11] concerning the constellation of symptoms and findings involved, and limited to the vulvar vestibule, consists of (a) severe pain on vestibular touch to attempted vaginal entry, (b) tenderness to pressure localized within the vulvar vestibule, and (c) physical findings confined to vulvar erythema of various degrees. This definition seems to be consistently valid only for (a) and (b), since many patients suffering from neuropathic pain may present an apparently normal mucosa without current signs of erythema. Indeed, there may be a more appropriate definition of vulvodynia for these cases. According to Bergeron et al.,[12] erythema does not appear to be a useful diagnostic criterion; in addition, no active inflammation was seen in biopsies obtained from the vestibular mucosa by analysing cyclooxygenase 2 and inducible nitric oxide synthase by the indirect immunohistochemistry method.

New therapy

A basic therapeutic approach to vulvar vestibulitis syndrome/vulvodynia is mandatory.[4] Hygienic and behavioral recommendations should be given in order to avoid chronic irritation and maceration of the fragile tissues, and improve perineal care. Prevention of yeast infection recurrence should be maintained with antimycotic oral treatment. Food intake should be qualitatively controlled as well, to reduce vestibular irritation during micturition, and to reduce recurrence of *Candida*. Relaxation of the pelvic floor should be obtained through self-massage, physiotherapy, and/or electromyographic feedback.[4,13] In fact, treatment of underlying causes of organic and psychologic etiologic specific factors in particular must be done before effective anthalgic therapy. The authors suggested specific guidelines for management of neuropathic pain due to vulvar vestibulitis syndrome/vulvodynia (Table 12.5.1).[14]

As a rule, patients with intractable (concerning the conventional therapy) neuropathic pain from vulvar vestibulitis syndrome/vulvodynia need the second (invasive, nonsurgical) stage of treatment. The pathophysiologic basis of this approach should be sought in the histologic alterations of vestibular innervation, which appears intraepithelially increased in the mucosa of vulvar vestibulitis syndrome/vulvodynia patients. If chronic aggressive factors can transform normal mucosa into an altered histologic picture (Fig. 12.5.1), a correct, *ad hoc* pathophysiologic treatment with periodic anesthetic blocks can restore the normal innervation. The persistent efficacy of nerve block therapy may be explained as follows. The anesthetic block of specific afferent fibers (especially neurovegetative) from an area involved in neuropathic transmission might induce a progressive self-reduction (neuroplasticity) of the hyperplastic peripheral nervous arborization in the intraepithelial field, with a parallel reduction of the neurogenically induced degranulation of the upregulated mast cells. In fact, even a transient anesthetic deafferentation repeated monthly should be sufficient to modify an altered (excessive) supply of nervous endings, func-

Table 12.5.1. Guidelines for nonsurgical management of neuropathic pain due to vulvar vestibulitis syndrome/vulvodynia. Stages of treatment (a multimodal, interdisciplinary treatment approach)

1. Conventional, noninvasive
   a. Pharmacologic
   b. Electromyographic biofeedback of pelvic floor musculature[13]
   c. TNS (transcutaneous nerve stimulation)
2. Invasive, nonsurgical
   a. Peripheral anesthetic blocks (impar ganglion; sacral, pudendal, and ilioinguinal nerves)[14]
   b. Sacral nerves stimulation by implantable catheters[15]

tionally producing allodynia and hyperalgesia as a result of reduced pain threshold. Therefore, we have employed monthly anesthetic nerve blocks of the impar ganglion,[4,14] which is the last ganglion of the sympathetic chain and has the task of transmitting sympathetic information to and from the perineal area. Regarding somatic deafferentation, repeated anesthetic blocks of some regional somatic nerves may complete the recovery of status quo ante.

As far as materials and methods are concerned, every session of blocks is currently composed of anesthetic blocks of sacral, pudendal (through perineal pathway), and ilioinguinal nerves, and finally of the impar ganglion (under the guidance of a finger rectally introduced) (Fig. 12.5.2), which is the main target. Plain 0.25% bupivacaine is used in a total volume of no more than 30 ml per session, delivered by 30–90-mm, 23-gauge, disposable needles.

The correct use of these anesthetic blocks offers a dramatic improvement in clinical conditions by controlling burning pain immediately (onset time less than 2 min). After the first sessions of anesthetic blocks, the duration of pain relief is limited to a

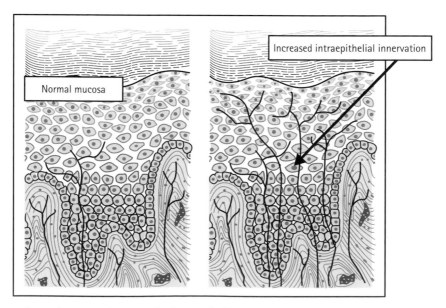

Figure 12.5.1. Schematic pictures of normal mucosa and mucosa of vulvar vestibulitis syndrome patients.

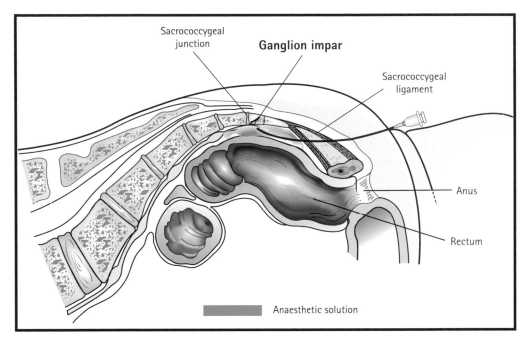

Figure 12.5.2. Anesthetic block of ganglion impar. Reproduced from Vincenti and Graziottin[14] with permission.

few hours or days. After 2–3 months, pain-free time becomes longer, up to a few weeks' duration. Within about 6 months, more than 80% of patients affected by intractable pain from vulvar vestibulitis syndrome/vulvodynia obtain persistent pain relief, rating more than 93% in comparison with the preblock period (Table 12.5.2). Follow-up of cases reported here are longer than 6 months.

For additional comfort when pain relief by block therapy is still incomplete, gabapentin and tricyclic antidepressant (amitriptyline) drugs are used. Dosage is adjusted by the principle of minimum effective dose, or of the dose allowing acceptable minor side effects. Parallel treatment of the predisposing, precipitating, and maintaining factors contributing to chronic agonist stimuli upregulating the mast-cell degranulation is recommended.

When the neuropathic pain has disappeared, therapy should be initiated to (re)gain sexual pleasure and satisfactory intimacy with adequate genital arousal. The shift from pain to pleasure may require parallel biologic and psychologic treatment, addressing the issues of both the woman and the couple.[4] The sexual prognosis is dependent upon the duration of sexual pain, the damage to the couple's intimate relationship, and the efficacy of the support in addressing pre-existing, concomitant, and persisting sexual health issues, such as low libido, poor mental and genital arousal, and fear of re-experiencing pain.

Early and appropriate management of pain associated with vulvar vestibulitis syndrome/vulvodynia is key for both the effectiveness of the anthalgic treatment and the successful outcome of the sexologic therapy.[4]

Conclusion

Current noninvasive treatment may be useful in a number of patients, but the most severe cases need a more aggressive approach, such as anesthetic nerve blocks. Monthly repeated blocks with bupivacaine of the impar ganglion and of the sacral, pudendal, and ilioinguinal nerves, complemented by ancillary therapy with antidepressant and anticonvulsant (e.g., gabapentin) drugs, in many patients may progressively reduce the intensity of pain and its extension until complete recovery. This invasive but nonsurgical therapy seems to be the most effective treatment for women affected by severe neuropathic pain caused by vulvar vestibulitis syndrome/vulvodynia and resistant to current noninvasive therapy.

Table 12.5.2. Casistics and results of anthalgic treatment with anesthetic nervous blocks in patients suffering from intractable pain caused by vulvar vestibulitis syndrome/vulvodynia (more than 6 months after completion of treatment)

Number of cases	57
age (years) (average, range)	37.7 (19–82)
Duration of time (years) (average, range) of intractable pain before invasive therapy	4.2 (1–28)
Number of anthalgic sessions (median value, range)	6 (2–18)
Percentage of cases with complete recovery	84.2
Pain before treatment (visual analog scale 0–100) (average value)	60.2
pain after treatment (visual analog scale 0–100) (average value)	3.9

References

1. Bohm-Starke N, Hilliges M, Falconer C et al. Neurochemical characterization of the vestibular nerves in women with vulvar vestibulitis syndrome. *Gynecol Obstet Invest* 1999; 48: 270–5.

2. Bohm-Starke N, Hilliges M, Blomgren B et al. Increased blood flow and erythema in posterior vestibular mucosa in vulvar vestibulitis. *Am J Obstet Gynecol* 2001; 98: 1067–74.

3. Bohm-Starke N, Hilliges M, Brodda-Jansen G et al. Psychophysical evidence of nociceptor sensitization in vulvar vestibulitis syndrome. *Pain* 2001; 94: 177–83.

4. Graziottin A, Brotto L. Vulvar vestibulitis syndrome: a clinical approach. *J Sex Marital Ther* 2004; 30: 125–39.

5. Woolf CJ. The pathophysiology of peripheral neuropathic pain: abnormal peripheral input and abnormal central processing. *Acta Neurochir Suppl* 1993; 58: 125–30.

6. Dickenson AH. A cute for wind up: NMDA receptors antagonists as potential analgesics. *Trends Pharmacol Sci* 1990; 11: 307–9.

7. Tsuda M, Mizokoshi A, Shigemoto-Mogami Y et al. Activation of p38 mitogen-activated protein kinase in spinal hyperactive microglia contributes to pain hypersensitivity following peripheral nerve injury. *Glia* 2004; 45: 89–95.

8. Imbe H, Okamoto K, Kadoya T et al. Galectin-1 is involved in the potentiation of neuropathic pain in the dorsal horn. *Brain Res* 2003; 993: 72–83.

9. Casey KL, Lorenz J, Minoshima S. Insights into the pathophysiology of neuropathic pain through functional brain imaging. *Exp Neurol* 2003; 184(Suppl 1): 80–8.

10. Merskey H, Bogduk N. *Classification of Chronic Pain.* Seattle: IASP Press, 1994.

11. Friedrich EG. Vulvar vestibulitis syndrome. *J Reprod Med* 1987; 32: 110–14.

12. Bergeron S, Binik YM, Khalifé S et al. Vulvar vestibulitis syndrome: reliability of diagnosis and evaluation of current diagnostic criteria. *Obstet Gynecol* 2001; 98: 45–51.

13. McKay E, Kaufman RH, Doctor U et al. Treating vulvar vestibulitis with electromyographic biofeedback of pelvic floor musculature. *J Reprod Med* 2001; 46: 337–42.

14. Vincenti E, Graziottin A. Neuropathic pain in vulvar vestibulitis: diagnosis and treatment. *Urodinamica* 2004; 14: 112–16.

15. Whiteside JL, Walters MD, Mekhail N. Spinal cord stimulation for intractable vulvar pain. A case report. *J Reprod Med* 2003; 48: 821–3.

12.6 Difficult cases: treatment of sexual pain disorders

Sophie Bergeron, Caroline F Pukall, Yitzchak M Binik

Why sexual pain disorders are inherently difficult to treat

Many health professionals do not enjoy treating women suffering from sexual pain disorders (i.e., dyspareunia and vaginismus) and find it difficult to deal with patients afflicted by these conditions. Why is this? First, the presence of a recurrent pain tends to elicit feelings of powerlessness in the health professional, which are due, on the one hand, to the chronic nature of this symptom, and, on the other hand, to the strong emotions generated by the experience of pain in the patients. Second, dyspareunia and vaginismus tend to have a negative impact on the entire sexual response cycle, generating other sexual dysfunctions that also require treatment and that strain the overall relationship of the couple. An additional deterrent for physicians is that in comparison with other sexual dysfunctions, little is known about the etiology or treatment of sexual pain.[1] Finally, there is great diagnostic confusion surrounding dyspareunia and vaginismus, since they are difficult to differentiate from one another.[2] More specifically, the distinctness of the two disorders from the point of view of treatment is not clear. Research, to date, indicates a more pronounced phobic component in women with vaginismus.[3] However, in view of the lack of definitive data pertaining to the treatment of vaginismus, this chapter will mainly focus on dyspareunia, with mention of vaginismus when relevant.

Chronic recurrent pain

Since intercourse is an activity associated with intense pleasure, the presence of pain is all the more in contrast with one's expectations. This experience is bound to elicit intense reactions in both members of the affected couple in their attempt to make sense of a condition that often takes years to diagnose.[4] Therefore, treating health professionals must deal not only with a difficult physical symptom – pain – for which there is no quick fix, but also sometimes with the feelings of hopelessness, despair, and anguish expressed by their patients.

Comorbid sexual dysfunctions

The pain affects all phases of sexual function (see Chapters 6.1–6.5, and 12.1–12.5 of this book). For example, women with dyspareunia and vaginismus have been shown to have less sexual desire and arousal, a lower frequency of intercourse, and less orgasmic capacity both during intercourse and manual stimulation than controls.[5-8] Clinically, the majority of these patients meet the diagnostic criteria of the *Diagnostic and Statistical Manual of Mental Disorders*, fourth edition,[9] for both inhibited sexual desire and sexual arousal disorder, and often for secondary anorgasmia as well. Inhibited sexual desire is generally viewed as one of the most difficult sexual dysfunctions to treat;[10] combined with chronic, recurrent pain during sex, sexual desire is unlikely to be any easier to restore. In dealing with cases of sexual pain, health professionals may have to treat the entire spectrum of female sexual dysfunction, with each new impairment adding to the burden of the previous one.

Lack of efficacious treatments

There is a paucity of adequate health-care services for women suffering from sexual pain, with at least two studies showing that many women with dyspareunia receive less than optimal relief from their pain.[11,12] One recent study found that approximately 60% of women suffering from vulvar pain complaints sought treatment for their pain, but 30% had to consult three or more physicians in order to obtain a diagnosis, and the condition remained undiagnosed in 40% of the women who had consulted.[12]

Since research interest in this area began to increase only in the early 1980s, many important clinical questions remain unanswered. Thus, current therapeutic options are largely based on trial and error, with few empirical outcome data to rely on to devise appropriate treatment plans. Empirically validated treatments are urgently needed: there are no randomized clinical trials for vaginismus, and only a few for dyspareunia.[4,13–15] Moreover, the results of these trials show that dyspareunia is difficult to treat: apart from vestibulectomy for vulvar vestibulitis syndrome – which has high success rates but involves more risk – medical interventions are not successful; behavioral interventions are generally successful in about 40% of patients. Although not confirmed by any controlled study, reported success rates in the treatment of vaginismus are high;[16] however, many clinicians find this condition just as difficult to treat as dyspareunia, perhaps because of the important avoidance component which renders adherence to any kind of intervention problematic, leading to high dropout rates. Unfortunately, for health professionals involved in the treatment of dyspareunia and/or vaginismus, the choice of interventions is largely driven by one's background and training, or by the patients' preferences, with multidisciplinary efforts still being the exception rather than the rule.

Diagnostic confusion

Two recent studies have demonstrated that the only factor differentiating women with dyspareunia from those with vaginismus is the avoidance of penetration by the latter.[8,17] In addition, these disorders overlap with what could be referred to as the vulvodynia spectrum, or idiopathic vulvar pain conditions. Such diagnostic confusion represents yet another factor contributing to the treatment challenges presented by the sexual pain disorders, as it inevitably leads to confusion among health professionals working together in an attempt to treat these patients – a confusion that is picked up by the women themselves and contributes to their distress.

As is the rule in this textbook, patients' right to privacy and confidentiality must be protected. Therefore, the material has been disguised and altered to protect privacy, while simultaneously maintaining the essential clinical problem. Interventions are unaltered and described by the authors.

The following case vignette describes a difficult sexual pain case and the challenges it presents for the physician. Karen, aged 26, has suffered from pain during intercourse for the last 3 years. She was referred by her general practitioner to a gynecologist because it was felt that he could be of more help to her. At the time of the first appointment with the gynecologist, Karen had consulted four physicians in her town and had been told by different clinicians that the problem was in her head, that a glass of wine would do the trick, and that there was nothing wrong with her physically. The fourth physician she consulted knew about sexual pain; he told her that she had vulvar vestibulitis

combined with vaginismus and prescribed a corticosteroid cream. When Karen reported 3 months later that the cream had not helped, he referred her to a gynecologist. When she arrived at her first appointment, the gynecologist was confronted with an emotional patient who suffered not only from painful sex but also from an absence of sexual desire and a romantic relationship that was falling apart. The gynecologist listened to Karen's story and, after explaining to her that he had no miracle cure to offer, suggested that an anesthetic gel might help to reduce her pain during intercourse and offered to see her every 3 months. Appointments involved providing support and encouragement to Karen while attempting to find the right medical treatment for her. Although she was discouraged by the lack of success of the various interventions, Karen did appear to appreciate the close medical follow-up. The gynecologist suggested she might want to join a sexual pain support group, which she did. Meanwhile, they tried three different creams over a 1-year period, including an estrogen cream, a stronger anesthetic cream, and cromolyn cream. After a few helpful sessions of physical therapy to reduce her muscle tension, Karen opted for a vestibulectomy. She still experiences some discomfort from time to time, but, overall, is quite happy with the outcome of her surgery.

The combination of (1) a complex and multisymptom clinical picture where all phases of sexual function are impaired and relationship adjustment is compromised, (2) a lack of appropriate and validated treatments, and (3) diagnostic confusion leads to patients being frustrated and skeptical of what health professionals have to offer. In addition, these factors may sometimes lead to health professionals avoiding difficult sexual pain treatment cases.

Predictors of treatment outcome

Although we have suggested that most sexual pain cases are difficult to treat, many factors can contribute to the varying degrees of complexity. In particular, the degree of pain intensity has been shown to influence treatment outcome only modestly. More interestingly, key psychosocial factors that affect not only pain but also other dimensions of outcome (e.g., sexual function) have now been identified. Other factors that may play a role in adding to the burden of sexual pain include whether the pain is provoked or unprovoked, the time of onset of the disorder (lifelong or acquired), past sexual trauma, and the presence of complicating medical and psychologic problems. All of the above predictors of treatment outcome have been studied in dyspareunia populations. To our knowledge, no predictors of outcome for vaginismus have been reported.

Pain intensity and related psychosocial factors

We tend to assume that women who are suffering from more intense pain will present additional challenges for the health professional. This assumption is supported by empirical findings which show that the higher the pretreatment pain intensity, the worse the therapeutic outcome for both surgical[18] and psychosocial interventions for chronic pain.[19] Although pain intensity should be taken into account when assessing the difficulty of a case, the psychosocial factors that influence it may be even more important. We have recently found that psychologic variables, such as high degrees of pain catastrophizing (negative self-talk or rumination about pain) and low levels of self-efficacy (one's sense of mastery over the pain), explained 44% of the variance in pain intensity in women with vulvar vestibulitis syndrome – the main cause of dyspareunia in premenopausal women (Desrochers et al.[20]). Interestingly, the relationship between catastrophizing and pain was mediated by anxiety, suggesting that the more women with sexual pain tend to catastrophize, the more anxious they become, and this, in turn, has a negative impact on their experience of pain. Other studies have shown that increased anxiety is significantly related to increased pain in women with dyspareunia, whereas high relationship adjustment is related to decreased pain.[21,22] Similarly, high pain catastrophizing and low self-efficacy have been found to be reliable predictors of negative outcomes in cognitive-behavioral pain management and biofeedback,[23,24] as well as in surgical interventions for chronic pain.

Finally, Meana et al.,[22] in a sample of 100 women with dyspareunia, found that those who attributed their pain to psychosocial factors (i.e., internal attributions) tended to report higher psychologic and dyadic distress, as well as higher levels of pain and sexual dysfunction, than women who attributed their pain to physical factors (i.e., external attributions). These results indicate the importance of health professionals' conceptualizations of sexual pain, indicating that when they send the message that the pain is in the woman's head, they may inadvertently be causing iatrogenic harm. In summary, psychosocial factors appear to play an important role in modulating pain intensity and should be taken into account when assessing the degree of difficulty of a sexual pain case.

Despite the fact that elevated pain intensity is associated with a more complex clinical presentation, an increasing number of studies suggest that pain and related disability may be distinct and partially independent phenomena.[25] Our own work shows that there is a significant correlation ($r = 0.30$) between pain during intercourse and sexual function, as is the case for the association between pain and disability in other chronic pain populations.[25] Nonetheless, current studies in the area of sexual pain are beginning to show that other factors are more important than pain intensity in determining the degree of sexual dysfunction experienced by patients. For example, we have found that after controlling for pain intensity, low levels of self-efficacy explained 24% of the variance in sexual dysfunction in women with vulvar vestibulitis syndrome, whereas relationship adjustment explained 28% of the variance (Desrochers et al.[20]; Jodoin et al.[26]). Along the same lines, a 2.5-year follow-up of women with vulvar vestibulitis who took part in a randomized treatment outcome study has shown that factors such as conservative sexual attitudes and low confidence

in the efficacy of the treatment received explained a larger proportion of the variance in negative outcome than pretreatment degree of pain, although higher pretreatment pain intensity was modestly predictive of a worse outcome.[27] These findings represent another line of evidence supporting the important role of psychosocial factors in the expression of sexual pain and in determining the relative difficulty of a given case.

Provoked versus unprovoked pain

Both clinical reports and empirical data demonstrate that women with unprovoked or chronic pain show higher levels of psychologic distress and respond less favorably to certain therapeutic approaches than those with provoked or recurrent pain. More specifically, women suffering from essential vulvodynia (i.e., unprovoked vulvar dysesthesia) report greater interference with their sexual function and more hypochondriasis, anxiety, and somatization than women suffering from other vulvar disorders.[28] However, these results may stem in part from the idiopathic nature of vulvodynia compared with the better-circumscribed vulvar disorders with which it was compared in this study. As for treatment, one study has shown that women with essential vulvodynia respond less favorably to a surgical approach than women with vulvar vestibulitis, thereby concluding that surgery should be proscribed for this group of patients.[29]

Lifelong versus acquired

It is also thought that a lifelong history of sexual pain may not result in as positive an outcome as an acquired problem, where episodes of painless sex have been experienced. This is intuitively appealing, as it might be harder for a woman to diminish her pain and penetration anxiety if she has never known intercourse without such pain. At least one study has shown that women suffering from vulvar vestibulitis and undergoing surgical intervention do not benefit as much from the procedure if they have had the condition since their first intercourse attempt.[29] Unfortunately, there are very few data to support the assumption that lifelong cases are more difficult to treat. Specifically, the number of years since the onset of the problem is not a predictor of treatment outcome for cognitive-behavioral therapy, biofeedback, or vestibulectomy in women with vulvar vestibulitis.[27]

Past sexual trauma

Recent empirical findings suggest that women with idiopathic vulvar pain – an important source of dyspareunia and vaginismus – are exposed to factors that influence their risk of developing genital pain well before menarche, as in early-childhood victimization.[30] Clinically, it is often found that cases where the woman presented a history of sexual trauma were somewhat more difficult to treat due to the additional time and work involved in processing the traumatic event. Although sexual trauma has not been investigated as a predictor of outcome in the treatment of the sexual pain disorders, studies focusing on psychosocial interventions for pain have found that a history of sexual abuse is a significant predictor of poorer outcome.[19] Interestingly, results from a recent study suggest that women diagnosed with vaginismus report significantly more sexual abuse than women with vulvar vestibulitis.[8]

Other medical and psychologic problems

Complicating medical problems include chronic dermatologic conditions leading to painful intercourse, such as lichen sclerosus and lichen planus, as well as vulvar fissures. Many of these conditions can be managed with topical ointments, such as strong corticosteroids, although they can never be cured. Thus, the therapeutic goal becomes one of helping the woman and her partner adjust to sex given a chronic genital condition, focusing on education regarding the impact of this condition on sexual function.

Certain psychologic problems, mainly personality disorders, clinical depression, or an anxiety disorder, can further complicate the clinical picture and modify the health professional's therapeutic goals and expectations. Studies on the predictors of surgical outcome in pain populations suggest not only that psychologic factors are the best predictors of outcome, but also that hypochondriasis and anxiety in particular are related to worse surgical outcomes, as is the presence of severe relationship distress.[18] In terms of psychologic predictors of treatment outcome for psychosocial pain treatment programs, somatization, depression, and anxiety have all been shown to be associated with poorer outcomes.[19] In the case of sexual pain disorders, lifelong vaginismus in particular is characterized by a strong phobic element associated with a significant avoidance of any form of attempt at vaginal penetration,[3] which tends to make the resolution of the pain problem more complicated. The following case vignette illustrates the difficulties involved in treating a case of lifelong vaginismus where the woman presented with other psychologic problems, and the couple struggled with issues such as poor communication, lack of trust, and ambivalence about having children.

A couple in their thirties were referred to a sex and couple therapy clinic by the woman's gynecologist for "fear of sex". Laurie and Tony had been married for 9 years, and had dated for 6 years prior to their marriage. They had no children and both came from a religious background. Tony worked in a family business, and Laurie was not working at the time of the assessment. She suffered from an anxiety disorder and had taken a sick leave from work in an attempt to reduce stress in her life.

Laurie was diagnosed with lifelong and generalized vaginismus. Neither Laurie nor Tony had had much sexual experience before they started dating. Laurie had never explored her body or masturbated, and had never experienced orgasm. She seemed uncomfortable discussing most aspects of sexuality, and lacked even the basic vocabulary to express sexual concepts.

It also became gradually obvious to the therapist that the couple did not communicate well, and that there remained trust issues from problems unrelated to the vaginismus. When confronted with this observation, they maintained that their communication was fine, and that they were not interested in working on it, even if it might help them work on the sexual problem. Laurie and Tony, very impatient for penetration to happen, decided to aim for penetration for the sake of conception. They wanted to conceive since they were now in their mid-thirties and "time was running out". They were also under much pressure from the family, who could not understand what was taking them so long to start a family. However, it became apparent that Laurie was ambivalent about having children and that this was impeding progress in therapy. Laurie made excuses as to why the therapy homework exercises were not done; she started canceling sessions and talking about issues other than the sexual problem. Treatment ended with Laurie having completed her first gynecologic examination but not having achieved vaginal penetration with her husband.

In summary, difficult cases can be conceptualized as ones in which there are multiple problem areas in addition to the sexual pain, rendering a resolution less likely both in the eyes of the patient and in those of the treating health professional(s). Psychosocial factors in particular, such as high catastrophizing, low self-efficacy, internal attributions, poor relationship adjustment, and past sexual trauma, appear to be important determinants of pain and related sexual function. In addition, confidence in the efficacy of treatment is a significant predictor of outcome for dyspareunia, highlighting the importance of how we approach what we consider to be difficult cases and the types of expectations that we foster in these patients.

Strategies for treating difficult cases

Considering the diagnostic confusion that prevails in the area of sexual pain, one of the first steps to facilitate the treatment of a difficult case is to conduct a careful evaluation in order to determine the appropriate diagnosis, and to devise an adequate treatment plan. This is ideally done in a multidisciplinary fashion, with a gynecologist or dermatologist establishing a medical diagnosis, and psychologists/sexologists and/or physical therapists assessing the cognitive, affective, behavioral and muscular dimensions of the condition.[31] A thorough description of the evaluative procedure is beyond the scope of this chapter.

Probably the single most important treatment strategy for dealing with difficult cases is the adoption of a multimodal perspective, independent of one's training background.[32] This model is currently the reference standard in the treatment of other pain problems and has proven successful in reducing pain and disability.[33] The advantages of working within such a conceptual framework are multiple; it is probably the only model that provides the ability to address the varied problem areas typically presented by difficult sexual pain cases. The multimodal approach also holds the potential to accelerate patient recovery, as it targets multiple symptoms simultaneously, early in the treatment process, symptoms such as pain and sexual function, which tend to be interdependent. Therefore, a change in one problem area usually brings about a change in another problem area, fostering patient hope and satisfaction with treatment. Initial therapeutic gains are also facilitated by patients having access to all relevant health professionals from the very beginning, an advantage that is not provided by the referral model, in which patients must wait many months between visits to different health professionals. Those currently using a multimodal approach for the treatment of dyspareunia resulting from vulvar vestibulitis have reported that, in addition to its being quite successful, it has the benefit of saving a large proportion of these women from surgical intervention.[34] However, no randomized treatment outcome study to date has compared a multimodal approach to a unimodal one in the treatment of sexual pain.

Adopting a multimodal, multidisciplinary model for patient care is associated with specific theoretic and clinical ramifications (see Chapter 17.6). First, in line with current conceptualizations of chronic and recurrent pain problems, this model emphasizes the interdependent roles of biologic, cognitive, affective, behavioral, and interpersonal factors that contribute to the development and maintenance of sexual pain,[35] suggesting that multiple etiologic pathways may lead to similar symptom presentations.[1]

Second, from a clinical point of view, a multimodal approach is based on the acknowledgment that no single discipline has all the answers and that one will not be able to manage a difficult case successfully without the close collaboration of trusted colleagues from other health-care professions. Thus, adopting a multimodal perspective necessarily involves working as a multidisciplinary team, albeit sometimes a virtual one. This is often the case in North America, since the organization of health services does not facilitate the application of this model of care. Nonetheless, a good way to apply this model is when a central team member is responsible for organizing and planning patient care, treatment decisions (in conjunction with the patient), and referrals to other health professionals.

The elaboration of goals constitutes a crucial step in instilling hope and stimulating faith in the proposed treatment, particularly short-term ones. Some types of goals tend to foster further disappointments while others strengthen the patient–health professional alliance and promote self-efficacy. In an attempt to create healthy, realistic expectations, it is preferable to avoid making the complete elimination of pain an absolute goal, but rather to provide detailed information concerning the multiple life areas that may improve after treatment, such as sexual function and relationship satisfaction. Additionally, it is helpful not to make the increase in frequency of sexual activities or intercourse a goal *per se*; that would only further stigmatize and alienate the woman suffering from a complicated case of sexual pain.[31] A useful alternative lies in having the partner participate in the treatment program – including all medical visits – and helping the couple regain enjoyment in nonpenetrative sexual activities. The following case vignette illustrates the use of a multimodal perspective in the treatment of a difficult case of dyspareunia involving other medical, psychologic, and relationship problems, but without a central team member coordinating patient care.

Lisa, aged 35, was referred to a sex and couple therapy clinic by her general practitioner, whom she had consulted for anxiety and depression following the development of dyspareunia and chronic vulvar pain. At the time of the assessment, she was taking antidepressants to manage her psychologic difficulties. Lisa had been married for 5 years and stated that she was unhappy and unfulfilled in her marriage. She reported never particularly enjoying sex and never having much sexual desire – even prior to the onset of the dyspareunia. She and her husband engaged in sexual activities without vaginal penetration about three to four times a year. Since the onset of her dyspareunia, she had no desire for sex and he had stopped initiating after her repeated refusals. Other issues present in the clinical picture included a profound dissatisfaction with her work, and strong dependency needs vis-à-vis her husband, coupled with resentment toward him for controlling most aspects of their marriage. The husband chose not to be a part of the therapy.

The goals that were established with Lisa were to (1) reduce her pain and its impact on her life, (2) increase her assertiveness with her husband, (3) break the avoidance pattern that they had developed surrounding the sexual pain problem by communicating about it, and (4) decrease her anxiety and depression. It was agreed that Lisa would continue seeing her general practitioner and gynecologist to facilitate the management of her psychologic symptoms and medical condition. However, there was no communication between the psychologist and the two physicians. Lisa had also tried physical therapy in the past, but felt she had not benefited from it. She had never done the recommended exercises and experienced some degree of guilt over what she qualified as an unsuccessful outcome.

It was difficult at first to establish a therapeutic alliance with Lisa, as she was generally skeptical of how a psychologist could help her alleviate her pain and improve her overall sexual and relationship satisfaction. Initial work focused on helping her reconceptualize her pain problem as a multidimensional one over which she had some degree of control, via a pain diary in which she noted what factors appeared to affect her pain and the distress it provoked. She was also taught breathing exercises and cognitive restructuring to learn to manage her pain. Despite initial efforts to work on the avoidance pattern and sexual dysfunction, this avenue appeared to lead nowhere. However, some improvements were noted, such as a reduction in Lisa's chronic vulvar pain and professional dissatisfaction.

Efforts were made to understand and confront Lisa's ambivalence about getting better and her inconsistent commitment to therapy. These efforts contributed to clarify what factors were holding her back and to address these in a more direct fashion. Shortly thereafter, Lisa began being more assertive with her husband regarding her needs in the relationship, to which he responded positively. Lisa broached the topic of sexual pain with him and realized that he was in fact feeling quite hurt and rejected by her lack of interest in sex. They then began to make changes in their sex life, with Lisa asserting her sexual needs, and this led to more satisfying sex and increased desire and arousal. Soon thereafter, Lisa's sexual desire developed significantly, and she and her husband began to engage in sexual activities once a week. Although intercourse was still painful, the couple had begun discussing having children. Lisa decided to start her physical therapy treatments again. The sex therapy work then focused on keeping her motivated to do the exercises and building a graded dilation hierarchy in collaboration with the physical therapist. The treatment ended prematurely due to the pregnancy leave of the therapist, but Lisa continued seeing her physical therapist, her general practitioner, and her gynecologist.

The following case is an example of how a well-coordinated, multimodal approach led by a gynecologist can maintain patient hope and treatment adherence despite an arduous process to recovery.

Julie, now 25, developed dyspareunia after a series of repeated yeast infections during her early twenties, which were alternately treated with prescription antifungal creams, over-the-counter ones without confirmation of a diagnosis, and an oral antifungal agent – none helped her pain. After these unsuccessful treatment attempts, Julie consulted a gynecologist, who specialized in the treatment of dyspareunia and vulvodynia. After a careful evaluation, he explained that the treatment of her problem might take many months and involve more than one health professional, since she had had the pain for a number of years, had tense circumvaginal muscles, and did not presently engage in intercourse out of fear of pain and lack of desire. After recommending medical visits at 3-month intervals and prescribing an anesthetic gel, he referred Julie to a sex therapist, with whom treatment focused on increasing her desire and arousal and reducing her fear of pain. Her comfort with sexuality and her romantic relationship improved, but her dyspareunia was only slightly alleviated. After discussing Julie's progress with the sex therapist and with the patient herself, the gynecologist referred her to a physical therapist, who worked on reducing the tension in her pelvic floor. Based on the biofeedback monitor and on the gynecologist's observations, Julie's muscles appeared less tense, but the patient was still rarely engaging in intercourse, since her pain was still present. Finally, the gynecologist suggested that he perform a vestibulectomy, which was successful in reducing her pain. However, Julie remained fearful of intercourse and went back to the sex therapist, upon recommendation of her physician, to increase her comfort with vaginal penetration. Julie now enjoys pain-free intercourse and is grateful to her gynecologist, who recently delivered her first baby.

Why work with difficult sexual pain cases?

The very issues that make sexual pain disorders so challenging are also the ones that make them one of the most interesting women's sexual dysfunctions to treat: the complexity of the clinical picture and the interrelation of the many etiologic factors involved, and the impact on several important areas of life all contribute to our interest in treating difficult sexual pain disorders.[31] More importantly, the high prevalence of sexual pain disorders, combined with the paucity of adequate treatments for this women's sexual health problem, makes this work all the more meaningful and valuable.

References

1. Binik YM, Meana M, Berkley K et al. The sexual pain disorders: is the pain sexual or is the sex painful? *Annu Rev Sex Res* 1999; 10: 210–35.
2. Van Lankveld JJDM, Brewaeys AMA, Ter Kuile MM et al. Difficulties in the differential diagnosis of vaginismus, dyspareunia and mixed sexual pain disorder. *J Psychosom Obstet Gynaecol* 1995; 16: 201–9.
3. Reissing ED, Binik YM, Khalifé S et al. Vaginal spasm, pain, and behavior: an empirical investigation of the diagnosis of vaginismus. *Arch Sex Behav* 2004; 33: 5–17.
4. Bergeron S, Binik YM, Khalifé S et al. A randomized comparison of group cognitive-behavioral therapy, surface electromyographic biofeedback, and vestibulectomy in the treatment of dyspareunia resulting from vulvar vestibulitis. *Pain* 2001; 91: 297–306.
5. Meana M, Binik YM, Khalifé S et al. Biopsychosocial profile of women with dyspareunia. *Obstet Gynecol* 1997; 90: 583–9.
6. Van Lankveld JJ, Weijenborg PT, Ter Kuile MM. Psychologic profiles of and sexual function in women with vulvar vestibulitis and their partners. *Obstet Gynecol* 1996; 88: 65–70.
7. Danielsson I, Sjoberg I, Wikman M. Vulvar vestibulitis: medical, psychosexual and psychosocial aspects, a case-control study. *Acta Obstet Gynecol Scand* 2000; 79: 872–8.
8. Reissing ED, Binik YM, Khalifé S et al. Etiological correlates of vaginismus: sexual and physical abuse, sexual knowledge, sexual self-schema, and relationship adjustment. *J Sex Marital Ther* 2003; 29: 47–59.
9. American Psychiatric Association. *Diagnostic and Statistical Manual of Mental Disorders*, 4th edn. (DSM-IV). Washington, DC: 1994.
10. Rosen RC, Leiblum SR. Treatment of sexual disorders in the 1990's: an integrated approach. *J Consult Clin Psychol* 1995; 63: 877–90.
11. Jamieson DJ, Steege JF. The prevalence of dysmenorrhea, dyspareunia, pelvic pain, and irritable bowel syndrome in primary care practices. *Obstet Gynecol* 1996; 87: 55–8.
12. Harlow BL, Wise LA, Stewart EG. Prevalence and predictors of lower genital tract discomfort. *Am J Obstet Gynecol* 2001; 185: 545–50.
13. Bornstein J, Livrat G, Stolar Z et al. Pure versus complicated vulvar vestibulitis: a randomized trial of fluconazole treatment. *Gynecol Obstet Invest* 2000; 50: 194–7.
14. Njirjesy P, Sobel JD, Weitz MV et al. Cromolyn cream for recalcitrant vulvar vestibulitis: results of a placebo controlled study. *Sex Transm Infect* 2001; 77: 53–7.

15. Weijmar Shultz WCM, Gianotten WL, Van Der Meijden WI et al. Behavioural approach with or without surgical intervention for the vulvar vestibulitis syndrome: a prospective randomized and non-randomized study. *J Psychosom Obstet Gynaecol* 1996; 17: 143–8.

16. Reissing ED, Binik YM, Khalifé S. Does vaginismus exist? A critical review of the literature. *J Nerv Ment Dis* 1999; 187: 261–74.

17. de Kruiff ME, ter Kuile MM, Weijenborg PThM et al. Vaginismus and dyspareunia: Is there difference in clinical presentation? *J Psychosom Obstet Gynaecol* 2000; 2: 149–55.

18. Block AR. Presurgical psychological screening in chronic pain syndromes: psychosocial risk factors for poor surgical results. In RJ Gatchel, DC Turk, eds. *Psychosocial Factors in Pain: Critical Perspectives.* New York: Guilford Press, 1999: 390–400.

19. Gatchel RJ, Epker J. Psychosocial predictors of chronic pain and response to treatment. In RJ Gatchel, DC Turk, eds. *Psychosocial Factors in Pain: Critical Perspectives.* New York: Guilford Press, 1999: 412–34.

20. Descrochers G, Bergeron S, Khalifé S et al. Vulvar vestibulitis syndrome: the consequences of pain anxiety and hypervigilance on pain and sexual impairment. Poster presented at the XVII World Congress of Sexology, July 2005; Montreal, Canada.

21. Meana M, Binik YM, Khalifé S et al. Affect and marital adjustment in women's rating of dyspareunic pain. *Can J Psychiatry* 1998; 43: 381–4.

22. Meana M, Binik YM, Khalifé S et al. Psychosocial correlates of pain attributions in women with dyspareunia. *Psychosomatics* 1999; 40: 497–502.

23. Nicholas MK, Wilson PH, Goyen J. Comparison of cognitive-behavioral group treatment and an alternative non-psychological treatment for chronic low back pain. *Pain* 1992; 48: 339–47.

24. Turner JA, Clancy S. Strategies for coping with chronic low back pain: relationship to pain and disability. *Pain* 1986; 24: 355–66.

25. Sullivan MJ, Stanish W, Waite H et al. Catastrophizing, pain, and disability in patients with soft-tissue injuries. *Pain* 1998; 77: 253–60.

26. Jodoin M, Bergeron S, Khalifé S et al. Attributions of responsibility for pain in vulvar vestibulitis syndrome. Poster presented at the XVII World Congress of Sexology, July 2005: Montreal, Canada.

27. Bergeron S, Binik YM, Khalifé S et al. Facteurs associés au succès thérapeutique dans le traitement de la vestibulite vulvaire. In J Levy, D Maisonneuve, DH Bilodeau et al., eds. *Enjeux psychosociaux de la santé.* Montréal: Presses de l'Université du Québec, 2003: 135–49.

28. Stewart DE, Reicher AE, Gerulath AH et al. Vulvodynia and psychological distress. *Obstet Gynecol* 1994; 84: 587–90.

29. Bornstein J, Goldik Z, Stolar Z et al. Predicting outcome of the surgical treatment of vulvar vestibulitis. *Obstet Gynecol* 1997; 89: 695–8.

30. Harlow BL, Stewart EG. A population-based assessment of chronic unexplained vulvar pain: have we underestimated the prevalence of vulvodynia? *J Am Med Womens Assoc* 2003; 58: 82–8.

31. Bergeron S, Meana M, Binik YM et al. Painful genital sexual activity. In SB Levine, CB Risen, S Althof, eds. *Handbook of Clinical Sexuality for Mental Health Professionals.* New York: Brunner-Routledge, 2003: 131–52.

32. Bergeron S, Binik YM, Khalifé S et al. The treatment of vulvar vestibulitis syndrome: Toward a multimodal approach. *Sex Marital Ther* 1997; 12: 305–11.

33. Flor H, Fydrich T, Turk DC. Efficacy of multidisciplinary pain treatment centers: a meta-analytic review. *Pain* 1992; 49: 221–30.

34. Weijmar Schultz WCM, van de Wiel HBM. Vulvar vestibulitis syndrome, care made to measure. *J Psychosom Obstet Gynaecol* 2002; 23: 5–7.

35. Melzack R, Wall PD. *The Challenge of Pain,* 2nd edn. London: Penguin, 1996.

HORMONAL TREATMENT OF FEMALE SEXUAL DYSFUNCTION

13.1 Available therapies and outcome results in premenopausal women

Susan R Davis

Introduction

Sexual activity in women is complex, involving biochemical, neurophysiologic, and cognitive processes. Psychologic functioning, past sexual history, the availability and presence of a partner, body image, life issues, and the culture and the society of a particular birth cohort contribute significantly to the multivariate nature of female sexuality (see Chapters 2.1–2.4 of this book). This chapter specifically focuses on the endocrine treatment of female sexual dysfunction in premenopausal women, with the assumption that the psychosocial aspects discussed in Chapters 3.1–3.4 and 9.3 are always addressed when any woman presenting with female sexual dysfunction is assessed.

The endogenous hormones that potentially influence female sexuality include estrogens, androgens, progesterone, prolactin, oxytocin, and glucocorticosteroids. These each interact with numerous neurochemicals within the central and peripheral nervous system. The latter include serotonin, catecholamines, dopamine, other neurotransmitters, and other hormones. The factors that determine the outcome of these complex interactions include the absolute levels of each hormone, their absolute receptor content, and the presence and levels of specific coactivator and corepressor proteins that modify the transcriptional response and the up- or down-regulation of receptor levels by other hormones (see Chapters 4.3, 5.3–5.5, and 6.1–6.3). Estrogens and androgens also influence vascular function by both endothelium-dependent and -independent mechanisms,[1] and thus have a vital role in maintenance of the health of the female genital tract as well as in arousal and orgasm. Research on female sexual dysfunction in premenopausal women has relied primarily on observational data, and in vitro and in vivo animal models (see Chapter 5.6), and few randomized, placebo-controlled trials have been published. Thus, insufficient data are available to support specific endocrine therapy for otherwise well, premenopausal women with female sexual dysfunction.

Endocrine and intracrine sources of sex steroids in women

Phylogenetic analysis of steroid receptors (see Chapter 5.5) indicates that the first steroid receptor was an estrogen receptor, followed by a progesterone receptor.[2] Specific regulation of physiologic processes by androgens and corticoids is a relatively recent innovation that emerged after these duplications.[2] Thus, in humans, androgens in ovaries are obligatory precursors of the biosynthesis of estrogens by the aromatase cytochrome P450 enzyme. Estrone is formed by the aromatization of androstenedione and estradiol by the aromatization of testosterone.

Throughout the reproductive years, the ovaries are a primary source of estradiol for action on peripheral target tissues under the control of follicle-stimulating hormone and inhibin. However, synthesis of estrogens from adrenal and ovarian androgen precursors within extragonadal compartments occurs throughout reproductive life.[3]

The primary source of circulating progesterone in premenopausal women is cyclic production by the ovaries. Serum progesterone concentrations are significantly correlated with brain tissue concentrations, suggesting that serum levels are a primary source for brain uptake,[4,5] although progesterone can also be synthesized within the brain.[6]

Androgens are 19-carbon steroid hormones that are associated with the induction of male secondary sexual characteristics. In women, androgens circulate in the concentration range nanomolar to micromolar, in contrast to the estrogens whose circulating concentrations are in the picomolar range. In descending order of their serum concentrations, the major androgens found in women include dehydroepiandrosterone sulfate, dehydroepiandrosterone, androstenedione testosterone, and dihydrotestosterone. Giving testosterone a reference potency of 100, the relative androgenic activities of the other members of the class are: dihydrotestosterone, 300; androstenedione, 10; and dehydroepiandrosterone and dehydroepiandrosterone sulfate, 5. Biosynthesis of the androgens takes place both in the adrenal and in the ovary. Dehydroepiandrosterone secretion is acutely stimulated by adrenocorticotropic hormone;[7,8] however, dehydroepiandrosterone sulfate, which has a long plasma half-life, may not acutely increase after adrenocorticotropic hormone administration.[9]

Changes in sex steroids during the menstrual cycle and with age

In premenopausal women with regular menstrual cycles, there is a rise in estradiol, testosterone, and androstenedione in the late follicular phase of the menstrual cycle and in the luteal phase.[10,11] There is also a diurnal variation in testosterone in women with the peak in the morning.[12] The luteal phase is characterized by the rise in progesterone. Estradiol and progesterone levels fall when ovulation ceases, as at menopause. In contrast, total and free testosterone levels fall from the third to the fifth decade in premenopausal women, such that women in their 40s have about half the circulating levels of women in their 20s.[13,14] Furthermore, in the late reproductive years, there is failure of the midcycle rise in free testosterone which characterizes the menstrual cycle in young ovulating women.[15]

The levels of dehydroepiandrosterone sulfate and dehydroepiandrosterone also fall with increasing age.[16] This may contribute significantly to the decline in total and free testosterone level with age, as dehydroepiandrosterone sulfate serves as a prehormone for about half of ovarian testosterone production[17] (see Chapter 6.3).

Metabolism and action of sex steroids

Traditionally, hormonal action has been understood as endocrine and paracrine, and measurement of circulating hormone levels has been used as a determinant of tissue exposure. However, more recently, the complexity of steroid action has been appreciated.[18] Labrie et al. defined intracrinology:

"Intracrine activity describes the formation of active hormones that exert their action in the same cells in which synthesis took place without release into the pericellular compartment."[19] Tissue sensitivity to androgens varies according to the amount and activity of the enzymes 5α-reductase and aromatase, which may vary considerably between individuals. Tissue responses may also vary with subtle differences in individual receptors. For example, the number of repeat sequences of cytosine, adenine, and guanine nucleotides, CAG repeats, in the deoxyribonucleic acid (DNA) molecule coding for the androgen receptor may vary in individuals. Thus, even with highly sensitive assays for sex steroids, the measurement of any sex steroid will provide only an indication of deficiency or excess, but not an absolute measure of tissue exposure or tissue sensitivity and responsiveness, and the clinical features will be the mainstay of diagnosis. This, unfortunately, limits much of the data pertaining to sex steroids and female sexual function.

Importance of sex hormone-binding globulin

Many steroids circulate tightly bound to sex hormone-binding globulin, which is a pivotal determinant of their bioavailability.[20] In normal, reproductive-aged women, 82% of the binding sites of sex hormone-binding globulin are unoccupied. For the occupied binding sites, androstendiol is the major sex hormone-binding globulin ligand, followed by dehydroepiandrosterone, testosterone, cortisol, cortisone, dihydrotestosterone, and androstenedione. Conversely, the binding affinity for steroids bound by sex hormone-binding globulin is dihydrotestosterone > testosterone > androstenediol > estradiol > estrone. Sex hormone-binding globulin also weakly binds dehydroepiandrosterone, but not dehydroepiandrosterone sulfate.[20] Because of its high affinity for sex hormone-binding globulin, only 1–2% of total circulating testosterone is free or biologically available under normal physiologic conditions in women.[20] Elevations in estradiol (as occurs during pregnancy), hyperthyroidism, and liver disease cause a marked increase in sex hormone-binding globulin levels, whereas hypothyroidism, obesity, and hyperinsulinemia are associated with decreased sex hormone-binding globulin levels. In addition, oral administration of steroid hormones and their analogs can alter sex hormone-binding globulin levels, whereas parenteral administration of these compounds typically has a much weaker influence. The standard dose of oral estrogen used in the oral contraceptive pill will increase sex hormone-binding globulin. Lower sex hormone-binding globulin levels enable increased clearance of testosterone, whereas higher sex hormone-binding globulin levels are associated with a decrease in clearance. Thus, women with high sex hormone-binding globulin, such as women on the oral contraceptive pill, have a greater total testosterone, and women with low sex hormone-binding globulin have little change in their total testosterone level with exogenous therapy. As total testosterone is a poor indicator of androgen exposure, the concentration of free testosterone or non-sex hormone-binding globulin-bound testosterone, so-called bioavailable testosterone, should be measured after testosterone therapy. Such assays may not always be reliable or available. As sex hormone-binding globulin levels may fall somewhat with increased circulating testosterone, baseline sex hormone-binding globulin may be a useful predictor of risk of excess androgenization with testosterone treatment, and should be measured in all women prior to such therapy. Sex hormone-binding globulin levels do not vary with age in premenopausal women.[14,21]

Hormones and hypoactive sexual desire disorder

As sexuality is multifactorial and mechanistic studies in humans cannot clearly elucidate the role of hormones in sexual function, rodent models of sexually receptive behaviors have been used to gain insight into some of the actions of sex steroids. There is, however, no animal model for female arousal or orgasm, and the influence of cognitive factors, such as fantasy, cannot be studied in animals. Vaginal plethysmography (see Chapter 10.1) has been used in human studies; however, the correlation between blood flow measures and verbal reports of arousal is poor.[22–24]

The central role of estrogens in sexual function

Estradiol and testosterone are both present in the human female brain, with the highest concentrations of estradiol measured in the hypothalamus and the preoptic area, and of testosterone, in the substantia nigra, hypothalamus, and preoptic area[25] (see Chapter 5.3). The concentration of testosterone is several times higher than estradiol in each of these regions, with the highest ratio of testosterone to estradiol demonstrated in the hypothalamus and preoptic area. This distribution corresponds with the high aromatase activity found in these regions in animals.[26] It is biologically plausible that within these regions testosterone is aromatized to estradiol, resulting in high estradiol concentrations that then modify sexual behavior.

Animal studies of hormones and female sexual function

Both estrogen receptors (estrogen receptors α and β) are expressed in the primate brain.[27] Estrogen exhibits widespread actions throughout the brain, both via its receptors, and non-genomically, with interactions with many neurotransmitter systems, including catecholaminergic, serotoninergic, cholinergic, and γ-aminobutyric acidergic systems.[28,29] Oophorectomized rats and mice exhibit no lordotic behavior, but they have no estrogens or androgens because their adrenals do not make C19 steroids. Estrogen therapy alone has little or no effect on restoration of lordosis in oophorectomized mice, but after estrogen priming, progesterone restores lordosis.[30]

To clarify the possible role of each of the estrogen receptors and estrogen action in sexual behaviors, mice in which each or both estrogen receptors have been knocked out, or in which the aromatase enzyme has been mutated (aromatase knockout), have been studied. In each of these models, serum testosterone is normal or elevated. Behavioral changes evaluated have included female sexual receptivity (lordosis posturing), aggression, and pup-caring behavior. Mice in which the estrogen receptor α has been knocked out (estrogen receptor knockout mice) exhibit no lordosis behavior, reduced pup caring, and increased aggression.[31] In contrast, the mice in which the estrogen receptor β has been knocked out (beta estrogen receptor knockout mice) exhibit normal sexual function.[31] In female aromatase knockout mice, which are completely estrogen deficient, there is marked loss of lordosis.[32] Residual lordotic behavior in the aromatase knockout mice indicates that neuronal pathways may be activated in a ligand-independent manner by the intact estrogen receptor. When both estrogen receptors α and β are knocked out, there is complete loss of sexual function in the animals despite the presence of normal testosterone levels.[31] Taken together, these data indicate that, in the mouse model, estrogen receptor α is crucial for lordotic behavior, and that, despite lack of a relationship between circulating estradiol levels and sexual parameters, estradiol and the estrogen receptors have an essential role in the neurobiology of sexual behavior in animal models.

There no evidence from randomized clinical trials that treatment of premenopausal women with estradiol improves sexual function.

Central effects of progesterone

The progesterone receptor exists in two different molecular forms, progesterone receptor-A and progesterone receptor-B. Progesterone receptors are also present in the brain.[33] The function and role of the two different isoforms in the brain have not been defined, and pharmacologic approaches using ligand antagonists and knockout models do not distinguish between the two isoforms. Progesterone, like estrogen, modulates gene expression in the rodent hypothalamus and thus regulates neuronal networks that control female sexual behavior. Estradiol increases the expression of progesterone receptor, which in turn functions as a critical coordinator of key regulator events associated with the sexual response.[33] The results of various studies using the progesterone antagonist RU 486, intracerebral administration of antisense nucleotides, and progesterone receptor knockout mice confirm that facilitation of sexual behavior of rodents by progesterone is mediated both by estradiol-induced genomic activation of neural progesterone receptor and by a process involving ligand-independent action of the progesterone receptor via the cell membrane dopamine$_1$ receptor (D$_1$).[33] It is believed that activation of cell membrane receptors results in a signal transduction cascade that leads to phosphorylation of the progesterone receptor or a specific coactivator, and hence neuronal effects. In animal models, progesterone facilitation of lordosis is also influenced by the cannabinoids.[34] There is no evidence from randomized clinical trials that treatment of premenopausal women with progesterone improves sexual function.

Adrenal preandrogens

Dehydroepiandrosterone is converted to both testosterone and estradiol; therefore, any positive effects of dehydroepiandrosterone on sexual function cannot distinguish between the role of dehydroepiandrosterone alone or as a precursor of testosterone and/or estradiol. The effects of oral dehydroepiandrosterone on the sexual function of women have been evaluated in a few placebo-controlled, randomized, clinical trials with inconsistent findings. In a crossover study of 24 women with adrenal insufficiency, sexual thoughts, interest, and satisfaction (mental and physical) increased significantly after 4 months of active treatment (50 mg/day).[35] In this study, serum testosterone was increased from below normal to the lower part of the normal range by the therapy. Two other studies of women with Addison's disease found no effect of the same dose of dehydroepiandrosterone on cognitive or sexual function.[36,37] Significant improvements in self-esteem, mood, and fatigue were observed.[36,37] In perimenopausal women without adrenal deficiency, a parallel-group, placebo-controlled, randomized, clinical trial did not show improvements in libido in 66 perimenopausal women treated with 50 mg/day dehydroepiandrosterone for 4 months.[38] However, an open-label study of dehydroepiandrosterone treatment (50 mg/day) in 113 healthy women with diminished desire, arousal, and orgasmic capacity showed improvement in desire, arousal, lubrication, orgasm, and satisfaction ($p < 0.05$).[39]

In summary, there are no strong data to show beneficial effects of exogenous dehydroepiandrosterone on sexual function in health or in adrenal insufficiency.

Role of testosterone in premenopausal women

Evidence from basic research and physiology

Androgen receptor message ribonucleic acid (mRNA)-containing neurons are widely distributed in the female rat brain, with the greatest densities in neurons in the hypothalamus, and in regions of the telencephalon that provide strong inputs in the medial preoptic and ventromedial nuclei, each of which is thought to play a key role in mediating the hormonal control of sexual behavior, as well as in the lateral septal nucleus, the medial and cortical nuclei of the amygdala, the amygdalohippocampal area, and the bed nucleus of the stria terminalis.[40] In the adult, male, cynomolgus monkey, high densities of P450 aromatase and androgen receptor mRNA-containing neurons were observed in discrete hypothalamic areas involved in the regulation of gonadotropin secretion and reproductive behavior.[41] All areas that contained P450 aromatase mRNA-expressing cells also contained androgen receptor mRNA-expressing cells. However, there were areas in which androgen receptor mRNA was expressed, but not P450 aromatase mRNA, suggesting that testosterone acts via different signaling mechanisms in specific brain regions.[41] No equivalent data are available for humans or female primates. In rodent models, as reviewed above, testosterone does not maintain normal sexual behavior in the absence of estrogen action.

Evidence from studies in humans

Studies examining the relationships between circulating endogenous testosterone levels and sexual activity in premenopausal women have produced varying results. In several small studies, low sexual desire had been associated with lower testosterone and dehydroepiandrosterone sulfate levels.[42-44] In contrast, other researchers have reported that decreased libido is associated with greater fluctuations in testosterone in the late reproductive years.[45] Cawood and Bancroft reported no relationship between androgens and sexual parameters in 141 volunteer non-hormone therapy users aged 40–60 years.[46]

As young women who undergo bilateral oophorectomy experience an approximately 50% reduction in circulating testosterone concentrations,[47] the study of young women after oophorectomy has provided one approach to evaluate the effects of low testosterone levels on sexual function. However, there are several confounders in such studies, including the benefit of treating the problem that required the surgery in the first place and possible adverse effects of the surgery. Overall, observational studies of oophorectomized women suggest that decreased testosterone levels may affect sexual function in some women, although many women report improved sexual well-being after bilateral oophorectomy.[48,49]

Only one randomized, clinical trial of testosterone therapy has been reported in premenopausal women.[50] This crossover study involved 45 premenopausal women presenting with low libido. Transdermal testosterone, administered as a cream, was reported to improve significantly sexual motivation, fantasy, frequency of sexual activity, pleasure, orgasm, and satisfaction.[50] In addition to the positive effects on sexual function, testosterone significantly improved the total score and all subscale scores of the Personal General Well-Being Index in premenopausal women.[50] The mean free androgen index was just above the proposed upper limit for young women, although no true range has been formally established for this estimate of free testosterone.

Hormones and sexual arousal

It is becoming clear that inadequate sexual arousal may in part be due to decreased blood flow to the sexually responsive organs. While atherosclerosis may be implicated in older women with vascular risk factors, it seems that hormonal changes may play a part in younger women.

Estrogen influences vascular function via genomic and nongenomic mechanisms.[1] Estrogen has direct effects on genital anatomy, enhancing peripheral blood flow and peripheral nerve function, and improving vaginal lubrication.[51]

Testosterone appears to be important for its vasomotor effects,[52] enhancing vaginal blood flow and lubrication.[53,54] These effects may be due to direct androgen actions or partly to estradiol biosynthesis from testosterone in the vascular bed.[55] Cellular research indicates that vaginal tissue may express a specific nuclear receptor for the very powerful androgen, $\Delta 5$-β androstenediol.[56]

In a randomized, clinical trial with a crossover design, acute testosterone administration at pharmacologic levels was found to increase vaginal pulse amplitude in eugonadal women, with a strong statistical correlation between vaginal pulse amplitude and self-reporting of genital sensations.[53] In a single-blind study, acute dehydroepiandrosterone had no significant effect on either vaginal pulse amplitude responses or subjective responses to erotic films 30 min postdose in 12 healthy, premenopausal women.[57] As sublingual testosterone did not have an effect until 1.5 h,[53] it is possible that evaluation of vaginal pulse amplitude may have been performed at too early a time point for a true effect to be measured, resulting in a type 1 error.

Hormones and dyspareunia

Dyspareunia has a number of causes, but lack of estrogenization is a common cause in women experiencing estrogen deficiency due to a variety of causes. Significant negative associations between androstenedione and testosterone levels and vaginal atrophy have also been reported.[54] Androgen receptors have been reported in the vagina, and these may play a role in vaginal health (see Chapter 12.4). Local estrogen therapy can be effectively used to treat vaginal atrophy. Although this is usually a treatment reserved for postmenopausal women, low-dose vaginal estrogen is worth considering when this is the presenting problem for premenopausal women.

Situations resulting in sex-steroid deficiency in premenopausal women

As long as women continue to ovulate regularly, estrogen and progesterone levels are maintained until the time of menopause. However, as described above, androgen levels decline with age from the young reproductive years. Thus, aging contributes to decline in androgens. Factors that interfere with cyclic sex steroid production will therefore interfere with sex-steroid levels. Such factors include rapid weight loss and anorexia nervosa, in which estrogen and progesterone levels fall, but testosterone levels are often maintained.

Hyperprolactinemia, when pathophysiologic or iatrogenic, results in hypogonadotropic hypogonadism, loss of libido, and distress.[58] These adverse effects have been attributed to loss of ovarian function. Lundberg and Hulter reported that 53 (84.1%) out of the 63 women with hypothalamic pituitary disorders who had hyperprolactinemia had diminished sexual desire, but only 15 (32.6%) out of the 46 women with normal serum prolactin had this symptom ($p < 0.001$).[59]

Adrenal insufficiency is associated with reductions in dehydroepiandrosterone sulfate and free and total testosterone.[60] Similarly, glucocorticosteroid excess, either endogenous or exogenous, leads to adrenal suppression and androgen insufficiency, and thus may indirectly inhibit sexual function.[61] However, no clinical data indicate that this is an effect independent of the disease process for which glucocorticosteroid therapy is being used.

Use of the oral contraceptive pill results in suppressed ovarian function, and hence suppressed estradiol and progesterone levels, suppressed ovarian testosterone production, and low pituitary gonadotropins (see Chapter 7.6). In addition, the oral estrogen in the oral contraceptive pill increases sex hormone-binding globulin and thus reduces free testosterone. It is often said that use of the oral contraceptive pill adversely affects libido, but evidence to support this hypothesis is lacking.

Other hormones influencing sexual behavior

Oxytocin

Circulating levels of the neuropeptide oxytocin have been reported to be increased during sexual arousal and orgasm in humans, and its receptor may have a role in sexual behavior. When oxytocin had been infused into the brains of estrogen-treated, female rats (which are not very sexually receptive), their sexual activity was considerably stimulated.[62] Estradiol increases the expression of oxytocin and its receptor in the ventromedial hypothalamus of the rat.[63] The author is unaware of any correlates to this finding in humans.

Dopamine

Apomorphine is a dopaminergic agonist with affinity for dopamine D_1, but mostly dopamine D_2, receptors within the brain that are believed to be involved in sexual function.[64] It has been hypothesized that apomorphine may improve sexual interest and arousal by a central mechanism.

A single, randomized, clinical trial of apomorphine, administered sublingually to premenopausal women with normal testosterone levels, presenting with arousal disorder with hypoactive sexual desire disorder, has been conducted. Apomorphine treatment improved sexual desire and arousal versus placebo.[65] The extent to which these effects are due to central versus peripheral drug action requires further research.

Hormonal evaluation of the premenopausal woman presenting with low libido

Evaluation of loss of libido requires a sensitive, multisystem approach, including both physical and psychosocial factors.

History and examination

It is critical to establish whether the woman has ever experienced satisfactory sexual activity, how long she has felt sexual well-being to be a problem, and the extent to which this is causing her distress. The quality of the current relationship should be discussed, and other psychosocial stressors considered. All women need to be screened for depression as a primary cause of their female sexual dysfunction.

A complete gynecologic history should be taken, and the possibility of iron deficiency, thyroid disease, or hyperprolactinemia addressed. In the presence of regular cycles (periods every 21–35 days), dysfunction of the hypothalamic-pituitary-ovarian axis is unlikely, excluding estrogen deficiency and hyperprolactinemia. Amenorrhea before age 40 years requires full assessment.

A general physical examination should include assessment of thyroid status, and presence of anemia or galactorrhea. Gynecologic examination should include a pelvic examination with attention to signs of vaginal atrophy; size of the introitus; presence of discharge; and evidence of infection, vulvodynia, and deep tenderness (see Chapters 9.2–9.5).

Laboratory assessment (see Chapter 6.3)

In women presenting with low libido and fatigue, one should routinely measure iron stores (which might be low despite normal hemoglobin) and thyroid-stimulating hormone, to exclude subclinical thyroid disease; on clinical suspicion, other investigations should be conducted for chronic fatigue. Measurement of estradiol and follicle-stimulating hormone is indicated only to diagnose premature ovarian failure in amenorrheic women. Prolactin should be measured in the setting of oligomenorrhea, amenorrhea, and/or galactorrhea.

Free or bioavailable (non-sex hormone-binding globulin-bound) testosterone measures are the most reliable indicators of tissue testosterone exposure. High levels do not predict higher libido; however, a level above average probably rules out androgen insufficiency as a cause of the problem. Timing of measurement to prevent misdiagnosis of low testosterone is critical. Blood should be drawn between 8 and 10 am because of the diurnal variation of testosterone, which has higher levels at this time.[12] Testosterone levels reach their nadir during the early follicular phase, with small but less significant variation across the rest of the cycle.[10,66] Thus, blood should be drawn after day 8 of the cycle, and preferably before day 20. A serum sample is preferred to plasma.

The reference standard method to measure free testosterone is considered by many investigators to be equilibrium dialysis. However, this method is labor-intensive and expensive, and not feasible in clinical practice. The Sodergard equation can be reliably used to calculate free testosterone if total testosterone, albumin, and sex hormone-binding globulin are known.[67,68] Measurement of free testosterone by analog assays is unreliable and should not be used in clinical practice.[69] The free androgen index (nmol/l total testosterone × 100/nmol/l sex hormone-binding globulin) has been used as a surrogate for free testosterone, but it is unreliable when sex hormone-binding globulin levels are low.[70]

The measurement of sex hormone-binding globulin is not controversial, is relatively simple to perform, and has good reproducibility.

Dehydroepiandrosterone is usually measured in the sulfated form, dehydroepiandrosterone sulfate, because the half-life is much longer, resulting in more stable levels. The immunoassay

---

Table 13.1.1.

A) Female androgen insufficiency syndrome: proposed pattern of clinical symptoms and signs of the presence of decreased bioavailable testosterone and normal estrogen status[85]
   Clinical symptoms
      Decreased libido, sexual receptivity, and pleasure
      Low energy – persistent, unexplained fatigue
      Dysphoric mood
      Diminished psychologic well-being
      Blunted motivation
   Clinical signs
      Decreased bone density
      Decreased muscle mass and strength
      Adipose tissue redistribution
      Decreased sexual hair
      Changes in cognition or memory

B) Evidence-based clinical estrogen deficiency syndrome
   Clinical symptoms
      Hot flushes
      Night sweats
      Sleep disruption
      Vaginal dryness
   Clinical signs
      Vasomotor episodes
      Vaginal atrophy
      Decreased bone mineral density

Table 13.1.2. Causes of low bioavailable testosterone in women

- Normal aging
  - Symptomatic pre/postmenopausal women with low bioavailable testosterone
- Ovarian insufficiency
  - Uni/bilateral oophorectomy
  - Hysterectomy
  - Premature ovarian failure
  - Postchemo/radiotherapy
- Adrenal insufficiency
  - Adrenal failure/surgery
- Combined
  - Hypopituitism
- Iatrogenic
  - Treatment with exogenous oral estrogen
  - Chronic glucocorticosteroid therapy

Table 13.1.3. Basic biochemical investigations for women presenting with low libido

General
- TSH, iron stores

Specific

"Premenopausal" and amenorrhea
- Estradiol plus FSH (for diagnosis of hypothalamic amenorrhea/premature ovarian failure)
- Prolactin

Androgen profile
- SHBG
- Free testosterone by equilibrium dialysis (reference standard)
  Or
  Total testosterone after organic solvent extraction and calculation of free testosterone*
  Or
  Total testosterone by radioimmunoassay (with awareness of limitations) and calculation of free testosterone*
  * (or calculation of free androgen index: total testosterone nM/SHBG nM 100 if SHBG in normal range)
- DHEA-S
- Early morning cortisol: if adrenal insufficiency suspected

DHEA-S: dehydroepiandrosterone sulfate; FSH: follicle-stimulating hormone; SHBG: sex hormone-binding globulin; TSH: thyroid-stimulating hormone.

for dehydroepiandrosterone sulfate is relatively robust and simple to perform. Dehydroepiandrosterone sulfate does not vary in concentration within the various phases of the menstrual cycle, and is not bound to dehydroepiandrosterone. It also does not seem to be affected by estrogen therapy at standard doses. A number of authors have shown normal, age-related decline curves for dehydroepiandrosterone sulfate, which are all quite compatible. If low levels are found, a morning cortisol level should be drawn to rule out adrenal insufficiency.

Hormonal therapies

It is inappropriate to treat premenopausal women with ovulatory cycles with estrogen therapy for female sexual dysfunction. Women found to be amenorrheic should have their underlying problem managed and, when indicated, receive estrogen-progestin therapy. There is no evidence that use of the oral contraceptive pill adversely affects sexual function in otherwise well women, or in women using the oral contraceptive pill to manage dysmenorrhea or menorrhagia. However, oral contraceptive pills containing antiandrogenic progestins may result in lowering of libido in some women.

Although testosterone levels clearly fall with age, and testosterone may prove to be a useful therapy for hypoactive sexual desire disorder in premenopausal women, at present, the use of testosterone therapy in premenopausal women remains highly controversial, as evidence for its efficacy is limited.

Potential adverse effects of testosterone therapy need to be considered, including hirsutism and acne, balding, voice deep-

ening, and cliteromegaly. Other symptoms associated with exogenous androgen excess may include menstrual disturbances and polycythemia. In the polycystic ovarian syndrome, androgen excess is also associated with abnormal carbohydrate metabolism. However insulin resistance may underlie the etiology of this disorder, such that it is inappropriate to extrapolate the metabolic consequences of polycystic ovarian syndrome to that of simple androgen excess. There is evidence that some women with adrenal androgen excess, as in congenital adrenal hyperplasia, have insulin resistance. Although oral testosterone therapy as methyltestosterone results in lowering of high-density lipoprotein cholesterol,[71] there is no evidence that parenteral testosterone therapy has adverse cardiovascular effects.[52,72-74] High doses of orally administered androgens, such as methyltestosterone and, to a lesser extent, testosterone undecanoate, may be associated with hepatoxicity (peliosis hepatis, hepatic neoplasms, and cholestatic jaundice), but this has not been a problem for lower-dose therapy.[71]

It is known that androgens may exert an effect on the endometrium via aromatization to estrogen locally within the endometrium. There is no evidence that exogenous testosterone increases the risk of endometrial cancer or endometriosis.

The greatest concern pertaining to the administration of testosterone to reproductive-aged women is the potential for harm to either the mother or fetus should pregnancy occur during therapy. Wolf et al. studied the effects of a range of doses of testosterone propionate administered subcutaneously to pregnant Sprague-Dawley rats.[75] Androgenic effects were seen at a dose of 0.5 mg, which elevated maternal levels of testosterone 10-fold but had no effect on fetal levels. Viability of the offspring was unaffected at any dose. Adverse fetal effects included increased anogenital distance, reduced number of areolas and nipples, cleft phallus, small vaginal orifice, and presence of prostatic tissue. The 0.1-mg dose, which would be estimated to have increased female serum levels about twofold, did not cause any adverse effects.

Many cases of virilization during pregnancy have been reported, usually associated with luteoma of pregnancy or hyperreactio luteinalis. Fuller et al. reported a case of adrenal androgen-producing adenoma causing virilization of a 33-year-old woman, who delivered a virilized, healthy, female fetus. Postpartum, the mother had 2–5-fold excess circulating testosterone, dehydroepiandrosterone sulfate, and androstenedione.[76] In contrast, other reports of significant maternal virilization due to a variety of causes have not been associated with fetal virilization.[77-79] That virilization of the fetus does not commonly occur and that high levels are required for maternal virilization to occur is consistent with the fact that normal pregnancy is a hyperandrogenic state.[79] Testosterone levels begin to rise in the first trimester, free testosterone peaking in the third trimester of normal pregnancy.[79] It is believed that high circulating sex hormone-binding globulin and progesterone (which binds the androgen receptor) may protect the mother and fetus from virilization unless androgens are massively elevated.[79-81]

In the USA, oral formulations of the androgen precursors dehydroepiandrosterone and A-dione are available without prescription as "dietary supplements". Vaginal and topical administration of dehydroepiandrosterone to women has also been shown to increase testosterone levels appreciably.[81,82] In comparison, 100 mg androstenedione administered orally to women raised testosterone levels by approximately 3.5 nmol/l (100 ng/dl) in one study[83] and by more than 25 nmol/l (720 ng/dl) in another,[84] the latter corresponding to the upper normal range for men. The disparity in results could reflect differences in the purity and formulation of the androstenedione products used in the studies. Safety issues for oral dehydroepiandrosterone include acne, hirsutism, possible hepatotoxicity, and a reduction in high-density lipoprotein-cholesterol and other hepatic proteins (including sex hormone-binding globulin).[35,38] In view of the markedly supraphysiologic testosterone levels attained with androstenedione, the risk of virilization during chronic use in women is considerable.[84]

Androgen precursors are also estrogen precursors and thus may raise both testosterone and estradiol/estrone levels. There are insufficient data to support their use for the purpose of managing female sexual dysfunction.

Any premenopausal woman treated with androgen therapy needs thorough counseling regarding contraception and risk of adverse effects on a fetus. Monitoring should include assessment for signs of androgen excess, regular breast and pelvic examination, monitoring of serum androgen levels, and, in the presence of abnormal bleeding, endometrial biopsy. When testosterone is administered, continuation for longer than 6 months should be contingent on a clear improvement in sexual function and satisfaction. Although no adverse effects on lipids have been found with short-term parenteral therapies, a lipid profile, and, in the presence of a family history of diabetes or significant obesity, fasting insulin and glucose levels should be considered. Additional biochemical investigations, such as liver function tests, should be based on clinical judgment.

Conclusions and recommendations

Although hormones have an important role in the maintenance of female sexual function, there is currently insufficient evidence to support the use of hormonal therapy in the general management of otherwise well premenopausal women with female sexual dysfunction. As testosterone levels decline prior to the menopause and do not vary with natural menopause, it is tempting to extrapolate from the increasing data from studies in postmenopausal women that support the use of testosterone therapy for female sexual dysfunction. However, before such therapy can be broadly recommended, further studies are needed. Such studies may support the preliminary evidence for the effectiveness of testosterone in increasing libido, arousal, and orgasm in premenopausal women. However, safety data for testosterone therapy for premenopausal women are lacking, and the long-term safety of exogenous testosterone in women requires study before long-term use can be recommended. The current evidence for the effectiveness of dehydroepiandrosterone and androstenedione is also inconclusive.

References

1. Mendelsohn ME, Karas RH. The protective effects of estrogen on the cardiovascular system. *N Engl J Med* 1999; 340: 1801–11.
2. Thornton J. Evolution of vertebrate steroid receptors from an ancestral estrogen receptor by ligand exploitation and serial genome expansions. *Proc Natl Acad Sci USA* 2001; 98: 5671–6.
3. Simpson E, Rubin G, Clyne C et al. The role of local estrogen biosynthesis in males and females. *Trends Endocrinol Metab* 2000; 11: 184–8.
4. Bixo M, Andersson A, Winblad B et al. Progesterone, 5α-pregnane-3,20-dione and 3α-hydroxy-5α-pregnan-20-one in specific regions of the human female brain in different endocrine states. *Brain Res* 1997; 764: 173–8.
5. Billiar R, Little B, Kline I et al. The metabolic clearance rate, head and brain extractions, and brain distribution and metabolism of progesterone in the anesthetised female monkey. *Brain Res* 1975; 94: 99–113.
6. Inoue T, Akahira J, Darnel A et al. Progesterone production and actions in the human central nervous system and neurogenic tumors. *J Clin Endocrinol Metab* 2002; 87: 5325–31.
7. Vaitukaitis JL, Dale SL, Melby JC. Role of ACTH in the secretion of free DHA and its sulphate ester in man. *J Clin Endocrinol Metab* 1969; 29: 1443–7.
8. Vermeulen A, Ando S. Prolactin and adrenal androgen secretion. *Clin Endocrinol (Oxf)* 1978; 8: 295–303.
9. Haning RV Jr, Cabot M, Flood CA et al. Metabolic clearance rate (MCR) of dehydroepiandrosterone sulfate (DS), its metabolism to dehydroepiandrosterone, androstenedione testosterone and dihydrotestosterone, and the effects of increased plasm DS concentration on DS MCR in normal women. *J Clin Endocrinol Metab* 1989; 69: 1047–52.
10. Sinha-Hakim I, Arver S, Beall G et al. The use of a sensitive equilibrium dialysis method for the measurement of free testosterone levels in healthy, cycling women and in human immunodeficiency virus-infected women. *J Clin Endocrinol Metab* 1998; 83: 1312–18.
11. Judd HL, Judd G, Lucas WE et al. Endocrine function of the postmenopausal ovary. Concentrations of androgens and estrogens in ovarian and peripheral venous blood. *J Clin Endocrinol* 1974; 39: 1020–5.
12. Vierhapper H, Nowotny P, Waldhausl W. Determination of testosterone production rates in men and women using stable isotope dilution and mass spectromety. *J Clin Endocrinol Metab* 1997; 82: 1492–6.
13. Zumoff B, Strain GW, Miller LK et al. Twenty-four hour mean plasma testosterone concentration declines with age in normal premenopausal women. *J Clin Endocrinol Metab* 1995; 80: 1429–30.
14. Davis S, Schneider H, Donarti-Sarti C et al. Androgen levels in normal and oophorectomised women. Climacteric 2002; Proceedings of the 10th International Congress on the Menopause, Berlin.

15. Mushayandebvu T, Castracane DV, Gimpel T et al. Evidence for diminished midcycle ovarian androgen production in older reproductive aged women. *Fertil Steril* 1996; 65: 721–3.

16. Labrie F, Belanger A, Cusan L et al. Physiological changes in dehydroepiandrosterone are not reflected by serum levels of active androgens and estrogens but of their metabolites: intracrinology. *J Clin Endocrinol Metab* 1997; 82: 2403–9.

17. Haning JRV, Hackett R, Flood CA et al. Plasma dehydro-epiandrosterone sulfate serves as a prehormone for 48% of follicular fluid testosterone during treatment with menotropins. *J Clin Endocrinol Metab* 1993; 76: 1301–7.

18. Labrie F. Intracrinology. *Mol Cell Endocrinol* 1983; 78: C113–18.

19. Labrie F, Luu-The V, Labrie C et al. Endocrine and intracrine sources of androgens in women: inhibition of breast cancer and other roles of androgens and their precursor dehydroepiandrosterone. *Endocr Rev* 2003; 24: 152–82.

20. Dunn JF, Nisula BC, Rodboard D. Transport of steroid hormones. Binding of 21 endogenous steroids to both testosterone-binding globulin and cortico-steroid-binding globulin in human plasma. *J Clin Endocrinol Metab* 1981; 53: 58–68.

21. Guay A, Munarriz R, Jacobson J et al. The spectrum of decreasing androgens with age using various testosterone measuring techniques in normal premenopausal (PM) women. ISSWSH Annual Meeting, Vancouver, Canada, 2000.

22. Meston C. The psychophysiological assessment of female sexual function. *J Sex Marital Ther* 2000; 25: 6–16.

23. Meston C, Gorzalka B. The effects of sympathetic activation on physiological and subjective sexual arousal in women. *Behav Res Ther* 1995; 33: 651–64.

24. Tuiten A, Laan E, Panhuysen G et al. Discrepancies between genital responses and subjective sexual function during testosterone substitution in women with hypothalamic amenorrhea. *Psychosom Med* 1996; 58: 234–41.

25. Bixo M, Backstrom T, Winblad B et al. Estradiol and testosterone in specific regions of the human female brain in different endocrine states. *J Steroid Biochem Mol Biol* 1995; 55: 297–303.

26. Roselli CE, Resko JA. Aromatase activity in the rat brain: hormone regulation and sex differences. *J Steroid Biochem Mol Biol* 1993; 44: 499–508.

27. Pau C, Pau K, Spies H. Putative estrogen receptor beta and alpha mRNA expression in male and female rhesus macaques. *Mol Cell Endocrinol* 1998; 146: 59–68.

28. Kelly M, Levin E. Rapid actions of plasma membrane estogen receptors. *Trends Endocrinol Metab* 2001; 12: 152–6.

29. McEwen BS. Estrogen action throughout the brain. *Recent Prog Horm Res* 2002; 57: 357–84.

30. Moss R, McCann S. Action of luteinizing hormone-releasing factor (LRF) in the initiation of lordosis behavior in the estrone-primed ovariectomized female rat. *Neuroendocrinology* 1975; 17: 309–18.

31. Ogawa S, Chester AE, Hewitt SC et al. Abolition of male sexual behaviours in mice lacking estrogen receptors alpha and beta. *Proc Natl Acad Sci USA* 2000; 97: 14737–41.

32. Bakkar J, Honda S-I, Harada H et al. The aromatase knock-out mouse provides new evidence that estradiol is required during development in the female for the expression of sociosexual behaviours in adulthood. *J Neurosci* 2000; 22: 9104–12.

33. Mani S, Blaustein J, O'Malley BW. Progesterone receptor function from a behavioral perspective. *Horm Behav* 1997; 31: 244–55.

34. Mani S, Mitchell A, O'Malley BW. Progesterone receptors and dopamine receptors are required in delta9-tetrahydrocannabinol modulation of sexual receptivity in female rats. *Proc Natl Acad Sci USA* 2001; 98: 1249–54.

35. Arlt W, Callies F, Van Vlijmen JC et al. Dehydroepiandrosterone replacement in women with adrenal insufficiency. *N Engl J Med* 1999; 341: 1013–20.

36. Lovas K, Gebre-Medhin G, Trovik T et al. Replacement of dehydroepiandrosterone in adrenal failure: no benefit for subjective health status and sexuality in a 9-month randomized parallel group clinical trial. *J Clin Endocrinol Metab* 2003; 88: 1112–18.

37. Hunt P, Gurnell E, Huppert F. Improvement in mood and fatigue after dehydroepiandrosterone replacement in Addison's disease in a randomized, double blind trial. *J Clin Endocrinol Metab* 2000; 85: 4650–6.

38. Barnhart K, Freeman E, Grisso JA et al. The effect of dehydro-epiandrosterone supplementation to symptomatic perimenopausal women on serum endocrine profiles, lipid parameters, and health-related quality of life. *J Clin Endocrinol Metab* 1999; 84: 3896–3902.

39. Munarriz R, Talakoub L, Flaherty E et al. Androgen replacement therapy with dehydroepiandrosterone for androgen insufficiency and female sexual dysfunction: androgen and questionnaire results. *J Sex Marital Ther* 2002; 28(Suppl 1): 165–73.

40. Simerley R, Muramatsu M, Swanson L. Distribution of androgen and estrogen receptor mRNA-containing cells in the rat brain: an in situ hybridization study. *J Comp Neurol* 1990; 294: 76–95.

41. Roselli CE, Klosterman S, Resko J. Anatomic relationships between aromatase and androgen receptor mRNA expression in the hypothalamus and amygdala of adult male cynomolgus monkeys. *J Comp Neurol* 2001; 439: 208–23.

42. Alexander G, Sherwin B, Bancroft J et al. Testosterone and sexual behavior in oral contraceptive users and nonusers: a prospective study. *Horm Behav* 1990; 24: 388–402.

43. Riley A, Riley E. Controlled studies on women presenting with sexual drive disorder. I. Endocrine status. *J Sex Marital Ther* 2000; 26: 269–83.

44. Guay AT, Jacobson J. Decreased free testosterone and dehydro-epiandrosterone-sulfate (DHEA-S) levels in women with decreased libido. *J Sex Marital Ther* 2002; 28(Suppl 1): 129–42.

45. Gracia C, Samuel M, Freeman EW et al. Predictors of decreased libido in women during the late reproductive years. *Menopause* 2004; 11: 144–50.

46. Cawood EHH, Bancroft J. Steroid hormone, the menopause, sexuality and well-being of women. *Psychol Med* 1996; 26: 925–36.

47. Judd HL, Lucas WE, Yen SSC. Effect of oopherectomy on circulating testosterone and androstenedione levels in patients with endometrial cancer. *Am J Obstet Gynecol* 1994; 118: 793–8.

48. Rhodes J, Kjerulff K, Lagenberg P et al. Hysterectomy and sexual functioning. *JAMA* 1999; 282: 1934–41.

49. Nathorst-Boos J, von Schoultz H. Psychological reactions and sexual life after hysterectomy with and without oophorectomy. *Gynecol Obstet Invest* 1992; 34: 97–101.

50. Goldstat R, Briganti E, Tran J et al. Transdermal testosterone improves mood, well being and sexual function in premenopausal women. *Menopause* 2003; 10: 390–8.

51. Semmens J, Tsai C, Semmens E et al. Effects of estrogen therapy on vaginal physiology during menopause. *Obstet Gynecol* 1985; 66: 15–18.

52. Worboys S, Kotsopoulos D, Teede H et al. Parental testosterone improves endothelium-dependent and independent vasodilation in postmenopausal women already receiving estrogen. *J Clin Endocrinol Metab* 2001; 86: 158–61.

53. Tuiten A, Von Honk J, Koppeschaar H et al. Time course of effects of testosterone administration on sexual arousal in women. *Arch Gen Psychiatry* 2000; 57: 149–53.

54. Leiblum S, Bachmann GA, Kemmann E et al. The importance of sexual activity and hormones. *JAMA* 1983; 249: 2195–8.

55. Harada N, Sasano H, Murakami H et al. Localized expression of aromatase in human vascular tissues. *Circ Res* 1999; 84: 1285–91.

56. Shao T, Castenada E, Rosenfeld R et al. Selective retention and formation of delta 5 androstenediol-receptor complex in cell nuclei of the rat vagina. *J Biol Chem* 1975; 250: 3095–3100.

57. Meston C, Heiman J. Acute dehydroepiandrosterone effects on sexual arousal in premenopausal women. *J Sex Marital Ther* 2002; 28: 53–60.

58. Buckman M, Kellner R. Reduction in distress of hyperprolactinemia with bromocriptine. *Am J Psychiatry* 1984; 6: 351–8.

59. Lundberg P, Hulter B. Sexual dysfunction in patients with hypo-thalamo-pituitary disorders. *Exp Clin Endocrinol* 1991; 98: 81–8.

60. Miller K, Sesmilo G, Schiller A et al. Androgen deficiency in women with hypopituitarism. *J Clin Endocrinol Metab* 2001; 86: 561–7.

61. Abraham GE. Ovarian and adrenal contribution to peripheral androgens during the menstrual cycle. *J Clin Endocrinol Metab* 1974; 39: 340–6.

62. Caldwell J, Pedersen C, Prange A. Oxytocin facilitates the sexual receptivity of estrogen-treated female rats. *Neuropeptides* 1984; 7: 175–89.

63. Etgen A, Ansonoff M, Quesda A. Mechanisms of ovarian steroid regulation of norepinephrine receptor-mediated signal transduction in the hypothalamus: implications for female reproductive physiology. *Horm Behav* 2001; 42: 169–77.

64. Lal S, Kiely M, Thavundayil JX et al. Effect of bromocriptine in patients with apomorphine-responsive erectile impotence: an open study. *J Psychiatry Neurosci* 1991; 16: 262–6.

65. Caruso S, Agnello C, Intelisano G et al. Placebo-controlled study on efficacy and safety of daily apomorphine SL intake in premeno-pausal women affected by hypoactive sexual desire disorder and sexual arousal disorder. *Urology* 2004; 63: 955–9.

66. Judd HL, Yen SSC. Serum and androstenedione and testosterone levels during the menstrual cycle. *J Clin Endocrinol Metab* 1973; 36: 475–81.

67. Vermeulen A, Verdonck L, Kaufman M. A critical evaluation of simple methods for the estimation of free testosterone in serum. *J Clin Endocrinol Metab* 1999; 84: 3666–72.

68. Sodergard R, Backstrom T, Shanhag V et al. Calculation of free and bound fractions of testosterone and estradiol-17 beta to human plasma proteins at body temperature. *J Steroid Biochem* 1982; 16: 801–10.

69. Klee GG, Heser D. Techniques to measure testosterone in the elderly. *Mayo Clin Proc* 2000; 75: S19–S25.

70. Davis S, Humberstone A, Milne R et al. Measurement of serum total testosterone levels after administration of testosterone can underestimate the amount of testosterone that has been absorbed. Proceedings of the Endocrine Society's 85th Annual Meeting, Philadelphia, 2003.

71. Barrett-Connor E, Young R, Notelovitz M et al. A two-year, double-blind comparison of estrogen-androgen and conjugated estrogens in surgically menopausal women. Effects on bone mineral density, symptoms and lipid profiles. *J Reprod Med* 1999; 44: 1012–20.

72. Bernini G, Sgro M, Moretti A. Endogenous androgens and carotid intimal-medial thickness in women. *J Clin Endocrinol Metab* 1999; 84: 2008–12.

73. Goodman-Gruen D, Barrett-Connor E. Total but not bioavailable testosterone is a predictor of central adiposity in postmenopausal women. *Int J Obes* 1995; 19: 293–8.

74. Davis SR, Walker KZ, Strauss BJ. Effects of estradiol with and without testosterone on body composition and relationships with lipids in post-menopausal women. *Menopause* 2000; 7: 395–401.

75. Wolf C, Hotchkiss A, Ostby J et al. Effects of prenatal testosterone propionate on the sexual development of male and female rats: a dose-response study. *Toxicol Sci* 2002; 65: 71–86.

76. Fuller P, Pettigrew I, Pike J et al. An adrenal adenoma causing virilization of mother and infant. *Clin Endocrinol* 1983; 18: 143–53.

77. Berger N, Repke J, Woodruff J. Markedly elevated serum testo-sterone in pregnancy without fetal virilization. *Obstet Gynecol* 1984; 63: 260–2.

78. Ito M, Tohya T, Yoshimura T et al. Theca lutein cysts with mater-nal virilization and elevated serum testosterone in pregnancy. *Acta Obstet Gynecol Scand* 1987; 66: 565–6.

79. Ben-Chetrit A, Greenblatt E. Recurrent maternal virilization during pregnancy associated with polycystic ovarian syndrome: a case report and review of the literature. *Hum Reprod* 1995; 10: 3057–60.

80. McClamrock H, Adashi E. Gestational hyperandrogenism. *Fertil Steril* 1992; 57: 257–70.

81. Casson PR, Straughn AB, Umost ES et al. Delivery of deyhdro-epiandrosterone to premenopausal women: effects of microniza-tion and non-oral administration. *Am J Obstet Gynecol* 1996; 174: 649–53.

82. Labrie F, Diamond P, Cusan L et al. Effect of 12-month dehydro-epiandrosterone replacement therapy on bone, vagina and endometrium in postmenopausal women. *J Clin Endocrinol Metab* 1997; 82: 3498–3505.

83. Leder BZ, Lelanc KM, Longcope C et al. Effects of oral androstenedione administration on serum testosterone and estra-diol levels in postmenopausal women. *J Clin Endocrinol Metab* 2002; 87: 5449–54.

84. Kicman A, Bassindale T, Cowan D et al. Effect of androstenedione ingestion on plasma testosterone in young women; a dietary sup-plement with potential health risks. *Clin Chem* 2003; 49: 167–9.

85. Bachmann GA, Bancroft J, Braunstein G et al. Female androgen insufficiency: the Princeton Consensus Statement on definition, classification and assessment. *Fertil Steril* 2002; 77: 665.

13.2 Available therapies and outcome results in transition and postmenopausal women

Alan M Altman, Dina M Deldon-Saltin

Introduction

The menopause, or last menstrual period, and the perimenopause, the transition leading up to and encompassing the last menstrual period, are not diseases. They are part of the natural transition from the reproductive years to postreproductive life. All women will experience this transition, with or without symptoms of hormonal change, if they live long enough. While the mean age of the menopause has remained around 51 years, the time women will live beyond their menopause has increased due to the extension of life expectancy to the mid-80s. Many women will now spend approximately one-third of their lives or more after the cessation of estradiol production by the ovaries. This leads to a change in the spectrum of diseases that women will suffer from as they age. Coronary heart disease, dementia, and osteoporotic fractures increase as women live further beyond the menopause.

Along with this life extension, there is an expectation of continuing sexual function beyond the menopause. This has been more pronounced of late due to three sociologic phenomena: the arrival of a more openly sexual generation to the perimenopausal years, the sexual emphasis in the media and entertainment industries, and the growing equality in the bedroom with women asking, "What about me?" While the sexual changes during the perimenopausal transition and after the menopause have been covered in earlier chapters, the endocrine therapies available for women with sexual dysfunction will be reviewed in this chapter. The postmenopausal period will be covered first. The perimenopausal transition, characterized by erratic ovarian function of almost certain unpredictability due to wide variations in estrogen levels, will then be discussed.

Estrogen

While 50% of men over 50, 60% of men over 60, and 70% of men over 70 have some degree of erectile dysfunction, 100% of women have some degree of genital atrophy at some point after the menopause due to the cessation of ovarian estradiol production. Estrogen production continues in postmenopausal women, however, through peripheral conversion of androstenedione to estrone. This conversion increases with increasing body weight due to the ability of adipose tissue to aromatize androgens into estrogens[1] (see Chapters 5.5 and 6.1–6.3 of this book).

Urogenital changes contributing to altered sexual function

Estrogen is required for normal blood flow to the tissues of the reproductive organs. It also acts on estrogen receptors in these organs, allowing successful intercourse by maintaining the vaginal epithelium, thereby supporting elasticity and lubrication capabilities. High concentrations of estrogen receptors in the vagina, vulva, and urethra suggest that these tissues require estrogen for maintenance of function and make these tissues highly susceptible to atrophy due to the diminished estrogen production that occurs after the menopause. Low estrogen levels cause thinning of vaginal mucosal epithelium, atrophy of vaginal smooth muscles, and vaginal dryness, which in turn can lead to dyspareunia. Atrophic changes in the genitourinary system can be detected within 6–8 weeks in an estrogen-reduced environment.[2,3] Sarrel found that vaginal dryness, burning, and dyspareunia were reported more often in women with levels of estradiol under 50 pg/ml than in those with higher levels[4] (see Chapter 7.2).

The vaginal lining is highly rugated or folded. Its epithelium has a unique microscopic structure, which is responsive to estrogen. The cells respond cyclically to monthly variations in hormone levels. The vaginal epithelium contains no glands. Lubrication is produced by fluid transudation from blood vessels with some contribution from endocervical and Bartholin's glands. Before menopause, the vaginal environment has a pH of 3.5–4.5. This low pH environment is maintained by breakdown of the glycogen provided by sloughed cells in the vaginal lumen. Glycogen is hydrolyzed into glucose, and the latter is metabolized to lactic acid by normal vaginal flora. This acidic environment discourages growth of pathogenic bacteria[5] (see Chapters 4.1–4.4).

Urogenital atrophy, also referred to as vaginal dryness or atrophic vaginitis, is common, affecting nearly 15% of perimenopausal and 10–40% of postmenopausal women. Atrophy begins in the perimenopausal period and continues over many years. Aging also contributes to thinning of the hair of the mons and shrinkage of the labia minora. The labia majora flatten as the subcutaneous fat and elasticity of the structures diminish. It is common for women to experience pruritis at the onset of atrophy, as tissues are shrinking. With estrogen loss, the vagina becomes pale and its epithelium thins, resulting in diminished distensibility and reduced secretions. The estrogen-deficient vagina is easily traumatized and can bleed. The estrogen deficiency also changes the vaginal environment into an alkaline one, predisposing the vagina to colonization by pathogenic bacteria. By the post-menopausal period, the endocervical glandular tissue produces less mucin, contributing to the overall vaginal dryness that is often the presenting complaint of the patient[6] (see Chapters 6.1–6.4).

These physiologic, vascular, and hormonal changes can cause dyspareunia. Women begin avoiding sexual relations with their partner secondary to the fear of painful intercourse. Dyspareunia can lead to avoidance, and avoidance can lead to further vaginal atrophy, which can cause worsening dyspareunia. Hence, the vicious cycle can ultimately lead to performance anxiety and loss of any sexual desire.

Treatment of urogenital atrophy

Nonpharmacologically, vaginal lubricants and moisturizers applied on a regular basis can be used to treat urogenital symptoms such as vaginal itching, irritation, and dyspareunia. Local use of vaginal lubricants to ease penetration and allow successful and pain-free intercourse can help treat symptoms and also allow some increase in blood flow, but has diminished ability to treat the source of the problem, namely, estrogen insufficiency. However, they can be offered to women as a first-line therapy, especially for those who wish to avoid the use of hormones. Lubricants should be pH neutral so as to not alter the vaginal environment and flora. Many varieties are available over-the-counter at local pharmacies or specialty stores. Water-based lubricants are easily absorbed, but silicone-based lubricants can leave the skin with an oily texture. It should be noted that some lubricants can decrease condom integrity, especially petroleum-based products and oils.

Vaginal moisturizers are promoted as providing long-term relief of vaginal dryness rather than being just sexual lubricants. Moisturizers are claimed to provide more than transient lubrication. A bioadhesive, polycarbophil-based polymer works by attaching to mucin and epithelial cells on the vaginal wall through anionic binding. The polycarbophil portion carries up to 60 times its weight in water and holds water in place against the vaginal epithelial surface until it is sloughed off, typically after 24 h. One such moisturizer was compared with a lubricant in a double-blind, randomized, crossover trial in 93 perimenopausal and postmenopausal women with vaginal dryness. After 5 days of daily use, the polycarbophil-based polymer produced a longer duration of lubrication and a significantly lower vaginal pH than the lubricant (baseline pH 5.6 ± 1.1, moisturizer 4.9 ± 1.1, lubricant 5.7 ± 1.0). More women reported product residue with the polycarbophil-based polymer (8%), but, overall, side effects were similar between the two groups.[5]

While the process of intercourse itself or, for that matter, masturbation can increase vaginal blood flow and help maintain vaginal health, it often takes the use of estrogen therapy to return function that can again lead to successful intercourse. The replenishment of estrogen results in increased vaginal compliance, decreased vaginal pH, increased vaginal blood flow and lubrication, and restored clitoral and vaginal vibration and pressure thresholds. In a recent study, 15% of women on hormone therapy reported vaginal dryness after a 5-year follow-up, compared to 30–40% of their non-hormone-therapy counterparts. Consequently, the degree of dyspareunia was also less among the hormone therapy than the non-hormone-therapy users.[7] With estrogen use, women report less vaginal irritation, pain, dryness, or burning during intercourse. Relief from these symptoms often leads to increased sexual desire and arousal.[2]

Oral versus nonoral estrogen use

Local estrogen therapy can be as effective as systemic estrogen for restoring vaginal epithelium and relieving atrophy.[2,8] Recent studies on local estrogen therapy have shown restoration of vaginal epithelium to its normal state within several months. Local therapy in the past has meant the use of vaginal estrogen creams. Conjugated equine estrogen, estradiol, and estriol creams administered intravaginally can partly or completely restore vaginal cytology to premenopausal levels, and improve or cure urogenital atrophy and dryness.[5] Creams, however, can be absorbed into the systemic circulation, higher dosages resulting in higher systemic estrogen concentrations. The cream form of estrogen is also more subject to irregular application intervals, bolus absorption, and low absorption capacity of the fat-based vehicle, as well as the overall messiness of the product.[9]

More recently, other forms of local estrogen vehicles have been developed, such as rings and tablets, which may have better efficacy as well as more convenience. An opaque vaginal ring containing 2 mg estradiol is now available. The ring is placed in the vagina for 3 months, during which time it slowly releases the hormone. Comparisons between estradiol released from a ring and estradiol in cream form have shown equivalent efficacy in studies. A randomized, open-label, crossover study of 165 postmenopausal women with atrophic vaginitis compared continuous low-dose estradiol released from a ring with estriol vaginal cream. Both treatments were shown to be equally effective in alleviating the feeling of vaginal dryness as well as improving vaginal atrophy. They were also both efficient in restoring the vaginal mucosa to an estrogen-rich state. Quantitative analysis of the vaginal smears showed no difference between the two treatments in the number of parabasal, intermediate, and superficial cells in the mucosal wall. In relation to preference, 106 (64%) of 165 women preferred treatment with the ring. No preference was shown in 8 women (5%), while 29 (18%) preferred cream. The estradiol ring was well-tolerated by patients and did not cause more severe local adverse events than other, existing treatments. Systemic effects were minimal, as very little estradiol reaches the systemic circulation.[9] However, the ring must fit the individual's vagina; otherwise, it is impractical to use, as too much atrophy does not allow enough room for the ring.

Local estrogen in the form of a tablet is also available for symptoms associated with vaginal dryness. A 17-beta-estradiol tablet in a 25-µg, single vaginal dose applicator is administered daily for the first 2 weeks of treatment, and then decreased to one vaginal tablet twice weekly as maintenance therapy. This product works locally and is not designed to help systemic symptoms of menopause.[10]

With respect to systemic use, estrogens can be divided into three groups: 17-beta-estradiol, conjugated equine estrogen, and estrone derivatives, which include the synthetic conjugated estrogens, esterified estrogens, and other estrogen derivatives. 17-beta-estradiol is the estrogen that is made in abundance by the ovaries prior to menopause. Estrone is the estrogen most abundant after menopause because its primary source is peripheral conversion of androstenedione in adipose and other tissue. Estradiol and estrone are interconverted, conversion of estradiol to estrone predominating. Estradiol can also be converted to estriol.[5,11] Conjugated equine estrogen is manufactured from pregnant mare's urine.

Oral administration has been the most common route of estrogen therapy. Oral estrogens have been available for many years. They are usually well tolerated and cost-effective, especially the older generic brands. Oral estrogens undergo first-pass metabolism in the liver. The most notable benefit of first-pass metabolism is improvement in lipid values, such as high-density lipoprotein and low-density lipoprotein cholesterol.

There are several drawbacks to the oral administration of estrogen, however. First-pass metabolism reduces the systemic availability of estradiol, after oral administration, to less than 20%, because most of the oral estradiol is metabolized to estrone and conjugates, resulting in a high estrone to estradiol ratio that does not reflect physiologic levels.[8,12] Oral estrogens also increase sex hormone-binding globulin, which binds free testosterone, thereby reducing the amount of biologically active testosterone. It is thought that this reduction in biologically active testosterone is one cause of decreased libido in postmenopausal women on oral estrogen therapy.

Oral estrogen is also associated with prothrombotic changes in hemostatic factors and an increase in inflammatory markers, such as C-reactive protein. The difference in C-reactive protein level may be due to the first-pass effect and a resultant stimulation of C-reactive protein synthesis in the liver.[13] In addition, there is an increased risk of having a venous thromboembolic event with oral estrogen therapy. The Estrogen and ThromboEmbolism Risk Study, an observational study, documented a 3.5-fold greater risk of venous thromboembolism in women using oral estrogen than in those using placebo (95% CI, 1.8–6.8).[14]

Transdermal hormone therapy provides more consistent blood hormone levels, and this translates into prevention of withdrawal symptoms. In addition to effectiveness at lower doses compared with oral administration, products administered by the nonoral route avoid first-pass hepatic effects.[12] This decreases some of the adverse events associated with oral estrogen use. The Estrogen and ThromboEmbolism Risk Study showed that the risk of venous thromboembolic events is not associated with transdermal estrogen use, finding no significant difference in venous thromboembolic event rates between the transdermal and the placebo groups.[14]

Systemic estrogen is also available in the form of a vaginal ring. The estradiol acetate vaginal ring is an off-white, soft, flexible ring with central core, which contains either 0.05 or 0.10 mg/day of estradiol acetate. It is placed intravaginally, where it remains for 90 days, steadily releasing hormone over that time. This ring has the added benefit of increasing local, as well as systemic, estradiol levels. In a 13-week, double-blind, placebo-controlled trial conducted to evaluate the efficacy of the two doses of the estradiol acetate ring, vaginal superficial cells were noted to increase by a mean of 16.0% for the 0.05 mg/day dose and 18.9% for the 0.10 mg/day dose, as compared to 1.11% for placebo.[15]

Heart and Estrogen/Progestin Replacement Study and Women's Health Initiative

There has been a decline of systemic hormone therapy use since the premature discontinuation and publication of the estrogen-progestin arm of the Women's Health Initiative Study in July 2002. In 1995, approximately 38% of postmenopausal women in the USA were taking hormone therapy. In 1997, hormone therapy was at its highest use in the USA with the rate of increase in use of 1% per quarter. After publication of the Heart and Estrogen/Progestin Replacement Study in 1998, the first decrease in hormone use occurred, with a decline of 1% per quarter.[16]

The Heart and Estrogen/Progestin Replacement Study was initiated in 1993 as a randomized, blinded, placebo-controlled, secondary prevention trial in which 2763 women with established coronary artery disease were randomly assigned to receive either 0.625 mg conjugated equine estrogen with 2.5 mg medroxyprogesterone acetate or placebo.[17] The women had a mean age of 66.7 years, were postmenopausal with an intact uterus, and were followed for an average of 4.1 years. Although there was no net difference in myocardial infarction rate between the two groups, a significant time trend was observed for the outcomes. There were more cardiovascular events in the hormone-treated group than the placebo group during year 1, and fewer in years 4 and 5, but no overall net benefit or detriment. Other findings included a statistically significant net decrease in low-density lipoprotein cholesterol and net increase in high-density lipoprotein cholesterol among hormone therapy users. There were also significantly more venous thromboembolic events and gallbladder disease in the active treatment group.

The Women's Health Initiative was designed as a primary prevention study, the primary outcome measuring the rate of nonfatal myocardial infarction or death due to myocardial infarction.[18,19] The study was a two-arm, randomized, double-blind, placebo-controlled study. It included healthy postmenopausal women aged 50–70 years, with a mean of 64 years. Women were an average of 12 years postmenopausal. They were divided into two groups, an estrogen-progesterone arm for those with intact uterus and an estrogen-only arm for women with prior hysterectomy. The estrogen-progesterone arm studied the use of conjugated equine estrogen plus medroxyprogesterone acetate versus placebo, while the estrogen arm studied only conjugated equine estrogen versus placebo.

The Women's Health Initiative was terminated after an average of 5.2 years of follow-up, as the stopping statistic for a greater risk of breast cancer in one of the treatment groups had been reached.[18] The estrogen-only arm of the Women's Health Initiative was terminated in March 2004 because of a slight increase in stroke risk among women in the conjugated equine estrogen treatment group.[19]

The data obtained from the Women's Health Initiative inform us of the risks and benefits of the use of oral systemic hormone therapy (conjugated equine estrogen with or without medroxyprogesterone acetate) in North American women that were, on average, 12 years postmenopausal. Women treated with conjugated equine estrogen and medroxyprogesterone acetate had a possible risk of coronary heart disease that was 29% higher than women in the placebo group (OR = 1.29; 95% CI, 1.02–1.63). The absolute rate of coronary heart disease events was 7 more cases per 10,000 person-years for the hormone-treated group than for the placebo group. There was an increased risk of coronary heart disease apparent at year 1, as seen with the Heart and Estrogen/Progestin Replacement Study, and a longitudinal trend toward overall benefit (p = 0.02).[18] In contrast, the estrogen-only arm demonstrated no increased or decreased risk of coronary heart disease in women treated with conjugated equine estrogen without medroxyprogesterone acetate (OR = 0.91; adjusted 95% CI, 0.72–1.15).[19]

Although the primary outcome measure of the Women's Health Initiative was the rate of nonfatal myocardial infarction or death due to myocardial infarction, several other outcomes measures were analyzed. The outcome measure of breast cancer was especially noted, as it was the outcome measure that stopped the estrogen/progestin arm of the study. However, this was a secondary endpoint and, in the final analysis, did not achieve statistical significance when correctly analyzed as such. There was no significant difference between the groups in the rate of *in situ* breast carcinoma, raising the question as to whether these excess tumors were promoted, as opposed to initiated. In addition, the invasive breast cancers were larger and more advanced at diagnosis in the active treatment arm (p = 0.04 for both).[18] In the estrogen-only arm, there was an opposite trend with a nonsignificant reduction in risk of breast cancer among women treated with conjugated equine estrogen (OR 0.77; adjusted 95% CI, 0.57–1.06).[19]

The risk of venous thromboembolic events was increased among women in the estrogen/progestin group of the Women's Health Initiative compared with the placebo group. The absolute risk attributable to treatment with estrogen/progestin was 8 additional cases of pulmonary embolism per 10,000 person-years.[18] The estrogen/progestin arm also showed an increased rate of ischemic stroke (OR = 1.44; 95% CI, 1.09–1.90), among women treated with hormone therapy, compared with those who received placebo. There was no increased risk of hemorrhagic stroke.[20] In the estrogen-only arm, the incidence of venous thromboembolic events, including both deep vein thrombosis and pulmonary embolism, was increased in women treated with estrogen compared with women who received placebo.[19] There was a slightly increased risk of stroke, equivalent to 12 additional events per 10,000 person-years among women treated in the estrogen-only arm of the Women's Health Initiative compared with women who received placebo.[20]

Both arms of Women's Health Initiative showed that hormone therapy significantly reduces the risk of spine, hip, and other fragility fracture in women not selected for increased fracture risk.

The results of the Women's Health Initiative Memory Study, a study within the Women's Health Initiative, showed that more women in the treatment group had smaller average increases in the Mini-Mental Status Examination scores than in the placebo group (p = 0.008).[21] This study had some methodological limitations, and the findings are not surprising, given that the women were aged over 65 years, a group in whom hormone therapy is not routinely commenced. When the data from this Women's Health Initiative subgroup were segmented by 5-year age groups, the only active treatment group with an increased risk of dementia was the one of women 75–79 years of age.[22] In the estrogen-only arm of the Women's Health Initiative an adverse effect of treatment was not demonstrated.

Because only one-third of women were younger than 60 years old, only 13% were 50–54 years old, and most importantly, only 16% were within five years of their final menstrual period, the WHI does not provide strong evidence about younger postmenopausal women who are closer to menopause; the women who are most likely to initiate hormone therapy for treatment of menopausal symptoms. Evaluating the subgroup of women in the WHI who were 50–54 years of age is risky, because the study was not designed to provide reliable data on these women. Thus, the WHI does not provide information on the benefits and risks of beginning hormone therapy at the time of the menopause. The WHI trials also only tested one drug regimen CEE 0.625 mg/day (plus MPA 2.5 mg/day in women with intact uterus). It does not provide information about the use of other doses, formulations, regimens, routes of administration or doses and duration of hormone therapy.

Lobo reported on results from two large, prospective, randomized control trials of over 4000 women with a mean age of 53.6 years and averaging 4.9 years from the final menstrual period, a good ten years younger than in the WHI study, in order to look at CHD risk in young, healthy postmenopausal women.[23] Several regimens of combined CEE and MPA were assessed. Results were reported for year one of the trials, as this was the event time for early harm demonstrated in both the HERS and WHI studies. The rates for CHD related death or MI were 0/1000 vs 3.01/1000 in the treatment and placebo groups respectively. He concluded that the results of early CHD risk observed in the WHI study may not be applicable to healthy postmenopausal women closer to their menopause, even with the use of CEE/MPA.

In response to the discontinuation of the estrogen/progestin arm of the Women's Health Initiative, professional societies and governmental agencies released statements or revised practice guidelines for hormone therapy. The American College of Obstetricians and Gynecologists published a response to the Women's Health Initiative on their website on 3 June 2003. In this response, the college stated that "the decision about use of hormone therapy requires evaluation of the risks and benefits for each individual woman. For women currently using hormone therapy, it is important to assess their reasons for use and to evaluate potential risks, benefits, and alternatives. Women who take hormone therapy for the management of vasomotor symptoms should be encouraged to take it for as short a time as needed, and to use the lowest effective dose."[24] Other societies, such as the National Association of Nurse Practitioners in Women's Health and the North American Menopause Society, and the US Food and Drug Administration have also recommended that the lowest dose and shortest duration of hormone therapy be used. However, there are no randomized, controlled clinical data showing that lower dose and shorter duration are as effective or safer. In fact, while the Women's Health Initiative and the Heart and Estrogen/Progestin Replacement Study showed a greater risk of coronary heart disease in year 1, longer-term use actually showed increased protection against coronary heart disease over time.[16,18,19]

It is obvious that since the publication of the Heart and Estrogen/Progestin Replacement Study and the Women's Health Initiative trials, hormone therapy usage has declined to a significant extent. It is, however, unclear how to weigh the menopausal symptom relief provided by hormone therapy and the significantly reduced fracture risk against the risks of coronary heart disease, venous thromboembolic events, stroke, and possible breast cancer with combined therapy.[25] Using a Markov decision-analysis model, a group of researchers designed a study which compared the quality-adjusted life expectancy with and without combination hormonal replacement therapy in three cohorts of women over a 20-year period. The women were at either high or low risk of breast cancer and coronary heart disease or at high risk of osteoporosis. The results of this study revealed that hormone therapy decreased life expectancy slightly compared with no hormone therapy if menopausal symptoms are not considered. However, if relief from menopausal symptoms is considered and the usefulness of life with symptoms is worth under 0.996 compared with life without symptoms, then 5 years of hormone therapy provides equivalent quality-adjusted life-years.[25] In essence, if the benefit of hormone therapy exceeds the risks, that is, if vaginal dyspareunia is improved, women should continue their hormone usage.

The use of estrogen must be individualized to each patient's needs and expectations. There is no "one-size-fits-all" recipe. What holds for women 10–20 years postmenopausal cannot be extrapolated to women recently postmenopausal, the largest population drawn to the health-care provider with questions and pending decisions about hormone therapy. What holds for oral estrogen therapy, and its thrombogenic potential, cannot be extrapolated to nonoral systemic estrogen or to use of vaginal estrogen for local therapy.

Systemic estrogen has been shown to improve vasomotor symptoms significantly, including hot flushes, night sweats, and sleep disturbance, all of which can affect a women's body image, mood, and sexual desire. Alleviation of such symptoms can often go a long way toward increasing both quality of life and, indirectly, the drive for intimate contact and sexual activity.

Progestogen use

In a woman with an intact uterus, the addition of progestogen to estrogen therapy is necessary to prevent endometrial hyperplasia and carcinoma. Progestogens are steroid compounds that help prevent endometrial hyperplasia and cancer in women on estrogen with an intact uterus, by downregulating estrogen receptors in the endometrium. There are two types of progestogens, natural and synthetic. Progesterone is the only natural progestogen, and it is poorly absorbed. However, a micronization process, breaking down the progesterone into minute particles, improves its absorption by increasing the surface area of the hormone, making it more likely to be dissolved in the intestine. The bioavailability of micronized progesterone, however, continues to be limited because of extensive hepatic metabolism. Thus, large doses or twice daily dosing is often required to achieve therapeutic levels.[11]

Synthetic progestogens are divided into those related to progesterone, and those related to testosterone.[11] The progestogens related to progesterone can be divided into two major groups: the pregnane group and the 19-non-pregnane group. Both can be further divided into acetylated and nonacetylated derivatives. The most widely used (in the USA) progestogen in this group is medroxyprogesterone acetate, which is an acetylated pregnane derivative. In the circulation, medroxyprogesterone acetate is bound nonspecifically to albumin and undergoes extensive metabolism by hydroxylation and conjugation. The half-life of the drug is approximately 24 h. The other major group of progestogens is related to testosterone. This group can be divided into two major subgroups: the ethinylated and nonethinylated groups. The ethinylated group can be subdivided into two additional groups. One is the estranes group, which includes nonethindrone (USA) or norethisterone (Europe). In the other subgroup, 13-ethylgonanes, levonorgestrel is one of the most potent and orally active progestogens. Other compounds belonging to this group are desogestrel, norgestimate, and gestodene.[11]

The addition of a progestogen to estrogen therapy is necessary in women with an intact uterus to eliminate the risk of endometrial cancer associated with unopposed estrogen. However, the addition of a progestogen can decrease both mood and libido.[26] It does this by downregulating the estrogen receptor, a desired result in the endometrium, but potentially undesirable in the brain, heart, bone, and genitalia. It is this decrease in mood and libido that may lead to poor compliance among women who would benefit from estrogen therapy. In a recent, double-blind, crossover study, the side effects of medroxyprogesterone acetate and norethindrone acetate were compared in women using postmenopausal hormone therapy. The women showed cyclic changes, with negative mood and physical symptoms culminating during the late progestogen phase, and positive mood during the estrogen-only phase. Symptoms declined with time but remained after 5 months. Women with a history of premenstrual syndrome responded more strongly than those without a history of premenstrual syndrome.[27]

Several studies in the literature have reported negative effects of progestogens on sexual function. The effects of estrogen alone or with medroxyprogesterone acetate on psychologic function and sexual behavior were evaluated in a study of 48 healthy, naturally menopausal women. The benefits of estrogen were diminished by medroxyprogesterone acetate coadministration.[28] Another report, comparing the use of estradiol alone or in combination with lynestrenol, a 19-norsteriod, revealed that women who used the combination therapy reported more negative mood symptoms than the estrogen-only group.[29] In a third study, women who were intolerant of a conjugated equine estrogen/medroxyprogesterone acetate regimen were switched to conjugated equine estrogen plus progesterone and reported better vasomotor, somatic, psychologic, cognitive, and sexual function.[30]

In a recent animal study, the potential for medroxyprogesterone acetate to antagonize the estradiol effects of the female social sexual behavior of ovariectomized pigtail macaques was examined. Six ovariectomized pigtail macaques were tested under the following conditions: (1) placebo; (2) 17-beta-estradiol alone; (3) estradiol plus progesterone; (4) estradiol plus medroxyprogesterone acetate. Each hormone treatment was administered for 1 week and was separated by a minimum 3-week washout period. Female sexual initiation rates varied significantly across the treatment conditions ($p < 0.001$). The estradiol-only treatment induced a rise in female sexual initiation rates relative to the placebo condition ($p = 0.016$). The addition of progesterone failed significantly to attenuate the effect of estradiol on female sexual initiations ($p = 0.276$). Although rates of behavior during the estradiol plus progesterone condition also failed to rise above those observed under the placebo condition ($p = 0.181$), the medroxyprogesterone acetate plus estradiol treatment significantly attenuated rates of female sexual behavior, both in comparison with the estradiol-only ($p = 0.001$) and the estradiol plus progesterone condition ($p = 0.038$).[31]

Progestogens, however, appear to produce a wide range of patient responsiveness and tolerability, suggesting that women who do not tolerate one regimen might be effectively switched to another and experience improvement. Bjorn et al. showed that medroxyprogesterone acetate induced more physical symptoms than norethindrone when compared in a double-blind, crossover study of postmenopausal women on hormone therapy.[27]

When added to estrogen for endometrial protection, progestogens can be administered in a variety of regimens. In a continuous combined regimen, patients receive daily doses of both estrogen and progesterone. There are also several different cyclic regimens in which progesterone is taken during only a portion of the cycle, such as the last 10–14 days of the hormone therapy cycle. In some instances, progesterone is given for only 10–14 days every 3–6 months, depending on the progestogen used and the bleeding response. If this regimen is chosen, a potent progestogen should be used to ensure sufficient endometrial shedding. A meta-analysis of the relative risk of endometrial cancer with hormone therapy found no difference between continuous and intermittent regimens.[32] In the Postmenopausal Estrogen/Progestin Interventions Study, the risk of endometrial hyperplasia was lower among women who received progestogens than those who took estrogen alone, whether these were administered in a continuous or sequential regimen.[33]

Androgens (see Chapter 13.1)

The question as to whether estrogen has a direct impact on sexual desire is complex. However, the question of whether androgens have a direct impact on sexual desire has been studied extensively. Historically, androgens have been identified with male sexual function. However, androgens not only are necessary for the development of reproductive function and hormonal homeostasis within a woman, but also represent the immediate precursors to the biosynthesis of estrogens.[34] A normal ovary produces relatively large amounts of androgen compared with estrogen across the female life span. The three main naturally occurring steroids responsible for androgen action are testosterone and dihydrotestosterone, formed from the precursors dehydroepiandrosterone and its sulfate (dehydroepiandrosterone-S), as well as androstenedione. In women, peripheral tissues convert androgen precursors into more potent androgens, and may also convert androgens to estrogens via aromatase activity.[35]

The extent to which the postmenopausal ovary produces androgens remains controversial. In the early postmenopausal time period, elevated gonadotropins (follicle-stimulating hormone, luteinizing hormone) drive the remaining stromal tissue of the ovary to produce testosterone. Despite this drive by the postmenopausal ovary to produce androgens, testosterone levels are still lower than they were premenopausally due to the significant age-related decline in testosterone and adrenal androgen production beginning in the mid-20s. Circulating testosterone falls by approximately 50% after bilateral oophorectomy.[36] Oral estrogen therapy increases the production of sex hormone-binding globulin by its first-pass effect through the liver. Sex hormone-binding globulin preferentially binds testosterone, but also binds estrogen, thereby reducing the amount of both bioavailable hormones. Hence, the use of oral estrogen postmenopausally (as well as its use premenopausally in oral contraceptive therapy) can diminish bioavailable testosterone and may affect sexual desire and arousal, as well as diminish bioavailable estrogen and allow relapse of vasomotor symptoms. Therefore, some have suggested that testosterone therapy, as an adjunct to estrogen therapy, is useful in the treatment of female sexual dysfunction and relapse of estrogen-withdrawal symptoms.

In a study of postmenopausal women by Laughlin et al.,[36] androstenedione levels in hysterectomized women were approximately 10% lower than nonhysterectomized women ($p = 0.039$), regardless of ovarian status. In women with an intact uterus, androstenedione levels declined with age and were 20% lower in women who were greater than 30 years postmenopausal. In addition, total and bioavailable testosterone levels were reduced 29% ($p < 0.001$) in hysterectomized women with ovarian conservation and 40% ($p < 0.001$) in women with bilateral oophorectomy, compared to women with an intact uterus. Interestingly, total, but not bioavailable, testosterone levels increased with chronologic age, most of the increase occurring during the fifth decade with stable levels thereafter. Both total and bioavailable testosterone levels were 40–50% lower in oophorectomized than in intact women. Plasma sex hormone-binding globulin adjusted for body mass index reportedly increased with age in women with an intact uterus, but did not vary, in regard to age or years since surgery, in oophorectomized women.[36]

Among the studies demonstrating the impact of testosterone on sexual function, Sarrel et al. showed significant improvement in sexual desire ($p < 0.05$) and in frequency of sexual intercourse ($p < 0.01$) in healthy, postmenopausal women receiving 1.25 mg estrogen plus 2.5 mg methyltestosterone versus estrogen alone and placebo.[37] Other studies have shown similar results with estrogen/testosterone combinations. Shifren et al. showed improvement in scores for the frequency of sexual activity and pleasure orgasm on the Brief Index of Sexual Functioning for Women for surgically postmenopausal women receiving conjugated equine estrogen 0.625 mg and transdermal testosterone 300 µg/day versus placebo ($p = 0.07$).[38,39]

Esterified estrogen and methyltestosterone 1.25 mg/2.5 mg is a combination estrogen and androgen pill approved for and utilized in the management of moderate to severe vasomotor symptoms associated with menopause in patients who do not respond to estrogen alone. This formulation also comes in a half-strength dose of esterified estrogen/methyltestosterone 0.625 mg/1.25 mg.[40] Although this formulation has not been approved for treatment of female sexual dysfunction, many researchers have shown success in the treatment of sexual dysfunction in postmenopausal women with these formulations.

Lobo et al. conducted a double-blind, randomized, controlled study of 218 women, measuring change in level of sexual interest or desire in women receiving esterified estrogen 0.625 mg versus those receiving esterified estrogen/methyltestosterone 0.625 mg/1.25 mg. The target population was healthy, postmenopausal women aged 40–65 years with hypoactive sexual desire associated with the onset of menopause. Women were required to be currently taking estrogen and to have had adequate sexual interest before the onset of menopause. Results showed that the mean serum concentration of bioavailable testosterone almost doubled in patients receiving esterified estrogen and methyltestosterone ($p < 0.010$). A significant decrease in sex hormone-binding globulin was also observed in this group ($p < 0.010$). Both treatments produced increases in the Sexual Intimacy Quotient sexual interest/desire score, the combination group showing consistently greater improvement and reaching significance at week 16.[41]

Because of the short half-life and ability of testosterone to permeate readily the layers of skin to become absorbed, transdermal administration of testosterone in women has a compelling biopharmaceutic rationale. In addition, nongenital skin contains low levels of 5α-reductase and aromatase, thereby decreasing the degree of metabolism into dihydrotestosterone and estradiol that occurs with oral administration.[42] Data obtained from surgically menopausal women receiving treatment with a testosterone matrix patch of 300 µg a day and either transdermal estradiol (0.05–0.10 mg daily) or oral conjugated equine estrogen (0.625 mg/day) indicated that women on conjugated equine estrogen had higher sex hormone-binding globulin levels. In addition, the calculated increments in total testosterone for a 300 μg/day patch would be 51.4 ng/dl with transdermal estradiol versus 69.2 ng/dl for oral conjugated equine estrogen. However, the calculated increments, for free testosterone, were 4.6 pg/ml for transdermal estradiol versus 3.0 pg/ml for oral conjugated equine estrogen. This indicates that for women who require treatment with both testosterone and estrogen, the use of transdermal estradiol results in greater levels of free (bioavailable) testosterone.[42]

Topical gels containing micronized testosterone are compounded and sold in specialized pharmacies in the USA. The big disadvantage of compounded pharmaceuticals is that there is no way to regulate the dose and purity of the product. Therefore, not all batches are equivalent, and the compounded formula may not be uniform throughout. Experimental testosterone transdermal patches are currently being developed for use in women. They are not yet approved by the Food and Drug Administration for treatment of low sexual desire, but researchers are getting promising results. They have been designed to deliver testosterone at rates of 150 and 300 μg/day, which are approximately 50% and 100%, respectively, of daily testosterone production in premenopausal women.[42]

Although a large body of data suggests that testosterone replacement can be effective in the treatment of female sexual dysfunction and the rush by pharmaceutic companies to develop the best testosterone delivery system, there is, as yet, no Food and Drug Administration approval for such use of androgens in women. Clinicians also have limited ability to test adequately for testosterone insufficiency due to the use of assays based on higher levels in males with reduced sensitivity at the lower levels where female levels lie. Furthermore, there is no evidence that any specific lower limit of measured free or total testosterone is diagnostic of a deficiency state. Presently, most off-label use of androgen therapy in the USA for sexual dysfunction in women is via empiric trial of therapy based on the patient's clinical history and presenting complaints, with or without verification by testing of blood levels.

As no androgen products are approved for use in women, off-label products from the male side have been utilized. However, testosterone is available in many forms. There are several varieties of oral androgens available from pharmacies currently. However, they require cautious use, as their 17-alkyl substitutions can lead to liver toxicity. Oral testosterone undeconate is generally thought to be safe, but it requires at least twice daily dosing, taken with food to enhance absorption.[43] Testosterone has also been administered as intramuscular injections of either testosterone enanthate or testosterone cypionate in doses of 200–250 mg every 2 weeks.[43] A testosterone implant is also currently available. The implant is inserted under the skin into the lower abdominal wall or buttock. The implant slowly releases testosterone over 4–5 months.[44] Recently, two transdermal gels have reached the market.[45,46] The gels are rubbed onto the skin daily. Both have proven effective and well tolerated, but are expensive. Skin patches have also been effective, but the adhesive can cause irritation.[43] The latest devel-

oped preparation, buccal tablets, has reached the market. The buccal system produces a steady-state testosterone level comparable to the gels.[47]

Dehydroepiandrosterone, a weak androgen, is available in the USA without prescription. Dehydroepiandrosterone is produced by both the adrenal glands and ovaries. Like other androgens, its production is decreased after the menopause. In the postmenopausal woman, production of dehydroepiandrosterone and dehydroepiandrosterone sulfate (the sulfated form) by the adrenals is the major source of serum testosterone.[48]

In 1994, a small, randomized, placebo-controlled, crossover trial of nightly oral dehydroepiandrosterone administered to 13 men and 17 women aged 40–70 over a 6-month period was conducted. In response to dehydroepiandrosterone administration, serum levels of dehydroepiandrosterone and dehydroepiandrosterone sulfate were elevated from placebo values (7.19 ± 0.5–16.13 ± 1.3 nmol/l; 1.78 ± 0.17–9.27 ± 0.76 μmol/l; $p < 0.001$). Between baseline and 12 weeks of dehydroepiandrosterone administration in women, serum androstenedione increased from 1.33 ± 0.13 to 3.0 ± 0.19 nmol/l ($p < 0.001$), serum testosterone from 0.72 ± 0.07 to 1.46 ± 0.14 nmol/l ($p < 0.001$), and serum dihydrotestosterone from 0.32 ± 0.03 to 0.9 ± 0.1 nmol/l ($p < 0.001$). Serum sex hormone-binding globulin concentrations exhibited a tendency to decline (105.5 ± 12.3 to 81.2 ± 10.6 nmol/l) that was not statistically significant. Serum levels of estrone and estradiol were not significantly altered (estrone, 256.2 ± 58.5 vs 268.2 ± 58.8 pmol/l; estradiol, 144.7 ± 35.2 vs 107.3 ± 20.6 pmol/l). Specific statements of well-being ranged from improved quality of sleep, more relaxed, increased energy to better ability to handle stress. No difference was noted in libido while subjects were receiving dehydroepiandrosterone compared to the placebo group.[49]

A more recent, retrospective, open-label study by Munarriz et al. showed that after a mean duration of 4 ± 2 months of dehydroepiandrosterone 50 mg (two subjects used 25 mg), serum values for dehydroepiandrosterone and dehydroepiandrosterone sulfate increased. The mean score for the sexual distress scale decreased from 35.7/48 to 19.6/48. The mean score for the Female Sexual Function Index increased from 41.3 ± 18.9 to 67.7 ± 16.1. The individual domain scores for desire increased from 3.3/10 to 5.9/10; arousal, 6.9/20 to 14.3/20; lubrication, 10.0/20 to 14.6/20; orgasm, 5.7/15 to 11.5/15; and satisfaction, 6.2/15 to 12.2/15.[50]

Data pertaining to the use of dehydroepiandrosterone remain inconclusive, and safety data for dehydroepiandrosterone therapy are clearly lacking.

Tibolone

Now used in Europe, Asia, and Australasia, tibolone is a synthetic steroid with therapeutic indications for the treatment of estrogen deficiency symptoms in postmenopausal women more than 1 year after menopause, as well as the prevention of osteoporosis in estrogen-deficiency states.[51] Tibolone has tissue-specific estrogenic, progestogenic, and androgenic properties. Treatment with tibolone does not require a separate progestogen to offset the risk of endometrial hyperplasia that is present with estrogens, because of its own progestogenic actions on the endometrium.

Upon oral administration, tibolone is metabolized into 3α-OH tibolone and 3β-OH tibolone. These metabolites bind to estrogen receptors. The 3β-OH tibolone metabolite and tibolone itself may be further metabolized to a Δ-4 isomer of tibolone, which has affinity for progesterone and androgen receptors. Furthermore, tibolone lowers sex hormone-binding globulin, such that the effects of tibolone with respect to sexual function may be due to lowering of sex hormone-binding globulin and direct effects of the Δ-4 isomer.[52]

The effects of tibolone 2.5 mg have been compared with both placebo and oral estrogen-progestin therapy. However, none of these studies distinguish whether any benefit of tibolone is due to a direct action or sex hormone-binding globulin lowering effect. In a study of tibolone versus 17-beta-estradiol 2 mg plus norethisterone acetate 1 mg on sexual life when tibolone was compared to estradiol/norethisterone acetate, higher scores were found regarding all items in favor of tibolone at 24 weeks as well as at 48 weeks. These differences reached significance for the items frequency, satisfaction and enjoyment. Unfortunately, there was no placebo group in this study with which to compare drug effect.[53]

The effects of tibolone versus conjugated equine estrogen 0.625 mg plus medroxyprogesterone acetate 2.5 mg on sexual performance in postmenopausal women was also studied.[54] Approximately 25 women were randomized to each group and treated for 1 year. At the end of the year, it was found that treatment with either preparation significantly improved subjective well-being, vasomotor symptoms, and vaginal dryness. Tibolone therapy increased sexual desire and coital frequency ($p = 0.001$, $p = 0.014$). The rates of side effects in both groups were not statistically significant ($p = 0.84$).[55]

A pilot study investigating the effect of a continuous combination of norethisterone acetate (1 mg) and estradiol valerate (2 mg) versus tibolone on memory, sexuality, and mood was performed by Albertozzi et al. in 2000. Both groups had improvements in sexuality, which was achieved mainly by an improvement of sexual desire ($p < 0.05$). Both drugs also showed an increase in semantic memory and no effect on mood.[54]

A randomized, double-blind, crossover study was conducted to compare the effects of tibolone versus placebo on sexual function and climacteric symptoms in postmenopausal women in 2001. Each of the 38 subjects that completed the study was randomized to receive oral tibolone 2.5 mg a day for 3 months followed by placebo for 3 months, or the reverse. Vaginal blood flow during erotic stimulation by fantasy and film was measured by vaginal photoplethysmograph. Subjective sexual satisfaction data were also collected from participants by sexual function questionnaires and daily diaries. The results showed that baseline phasic changes in vaginal pulse amplitude levels were significantly higher on tibolone than on placebo ($p < 0.001$), indicating that tibolone enhanced vaginal blood flow independently of sexual stimulation. After exposure to two periods of sexual fantasy, a significantly greater increase in vaginal pulse amplitude was noted with tibolone than with placebo ($p < 0.05$). Subjective assessment of vaginal lubrication after erotic stimulation showed significantly more lubrication with tibolone than with placebo ($p < 0.001$). Analysis of sexual function based on subjects' daily diaries revealed that the mean frequency of sexual fantasies, the mean frequency of arousability, and mean frequency of desire for sex were higher with tibolone than with placebo, with p values of < 0.03, < 0.01, and 0.08 respectively. Significantly more vaginal lubrication during sexual intercourse was reported with tibolone than with placebo ($p < 0.01$), and there was also a trend in favor of tibolone for less dyspareunia ($p = 0.08$). According to the Greene climacteric scale, vasomotor symptoms were significantly reduced with tibolone treatment compared with placebo ($p < 0.0005$).[56]

Other over-the-counter therapies

The recent fear of hormones has led many women to pursue herbal therapies because they are "natural" and therefore assumed to be safer. In the USA, this is a totally unregulated, multibillion-dollar industry. What is on the label is not necessarily in the jar, and what is in the jar is not necessarily on the label. All sorts of claims are made for these products, especially when it comes to sexual improvement effects. Health-care providers should caution patients about use of such products and to be wary of the claims of effect on sexual function.

Perimenopause

The years prior to menopause that encompass the change from normal ovulatory cycles to cessation of menses are known as the perimenopausal transition years.[57] The perimenopausal transition period is characterized by erratic production of estradiol by the ovaries. Estrogen levels in women during this transition can be high, normal, or low at any given time. This fluctuation in blood levels of estrogen can persist until full ovarian failure occurs. Menstrual cycle length is determined by the rate and quality of follicular growth and development, and it is normal for the cycle to vary in individual women. In perimenopausal women, cycles can become progressively shorter, primarily because of the shortening of the follicular phase. A decrease in the production of inhibin B by the ovarian granulosa cells leads to an increase in production of follicle-stimulating hormone by the pituitary, leading to accelerated development of the predominant ovarian follicle, a shorter follicular phase, and increased levels of estradiol.

These fluctuating levels of hormones may cause perimenopausal women to experience insomnia, hot flushes, and changes in mood. They also begin experiencing dyspareunia from a reduction in vaginal lubrication and elasticity. Both the changes in sleep patterns and mood, and increases in dyspareunia can lead to an overall loss of libido.

While education is the first-line therapy for perimenopausal women, some may ultimately require hormonal therapy of some kind. Unlike their postmenopausal counterparts, however, traditional hormone replacement therapy is not the best option for these women. The low doses of estrogen utilized in hormone replacement do not suppress the ovary and the fluctuating levels of estrogen continue. The addition of hormonal therapy can augment or exaggerate problems instead of modifying them. Appropriate hormone therapy should first suppress the erratically functioning ovaries and then provide a stable level avoiding the fluctuations and hence symptoms. The use of oral contraceptive therapy has remained the reference standard for perimenopausal hormone therapy when it is needed due to the suppression provided. While perimenopausal decreases in sexual desire can stem from diminishing levels of testosterone, low-dose oral contraceptive therapy is more frequently the culprit. Such therapy can increase sex hormone-binding globulin levels, decrease bioavailable testosterone by decreased ovarian production as well as increased binding by sex hormone-binding globulin, and delete the midcycle surge of testosterone involved in increased sexual drive at the time of ovulation. Other perimenopausal therapeutic interventions, such as the use of antidepressant therapies, can have a negative impact on sexual function, including decreased desire and arousal capabilities.

Thus, while the treatment of sexual dysfunction in perimenopausal women is not very different from its treatment in premenopausal women, the variables presented by the unique pathophysiology of this transition and the kinds of therapies available for perimenopausal symptoms can have a negative impact on sexual function. Any therapeutic intervention must take into account these variables, and adjustments of such therapies may be necessary.

References

1. Meldrum DR, Davidson BJ, Tataryn IV et al. Changes in circulating steroids with aging in postmenopausal women. *Obstet Gynecol* 1981; 57: 624–8.
2. Bachmann GA, Leiblum SR. The impact of hormones on menopausal sexuality: a literature review. *Menopause* 2004; 11: 120–30.
3. Freedman MA. Quality of life and menopause: the role of estrogen. *J Womens Health* 2002; 11: 703–18.
4. Sarrel PM. Effects of hormone replacement therapy on sexual psychophysiology and behavior in postmenopause. *J Womens Health Gend Based Med* 2000; 9(S1): S25–32.
5. Willhite LA, O'Connell MB. Urogenital atrophy: prevention and treatment. *Pharmacotherapy* 2001; 21: 464–80.
6. Scott JR, DiSaia PJ, Hammond CB et al. Genitourinary atrophy. In *Danforth's Obstetrics and Gynecology*, 8th edn. New York: Lippincott, Williams & Wilkins, 1999: 682–3.
7. Vestergaard P, Hermann AP, Stilgren L et al. Effects of 5 years of hormonal replacement therapy on menopausal symptoms and blood pressure – a randomized controlled study. *Maturitas* 2003; 46: 123–32.
8. Buckler H, Al-Azzawi F, the UK VR Multicentre Trial Group. The effect of a novel vaginal ring delivering oestradiol acetate on climacteric symptoms in postmenopausal women. *Br J Obstet Gynaecol* 2003; 110: 753–9.
9. Barentsen R, van de Weijer PHM, Schram JHN. Continuous low dose estradiol released from a vaginal ring versus estriol vaginal cream for urogenital atrophy. *Eur J Obstet Gynecol Reprod Biol* 1997; 71: 73–80.
10. Vagifem [package insert]. Bagsvaerd, Denmark: Novo Nordisk, 2004.
11. Shoham Z, Kopernik G. Tools for making correct decisions regarding hormone therapy. I. Background and drugs. *Fertil Steril* 2004; 81: 1447–57.
12. Slater CC, Hodis HN, Mack WJ et al. Markedly elevated levels of estrone sulfate after long-term oral, but not transdermal, administration of estradiol in postmenopausal women. *Menopause* 2001; 8: 200–3.
13. Decensi A, Omodei U, Robertson C et al. Effect of transdermal estradiol and oral conjugated estrogen on C-reactive protein in retinoid-placebo trial in healthy women. *Circulation* 2002; 106: 1224–8.
14. Scarabin PY, Oger E, Plu-Bureau G, for the Estrogen and ThromboEmbolism Risk (ESTHER) Study Group. Differential association of oral and transdermal oestrogen-replacement therapy with venous thromboembolism risk. *Lancet* 2003; 362(9382): 428–32.
15. Femring [package insert]. Rockaway, NY: Warner Chilcott Inc., 2004.
16. Haas JS, Kaplan CP, Gerstenberger EP et al. Changes in the use of postmenopausal hormone therapy after the publication of clinical trial results. *Ann Intern Med* 2004; 140: 184–8.
17. Hulley S, Grady D, Bush T et al. Randomized trial of estrogen plus progestin for secondary prevention of coronary heart disease in postmenopausal women. Heart and Estrogen/Progestin Replacement Study (HERS) Research Group. *JAMA* 1998; 280: 605–13.
18. Rossouw JE, Anderson GL, Prentice RI et al. Risks and benefits of estrogen plus progestin in healthy postmenopausal women; principal results from the Women's Health Initiative randomized controlled trial. *JAMA* 2002; 299: 321–33.
19. Anderson GL, Limacher M, Assaf AR et al. Effects of conjugated equine estrogen in postmenopausal women with hysterectomy. *JAMA* 2004; 291: 1701–12.
20. Wassertheil-Smoller S, Hendrix SL, Limacher M et al. Effect of estrogen plus progestin in stroke in postmenopausal women: the Women's Health Initiative: a randomized trial. *JAMA* 2003; 289: 2673–84.
21. Rapp SR, Espeland MA, Shumakaer SA et al. Effect of estrogen plus progestin on global cognitive function in postmenopausal women: the Women's Health Initiative Memory Study: a randomized controlled trial. *JAMA* 2003; 289: 2663–72.
22. Shumaker SA, Legault C, Rapp SR et al. Estrogen plus progestin and the incidence of dementia and mild cognitive impairment in postmenopausal women: the Women's Health Initiative Memory Study: a randomized controlled trial. *JAMA* 2003; 289: 2651–62.
23. Lobo R. Evaluation of cardiovascular event rates with hormone therapy in healthy, early postmenopausal women. *Arch Int Med* 2004; 164: 482–4.

24. American College of Obstetrics and Gynecology. Response to Women's Health Initiative Study Results by the American College of Obstetricians and Gynecologists. 2003. Available at: www.acog.org/member_access/misc/whiResponse.cfm?printerFriendly=yes. Accessed 20 July 2004.

25. Kim C, Kwok YS. Decision analysis of hormone replacement therapy after the Women's Health Initiative. Am J Obstet Gynecol 2003; 189: 1228–33.

26. Myers LS, Dixen J, Morrisette D et al. Effects of estrogen, androgen, and progestin on sexual psychophysiology and behavior in postmenopausal women. J Clin Endocrinol Metab 1990; 70: 1124–31.

27. Bjorn I, Bixo M, Strandberg K et al. Negative mood changes during hormone replacement therapy: a comparison between two progestogens. Am J Obstet Gynecol 2000; 183: 1419–26.

28. Sherwin BB. The impact of different doses of estrogen and progestin on mood and sexual behavior in postmenopausal women. J Clin Endocrinol Metab 1991; 72: 336–43.

29. Holst J, Backstom T, Hammarback S et al. Progesterone addition during oestrogen replacement therapy – effects on vasomotor symptoms and mood. Maturitas 1989; 11: 13–20.

30. Fitzpatrick LA, Pace C, Wiita B. Comparison of regimens containing oral micronized progesterone or medroxyprogesterone acetate on quality of life in postmenopausal women: a cross-sectional survey. J Womens Health Gend Based Med. 2000; 9: 381–7.

31. Pazol K, Wilson ME, Walen K. Medroxyprogesterone acetate antagonized the effects of estrogen treatment on social and sexual behavior in female macaques. J Clin Endocrinol Metab 2004; 89: 2998–3006.

32. Grady D, Gebretsadik T, Kerlikowske K et al. Hormone replacement therapy and endometrial cancer risk: a meta-analysis. Obstet Gynecol 1995; 85: 304–13.

33. PEPI Investigators. Effects of estrogen or estrogen/progestin regimens on heart disease risk factors in postmenopausal women: the Postmenopausal Estrogen/Progestin Interventions (PEPI) Trial. JAMA 1995; 273: 199–208.

34. Bachmann G, Bancroft J, Braunstein G et al. Female androgen insufficiency: the Princeton consensus statement of definition, classification, and assessment. Fertil Steril 2002; 77: 660–5.

35. Schneider HPG. Androgens and antiandrogens. Ann N Y Acad Sci 2003; 997: 292–306.

36. Laughlin GA, Barrett-Connor E, Kritz-Silverstein D et al. Hysterectomy, oophorectomy, and endogenous sex hormone levels in older women: the Rancho Bernado Study. J Clin Endocrinol Metab 2000; 85: 645–51.

37. Sarrel P, Dobay B, Wiita B. Estrogen and estrogen-androgen replacement in postmenopaual women dissatisfied with estrogen-only therapy; sexual behavior and neuroendocrine responses. J Reprod Med 1998; 43: 847–56.

38. Shifren JL, Braunstein GD, Simon JA et al. Transdermal testosterone treatment in women with impaired sexual function after oophorectomy. N Engl J Med 2004; 343: 682–8.

39. Buster J. Large phase III study confirms that transdermal testosterone patch 300 mg/day significantly improves sexual function with minimal side effects in surgically menopausal women. Presented at Endocrine 86th Annual Meeting, New Orleans, 16–19 June 2004.

40. Estratest and Estratest H.S. [package insert]. Marietta: Solvay Pharmaceuticals, Inc., 2004.

41. Lobo RA, Rosen RC, Yang HM et al. Comparative effects of oral esterified estrogens with and without methyltestosterone on endocrine profiles and dimensions of sexual function in postmenopausal women with hypoactive sexual desire. Fertil Steril 2003; 79: 1341–52.

42. Mazer NA, Shifren JL. Transdermal testosterone for women: a new physiological approach for androgen therapy. Obstet Gynecol Surv 2003; 58: 489–500.

43. Bremner WJ. Therapeutic efficacy of androgen delivery systems. Updates in Infertility Treatment 2004. Marco Island, FL. 22–24 January 2004.

44. Testosterone Implant 50, 100 or 200 mg [package insert]. Roseland: Organon Laboratories Ltd, 2004.

45. Testim 1% [package insert]. Norristown: Auxilium Pharmaceuticals, Inc., 2003.

46. AndroGel 1% [package insert]. Marietta: Solvay Pharmaceuticals, Inc., 2004.

47. Dobs AS, Matsumoto AM, Wang C et al. Short-term pharmacokinetic comparison of a novel testosterone buccal system and a testosterone gel in testosterone deficient men. Curr Med Res Opin 2004; 20: 729–38.

48. Kovalevsky G. Hormones and female sexual dysfunction in postmenopasual women. Menopausal Med 2004; 12: 1–5.

49. Morales AJ, Nolan JJ, Nelson JC et al. Effects of replacement dose of dehydroepiandrosterone in men and women of advancing age. J Clin Endocrinol Metab 1994; 78: 1360–7.

50. Munarriz R, Talakoub L, Flaherty E et al. Androgen replacement therapy with dehydroepiandrosterone for androgen insufficiency and female sexual dysfunction: androgen and questionnaire results. J Sex Marital Ther 2002; 28(s): 165–73.

51. Livial [package insert]. Roseland: Organon Laboratories Ltd, 2004.

52. Davis SR. The effects of tibolone on mood and libido. Menopause 2002; 9: 162–70.

53. Nathorst-Boos J, Hammar M. Effect on sexual life – a comparison between tibolone and a continuous estradiol-northisterone acetate regimen. Maturitas 1997; 26: 15–20.

54. Albertazzi P, Natale V, Barboline C et al. The effect of tibolone versus continuous combined norethisterone acetate and oestradiol on memory, libido, and mood of postmenopausal women: a pilot study. 2000; 36: 223–9.

55. Kokcu A, Cetinkaya MB, Yanik F et al. The comparison of effects of tibolone and conjugated estrogen-medroxyprogesterone acetate therapy on sexual performance in postmenopausal women. Maturitas 2000; 36: 75–80.

56. Laan E, van Lunsen RHW, Everaerd W. The effects of tibolone on vaginal blood flow, sexual desire and arousability in postmenopausal women. Climacteric 2001; 4: 28–41.

57. Speroff L, Glass RH, Kase NG. The perimenopausal transition. In Clinical Gynecologic Endocrinology and Infertility, 6th edn. Baltimore: Lippincott, Williams & Wilkins, 1999: 651–6.

13.3 Difficult cases: hormonal treatment of desire, arousal and orgasm disorders

Bronwyn G A Stuckey

Menopause is universal and leads to dramatic changes in estrogen status and corresponding changes in female sexual function (see Chapters 6.1–6.3 of this book). However, there are other, less common conditions associated with disturbances in hormones which may require specific management, constituting difficult endocrine management problems.

As in other portions of this textbook relating to difficult case management, all efforts have been made to protect the privacy of patients and to maintain the management strategies utilized in the case for teaching purposes.

Hypogonadotropic hypogonadism

Case history

An 18-year-old woman presented with failure of progression into puberty and the accompanying sign of anosmia. The history was consistent with Kallmann's syndrome, and subsequent genetic studies have confirmed this diagnosis. Gonadotropins and estradiol were undetectable. The free androgen index was within the low normal range. Puberty and menses were induced by exogenous estrogen and progestin therapy. The patient married and returned at age 25 years with a request for ovulation induction to achieve pregnancy. There had been no complaint from the patient of impaired sexual function. Ovulation induction was attempted first with pulsatile gonadotropin-releasing hormone and subsequently with exogenous gonadotropins. After several cycles of therapy, pregnancy was achieved. The patient reported, in retrospect, markedly improved sexual function during ovarian stimulation with both gonadotropin-releasing hormone and gonadotropins compared to that experienced on exogenous estrogen and progestin therapy. When she returned to the former estrogen/progestin regimen, she was concerned by the fall in her feelings of sexual interest.

Question: is there an indication for androgen therapy, together with estrogen and progestin, in such patients?

Isolated hypogonadotropic hypogonadism is associated with lack of pituitary drive to the ovaries while the pituitary-adrenal axis remains intact. It may be secondary to congenital conditions such as Kallmann's syndrome; to drug therapy such as opioids, especially when administered intrathecally; or to hyperprolactinemia.[1-3] Central or secondary hypogonadism is associated with greater deficiency of ovarian sex hormone secretion, particularly androgen secretion, than is associated with normal menopausal aging.[4] Although this is recognized, it has not been addressed in clinical studies of combined estrogen and androgen therapy in this patient group, with sexual function as an endpoint. This may be partly because of the difficulty in recruiting adequate numbers of patients in this category.

Panhypopituitarism is associated with a lack of stimulatory drive, not only to the ovaries, but also the adrenal gland, the other major site of sex hormone production.[4] Despite demonstrated sex hormone deficiency, including androgen deficiency, there is a paucity of data addressing sexual function in this group. In one study of 38 women with hypopituitarism, dehydroepiandrosterone was used in doses of 30 mg daily for those younger than 45 years and 20 mg daily for older women.[5] Patients were asked to report sexual interest and activity as reduced, unchanged, or increased. No significant effect of dehydroepiandrosterone was observed in the 6-month randomized part of the study.

Hyperprolactinemia

Case history

A 45-year-old woman presented with galactorrhea, insomnia, and dyspareunia. She had had a hysterectomy 16 years previously for menorrhagia. Prolactin was 3000 mU/l (< 500). Gonadotropins and estrogen were suppressed. Magnetic resonance imaging scan showed a small pituitary microadenoma consistent with a prolactinoma. Dopamine agonist therapy in the form of cabergoline was commenced, with rapid suppression of her prolactin, a return of biochemical evidence of ovulation, and an improvement in sexual function. At the age of 51, she became postmenopausal and commenced estrogen and progestin hormone therapy for menopausal symptoms. Dopamine agonist therapy was continued for the next 3 years. Since the pituitary tumor was small and the patient was postmenopausal, a decision was made by her physician that the dopamine agonist was serving no purpose and could be withdrawn. There was a subsequent rise in serum prolactin to 2000 mU/l (< 500) and a fall in sexual interest and response. Sexual function improved with the reinstitution of dopamine therapy.

Question: does high prolactin adversely affect sexual function, independently of changes in sex hormones, in such patients?

Hyperprolactinemia may be caused by prolactin-secreting pituitary tumor (prolactinoma), pituitary stalk disruption by space-occupying lesions, psychotropic medication, or renal failure. The secretion of prolactin is under inhibitory control by hypothalamic dopamine, which binds to D_2 receptors on lactotrophs. Increased prolactin secretion by the pituitary inhibits release of hypothalamic gonadotropin-releasing hormone and, consequently, of gonadal sex hormones.

Hyperprolactinemia caused by a prolactinoma produces menstrual disturbance, leading to an earlier diagnosis in women than in men.[6] Both menstrual disturbance and decreased libido have been documented with high prevalence in women with a prolactinoma.[7,8] Treatment with a dopamine agonist such as bromocriptine or cabergoline will usually restore normal endocrine function and induce tumor shrinkage. Studies of dopamine agonist therapy in men confirm a brisk response of sexual dysfunction to therapy.[9] Whether the early response relates to the fall in prolactin or the institution of dopamine is not known. No such confirmatory studies exist in women partly because of the small numbers of study participants.[8]

Case history

A 29-year-old woman with schizophrenia presented with amenorrhea, galactorrhea, dyspareunia, and loss of libido. She had required hospitalization and was being treated with thioridazine. Soon after commencing this medication, she had experienced amenorrhea. She became aware of decreased sexual function and galactorrhea. Serum prolactin was 2674 mU/l (< 500), and gonadotropins and estradiol were suppressed. Her attending physician treated her with cabergoline, resulting in a fall of prolactin, return of menses, and improvement in sexual interest. However, she experienced a relapse in her psychiatric symptoms, and the dopamine agonist was withdrawn, with subsequent return of her sexual symptoms.

Question: what is the optimal management of psychotropic-induced hyperprolactinemia and sexual dysfunction?

Hyperprolactinemia induced by psychotropic medication is commonly associated with sexual dysfunction in both men and women. The mechanism of antipsychotic therapy is to block dopaminergic action in the mesolimbic system. Side effects of the blockade of dopaminergic action elsewhere include movement disorders, caused by blockade of dopamine action in the striatum, and hyperprolactinemia, caused by blockade of dopamine D_2 receptors in the pituitary. All conventional antipsychotic medications cause elevation in prolactin.[10,11] Among the newer antipsychotic agents, risperidone also causes significant hyperprolactinemia, but other agents, such as clozapine, olanzapine, quetiapine, and aripiprazole, cause very little, if any, elevation of prolactin.[12]

Again, the effects of psychotropic-induced hyperprolactinemia have been more widely studied in men than in women. However, the rise in prolactin is more marked in women and is associated with galactorrhea, amenorrhea, hypoestrogenism, vaginal dryness, and reduced libido.[13,14] In a study of sexual dysfunction in men and women taking conventional psychotropic medication, hyperprolactinemia was found to be strongly related to sexual dysfunction in females.[15] However, it is unclear whether the sexual side effects are secondary to the elevation of prolactin or to the dopamine blockade.

It is conventional wisdom that the institution of dopamine agonists to treat hyperprolactinemia in such patients is contraindicated because it may lead to loss of psychotropic control. This view is supported by data showing increased dopaminergic activity in schizophrenia and by evidence of dopamine-induced psychosis in patients treated for Parkinson's disease.[16,17] Despite this belief, small studies have reported a low incidence of deleterious psychiatric effects of dopamine agonists used to treat psychotropic-induced hyperprolactinemia.[18–21]

Nevertheless, newer selective, "prolactin-sparing" antipsychotic agents are preferred when hyperprolactinemia and its side effects, including sexual dysfunction, are recognized. In a study of 20 female patients with risperidone-induced hyperprolactinemia, amenorrhea, and sexual dysfunction, the change to olanzapine produced a significant fall in prolactin and improvement in sexual function.[22] In a smaller study of five patients, four of whom were female, a switch to quetiapine produced improvements in hyperprolactinemia and in sexual side effects associated with conventional antipsychotic therapy.[23]

Sexual dysfunction associated with hyperprolactinemia induced by antipsychotic medication may be unreported by patients unless sought in the clinical history, and may be an important cause of noncompliance with medication. However, studies of therapeutic intervention with change of antipsychotic therapy or dopamine agonist therapy are very few and uncontrolled.

Case history

A 33-year-old woman had a history of acute renal failure after exposure to a plant-derived nephrotoxin. She rapidly required dialysis and had been having dialysis for 9 years when she presented. Initially, she had felt so unwell that sexual activity was not considered a priority for her or her husband. However, her feeling of well-being had improved, and she sought help for her lack of sexual drive and response. She had had no menses since she had been on dialysis. Her creatinine (predialysis) was 600 μmol/l (50–95). Serum prolactin was 2900 mU/l (< 500), luteinizing hormone was < 1 mU/l, and estradiol was < 100 pmol/l. Cabergoline was prescribed, but it was not tolerated and led to no decrease in serum prolactin.

Question: what is the mechanism and the management of hyperprolactinemia in renal failure?

Hyperprolactinemia is also common in patients with renal failure, secondary to increased production more than impaired clearance.[24] Hyperprolactinemia appears to worsen, rather than improve, after the institution of peritoneal or hemodialysis.[25] Women with advanced renal failure usually have amenorrhea and hypoestrogenemia, especially if there is hyperprolactinemia present, and studies have identified reduced sexual function in patients undergoing dialysis.[26,27] Although the debility of the disease may be responsible for diminution in sexual interest and drive, this may be at least partly attributable to hypogonadism and hyperprolactinemia.[28]

The mechanism of the rise in prolactin and its role in sexual function in renal failure have been poorly understood. Although a fall in prolactin with bromocriptine therapy had been reported, prolactin in chronic renal failure appears to be less responsive to either stimulation or suppression than it is in patients without uremia.[29,30] Recent studies have focused on the role of the prolactin receptor as a member of the cytokine/hemopoietin receptor superfamily. Prolactin promotes expression of the erythropoietin receptor and thereby promotes erythropoiesis. It has been suggested that, in renal failure, hyperprolactinemia is a compensatory response to the reduced

availability of renal-derived erythropoietin.[31] This hypothesis is supported by studies showing a fall in prolactin with erythropoietin therapy, although not all are confirmatory.[32–34] Improvements in gonadal and sexual function, together with a fall in prolactin, have also been reported in patients with renal failure after commencement of erythropoietin therapy.[35,36] However, it is not clear that these improvements are dependent on changes in prolactin rather than improved well-being.[37,38]

In a nonblinded study, estrogen and progestin therapy has been shown to improve sexual function in amenorrheic, hypoestrogenic women on renal dialysis, compared with women receiving no sex hormone therapy.[39] This study reported an increase in frequency of intercourse, sexual satisfaction, and libido. Interestingly, prolactin fell in those patients treated with estrogen and progestin, and the relative contribution of these changes to the improvement is unclear.

Finally, renal transplantation is associated with a fall in prolactin and an improvement in sexual function in women undergoing dialysis.[40–42] The contribution of the fall in prolactin after transplant is undoubtedly a small part of the overall improvement in quality of life and sexual function.

Adrenal insufficiency

Case history

A 40-year-old woman developed fatigue, weight loss, and skin pigmentation. Plasma cortisol was low and did not rise with synthetic ACTH (1–24) (cosyntropin) stimulation. Addison's disease was diagnosed, and she was treated with replacement glucocorticoid and mineralocorticoid therapy. A few years later, she entered early menopause, and combined estrogen and progestin therapy was prescribed. She complained of dwindling sexual interest. Serum dehydroepiandrosterone sulfate was low, consistent with adrenal failure and reduced adrenal androgen production.

Question: what evidence supports dehydroepiandrosterone therapy for the treatment of sexual dysfunction in patients with adrenal failure?

Several studies have shown impaired quality-of-life measures, including measures of sexual function, in patients with adrenal insufficiency, despite adequate glucocorticoid and mineralocorticoid replacement.[43,44] This impairment seems to be greater for females than for males, and it is proposed that dehydroepiandrosterone therapy is an important factor missing in conventional adrenal replacement regimens.[45]

Dehydroepiandrosterone and dehydroepiandrosterone sulfate are major secretory products of the adrenal and are low in adrenal insufficiency of either primary or secondary origin. In the periphery, dehydroepiandrosterone functions as a prohormone, being converted to testosterone via hydroxysteroid dehydrogenase, or to estradiol by aromatase.[46] In women, it leads to a rise in circulating testosterone. However, there is also evidence of dehydroepiandrosterone synthesis and metabolism in the brain, where it appears to exert effects on neuronal growth.[47]

Four studies of dehydroepiandrosterone therapy in adrenal insufficiency have directly addressed sexual function in women. There is variability in the adequacy of the measures of sexual function used. The study by Johannsson et al., showing no benefit of dehydroepiandrosterone in women with adrenal insufficiency secondary to pituitary disease, has been discussed above.[5] Arlt et al. demonstrated a significant effect of dehydroepiandrosterone 50 mg daily on sexual thoughts, interest, and mental and physical satisfaction.[48] This study included 24 patients with both primary and secondary adrenal failure in a crossover design with a visual analog scale to assess sexual function. However, these findings could not be replicated in a similar crossover design study, using the same dose in 24 women with primary adrenal failure.[49] Similarly, a parallel-group, placebo-controlled study, using dehydroepiandrosterone 25 mg daily in 36 women with predominantly primary adrenal failure, also failed to show any benefit of treatment.[50]

The lack of uniformity of findings in studies of dehydroepiandrosterone replacement in a condition where there is documented deficiency highlights the complexity surrounding all studies of female sexuality. Moreover, it suggests that uniformity is not likely to be found in studies of dehydroepiandrosterone in patients without documented deficiency.

This group of conditions encompasses difficult cases of endocrine causation of female sexual dysfunction. They include diseases, such as hypoadrenalism, either primary or secondary, where deficiencies of hormones or prohormones have been identified, but therapeutic trials of replacement have failed to provide conclusive evidence of benefit. They also include conditions, such as drug-induced or uremia-associated hyperprolactinemia, where conventional therapeutic intervention is either contraindicated or ineffective. In all of these conditions there is a lack of recognition by practitioners and a lack of quality data on best-practice management.

References

1. Seminara SB, Hayes FJ, Crowley WF Jr. Gonadotropin-releasing hormone deficiency in the human (idiopathic hypogonadotropic hypogonadism and Kallmann's syndrome): pathophysiological and genetic considerations. *Endocr Rev* 1998; 19: 521–39.

2. Finch PM, Roberts LJ, Price L et al. Hypogonadism in patients treated with intrathecal morphine. *Clin J Pain* 2000; 16: 251–4.

3. Rolland R, Corbey RS. Hyperprolactinemia and hypogonadism in the human female. *Eur J Obstet Gynecol Reprod Biol* 1977; 7: 337–48.

4. Miller KK, Sesmilo G, Schiller A et al. Androgen deficiency in women with hypopituitarism. *J Clin Endocrinol Metab* 2001; 86: 561–7.

5. Johannsson G, Burman P, Wiren L et al. Low dose dehydroepiandrosterone affects behavior in hypopituitary androgen-deficient women: a placebo-controlled trial. *J Clin Endocrinol Metab* 2002; 87: 2046–52.

6. Colao A, Sarno AD, Cappabianca P et al. Gender differences in the prevalence, clinical features and response to cabergoline in hyperprolactinemia. *Eur J Endocrinol* 2003; 148: 325–31.

7. Lundberg PO, Hulter B. Sexual dysfunction in patients with hypothalamo-pituitary disorders. *Exp Clin Endocrinol* 1991; 98: 81–8.

8. Koppelman MC, Parry BL, Hamilton JA et al. Effect of bromocriptine on affect and libido in hyperprolactinemia. *Am J Psychiatry* 1987; 144: 1037–41.

9. De Rosa M, Zarrilli S, Vitale G et al. Six months of treatment with cabergoline restores sexual potency in hyperprolactinemic males: an open longitudinal study monitoring nocturnal penile tumescence. *J Clin Endocrinol Metab* 2004; 89: 621–5.

10. Wieck A, Haddad PM. Antipsychotic-induced hyperprolactinaemia in women: pathophysiology, severity and consequences. Selective literature review. *Br J Psychiatry* 2003; 182: 199–204.

11. Kleinberg DL, Davis JM, de Coster R et al. Prolactin levels and adverse events in patients treated with risperidone. *J Clin Psychopharmacol* 1999; 19: 57–61.

12. Compton MT, Miller AH. Antipsychotic-induced hyperprolactinemia and sexual dysfunction. *Psychopharmacol Bull* 2002; 36: 143–64.

13. Ghadirian AM, Chouinard G, Annable L. Sexual dysfunction and plasma prolactin levels in neuroleptic-treated schizophrenic outpatients. *J Nerv Ment Dis* 1982; 170: 463–7.

14. Knegtering H, van der Moolen AE, Castelein S et al. What are the effects of antipsychotics on sexual dysfunctions and endocrine functioning? *Psychoneuroendocrinology* 2003; 28: 109–23.

15. Smith SM, O'Keane V, Murray R. Sexual dysfunction in patients taking conventional antipsychotic medication. *Br J Psychiatry* 2002; 181: 49–55.

16. Davis KL, Kahn RS, Ko G et al. Dopamine in schizophrenia: a review and reconceptualization. *Am J Psychiatry* 1991; 148: 1474–86.

17. Wolters EC. Dopaminomimetic psychosis in Parkinson's disease patients: diagnosis and treatment. *Neurology* 1999; 52(Suppl 3): S10–3.

18. Tollin SR. Use of the dopamine agonists bromocriptine and cabergoline in the management of risperidone-induced hyperprolactinemia in patients with psychotic disorders. *J Endocrinol Invest* 2000; 23: 765–70.

19. Cohen LG, Biederman J. Treatment of risperidone-induced hyperprolactinemia with a dopamine agonist in children. *J Child Adolesc Psychopharmacol* 2001; 11: 435–40.

20. Cavallaro R, Cocchi F, Angelone SM et al. Cabergoline treatment of risperidone-induced hyperprolactinemia: a pilot study. *J Clin Psychiatry* 2004; 65: 187–90.

21. Smith S. Neuroleptic-associated hyperprolactinemia. Can it be treated with bromocriptine? *J Reprod Med* 1992; 37: 737–40.

22. Kim KS, Pae CU, Chae JH et al. Effects of olanzapine on prolactin levels of female patients with schizophrenia treated with risperidone. *J Clin Psychiatry* 2002; 63: 408–13.

23. Keller R, Mongini F. Switch to quetiapine in antipsychotic agent-related hyperprolactinemia. *Neurol Sci* 2002; 23:233–5.

24. Sievertsen GD, Lim VS, Nakawatase C et al. Metabolic clearance and secretion rates of human prolactin in normal subjects and in patients with chronic renal failure. *J Clin Endocrinol Metab* 1980; 50: 846–52.

25. Gomez F, de la Cueva R, Wauters JP et al. Endocrine abnormalities in patients undergoing long-term hemodialysis. The role of prolactin. *Am J Med* 1980; 68: 522–30.

26. Handelsman DJ. Hypothalamic-pituitary gonadal dysfunction in renal failure, dialysis and renal transplantation. *Endocr Rev* 1985; 6: 151–82.

27. Mastrogiacomo I, De Besi L, Serafini E et al. Hyperprolactinemia and sexual disturbances among uremic women on hemodialysis. *Nephron* 1984; 37: 195–9.

28. Steele TE, Wuerth D, Finkelstein S et al. Sexual experience of the chronic peritoneal dialysis patient. *J Am Soc Nephrol* 1996; 7: 1165–8.

29. Ermolenko VM, Kukhtevich AV, Dedov II et al. Parlodel treatment of uremic hypogonadism in men. *Nephron* 1986; 42: 19–22.

30. Peces R, Horcajada C, Lopez-Novoa JM et al. Hyperprolactinemia in chronic renal failure: impaired responsiveness to stimulation and suppression. Normalization after transplantation. *Nephron* 1981; 28: 11–16.

31. Bellone G, Rollino C, Borsa S et al. Association between elevated prolactin levels and circulating erythroid precursors in dialyzed patients. *Proc Soc Exp Biol Med* 2000; 223: 367–71.

32. Ramirez G, Bittle PA, Sanders H et al. Hypothalamo-hypophyseal thyroid and gonadal function before and after erythropoietin therapy in dialysis patients. *J Clin Endocrinol Metab* 1992; 74: 517–24.

33. Kokot F, Wiecek A, Schmidt-Gayk H et al. Function of endocrine organs in hemodialyzed patients of long-term erythropoietin therapy. *Artif Organs* 1995; 19: 428–35.

34. Watschinger B, Watzinger U, Templ H et al. Effect of recombinant human erythropoietin on anterior pituitary function in patients on chronic hemodialysis. *Horm Res* 1991; 36: 22–6.

35. Schaefer RM, Kokot F, Kuerner B et al. Normalization of serum prolactin levels in hemodialysis patients on recombinant human erythropoietin. *Int J Artif Organs* 1989; 12: 445–9.

36. Yeksan M, Tamer N, Cirit M et al. Effect of recombinant human erythropoietin (r-HuEPO) therapy on plasma FT3, FT4, TSH, FSH, LH, free testosterone and prolactin levels in hemodialysis patients. *Int J Artif Organs* 1992; 15: 585–9.

37. Schaefer RM, Kokot F, Wernze H et al. Improved sexual function in hemodialysis patients on recombinant erythropoietin: a possible role for prolactin. *Clin Nephrol* 1989; 31: 1–5.

38. Steffensen G, Aunsholt NA. Does erythropoietin cause hormonal changes in haemodialysis patients? *Nephrol Dial Transplant* 1993; 8: 1215–18.

39. Matuszkiewicz-Rowinska J, Skorzewska K, Radowicki S et al. The benefits of hormone replacement therapy in pre-menopausal women with oestrogen deficiency on haemodialysis. *Nephrol Dial Transplant* 1999; 14: 1238–43.

40. Toorians AW, Janssen E, Laan E et al. Chronic renal failure and sexual functioning: clinical status versus objectively assessed sexual response. *Nephrol Dial Transplant* 1997; 12: 2654–63.

41. Saha MT, Saha HH, Niskanen LK et al. Time course of serum prolactin and sex hormones following successful renal transplantation. *Nephron* 2002; 92: 735–7.

42. Chen Y, Chu SH, Lin MH et al. Impact of renal transplantation on sexual function in female recipients. *Transplant Proc* 2003; 35: 313–14.

43. Rosen T, Wiren L, Wilhelmsen L et al. Decreased psychological well-being in adult patients with growth hormone deficiency. *Clin Endocrinol* 1994; 40: 111–16.

44. Lovas K, Loge JH, Husebye ES. Subjective health status in Norwegian patients with Addison's disease. *Clin Endocrinol* 2002; 56: 581–8.

45. Arlt W. Quality of life in Addison's disease – the case for DHEA replacement. *Clin Endocrinol* 2002; 56: 573–4.

46. Allolio B, Arlt W. DHEA treatment: myth or reality? *Trends Endocrinol Metab* 2002; 13: 288–94.

47. Baulieu EE, Robel P. Dehydroepiandrosterone (DHEA) and dehydroepiandrosterone sulfate (DHEAS) as neuroactive neurosteroids. *Proc Natl Acad Sci USA* 1998; 95: 4089–91.

48. Arlt W, Callies F, van Vlijmen JC et al. Dehydroepiandrosterone replacement in women with adrenal insufficiency. *N Engl J Med* 1999; 341: 1013–20.

49. Hunt PJ, Gurnell EM, Huppert FA et al. Improvement in mood and fatigue after dehydroepiandrosterone replacement in Addison's disease in a randomized, double blind trial. *J Clin Endocrinol Metab* 2000; 85: 4650–6.

50. Lovas K, Gebre-Medhin G, Trovik TS et al. Replacement of dehydroepiandrosterone in adrenal failure: no benefit for subjective health status and sexuality in a 9-month, randomized, parallel group clinical trial. *J Clin Endocrinol Metab* 2003; 88: 1112–18.

NONHORMONAL MEDICAL TREATMENT OF FEMALE SEXUAL DYSFUNCTION

14.1 Nonhormonal medical treatment options for female sexual dysfunction

Salvatore Caruso

Introduction

Sexual disorders have recently attracted much attention, generating new research in the epidemiology, pathophysiology, and pharmacotherapy of female sexual dysfunction. Such interest, paradoxically, was stimulated when scientific research defined the efficacy of oral medication to inhibit the enzyme phosphodiesterase type 5. This class of drug was initially used experimentally in cardiology and, "by chance and unexpectedly", displayed side effects that produced erection in male test subjects.[1]

The success of selective phosphodiesterase type 5 inhibitors in the treatment of erectile dysfunction raised the question of whether similar medication could also be efficacious in the treatment of female sexual dysfunction.[2] One of the impediments to research and clinical development in the female sexual dysfunction field has been the lack of definite diagnostic procedures and limited basic science research.[3] Specifically, the biologic mechanism of sexual excitement and orgasm is not yet well defined,[4] although it has become increasingly evident that female sexual dysfunction can have an organic basis secondary to medical problems, even if risk factors for female sexual dysfunction are both psychologic and physiologic.[5]

The availability of selective phosphodiesterase type 5 inhibitors to treat erectile dysfunction in men has spurred new interest and attention in medical research for the treatment of sexual dysfunction in women. This recent attention to medical research in female sexual dysfunction will shed light on possible causes of problems, and describe potential therapeutic approaches. Furthermore, clinicians who treat women suffering from female sexual dysfunction have begun to consider a possible role of selective phosphodiesterase type 5 inhibitors in treating female sexual arousal disorder.

Selective phosphodiesterase type 5 inhibitors have revolutionized sexology, which, until the 1990s, was almost dormant. At that time, there was a clear dichotomy between biologic attempts at treatment, which were often rudimentary and fundamentally ill-founded, and psychotherapeutic methods, which were widely espoused for female sexual disorders.

The considerations that led to diametrically opposite treatments between men and women were based on clinical speculation that female sexuality was more expressive than male sexuality. The ignorance of female pathophysiology has produced major difficulties in defining medical treatment. It is easier to define female sexuality as more complex, less accessible, and thus psychologic. The heirs of the Freudian culture managed female sexology with the complicity of a medical community that was ignorant of female sexual pathophysiology.

Today three schools of thought on female sexual dysfunction treatment exist. These include purely psychologic, purely biologic, and a hybrid of psychologic-biologic. The psychologic and biologic cultures are opposed, and often clash. The former affirms that it would be an oversimplification to treat a women affected by sexual dysfunction pharmacologically; the latter, in contrast, sees a therapeutic option aimed at reducing the time under therapy. However, psychotherapists have always tried to use short-term therapy aimed at triggering behavioral change.[6]

Currently, medical and physiologic factors are considered to cause female sexual dysfunction, including reduction of the vaginal and clitoral blood flow, previous gynecologic operations, alterations of the pelvic floor due to childbirth, or disorders secondary to hormonal alterations[7] (see Chapters 6.1–6.5). Magnetic resonance imaging showed that during female sexual arousal, changes occur in the anterior vaginal wall and the clitoris[8] (see Chapter 10.2). It is accepted that the clitoris plays a functional role during sexual arousal.[9–16] All these aspects constitute the biologic pathways that could be treated with pharmacologic agents.

Improved understanding of the structures involved in normal sexual function, as well as of age-related changes, help practitioners evaluate and manage women with female sexual dysfunction. The continued quest to understand female sexual function and dysfunction requires more education and research on the treatment of underlying medical conditions and the use of pharmacologic therapies.[17,18]

Sexual arousability largely depends on the sympathetic nervous system and nonadrenergic/noncholinergic neurotransmitters. For instance, vasoactive intestinal polypeptide and nitric oxide are involved in smooth muscle relaxation and enhancement of genital blood flow, while various hormones may influence female sexual function[19–21] (see Chapters 5.1–5.5).

Today there are no drugs approved for the safe and effective treatment of female sexual dysfunction.[22] There are independent studies supported by pharmaceutic companies investigating the efficacy and safety of hormonal and nonhormonal agents that act on genital tissues, the vascular system, and the peripheral and/or central sexual pathways. Phosphodiesterase type 5 inhibitors are a commonly studied nonhormonal pharmacologic agent.

Selective phosphodiesterase type 5 inhibitors

The introduction of selective phosphodiesterase type 5 inhibitors[23] for the treatment of men affected by erectile dysfunction represented a major advance in understanding and managing the neurovascular mechanisms of the male sexual response.

In the female clitoral corpus cavernosum, the release of nitric oxide from the nonadrenergic, noncholinergic nerves and/or the endothelium activates guanylyl cyclase and increases intracellular cyclic guanosine monophosphate levels. Cyclic guanosine monophosphate modulates intracellular calcium and, in turn, regulates smooth muscle contractility and erectile function.[20] Phosphodiesterase type 5 plays an important physiologic role by regulating the intracellular levels of cyclic nucleotides.[24] Selective phosphodiesterase type 5 inhibitors can inhibit cyclic guanosine monophosphate hydrolysis by high-affinity, selective action in intact cells and in soluble extracts of human clitoral corpus cavernosum smooth muscle cells.[25] In addition, phosphodiesterase type 5 has been found in clitoral and vaginal tissue[26,27] (see Chapters 5.1–5.6).

Clinical trials suggest that selective phosphodiesterase type 5 inhibitors could be an effective treatment for female sexual dysfunction.[28,29] On the basis of these observations that human clitoral corpus cavernosum smooth muscle tone may be regulated by synthesis and release of nitric oxide,[30] and that this pathway is dependent on phosphodiesterase type 5 activity, researchers in the sexual field hypothesized that selective phosphodiesterase type 5 inhibitors could have beneficial clinical effects for women affected by sexual arousal disorders.

In a clinical setting, selective phosphodiesterase type 5 inhibitors were shown to enhance genital blood flow and vaginal and clitoral engorgement in women affected by female sexual arousal disorder. There have been many studies on selective phosphodiesterase type 5 inhibitors over the last few years, conducted with either premenopausal or postmenopausal women, as well as healthy women without sexual dysfunction, to study female sexual pathways, and on subjects with psychotropic-induced sexual dysfunction, and the results of these studies follow.

Premenopausal studies

A pilot study on the effect of the selective phosphodiesterase type 5 inhibitor sildenafil on subjective and physiologic parameters of the female sexual response determined its safety and efficacy for use in women with sexual arousal disorder.[31] Physiologic measurements, including genital blood flow, vaginal lubrication, intravaginal pressure-volume changes, and genital sensation, were recorded before and after sexual stimulation at baseline and after administration of 100 mg sildenafil. Poststimulation physiologic measurements improved significantly. Subjective sexual function complaints, including reduced arousal, low desire, diminished sexual satisfaction, difficulty in achieving orgasm, decreased vaginal lubrication, and dyspareunia, also improved significantly.

The major findings of a double-blind, crossover, placebo-controlled study on premenopausal women with normal ovulatory cycles and normal levels of steroid hormones, affected by female sexual arousal disorder without hypoactive sexual desire disorder, were that subjects may benefit from treatment with the selective phosphodiesterase type 5 inhibitor, showing improvement in arousal, and indirectly in orgasm, and frequency and enjoyment of sexual intercourse.[32] These aspects could explain the differences in the results from studies treating postmenopausal women that showed little or no improvement.

Postmenopausal studies

Another study treated postmenopausal women with sexual dysfunction, based on history, with an open-label, nonrandomized study.[33] Overall, only 18.1% had a significant therapeutic response, while clitoral discomfort and hypersensitivity occurred in 21%. Side effects included headache, dizziness, and dyspepsia. The data suggest that the selective phosphodiesterase type 5 inhibitor sildenafil is well tolerated in postmenopausal women with sexual dysfunction, but overall sexual function did not improve significantly, although there were changes in vaginal lubrication and clitoral sensitivity. It must be noted that vaginal engorgement insufficiency and clitoral erectile insufficiency in postmenopausal women resulted from organic vasculogenic dysfunction due to pathophysiologic variations in endogenous hormones, as in estrogen deprivation. An important point in treating postmenopausal women with female sexual arousal disorder is that they also need an adequate testosterone level to receive benefits from selective phosphodiesterase type 5 inhibitor treatment.

In a randomized trial of selective phosphodiesterase type 5 inhibitor in postmenopausal women with female sexual arousal disorder that were receiving estrogen but not androgen therapy, no significant improvement in sexual arousal was found.[34] To assess efficacy, patients completed the Global Efficacy Questions, the Life Satisfaction Checklist, an event log of sexual activity, and a 31-item sexual function questionnaire. To assess safety, adverse event data were recorded. Estrogenized and estrogen-deficient women were diagnosed with female sexual arousal disorder, but it was the primary presenting symptom in only 46% and 50% of the women, respectively. It was concluded that any genital physiologic effect of selective phosphodiesterase type 5 inhibitor was not perceived as improving the sexual response in estrogenized or estrogen-deficient women with a broad spectrum of sexual dysfunction that included female sexual arousal disorder. Estrogenized postmenopausal women with female genital sexual arousal disorder and orgasmic impairment based only on clinical assessment do not benefit from selective phosphodiesterase type 5 inhibitor. However, photoplethysmography could have a predictive value: those women showing low vaginal pulse amplitude response benefited from selective phosphodiesterase type 5 inhibitor compared with women with a higher response. Thus, estrogenized women diagnosed with acquired female genital sexual arousal disorder may be a heterogeneous group, and photoplethysmography might be useful in their further characterization.[35] It is well known that hormone therapies usually improve vaginal epithelial thickness and engorgement in postmenopausal women, but also decrease serum androgen levels due to decreased luteinizing hormone-driven, ovarian, stromal steroidogenesis.[36] Thus, sexual arousal in postmenopausal woman and other aspects of female androgen-dependent sexuality are unlikely to be improved by exclusive treatment with selective phosphodiesterase type 5 inhibitor.

Selective phosphodiesterase type 5 inhibitor efficacy in postmenopausal women with female sexual arousal disorder who had adequate estradiol and free testosterone concentrations, or were receiving estrogen and/or androgen therapy, was assessed by a double-blind, placebo-controlled study.[37] Women with female sexual arousal disorder without hypoactive sexual desire disorder had a significantly greater improvement in sexual arousal, orgasm, intercourse, and overall satisfaction with sexual life during sildenafil intake compared with placebo,

while no efficacy was shown for women with concomitant hypoactive sexual desire disorder.

Efficacy studies in healthy women

To determine the changes in female sexual pathways with selective phosphodiesterase type 5 inhibitor, and to verify the safety, a randomized, double-blind crossover, placebo-controlled study was conducted with premenopausal women asymptomatic for sexual disorders, with normal ovulatory cycles and with normal levels of steroid hormones.[38] The selective phosphodiesterase type 5 inhibitor sildenafil improved arousal, orgasm, and enjoyment with respect to placebo. The major finding of the study was that a selective phosphodiesterase type 5 inhibitor could improve general sexual behavior. The benefits that the group felt were above the physiologic peripheral dimensions of sexuality, confirming what has been found by using selective phosphodiesterase type 5 inhibitors on males affected by erectile dysfunction. As a consequence, this study showed that the qualitative aspects of sexuality and the quantitative aspects, such as multiple orgasms, are significantly improved with respect to the pretest baseline values. The majority of the adverse events associated with the use of selective phosphodiesterase type 5 inhibitors were related to vasodilation, such as headache; or to gastrointestinal events, such as nausea; or to visual effects. Each of these adverse events reflects the well-known pharmacologic properties of selective phosphodiesterase type 5 inhibitors, which usually increase in incidence with increasing drug dose. The study suggested that selective phosphodiesterase type 5 inhibitors act on different sexual pathways in healthy women, improving their sexual experience.

Selective phosphodiesterase type 5 inhibitors were also found to be effective in enhancing vaginal engorgement during erotic stimulus conditions in healthy women without sexual dysfunction, but were not associated with an effect on subjective sexual arousal.[39] Women without sexual dysfunction were randomly assigned to receive either sildenafil or placebo. Subjective measurements of sexual arousal were assessed after participants had been exposed to erotic stimulus. Vaginal vasocongestion was recorded continuously during baseline, neutral, and erotic stimulus. At the end of each session, subjects were asked to specify which treatment they suspected they had received. Significant increases in vaginal vasocongestion were found with the selective phosphodiesterase type 5 inhibitor treatment compared with placebo. There were no differences between treatments on subjective sexual arousal experience. Analyses by "suspected treatment received" found that significantly stronger sexual arousal and vaginal wetness were reported for the treatment that was believed to be selective phosphodiesterase type 5 inhibitor than the treatment that was believed to be placebo.

Recently, the effect of a single oral dose of 50 mg sildenafil on the uterine and clitoral arterial blood flow in healthy, naturally postmenopausal women was studied. Color Doppler sonography, performed before and 1 h after sildenafil administration, showed clitoral and uterine blood flow improvement without erotic stimulus.[40]

Sildenafil for psychotropic-induced sexual dysfunction

Women reported significant improvements in all domains of sexual function, with improvement in overall sexual satisfaction, after selective phosphodiesterase type 5 inhibitor treatment. Significant improvements were reported regardless of psychotropic medication type. Patients taking selective serotonin reuptake inhibitors reported less improvement in arousal, libido, and overall sexual satisfaction than did other patients, whereas patients taking benzodiazepines reported significantly more improvement in libido and overall sexual satisfaction.[41]

Patients who had normal premorbid sexual function and who had developed sexual dysfunction, particularly anorgasmia with or without other sexual disturbances, i.e., loss of libido, lubrication difficulties, and uncomfortable or painful intercourse, were treated with a selective phosphodiesterase type 5 inhibitor. The subjects showed improvement of the presenting condition, usually depression, anxiety, or both, and experienced sexual side effects continuously for more than 4 weeks. Patients took selective phosphodiesterase type 5 inhibitors and reported a complete or very significant reversal of their sexual dysfunction. This included return of effective duration and intensity of adequate arousal, lubrication, and orgasmic function.[28]

In conclusion, selective phosphodiesterase type 5 inhibitors seem to be more effective in premenopausal women with sexual arousal disorder than in postmenopausal women. This could be explained by the important role played by sexual steroids in genital trophism. In fact, the best efficacy of sildenafil was in women affected by genital arousal dysfunction. These studies show that subjects with other sexual dysfunctions, such as hypoactive sexual desire disorder, do not benefit from sildenafil. Consequently, defining specific subgroups of women is the first step in treating their dysfunction.

Table 14.1.1 summarizes selective phosphodiesterase type 5 inhibitor use with sildenafil as a treatment for women with female sexual dysfunction.

D1/D2 dopamine receptor agonist

The use of a D1/D2 dopamine receptor agonist, such as sublingual apomorphine, for the treatment of erectile dysfunction provides strong evidence of the participation of the dopaminergic system in the control of sexual function.[42] The use of apomorphine to treat erectile dysfunction has not always been effective, as the exact involvement of dopamine in sexual motivation and in the control of genital arousal in humans is unknown. However, the daily intake of apomorphine seems to be effective,[43] even if multicenter and multiethnic studies need to confirm evidence obtained by studying small numbers of

Table 14.1.1. Summary of sildenafil treatment in women with female sexual dysfunction and in healthy women

Authors	Sexuality	Number of patients	Type of study	Measurement	Sildenafil mg	Female sexual response (FSR)
Berman et al.[31]	FSAD	48 postmenopausal	Prospective	Physiologic	100	Improvement
Caruso et al.[32]	FSAD	51 postmenopausal	Double-blind, crossover, placebo	PEQ	25–50	Improvement
Kaplan et al.[33]	Sexual disorders	30 postmenopausal	No randomly, Open-label	IFSF	50	Insufficient
Basson et al.[34]	FSAD	577 estrogenized and 204 control postmenopausal	Randomized, placebo-controlled	GEQ and PSQ	10–100	Not effective
Berman et al.[37]	FSAD	202 postmenopausal E-A treated	Double-blind, placebo-controlled	FIEI	25–50–100	Improvement
Caruso et al.[38]	Healthy women	50 postmenopausal	Double-blind, crossover, placebo	PEQ	50	Improvement
Laan et al.[39]	Healthy women	12 postmenopausal	Randomized, placebo-controlled	Physiologic	50	Enhancing vaginal engorgement
Alataş et al.[40]	Healthy women	25 postmenopausal	Open-label	Color Doppler sonography	Single dose 50	Improved clitoral blood flow

FIEI = Female intervention efficacy index; FSAD = Female sexual arousal disorder; GEQ = Global efficacy question; IFSF = Index of female sexual function; PEQ = Personal experiences questionnaire; PSQ = Perceived stress questionnaire.

subjects. In contrast, experimental data suggest an implication of dopamine at all these stages of the copulatory behavior in rodents.[44] Apomorphine induces a patterned behavioral sexual arousal response and obvious genital vasocongestive engorgement in female rats. The frequency of the apomorphine-induced responses varied during the estrous cycle and decreased after oophorectomy, revealing the hormonal dependency.[45]

The release of dopamine at the level of the nucleus accumbens, which is innervated by the mesolimbic dopaminergic pathway originating in the ventral segmental area, is positively implicated in the precopulatory or appetitive phase in male rats. There is also a permissive role in the copulatory or consumatory phase for dopamine released at the level of the median preoptic area, which receives projection from the dopaminergic hypothalamic pathway within the hypothalamus. It is noteworthy that the participation of the dopaminergic system is not specific to sexual behavior but rather reflects the more general involvement of dopamine in the regulation of cognitive, integrative, and reward processes. Due to its role in the control of locomotor activity, the integrity of the nigrostriatal dopaminergic pathway is also essential for the display of copulatory behavior. More specifically to sexual function, it is likely that dopamine can trigger genital arousal by acting on oxytocinergic neurons located in the paraventricular nucleus of the hypothalamus, and perhaps on the proerectile sacral parasympathetic nucleus within the spinal cord.

The regulation of genital arousal by dopamine has not yet been well established in females. However, a placebo-controlled study was performed to verify whether a D1/D2 dopamine receptor agonist was effective in premenopausal women affected by arousal disorder with hypoactive sexual desire disorder.[46] Women were randomly allocated to treatment in one of six possible sequences of three 2-week double-blind, crossover study periods with the D1/D2 dopamine receptor agonist apomorphine 2 mg or 3 mg, washout, and placebo. The daily intake of the drug was effective with both the 2-mg and 3-mg dosages compared with placebo for arousal and desire. The effects of 3 mg apomorphine were better than those obtained with 2 mg. The orgasm, enjoyment, and satisfaction with frequency scores improved during treatment with daily D1/D2 dopamine receptor agonist compared with baseline and placebo. Adverse events were mild or moderate, occurring both during the "as required" part and during daily usage, and were mainly nausea, vomiting, dizziness, or headache. However, during the placebo period, two women had adverse events, mainly headache.

Recently, a randomized, double-blind, placebo-controlled study was performed to evaluate changes in female sexual response in premenopausal women with orgasmic sexual dysfunction treated with 3 mg sublingual apomorphine. Sexual response was evaluated objectively by Doppler sonography, and subjectively by self-reported questionnaire, after vibrator stimuli with the addition of apomorphine or placebo. Clitoral hemodynamic changes were higher with the D1/D2 dopamine receptor agonist than placebo, even when there were no differences between D1/D2 dopamine receptor agonist and placebo in regard to orgasm, probably due to confounding factors such as study situation, lack of intimacy, and a single apomorphine dose.[47]

In conclusion, a D1/D2 dopamine receptor agonist could be efficacious in treating women affected by sexual arousal disorder and hypoactive sexual desire disorder because of its action on the dopaminergic system. At present, an intranasal formulation of D1/D2 dopamine receptor agonist for treating female sexual dysfunction is being studied. Dopamine agonists in sexual dysfunction could be a promising research area in the development of treatment for female sexual dysfunction.

Other medications

There have been few studies of drugs targeting the central nervous system to date. Bupropion may have a beneficial effect on premenopausal women with hypoactive sexual desire disorder.[48] Bupropion can also be an effective antidote to selective serotonin reuptake inhibitor-induced sexual dysfunction. In a placebo-controlled trial, bupropion produced an increase in desire and frequency of sexual activity compared with placebo. However, frequency was correlated to total testosterone level at baseline and during treatment.[49]

The efficacy of various medications, such as L-arginine, yohimbine, phentolamine, and prostaglandin E_1, in the treatment of female sexual dysfunction is still under investigation.[50] In a randomized, double-blind, three-way crossover study, the combined oral administration of the nitric oxide-precursor L-arginine and the alpha 2-blocker yohimbine for subjective and physiologic sexual arousal in postmenopausal women with female sexual arousal disorder increased vaginal pulse amplitude responses to erotic stimuli compared with placebo.[51]

Phentolamine is a combined alpha 1- and alpha 2-adrenoceptor antagonist that has been used to treat erectile dysfunction by intracavernosal injection. Results of a pilot study with a single-blind, dose-escalation design indicated a mild, positive effect of oral phentolamine across all measurements of arousal, with significant changes in self-reported lubrication and pleasurable sensations in the vagina.[52] All subjects had received a single dose of 40 mg oral phentolamine and placebo. Dependent variables for the study included vaginal pulse amplitude, as measured by vaginal photoplethysmography, self-reported measures of sexual response, and patient- and physician-based assessments of adverse events. In another study, physiologic readings by vaginal photoplethysmography were significantly different from placebo in the women using hormone therapy with 40 mg phentolamine.[53] No significant differences were found among women not receiving hormone therapy, so that phentolamine may show promise as a treatment for female sexual arousal disorder in estrogenized postmenopausal women.

Currently, intravaginal application of prostaglandin E_1 is under investigation to determine its efficacy in the treatment of female sexual dysfunction. In a study conducted to evaluate the efficacy of topical alprostadil cream in women with sexual arousal disorder, each subject was administered a single intra-vaginal dose of placebo followed by three escalating intra-vaginal doses of active drug at 2-week intervals. However, photoplethysmography measurement of vaginal pulse amplitude was not able to demonstrate treatment sensitivity.[54] Similarly, in a randomized, double-blind, placebo-controlled study, women with sexual arousal disorder were enrolled to use 500-, 1000-, or 1500-g doses of alprostadil or placebo cream to be applied to the vulvar area prior to vaginal intercourse for a period of 6 weeks. The arousal success rate was highest in the alprostadil 1000-g group and lowest in the 500-g group, but the responses were not different from that of the placebo cream for any of the three doses of the drug.[55] In contrast, a study conducted with color Doppler ultrasonography to measure clitoral hemodynamic changes showed improvement in peak systolic velocity and end diastolic velocity after topical application of 1 g of 0.2% alprostadil gel, and labial and clitoral engorgement.[56] Furthermore, women with sexual arousal and orgasmic disorders seem to have better clitoral cavernosal arterial hemodynamics after topical administration of alprostadil.[57]

A summary of drug treatments in women with female sexual dysfunction can be found in Table 14.1.2.

Conclusions

Female sexual dysfunction is a combination of problems with both biologic and psychologic components, and is multifactorial in etiology.

The studies that have been carried out with selective phosphodiesterase type 5 inhibitors and a D1/D2 dopamine receptor agonist show that these drugs are potentially useful in treating women with a specific sexual dysfunction. We are only at the beginning of a new era in treating female sexual dysfunction, and the development of new drugs in this field can only improve the situation.

There are currently potential therapeutic options for the treatment of female sexual dysfunction that include both hormonal and nonhormonal pharmacologic therapies. However, sex therapists are discovering that integrating adjunctive use of drugs with sex therapy can accelerate the therapeutic process and improve outcome. As new pharmaceuticals are developed and approved, opportunities for medical and non-medical sex therapies will increase.[58] To date, the results of the studies on women affected by sexual dysfunction who received drug treatments have not reached uniformity of efficacy. This could be a result of the multifactorial aspect of female sexual dysfunction.[59] Specific subgroups obviously need to be diagnosed

Table 14.1.2. Summary of drug treatments in women with female sexual dysfunction

Authors	Sexuality	Type of study	Measurement	Drug	Female sexual response (FSR)
Caruso et al.[47]	HSDD FSAD	Double-blind, crossover, placebo	PEQ	Apomorphine	Improvement
Bechara et al.[48]	FSOD	Double-blind, randomized, placebo-controlled	FSFI and color Doppler sonography	Apomorphine	Improvement
Segraves et al.[49]	HSDD	Open label	Questionnaires	Bupropion	Improvement
Clayton et al.[50]	FSD due to SSRI	Placebo-controlled	Questionnaires	Bupropion	Improvement
Meston and Worcel[52]	FSAD	Double-blind, randomized, crossover, placebo-controlled	Photoplethysmography	Yohimbine plus L-arginine	Improvement
Rosen et al.[53]	FSAD	Single-blind, placebo-controlled	Photoplethysmography	Phentolamine	Improvement
Rubio-Aurioles et al.[54]	FSAD	Placebo-controlled	Photoplethysmography	Phentolamine	HTR dependent
Islam et al.[55]	FSAD	Double-blind, crossover, placebo	Photoplethysmography	Alprostadil	Not effective
Padma-Nathan et al.[56]	FSAD	Double-blind, randomized, placebo-controlled	FSEP and FSFI	Alprostadil	Dose-response effect
Becher et al.[57]	Healthy women	Open label	Color Doppler sonography	Alprostadil	Improved labial and clitoral blood flow
Bechara et al.[58]	FSAD and FSOD	Open label	Color Doppler sonography	Alprostadil	Improved clitoral blood flow

FSAD = Female sexual arousal disorder; FSD = Female sexual disorder; FSEP = Female sexual encounter profile; FSFI = Female sexual function index; FSOD = Female sexual orgasm disorder; HSDD = Hypoactive sexual desire disorder; PEQ = Personal experiences questionnaire; SSRI = Selective serotonin reuptake inhibitor.

exactly, as treating all sexual dysfunctions with drugs is not always effective. Finally, we are beginning to consider sexual dysfunction treatment rather than symptomatic therapy, preferably in an integrative setting.

References

1. Shabsigh R. Prevalence of and recent developments in female sexual dysfunction. *Curr Psychiatry Rep* 2001; 3: 188–94.

2. Basson R. Female sexual response: the role of drugs in the management of sexual dysfunction. *Obstet Gynecol* 2001; 98: 350–3.

3. Leiblum SR. Definition and classification of female sexual disorders. *Int J Impot Res* 1998; 10(Suppl 2): S104.

4. Pfaus JG. Neurobiology of sexual behaviour. *Curr Opin Neurobiol* 1999; 9: 751–8.

5. Davis AR. Recent advances in female sexual dysfunction. *Curr Psychiatry Rep* 2000; 2: 211–14.

6. Balint M, Ornstein PH, Balint E. *Focal Psychotherapy, an Example of Applied Psychoanalysis.* London: Tavistock, 1972.

7. Goldstein I. Female sexual arousal disorder: new insights. *Int J Impot Res* 2000; 12: S152–7.

8. Schulz WW, van Andel P, Sabelis I et al. Magnetic resonance imaging of male and female genitals during coitus and female sexual arousal. *Br Med J* 1999; 319: 1596–1600.

9. Sadeghi-Nejad H, Moreland RB, Traish AM et al. Preliminary report on the development and characterization of rabbit clitoral smooth muscle cell culture. *Int J Impot Res* 1998; 10: 165–9.

10. Levin RJ. The physiology of sexual function in women. *Clin Obstet Gynaecol* 1980; 7: 213–52.

11. Park K, Goldstein I, Andry C et al. Vasculogenic female sexual dysfunction: the hemodynamic basis for vaginal engorgement insufficiency and clitoral erectile insufficiency. *Int J Impot Res* 1997; 9: 27–37.

12. Goldstein I, Berman JR. Vasculogenic female sexual dysfunction: vaginal engorgement and clitoral erectile insufficiency syndromes. *Int J Impot Res* 1998; 10(Suppl 2): S84–90.

13. Van Turnhout AA, Hage JJ, van Diest PJ. The female corpus spongiosum revisited. *Acta Obstet Gynecol Scand* 1995; 74: 767–71.

14. Baskin S, Erol A, Li YW et al. Anatomical studies of the human clitoris. *J Urol* 1999; 162 (3 Pt 2): 1015–20.

15. Ingelman-Sundberg A. The anterior vaginal wall as an organ for the transmission of active forces to the urethra and the clitoris. *Int Urogynecol J Pelvic Floor Dysfunct* 1997; 8: 50–1.

16. Toesca A, Stolfi VM, Cocchia D. Immunohistochemical study of the corpora cavernosa of the human clitoris. *J Anat* 1996; 188: 513–20.

17. Bancroft J. The medicalization of female sexual dysfunction: the need for caution. *Arch Sex Behav* 2002; 31: 451–5.

18. Walton B, Thorton T. Female sexual dysfunction. *Curr Womens Health Rep* 2003; 3: 319–26.

19. Argiolas A. Neuropeptides and sexual behaviour. *Neurosci Biobehav Rev* 1999; 23: 1127–42.

20. Hauser-Kronberger C, Cheung A, Hacker GW et al. Peptidergic innervation of the human clitoris. *Peptides* 1999; 20: 539–43.

21. Marthol H, Hilz MJ. Female sexual dysfunction: a systemic overview of classification, pathophysiology, diagnosis and treatment. *Fortschr Neurol Psychiatr* 2004; 72: 121–35.

22. Furcroy JL. Female sexual dysfunction: potential for pharmacotherapy. *Drugs* 2003; 63: 1–12.

23. Boolell M, Gepi-Attee S, Gingell JC et al. Sildenafil, a novel effective oral therapy for male erectile dysfunction. *Br J Urol* 1996; 78: 257–61.

24. Moreland RB, Goldstein I, Traish A. Sildenafil, a novel inhibitor of phosphodiesterase type 5 in human corpus cavernousum smooth muscle cells. *Life Sci* 1998; 62: 309–18.

25. Park K, Moreland RB, Goldstein I et al. Sildenafil inhibits phosphodiesterase type 5 in human clitoral corpus cavernosum smooth muscle. *Biochem Biophys Res Commun* 1998; 249: 612–17.

26. Traish A, Moreland RB, Huang YH et al. Development of human and rabbit vaginal smooth muscle cell cultures: effects of vasoactive agents on intracellular levels of cyclic nucleotides. *Mol Cell Biol Res Commun* 1999; 2: 131–7.

27. d'Amati G, Di Gioia CR, Bologna M et al. Type 5 phosphodiesterase expression in the human vagina. *Urology* 2002 60: 191–5.

28. Nurnberg HG, Lauriello J, Hensley PL et al. Sildenafil for sexual dysfunction in women taking antidepressants. *Am J Psychiatry* 1999; 156: 1664.

29. Rosenberg KP. Sildenafil. *J Sex Marital Ther* 1999; 25: 271–9.

30. Burnett AL, Calvin DC, Silver RI et al. Immunohistochemical description of nitric oxide syntheses isoforms in human clitoris. *J Urol* 1997; 158: 75–8.

31. Berman JR, Berman LA, Lin H et al. Effect of sildenafil on subjective and physiologic parameters of the female sexual response in women with sexual arousal disorder. *J Sex Marital Ther* 2001; 27: 411–20.

32. Caruso S, Intelisano G, Lupo L et al. Premenopausal women affected by sexual arousal disorder treated with sildenafil: a double-blind, crossover, placebo-controlled study. *Br J Obstet Gynaecol* 2001; 108: 623–8.

33. Kaplan SA, Reis RB, Kohn IJ et al. Safety and efficacy of sildenafil in postmenopausal women with sexual dysfunction. *Urology* 1999; 53: 481–6.

34. Basson R, McInnes R, Smith MD et al. Efficacy and safety of sildenafil citrate in women with sexual dysfunction associated with female sexual arousal disorder. *J Womens Health Gend Based Med* 2002; 11: 367–77.

35. Basson R, Brotto LA. Sexual psychophysiology and effects of sildenafil citrate in oestrogenised women with acquired genital arousal disorder and impaired orgasm: a randomised controlled trial. *Br J Obstet Gynaecol* 2003; 110: 1014–24.

36. Casson PR, Elkind-Hirsch KE, Buster JE et al. Effect of postmenopausal oestrogen replacement on circulating androgen. *Obstet Gynecol* 1997; 90: 995–8.

37. Berman JR, Berman LA, Toler SM et al. Safety and efficacy of sildenafil citrate for the treatment of female sexual arousal disorder: a double-blind, placebo-controlled study. *J Urol* 2003; 170: 2333–8.

38. Caruso S, Intelisano G, Farina M et al. The function of sildenafil on female sexual pathways: a double-blind, cross-over, placebo-controlled study. *Eur J Obstet Gynecol* 2003; 110: 201–16.

39. Laan E, van Lunsen RH, Everaerd W et al. The enhancement of vaginal vasocongestion by sildenafil in healthy premenopausal women. *J Womens Health Gend Based Med* 2002; 11: 357–65.

40. Alatas E, Yagci AB. The effect of sildenafil citrate on uterine and clitoral arterial blood flow in postmenopausal women. *MedGenMed* 2004; 6: 51. www.medscape.com.

41. Salerian AJ, Deibler WE, Vittone BJ et al. Sildenafil for psychotropic-induced sexual dysfunction in 31 women and 61 men. *J Sex Marital Ther* 2000; 26: 133–40.

42. Giuliano F, Allard J. Dopamine and male sexual function. *Eur Urol* 2001; 40: 601–8.

43. Caruso S, Intelisano G, Farina M et al. Efficacy and safety of daily intake of apomorphine SL in men affected by erectile dysfunction and mild hyperprolactinemia: a prospective, open-label, pilot study. *Urology* 2003; 62: 922–7.

44. Foreman MM, Hall JL. Effects of D2-dopaminergic receptor stimulation on male rat sexual behaviour. *J Neural Transm* 1987; 68: 153–70.

45. Beharry R, Hale T, Heaton J et al. Evidence for centrally initiated genital vasocongestive engorgement in the female rat: findings from a new model of female sexual arousal response. *Int J Impot Res* 2003; 15: 122–8.

46. Caruso S, Agnello C, Intelisano G et al. Placebo-controlled study on efficacy and safety of daily apomorphine SL intake in premenopausal women affected by hypoactive sexual desire disorder and sexual arousal disorder. *Urology* 2004; 63: 955–9.

47. Bechara A, Bertolino MV, Casabè A et al. A double-blind randomized placebo control study comparing the objective and subjective changes in female sexual response using sublingual apomorphine. *J Sex Med* 2004; 1: 209–14.

48. Segraves RT, Clayton A, Croft H et al. Bupropion sustained release for the treatment of hypoactive sexual desire disorder in premenopausal women. *J Clin Psychopharmacol* 2004; 24: 339–42.

49. Clayton AH, Warnock JK, Kornstein SG et al. A placebo-controlled trial of bupropion SR as an antidote for selective serotonin reuptake inhibitor-induced sexual dysfunction. *J Clin Psychiatry* 2004; 65: 62–7.

50. Marthol H, Hilz MJ. Female sexual dysfunction: a systemic overview of classification, pathophysiology, diagnosis and treatment. *Fortschr Neurol Psychiatr* 2004; 72: 121–35.

51. Meston CM, Worcel M. The effects of yohimbine plus L-arginine glutamate on sexual arousal in postmenopausal women with sexual arousal disorder. *Arch Sex Behav* 2002; 31: 323–32.

52. Rosen RC, Phillips NA, Gendrano NC 3rd et al. Oral phentolamine and female sexual arousal disorder: a pilot study. *J Sex Marital Ther* 1999; 25: 137–44.

53. Rubio-Aurioles E, Lopez M, Lipezker M et al. Phentolamine mesylate in postmenopausal women with female sexual arousal disorder: a psychophysiological study. *J Sex Marital Ther* 2002; 28(Suppl 1): 205–15.

54. Islam A, Mitchel J, Rosen R et al. Topical alprostadil in the treatment of female sexual arousal disorder: a pilot study. *J Sex Marital Ther* 2001; 27: 531–40.

55. Padma-Nathan H, Brown C, Fendl J et al. Efficacy and safety of topical alprostadil cream for the treatment of female sexual arousal disorder: a double-blind, multicenter, randomized, and placebo-controlled clinical trial. *J Sex Marital Ther* 2003; 29: 329–44.

56. Becher EF, Bechara A, Casabe A. Clitoral hemodynamic changes after a topical application of alprostadil. *J Sex Marital Ther* 2001; 27: 405–10.

57. Bechara A, Bertolino MV, Casabe A et al. Duplex Doppler ultrasound assessment of clitoral hemodynamics after topical administration of alprostadil in women with arousal and orgasmic disorders. *J Sex Marital Ther* 2003; 29(Suppl 1): 1–10.

58. Perelman MA. The impact of the new sexual pharmaceuticals on sex therapy. *Curr Psychiatry Rep* 2001; 3: 195–201.

59. Basson R. The complexities of female sexual arousal disorder: potential role of pharmacotherapy. *World J Urol* 2002; 20: 119–26.

14.2 Difficult cases: medical treatment of female sexual dysfunction

Edgardo F Becher, Andrea Salonia, Irwin Goldstein

According to the National Health and Social Life Survey,[1] approximately 43% of American women suffer from sexual health concerns that, in some cases, cause significant personal and couple distress (see Chapter 2.1). Sexual dysfunction in women is a multifactorial syndrome with interrelated medical, psychologic, and interpersonal components.[2-4] Thus, the best model to manage women with sexual problems would be a multidisciplinary setting staffed with sexual medicine psychologic- and biologic-focused health-care professionals. Management of women with sexual health concerns should be considered in a step care paradigm in which the selected therapies progress from least invasive to progressively more invasive, depending, in part, upon patient outcome[2-4] (see Chapters 13.1–13.3, 14.1, 15.1, and 15.2).

In many cases, the female sexual dysfunction is based, in part, on an unrecognized medical condition.[4-7] Possible medical problems include hormonal, neurologic, vascular, pharmacologic, inflammatory, infectious, and other nonpsychologic pathophysiologies.[5-7] The aim of this chapter is to review difficult medical cases in women with sexual dysfunction. This chapter will review seven cases of women who presented for management of a sexual dysfunction in a multidisciplinary setting and ultimately required medical intervention as part of the care provided to manage the sexual complaint. This medical care was provided, in all cases, in addition to other interventions, including psychologic counseling and physical therapy as indicated. The purpose of the chapter is to illustrate some typical cases in which medical intervention strategies were utilized in the management of women with sexual health problems.

In this textbook on women's sexual health, in which patient management is discussed, it is important to emphasize that evidence-based medical management in this field is still in its infancy.[4] At the time of writing, there are no government agency-approved pharmaceutic agents indicated specifically for the treatment of a women's sexual health disorder. Similarly, there are few recognized medical conditions that predictably interfere with women's desire, arousal, or orgasm function. It is *not* the purpose of this chapter to illustrate anecdotal medical care. To the best of the authors' abilities, each case is founded on peer review medical evidence.

As in other portions of this textbook relating to difficult case management, every effort has been made to protect the privacy of patients and to maintain the management strategies utilized in the case for teaching purposes.

Case 1

SR, aged 23, while inserting a tampon, noted something unusual "down there". It felt like a series of clusters of small bumps on the left labium of her labia majora. She also felt a small "lump" near her clitoris. Once or twice a day, SR complained of itching in the area. SR tried to inspect this herself with a mirror but did not know what to look for.

SR is an au pair providing live-in child care for a family with three young children. She had limited sexual activity as a teenager and used condoms for contraception. For the last 2 years, she has used the combined oral contraceptive pill, in part, to control cramping and excessive menstrual bleeding. SR has little free time for dating and relationships, but she did meet someone at a party and they "hit it off". SR was sexually active in this new relationship and they did not always use a condom. She did arouse and experience orgasm primarily through clitoral stimulation. SR believed that compared to the time when she was not using the combined oral contraceptive, her sexual responses were somewhat blunted.

SR was worried about the new "masses down there" and in particular was frightened about sexually transmitted diseases. As a result, she stopped sexual activity, including self-stimulation, until she could find out what was wrong. The decision to stop sexual activity caused stress in the relationship and caused her great personal anxiety and frustration. SR went to her primary care physician, but no abnormality was found during repeated internal pelvic examination. Pap smears were negative. SR was frustrated and determined to get a second opinion. After 6 months of abstinence and worry about the lumps, she self-referred herself to a multidisciplinary sexual medicine clinic.

She was evaluated by the psychologist as follows. SR is a 23-year-old single woman with a history of "finding something that feels different" on her genitals. The patient is very unhappy about this situation, feels guilty, and reports conflict in her relationship. The patient reports that this has been a frustrating issue for more than 6 months. There is no history of depression, substance abuse, or other mental health issues. There is no history of trauma or sexual abuse.

SR underwent physical examination under bright light with the examiner wearing magnifying surgical loupes. Upon clitoral hood retraction, a single 0.5 × 0.33 cm genital wart was noted on the left side of the prepuce (Fig. 14.2.1). In addition, within the hairs on the labia majora, a series of conylomata, 30–45 mm in size, some flat and some raised, were noted on the left labium of the labia majora and in the sulcus between the left labium of the labia majora and the labia minora.

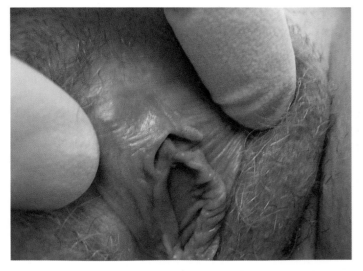

Figure 14.2.1. Physical examination was performed under bright light with the examiner wearing magnifying surgical loupes. Upon clitoral hood retraction, a single 0.5 × 0.33 cm genital wart was noted on the left side of the prepuce.

SR agreed to undergo a minor surgical excision of the lesion on the frenulum under local anesthesia. A course of imiquamod was administered over 1 month for the lesions on the labia majora and in the sulcus. She received counseling on "safe sex" with condoms. She has stopped the combined oral contraceptive agents and has noted a restoration of the previous level of sexual desire, arousal, and orgasm that she experienced as a teenager. She has been advised to have annual Pap smears.

Comments

Genital warts, condylomata acuminata, caused by human papillomavirus infection are frequently encountered in sexual medicine care, as genital warts are one of the most common sexually transmitted diseases[8] (see Chapter 7.7). Genital warts are caused, in part, by direct, skin-to-skin transmission of the human papillomavirus during sex with an infected person. Genital warts may be flesh-colored, painless, raised or flat, single or multiple, and small or large (often appearing cauliflower-like), and may appear in and around the vulva, vestibule, vagina, or cervix. The various treatments for genital warts include topical chemicals (e.g. podofilox, imiquimod[9]), cryotherapy (liquid nitrogen), laser therapy, and surgical excision. The choice of therapy is based on multiple variables such as the quantity, dimension, and location of the lesions, as well as patient choice, cost, convenience, risks, and clinician experience. Human papillomavirus can cause genital warts and cervical cancer; thus, it is important that individuals with genital human papillomavirus be diagnosed and treated, and get annual follow-up, including Pap smears. Because the human papillomavirus remains dormant in the body, genital warts may reappear at any time after treatment. The goal of treatment is clearance of visible warts. Some evidence exists that treatment reduces infectivity, but there is no objective evidence yet that treatment reduces the incidence of cervical cancer.[8,9]

Case 2

FG, aged 57, complained of diminished arousal response for the last 4 years since entering menopause. She had "great sexual activity" from her teens to just before menopause. "I am interested in sex, I have always been and I maintain the drive. Sex is important for me and I love my husband very much." Since starting menopause, "I'm dry as a bone" and "sex is most uncomfortable". "I don't even want to touch myself anymore." "I am rarely able to achieve orgasm during intercourse." "It just takes much more effort to have orgasm and the orgasms I achieve are very muffled." FG tried eating soy supplements and a variety of herbals without success. She even tried sildenafil, obtained from a friend, but all this provided was a headache and facial flushing. The lubricants that she tried were messy and not very satisfactory.

FG was evaluated by her local gynecologist. She was referred to a sex therapist and started on low-dose, systemic estrogen and progesterone, and she was advised to purchase vibrators and lubricants. Since FG has a sister with breast cancer, FG discontinued the hormone treatment after several weeks after exposure to recent media discussion relating systemic estrogen use to increased breast cancer risk. FG referred herself to a multidisciplinary sexual medicine clinic.

FG was evaluated by the psychologist as follows. This 57-year-old married woman reports a chief complaint of diminished vaginal lubrication and discomfort during sexual intercourse for approximately 4 years. She states that she is unable to have a satisfying orgasm with her husband. Over recent years, this has become an increasing problem both for her and her husband. The patient does have some history of sexual abuse as a child, but she is reluctant to discuss this and feels that it is irrelevant. She denies that her past history has negatively affected her relationship with her husband. By nature, the patient is a positive, optimistic woman who appears pleased with the quality of her life. She has no history of depression or other psychologic issues. She drinks alcohol on social occasions and has no tobacco or illegal substance history.

FG underwent a history and physical examination. FG undergoes routine Pap smears and breast examination. She denies any history of sexually transmitted diseases, endometriosis, cervical dysplasia, or interstitial cystitis. Her last menstrual period was 4 years ago. There has been no history of breakthrough bleeding. She has occasional night sweats and hot flushes but is not disabled by them. Physical examination revealed a normal glans clitoris. Approximately two-thirds of the posterior aspect of the right and left labia minora were fused to the labia majora. The thickness of the upper third of the labia minora was several millimetres. The vagina lacked rugae and lubrication was absent on the vaginal walls (Fig. 14.2.2). There was positive Q-tip testing, grade 2–4/10, in multiple locations around the labial-hymenal junction. There was minimal vaginal wall bleeding with Q-tip contact. Biothesiometry studies revealed that the vibration perception threshold was 3 V in the right and left pulp index fingers, and 13–15 V in the labia, clitoris, frenulum, and urethral meatus. Hormone studies revealed the following values: thyroid-stimulating hormone 2.4 (0.4–5.50 µIU/ml), follicle-stimulating hormone 72 (23–116 mIU/ml), luteinizing hormone 33 (16–54 mIU/ml), prolactin 9.7 (1.8–20.3 ng/ml), dehydroepiandrosterone sulfate 93 (35–430 µg/ml), androstenedione 1.0 (0.2–3.1 ng/ml), total testosterone 33 (15–70 ng/dl), free testosterone 0.9 (0.3–1.9 ng/dl), sex hormone-binding globulin 49 (17–120 nmol/l), and estradiol <20 (11–526 pg/ml).

The patient was notified that her diagnoses were diminished arousal and orgasm, dyspareunia, diminished genital sensation, genital atrophy, atrophic vaginitis, and diminished estradiol. We discussed the various treatments of her atrophic vaginitis by estradiol administration. We suggested that as a safer alternative, especially as it concerns breast cancer risk, low-dose local estradiol was probably associated with less risk than systemic estradiol administration. FG began treatment with local estradiol to the vestibule and the vagina. Within

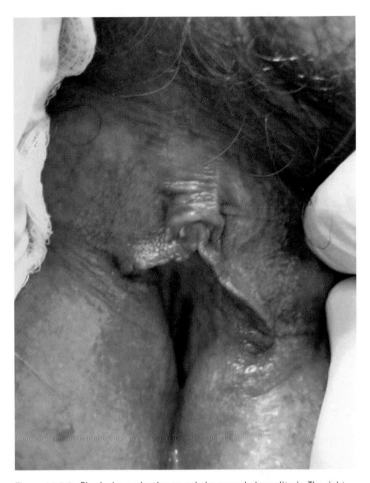

Figure 14.2.2. Physical examination revealed a normal glans clitoris. The right and left labia minora were fused to the labia majora for two-thirds of the posterior aspect. The thickness of the upper third of the labia minora was several millimetres. The vagina lacked rugae, and lubrication was absent on the vaginal walls.

weeks, FG noticed a real difference in lubrication and diminished discomfort. "I love this treatment." She could not believe that it took her 4 years to get effective treatment for this problem, and she thinks that all postmenopausal women should be aware of local vaginal and vestibular low-dose estradiol therapy.

Comments

Basic science research has shown that the sex steroid hormone, estradiol, is critical for vaginal structure and function, such as lubrication, blood flow, and sensitivity[10] (see Chapters 5.5, 5.6, 6.3, 7.2, and 13.1–13.3). In postmenopausal women, vaginal atrophy is a frequent complaint with symptoms of vaginal dryness, itching, discomfort, and painful intercourse. Systemic estrogen treatment via oral or patch hormone therapy for symptoms of atrophic vaginitis is not necessary in all cases. A substitute strategy involves use of various local estradiol delivery systems, including low-dose estradiol creams, ointments, intravaginal tablets, suppositories, and silicone rubber rings. The low risk of systemic absorption of estradiol with local vaginal and vestibular low-dose estradiol administration has been assessed. In a recent study of 1472 women with histologically confirmed breast cancer, 69 had bothersome vaginal atrophy and were treated with topical vaginal estrogen. Topical estrogen usage did not appear to be associated with increased risk of recurrence of breast cancer.[11] Most investigations show no major estrogen-related side effects or endometrial proliferation.[12-14] In postmenopausal women, the efficacy of low-dose estradiol local vaginal and vestibular delivery systems for estrogen deficiency has been established. Local estradiol has been shown to alleviate numerous subjective symptoms (discomfort, dryness, and diminished sensitivity) and to have various objective outcomes, such as vaginal mucosal health, induction of a high maturation index of vaginal mucosal cells, and reduction of vaginal pH below 5.5. It may be necessary to try different delivery systems for some postmenopausal women, as individuals using topical estradiol can complain of uterine bleeding, breast pain, allergy to the vehicle, and perineal pain.[11-14]

Case 3

RH, aged 32, has been married for 10 years to her high-school sweetheart. RH is a teacher and during the summer, she works as a camp counselor. She has two children and always seems busy with community, education, and religious activities. She has had sexual activity only with her husband, and they waited until after they were married for sexual intercourse. She has never had orgasm during sexual intercourse, leading to frustration and anxiety concerning the couple's sexual activities in general. As a result, she tends to avoid intimacy.

RH discussed the sexual problem with her gynecologist at a recent examination. Her physical examination was normal and she was advised to see a sex therapist. RH wanted to see the therapist with her husband, but he did not cooperate.

Over the next few years, the problem persisted and the frustration intensified. RH eventually sought help at a multidisciplinary sexual medicine clinic.

She was seen by the psychologist, who reported as follows. This is a 32-year-old woman who has been married for the past 10 years. She notes that she has a lifelong orgasm disorder. She continues to be sexually active but feels that any sexual contact is related to guilt and a sense of obligation. She reports that sex at this time feels like a task that needs to be completed. She has no sexual abuse history and no psychologic trauma. She has had some mild depression as an adult, but this seems insignificant for her sexual dysfunction. She feels pressure from her husband to be sexually active but describes him as minimally supportive. She drinks alcohol on a social basis, uses no illegal substances, and has not smoked since college.

On history taking, RH revealed that while she had limited interest in masturbation, she was able to have orgasmic release by herself. She was able to lubricate vaginally once she got

involved in the sexual activity. There was some discomfort during penetration but there was no overt pain or tenderness. She had normal menses and never any sexually transmitted diseases. She never used oral contraceptive pills.

Physical examination revealed that the clitoris, frenulum, urethral meatus, labia minora, and hymenal tissues were unremarkable (Fig. 14.2.3). Biothesiometry studies revealed that the vibration perception threshold was 3 V in the right and left pulp index fingers and 7 V in the labia, clitoris, frenulum, and urethral meatus. Hormone studies revealed the following values: thyroid-stimulating hormone 1.1 (0.4–5.50 µIU/ml), follicle-stimulating hormone 2.5 (1.5–33.4 mIU/ml), luteinizing hormone 6.3 (0.5–76.3 mIU/ml), prolactin 11.3 (2.8–29.2 ng/ml), dehydroepiandrosterone sulfate 236 (35–430 µg/ml), androstenedione 2.5 (0.2–3.1 ng/ml), total testosterone 62 (15–70 ng/dl), free testosterone 1.3 (0.3–1.9 ng/dl), sex hormone-binding globulin 27 (17–120 nmol/l), and dihydrotestosterone 136 (50–250 pg/ml). The patient was notified that all hormonal testing was unremarkable.

Further history taking was performed in the presence of the husband. On careful questioning, it became apparent that he suffered from lifelong premature ejaculation. The estimated

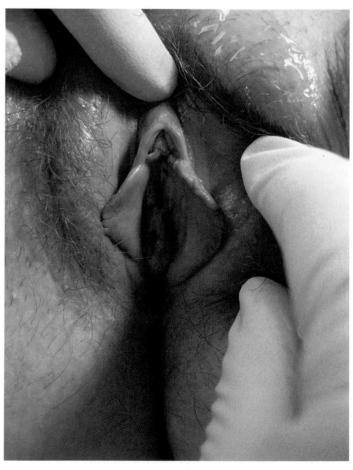

Figure 14.2.3. Physical examination revealed that the clitoris, frenulum, urethral meatus, labia minora, and hymenal tissues were unremarkable.

intravaginal ejaculatory latency time was consistently 1–2 min. The husband had a limited sexual repertoire and was completely unaware of the premature ejaculation, since this was how he always ejaculated.

Medical treatment in this case was directed to the husband and included selective serotonin reuptake inhibitors, topical anesthetics, and oral phosphodiesterase type 5 inhibitors. Medical treatment, in conjunction with the couple's sex therapy was successful. The follow-up intravaginal ejaculatory latency time more than doubled to 4 min. He learned how to become more attentive to her sexual needs and broadened his foreplay repertoire. RH has, for the first time, experienced orgasm during sexual activity with her husband including sexual intercourse. The couple are more satisfied with their sexual activity and have increased the frequency to several times per week.

Comments

It is important to be aware that a sexual problem in one member of the couple may be caused by the partner (see Chapter 8.2). One classic example is dyspareunia resulting from severe penile curvature associated with Peyronie's disease.[15] Another standard example is anorgasmia in the woman secondary to premature ejaculation in the man.[16] Premature ejaculation is one of the most common male sexual dysfunctions.[17] The most important method of diagnosing premature ejaculation is by intravaginal ejaculatory latency time defined as the time, measured by stopwatch, between the start of vaginal intromission and the start of intravaginal ejaculation. An intravaginal ejaculatory latency time of 2 min or less is a common inclusion criterion for clinical studies in premature ejaculation. Premature ejaculation may also be assessed by subject assessment of ejaculatory control, satisfaction with ejaculatory control, sexual satisfaction, and partner sexual satisfaction. Most physicians do not inquire about the existence of premature ejaculation of the partner when the female patient has other sexual complaints (diminished interest, diminished arousal) or when the patient has orgasmic dysfunction. Since premature ejaculation in the male often adversely affects partner sexual satisfaction, partner distress is a common motivation for afflicted men to seek treatment. Treatment for premature ejaculation may include sex therapy, selective serotonin reuptake inhibitors, topical anesthetics, and phosphodiesterase type 5 inhibitors.[18–21]

Case 4

LA, a healthy, 38-year-old woman, married 5 years ago. She had an excellent previous sex life with good interest, arousal, and orgasmic function. She experienced no pain during sexual activity. The couple decided to have a child together, but, after several years of failure to achieve pregnancy, LA underwent evaluation for infertility. She took leuprolide acetate self-injections for one and a half years during infertility treatment and *in vitro* fertilization cycles. Since the infertility treatment,

LA claims to have lost her sexual desire. Compared to previous capabilities, she describes 10% desire, 10% arousal, and 10% orgasmic function. She also notes there is a moderate discomfort during initial penetration but this soon disappears. She states, "I want my sex life back, I want to have a family, but now I have to force myself to have sex."

LA had sought advice from her gynecologist. She was told that all looked normal on physical examination and a serum testosterone blood test was "within normal limits". Due to persistence of the sexual problem, LA was referred to a multidisciplinary sexual medicine clinic.

LA was initially evaluated by the psychologist, who reported as follows. This 38-year-old woman was seen today with her husband of 5 years. The patient is undergoing infertility evaluation. She reports that ever since the infertility treatment began, she experiences marked diminished desire, arousal, and orgasm and painful intercourse. As a result, the couple have been sexually active virtually exclusively to achieve pregnancy. Although this has been difficult and frustrating for them, they have remained close, open to communicating about the situation, and committed to finding a solution for both the infertility and sexual problems. The patient herself has a difficult early history with emotional and sexual abuse. Her mother died when she was 12 years old, and the patient began a difficult adolescence with alcohol and substance abuse. She then entered her first marriage, which lasted 4 years because of her abusive husband. She now seems stabilized, and denies any depression or other mental health-related issues. She has never been in psychotherapy. Some behavioral relaxation may be an important adjunct to her medical treatment.

LA underwent history taking and physical examination. There was no additional contributory medical or surgical history. Physical examination revealed a clitoris diminished in size and a partially phimotic prepuce. The urethral meatus was normal. The labia minora was fused to the labia majora bilaterally in the posterior 20%. There were multiple areas of erythema overlying ostia of minor vestibular glands (Fig. 14.2.4). Q-tip testing was positive in many of these locations. Biothesiometry studies revealed that the vibration perception threshold was 3 V in the right and left pulp index fingers and 15–18 V in the labia, clitoris, frenulum, and urethral meatus. Hormone studies revealed the following values: thyroid-stimulating hormone 1.6 (0.4–5.50 µIU/ml), follicle-stimulating hormone < 1.5 (1.5–33.4 mIU/ml), luteinizing hormone < 0.5 (0.5–76.3 mIU/ml), prolactin 8.8 (2.8–29.2 ng/ml), dehydroepiandrosterone sulfate 101 (35–430 µg/ml), androstenedione 1.2 (0.2–3.1 ng/ml), total testosterone 12 (15–70 ng/dl), free testosterone 0.3 (0.3–1.9 ng/dl), sex hormone-binding globulin 49 (17–120 nmol/l), and dihydrotestosterone 34 (50–250 pg/ml).

The overall impression was sexual dysfunction, including low desire, arousal, and orgasm; mild genital atrophy; diminished genital sensation; and dyspareunia with vestibular adenitis. The sex steroid blood tests revealed low gonadotropins, low total and free testosterone, and low dihydrotestosterone. Discussion ensued to communicate directly with

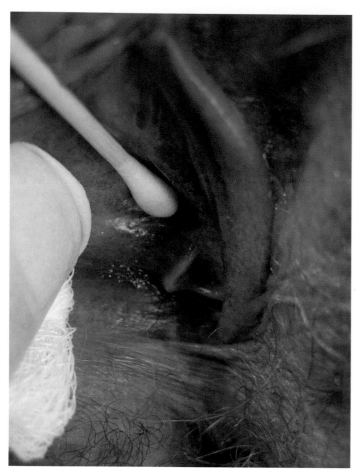

Figure 14.2.4. Physical examination revealed areas of erythema overlying ostia of minor vestibular glands.

the infertility specialists and consider the leuprolide acetate as a direct cause of the endocrine milieu disturbance. The patient sought second opinions concerning infertility management and presently is off leuprolide. Her testosterone values have remained abnormally low, as found at the 2-year follow-up. She has started to receive counseling from the sex therapist.

Currently, the couple is considering an international adoption. The patient started systemic testosterone therapy with marked improvement in sexual function and diminished pain symptoms after 6 months of therapy. She has remained in psychologic therapy.

Comments

Androgens, like other sex steroids such as estrogens, are critical for sexual function and genital tissue structure[10] (see Chapters 5.5, 6.1–6.3, and 13.1). Leuprolide acetate is approved for treatment of men with advanced prostate cancer.[22] Leuprolide acetate is also used by gynecologists to treat women with endometriosis,[23] uterine fibroids,[24] and infertility.[25] Leuprolide acetate is a gonadotropin-releasing hormone agonist that suppresses ovarian function, induces a "temporary" menopause

state, and interrupts estrogen output. The use of leuprolide acetate for infertility is based on the observation that suppression of estrogen enables other hormonal preparations to induce multiple ovum development.[25] Leuprolide acetate also significantly interferes with ovarian synthesis of testosterone.[26] There are few well-controlled data on the long-term adverse effects of leuprolide acetate on androgen biosynthesis in women.

Case 5

GS, aged 43, consulted her primary care physician for increasingly disturbing and worsening localized itching and burning in the clitoris, a condition that she had had since 38 years of age. The clitoral pain symptoms have prevented her from wearing tight clothing. The itching and burning has increased significantly during the past year, adversely affecting her personal, social, and work life. She avoids relationships for fear that the interaction will lead to sexual activity. She has never had sexual intercourse. She performed clitoral masturbation on occasion as a young teenager but now avoids any clitoral contact. Her past medical history is negative for trauma or infections in the clitoral area.

GS was referred to several gynecologists and psychologists. She was managed with topical xylocaine and topical estrogen creams. She was also treated for yeast infections. Due to persistence of the clitoral pain, GS was referred to a multidisciplinary sexual medicine clinic.

GS was evaluated by the psychologist as follows. This 43-year-old, single woman presents with complaints of clitoral pain preventing her from engaging in sexual activity. The patient states that she is unable to achieve orgasm and doubts whether she has ever been orgasmic. She denies any significant psychologic history. She recently began taking a sleep medication since the symptoms interfered with sleep. The patient has never been abused or experienced any psychologic trauma. She has no history of substance or alcohol abuse. The patient is not currently in a relationship and reports that her clitoral pain is increasingly becoming an issue in possible relationships. She adds that men often perceive her clitoral pain as a personal failure. GS has seen therapists in the past, but no psychologic issues have been uncovered.

GS underwent a history and physical examination. She had normal menses, used no medications, and had no urinary tract symptoms. Physical examination revealed a white color patch and a pale, nonpigmented, skin-wrinkled area with scaling and cracking involving the entire clitoral hood, the left frenulum and the region between the posterior fourchette and the anus (Fig. 14.2.5). The rest of the vestibular examination revealed fusion of the labia minora onto the labia majora.

The diagnosis of lichen sclerosus was suspected. A biopsy of the clitoral hood was offered to define the disorder, but the patient refused. She was treated with twice daily topical clobetasol. After 8 weeks, she reported complete reversal of the itching, burning, and pain. Physical examination failed to identify

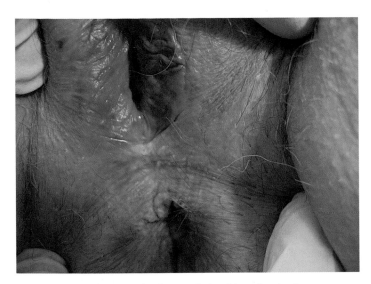

Figure 14.2.5. Physical examination revealed a white-colored, pale, nonpigmented, skin-wrinkled area with scaling and cracking involving the region between the posterior fourchette and the anus.

any suspicious dermatitis lesions on the clitoral hood, clitoris or region between the posterior fourchette and anus. There was no obvious residual scarring of the clitoris, clitoral hood or region between the posterior fourchette and anus. She has noted improvement of her mood and general well-being, and feels ready to start new relationships. She was advised to continue counseling by the sex therapist.

Comments

Lichen sclerosus is a chronic genital dermatitis condition associated with visible signs of small white patches on the genitals[27,28] and a wide variation in presentation symptoms, including, itching, burning, and pain with sex (see Chapters 9.5 and 12.2). In some women, the symptoms can interfere with sexual activity, routine activities, and sleep. The diagnosis of lichen sclerosus is suggested by physical examination showing white-colored genital, vulvar, and vestibular tissue with paleness, loss of pigmentation, and characteristic "cigarette paper" wrinkling. Diagnosis is conformed by biopsy. Genital lichen sclerosus is presently managed by the ultrapotent fluorinated steroid, clobetasol.[28]

Case 6

BC, a 37-year-old, single, Caucasian woman, complained primarily of severe pain localized to the genital region during heterosexual or self-masturbation, and during coital thrusting. This pain has affected her since age 26. BC described the genital sexual pain as starting as a localized discomfort at the anterior vaginal wall, and then becoming an actual pain at the clitoris, labia minora, urethral meatus, and region surrounding the urethral meatus. BC reported that the pain developed suddenly,

without obvious cause. During the last several years, the genital sexual pain increased significantly, and she currently has diminished ability to have orgasm. BC has tried many over-the-counter analgesic agents without success. The overall condition has been very distressing and has adversely affected her sexual relationships.

Two to three months before the beginning of the genital sexual pain disorder at age 26, she complained of urinary urgency, frequency (10 times per day) and nocturia (three times per night), burning during voiding, and suprapubic discomfort during and after voiding. There was some relation between the genital sexual pain disorder and the irritative urinary symptoms, especially after coitus or just prior to menses. BC had multiple negative urine culture and sensitivity tests performed by her primary care physician.

BC was in a stable relationship with regular and satisfactory sexual intercourse for 5 years before the genital sexual pain disorder. BC has performed self-masturbation since she was 15 years old. Masturbation was never painful until she was 26 years of age. For the genital sexual pain disorder, BC had been treated with topical estrogen, local anesthetics, baclofen, alpha-blockers, and diazepam. BC reported that after having sex, significant amelioration of the local discomfort was achieved by bed rest in a face-down position.

BC was advised to seek a second opinion at a multidisciplinary sexual medicine clinic. BC was seen by the psychologist, who reported as follows. This 37-year-old, single woman has a chief complaint of genital sexual pain, urinary irritative and dysuria symptoms, and suprapubic discomfort. Over the last several years, this has become an increasing problem for both her and her partners. She is currently in a stable relationship. The patient has a history of sexual abuse as a child, but she is reluctant to discuss this. She denies that her past history has negatively affected her relationships or her ability to trust men. She does recall in her youth that her father and brother often looked at pornography, and she found this very embarrassing. By nature, the patient is a negative, pessimistic woman who is very cautious in decision making and in her relationships. She has no history of overt depression or other psychologic disorders. She consumes six alcohol drinks per week and used illegal substances during her teenage and early adult years.

Physical examination was negative for vaginitis, urethritis, or herpes. Bimanual examination revealed tenderness just under the posterior bladder wall and above the pubic bone. BC's pelvic floor muscles were rigid. Because of suspicion of interstitial cystitis, BC underwent urodynamic testing. The first sensation of bladder filling occurred at 50 ml. The first strong desire to void occurred at 75 ml. BC's irritative symptoms were reproduced during filling. Cystoscopy with hydrodistention was performed and verified the presence of Hunner's ulcers, linear scarring, hypervascularity, and bloody effluent and glomerulations after hydrodistention. Potassium sensitivity testing showed increased epithelial permeability with the instillation of a mild potassium chloride solution, with exacerbation of the symptoms of urgency and pain.

BC underwent multimodal treatment for interstitial cystitis, including behavioral, pharmacologic, and surgical therapies. Behavioral therapies included dietary modification, bladder training, and pelvic floor physical therapy. Pharmacologic therapy involved pentsosan polysulfate, antihistamines, tricyclic antidepressants, anticholinergics, antiepileptics, muscle relaxants and anti-inflammatory agents, and narcotics for symptom relief. Surgical therapy included hydrodistention and intravesical instillations of dimethyl sulfoxide on a weekly basis.

After the first 4 weeks of interstitial cystitis treatment, BC reported a significant reduction of the sexual pain along with a major reduction of the "cystitis symptoms" previously described. BC also continued with the sexologic management.

Comments

Interstitial cystitis is a chronic, often severe, inflammation and hypersensitivity disorder of the bladder wall[29-34] (see Chapters 7.3 and 17.4). Interstitial cystitis affects mainly middle-aged Caucasian women. It is estimated that there are 450,000 cases in the USA. Primary symptoms include urinary frequency and urgency, and lower abdominal or perineal pain. More than half of interstitial cystitis patients have pain while riding in car, and approximately two of three interstitial cystitis patients are unable to work full time because of the symptoms. Interstitial cystitis can produce pain that is perceived in any location in the pelvis in any combination with or without urinary frequency/urgency and sexual pain disorders. Interstitial cystitis and vulvodynia may coexist. The diagnosis of interstitial cystitis is based upon symptoms, excluding other conditions such as urinary tract infections, urethral diverticulum, or urethral stricture. Conclusive diagnosis of interstitial cystitis is made by cystoscopy during bladder distention that reveals small petechial hemorrhages or glomerulations) and/or larger Hunner's ulcers, and by positive potassium testing. Treatment is multimodal, including behavioral, pharmacologic, and surgical interventions.[29-34]

Case 7

WA, a 33-year-old married woman, complained for 5 years of localized pain and burning in the introitus during penetration that persists after the sexual intercourse. WA noted that the pain was 10/10 on an analog visual pain scale, was present on every occasion, and caused her to stop the intercourse activity about half of the times. WA also noted a progressive decrease in sexual desire and arousal for the last 7 years. Compared to previous capabilities, WA has 20% desire, 20% arousal, and 80% orgasmic function. The sexual problem has generated considerable personal distress and interfered with the couple's relationship. The husband believes that WA does not love him or find him sexually attractive. WA has had two normal pregnancies and vaginal deliveries. The last delivery at age 26 was followed by postpartum depression, for which she was treated with selective serotonin reuptake inhibitors for 2 years. She uses no medication at present other than combined oral contraceptives for the last 6 years.

WA was examined by various psychologists, primary care physicians, and her local gynecologist. No abnormalities were identified and no treatments have thus far proved effective. WA was referred to a multidisciplinary sexual medicine clinic.

WA's psychologic evaluation was as follows. This is a 33-year-old woman who has been married for 11 years. The couple report a decline in sexual interest and satisfaction shortly after the birth of their second child 7 years ago. The couple are both very frustrated, and neither husband nor wife tend to initiate any sexual contact. The patient presents as having some mild agitated depression as well as chronic fatigue and stress secondary to her busy schedule and parenting duties. There is a past psychologic history of postpartum depression, but no history of sexual trauma or abuse. The couple have had marital counseling, although their communication is diminished due to lack of privacy and the inability to reach a resolution about the sexual issues.

WA underwent history taking and physical examination. She denied any past medical history, including high cholesterol, hypertension, diabetes mellitus, and cancer, as well as urinary tract infections, endometriosis, and interstitial cystitis. Physical examination revealed 30% clitoral phimosis, and normal labia and urethral meatus. At the labial–hymenal junction, there were regions of erythema overlying the ostia of the minor vestibular glands (Fig. 14.2.6). Q-tip testing was positive with an intensity of 4–8/10. The vagina had rugae and normal mucosa. Biothesiometry revealed vibration perception threshold testing of 3 V in the pulp index fingers and 10–13 V in the clitoris, frenulum, urethral meatus, and labia minora. Hormone studies revealed the following values: thyroid-stimulating hormone 2.1 (0.4–5.50 µIU/ml), follicle-stimulating hormone 1.5 (1.5–33.4 mIU/ml), luteinizing hormone 0.5 (0.5–76.3 mIU/ml), prolactin 12.3 (2.8–29.2 ng/ml), dehydroepiandrosterone sulfate 75 (35–430 µg/ml), androstenedione 0.9 (0.2–3.1 ng/ml), total testosterone 24 (15–70 ng/dl), free testosterone < 0.3 (0.3–1.9 ng/dl), sex hormone-binding globulin 176 (17–120 nmol/l), and dihydrotestosterone 55 (50–250 pg/ml).

WA was diagnosed as having diminished desire and arousal, diminished genital sensation, vestibular adenitis, and androgen insufficiency. We advised WA to discontinue the oral contraceptives and initiate birth control by barrier method or encourage her husband to undergo vasectomy. We initiated a series of consultations for pelvic floor physical therapy and encouraged couple's sex therapy. Gabapentin was administered to help diminish the sexual pain, and local anesthetics were prescribed to provide pain relief. Androgens were administered with dehydroepiandrosterone and local testosterone gel. At 3 months, laboratory results showed recovery of all hormonal parameters to the upper third of the reference values, with virtual complete elimination of the sexual pain and the beginning of sexual dreams, thoughts, and fantasies. All treatments continued, and hormonal blood tests evaluations were carried

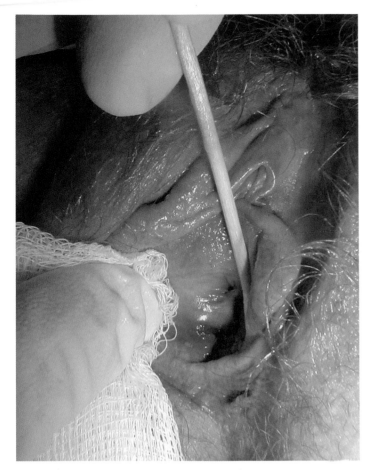

Figure 14.2.6. At the labial-hymenal junction, regions of erythema overlay the ostia of the minor vestibular glands.

of patients with vulvar vestibulitis when compared with a healthy control group.[39] Sutherland found that women with vulvar vestibulitis syndrome and concomitant hypogonadism reveal a significant decrease in the concentration of androgenic receptors in the minor vestibular glands when compared with a control group.[40] There is a relationship between use of oral contraceptives and vulvar vestibulitis syndrome, and it is probably related, in part, to the androgen insufficiency observed in women on the combined oral contraceptives.[41-43] The treatment of vulvar vestibulitis syndrome includes: topical anesthetics, physical therapy, behavioral therapy, hormone therapy, and surgical excision.

Conclusion

Numerous psychologic and biologic pathophysiologies adversely affect women's sexual health. This chapter focused on several biologic conditions, such as infection, partner sexual dysfunction, pain syndromes, hormonal aberrations, genital tissue atrophy, and adverse pharmacologic consequences. As the field of women's sexual health matures and research investigations concerning biologic pathophysiologies become commonplace, it is hoped that evidence-based data will accumulate to support the safe and effective utilization of medical management alongside the traditional treatment by psychologic intervention.

Acknowledgments

Dr Edgardo Becher is grateful to Dr Sandra García for her contribution. Dr Andrea Salonia is grateful to Dr Alberto Briganti, Dr Elena Longhi, Dr Giuseppe Zanni, Prof. Patrizio Rigatti, and Prof. Francesco Montorsi for their contributions.

out every 3 months. At 9-month follow-up, the patient noted improvement of her mood and general well-being in addition to resolution of the genital symptoms. She has discontinued the gabapentin and no longer uses the topical xylocaine. She has noted some mild acne and increased facial hair that she refers to as "fuzzies" on her face cheeks.

Comments

Vulvar vestibulitis syndrome was described by Friedrich[35] in 1987 and is characterized by: 1) severe pain upon palpation in the vestibular area or in the introitus; 2) pain upon pressure localized in the vestibule; and 3) evident vestibular erythema of variable intensity for at least 6 months (see Chapters 12.1–12.6). Vulvar vestibulitis syndrome is associated with inflammatory involvement of the minor vestibular glands, revealing significant squamous metaplasia surrounded by inflammatory cells that form follicles of T lymphocytes and plasmatic cells.[36,37] Eva et al. reported an abnormal expression of estrogenic receptors in vestibular tissue on patients with vulvar vestibulitis syndrome.[38] Hodgins et al. found a significant decrease in the concentration of estrogenic receptors in biopsies

References

1. Laumann EO, Paik A, Rosen RC. Sexual dysfunction in the United States. Prevalence and predictors. JAMA 1999; 281: 537–44.
2. Lewis RW, Fugl-Meyer KS, Bosch R et al. Epidemiology/risk factors of sexual dysfunction. J Sex Med 2004; 1: 35–9.
3. Basson R, Althof S, Davis S et al. Summary of the recommendations on sexual dysfunctions in women. J Sex Med 2004; 1: 24–34.
4. Hatzichristou D, Rosen RC, Broderick G et al. Clinical evaluation and management strategy for sexual dysfunction in men and women. J Sex Med 2004; 1: 49–57.
5. Meston CM, Hull E, Levin RJ et al. Disorders of orgasm in women. J Sex Med 2004; 1: 66–8.
6. Davis SR, Guay AT, Shifren JL et al. Endocrine aspects of female sexual dysfunction. J Sex Med 2004; 1: 82–6.
7. Nappi R, Salonia A, Traish AM et al. Clinical biologic pathophysiologies of women's sexual dysfunction. J Sex Med 2005; 2: 4–25.

8. Kodner CM, Nasraty S. Management of genital warts. *Am Fam Physician* 2004; 70: 2335–42.

9. Sauder DN, Skinner RB, Fox TL et al. Topical imiquimod 5% cream as an effective treatment for external genital and perianal warts in different patient populations. *Sex Transm Dis* 2003; 30: 124–8.

10. Giraldi A, Marson L, Nappi R et al. Physiology of female sexual function: animal models. *J Sex Med* 2004; 1: 237–53.

11. Dew JE, Wren BG, Eden JA. A cohort study of topical vaginal estrogen therapy in women previously treated for breast cancer. *Climacteric* 2003; 6: 45–52.

12. Suckling J, Lethaby A, Kennedy R. Local oestrogen for vaginal atrophy in postmenopausal women. *Cochrane Database Syst Rev* 2003; CD001500.

13. Crandall C. Vaginal estrogen preparations: a review of safety and efficacy for vaginal atrophy. *J Womens Health* 2002; 11: 857–77.

14. Eriksen PS, Rasmussen H. Low-dose 17 beta-estradiol vaginal tablets in the treatment of atrophic vaginitis: a double-blind placebo controlled study. *Eur J Obstet Gynecol Reprod Biol* 1992; 44: 137–44.

15. Wabrek AJ, Wabrek CJ. Dyspareunia. *J Sex Marital Ther* 1975; 1: 234–41.

16. Pierce AP. The coital alignment technique (CAT): an overview of studies. *J Sex Marital Ther* 2000; 26: 257–68.

17. McMahon CG, Abdo C, Incrocci L et al. Disorders of orgasm and ejaculation in men. *J Sex Med* 2004; 1: 58–65.

18. Lue TF, Giuliano F, Montorsi F et al. Summary of the recommendations on sexual dysfunctions in men. *J Sex Med* 2004; 1: 6–23.

19. Hatzichristou D, Rosen RC, Broderick G et al. Clinical evaluation and management strategy for sexual dysfunction in men and women. *J Sex Med* 2004; 1: 49–57.

20. Rowland D, Perelman M, Althof S et al. Self-reported premature ejaculation and aspects of sexual functioning and satisfaction. *J Sex Med* 2004; 1: 225–32.

21. Waldinger MD, Schweitzer DH, Olivier B. On-demand SSRI treatment of premature ejaculation: pharmacodynamic limitations for relevant ejaculation delay and consequent solutions. *J Sex Med* 2005; 2: 121–31.

22. D'Amico AV, Manola J, Loffredo M et al. 6-month androgen suppression plus radiation therapy vs radiation therapy alone for patients with clinically localized prostate cancer: a randomized controlled trial. *JAMA* 2004; 292: 821–7.

23. Maitoko K, Sasaki H. Gonadotropin-releasing hormone agonist inhibits estrone sulfatase expression of cystic endometriosis in the ovary. *Fertil Steril* 2004; 82: 322–6.

24. Palomba S, Orio F Jr, Russo T et al. Long-term effectiveness and safety of GnRH agonist plus raloxifene administration in women with uterine leiomyomas. *Hum Reprod* 2004; 19: 1308–14.

25. Check ML, Check JH, Choel JK et al. Effect of antagonists vs agonists on in vitro fertilization outcome. *Clin Exp Obstet Gynecol* 2004; 31: 257–9.

26. Garcia-Velasco JA, Isaza V, Vidal C et al. Human ovarian steroid secretion in vivo: effects of GnRH agonist versus antagonist. *Hum Reprod* 2001; 16: 2533–9.

27. Carlson JA, Lamb P, Malfetano J et al. Clinicopathologic comparison of vulvar and extragenital lichen sclerosus: histologic variants, evolving lesions, and etiology of 141 cases. *Mod Pathol* 1998; 11: 844–54.

28. Bracco GL, Carli P, Sonni L et al. Clinical and histologic effects of topical treatments of vulval lichen sclerosus. A critical evaluation. *J Reprod Med* 1993; 38: 37–40.

29. Nordling J. Interstitial cystitis: how should we diagnose it and treat it in 2004? *Curr Opin Urol* 2004; 14: 323–7.

30. Parsons CL. Successful downregulation of bladder sensory nerves with combination of heparin and alkalinized lidocaine in patients with interstitial cystitis. *Urology* 2005; 65: 45–8.

31. Nguan C, Franciosi LG, Butterfield NN et al. A prospective, double-blind, randomized cross-over study evaluating changes in urinary pH for relieving the symptoms of interstitial cystitis. *BJU Int* 2005; 95: 91–4.

32. Selo-Ojeme DO, Onwude JL. Interstitial cystitis. *J Obstet Gynaecol* 2004; 24: 216–25.

33. Dell JR. Chronic pelvic pain of bladder origin: a focus on interstitial cystitis. *Int J Fertil Womens Med* 2003; 48: 154–62.

34. Buffington CA. Comorbidity of interstitial cystitis with other unexplained clinical conditions. *J Urol* 2004; 172: 1242–8.

35. Friedrich EG. Vulvar vestibulitis syndrome. *J Reprod Med* 1987; 32: 110–14.

36. Witkin S. Differential characterization of women with vulvar vestibulitis syndrome. *Am J Obstet Gynecol* 2002; 187: 589–94.

37. Woodruff J. Infection of the minor vestibular gland. *Obstet Gynecol* 1983; 62: 609–12.

38. Eva LJ, MacLean AB, Reid WM et al. Estrogen receptor expression in vulvar vestibulitis syndrome. *Am J Obstet Gynecol* 2003; 189: 458–61.

39. Hodgins MB, Spike RC, Mackie RM et al. An immunohistochemical study of androgen, estrogen, and progesterone receptors in the vulva and vagina. *Br J Obstet Gynaecol* 1998; 105: 216–22.

40. Sutherland S. Female sexual dysfunction due to pain: androgenic influence on the pathophysiology of vulvar vestibulitis syndrome. *J Urol* 2004; 171 (Suppl): 428.

41. Bouchard C, Brisson J, Fortier M et al. Use of oral contraceptive pills and vulvar vestibulitis: a case-control study. *Am J Epidemiol* 2002; 156: 254–61.

42. del Marmol V, Teichmann A, Gertsen K. The role of combined oral contraceptives in the management of acne and seborrhea. *Eur J Contracept Reprod Health Care* 2004; 9: 107–24.

43. Sutherland SE, Munarriz RM, Goldstein I. Combined estrogen-progestin oral contraceptives. *N Engl J Med* 2004; 350: 307–8.

SURGICAL TREATMENT OF
FEMALE SEXUAL DYSFUNCTION

15.1 Sexual pain disorders involving pathology within the vestibule: current techniques

Andrew T Goldstein, Irwin Goldstein

Introduction

It is estimated that 10–15% of women are afflicted with sexual pain disorders that, in many, greatly interfere with quality of life, cause significant distraction, and often preclude satisfactory sexual activity[1–3] (see Chapters 12.1–12.6 of this book). There are multiple hypotheses of the pathophysiologies of these sexual pain syndromes, and, accordingly, multiple management options delivered by various health-care professionals. Women afflicted with sexual pain disorders frequently consult numerous health-care providers. After undergoing history taking and physical examination, patients often receive multiple, conservative, medical and behavioral focused treatments, with few evidence-based outcome reports supporting their use.[4] There are more than 20 different treatments reported in the medical literature, including topical and intralesional steroids,[5] interferon,[6] biofeedback,[7] capsaicin,[8] lidocaine,[9] intravaginal physical therapy,[10] amitriptyline,[11] cognitive-behavioral therapy,[12] acupuncture,[13] and dietary changes.[14] Safety and efficacy data concerning these treatment regimens are published, for the most part, in small case series that are neither randomized nor placebo-controlled.

A step-care process is rational for the management of women with sexual pain disorders. Such a step-care process should first engage strategies that are the least invasive and end, if conservative treatments are unsuccessful, with strategies that are the most invasive, such as surgery. It is important that there are available published data concerning safety and efficacy outcome with surgical management of sexual pain disorders. Such data will provide worried patients with the information to make informed management choices.

This chapter will consider those women whose sexual pain disorder can be attributed to disorders of organs and tissues within the vestibule. Conditions involving vestibular contents include disorders of the clitoris, prepuce, frenulum, labia majora, labia minora, urethral meatus, major vestibular glands, minor vestibular glands, and hymen. The aim of this chapter is to provide information to health-care practitioners treating women with sexual pain disorder secondary to vestibular disorder that fail conservative treatment options and electively consider surgery.

Anatomy and embryology of the vestibule

The vulvar vestibule is defined as the tissue between Hart's line and the hymen. Hart's line marks the transition from the squamous mucosa of the vestibule to more keratinized mucosa of the labia minora (see Chapters 4.1–4.3). The vestibule extends from the frenulum of the clitoris anteriorly to the fourchette posteriorly (Fig. 15.1.1).

The embryonic origins of the various women's genital tissues are important and are therefore reviewed in this chapter. By week 6 of embryonic life, female embryos start to develop the genital ridge, the Wolffian duct lateral to the genital ridge, and the Müllerian duct. The lower part of the Müllerian duct fuses with the opposite Müllerian duct to form the uterovaginal canal. The upper part forms the body and cervix of the uterus, while the lower part forms the upper four-fifths of the vagina.

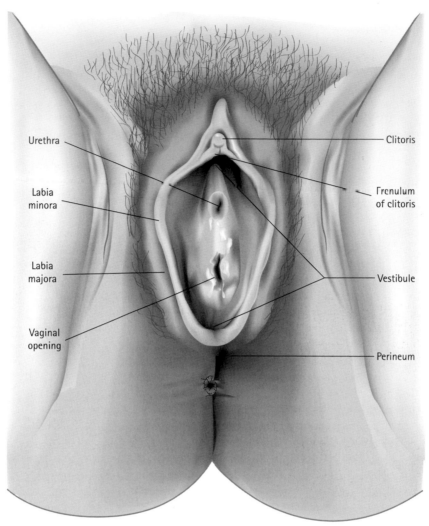

Figure 15.1.1. Anatomy of the vestibule: Hart's line laterally, the hymenal ring medially, the frenulum anteriorly, and the posterior fourchette.

The lower fifth of the vagina develops from the urogenital sinus. The Müllerian duct reaches down to the urogenital sinus and, at the meeting point, forms the Müllerian tubercle. The lower portion of the uterovaginal canal is canalized by a process of central desquamation, and the peripheral cells become the vaginal epithelium. The clitoris develops from the genital tubercle. The labia majora develop from the genital swellings. The labia minora develop from the genital folds.

The vestibule, the topic of focus for this chapter, develops from the lower most part of the urogenital sinus. The mucosa of the vestibule is thus embryonically derived from the urogenital sinus. This makes the tissue of the vestibule similar to the mucosa of the urethra and bladder, which is also derived from the urogenital sinus. This also differentiates the vestibule from the vaginal mucosa, which is derived from Müllerian tissue. This further differentiates the clitoris and labia from the vestibule, since the former are derived from the genital tubercle.

Sexual pain disorders of the vestibule

There are women whose sexual pain disorder can be attributed to pathologic conditions involving organs and tissues within the vestibule. Such women may have sexual pain disorders of the vestibule involving the clitoris, prepuce, frenulum, labia majora, labia minora, urethral meatus, major vestibular glands, minor vestibular glands, and hymen.

The most common vestibular pathology is vulvar vestibulitis syndrome, otherwise known as vestibulodynia or vestibular adenitis. Vulvar vestibulitis syndrome is thought to be the most frequent cause of dyspareunia in premenopausal women.[1,2] Vulvar vestibulitis syndrome was first described in the medical literature in 1880 by Thomas, as a medical syndrome in which there is "excessive sensibility of the nerves supplying the mucous membranes of some portions of the vulva; sometimes … confined to the vestibule".[15] Vulvar vestibulitis syndrome is characterized by three criteria described by Friedrich[3] in 1987: exquisite tenderness when the vestibule is palpated with a cotton swab, vestibular erythema (often at the ostia of the major and minor vestibular glands), and severe pain at attempted vaginal entry with a penis, speculum, tampon, etc.

Pathophysiology of vulvar vestibulitis syndrome

Although millions of women around the world are afflicted by vulvar vestibulitis syndrome, limited research has been performed on the underlying pathophysiology. Recently, with US National Institutes of Health funding, new information has become available and progress has been made in understanding pathologic changes in vulvar vestibulitis syndrome. Bohm-Starke and colleagues used PGP 9.5 immunohistochemistry to demonstrate a proliferation of intraepithelial nerve endings in the vestibular mucosa in women with vulvar vestibulitis syndrome. In addition, they further characterized these nerve endings by showing calcitonin gene-related peptide, which is known to exist only in C-afferent nociceptors, to be the only neuropeptide detected in these nerve endings.[16] Bornstein and colleagues confirmed these results and used computer-assisted histomorphometry to show that the total nerve fiber area in women with vulvar vestibulitis syndrome is 10 times higher than in controls.[17] This increased density of C-afferent nociceptors may explain the allodynia and hyperpathia that women with vulvar vestibulitis syndrome experience with vestibular touch (see Chapter 12.1).

Surgery for vulvar vestibulitis syndrome

Woodruff et al. first described surgery for vulvar vestibulitis syndrome in 1983, calling it "modified perineoplasty".[19] Since then, there have been 33 different case series compromising a total of 1159 patients. These reports represent several different surgical procedures, as there have evolved variations and modifications of the basic surgical excision and reconstructive procedure for management of vulvar vestibulitis syndrome.

In the original procedure, Woodruff et al. excised a semicircular segment of perineal skin, the mucosa of the posterior vulvar vestibule, and the posterior hymeneal ring. Over time, modifications have emerged to limit the invasiveness of Woodruff's original surgical technique. Specifically, in a procedure known as vulvar vestibulectomy, the posterior incision extends only to the posterior fourchette and does not include excision of perineal skin (Fig. 15.1.2). Three centimeters of the vaginal mucosa is then undermined (Fig. 15.1.3) and approximated to the perineum (Fig. 15.1.4). A complete vulvar vestibulectomy includes excision of the mucosa adjacent to the urethra, whereas, in a modified vestibulectomy, the excision of mucosa is limited to the posterior vestibule.

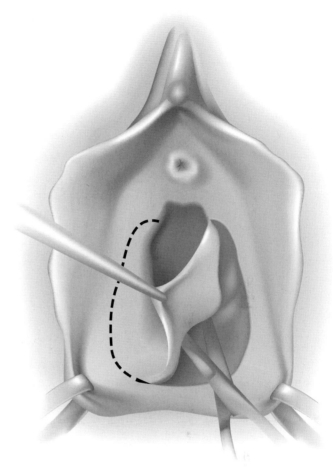

Figure 15.1.2. Vulvar vestibulectomy: excision of the vestibular mucosa.

In a further attempt to minimize the invasiveness of surgery for vulvar vestibulitis syndrome, some surgeons have recommended vestibuloplasty; excision of localized painful areas of vestibular mucosa without vaginal advancement.[20] Whereas vestibulectomy or perineoplasty is performed under general or regional anesthesia in an operative suite, vestibuloplasty can be performed with local anesthesia. Prior to the procedure, a cotton swab is used to delineate painful areas of the vestibule. These areas are outlined with a marking pen and then injected with lidocaine 1% with epinephrine. A scalpel is used to excise the tender superficial mucosa, including the tissue at the base of the hymen. The defects are closed with interrupted sutures of 4–0 Vicryl.

During perineoplasty and vestibulectomy, the vaginal advancement covers the ostia of the Bartholin glands, thereby increasing the risk of postoperative Bartholin gland cysts. Some authors recommend surgical excision of Bartholin's glands during perineoplasty or vestibulectomy. However, other authors specifically reject prophylactic Bartholin gland excision, as the risk of Bartholin gland cyst is only 1%, and excision increases intraoperative blood loss and scar tissue formation.[21]

Several studies have utilized laser surgery for treatment of vulvar vestibulitis syndrome. In one study, a carbon dioxide laser was used to ablate the vestibular mucosa up to a depth of

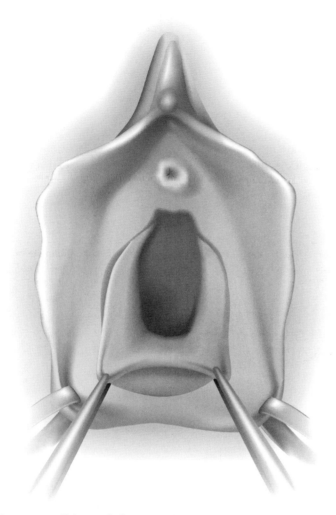

Figure 15.1.3. Vulvar vestibulectomy: vaginal mucosa is separated from the fascia of the rectovaginal septum to create an advancement flap.

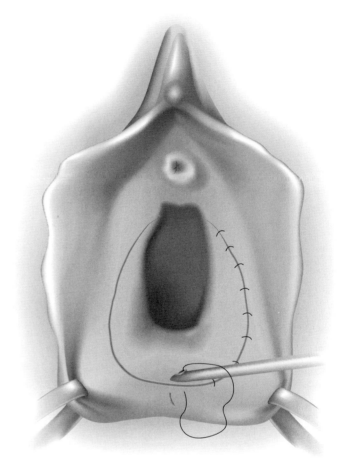

Figure 15.1.4. Vulvar vestibulectomy: the vaginal advancement flap is approximated to the perineum to complete the procedure.

1 cm.[22] This technique had limited success and often caused exacerbations of symptoms. More recently, a less invasive laser, the flashlamp-excited dye laser, has been used with a lower complication rate and a slightly higher success rate.[23] In general, the results of laser surgery are less successful than surgical techniques as previously described.

Most authors suggest that no one surgical technique is appropriate for all women with vulvar vestibulitis syndrome. It is suggested that the surgeon choose the least invasive procedure that adequately treats an individual patient's symptoms. For example, if a patient has tenderness confined to a small portion of the vestibule, vestibuloplasty would be the most appropriate procedure. However, if a woman has allodynia in her entire vestibule and recurrent fissuring at the posterior fourchette, perineoplasty would be the correct procedure.

Closure techniques vary between different studies and surgeons. However, modifications of closure technique have been used to limit the risk of hematoma, scar tissue, vaginal stenosis, and wound dehiscence. Marinoff and others have described several changes to vestibulectomy that have reduced complications

and improved the success rates of this procedure.[26] Specifically, the vaginal advancement flap should be anchored in an advanced position by several mattress sutures of 3–0 Vicryl. These mattress sutures minimize tension along the suture line, thereby limiting the risk of wound dehiscence. The mattress stitches should be thrown in an anterior–posterior direction to prevent compromise of the vaginal diameter. In addition, the vaginal advancement flap should be approximated to the perineum with interrupted stitches of 4–0 Vicryl to help prevent hematoma and wound disruption.

Success of surgical correction of vulvar vestibulitis syndrome also depends on appropriate postoperative care. In the immediate postoperative period, liberal use of ice packs prevents swelling and helps with pain. Sitz baths starting several days after the surgery can help with postoperative pain and may help prevent infection. Physical activity should be limited for the first 4–8 weeks required for the surgical site to heal, to help prevent wound dehiscence. Close communication and frequent visits to a certified woman's physical therapist specializing in such pelvic floor disorders are encouraged. Under monitoring by the physical therapist and biofeedback pelvic floor electromyography, vaginal dilators can be used after the surgical site has healed to help the postoperative patient resume normal sexual functioning.

Complications of surgery

Patients considering surgery need to be informed that complications of vestibuloplasty, vestibulectomy, and perineoplasty do occur, although they are infrequent. The risks of surgery increase with the invasiveness of the procedure performed. Specifically, complications include bleeding, infection, increased pain, hematoma, wound dehiscence, vaginal stenosis, scar tissue formation, and Bartholin duct cyst formation.[27] The risk of these complications can be reduced if appropriate surgical techniques are utilized. Surgical intervention is offered as a treatment alternative in women who have failed conservative medical, psychologic, and/or physical therapy.[26,28]

Review of the literature on surgical treatment of vulvar vestibulitis syndrome

Evaluation of the risks and benefits among the various surgical strategies is difficult because there is no standardized terminology, nor have any comparison trials been performed.[18]

Table 15.1.1. Summary of papers on vulvar vestibulitis syndrome

Authors	Procedure	Number of patients	Length of follow-up (in months)	Complete resolution of pain	Partial (significant) resolution of pain	No significant resolution of pain	Complete or significant reduction in pain
Woodruff et al.[19]	Perineoplasty	18	6–60	18	0	0	100%
Woodruff et al.[19]	Perineoplasty	14	6–36	12	2	0	100%
Woodruff and Friedrich[30]	Perineoplasty	44	NS*	36	6	2	95%
Peckham et al.[31]	Perineoplasty	9	NS	9	0	0	100%
Friedrich[3]	Perineoplasty	38†	NS	23		15	60%
Michlewitz et al.[32]	Perineoplasty	16	NS	16			100%
Bornstein and Kaufman[33]	Perineolpasty (modified)	20	6–36	14	4	2	90%
Marinoff and Turner[27]	Perineoplasty	73	12–36	60	11	2	97%
Westrom[34]	Modified vestibulectomy	12	15–19	10	1	1	92%
Schover et al.[35]	Vestibuloplasty	38	1–24	18	14	6	84%
Mann et al.[36]	Perineoplasty	56	6–54	37	12	7	88%
Barbaro et al.[37]	Modified vestibulectomy	21	1–3	19	2		100%
Abramov et al.[38]	Vestibulectomy	7	12	7			100%
Bornstein et al.[39]	Perineoplasty	11	6	9	1	1	91%
Foster et al.[40]	Perineoplasty	93	>48	51	31	11	88%
Chaim et al.[41]	Perineoplasty (modified)	16	10–70	15		1	94%
de Jong et al.[42]	Perineoplasty	14	36–84	3	3	8	43%
Baggish and Miklos[43]	Vestibulectomy	15	12	13		2	87%
Goetsch[20]	Vestibuloplasty	12	6–72	10	2		100%
Kehoe and Luesley[44]	Modified vestibulectomy	37	3–34	22	11	4	89%
Weijmar Schultz et al.[45]	Vestibulectomy	13	2–36	7	4	2	85%
Bergeron et al.[46]	Vestibulectomy	38	13–120	24		14	68%
Bergeron et al.[12]	Vestibulectomy	22	6	15		7	68%
Bornstein et al.[47]	Perineoplasty	79	12	60	19		100%
Berville et al.[48]	Vestibulectomy	12	8	6	4	2	83%
Marinoff[26]	Perineoplasty	107	3–48	70	18	19	82%
Westrom and Willen[49]	Modified vestibulectomy	42	6	33	5	4	90%
Kehoe and Luesley[50]	Vestibulectomy	54	2–42	33	15	6	89%
Hopkins[51]	Perineoplasty	21	NS	19		2	90%
McKormack and Spence[52]	Perineoplasty	42	12–120	16	19	7	83%
Schneider et al.[53]	Vestibulectomy	54	6	30	15	9	83%
Gaunt et al.[54]	Vestibulectomy	42	6–24	28	10	4	90%
Goldstein and Klingman[28]	Vestibulectomy	69	12–60	31	30	7	88%
Total		1159					

*NS: length of follow-up not stated.
†Includes 13 patients who had a previous surgical failure by another surgeon

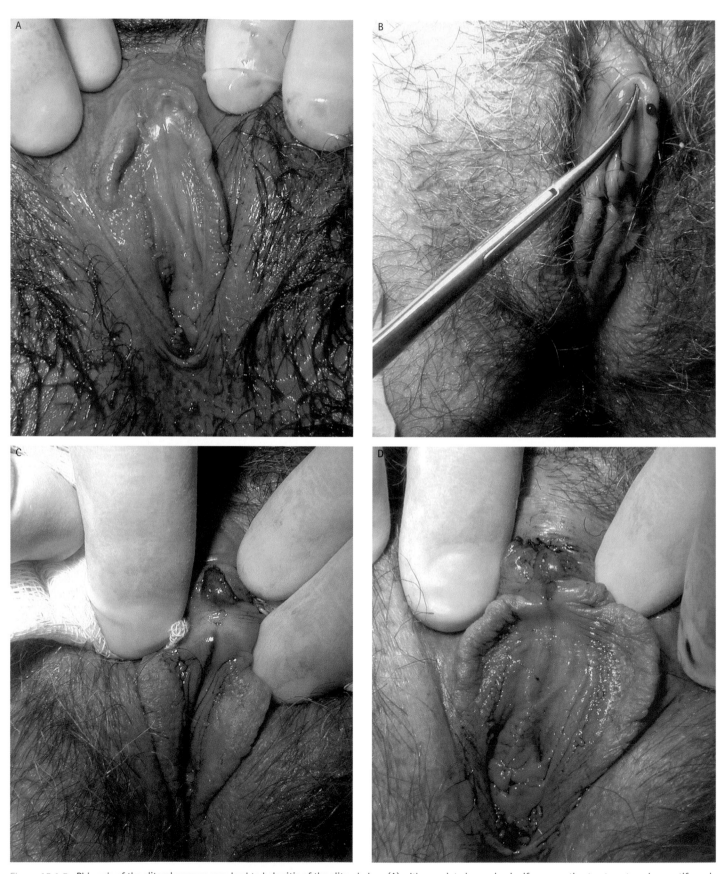

Figure 15.1.5. Phimosis of the clitoral prepuce may lead to balanitis of the clitoral glans (A) with associated sexual pain. If conservative treatment, such as antifungal treatment, fails, a dorsal slit procedure may be performed (B–D).

This chapter will review 33 papers in the English literature regarding the surgical management of vulvar vestibulitis syndrome (Table 15.1.1). This review reveals that the surgical success rate was greater than 80% in 29 of the studies cited. However, it is difficult to compare these studies. Techniques and terminology used to describe the various procedures varied significantly. Different authors referred to widely different surgeries characterized by the same name. Often there are changes to the techniques employed even within the same series of patients. The outcome criteria for "surgical success" are often poorly defined, and rarely are standard procedures employed to assess success. The evaluation of success is always nonblinded, rendering it biased and highly subjective. Patient selection criteria are usually not mentioned within a given series. Most studies did not distinguish between various forms of vestibulitis (primary or secondary vestibulitis, constant pain, or pain only with provocation). There is a great degree of variability in the length of follow-up even within a given series, and follow-up is rarely long-term. Therefore, determining the rate of recurrence of vulvar vestibulitis syndrome after surgery is very difficult to assess.

The rationale for performing surgery is based on the underlying pathology. One hypothesis of the pathophysiology of vulvar vestibulitis syndrome is that there is extreme hypersensi-

tivity of the vestibular tissue associated with increased nerve density in the vestibular mucosa. Surgery is successful because excision of the mucosa removes the neuronal hyperplasia. The fact that the vestibule is embryonically derived from tissue different than the vagina may explain why there is very little recurrence of symptoms after surgical resection of the vestibule with vaginal advancement.

Surgical treatment of vulvar vestibulitis syndrome results in significant resolution of dyspareunia in more than half of the patients operated. In addition, a clinically meaningful reduction in dyspareunia is reported in approximately two-thirds of the remaining patients. There is a high degree of patient satisfaction with surgical treatment of vulvar vestibulitis syndrome.

Surgery for other sexual pain disorders within the vestibule

Disorders of the various tissues within the vestibule may cause sexual pain. For example, phimosis of the clitoral prepuce may lead to balanitis of the clitoral glans with associated sexual pain. If conservative treatment fails, such as antifungal treatment, a

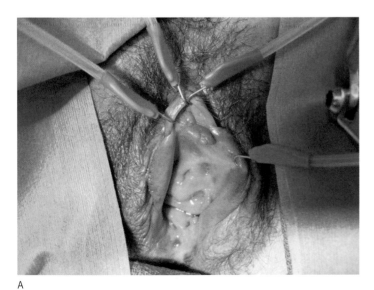

A

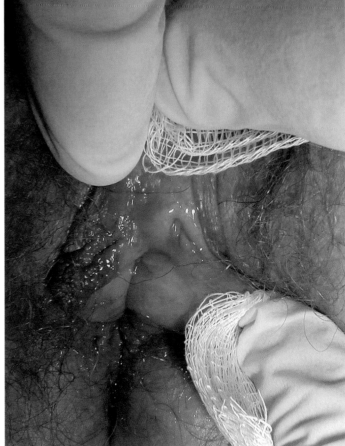

B

Figure 15.1.6. A clitoral tumor, such as a clitoral fibroepithelioma, may also cause pain. Treatment is by surgical excision.

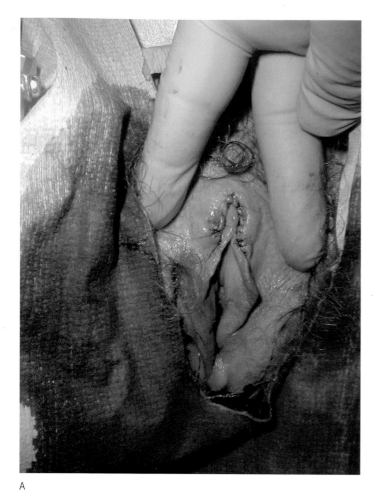

A

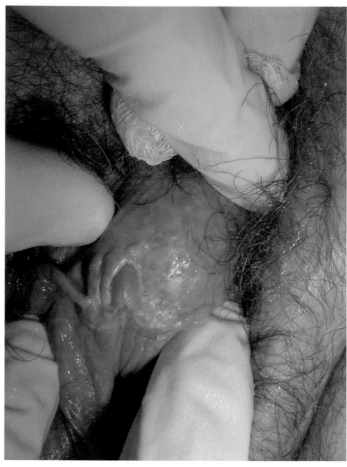

B

Figure 15.1.7. A sebaceous cyst may involve the prepuce and lead to severe pain and swelling of the prepucial tissue. Incision and drainage of the abscess may be required. A shows an intra-operative photo at the completion of the dorsal slit procedure. B is an office photograph at 6 months follow-up showing healing of the incision with the exposed glans clitoris.

dorsal slit procedure may be performed (Fig. 15.1.5). A clitoral tumor may also cause pain. We have performed multiple excisions of clitoral fibroepitheliomas (Fig. 15.1.6). A sebaceous cyst may involve the prepuce and lead to severe pain and swelling of the prepucial tissue. Incision and drainage of the abscess may be required (Fig. 15.1.7).

Dermatologic conditions of the vestibule or vulva may require surgical intervention when conservative treatment with ultrapotent topical steroids fails. Perineoplasty surgery can be used for treatment of lichen sclerosus, a chronic cutaneous disorder with a predilection for the vulva. The chronic inflammation associated with lichen sclerosus often causes destruction of the vulvar architecture with scarring of the posterior fourchette and perineum. Rouzier et al. described a series of 62 women with introital stenosis caused by lichen sclerosus who underwent perineoplasty.[24] Ninety percent of these women had significant improvement in their sexual function after surgery. Perineoplasty can also be used successfully for women who have recurrent idiopathic fissuring at the posterior fourchette, especially since perineoplasty widens the introitus. While simple excision of recurrent fissures is a less invasive procedure,

narrowing of the introitus may result.[25] Urethral prolapse may be a cause of vestibular pain. Should conservative treatments, such as local estrogen therapy, fail, surgery may be a management option (Fig. 15.1.8). Bartholin's cysts may present as vestibular pain. Marsupialization of the cyst can be performed to obviate the sexual pain (see Chapter 22.2).

Conclusion

In the step-care process of the management of women with sexual pain, conservative treatments are performed first. Should psychologic, medical, and/or psychologic management fail, surgery is a safe and effective treatment for women with sexual pain disorder.[18,29] The most common disorder in women with sexual pain is vulvar vestibulitis syndrome. There are limitations of the surgical safety and efficacy outcome data. Nevertheless, there are also limited outcome studies showing the safety and efficacy of conservative (psychologic, medical, or physical therapy) treatment approaches for vulvar vestibulitis syndrome. While surgery poses risks of infection, scar tissue, increased pain, Bartholin's

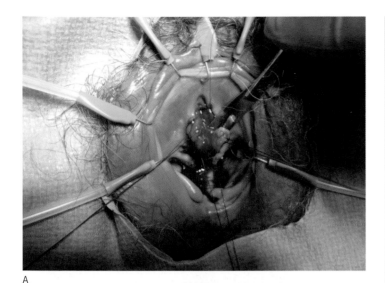

A

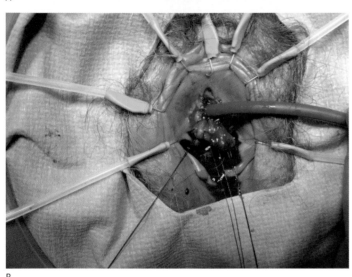

B

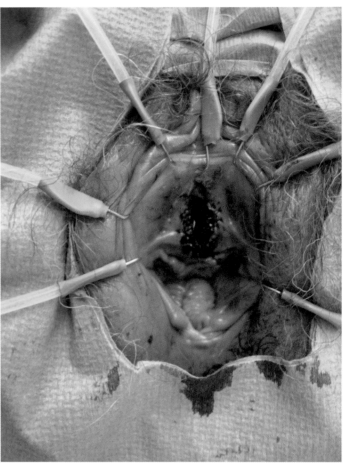

C

Figure 15.1.8. Urethral prolapse may be a cause of vestibular pain. Should conservative treatments, such as local estrogen therapy, fail, surgery may be a management option.

cysts, disfigurement, and recurrence of symptoms after surgery, contemporary literature reveals that these risks are low.

References

1. Bergeron S, Binik YM, Khalife S et al. Vulvar vestibulitis syndrome: a critical review. *Clin J Pain* 1997; 13: 27–42.

2. Meana M, Binik YM, Khalife S et al. Biopsychosocial profile of women with dyspareunia. *Obstet Gynecol* 1997; 90(4 Pt 1): 583–9.

3. Friedrich EG Jr. Vulvar vestibulitis syndrome. *J Reprod Med* 1987; 32: 110–14.

4. Harlow BL, Stewart EG. A population-based assessment of chronic unexplained vulvar pain: have we underestimated the prevalence of vulvodynia? *J Am Med Womens Assoc* 2003; 58: 82–8.

5. Murina F, Tassan P, Roberti P et al. Treatment of vulvar vestibulitis with submucous infiltrations of methylprednisolone and lidocaine. An alternative approach. *J Reprod Med* 2001; 46: 713–16.

6. Marinoff SC, Turner ML, Hirsch RP et al. Intralesional alpha interferon. Cost-effective therapy for vulvar vestibulitis syndrome. *J Reprod Med* 1993; 38: 19–24.

7. Glazer HI, Rodke G, Swencionis C et al. Treatment of vulvar vestibulitis syndrome with electromyographic biofeedback of pelvic floor musculature. *J Reprod Med* 1995; 40: 283–90.

8. Friedrich EG Jr. Therapeutic studies on vulvar vestibulitis. *J Reprod Med* 1988; 33: 514–18.

9. Zolnoun DA, Hartmann KE, Steege JF. Overnight 5% lidocaine ointment for treatment of vulvar vestibulitis. *Obstet Gynecol* 2003; 102: 84–7.

10. Bergeron S, Brown C, Lord MJ et al. Physical therapy for vulvar vestibulitis syndrome: a retrospective study. *J Sex Marital Ther* 2002; 28: 183–92.

11. McKay M. Dysesthetic ("essential") vulvodynia. Treatment with amitriptyline. *J Reprod Med* 1993; 38: 9–13.

12. Bergeron S, Binik YM, Khalife S et al. A randomized comparison of group cognitive-behavioral therapy, surface electromyographic biofeedback, and vestibulectomy in the treatment of dyspareunia resulting from vulvar vestibulitis. *Pain* 2001; 91: 297–306.

13. Danielsson I, Sjoberg I, Ostman C. Acupuncture for the treatment of vulvar vestibulitis: a pilot study. *Acta Obstet Gynecol Scand* 2001; 80: 437–41.

14. Solomons CC, Melmed MH, Heitler SM. Calcium citrate for vulvar vestibulitis. A case report. *J Reprod Med* 1991; 36: 879–82.

15. Thomas TG. *Practical Treatise on the Diseases of Women.* Philadelphia: Henry C. Lea's Son & Co., 1880.

16. Bohm-Starke N, Hilliges M, Falconer C et al. Neurochemical characterization of the vestibular nerves in women with vulvar vestibulitis syndrome. *Gynecol Obstet Invest* 1999; 48: 270–5.

17. Bornstein J, Goldschmid N, Sabo E. Hyperinnervation and mast cell activation may be used as histopathologic diagnostic criteria for vulvar vestibulitis. *Gynecol Obstet Invest* 2004; 58: 171–8.

18. Haefner HK. Critique of new gynecologic surgical procedures: surgery for vulvar vestibulitis. *Clin Obstet Gynecol* 2000; 43: 689–700.

19. Woodruff JD, Genadry R, Poliakoff S. Treatment of dyspareunia and vaginal outlet distortions by perineoplasty. *Obstet Gynecol* 1981; 57: 750–4.

20. Goetsch MF. Simplified surgical revision of the vulvar vestibule for vulvar vestibulitis. *Am J Obstet Gynecol* 1996; 174: 1701–5; discussion 5–7.

21. Peters WA 3rd. Bartholinitis after vulvovaginal surgery. *Am J Obstet Gynecol* 1998; 178: 1143–4.

22. Tschanz C, Salomon D, Skaria A et al. Vulvodynia after CO_2 laser treatment of the female genital mucosa. *Dermatology* 2001; 202: 371–2.

23. Reid R, Omoto KH, Precop SL et al. Flashlamp-excited dye laser therapy of idiopathic vulvodynia is safe and efficacious. *Am J Obstet Gynecol* 1995; 172: 1684–96; discussion 96–701.

24. Rouzier R, Haddad B, Deyrolle C et al. Perineoplasty for the treatment of introital stenosis related to vulvar lichen sclerosus. *Am J Obstet Gynecol* 2002; 186: 49–52.

25. Edwards L. Vulvar fissures: causes and therapy. *Dermatol Ther* 2004; 17: 111–16.

26. Marinoff SC. Surgical treatment of vulvar vestibulitis. In *Vulvodynia Workshop: Current Knowledge and Future Direction*, National Institutes of Health, 1997: 28–32.

27. Marinoff SC, Turner ML. Vulvar vestibulitis syndrome: an overview. *Am J Obstet Gynecol* 1991; 165(4 Pt 2): 1228–33.

28. Goldstein A, Klingman D. Long-term patient satisfaction with vulvar vestibulectomy with vaginal advancement for vulvar vestibulitis syndrome. In *Vulvodynia and Sexual Pain Disorders in Women: A State of the Art Conference*, Atlanta: 27 October 2004.

29. Edwards L. New concepts in vulvodynia. *Am J Obstet Gynecol* 2003; 189(Suppl 3): S24–30.

30. Woodruff JD, Friedrich EG Jr. The vestibule. *Clin Obstet Gynecol* 1985; 28: 134–41.

31. Peckham BM, Maki DG, Patterson JJ et al. Focal vulvitis: a characteristic syndrome and cause of dyspareunia. Features, natural history, and management. *Am J Obstet Gynecol* 1986; 154: 855–64.

32. Michlewitz H, Kennison RD, Turksoy RN et al. Vulvar vestibulitis – subgroup with Bartholin gland duct inflammation. *Obstet Gynecol* 1989; 73(3 Pt 1): 410–13.

33. Bornstein J, Kaufman RH. [Perineoplasty for vulvar vestibulitis]. *Harefuah* 1989; 116: 90–2.

34. Westrom L. Vulvar vestibulitis. *Lancet* 1991; 338(8774): 1088.

35. Schover LR, Youngs DD, Cannata R. Psychosexual aspects of the evaluation and management of vulvar vestibulitis. *Am J Obstet Gynecol* 1992; 167: 630–6.

36. Mann MS, Kaufman RH, Brown D Jr et al. Vulvar vestibulitis: significant clinical variables and treatment outcome. *Obstet Gynecol* 1992; 79: 122–5.

37. Barbero M, Micheletti L, Valentino MC et al. Membranous hypertrophy of the posterior fourchette as a cause of dyspareunia and vulvodynia. *J Reprod Med* 1994; 39: 949–52.

38. Abramov L, Wolman I, David MP. Vaginismus: an important factor in the evaluation and management of vulvar vestibulitis syndrome. *Gynecol Obstet Invest* 1994; 3: 94–7.

39. Bornstein J, Zarfati D, Goldik Z et al. Perineoplasty compared with vestibuloplasty for severe vulvar vestibulitis. *Br J Obstet Gynaecol* 1995; 102: 652–5.

40. Foster DC, Butts C, Shah KV et al. Long term outcome of perineoplasty for vulvar vestibulitis. *J Womens Health* 1995; 4: 669–75.

41. Chaim W, Meriwether C, Gonik B et al. Vulvar vestibulitis subjects undergoing surgical intervention: a descriptive analysis and histopathological correlates. *Eur J Obstet Gynecol Reprod Biol* 1996; 68(1–2): 165–8.

42. de Jong JM, van Lunsen RH, Robertson EA et al. Focal vulvitis: a psychosexual problem for which surgery is not the answer. *J Psychosom Obstet Gynaecol* 1995; 16: 85–91.

43. Baggish MS, Miklos JR. Vulvar pain syndrome: a review. *Obstet Gynecol Surv* 1995; 50: 618–27.

44. Kehoe S, Luesley D. An evaluation of modified vestibulectomy in the treatment of vulvar vestibulitis: preliminary results. *Acta Obstet Gynecol Scand* 1996; 75: 676–7.

45. Weijmar Schultz WC, Gianotten WL, van der Meijden WI et al. Behavioral approach with or without surgical intervention to the vulvar vestibulitis syndrome: a prospective randomized and nonrandomized study. *J Psychosom Obstet Gynaecol* 1996; 17: 143–8.

46. Bergeron S, Bouchard C, Fortier M et al. The surgical treatment of vulvar vestibulitis syndrome: a follow-up study. *J Sex Marital Ther* 1997; 23: 317–25.

47. Bornstein J, Goldik Z, Stolar Z et al. Predicting the outcome of surgical treatment of vulvar vestibulitis. *Obstet Gynecol* 1997; 89(5 Pt 1): 695–8.

48. Berville S, Moyal-Barracco M, Paniel BJ. [Treatment of vulvar vestibulitis by posterior vestibulectomy. Twelve case reports]. *J Gynecol Obstet Biol Reprod (Paris)* 1997; 26: 71–5.

49. Westrom LV, Willen R. Vestibular nerve fiber proliferation in vulvar vestibulitis syndrome. *Obstet Gynecol* 1998; 91: 572–6.

50. Kehoe S, Luesley D. Vulvar vestibulitis treated by modified vestibulectomy. *Int J Gynaecol Obstet* 1999; 64: 147–52.

51. Hopkins M. Perineoplasty for the treatment of vulvar vestibulitis. In *Operative Techniques in Gynecologic Surgery*. London: WB Saunders, 1998: 228–30.

52. McCormack WM, Spence MR. Evaluation of the surgical treatment of vulvar vestibulitis. *Eur J Obstet Gynecol Reprod Biol* 1999; 86: 135–8.

53. Schneider D, Yaron M, Bukovsky I et al. Outcome of surgical treatment for superficial dyspareunia from vulvar vestibulitis. *J Reprod Med* 2001; 46: 227–31.

54. Gaunt G, Good A, Stanhope CR. Vestibulectomy for vulvar vestibulitis. *J Reprod Med* 2003; 48: 591–5.

15.2 Difficult cases: surgical treatment of female sexual dysfunction

Irwin Goldstein

Introduction

Sexual dysfunction in women is common and may interfere with quality of life[1,2] (see Chapters 2.1–2.4 of this book). Sexual dysfunctions are the result of interactions among numerous mind, body, and relationship factors.[3] Therefore, ideal management of women with sexual problems would be in a multidisciplinary setting with psychologic- and biologic-focused health-care professionals.[4,5] Management of women with sexual dysfunction should be performed in a step-care paradigm in which treatments selected evolve from the least invasive to progressively more invasive management strategies.[1,3–6] Surgery for the treatment of a woman's sexual dysfunction should be considered only as the last resort.

This chapter reviews difficult surgical cases of sexual dysfunction, comprising five cases of women who presented for management of sexual dysfunction in a multidisciplinary setting, and who ultimately required surgical intervention as part of the care provided to manage the sexual complaint. This surgical care was provided, in all cases, in addition to other biologic and psychologic interventions. The purpose of the chapter is to illustrate some typical cases in which surgical intervention strategies are utilized in the management of women with sexual health problems. When appropriate, photographs are provided. As with all medical conditions, in cases of failed conservative interventions, not only is surgery indicated, but also it is the one therapy that may resolve the overall sexual dysfunction. As in other portions of this textbook relating to difficult case management, all efforts have been made to protect the privacy of patients and to maintain the management strategies utilized in the case for teaching purposes.

Case 1

KS is a 26-year-old, healthy, sexually active woman who has no health problems and takes no medication. She states that, when she was a teenager, during sexual arousal, her vagina produced a significant amount of clear, viscous, slimy, "egg white-like" lubrication that soaked through her clothes. In college, she noticed that during sexual stimulation the inside of her vaginal walls would produce some fluid, but not the same volume and quality of lubrication she had experienced as a teenager. In her second year of college, she noticed a small red bubble on the labia minora. When KS touched this bubble, it burst, and a small amount of fluid came out. She went to her gynecologist, but nothing abnormal was observed. During KS's final years of college, her labia minora would generally become swollen when she was aroused, and it would take days for the swelling to go away.

For the 4 years following her graduation from college, when KS became sexually aroused, the labia minora would swell within minutes, and it felt as if "there were water balloons inside the flesh of my labia". The swelling, especially on the left labium, increased to a volume larger than a "pecan in its shell". She observed that the membrane of the "water balloon" surrounding the fluid was easily palpable inside the skin of the labia minora. On the right side, the swelling was located just inside the vaginal introitus. After sexual stimulation, when the swelling developed, KS felt a burning discomfort. Although the bilateral swelling occurred within minutes, it could take weeks for it to dissipate completely. If KS was frequently sexually aroused, the swelling got larger and larger. This condition was very painful because "the swelling distended the delicate labia", and anything that contacted the labia caused pain, including her clothing. It could even be painful to sit. If the labia remained swollen for a long time, the skin became desensitized, and there was more of a distressing discomfort than pain. Despite having a healthy sexual interest, KS avoided relationships and sexual experiences because of this problem.

KS had been to a series of physicians, and she had many different diagnoses, but none helped to alleviate the problem. One gynecologist told her the swelling was "trauma from oral sex". The physician used a syringe to aspirate the fluid, giving significant relief. KS's boyfriend then "shaved his beard", but that made no difference. Another physician biopsied the membrane of the "water balloon". Another physician surgically removed the cyst from her left labium, but the swelling started to recur, dramatically related to sexual arousal but to no other time. KS was frustrated that the relationship of the swelling to sexual arousal remained unexplained. KS would seek relief by repeated office visits for needle aspiration until she started to do this by herself. When she touched the aspirated fluid, it felt exactly like the vaginal lubrication she had been "missing since college".

KS decided to seek a new opinion, going for the first time to a multidisciplinary sexual medicine clinic. She was initially evaluated by the psychologist as follows. KS is currently emotionally stable without medication. There is no history of sexual abuse, substance abuse, or trauma. She is concerned about the long-term implications of this problem.

KS subsequently underwent history taking and physical examination, but this failed to reveal the disorder. She was advised to undergo duplex Doppler ultrasonography before and after audiovisual and vibratory sexual stimulation (see Chapter 14.3). This study revealed 3.5×5 cm right and 2.8×6 cm left, fluid-filled, irregular spaces with septa, consistent with Bartholin's cysts (Fig. 15.2.1). KS was advised to undergo marsupialization of both Bartholin's cysts. At the time, she was not sexually involved with anyone, so there was no problem. As KS felt that there were no appropriate means to "remove the cysts that weren't there", she decided to wait until she was in a relationship to have the problem corrected.

Approximately 1½ years later, KS was in a new relationship and sought definitive surgical treatment. She presented to the operating room, having undergone sexual stimulation the night before. Under intraoperative ultrasound control, both cysts were localized, punctured, filled with saline, and marsupialized (Fig. 15.2.2). Postoperatively, KS happily stated that her fluid now flowed right out, as it did in high school. She had forgotten what she was missing. "It's been so long since I self-lubricated like that – I am very, very glad it works."

Comments

It is important to understand the anatomy, structure, and function of the multiple organs within the vestibule (see Chapters 4.1 and 4.2). A careful and detailed inspection of the vestibule is critical in women with sexual dysfunction. In this case, the sexual medical disorder was present only during sexual arousal. In such situations, we have found duplex Doppler ultrasonography before and after audiovisual and vibratory sexual stimulation to be very useful in observing the arousal-related disorder.

Sexual medicine physicians can be expected to encounter Bartholin's duct cysts or gland abscesses in their female patients with sexual dysfunction, especially those who present with labial tissue swelling at the vaginal introitus associated with sexual stimulation and arousal causing local vaginal and intercourse discomfort. Bartholin's glands are homologs of Cowper's glands in males. Bartholin's glands, which provide lubricant for the labia minora and vestibule, are located bilaterally at the base of the labia minora and drain through 2–2.5-cm-long ducts that empty into the vestibule at about the 4 o'clock and 8 o'clock positions. The glands rarely exceed 1 cm in size and are not palpable except in the presence of abnormal gland drainage. Bartholin's duct cysts are the most common cystic growth in the vulva and occur in the labia majora. It is likely that Bartholin's glands involute as a woman ages, so that Bartholin's duct cysts are more common at 20–29 years of age. Obstruction of the distal Bartholin's duct may result in the retention of secretions, with resultant dilation of the duct and formation of a cyst. The cyst may become infected, and an abscess may develop in the gland. The treatment of Bartholin's duct cyst depends on the patient's symptoms. An asymptomatic cyst may require no treatment, but symptomatic Bartholin's duct cysts and gland abscesses require drainage by marsupialization.[7,8]

Case 2

FI, aged 25, with satisfactory sexual activity, had, since her teens, complained of episodes, once or twice a year, of painful swelling of the clitoris. Most of these episodes lasted hours to days and ultimately resolved spontaneously. The swelling episodes appeared unrelated to either self-stimulation or penetrative sexual activity. These occurrences were also unrelated to her menstrual cycle or to any physical activity. She took no medication other than an oral contraceptive that she had been using since college. She did not ride bicycles or horses and could not recall any episode of obvious blunt perineal trauma. During the episodes of clitoral swelling, the discomfort completely prevented sexual activity and the use of any clothing that would contact the tender region. FI mentioned these episodes to her gynecologist, but she was told all was normal on examination.

One year ago, FI had one episode of painful clitoral swelling that persisted beyond the usual few days. For the first time, FI went to a gynecologist with this condition in an active state. She was again informed that the examination was normal. FI was treated with a 5-day course of oral antibiotics, and over the next few days the swelling and discomfort resolved.

Approximately 6 months later, FI experienced another

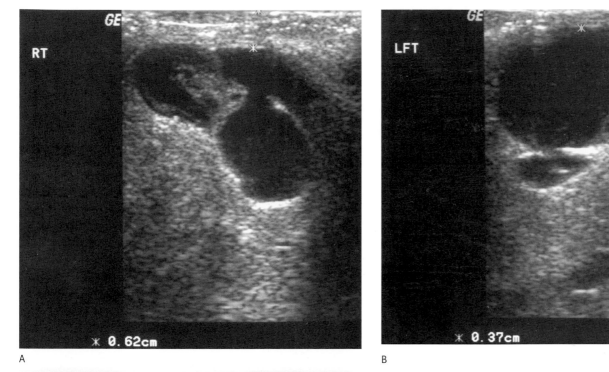

A

B

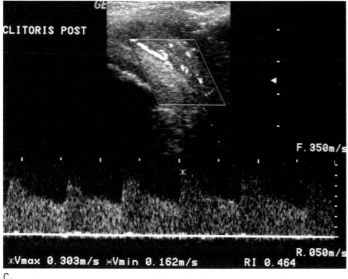

C

Figure 15.2.1. Duplex Doppler ultrasound revealed a 3.5 × 5 cm right and 2.8 × 6 cm left, fluid-filled, irregular space with septa consistent with Bartholin's cysts. Since the disorder is evident only after sexual stimulation, as shown by the clitoral ultrasound study, the ultrasound was performed before and after audiovisual and vibratory stimulation.

episode of painful clitoral swelling that again developed for no apparent reason. This episode also persisted and worsened over the next few days, preventing her from engaging in any form of sexual activity. FI contacted her gynecologist, who prescribed the same oral antibiotics. Unfortunately, despite 5 days of antibiotic treatment, the symptoms of clitoral swelling and pain persisted. FI was referred to a new gynecologist, who noted severe clitoral swelling of unknown etiology. FI wanted to know what the problem was. She was admitted to the hospital for intravenous antibiotics, observation, and pelvic ultrasound examination. The radiologist performing the examination could not rule out clitoral priapism.

FI was transferred for emergency opinion to a multidisciplinary sexual medicine clinic. Upon admission, FI underwent history taking and physical examination. The clitoral prepuce was markedly swollen and tender, and the glans clitoris could not be visualized by prepucial retraction (Figs 15.2.3 and 15.2.4). The preliminary psychologic interview failed to identify any history of trauma or abuse, or any contributing psychologic problems. FI was frustrated and anxious over the inability to understand what was happening "down there", but she was happily married with a very supportive husband. FI had had a marked loss of interest, arousal, and orgasm after the birth of her two daughters. Sexual activity had become limited and was now

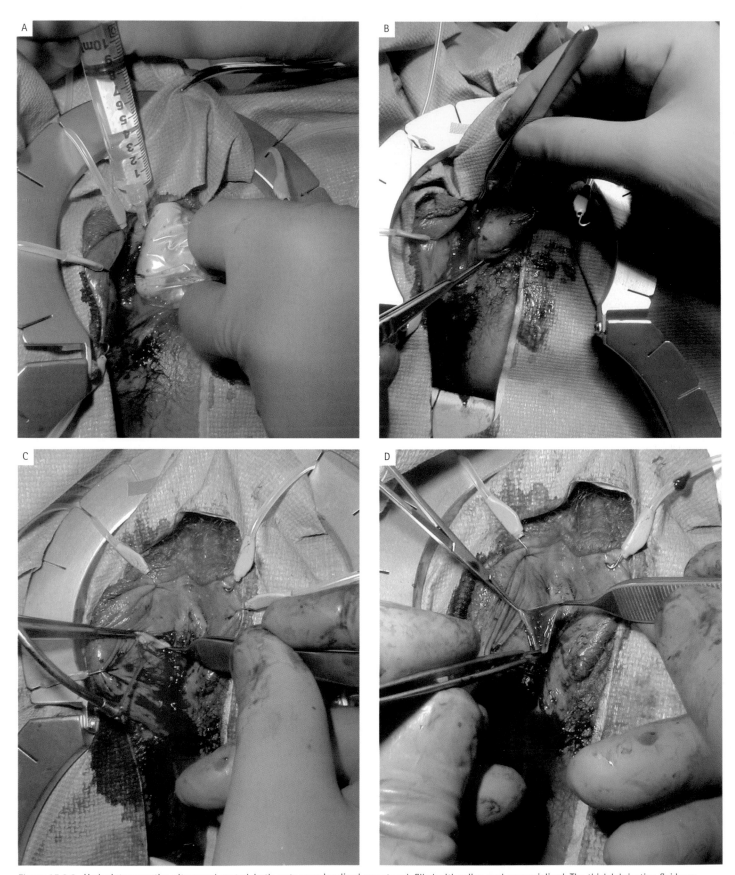

Figure 15.2.2. Under intraoperative ultrasound control, both cysts were localized, punctured, filled with saline, and marsupialized. The thick lubricating fluid was noted to emanate from the Bartholin's cyst.

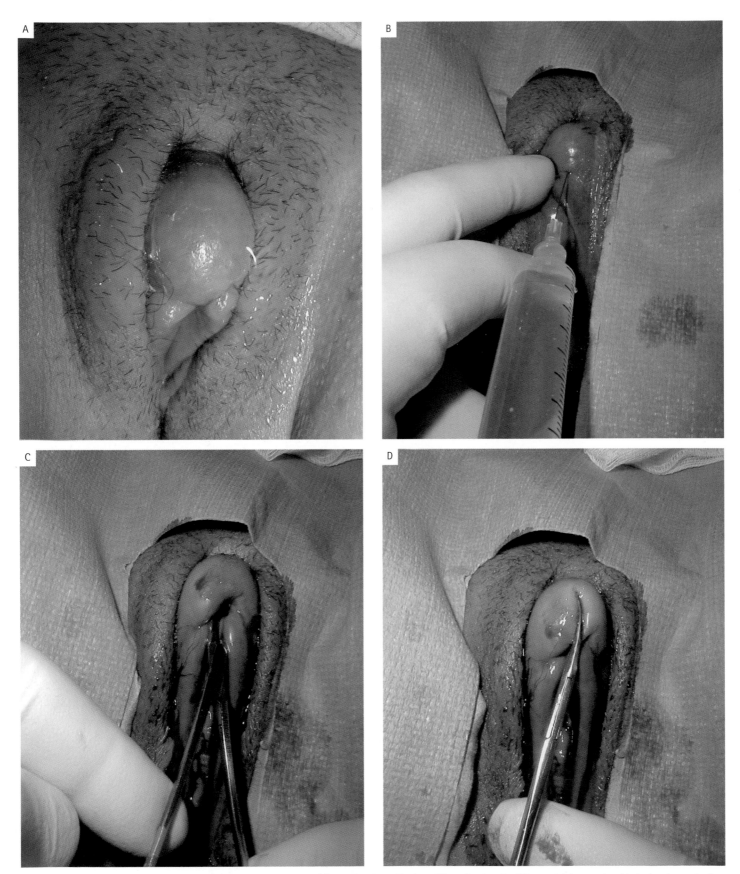

Figure 15.2.3. The clitoral prepuce was markedly swollen and tender (A), and the glans clitoris could not be visualized by prepucial retraction. Under local anesthesia with sedation (B), a dorsal slit of the prepuce was utilized to gain clitoral glans exposure (C, D).

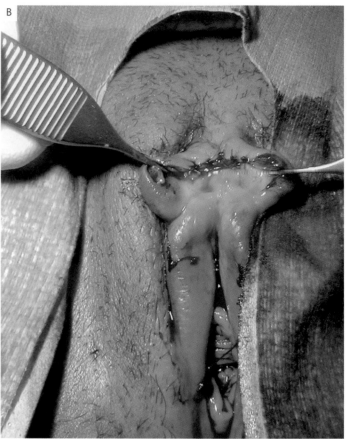

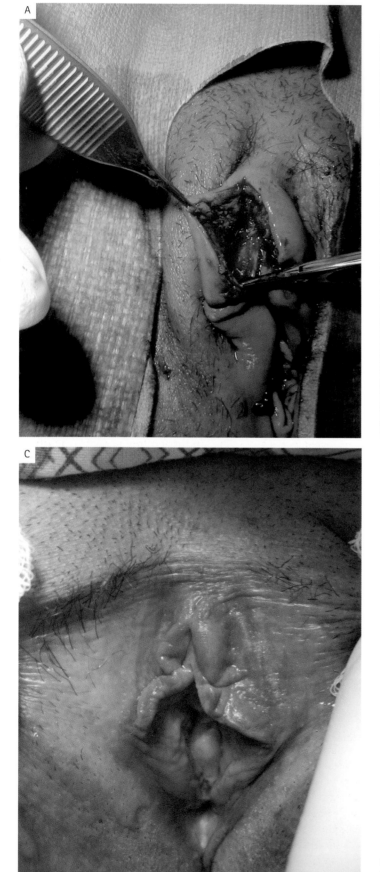

Figure 15.2.4. Emergency incision and drainage of the abscess was performed (A, B). At 6-month follow-up, the anatomy of the vestibule appeared normal (C).

associated with mild to moderate discomfort during penetration.

FI was advised to undergo duplex Doppler ultrasound examination of the clitoris. The peak systolic velocity in the right and left clitoral cavernosal arteries was 10–15 cm/s, and the end diastolic velocity was 5–7 cm/s. The right and left clitoral shaft diameters were 1.1 and 1.0 cm, respectively. There was evidence of a hypoechoic, fluid-filled space of 3.1 × 2.3 cm, underlying the right aspect of the prepuce, that appeared contiguous with pubic subcutaneous tissue and consistent with a prepucial abscess. Under local anesthesia with sedation, FI underwent emergency incision and drainage of the abscess, as well as a dorsal slit of the prepuce to gain clitoral glans exposure (Figs 15.2.3 and 15.2.4). FI did well postoperatively and was seen at 1-, 2-, and 6-month follow-up (Fig. 15.2.4). Her physical examination was unremarkable. She was informed that the recurrent symptoms she experienced were probably secondary to a repeated, intermittent, subcutaneous tissue infection, probably of a sebaceous cyst underlying the prepuce. FI was notified that if she was distressed or bothered by her changed sexual function since childbirth, she could undergo an evaluation, including sex steroid hormones.

Comments

Sebaceous cysts are often found in the genital area (see Chapters 9.5 and 12.2). Sebaceous cysts are formed when the release of the relatively thick fluid sebum produced by the sebaceous glands in the skin is obstructed. If cysts become infected or grow to a bothersome size, surgical intervention may be necessary. Sebaceous cysts can recur if they are not removed completely. In women with clitoral pain syndromes, careful physical examination of the clitoris and prepuce is aided by magnification with surgical loupes. Proper examination involves elevation of the lateral aspect of the clitoral shaft in a cephalic direction. The clitoral glans should be exposed fully. Nearby sebaceous cysts occur under the skin, vary in size, and tend to be smooth to the touch.[9]

Case 3

BT, aged 33, a healthy, single nurse, has been in a relationship for the last 8 years. At age 25, BT was prescribed the combined oral pill for contraception and control of irregular and painful menstrual periods. She has remained on the combined oral contraceptive for the last 8 years. From age 19 to 27, BT was interested in sexual activity, easily aroused, and enjoyed excellent quality orgasmic release. Over the last 6 years, BT noted progressively diminished interest in sexual activity, which had worsened significantly over the last 2 years. During the last 24 months, BT also suffered a raw, burning discomfort during penetration, described as like rubbing on sandpaper, that hurt for a day or two after a sexual encounter. She experienced the same discomfort when she wore tight clothing that contacted her genital area. BT also noted that during sexual activity she had less genital feeling, was drier, and did not lubricate as much any more. The sexual problems have been a huge predicament in the relationship, as her partner feels that BT is no longer attracted to him.

BT had sought advice from her local primary care physician. Physical examinations were always unremarkable and she was ultimately advised to "be a good actress". She went to several gynecologists and was managed with topical estrogen creams and with oral and topical treatments for yeast infections. Due to persistence of the sexual problem, BT was referred to a multidisciplinary sexual medicine clinic.

BT was initially evaluated by the psychologist. She provided a history of abuse by an alcoholic father during adolescence. Her mother had divorced and remarried, and BT lived with her mother and stepfather for 7 years before moving in with her current boyfriend. BT had a problem with alcohol in her teens but underwent rehabilitation, went to nursing school, and enjoys her health-care profession. She does not use recreational drugs and is in a committed relationship. She hopes to have a family and continue with her nursing career.

BT underwent history taking and physical examination. She provided the above history and added that, compared to previous capabilities, her current sexual desire was estimated to be only 10%; peripheral arousal, lubrication, and engorgement only 25%; and orgasmic release, now only occurring rarely with deep penetration, was approximately 20%. Physical examination revealed a 1.5-cm mass on the left frenulum that involved the posterior aspect of the clitoral glans (Fig. 15.2.5). The urethral meatus was without lesion. There was 20% fusion of the posterior aspect of the labia minora to the labia majora bilaterally. There were multiple areas of erythema overlying ostia of minor vestibular glands. Q-tip testing was positive in multiple areas overlying the ostia of the minor vestibular glands.

Biothesiometric studies revealed that the vibration perception threshold was 3 V in the right and left pulp index fingers, and 12 V in the right and left labia. The clitoris was too tender for assessment. The overall impression was a history of sexual abuse and ethanol use; sexual dysfunction including low desire, arousal, and orgasm; mild genital atrophy; mild diminished genital sensation; and dyspareunia with a 1.5-cm clitoral-frenular mass and vestibular adenitis. The plan was to observe the mass over the next month, consider sex steroid blood testing, develop psychologic coping strategies with the psychologist, and engage in physical therapy consultation for the vestibular pain.

One month later, BT returned to review the blood-test results. Hormone studies revealed the following values: thyroid-stimulating hormone 2.1 (0.4–5.50 µIU/ml), follicle-stimulating hormone 0.2 (1.5–33.4 mIU/ml), luteinizing hormone 0.6 (0.5–76.3 mIU/ml), prolactin 13.7 (1.8–20.3 ng/ml), dehydroepiandrosterone sulfate 58 (35–430 µg/ml), androstenedione 1.0 (0.2–3.1 ng/ml), total testosterone 14 (15–70 ng/dl), free testosterone <0.5 (0.3–1.9 ng/dl), sex hormone-binding globulin 249 (17–120 nmol/l), and estradiol <20 (11–526 pg/ml).

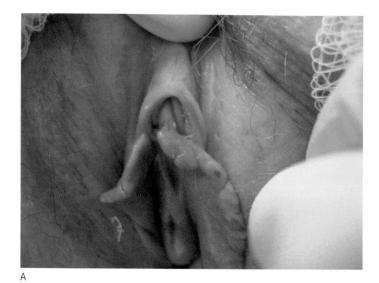

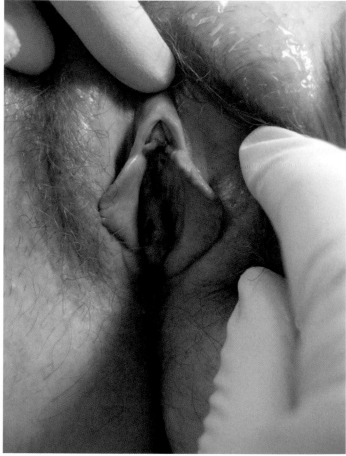

Figure 15.2.5. Physical examination revealed a 1.5 cm mass on the left frenulum that involved the posterior aspect of the clitoral glans (A). At 6-month postoperative follow-up (B), physical examination revealed no evidence of tumor recurrence.

Repeat physical examination showed the clitoral-frenular mass to be potentially more tender. After discussion, it was decided to perform an excisional biopsy of the mass and, in the postoperative period, discontinue the oral contraceptive pill, consider alternative contraception, and contemplate beginning androgen therapy.

BT underwent excisional biopsy under local anesthesia, preserving as much clitoral and frenular tissue as possible. The diagnosis was fibroepithelioma. Although this is a benign tumor, it may recur. At 6-month postoperative follow-up, physical examination revealed no evidence of tumor recurrence (Fig. 15.2.5). BT had utilized androgen therapy and normalized many of the abnormal sex steroid blood test values, except for a persistent sex hormone-binding globulin value. She experienced marked improvement in sexual interest and arousal. Orgasm was now possible by both clitoral and internal stimulation. Concerning the fibroepithelioma, BT will continue to undergo surveillance physical examination on a regular basis.

Comments

In women with sexual dysfunction, a full physical examination involves examination of the entire vestibule under magnification with surgical loupes (see Chapters 9.5 and 12.2). Clitoral disorders, such as fibroepithelioma, are not always identified (BT had at least four pelvic examinations in the last 2 years) because most health-care professionals do not retract the prepuce and examine the glans clitoris.

Fibroepitheliomas are characterized histologically by a mix of primordial follicular epithelium with more mature follicular epithelium within nodular collections of stroma. Fibroepitheliomas are usually found in the lower abdominal and perineal regions, or in the upper aspects of the lower extremities. Fibroepitheliomas can be precursors to basal cell carcinoma, but aggressive behavior in fibroepitheliomas is unusual.[10]

Case 4

NH, a 51-year-old, single, biotechnology consultant, was healthy until 6 years ago, and took only thyroid replacement for a hypothyroid condition that developed after an earlier pregnancy. NH had an excellent sex life with 100% desire, 100% arousal, and 100% orgasm from her teens until 6 years ago, when she was found to have a melanoma. She underwent surgical excision and, several weeks later, prophylactic chemotherapy. NH entered chemotherapy-induced menopause at age 46. She was happy before the chemotherapy and met a man with whom she had great sexual activity and satisfaction. Since the menopause, however, she has lost interest, and there has been significant pain and discomfort during penetration. On a business trip to London a year ago, she met another man and was very attracted to him. One month later, when they rendezvoused in Italy, NH was just not interested, and the sexual activity was very poor and painful. When premenopausal and performing self-stimulation, she would predictably reach orgasm in 15 min or less. Now it often takes more than 1 h and the orgasm is muted. NH is not even interested in trying. She is afraid of being alone, being one-dimensional, and never having or wanting to have passion again. The sexual problem is affecting her work, her relationships, and her self-image.

NH informed her gynecologist of the sexual dysfunction. She was advised to initiate hormone therapy. After learning of the risks and benefits, NH chose to use an estrogen and proges-terone patch. Unfortunately, while this made her feel better in general, the sexual symptoms persisted. NH was referred to a multidisciplinary sexual medicine clinic.

NH was seen initially by the psychologist. During chemo-therapy, she became menopausal and began to experience severe hot flashes, claustrophobia, fatigue, loss of interest in many activities, poor concentration, and insomnia. She is cur-rently on paroxetine, which helps to reduce her phobic reac-tions and hot flashes. She is feeling very distressed by her present situation, and is struggling with many life issues such as career and finances. She is currently not in a relationship, as initiating relationships is now difficult and her moods are very variable. She is able to experience orgasms of reduced intensity and lubricates to some degree when aroused, but still has low interest. She experiences "significant discomfort", described as feeling like rubbing burnt tissue, when sexually active.

NH's history was as above. In addition, she noted that, compared to previous capabilities, she had 20% desire, 20% arousal, and 10% orgasmic function. NH's physical examination revealed a decrease in size and thickness of the clitoris glans and prepuce. The urethral meatus revealed no prolapse There was marked atrophy of the labia minora, with 90% fusion to the labia majora bilaterally. There were multiple areas of erythema overlying ostia of Skene's glands/minor vestibular glands at 1, 2, 10, and 11 o'clock at the labial-hymenal junction (Fig. 15.2.6). Q-tip testing was markedly positive at all the sites of erythema with the patient describing pain intensity at a level of 5–10/10 at the various introital locations. The posterior fourchette of the

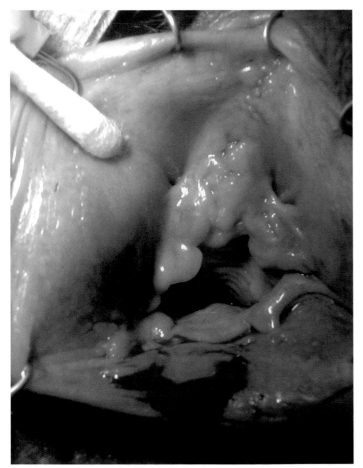

A

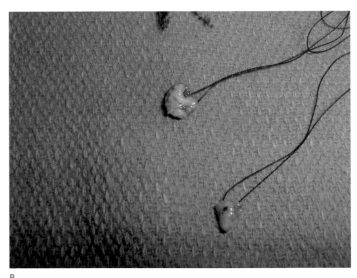

B

Figure 15.2.6. There were multiple areas of erythema overlying ostia of Skene's glands/minor vestibular glands at 1, 2, 10, and 11 o'clock at the labial-hymenal junction. Modification of the classic vestibulectomy involved excision exclusively of erythematous Skene's glands/minor vestibular glands at the 1, 2, 10, and 11 o'clock positions at the labial-hymenal junction. The outpatient surgery was performed under local anesthesia with sedation.

vestibule was free of pain. The vagina was consistent with mild atrophic vaginitis, revealing a relatively dry mucosa and decreased rugae formation. Biothesiometric studies revealed a vibration perception threshold of 4 V at the right and left pulp index fingers, with 14 V noted for the right and left labia minora and clitoris. Hormone studies revealed the following values: thyroid-stimulating hormone 2.3 (0.4–5.50 µIU/ml), follicle-stimulating hormone 39.6 (1.5–33.4 mIU/ml), luteinizing hormone 63.8 (0.5–76.3 mIU/ml), prolactin 11.2 (2.8–29.2 ng/ml), dehydroepiandrosterone sulfate 46 (35–430 µg/ml), androstenedione 0.7 (0.2–3.1 ng/ml), total testosterone 12 (15–70 ng/dl), free testosterone 0.4 (0.3–1.9 ng/dl), sex hormone-binding globulin 73 (17–120 nmol/l), dihydrotestosterone 63 (50–250 pg/ml), and estradiol 28 (11–526 pg/ml).

The impression was menopause following chemotherapy, mild depression, anxiety, high stress, decreased genital sensation, genital atrophy, atrophic vaginitis, and sexual dysfunction including marked diminished desire, arousal, orgasm with vulvar vestibulitis syndrome (primarily Skene's glands). The plan was to initiate psychologic consultation; physical therapy consultation in conjunction with local vestibular and intravaginal estrogen therapy; and systemic estrogen, progesterone, and androgen therapy.

At 3-month follow-up, NH was cautiously optimistic. She was found to have marked improvement in hormone blood tests. There was concomitant minor improvement in sexual interest, lubrication, and orgasmic intensity. The genital sexual pain persisted. Despite treatments, physical examination revealed persistence of the multiple areas of erythema overlying the ostia of multiple minor vestibular glands at the labial-hymenal junction. Q-tip testing was focally positive, overlying only the erythematous ostia with a range of pain of 5–10/10. She was placed on oral gabapentin but could not tolerate the medication due to drowsiness. She was then administered amitriptyline but realized only limited benefit.

At 1-year follow-up, despite ongoing psychologic counseling, biofeedback physical therapy, and systemic and local hormone therapy, NH was desperate for relief from the disabling genital sexual pain. The physical examination was essentially unchanged. She was advised to consider vestibulectomy. She underwent a diagnostic nerve block with 1% lidocaine, using a 31-gauge, 1-ml, 5/16-inch insulin syringe. After preparation with betadine, the injection revealed that Q-tip testing in the labial-hymenal junction was now negative.

NH was offered a modification of the complete vestibulectomy, involving excision exclusively of erythematous Skene's glands/minor vestibular glands at the 1, 2, 10, and 11 o'clock positions at the labial-hymenal junction. The outpatient surgery was performed under local anesthesia with sedation (Fig. 15.2.6). Pathologic analysis revealed a chronic inflammatory infiltrate surrounding the excised vestibular glands, with replacement of the columnar epithelium of the vestibular gland by squamous metaplasia. At 4 weeks postoperatively, NH returned to the physical therapist to undergo slow, progressive, vaginal introital dilation under supervision. At 3 months postoperatively, NH was

completely free of pain, and, as she maintained hormonal management throughout this period, she had improved desire, arousal, and orgasm to 75% of previous capabilities.

Comments

Rational health-care delivery for women with sexual dysfunction involves coordination and integration of mind, body and relationship factors (see Chapters 12.1–12.6). As it concerns biologic management, conservative treatment options should always be utilized first. If, however, conservative treatment applied for a "sufficient" period of time does not improve symptoms, invasive treatments should be considered. Of the various treatments for dyspareunia, surgery is associated with safe and effective treatment outcome.[11]

Case 5

NI, aged 28, and married for 5 years, has complained of severe vestibular pain since the delivery of her child 4 years ago. The birth involved a prolonged forceps delivery that was complicated by chronic pudendal neuropathy, leading to disabling left leg spasms and diminished genital sensation. The childbirth was also associated with a stage 3 perineal tear that was treated with a difficult repair of the posterior fourchette and perineum. Postpartum, NI underwent cauterization of granulation tissue at the perineal repair on four separate occasions, but the final cauterization led to chronic, severe pain in the vestibular region.

The 10/10 relentless pain in the vestibule in conjunction with the pudendal neuropathy has resulted in significant function impairment. NI is prevented from sitting for longer than 10 min, walking more than a quarter of a mile, or climbing stairs. She has painful defecation as well as a mild urinary and fecal incontinence. She cannot bend or twist, or carry her child. She cannot work in her capacity as an engineer. As a result, over the next 2 years, NI underwent several revisions of the posterior fourchette, treatment by pudendal nerve blocks, steroid injections, physical therapy, psychologic counseling, and oral gabapentin and amitriptyline. Her last good sexual intercourse was prior to the childbirth. She has distinct changes in desire, arousal, and, with the marked diminished genital sensation, she cannot achieve orgasm.

NI was referred to a multidisciplinary sexual medicine clinic. She was first seen by the psychologist, who reported as follows. This 28-year-old woman has significant vestibular pain since childbirth and posterior repair. She remains sexually active in a limited fashion but with severe pain during penetration. She is depressed, sees a therapist, and takes selective serotonin reuptake inhibitors. She is tearful during the interview. She is overwhelmed with the chronic pain and the significant reduction in functioning.

NI's history was as above. In addition, she noted that compared to previous capabilities, she had 10% desire, 10% arousal, and 10% orgasmic function. Physical examination revealed a normal appearing clitoris and labia minora. There was positive Q-tip testing at focal locations at 5 and 7 o'clock. The entire posterior fourchette was tender and the skin surface appeared to be burgundy-colored, erythematous, and beefy-appearing consistent with chronic inflammation (Fig. 15.2.7). Biothesiometric studies revealed a vibration perception threshold of 3 V for the right and left pulp index fingers, with 24 V noted for the right and left labia minora and 30 V for the clitoris. Hormone studies, obtained 1 month prior to the sexual medicine evaluation, revealed mild androgen insufficiency. The impression was postpartum depression; diminished desire, arousal, and orgasm; severe vestibular pain; pudendal neuropathy; severe diminished genital sensation; and mild androgen insufficiency. The plan was psychologic counseling, physical therapy consultation, pudendal nerve blocks (using intravaginal ultrasound guided nerve blocks), and androgen therapy.

Concerning the severe pain, one option was wide excision of the chronically inflamed vestibular and subcutaneous tissue of the posterior fourchette, and repair of the area by developing and advancing a vaginal flap closure (Fig. 15.2.7). The procedure was eventually performed, taking approximately 90 min. Intraoperative findings revealed chronically scarred vestibular tissue.

At 3-, 6-, and 12-month follow-up, NI showed a dramatic reduction in vestibular pain. Rehabilitation with multiple disciplines, including androgen therapy, physical therapy, and psychologic counseling, has resulted in improved sexual and physical functioning. NI now has improved desire and sexual thoughts "on the radar screen", resulting in her initiating sexual activity for the first time since the childbirth. NI still has not yet achieved a good orgasm, but treatment strategies are continuing.

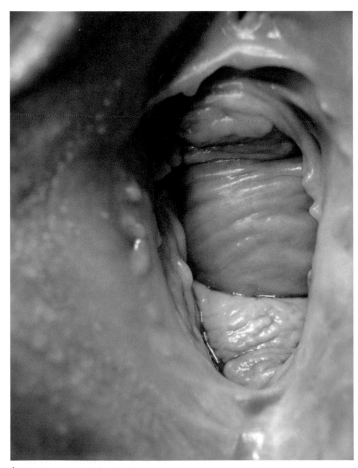

A

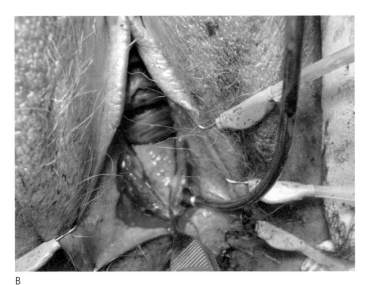

B

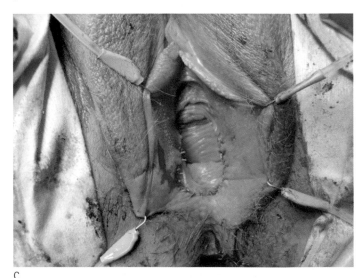

C

Figure 15.2.7. Physical examination revealed a normal-appearing clitoris and labia minora. There was positive Q-tip testing at focal locations at 5 and 7 o'clock. The entire posterior fourchette was tender and the skin surface appeared to be burgundy-colored, erythematous, and beefy-appearing, consistent with chronic inflammation. Wide excision of the chronically inflamed vestibular and subcutaneous tissue of the posterior fourchette was performed, and the area was repaired by developing and advancing a vaginal flap closure.

Comments

In complicated cases such as above, surgical intervention can be very effective (see Chapters 12.1–12.6).

Discussion

Chapter 15.2 reviews some of the various surgical treatment strategies for women with sexual dysfunction. As can be seen from these highly selected cases, surgical intervention can result in a discernible improvement in an individual woman's sexual function. In the management of women's sexual health, treatment is stepwise, starting from the most noninvasive and advancing, if needed, to surgical intervention. In the field of sexual medicine, it will always be relevant to train specialists who are skilled in the performance of surgical strategies for selected women with sexual health concerns not responsive to conservative management.

References

1. Basson R, Althof S, Davis S et al. Summary of the recommendations on sexual dysfunctions in women. *J Sex Med* 2004; 1: 24–35.

2. Lewis RW, Fugl-Meyer KS, Bosch R et al. Epidemiology/risk factors of sexual dysfunction. *J Sex Med* 2004; 1: 35–9.

3. Hatzichristou D, Rosen RC, Broderick G et al. Clinical evaluation and management strategy for sexual dysfunction in men and women. *J Sex Med* 2004; 1: 49–57.

4. Meston CM, Hull E, Levin RJ et al. Disorders of orgasm in women. *J Sex Med* 2004; 1: 66–8.

5. Davis SR, Guay AT, Shifren JL et al. Endocrine aspects of female sexual dysfunction. *J Sex Med* 2004; 1: 82–6.

6. Nappi R, Salonia A, Traish AM et al. Clinical biologic pathophysiologies of women's sexual dysfunction. *J Sex Med* 2005; 2: 4–25.

7. Eilber KS, Raz S. Benign cystic lesions of the vagina: a literature review. *J Urol* 2003; 170: 717–22.

8. Omole F, Simmons BJ, Hacker Y. Management of Bartholin's duct cyst and gland abscess. *Am Fam Physician* 2003; 68: 135–40.

9. Guelinckx PJ, Sinsel NK. An unusual case of clitoral enlargement: its differential diagnosis and surgical management. *Acta Chir Belg* 2002; 102: 192–5.

10. Val-Bernal JF, Gomez-Ortega JM, Fernandez-Llaca H et al. Fibroepithelioma of pinkus with tumor giant cells. *Am J Dermatopathol* 2002; 24: 336–9.

11. Gaunt G, Good A, Stanhope CR. Vestibulectomy for vulvar vestibulitis. *J Reprod Med* 2003; 48: 591–5.

SPECIAL ISSUES IN THE MANAGEMENT OF FEMALE SEXUAL DYSFUNCTION

16.1 Clinical trials in female sexual dysfunction

Raymond C Rosen, Jennifer L Barsky, David M Ferguson

Overview of clinical trials in female sexual dysfunction

While the conduct of clinical trials in male sexual dysfunctions (e.g., erectile dysfunction, premature ejaculation) is accepted and well established, the design and implementation of clinical trials in female sexual dysfunction is a more recent phenomenon and is not adequately defined or systematized. In contrast to the large literature on randomized, placebo-controlled trials of erectile dysfunction, which proliferated in the late 1990s and early 2000s, equivalent clinical trials in sexual arousal disorder in women have been few and far between, and have yielded much less consistent or clear-cut findings. This may be due to several factors, including differences in the relative stages of development of male and female sexual dysfunction research, as well as the complex nature of female sexual arousal. Substantial challenges also face investigators in the design of adequate clinical trials for sexual dysfunction in women. For example, large placebo effects have been noted in many studies, and discrepancies among different measures of outcome are apparent both across and within studies.

This chapter will consider the design of clinical trials for female sexual dysfunction, selection of the optimal patient population, assessment of relevant outcome measures in a standardized and clinically relevant way, and definition of treatment response criteria that are best suited to the domain of interest. The presence of multiple methodological and design issues underscores a range of problems in the conceptualization of sexual function in women, the current paradigm of clinical trials for studying female sexual dysfunction, and the current approach to diagnosis that guides much of the clinical research in female sexual dysfunction today.

The complexity of etiologic factors underlying sexual dysfunctions in women and the lack of adequate understanding of the pathophysiology or development of these disorders create a major challenge in defining a study population well suited for pharmacotherapeutic (or other) intervention. The task is complicated by culturally embedded notions of healthy female sexuality and sexual dysfunction in women,[1,2] making stable conceptualizations of "sexual dysfunction" difficult to achieve. Furthermore, despite increasing evidence of the overlap in symptoms within and across sexual dysfunctions in women,[3] most clinical trials of female sexual dysfunction tend to focus on a specific dysfunction, such as hypoactive desire disorder or female sexual arousal disorder. This implies that it is possible to identify a specific study population by validated diagnostic criteria. However, the artificial classification of these disorders in trials of female sexual dysfunction may pose a problem for generalizability of the study results, and may contribute to a lack of clear-cut treatment differences.

A key aspect of clinical trial design is the ability to detect a significant improvement in performance as a result of treatment. Currently, it is difficult for investigators in clinical trials of female sexual dysfunction to assess treatment outcomes and define treatment responders in a standardized way. Lack of agreement on the selection of suitable outcome measures in clinical trials of female sexual dysfunction is a major obstacle at present.[4] The role of physiologic measures, such as vaginal photoplethysmography (see Chapter 10.1 of this book) or functional magnetic resonance imaging of the brain (see Chapter 10.2), is controversial and also not well established. Whereas improved physiologic function may be a more obvious goal of treatment for men (e.g., increased frequency of erections), it is unclear what role comparable physiologic measures (e.g., increased lubrication) should play as biologic markers or endpoints in a clinical trial of female sexual dysfunction.

A US Food and Drug Administration guidance document[5] recommended the use of daily diary or event log frequency measures as preferable to self-administered questionnaires for assessing female sexual dysfunction outcomes in clinical trials. However, the clinical significance of behavioral frequency outcomes has been challenged.[6] Recent considerations of subjective outcomes in female sexual dysfunction, including distress,[7] indicate a need for increased focus on subjective issues in assessing improved sexual function in women. While there is little disagreement regarding the convergence of physiologic and subjective measures of outcome in men, available evidence suggests that physiologic and subjective measures of sexual response in women are not as strongly associated.[8]

Cultural and psychosocial determinations of women's sexual function further complicate the process of defining a treatment responder in clinical trials of female sexual dysfunction. If a study includes members of a cultural or other subgroup of women who have low expectations of sexual pleasure or satisfaction, it is unclear whether or how the definition of a treatment response or successful trial outcome should be adjusted. More culturally sensitive endpoints or assessment procedures may better incorporate subjects' expectations into the assessment of treatment outcomes, but this issue has not been addressed in recent trials of female sexual dysfunction.

Finally, the role of qualitative research in defining issues and endpoints to be addressed in clinical trials of female sexual dysfunction has not been adequately considered. In the past, qualitative and quantitative methods have been viewed as competing or rival approaches, and it was not uncommon for quantitative researchers to disregard evidence obtained from qualitative observations or interviews. More recently, however, "the classic qualitative-quantitative debate has been largely resolved with recognition that a variety of methodological approaches are needed and credible, that mixed methods can be especially valuable, and that the challenge is to appropriately match methods to questions rather than adhering to some narrow methodological orthodoxy."[9] Qualitative methods can be used specifically to assess the clinical relevance of specific measures and endpoints, and to determine whether current definitions of distress and sexual function are applicable in the clinical population.

Many of the challenges associated with conducting clinical trials for female sexual dysfunction may be attributed to the lack of a clearly defined, empirically supported model of female sexual response and satisfaction, despite recent advances in the classification of women's sexual dysfunctions.[10] The current model for clinical trials in male sexual dysfunction may not be sensitive to the complex and ill-defined scope of sexual response in women. In the post-Masters and Johnson era, it is unclear whether any one model should be used as the standard guide for diagnostic decision making. Psychosocial and cultural factors, furthermore, are not adequately measured or controlled for in these trials. Despite these limitations, the randomized, controlled trial remains the reference standard for clinical trial investigation and must necessarily be considered in detail for use in clinical trials of female sexual dysfunction.

Regulatory and medical perspectives

A variety of drugs, hormonal agents, and topical and transdermal formulations for female sexual dysfunction are currently in development, based on a broad range of hormonal and pharmacologic mechanisms (see Chapter 14.1). Along with the introduction of novel methods for the treatment of female sexual dysfunction, a wide range of new measurement approaches and assessment tools have been developed (see Chapter 11.2). These new tools have permitted more precise and reliable measurement of various aspects of sexual response in women. The use of valid and reliable outcome measures in the context of a well-controlled clinical trial is the sine qua non for medical acceptance and regulatory approval of any new drug or treatment.[11]

A major goal of this chapter is to review current standards of practice in the design and conduct of clinical trials in female sexual dysfunction. Many of these standards represent general concepts or principles in the design of clinical trials, although specific issues in the evaluation of new treatments for female sexual dysfunction are also addressed. These include the use of objective (physiologic) versus self-report (questionnaire) measures of sexual function, assessment of other domains of function, global patient and investigator assessments, and the use of disease-specific quality-of-life measures. Although much of the focus in recent years has been on the development of new pharmacologic or hormonal agents, similar standards of research should be applied in the evaluation of other methods of treatment, such as devices or nonpharmacologic therapies generally.

Design of clinical trials in female sexual dysfunction

The clinical trial process in most therapeutic areas, including female sexual dysfunction, is usually described as occurring in four phases (phases I, II, III, and IV), each of which is discussed below. These stages were described in detail for erectile dysfunction[11] and, more recently, in the Second Consultation on Sexual Medicine for female sexual dysfunction.[8] Beyond the immediate goal of obtaining regulatory approval, clinical trials are intended to predict the likely risk/benefit outcomes when the drug or device enters widespread clinical use.[11]

Phase I

These studies represent the first exposure in humans of the novel agent or device and are typically conducted in healthy individuals. The full range of phase I studies potentially relevant to female sexual dysfunction is shown in Table 16.1.1.

Initial studies in healthy volunteers typically involve administration of a single dose of the new agent. The first dose is selected on the basis of acute and chronic animal studies and, if available, data from human liver metabolism *in vitro*. The

Table 16.1.1. Phase I drug development in healthy volunteers

Study type	Rationale
Single dose	Assessment of tolerability after single-dose administration
Multiple dose	Assessment of tolerability over likely dosing period
Pharmacokinetics	Assess if preclinical studies predict kinetics and metabolites
Clinical pharmacology	Indirect assessment of efficacy; ensure adequate pharmacodynamic and pharmacokinetic relationships
Special populations	Children, elderly, and medical populations may display different tolerability/pharmacokinetics

Adapted from Rosen et al.[11]

initial dose selected may be 30–100 times lower than the predicted threshold efficacy dose in adults. Should this be well tolerated, additional doses will usually be evaluated at regular dose increments. Escalating dose studies may employ successive naive cohorts, but frequently use the same cohort with successive doses administered between estimated washout periods. The estimate of an appropriate washout period and the potential for confounding subsequent responses are, of course, problematic. Signs of poor tolerance or reaching a predetermined dose level will normally conclude this stage of development. Whenever possible, these studies involve concomitant assays of plasma drug levels.[8]

To ensure that tolerability is not affected by administration of subsequent doses of the drug, multiple dose studies are also typical. The frequency of dosing depends on the predicted dosing regimen of the novel agent. Again, plasma drug levels are monitored whenever possible. Formal pharmacokinetic and drug metabolism studies are usually initiated after single- and multiple-dose tolerability studies. It is important to ensure that there is no dose-dependent tissue drug accumulation, and that the metabolic pathway and potential for major drug interactions are known.[11]

The value of equal numbers of placebo subjects in these safety studies should be emphasized. Incorrectly attributing adverse events to active treatment at this stage may haunt the rest of clinical development and even affect labeling for an approved product. Inclusion of adequate numbers of placebo subjects allows better discrimination of treatment-related effects from effects common to the site or the methodology of the study.

Phase II

Efficacy assessment is first formally undertaken in phase II. Treatment assessment during this phase typically involves a mixture of objective measures (e.g., vaginal photoplethysmography) and self-report assessments (e.g., daily diaries, questionnaires). These measures are likely to be similar to, or serve as a pilot test for, the measures to be selected in the more extensive phase III studies. However, the primary objective of phase II efficacy studies is the identification of an effective dose range to be evaluated in phase III (dose setting). The range of doses in phase II studies is usually more limited than in phase I, since the

maximum tolerability of the drug has been established. A starting dose of 5–10% of the maximum tolerated dose may be initially studied. Additional information on drug tolerability is also obtained during this stage of clinical development, allowing calculation of potential benefit/risk ratio.[11] Early phase II studies frequently serve as "proof-of-principle" to justify further research. Mid-phase II studies may establish a clear dose–response curve, and late phase II studies serve as "mini-pivotal" trials, testing issues of population definition, recruitment, and outcome measures. Preferably, both mid- and late phase II studies are parallel designs.

Crossover designs, in which each patient serves as her own control, are often used in early phase II trials. The major advantage of this design is the availability of within-subject comparisons and the associated reduction in patient variability and increased statistical power. Heiman et al.[8] also note that various subject variables in women may be difficult to control (e.g., diet, body-mass index, alcohol intake, mood variability, menstrual cycle phase, precise hormonal status, and psychologic variables), but crossover designs minimize the potential error due to the variability from these factors. Potential problems are the likelihood of carryover and sequence effects from one treatment phase to the next and susceptibility to patient dropouts. These problems may be exacerbated if three or more treatment arms are included in the study design. The duration of treatment needed in each arm and potential for carryover effects are the major limitations, overall, of this type of design. Despite these limitations, crossover designs are frequently preferred in early phase II dose-setting studies. Different pharmacologic agents present different challenges in crossover designs. Those agents that are used "on-demand" and have a short pharmacokinetic and pharmacodynamic half-life (such as intranasal products) are best suited to this design. Hormone treatments, on the other hand, may have a pharmacodynamic half-life of weeks or months, and thus the washout period would be unwieldy.

When using a design that allows for "on-demand" treatment, it is important to recognize that outcome measures generally will reflect the patient's attitude toward the treatment, rather than observations of specific episodes of treatment. Thus, the number of exposures to treatment needed to effect a stable change in a patient's self-report may exceed the number of exposures required to demonstrate initial improvement. In effect, the half-life of an attitude is a major concern.[12]

Phase III

Prior to regulatory approval, it is necessary to conduct two or more large-scale pivotal outcome studies in appropriately selected patient groups. Phase III trials are usually designed as multicenter, randomized, prospective studies with two or more dose levels of the study drug and a double-blind placebo control condition. In the field of female sexual dysfunction assessment, relatively long periods (e.g., 6 months) have been used for treatment arms in large-scale phase III trials. Since irreversible changes may occur during treatment periods of such long duration, crossover designs are typically not recommended for use in phase III studies.

Parallel designs are typically employed in phase III trials. In the simplest parallel design study, patients are randomly assigned to two or more parallel treatment arms for the duration of the study period (usually 4–6 months). Each patient is exposed to one treatment condition only, and comparisons are made between treatment groups at various time points. Treatment-induced changes are assessed by analysis of between-group differences after treatment. Results can also be analyzed relative to changes in baseline. Baseline assessments are necessary to ensure that the treatment groups are equivalent prior to randomization.[11]

The parallel treatment period, usually double-blind, is sometimes preceded by a single-blind placebo or "no treatment" run-in period to establish a reproducible baseline prior to randomization. This run-in period can also be used to screen out patients who are most susceptible to placebo effects or are unable to follow the protocol procedures. Following this stage, patients are assigned to the double-blind, randomized phase of the study. Large placebo effects (30–70% response rates) are commonly observed in clinical trials of female sexual dysfunction. The magnitude of placebo effects might be reduced through the use of single-blind, lead-in procedures with exclusion of identified placebo responders. However, this approach has not been widely employed in female sexual dysfunction trials to date, and thus it is unknown whether or how the exclusion of placebo responders after a run-in period would actually influence placebo effect sizes in the randomized trial period. Moreover, eliminating placebo responders may bias the selection of subjects to those who potentially have no responsiveness of any kind.

Phase IV

Phase IV studies are undertaken either during the approval process or subsequent to approval.[11] One component involves "postmarketing surveillance" studies designed to expand the safety database through long-term tracking of patients on the active treatment. Special population studies may also be conducted during this phase. In general, phase IV studies are designed to increase understanding of the overall treatment profile in the target population(s). These studies may not include all of the controls (e.g., placebo-blinding and baseline assessment) utilized in phases II and III, although comparison treatments and special population groups are more likely to be included in the trial design during this phase.

Drug interaction studies

Women with sexual dysfunctions are likely in many cases to be receiving drug therapy for associated comorbidities (e.g., depression, menopausal symptoms, osteoporosis) (see Chapter 7.2). For this reason, it is important in the phase I and phase II studies that key drug interactions be examined. The interaction studies fall into two major categories: pharmacokinetic and pharmacodynamic interactions.

Pharmacokinetic drug interaction studies are designed to evaluate acute effects of the new agent on the plasma levels of other commonly used drugs that are concomitantly administered. Specific drug interaction studies may be required should the novel agent be known to induce or inhibit cytochrome-dependent liver metabolizing systems. Also important is the potential for pharmacodynamic interactions. Of particular relevance is the potential of novel drugs or hormonal preparations to influence the effects of other drugs. Alterations in blood pressure control in a woman with controlled hypertension and endocrine control in a diabetic woman, for example, would be undesirable features, and should be carefully evaluated during early phase I or phase II studies (see Chapter 7.3). Specific pharmacodynamic interactions relevant to the mechanism of action (e.g., centrally acting, peripherally acting) should be carefully assessed.

Study populations

General principles

All clinical trials require a precise definition of which patients are and are not eligible for inclusion in the trial. The most important underlying principle guiding this definition is that the study population should represent the overall patient population for whom the treatment under investigation is intended. If the study population is truly representative of the intended treatment population, the results of a well-designed controlled trial are likely to predict the "real-world" effect. On the contrary, if the study population is too narrowly defined, the trial results may not generalize to the broader population. Therefore, when conducting "pivotal" phase III trials in female sexual dysfunction, it is important for the investigator to define a group of patients that will be as representative as possible of the intended patient population at large. This is accomplished by taking into account such factors as age, overall health status, concomitant medications, and the severity and duration of the disorder.

Careful patient selection using unambiguous inclusion and exclusion criteria should be sufficient to delineate a study population that is easily recognized by all those who assess the study results. The US Food and Drug Administration guidance document on clinical trials in female sexual dysfunction[5] emphasizes the importance of specifying the hormonal status of the women (e.g., pre- or postmenopausal) in a clinical trial, as well as their specific sexual concern (e.g., female sexual arousal disorder, hypoactive sexual desire disorder). These factors should be controlled in any large-scale, clinical trial in women with female sexual dysfunction.

A third principle is that a logical and reasonable balance must be struck between the likely efficacy and safety of the treatment among enrolled patients and the "openness" of the entrance criteria. Specifically, the trial population should be sufficiently broad to represent the larger group of female patients who may eventually benefit from treatment, although it should not be so broad as to include patients who are clearly at direct high risk of injury from the study treatment or procedures.[11] It should also be expected that treatments intended for broader clinical populations will be associated with broader variance in responsiveness, potentially jeopardizing the power of a study.[12]

Specific study population issues in female sexual dysfunction: representative patient population

The phase III study population should include women with clearly defined subtypes of female sexual dysfunction, including or excluding hypoactive sexual desire disorder, sexual arousal disorder, orgasm disorder, or sexual pain disorder, depending on the desired indication. These sexual problems are frequently comorbid. Overlapping symptoms or comorbidities may weaken the diagnostic precision of the inclusion criteria for the study. Heiman et al.[8] suggested that an alternative strategy is to select a group of women who meet diagnostic criteria for one disorder and have subsyndromal levels of another sexual disorder.

The phase III study population should provide a representative mixture of the various degrees of severity that can be expected in the target population. Ideally, this should be assessed by well-validated and treatment-sensitive instruments. These are reviewed in detail in Chapter 11.2. Stratified assignment of subjects to treatment by severity may be necessary to avoid a decrease in sensitivity due to the heterogenity of symptom severities between groups.

According to the recent review by Heiman et al.,[8] the Female Sexual Function Index (FSFI)[13] is the self-administered questionnaire of choice for clinical trials of female sexual dysfunction. The Food and Drug Administration guidance document,[5] however, recommends the use of daily diary or event log measures to assess the frequency of satisfactory sexual events. Other female sexual dysfunction assessment tools are currently in development and advanced stages of testing.

Defining the disorder: inclusion and exclusion criteria

Inclusion criteria

Phase III studies of female sexual dysfunction need to identify specific sexual function criteria for inclusion in the clinical trial.

Ideally, this assessment should be performed in a standardized way using a validated diagnostic tool. Questionnaire measures are not ideally suited for this, and a structured diagnostic interview is preferable. Several versions of this are in development, particularly for the assessment of hypoactive sexual desire disorder. A valid diagnosis requires that the patient demonstrate personal distress regarding her sexual function. This may be assessed by a validated instrument such as the Female Sexual Distress Scale.[14] Since female sexual dysfunctions may be either primary (lifelong) or acquired, it is prudent to stipulate which situation applies in patient selection. Patients who were previously functional may have a higher probability of response to an intervention.

Hormonal status of the subjects must be addressed and may be defined by several factors: pre-, peri-, post-, or surgically menopausal status; the use of hormonal contraception; and the use of hormone therapy (including estrogens, progesterone, and androgens). Additionally, since the human teratogenic potential of a treatment may not be known, provisions for avoiding pregnancy during the study must be addressed.

Psychosexual and relational issues affect women's sexuality and should be addressed in clinical trials. The quality of a patient's relationship with her partner may greatly influence her response to interventions and satisfaction with her sexual function during treatment. The presence of sexual dysfunction in the partner may have serious confounding effects. The quality of the relationship should be addressed as part of the initial sexual history, and the presence of sexual dysfunction in the partner may be assessed by a validated instrument such as the Single Question Assessment of Erectile Dysfunction[15] or a standardized, multidimensional measure such as the International Index of Erectile Function.[16] The partner's willingness to comply with the study requirements is another important variable to consider for the inclusion criteria.

Finally, inclusion criteria must specify the age range of participants, ability and willingness to provide informed consent, and ability to comply with study requirements. For example, if participants must attempt or engage in intercourse at regular intervals to determine the efficacy of a treatment, a trial may specify that participants be in a stable relationship with a person of the opposite sex. It is unknown whether including non-heterosexual women in a study might lead to higher variances in the study endpoints, and thus less sensitivity to detect treatment effects.

Exclusion criteria

The major exclusion criteria in clinical trials of female sexual dysfunction typically include the following:

1. evidence of unresolved sexual trauma or abuse
2. female sexual dysfunction caused by *untreated* endocrine disease (e.g., hypopituitarism, hypothyroidism, diabetes mellitus)
3. pregnancy or breast-feeding

4. history of sensitivity to any of the ingredients in the test article

5. history or evidence of chronic or complicated urinary tract or vaginal infections within previous 12 months

6. history or evidence of pelvic inflammatory disease within previous 12 months

7. evidence of currently active sexually transmitted disease

8. history or evidence of currently active, moderate to severe vaginitis

9. history or evidence of current cervical dysplasia

10. history or evidence of current significant cervicitis as manifested by mucopurulent discharge from the cervix

11. history or evidence of significant gynecologic conditions such as uterine fibroids, vulvar vestibulitis, or vaginismus that may interfere with the patient's ability to comply with study procedures

12. psychoses and bipolar disorder

13. use of neuroleptics or lithium, or any medications, herbal treatments, or dietary supplements intended to enhance sexual function within previous 3 months

14. history of myocardial infarction within previous 6 months

15. history or evidence of significant renal or hepatic disease within previous 6 months

16. significant central nervous system diseases within the last 6 months, such as stroke, spinal cord injury, or multiple sclerosis

17. any condition which, in the investigator's opinion, would interfere with the patient's ability to provide informed consent or comply with study instructions, or which might confound the interpretation of the study results

18. any condition which would endanger the participant if she participated in this trial.

Clinical trial endpoints and outcomes in female sexual dysfunction trials

Specific outcome measures or endpoints in clinical trials of female sexual dysfunction can be divided into four major categories or types. These usually include the following.

Self-administered questionnaires

At present, several self-administered questionnaires are available, including the Brief Index of Sexual Functioning for Women[17,18] and the Female Sexual Function Index.[13] These questionnaires assess sexual function across a number of domains (e.g., sexual desire, arousal, orgasm, satisfaction) and measure average responses over a specified time period (e.g., 4 weeks). Scoring algorithms are provided for computing average responses in each of the specified sexual function domains. Both have demonstrated good reliability and validity. Chapter 11.2 describes these measures and other self-administered questionnaires in more detail.

Event logs and daily diaries

A variety of event logs and daily diaries have been used in clinical trials of male and female sexual dysfunction. These diaries or event logs are completed immediately after each episode of sexual activity and are designed to assess sexual function and satisfaction during each sexual episode. The Female Sexual Encounter Profile[12] has been employed in many studies. Several other event logs and diaries are under development. Data obtained from the sexual event log are typically regarded as primary or secondary endpoints from a regulatory perspective. Event logs are currently favored by the Food and Drug Administration to assess "satisfactory sexual events".[5]

Interview assessments

Although interview protocols have been developed for in-depth assessment of sexual function,[19] these methods have not been used extensively in clinical trials of male or female sexual dysfunction. Other interview tools currently under development may result in greater diagnostic precision for female sexual dysfunction, and greater specificity in the inclusion criteria.

Physiologic measures

Current physiologic measures, such as vaginal photoplethysmography, lack adequate standardization or clinical validation, and are not widely used in multicenter, large-scale treatment studies. These measures may be useful, however, in early phase II studies, or in mechanistic or early dose-finding studies. However, the predictive value of these studies from the laboratory setting to the at-home phase with self-report measures is not well established.

Primary and secondary endpoints should be specified in advance of the study. Secondary endpoints typically include other domains of sexual function (e.g., sexual desire, orgasmic satisfaction) and/or quality-of-life measures (e.g., relationship satisfaction, overall satisfaction). These measures have been recently described in detail elsewhere.[8]

Clinical and statistical significance

Clinical trials are typically powered to show a statistical difference between the active drug and placebo on the primary endpoint at the 0.05 level of significance or higher. When a large number of subjects are included in each arm of the study (e.g., 100 per treatment arm), a high degree of statistical significance may be obtained (e.g., $p < 0.001$) with relatively small mean differences between groups on the primary study endpoint. For example, a 1- or 2-point change on a self-report (self-administered questionnaire) scale might be statistically significant in a well-powered study, but may nonetheless represent a very slight difference or change in actual behavior. In the absence of clear-cut norms for determining clinical relevance, the interpretation of clinically meaningful change presents a serious challenge in the field. At present, the interpretation of clinically relevant change is highly variable from one study to another, and no published standards or norms are available. This is an important scientific and regulatory question that warrants attention.

Discussion

Sexual dysfunction in women is characterized by multiple, diverse etiologic determinants, a high degree of overlap between disorders, and a high frequency of comorbidity with mood disorders and other medical and mental health disorders. These factors complicate both the design of clinical trials and the interpretation of treatment effects. Although the elimination of women with comorbid disorders may be an appealing means of controlling for confounding variables, this can easily limit the generalizability of the findings. In designing a clinical trial for female sexual dysfunction, investigators need to consider the multiple etiologies and determinants of female sexual function, including hormonal status, psychologic factors, and issues pertaining to the relationship with the sexual partner. Each of these domains of influence affects the selection of subjects and assessment measures for a trial, and may influence the baseline levels of key endpoints. These issues should be carefully considered in planning the statistical analytic strategy for the trial.[20]

Diverse influences on sexual function in women require assessing treatment outcomes and satisfaction by multidimensional measures with sufficient breadth and sensitivity of measurement.[4] Some controversy surrounds methodological approaches to the assessment of treatment outcomes in clinical trials of female sexual dysfunction. Although the Food and Drug Administration has recommended the use of daily diary or event log measures to assess "satisfactory sexual events",[5] this position has recently been challenged in a consensus white paper on selection of endpoints in clinical trials of female sexual dysfunction: "Counting events is simple; what determines a woman's satisfaction or success with an event is less clear. Moreover, the judgment is entirely subjective, more nuanced and best captured by a self-administered questionnaire."[6]

We have emphasized the role of psychologic and relationship factors throughout as etiologic and maintaining factors in female sexual dysfunction. These factors very often are unaddressed or not controlled for in clinical trials of female sexual dysfunction, but are typically assumed to be operating in a constant state or level throughout the study. In fact, changes in sexual function in the woman are likely to initiate responses or changes in the couple's relationship, as well as in the woman's self-image or sexual self-schema.[21] These psychologic changes are likely to be determining factors in whether or not treatment changes are maintained during and after a clinical trial of female sexual dysfunction. Relationship factors and changes in the woman's partner may mediate her response in important ways. Typically, clinical trials in female sexual dysfunction have neither controlled for nor assessed these factors in the design or outcomes components of the trial.

In summary, despite the high prevalence of sexual problems in women, clinical trials in female sexual dysfunction have lagged significantly behind comparable treatment studies in male sexual dysfunction. The study design and choice of outcome measures have created opportunities and challenges for clinical investigators in this area. The lack of a common pathophysiologic model or clear-cut consensus regarding the diagnostic classification of female sexual dysfunction, and the determination of inclusion and exclusion criteria for clinical trials, has made it difficult to develop consistent standards for clinical trials. Finally, the difficulty in defining a treatment responder and the related need to establish clinically meaningful change criteria have been addressed in this chapter. Despite these current areas of challenge, major advances are anticipated in the clinical trial aspects of female sexual dysfunction diagnosis and treatment in the near future. This should lead to the eventual development of safe and effective long-term treatments.

Acknowledgments

The authors of this chapter acknowledge in particular the contributions of the First International Consultation on Erectile Dysfunction and the Second International Consultation on Sexual Medicine committees, and for permission received from the Consultations to adapt or reprint source material from their proceedings.

References

1. Tiefer L, Hall M, Tavris C. Beyond dysfunction: a new view of women's sexual problems. *J Sex Marital Ther* 2002; 23: 225–32.
2. Segraves RT. Historical and international context of the nosology of female sexual dysfunction. *J Sex Marital Ther* 2001; 27: 205–7.
3. Basson R. A model of women's sexual arousal. *J Sex Marital Ther* 2002; 28: 1–10.
4. Meston CM, Derogatis LR. Validated instruments for assessing female sexual function. *J Sex Marital Ther* 2002; 28: 155–64.
5. US Food and Drug Administration, Center for Drug Evaluation and Research. Female sexual dysfunction: clinical development of drug products for treatment. Rockville, MD: US Department of Health and Human Services, 2000.
6. Althof SE, Rosen RC, DeRogatis L, Corty E, Quirk F, Symonds T. Outcome measurement in female sexual dysfunction clinical trials: review and recommendations. *J Sex Marital Ther* 2005 Mar–Apr; 31(2): 153–66.
7. Bancroft J, Loftus J, Long JS. Distress about sex: a national survey of women in heterosexual relationships. *Arch Sex Behav* 2003: 32: 193–208.
8. Heiman JR, Guess MK, Connell K et al. Standards for clinical trials in sexual dysfunctions of women: research designs and outcomes assessment. In TF Lue, R Basson, R Rosen et al., eds. *Sexual*

Medicine: Sexual Dysfunctions in Men and Women. 2nd International Consultation on Sexual Dysfunctions. Paris: Éditions 21, 2004.

9. Patton MQ. *Qualitative Research and Evaluation Methods*, 3rd edn. Thousand Oaks: Sage, 2002.

10. Basson R, Berman J, Burnett A et al. Report of the international consensus development conference on female sexual dysfunction: definitions and classifications. *J Urol* 2000; 163: 888–93.

11. Rosen R, Bennett A, Ferguson D et al. Standards for clinical trials in erectile dysfunction: research designs and outcomes assessment. In A Jardin, G Wagner, S Khoury et al., eds. *Erectile Dysfunction*. Plymouth: Health Publications, 2000.

12. Ferguson DM. Clinical trial development in female sexual dysfunction. *J Sex Marital Ther* 2002; 28: 77–83.

13. Rosen RC, Brown C, Heiman J et al. The Female Sexual Function Index (FSFI): a multidimensional self-report instrument for the assessment of female sexual function. *J Sex Marital Ther* 2000; 26: 191–208.

14. Derogatis LR, Rosen R, Leiblum S et al. The Female Sexual Distress Scale (FSDS): initial validation of a standardized scale for assessment of sexually relevant personal distress in women. *J Sex Marital Ther* 2002; 28: 317–30.

15. Derby CA, Araujo AB, Johannes CB et al. Measurement of erectile dysfunction in population-based studies: the use of a single question self-assessment in the Massachusetts Male Aging Study. *Int J Impot Res* 2000; 12: 197–204.

16. Rosen RC, Riley A, Wagner G et al. The International Index of Erectile Function (IIEF): a multidimensional scale for assessment of erectile dysfunction. *Urology* 1997; 49: 822–30.

17. Taylor JE, Rosen RC, Leiblum SR. Self-report assessment of female sexual dysfunction: psychometric evaluation of the Brief Index of Sexual Functioning for Women. *Arch Sex Behav* 1994; 23: 627–43.

18. Mazer NA, Leiblum SR, Rosen RC. The Brief Index of Sexual Functioning for Women (BISF-W). A new scoring algorithm and comparison of normative and surgically menopausal populations. *Menopause* 2000; 7: 350–63.

19. Derogatis LR. The Derogatis Interview for Sexual Functioning (DISF/DISF-SR): an introductory report. *J Sex Marital Ther* 1997; 23: 291–304.

20. Islam A, Mitchel J, Hays J et al. Challenges in conducting multicenter clinical trials in female sexual dysfunction: baseline differences between study populations. *J Sex Marital Ther* 2001; 27: 525–30.

21. Cyranowski JM, Andersen BL. Schemas, sexuality, and romantic attachment. *J Pers Soc Psychol* 1998; 74: 1364–79.

16.2 Depression

Paula L Hensley, H George Nurnberg

Introduction

As the indications for antidepressant medications have expanded to conditions other than depression, there has been increased recognition of the problem of sexual dysfunction due to major depressive disorder, antidepressant use, or a combination of both the disorder and the treatment. Decreased libido has long been recognized as a symptom of depression, but patients with major depressive disorder also describe other forms of sexual dysfunction. The *Physician's Desk Reference* cites low rates of female sexual dysfunction due to antidepressants, since the rates listed rely on spontaneous reports from subjects in clinical trials. Rates of sexual dysfunction due to antidepressants in the psychiatric literature are much higher, some approaching 70–80%. The difficulty of determining the source of sexual dysfunction will be explored in this chapter (see Chapters 7.1–7.7 of this book). In addition, we will review the literature linking antidepressants to sexual dysfunction. Then, we will describe management strategies for this troublesome side effect. Recognition and management of sexual dysfunction is especially critical in women, since women have two to three times the rate of depressive and anxiety disorders of men and are prescribed the majority of antidepressants in the USA.

Rates of sexual dysfunction in the general population

The National Health and Social Life Survey reports that sexual dysfunction is rather common in the general population[1] (see Chapters 2.1–2.4). In the 18–59-year age group, women report a higher overall rate of sexual dysfunction than men – 43% versus 31%. Women describe complaints of low sexual desire (32%), inability to achieve orgasm (26%), and absence of pleasure in sex (23%). A survey of individuals aged 18–75 years in the UK reveals similar rates (41% of women and 34% of men report a current sexual problem); of the specific forms of sexual dysfunction reported, women were most dissatisfied if they had arousal problems and dyspareunia.[2] Age and general health can certainly play a role in sexual function. In a study examining the relationship between sexual dysfunction and physical, social,

and psychologic complaints, Dunn et al. report that arousal difficulty increases with age in women, while dyspareunia decreases with age.[3] In a random sample of community-dwelling women, however, Hawton et al. found that satisfaction with the sexual relationship was most closely related to marital adjustment, and was not related to age.[4] A good understanding of the base rates of sexual dysfunction in a general population assists in the assessment of depression-related sexual dysfunction and should help avoid misattribution of pre-existing symptoms to a subsequently diagnosed illness.

Depression and sexual dysfunction

Untreated depressed patients report high rates of abnormal sexual function. Up to 70% of unipolar depressed patients complain of decreased sexual desire.[5] Rates of sexual activity in depressed patients seem quite low. In a depressed population, reports of complete sexual inactivity in the preceding month were greater in women, at 49%, than in men (26%).[6] Sexual dysfunction in these depressed patients was examined prospectively and followed during treatment. For the women in the study, 72% had recurrent depression and the mean duration of the current episode was 62.2 weeks (standard deviation = 64.9). Prior to treatment, Kennedy et al. report the following rates of sexual dysfunction in women: decreased sexual drive (50%), decreased sexual arousal (50%), difficulty obtaining vaginal lubrication (40%), and difficulty in achieving orgasm (15%).[6] The authors suggest that depressed women are more likely to have difficulty with the early stages of sexual activity, desire and arousal, rather than with orgasm or resolution.[6] Longer periods of untreated depression and recurrent depression (which may indicate poor recovery between episodes) may predispose patients to high rates of sexual dysfunction.

In the past, few studies gathered data about sexual dysfunction prospectively. But with greater recognition of antidepressant-induced sexual dysfunction, some researchers are asking more specific questions regarding sexual function prior to initiating treatment for depression, yielding some important epidemiologic data. In a three-arm clinical trial (nefazodone vs a specialized form of cognitive-behavioral therapy called "cognitive-behavioral analysis system of psychotherapy" vs combined treatment with these two modalities) of the treatment of major depressive disorder, baseline measures of sexual dysfunction found that 16% of subjects described a history of sexual dysfunction while taking prior antidepressants.[7] However, few had been evaluated (1.8%) or received treatment (1.7%) for sexual dysfunction in the past.[8] Of the women, 48% reported at least one symptom of sexual dysfunction at baseline; specific complaints included difficulty in achieving orgasm (30%), inability to achieve orgasm (21%), decreased intensity of orgasm (19%), inadequate swelling or vaginal lubrication during sexual arousal (18%), and decreased sensitivity in genitals upon physical contact (10%). According to the protocol, patients previously treated with antidepressants could enter the study if they were medication-free for 2 weeks, or 4 weeks if treated with fluoxetine or monoamine oxidase inhibitors. As Zajecka et al. do not note how many of their subjects stopped antidepressants prior to the baseline assessments, it is possible that the high rates of sexual dysfunction at baseline were in part secondary to residual effects of discontinued antidepressants or major depressive disorder.[7,8]

Ekselius and von Knorring assessed 308 depressed patients (221 women and 87 men) for pre-existing sexual dysfunction prior to initiation of medication, using the Udvalg for Kliniske Undersogelser (UKU) Side Effect Rating Scale for psychotropic drugs.[9] The subjects were randomized to one of two selective serotonin reuptake inhibitors, sertraline or citalopram. Prior to treatment, 49% of the women in the sertraline group and 46% of the women in the citalopram group complained of decreased sexual desire. In addition, at baseline, 21% of the women in the sertraline group and 23% of the women in the citalopram group reported orgasmic dysfunction. In this study, the medication washout period was 1 week; the authors do not include data on the number of patients who discontinued another antidepressant prior to randomization.

Antidepressant effects

The selective serotonin reuptake inhibitors advanced the treatment of depressive and anxiety disorders by offering improved tolerability, easier titration, and safety in overdose compared to tricyclic and monoamine oxidase inhibitor antidepressants. Selective serotonin reuptake inhibitors seem to cause similar rates and types of sexual dysfunction; few statistically significant differences are found among the different medications. Studies that compare selective serotonin reuptake inhibitors for propensity to cause sexual dysfunction usually do not include prospective, systematic evaluation of sexual function.[10] Moreover, antidepressant-induced sexual dysfunction appears to be a dose-related phenomenon, and determining equivalency of doses used in such studies is difficult.[10,11] Selective serotonin reuptake inhibitors cause impairment in arousal (lubrication/engorgement) and orgasm (delayed or absent). Men report higher rates of antidepressant-induced sexual dysfunction, but women describe greater severity.[12,13]

The largest epidemiologic study of antidepressant-induced sexual dysfunction to date is a cross-sectional, observational study (n = 6297) conducted by Clayton et al.[14] In this data set, immediate-release bupropion, an antidepressant without effect at serotonin receptors, was the least likely to cause sexual dysfunction, at 22%, and paroxetine, a selective serotonin reuptake inhibitor, had the highest rate of sexual dysfunction, at 43%.[14] The authors identified a group of 798 people who were unlikely to develop antidepressant-related sexual dysfunction; some key features were that these subjects were younger and had no history of sexual side effects with antidepressants. In this target group, the prevalence of sexual dysfunction ranged from 7% for sustained-release bupropion to 30% for citalopram, a selective serotonin reuptake inhibitor, and extended-release venlafaxine, a serotonin and norepinephrine reuptake inhibitor. So in both the target group and the entire study population, selective serotonin reuptake inhibitors and selective serotonin and norpeinephrine reuptake inhibitors were associated with greater rates of sexual dysfunction than nonserotonergic antidepressants.

Montejo-Gonzalez et al. reported higher rates of treatment-emergent sexual dysfunction in a group of outpatients (192 women and 152 men) treated in open-label fashion with selective serotonin reuptake inhibitor antidepressants.[12] Of the 344 patients, 200 complained of some form of sexual dysfunction. Although the differences were not statistically significant, the overall rates of sexual dysfunction for the various selective serotonin reuptake inhibitors were as follows: fluoxetine, 54.38%; sertraline, 56.4%; fluvoxamine, 58.94%; and paroxetine, 64.71%.[12] The only statistically significant differences found among the selective serotonin reuptake inhibitors for specific types of sexual dysfunction were that paroxetine caused more delay of orgasm/ejaculation and more impotence/inadequate lubrication than fluvoxamine, fluoxetine, or sertraline (p < 0.05).[12] No significant differences emerged for loss of libido or delayed orgasm/ejaculation. In this sample, men had a higher incidence of treatment-emergent sexual dysfunction, but women had greater severity of symptoms.[12]

A subsequent report by Montejo et al. provides additional data, with 1022 outpatients (610 women and 412 men) followed prospectively and treated in an open-label fashion with various antidepressants, not limited to selective serotonin reuptake inhibitors.[13] In this sample, 604 patients (59.1%) overall reported treatment-emergent sexual dysfunction. Rates with the various antidepressants were moclobemide (a short-acting reversible inhibitor of monoamine oxidase), 3.9%; amineptine (a tricyclic antidepressant with dopamine reuptake-blocking actions), 6.9%; nefazodone (a phenylpiperazine antidepressant which blocks neuronal reuptake of serotonin and norepinephrine and blocks postsynaptic serotonin type-2 (5-HT$_2$) receptors), 8%; mirtazapine (a tetracyclic compound which blocks alpha-2 autoreceptors, 5-HT$_2$ receptors, and 5-HT$_3$ receptors), 24.4%; fluoxetine, 57.7%; fluvoxamine, 62.3%; sertraline, 62.9%; venlafaxine, 67.3%; paroxetine, 70.7%; and citalopram, 72.7%.[13] The medications with the two lowest rates of sexual dysfunction, moclobemide and amineptine, are not available in the USA. The third best, nefazodone, was withdrawn from the

US market in June 2004. Paroxetine caused a significantly greater incidence of erectile dysfunction and decreased vaginal lubrication when compared to fluoxetine, fluvoxamine, sertraline, citalopram, venlafaxine, mirtazapine, and nefazodone ($p < 0.05$).[13] When intensity of sexual dysfunction was analyzed, no statistically significant differences were observed between the selective serotonin reuptake inhibitors and venlafaxine for decreased libido. However, mirtazapine caused less intense delayed orgasm and anorgasmia than fluoxetine, fluvoxamine, sertraline, citalopram, venlafaxine, and paroxetine ($p < 0.005$).[13] Use of paroxetine led to greater intensity of delayed orgasm than mirtazapine, fluoxetine, fluvoxamine, sertraline, citalopram, and venlafaxine ($p < 0.005$), and to greater intensity of decreased vaginal lubrication than fluoxetine, fluvoxamine, and sertraline ($p < 0.005$).[13] As in the group's earlier report, more men than women reported sexual dysfunction (62.4% of men vs 56.9% of women).[13] Women reported greater intensity of decreased libido, delayed orgasm, and anorgasmia than did men ($p < 0.005$).[13]

Antidepressants may improve sexual function in some individuals, especially women. Piazza et al. compared the sexual function of depressed subjects, both men and women, before and during treatment with a selective serotonin reuptake inhibitor (sertraline or paroxetine).[15] Prior to treatment, women reported statistically significantly greater impairment in sex drive, psychologic arousal, ease of orgasm, and orgasm satisfaction than men. After completing 6-week treatment with a selective serotonin reuptake inhibitor, women reported significant improvements in sex drive and psychologic arousal, although no changes were appreciated in physiologic arousal, ease of orgasm, or orgasm satisfaction. In contrast, treated depressed men reported worsening of ease of orgasm and orgasm satisfaction, and there was a trend toward worsening of sex drive. Men reported no change in psychologic or physiologic arousal. Thus, depressed women appear to experience greater rates of sexual dysfunction at baseline and show improvement of function when treated. Men had lower rates of sexual dysfunction at baseline and found their function worsened with treatment.

The determination of whether a sexual disorder is primary or secondary, or whether it is due to depression or antidepressant treatment is difficult. Obtaining a complete sexual history prior to initiating treatment is important, but some people have difficulty in recalling which symptom started first. The typical pattern reported clinically is that a depressed patient suffers loss of libido as a symptom of depression, is not as sexually active as before, and then starts to take an antidepressant, regains some interest, but finds that arousal and/or orgasm is now impaired. Little rigorous study, however, has been done to define the pattern of dysfunction initiated by antidepressants. In addition, the interrelationships between the phases of sexual function potentially cause halo effects and the opposite, an undermining of one phase by difficulties in another. For example, impairment in arousal or orgasm can clearly have secondary effects on libido. This is just one of many potential confounds in evaluating sexual dysfunction.

Management of antidepressant-induced sexual dysfunction

The treatment of antidepressant-associated sexual dysfunction falls into four general treatment categories: (1) use of antidotes to reverse sexual dysfunction; (2) avoidance by use of antidepressants with fewer adverse sexual effects; (3) augmentation with or switching to an antidepressant with fewer adverse sexual effects after sexual dysfunction has emerged with another antidepressant; and (4) adaptation or tolerance by waiting, dose adjustment, or drug holiday.[16, 17]

Antidotes

Few reports of medications used as antidotes for sexual dysfunction focus on women. Most of the evidence for antidotes comes in the form of single case reports or case series. Some initially promising antidotes fail to separate from placebo in controlled trials. Open-label reports present evidence for the use of the following medications for antidepressant-induced sexual dysfunction: mianserin (7.5–15 mg/day),[18–20] cyproheptadine (4–12 mg 1–2 h before sexual activity, or 4–12 mg/day),[21–25] Ginkgo biloba (60–900 mg/day),[26–29] amantadine (100–200 mg/day),[30–32] loratadine (2.5–15 mg/day),[33] bethanechol (10 mg 30 min before sexual activity),[34,35] yohimbine (5.4 mg three times daily),[36,37] and methylphenidate (10–40 mg/day).[38,39]

Open-label reports of the use of bupropion as an adjunct to selective serotonin reuptake inhibitors seem promising; recommended dosing varies from as-needed 1–2 h before sexual activity (75–150 mg) to a standing daily dose.[40–43] However, the first published randomized, double-blind, placebo-controlled study (31 subjects, gender breakdown not reported) of patients treated for 3 weeks with either sustained-release bupropion 150 mg/day or placebo added to a selective serotonin reuptake inhibitor did not show a difference between the groups.[44] More recently, a 4-week, double-blind study of sustained-release bupropion, 150 mg twice daily, versus placebo added to a selective serotonin reuptake inhibitor in 48 women and seven men, found that bupropion increased both the desire for and frequency of sexual activity.[45] However, bupropion did not do better than placebo in improving ratings of global sexual function, sexual interest, arousal, and orgasm.[45]

Michelson et al. enrolled 61 women with fluoxetine-induced sexual dysfunction and randomized them to buspirone (10 mg twice daily), amantadine (50 mg/day), or placebo.[46] All three groups improved similarly; reported rates of improvement in sexual function were 20–50%.[46] In another placebo-controlled study of 27 women and 20 men treated with a selective serotonin reuptake inhibitor, subjects were randomized to buspirone, 20–60 mg/day, or placebo and treated for 4 weeks; 58% of the buspirone-treated subjects and 30% of the placebo-treated subjects reported improvement in sexual function, a non-statistically significant difference ($p = 0.07$).[47] Granisetron, a serotonin 5-HT$_3$ receptor antagonist that also has affinity for the serotonin 5-HT$_{1A}$ receptor, showed promising initial results in an open-label trial.[48] However, a placebo-controlled, crossover trial of 31 patients with sexual dysfunction secondary to selective serotonin reuptake inhibitors, randomly assigned to adjunctive granisetron (1–1.5 mg) or placebo 1–2 h before sexual activity, showed an improvement in sexual function from baseline with no differences between the groups.[49] In 148 women on fluoxetine, a double-blind, placebo-controlled trial of mirtazapine (15 mg/day), yohimbine (5.4 mg/day), olanzapine (2.5 mg/day), and placebo found moderate improvement in most sexual function measures in all the groups; no medication did better statistically than placebo.[50]

Avoidance and switching

A survey of clinical psychiatrists indicates that 79% would augment with or switch to a novel antidepressant for selective serotonin reuptake inhibitor-induced sexual dysfunction.[51] The underlying premise of switching for side-effect control is flawed because antidepressants are not interchangeable. The odds ratio of switching a true medication responder/remitted patient to another antidepressant and maintaining efficacy with a second agent is 0.64–1.2 – approximately a coin flip. The older antidepressants, such as tricyclic antidepressants and monoamine oxidase inhibitors, have sexual side effects, although their other side effects (such as weight gain, sedation, and orthostatic hypotension) usually eclipse sexual dysfunction. Three newer antidepressants, bupropion, mirtazapine, and nefazodone (recently withdrawn from the US market), may have fewer sexual side effects than serotonergic antidepressants.[14] Of these three medications, bupropion has consistently shown the lowest incidence of sexual dysfunction, and may improve sexual desire in depressed patients.

Tolerance, dose adjustment, and drug holiday

Some patients' antidepressant-induced sexual dysfunction remits over time. Indirect empirical evidence of the development of tolerance comes from antidote studies that used placebo groups or studies that followed patients longitudinally; these reports suggest a range of remission of 35–70%.[47,52–60] Other investigators have reported lower rates of tolerance of 6–20%.[10,13,47,52–63]

Because the dosage of medication required to attain depressive remission is the same as is needed to maintain remission,[64] dose reduction to re-establish sexual function may result in relapse or recurrence of depression or another treated disorder. Therefore, it is not a practical strategy in most cases.

Another less practical approach is the "drug holiday". The only published report is an uncontrolled study that described favorable results after subjects discontinued their selective serotonin reuptake inhibitor after their Thursday morning dose and restarted the medication at the usual dosage on the following Sunday at noon.[65] Subjects who were taking sertraline and paroxetine noted considerable improvement in sexual function without a significant return of depressive symptoms, but those using fluoxetine did not experience improvement in sexual function, presumably due to fluoxetine's long half-life. However, such intermittent dosing puts patients at risk of developing serotonergic discontinuation syndrome, which is more likely with the shorter half-life agents,[66] and may occur within 24 h of the last dose of medication.[67,68] Additional difficulties with this approach are that it hinders spontaneity and encourages noncompliance with medication.

Selective phosphodiesterase type 5 inhibitors for antidepressant-associated sexual dysfunction

Although sexual dysfunction is reversible in some individuals, patients who have recovered from depression and are experiencing increased interest in sexual activity may choose not to wait an indeterminate period of time for tolerance to occur. Use of a selective phosphodiesterase type 5 inhibitor to treat antidepressant-induced sexual dysfunction offers advantages – it is taken as needed, has a short duration of action, and has no central nervous system effects to interact with the primary antidepressant agent. Our research group postulated that a selective phosphodiesterase type 5 inhibitor could effectively assist patients to bridge the interval of waiting for full recovery of sexual function. In addition, for patients where sexual dysfunction does not remit over time, selective phosphodiesterase type 5 inhibitors can manage iatrogenic sexual dysfunction for the duration of antidepressant treatment.

Treatment studies

Most of the evidence supporting use of selective phosphodiesterase type 5 inhibitors in antidepressant-associated sexual dysfunction comes from studies that used samples of male subjects. Price reported efficacy for sildenafil (76%) compared to placebo (11%) in male erectile dysfunction associated with major depressive disorder.[69] Seidman et al. evaluated flexible-dose sildenafil treatment in men with erectile dysfunction and mild to moderate depressive symptoms (major depressive disorder was excluded) in a 12-week, randomized, double-blind, placebo-controlled trial.[70] Sildenafil was strongly associated with response of erectile dysfunction and a mean Hamilton Rating Scale for Depression score decrease (–10.6) in erectile dysfunction responders compared with (–2.3) in erectile dysfunction nonresponders ($p < 0.001$).[70] In a retrospective analysis of combined data from 10 phase II and III sildenafil double-blind, placebo-controlled, fixed and flexible dose studies, Nurnberg et al. identified a subgroup of 93 men among 3414 with erectile dysfunction taking concomitant selective serotonin reuptake inhibitor and assigned to either sildenafil 25–200 mg ($n = 62$) or placebo ($n = 31$).[71] Ratings for erectile function, orgasm, and sexual satisfaction demonstrated significant improvement for all men with erectile dysfunction receiving sildenafil and concomitant selective serotonin reuptake inhibitor therapy ($p < 0.0001$).[71] A similar retrospective analysis of the use of tadalafil (10–20 mg) (vs placebo) in 111 men taking antidepressants indicates statistically significant improvement in erectile function scores, rate of successful intercourse, and percentage of patients with improved erections in those subjects taking tadalafil when compared with those taking placebo.[72] Rosen and colleagues recently reported on the use of vardenafil in men with untreated mild to moderate major depressive disorder and erectile dysfunction.[73] Compared to placebo, men taking vardenafil reported improved erectile function, lower Hamilton Rating Scale for Depression scores, and improved self-esteem.[73]

In a prospective, double-blind, placebo-controlled, flexible-dose study of sildenafil for the management of serotonergic anti-depressant-associated sexual dysfunction in 90 men, Nurnberg et al. reported that sildenafil significantly improved sexual function on the primary measure, the Clinical Global Improvement Scale ($p < 0.001$).[74] A categoric improvement of "much improved" or "very much improved" was reported by 54.5% of sildenafil-treated subjects and 4.4% of the placebo-treated subjects.[74] In addition, the secondary sexual function inventory measures, the International Index of Erectile Function, the Arizona Sexual Experience Scale, and Massachusetts General Hospital-Sexual Functioning Questionnaire, all showed improvement from baseline to endpoint in subjects receiving sildenafil compared to those receiving placebo ($p < 0.001$).[74] Subjects had to be free from pre-existing sexual dysfunction, to be taking a minimum of 8 weeks' stable dose antidepressant, to maintain the dose throughout the duration of the study, and to have scores on the Hamilton Rating Scale for Depression and Hamilton Rating Scale for Anxiety both less than 10. Depression remained in remission for both groups; in addition, subjects continued the antidepressant and dose that effectively treated their depression, uninterrupted, and without relapse of major depressive disorder.[74]

At this time, there are insufficient comparative data to suggest that any one selective phosphodiesterase type 5 inhibitor medication is more efficacious than any other.

Selective phosphodiesterase type 5 inhibitor use for antidepressant-associated sexual dysfunction in women

It must be underscored that, at present, the use of selective phosphodiesterase type 5 inhibitors for antidepressant-induced sexual dysfunction in women is off-label and without Food and Drug Administration-approved indication. Women have greater prevalence of major depression and more severe treatment-emergent sexual dysfunction, and use more selective serotonin reuptake inhibitors than men. Consequently, it is to be expected that interest and questions regarding the efficacy of selective phosphodiesterase type 5 inhibitors in women would arise.

Increased understanding of the mechanisms of sexual function suggest that mechanisms analogous to men apply in female sexual dysfunction. Phosphodiesterase type 5 is present in the female genital tract, and nitric oxide synthase isoforms occur in human clitoral cavernosal tissue.[75] That suggests that female erectile tissue can respond to the enhancement of the nitric oxide–cyclic guanosine monophosphate axis, specifically in clitoral erection, labial swelling, and vaginal lubrication upon sexual stimulation.

Reports of sildenafil treatment in women describe increased vaginal vascular engorgement, enhanced clitoral responsiveness, and improved lubrication.[76] Case reports for primary female sexual dysfunction treatment describe potential benefit.[77] However, there have also been equivocal reports of efficacy in female sexual dysfunction of various etiologies.[78–80] In a double-blind, placebo-controlled, crossover study of postmenopausal and posthysterectomy women, Berman et al. report that sildenafil 100 mg enhanced female sexual response physiologic parameters with visual and vibratory sexual stimulation.[76] Use of sildenafil led to significant increases in vaginal pH compared with baseline and placebo ($p < 0.05$).[76] Genital blood flow and vaginal compliance increased with sildenafil, but were not statistically greater than with placebo.[76]

The established safety and tolerability provided an opportunity to examine sildenafil for serotonergic antidepressant-associated sexual dysfunction in women. Open-label reports by Nurnberg et al.[81] and Fava et al.[82] included women who experienced sexual dysfunction improvements comparable to men. A second open-label study by Nurnberg et al. reported on 10 women with major depressive disorder in remission, without pre-existing sexual dysfunction, and serotonergic antidepressant-induced anorgasmia.[83] Nine of 10 women had reversal of sexual dysfunction; dosing ranged from 50 to 100 mg taken 1–2 h before sexual activity.[83] Additional open studies and case reports support these findings.[81 86] It appears that sildenafil use improves arousal with increased sensitivity, clitoral tumescence, genital vascular engorgement, and lubrication in women with antidepressant-induced sexual dysfunction. Preliminary reports from the first double-blind, placebo-controlled trial of flexible-dose, sildenafil for serotonergic antidepressant-associated sexual dysfunction in 150 women indicate comparable efficacy to the male double-blind, placebo-controlled studies, with overall response rates over 80%.[87] The data on treating women with antidepressant-induced sexual dysfunction are more complicated due to the importance of hormonal factors.

Conclusions

The last 10–15 years has seen a revolution in the treatment of depression and related disorders. Although newer medications have fewer side effects overall, it is clear that sexual dysfunction is an important, prevalent, and potentially quite distressing adverse event for patients. We are also more aware of the effects of depression on the individual's sexual function. A variety of suggested treatment strategies exist for sexual dysfunction, but none show universal efficacy. Oral selective phosphodiesterase type 5 inhibitors appear to demonstrate a clear role for effectively managing antidepressant-associated treatment-emergent sexual dysfunction in men, but we await more data on women. Previous treatments were essentially random pharmacology. The physician in practice needs to make patients aware of the possibility of this side effect, assess for sexual dysfunction, and keep the lines of communication open so that patients do not prematurely discontinue their antidepressant, placing them at risk of relapse of their depression.

References

1. Laumann EO, Paik A, Rosen RC. Sexual dysfunction in the United States: prevalence and predictors. JAMA 1999; 281: 537–44.
2. Dunn KM, Croft PR, Hackett GI. Satisfaction in the sex life of a general population sample. J Sex Marital Ther 2000; 26: 141–51.
3. Dunn KM, Croft PR, Hackett GI. Association of sexual problems with social, psychological, and physical problems in men and women: a cross sectional population survey. J Epidemiol Community Health 1999; 53: 144–8.
4. Hawton K, Gath D, Day A. Sexual function in a community sample of middle-aged women with partners: effects of age, marital, socioeconomic, psychiatric, gynecological, and menopausal factors. Arch Sex Behav 1994; 23: 375–95.
5. Casper RC, Redmond DE Jr, Katz MM et al. Somatic symptoms in primary affective disorder. Presence and relationship to the classification of depression. Arch Gen Psychiatry 1985; 42: 1098–1104.
6. Kennedy SH, Dickens SE, Eisfeld BS et al. Sexual dysfunction before antidepressant therapy in major depression. J Affect Disord 1999; 56(2–3): 201–8.
7. Zajecka J, Dunner DL, Gelenberg AJ et al. Sexual function and satisfaction in the treatment of chronic major depression with nefazodone, psychotherapy, and their combination. J Clin Psychiatry 2002; 63: 709–16.
8. Zajecka J, Dunner DL, Hirschfeld RM et al. Sexual function and satisfaction in the treatment of chronic major depression with nefazodone, CBAS-psychotherapy (CBASP) and their combination. Paper presented at American College of Neuropsychopharmacology, 2000, San Juan, Puerto Rico.
9. Ekselius L, von Knorring L. Effect on sexual function of long-term treatment with selective serotonin reuptake inhibitors in depressed patients treated in primary care. J Psychopharmacol 2001; 21: 154–60.
10. Rosen RC, Lane RM, Menza M. Effects of SSRIs on sexual function: a critical review. J Clin Psychopharmacol 1999; 19: 67–85.
11. Altman CA. Effects of selective serotonin reuptake inhibitors on sexual function. J Clin Psychopharmacol 2001; 21: 241–2.
12. Montejo-Gonzalez AL, Llorca G, Izquierdo JA et al. SSRI-induced sexual dysfunction: fluoxetine, paroxetine, sertraline, and fluvoxamine in a prospective, multicenter, and descriptive clinical study of 344 patients. J Sex Marital Ther 1997; 23: 176–94.
13. Montejo AL, Llorca G, Izquierdo JA et al. Incidence of sexual dysfunction associated with antidepressant agents: a prospective multicenter study of 1022 outpatients. Spanish Working Group for the Study of Psychotropic-Related Sexual Dysfunction. J Clin Psychiatry 2001; 62(Suppl 3): 10–21.
14. Clayton AH, Pradko JF, Croft HA et al. Prevalence of sexual dysfunction among newer antidepressants. J Clin Psychiatry 2002; 63: 357–66.
15. Piazza LA, Markowitz JC, Kocsis JH et al. Sexual functioning in chronically depressed patients treated with SSRI antidepressants: a pilot study. Am J Psychiatry 1997; 154: 1757–9.
16. Nurnberg HG, Hensley PL, Lauriello J. Sildenafil in the treatment of sexual dysfunction induced by selective serotonin reuptake inhibitors – an overview. CNS Drugs 2000; 13: 321–35.
17. Nurnberg HG. Managing treatment-emergent sexual dysfunction associated with serotonergic antidepressants: before and after sildenafil. J Psychiat Pract 2001; 7: 92–108.
18. Aizenberg D, Gur S, Zemishlany Z et al. Mianserin, a 5-HT2a/2c and alpha 2 antagonist, in the treatment of sexual dysfunction induced by serotonin reuptake inhibitors. Clin Neuropharmacol 1997; 20: 210–14.
19. Aizenberg D, Naor S, Zemishlany Z et al. The serotonin antagonist mianserin for treatment of serotonin reuptake inhibitor-induced sexual dysfunction in women: an open-label add-on study. Clin Neuropharmacol 1999; 22: 347–50.
20. Dolberg OT, Klag E, Gross Y et al. Relief of serotonin selective reuptake inhibitor induced sexual dysfunction with low-dose mianserin in patients with traumatic brain injury. Psychopharmacology 2002; 161: 404–7.
21. Aizenberg D, Zemishlany Z, Weizman A. Cyproheptadine treatment of sexual dysfunction induced by serotonin reuptake inhibitors. Clin Neuropharmacol 1995; 18: 320–4.
22. Lauerma H. Successful treatment of citalopram-induced anorgasmia by cyproheptadine. Acta Psychiatr Scand 1996; 93: 69–70.
23. McCormick S, Olin J, Brotman AW. Reversal of fluoxetine-induced anorgasmia by cyproheptadine in two patients. J Clin Psychiatry 1990; 51: 383–4.
24. Steele TE, Howell EF. Cyproheptadine for imipramine-induced anorgasmia. J Clin Psychopharmacol 1986; 6: 326–7.
25. Arnott S, Nutt D. Successful treatment of fluvoxamine-induced anorgasmia by cyproheptadine. Br J Psychiatry 1994; 164: 838–9.
26. Ashton AK, Ahrens K, Gupta S et al. Antidepressant-induced sexual dysfunction and Ginkgo biloba. Am J Psychiatry 2000; 157: 836–7.
27. Ellison JM, DeLuca P. Fluoxetine-induced genital anesthesia relieved by Ginkgo biloba extract. J Clin Psychiatry 1998; 59: 199–200.
28. Cohen AJ, Bartlik B. Ginkgo biloba for antidepressant-induced sexual dysfunction. J Sex Marital Ther 1998; 24: 139–43.
29. Balon R. Ginkgo biloba for antidepressant-induced sexual dysfunction? J Sex Marital Ther 1999; 25: 1–2.
30. Balogh S, Hendricks SE, Kang J. Treatment of fluoxetine-induced anorgasmia with amantadine. J Clin Psychiatry 1992; 53: 212–13.
31. Balon R. Intermittent amantadine for fluoxetine-induced anorgasmia. J Sex Marital Ther 1996; 22: 290–2.

32. Shrivastava RK, Shrivastava S, Overweg N et al. Amantadine in the treatment of sexual dysfunction associated with selective serotonin reuptake inhibitors. *J Clin Psychopharmacol* 1995; 15: 83–4.

33. Brubaker RV. Fluoxetine-induced sexual dysfunction reversed by loratadine. *J Clin Psychiatry* 2002; 63: 534.

34. Gross MD. Reversal by bethanechol of sexual dysfunction caused by anticholinergic antidepressants. *Am J Psychiatry* 1982; 139: 1193–4.

35. Segraves RT. Reversal by bethanechol of imipramine-induced ejaculatory dysfunction. *Am J Psychiatry* 1987; 144: 1243–4.

36. Segraves RT. Reversing anorgasmia associated with serotonin uptake inhibitors. *JAMA* 1991; 266: 2279.

37. Jacobsen FM. Fluoxetine-induced sexual dysfunction and an open trial of yohimbine. *J Clin Psychiatry* 1992; 53: 119–22.

38. Bartlik BD, Kaplan P, Kaplan HS. Psychostimulants apparently reverse sexual dysfunction secondary to selective serotonin reuptake inhibitors. *J Sex Marital Ther* 1995; 21: 264–71.

39. Stoll AL, Pillay SS, Diamond L et al. Methylphenidate augmentation of serotonin selective reuptake inhibitors: a case series. *J Clin Psychiatry* 1996; 57: 72–6.

40. Labbate LA, Grimes JB, Hines A et al. Bupropion treatment of serotonin reuptake antidepressant-associated sexual dysfunction. *Ann Clin Psychiatry* 1997; 9: 241–5.

41. Bodkin JA, Lasser RA, Wines JD Jr et al. Combining serotonin reuptake inhibitors and bupropion in partial responders to antidepressant monotherapy. *J Clin Psychiatry* 1997; 58: 137–45.

42. Clayton AH, McGarvey EL, Abouesh AI et al. Substitution of an SSRI with bupropion sustained release following SSRI-induced sexual dysfunction. *J Clin Psychiatry* 2001; 62: 185–90.

43. Ashton AK, Rosen RC. Bupropion as an antidote for serotonin reuptake inhibitor-induced sexual dysfunction. *J Clin Psychiatry* 1998; 59: 112–15.

44. Masand PS, Ashton AK, Gupta S et al. Sustained-release bupropion for selective serotonin reuptake inhibitor-induced sexual dysfunction: a randomized, double-blind, placebo-controlled, parallel-group study. *Am J Psychiatry* 2001; 158: 805–7.

45. Clayton AH, Warnock JK, Kornstein SG et al. A placebo-controlled trial of bupropion SR as an antidote for selective serotonin reuptake inhibitor-induced sexual dysfunction. *J Clin Psychiatry* 2004; 65: 62–7.

46. Michelson D, Bancroft J, Targum S et al. Female sexual dysfunction associated with antidepressant administration: a randomized, placebo-controlled study of pharmacologic intervention. *Am J Psychiatry* 2000; 157: 239–43.

47. Landen M, Eriksson E, Agren H et al. Effect of buspirone on sexual dysfunction in depressed patients treated with selective serotonin reuptake inhibitors. *J Clin Psychopharmacol* 1999; 19: 268–71.

48. Nelson EB, Keck PE Jr, McElroy SL. Resolution of fluoxetine-induced sexual dysfunction with the 5-HT3 antagonist granisetron. *J Clin Psychiatry* 1997; 58: 496–7.

49. Nelson EB, Shah VN, Welge JA et al. A placebo-controlled, crossover trial of granisetron in SRI-induced sexual dysfunction. *J Clin Psychiatry* 2001; 62: 469–73.

50. Michelson D, Kociban K, Tamura R et al. Mirtazapine, yohimbine or olanzapine augmentation therapy for serotonin reuptake-

associated female sexual dysfunction: a randomized, placebo controlled trial. *J Psychiatr Res* 2002; 36: 147–52.

51. Dording CM, Mischoulon D, Petersen TJ et al. The pharmacologic management of SSRI-induced side effects: a survey of psychiatrists. *Ann Clin Psychiatry* 2002; 14: 143–7.

52. Nurnberg HG, Levine PE. Spontaneous remission of MAOI-induced anorgasmia. *Am J Psychiatry* 1987; 144: 805–7.

53. Harrison WM, Rabkin JG, Ehrhardt AA et al. Effects of antidepressant medication on sexual function: a controlled study. *J Clin Psychopharmacol* 1986; 6: 144–9.

54. Kavoussi RJ, Segraves RT, Hughes AR et al. Double-blind comparison of bupropion sustained release and sertraline in depressed outpatients. *J Clin Psychiatry* 1997; 58: 532–7.

55. Clayton AH, Owens JE, McGarvey EL. Assessment of paroxetine-induced sexual dysfunction using the Changes in Sexual Functioning Questionnaire. *Psychopharmacol Bull* 1995; 31: 397–413.

56. Feiger A, Kiev A, Shrivastava RK et al. Nefazodone versus sertraline in outpatients with major depression: focus on efficacy, tolerability, and effects on sexual function and satisfaction. *J Clin Psychiatry* 1996; 57(Suppl 2): 53–62.

57. Zajecka J, Mitchell S, Fawcett J. Treatment-emergent changes in sexual function with selective serotonin reuptake inhibitors as measured with the Rush Sexual Inventory. *Psychopharmacol Bull* 1997; 33: 755–60.

58. Labbate LA, Grimes J, Hines A et al. Sexual dysfunction induced by serotonin reuptake antidepressants. *J Sex Marital Ther* 1998; 24: 3–12.

59. Labbate LA, Grimes JB, Arana GW. Serotonin reuptake antidepressant effects on sexual function in patients with anxiety disorders. *Biol Psychiatry* 1998; 43: 904–7.

60. Reimherr FW, Chouinard G, Cohn CK et al. Antidepressant efficacy of sertraline: a double-blind, placebo- and amitriptyline-controlled, multicenter comparison study in outpatients with major depression. *J Clin Psychiatry* 1990; 51(Suppl B): 18–27.

61. Monteiro WO, Noshirvani HF, Marks IM et al. Anorgasmia from clomipramine in obsessive-compulsive disorder. A controlled trial. *Br J Psychiatry* 1987; 151: 107–12.

62. Ashton AK, Rosen RC. Accommodation to serotonin reuptake inhibitor-induced sexual dysfunction. *J Sex Marital Ther* 1998; 24: 191–2.

63. Shen WW, Hsu JH. Female sexual side effects associated with selective serotonin reuptake inhibitors: a descriptive clinical study of 33 patients. *Int J Psychiatry Med* 1995; 25: 239–48.

64. Hirschfeld RM, Schatzberg AF. Long-term management of depression. *Am J Med* 1994; 97(6A): 33S–8.

65. Rothschild AJ. Selective serotonin reuptake inhibitor-induced sexual dysfunction: efficacy of a drug holiday. *Am J Psychiatry* 1995; 152: 1514–16.

66. Rosenbaum JF, Fava M, Hoog SL et al. Selective serotonin reuptake inhibitor discontinuation syndrome: a randomized clinical trial. *Biol Psychiatry* 1998; 44: 77–87.

67. Coupland NJ, Bell CJ, Potokar JP. Serotonin reuptake inhibitor withdrawal. *J Clin Psychopharmacol* 1996; 16: 356–62.

68. Lane RM. Withdrawal symptoms after discontinuation of selec-

tive serotonin reuptake inhibitors (SSRIs). *J Serotonin Res* 1996; 3: 75–83.

69. Price D. Sildenafil citrate (Viagra) efficacy in the treatment of erectile dysfunction in patients with common concomitant conditions. Sildenafil Study Group. *Int J Clin Pract Suppl* 1999; 102: 21–3.

70. Seidman SN, Roose SP, Menza MA et al. Treatment of erectile dysfunction in men with depressive symptoms: results of a placebo-controlled trial with sildenafil citrate. *Am J Psychiatry* 2001; 58: 1623–30.

71. Nurnberg HG, Gelenberg A, Hargreave TB et al. Efficacy of sildenafil citrate for the treatment of erectile dysfunction in men taking serotonin reuptake inhibitors. *Am J Psychiatry* 2001; 158: 1926–8.

72. Segraves RT, Stevenson R, Lee J et al. Tadalafil for treatment of erectile dysfunction in men on antidepressants. New Research Poster presented at American Psychiatric Association, 3 May 2004, New York.

73. Rosen R, Montorsi F, Assalian P et al. Efficacy and tolerability of vardenafil in men with mild depressive disorder and erectile dysfunction: the Depression Related Improvement with Vardenafil for Erectile Response (DRIVER) study. Paper presented at 19th Congress of the European Association of Urology, 26 March 2004, Vienna, Austria.

74. Nurnberg HG, Hensley PL, Gelenberg AJ et al. Treatment of antidepressant-associated sexual dysfunction with sildenafil: a randomized controlled trial. *JAMA* 2003; 289: 56–64.

75. Park K, Moreland RB, Goldstein I et al. Sildenafil inhibits phosphodiesterase type 5 in human clitoral corpus cavernosum smooth muscle. *Biochem Biophys Res Commun* 1998; 249: 612–17.

76. Berman J, Goldstein I, Werbin T et al. Double blind placebo controlled study with crossover to assess effect of sildenafil on physiological parameters of the female sexual response. *J Urol* 1999; 161(Suppl 210): 210.

77. Bartlik B, Kaplan P, Kaminetsky J et al. Medications with the potential to enhance sexual responsivity in women. *Psychiatr Ann* 1999; 29: 46–52.

78. Kaplan SA, Reis RB, Kohn IJ et al. Safety and efficacy of sildenafil in postmenopausal women with sexual dysfunction. *Urology* 1999; 53: 481–6.

79. Basson R, McInnes R, Smith MD et al. Efficacy and safety of sildenafil in estrogenized women with sexual dysfunction associated with female sexual arousal disorder. *Obstet Gynecol* 2000; 95(4 Suppl 1): S54.

80. Sipski ML, Rosen RC, Alexander CJ et al. Sildenafil effects on sexual and cardiovascular responses in women with spinal cord injury. *Urology* 2000; 55: 812–15.

81. Nurnberg HG, Lauriello J, Hensley PL et al. Sildenafil for iatrogenic serotonergic antidepressant medication-induced sexual dysfunction in 4 patients. *J Clin Psychiatry* 1999; 60: 33–5.

82. Fava M, Rankin MA, Alpert JE et al. An open trial of oral sildenafil in antidepressant-induced sexual dysfunction. *Psychother Psychosom* 1998; 67: 328–31.

83. Nurnberg HG, Hensley PL, Lauriello J et al. Sildenafil for women patients with antidepressant-induced sexual dysfunction. *Psychiatr Serv* 1999; 50: 1076–8.

84. Ashton AK. Sildenafil treatment of paroxetine-induced anorgasmia in a woman. *Am J Psychiatry* 1999; 156: 800.

85. Rosenberg KP. Sildenafil citrate for SSRI-induced sexual side effects. *Am J Psychiatry* 1999; 156: 157.

86. Shen WW, Urosevich Z, Clayton DO. Sildenafil in the treatment of female sexual dysfunction induced by selective serotonin reuptake inhibitors. *J Reprod Med* 1999; 44: 535–42.

87. Nurnberg HG, Hensley PL, Croft H et al. Sildenafil citrate treatment for SRI-associated female sexual dysfunction. Poster presented at American Psychiatric Association, 21 May 2003, San Francisco.

16.3 Dermatologic disorders resulting in sexual dysfunction

Peter J Lynch

Rick was kissing his way from my shoulder down my arm. I could feel his lips hovering above the crease in my arm. I waited but he didn't continue. "Um, Ella," he said at last. I opened my eyes. He was staring at the crease…. "What is it?" "Psoriasis. I had it once when I was thirteen." Rick looked at it, then leaned over and kissed my eyelids shut. When I opened my eyes again I just caught a flicker of distaste cross his face.[1]

The adverse impact of disease affects society primarily in terms of economic cost[2] and affects individuals primarily in terms of physical, psychologic, social, and sexual function. The impact of disease in these four areas is collectively known as impact on quality of life[3,4] (see Chapter 2.4 of this book). In the past, it was thought that physician-assessed severity of disease would accurately measure the effect of a disease on a patient's quality of life. It was also thought that physician assessment would correlate well with patient assessment of impact on his or her quality of life. Unfortunately, objective assessment of disease severity correlates very poorly with the patient's own perception of disease impact, and, for that reason, patient-provided data represent the main source for quality of life assessment[5] (see Chapter 11.2). Thus, quality of life is generally measured through the use of questionnaire surveys provided to individual patients. This approach allows patients, rather than just their care providers, to provide input on what the presence of disease means to them.[4]

Quality-of-life assessment

Generic assessment

Generic assessment of quality of life considers all types of disease (infections, malignancy, etc.) and disease in all types of organs. This approach, for example, would allow the effect of a skin disease on quality of life to be compared to the effect of a pulmonary disease. In order to keep the surveys short and simple, the amount of detail that can be collected particular to any one disease is necessarily limited. Moreover the results obtained depend greatly on the group surveyed. Thus, in an underdeveloped country, skin disease may seem unimportant compared to gastrointestinal disease.[6,7] On the other hand, in the affluent, appearance-obsessed Western world, the effect of skin disease might be viewed as much more problematic.[8] The most widely used generic survey instrument is the 36-item, short-form survey of health status (Medical Outcomes Study). This survey is designed for use in clinical practice and research and includes a multi-item scale assessing the following: (1) limitations in physical activities because of health problems; (2) limitations in social activities because of physical or emotional problems; (3) limitations in usual role activities because of physical health problems; (4) bodily pain; (5) general mental health (psychologic distress and well-being); (6) limitations in usual role activities because of emotional problems; (7) vitality (energy and fatigue); and (8) general health perceptions.[9] It has been used to study the effect of acne, psoriasis, atopic dermatitis, and hand dermatitis on quality of life.[10]

Discipline-specific assessment

Assessment specific to a single discipline retrieves much more data pertinent to a given disease and thus allows excellent comparison among diseases referable to that discipline. Several instruments have been developed to assess quality of life for patients with dermatologic disease.[4] The first, and most widely used, is the Dermatology Life Quality Index, developed in 1994 by Findlay and Khan.[11] It is a short, 10-question questionnaire. Importantly for the purposes of this chapter, question 9 specifically inquires about the effect of disease on sexual function. Since each of the 10 questions can be answered with four degrees of effect (not at all, a little, a lot, very much), the maximum Dermatology Life Quality Index score is 40 points – the higher the score, the greater the impairment in quality of life. Patients with skin disease generally have scores between 5 and 20 points.[11]

A second questionnaire, Skindex, was developed in 1996.[5] This was a 61-item survey that was shortened the following year to 29 items (Skindex-29).[12] Two items regarding sexuality are included. An even shorter version, Skindex-16, was developed in 2001.[13] Skindex has been used to assess only a few dermatologic problems. Two other survey instruments for dermatologic problems have been formulated, the Dermatology-Specific Quality of Life[14] and the Dermatology Quality of Life scales.[15] Neither has been used for comparative purposes.

Disease-specific studies

Multiple studies have employed instruments developed for the sole purpose of evaluating either a single disease or a limited group of closely related diseases (e.g., Scalpdex). These provide very detailed information, but, because they are formulated specifically for each disease, they cannot be used to compare the effect on quality of life among various diseases. They are used primarily in therapeutic trials to measure the effect of treatment on disease severity and patients' quality of life.

The general impact of skin disease on quality of life and sexuality

Skin disease is ubiquitous and is associated with appreciable impact on the lives of those afflicted. In 1979, dermatologic examination of over 20 000 unselected American individuals found "significant" skin problems in about one-third of all those examined.[16] One-third of these (about 10% of the total population) described some social handicap as a result of their skin disease. A more recent survey of over 18 000 Norwegian adults reported a 25% prevalence rate for self-reported skin problems.[17] In this survey, the odds ratio for the presence of depression in those with skin problems was impressively high at 2.26. Finally, a survey of 10 000 French households revealed a 43%, 2-year incidence of self-reported skin disease. More than half of these patients indicated that their skin problems adversely affected their daily lives.[18]

The published data on the impact of skin disease in the specific area of sexual function are extremely limited.[19] However, in spite of the paucity of data, common sense tells us that any disease affecting the appearance, touch, and/or odor of a body is highly likely to cause anxiety, depression, diminution of self-image, attenuation of self-worth, and difficulty in social interaction. This, in turn, will surely lead to some degree of sexual dysfunction whether it has been measured or not.

The impact of individual dermatologic disorders on quality of life and sexual function

Most dermatologic disorders have an adverse effect on appearance, touch, and/or odor, and thus are likely to have an impact on sexual function. Not surprisingly, the most important and best studied of these conditions (genital warts, genital herpes, lichen sclerosus, and erosive lichen planus) directly affect the genitalia and are often limited to that site. These diseases are discussed in detail in Chapter 12.2 and will not be covered here. Instead, I will review six other conditions that either do not directly involve the genitalia or are not confined solely to the genitalia. The effect of these disorders on sexuality is more indirect and in many instances has not been well studied. Thus, for some disorders, a putative effect on sexual function has to be derived from data on disease effect in other closely related areas such as social and psychologic function. Information regarding the effect of additional skin diseases on quality of life can be found elsewhere.[4,11,20,21]

Acne

Clinical aspects

The prevalence of acne in young people is about 90% in males and 80% in females. After age 25, gender predominance switches to a prevalence of approximately 20% in women and 8% in men. Mild acne consists of open comedones ("blackheads") and small, skin-colored papules ("closed comedones") confined to the face. As severity increases, red papules and white-topped pustules appear. In very severe acne, red nodules and cysts are intermingled with numerous inflammatory papules. These may be located on the upper trunk as well as on the face (Fig. 16.3.1). The prevalence of acne, and possibly its severity, are increased in patients with polycystic ovarian disease, adrenal hyperplasia, and other conditions that affect the hormonal milieu.

Mild acne is treated with topically applied benzoyl peroxide, antibiotics, and retinoids. Orally administered antibiotics (tetracycline, erythromycin, doxycycline, or minocycline) are added in instances of moderate severity. Severe acne requires orally administered antiandrogens, such as oral contraceptives, and retinoids, such as isotretinoin.

Quality of life: social, psychologic, and sexual aspects

Probably because of sensitivity regarding sexual issues in adolescents and their families, the available quality of life data do not contain information on sexual function. What the data do indicate is that acne has a profound effect on social and psychologic function. One study of teenagers demonstrated that 58% were dissatisfied with their facial appearance and that this dissatisfaction correlated directly with feelings of embarrassment and social inhibition.[22] Another study indicated that girls have

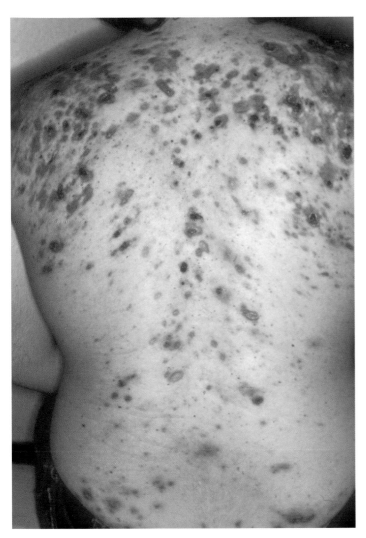

Figure 16.3.1. Cystic acne of the back. This is an example of how severe acne can be. Lesions are in various stages of development. Some are boil-like nodules, some are draining sinuses, and others are resolving with scar formation.

higher levels of emotional and behavioral dysfunction than boys.[23] Several studies found that the detrimental effect on function and emotion in patients with acne was as great as for patients with psoriasis.[24] It has also been shown that the effect of acne on psychologic and emotional function was as great for patients with acne as it was for patients with serious systemic disorders such as chronic disabling asthma, epilepsy, diabetes, and arthritis.[25] Similarly, Yazici et al. demonstrated that 26% and 30% of acne patients, versus 0% and 7% of controls, had significant anxiety and depression.[26] While no study has reported directly on sexual function, the severe effect of acne on social and psychologic function strongly suggests that sexual problems are present in many, if not most, patients with moderate to severe acne.

Female androgenetic alopecia

Clinical aspects

Female androgenetic alopecia (female pattern hair loss) is the counterpart to androgenetic alopecia in men. Hair loss occurs less commonly (and is usually less severe) in women than in men. Female androgenetic alopecia occurs in about 15% of premenopausal and 40% of postmenopausal women. The hair loss develops insidiously, sometimes diffusely, but most often the vertex is predominantly affected. No inflammation is found, but hair shafts are minaturized and the ostia of hair follicles gradually disappear. Genetic factors (both paternal and maternal) and sex hormones are important. However, as is also true for men, most women with female androgenetic alopecia have normal levels of sex hormones, and there is only little or no response to antiandrogen therapy. The use of topical minoxidil (2% or 5%) leads to partial, but clinically important, regrowth in about a quarter of women; the others usually note a decrease in the rate of hair loss.

Quality of life: social, psychologic, and sexual aspects

Much nonmedical literature (e.g., the biblical story of Samson and Delilah), and common sense, suggest that the presence of normal scalp hair is important for social function. The significance of hair loss in terms of quality of life has been well studied in men; much less is known about the effect of this disease on women. Cash et al. investigated 96 women with female androgenetic alopecia and compared their psychologic function with 60 balding men and 56 control women.[27] Women with female androgenetic alopecia, when compared both to the men and the female controls, possessed a more negative body image and reported higher social anxiety, lower self-esteem, and decreased life satisfaction. In another study, van der Donk et al.[28] found that the degree of psychologic dysfunction in women with female androgenetic alopecia was similar to that in patients with acne, psoriasis, and eczema. Similarly, Williamson et al.[29] and Schmidt et al.[30] also found that the decrease in quality of life in women was approximately the same as occurred in women with psoriasis. In addition, Schmidt et al.[30] noted that women who perceived their hair loss as severe (but for whom medical assessment revealed no visible loss) had psychologic dysfunction severe enough to approach a diagnosis of dysmorphophobia (body dysmorphic syndrome). Dolte et al. reported that 50% of women with female androgenetic alopecia had problematic interaction with those of the opposite sex.[31] One small study noted that, of 32 patients with female androgenetic alopecia, seven had severe, long-standing marital and sexual problems.[32]

Vitiligo

Clinical aspects

Vitiligo is an acquired depigmentation of the skin affecting 1–2% of the population. The patches of vitiligo are bright white with sharp demarcation from the adjacent normal skin. There is no inflammation, scale, or textural change. In the most common form of vitiligo, depigmentation involves the face and hands (Fig. 16.3.2). Pigment loss also occurs in the axillae and anogenital region in about 40% of these patients. Genetic factors and autoimmune dysfunction are important in the pathophysiology of vitiligo, which is slowly progressive, but it is uncommon for more than 20–25% of the skin to become depigmented. Topically applied steroids and calcineurin inhibitors are sometimes effective. Ultraviolet light therapy can be tried, but cosmetically pleasing results are unlikely to be achieved. For most patients, the application of skin dyes, "quick-tanning" agents, or pigmented cosmetic cover-up products represents the best approach.

Quality of life: social, psychologic, and sexual aspects

One study demonstrated that vitiligo patients scored lower on self-esteem than did matched controls.[33] Two newer studies[34,35] showed only a moderate effect on quality of life, less than that seen in acne, hair loss, atopic dermatitis, and psoriasis. However, a study from India, where vitiligo has tremendous social and religious meaning, reported a more marked decrement in quality of life.[36] A more recent study demonstrated dysfunction in the "emotions" and "functioning" domains.[37] Only one study has specifically examined the effect of vitiligo on sexual function.[38] In it, questionnaire results from 158 respondents indicated that 25% of the patients believed that their vitiligo interfered with their sexual relationships. Interestingly, of those adversely affected, about 50% indicated that the difficulty was due to their own embarrassment, and only 13% felt that the problem was due to their partner's reaction. Not surprisingly, sexual dysfunction correlated highly with low self-esteem.

Hidradenitis suppurativa

Clinical aspects

Hidradenitis suppurativa is a sterile, inflammatory folliculitis involving only those hair follicles with attached apocrine sweat glands. The prevalence rate is 0.5–1.0%, and it is more common in women, especially those of African-American background, and in those who are overweight. Tender red papules appear along the milk line, most lesions occurring in axillary, mammary, and anogenital sites (Fig. 16.3.3). The papules characteristically enlarge to form painful, boil-like nodules that often break down and drain purulent fluid. Most patients develop only a few lesions each month, but some may have dozens of lesions at a time. Lesions occurring in the anogenital region may be accompanied by edema and distortion of the genitalia. The pathophysiology is analogous to that of cystic acne. Genetics

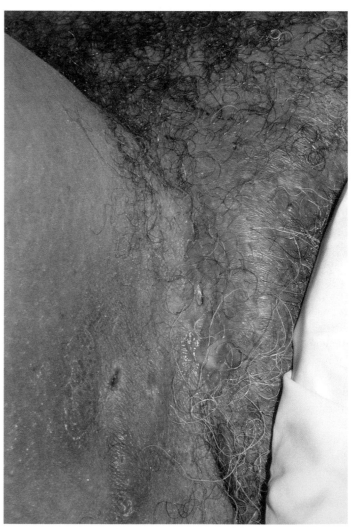

Figure 16.3.3. Hidradenitis suppurativa of the upper inner thigh and labium majus. The labium majus is red, painful, and swollen. The intensity of red color is somewhat obscured by the natural dark pigmentation in this African-American woman. An inflamed nodule on the upper, inner thigh has broken down and is draining pus.

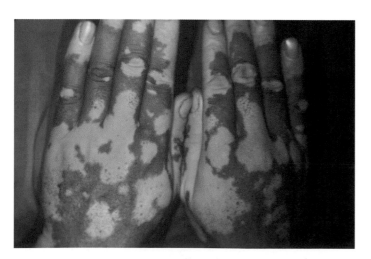

Figure 16.3.2. Vitiligo in an African-American woman. The significant color abnormalities on the dorsal hands make all types of social interactions problematic.

and hormonal factors are important, but levels of sex hormones are usually normal. Mild cases are treated as for cystic acne. More severe cases require surgical excision of involved tissue. Liposuction to remove, and laser therapy to destroy, the apocrine gland-related follicles are sometimes used. Orally administered retinoids and oral contraceptives, in contrast to their usefulness in acne, are of little help.

Quality of life: social, psychologic, and sexual aspects

Involvement of the breasts and anogenital region with unsightly, odorous, painful, draining lesions will certainly disrupt quality of life. However, only two studies on quality of life have been published. In the first, involving 98 women, the mean Dermatology Life Quality Index score was 8.9, patients expressing modest to moderate concern regarding social interaction with their partners, friends, and relatives.[39] This score is among the highest (indicating greater decrement in quality of life) reported for the 30 dermatologic diseases that have been studied with this instrument.[11] In the second study, inquiry was made about the effect of hidradenitis on sexuality; 26 of 58 women (45%) indicated that their disease adversely affected sexual function.[40]

Psoriasis

Clinical aspects

Psoriasis, which has a prevalence rate of approximately 1–2.5%, can begin at any age, but onset peaks in young adult life. In plaque-type psoriasis, red, scaling plaques most frequently develop on the knees, elbows, scalp, umbilicus, and gluteal cleft. Involvement of the external genitalia is fairly common, occurring in 20–30% of patients with moderate or severe psoriasis (Fig. 16.3.4). Fingernails and toenails are often dystrophic, and arthritis of mild or moderate severity sometimes occurs. Genetics and autoimmune dysfunction are important in the pathophysiology. Topically applied, mid- to high-potency corticosteroids are the mainstay of therapy. Topical retinoids, calcipotriol, and the calcineurin blockers (tacrolimus and pimecrolimus) may be added. Natural sunlight and ultraviolet light, especially in conjunction with oral psoralens and ultraviolet A therapy, are a widely used and effective treatment for psoriasis. Patients with severe disease may require systemically administered methotrexate, cyclosporine, or other agents.

Quality of life: social, psychologic, and sexual aspects

The lesions of psoriasis frequently occur in sensitive areas such as the scalp, hands, and genitalia. These are associated with shedding of scale, roughness on palpation, and malodor. Thus, it is not surprising that patients with psoriasis experience very poor, health-related quality of life. The problems of living with psoriasis have been poignantly described by John Updike. He has not only masterfully detailed his own personal distress[41] but has also created outstanding fictional depictions of individuals with psoriasis.

Many general reviews of quality of life in psoriasis have

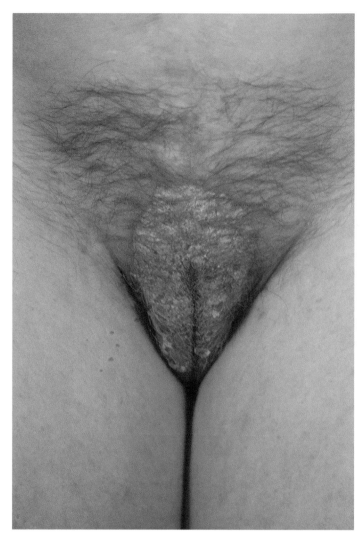

Figure 16.3.4. Psoriasis of the mons pubis and labia majora. The sharp margination and typical large silver–white scale of the involved tissue help to differentiate this disease from atopic dermatitis.

been published,[42–44] and these contain a few pertinent points. First, among approximately 15 studies on quality of life in psoriasis, the range of Dermatology Life Quality Index scores is larger than for any other skin disease.[11] This reflects the wide range of assessed and perceived severity. In these studies, the median score is about 12, placing psoriasis among the worst two or three common skin problems.[11] Second, in a study using the 36-item, short-form survey, the quality of life for psoriasis was found to be decreased to the same degree as for patients with cancer, arthritis, hypertension, diabetes, and depression.[44] For most dermatologic problems, impairment of quality of life is more severe in women than in men. But psoriasis seems to affect both sexes equally.[45]

A number of studies have examined the impact of psoriasis on sexual function. In 1988, Ramsay and O'Reagan surveyed 104 patients and found that 50% of the respondents affirmatively answered the question, "Do you feel having psoriasis has inhibited your sexual relationships?"[46] Of note, 65% of those experiencing sexual dysfunction had plaques in the genital area compared to only 35% of those who were not sexually affected. In 1989, Ginsburg and Link surveyed 100 adult psoriatic patients and found that 70% "agreed", or "strongly agreed" with the statement, "I feel physically unattractive and sexually undesirable when [my] psoriasis is bad."[47] Moreover, 46% "agreed" or "strongly agreed" with the statement, "When the psoriasis is severe, I am too ashamed to engage in sexual activity." Finlay and Coles reviewed 369 survey questionnaires in which the question was asked: "Has your psoriasis resulted in sexual difficulties over the last 4 weeks?"[48] About 30% of psoriatic patients answered "very much" or "a lot" to this question. Gupta and Gupta reviewed questionnaires completed by 120 hospitalized patients with moderate or severe psoriasis.[49] Of these, 41% answered affirmatively to the question, "Do you believe that, since the onset of psoriasis, your sexual activity has declined?" Of those patients reporting a decline in sexual activity, 43% indicated the decline was due to a decrease in their own sexual drive, whereas only 15% believed that the decline was due to a decrease in the sexual drive of their partner.[49] In 2001, questionnaires were mailed to the more than 40 000 members of the National Psoriasis Foundation.[50] Of those responding, 27% indicated that sexual activities were negatively affected. Finally, in a survey of 599 patients, the effect of psoriasis on sexual function was directly related to the severity of the disease as perceived by the patient.[51] Specifically, on a scale of 0 (not at all) to 10 (very much), the impact on sexuality was found to be 1.2, 1.9, and 3.7, respectively, for those with mild, moderate, or severe disease.

Atopic dermatitis

Clinical aspects

Atopic dermatitis (atopic eczema, neurodermatitis) has a prevalence of about 10%. Males and females are involved equally. The characteristic clinical feature is itching, usually described as severe. Nighttime scratching is notably troublesome. Mild disease demonstrates tiny (1–2 mm), follicular, red papules, but consequent scratching results in excoriation, weeping, and crusting. Patients who rub as well as scratch, develop lichenification (palpable skin thickening and exaggeration of the skin markings).

In children and adolescents, lesions are most often found in the antecubital and popliteal fossae. In adults, lesions occur most frequently on the dorsal feet (men), dorsal hands (women), occiput (women), and the anogenital region (both sexes) (Figs 16.3.5 and 16.3.6). Genetic factors, disordered development of inflammation, and possibly environmental allergens are important in the pathophysiology. Psychologic factors seem to play an adjuvant role in the timing and severity of the disease.

Topically applied lubricants and corticosteroids are sufficient for mild disease. Topically applied calcineurin inhibitors (tacrolimus and pimecrolimus) are used for facial and anogenital lesions. Sedating-type antihistamines (hydroxyzine or

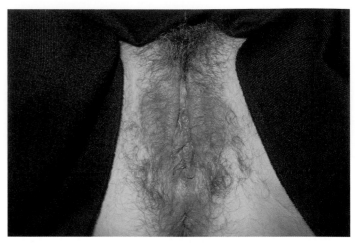

Figure 16.3.5. Atopic dermatitis of the vulva and perivulvar skin. Bright red inflammation is present. The margins of the involved lesions are not as distinct as those in psoriasis.

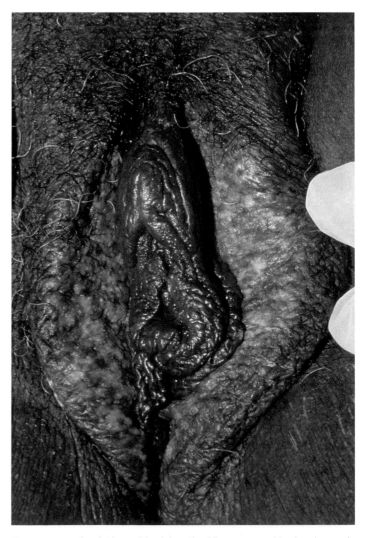

Figure 16.3.6. Atopic dermatitis of the vulva. Vigorous scratching has damaged the epidermal melanocytes and has led to both hyper- and hypopigmentation.

doxepin) may be used to control nighttime scratching. Systemically administered corticosteroids or cyclosporine may be necessary, on a short-term basis, for patients with severe disease.

Quality of life: social, psychologic, and sexual aspects

Six studies have reported Dermatology Life Quality Index scores of 4.1,[52] 5.5,[53] 6.6,[54] 7.3,[55] 11.0,[19] and 12.5.[56] An additional study, involving more severely affected, hospitalized patients reported a notably high Dermatology Life Quality Index score of 16.2.[57] Three of the above studies compared Dermatology Life Quality Index scores between patients with psoriasis and those with atopic dermatitis. In each instance, the impairment in quality of life was greater for atopic dermatitis.[57] Two other studies used instruments other than the Dermatology Life Quality Index. One noted that patients with atopic dermatitis had high anxiety levels.[58] The other, using the SF-36 questionnaire, found that patients with atopic dermatitis had significantly greater impairment in mental health than did patients with hypertension, type 2 diabetes, and psoriasis.[54]

Sexual issues were examined in several studies. Question 9 in the Dermatology Life Quality Index survey asks, "Over the last week, how much has your skin caused any sexual difficulties?" The range of possible answers is 0 ("none") to 4 ("very much"). In three studies, the mean scores for this question were 0.05, 0.4, and 0.5, indicating only a minor effect.[19,53,56] However, Drake et al. noted that nearly 40% of patients responding to question 9 experienced at least some sexual impairment.[59] Linnet and Jemec noted sexual problems in many patients with atopic dermatitis and found that these were correlated with the patient's anxiety levels rather than with physician-assessed severity of disease.[58] Two older studies considered patients with atopic dermatitis and psoriasis as a group. Van Dorssen et al. found that about one-third of these grouped patients had sexual problems,[60] and Niemeier et al. simply indicated that there was significant sexual impairment.[61]

Conclusions

From common sense and the quoted quality-of-life studies, we may conclude that skin problems frequently impair self-image and are often accompanied by anxiety and depression. This, in turn, adversely affects perception of sexual attractiveness, reduces libido, and leads to varying degrees of sexual dysfunction. Since so many skin diseases are readily visible, malodorous, and associated with scale and crust, it is likely that dermatologic disorders adversely affect sexual function more often, and more severely, than disease in most other organs. And, because our Western society specifically emphasizes physical appearance in women, the effect on sexuality will likely be more prominent in women than in men.

Importantly, the extent and severity of the skin disease, as determined by health professionals, are not good predictors of decreased quality of life. Moreover, medically achieved improvement in the severity of the disease usually restores only a portion of the patient's original quality of life. For this reason, we must remember that it is the patient's perception of quality-of-life impairment that is of utmost importance. Unfortunately, the patient's perception of his or her disease and its effect on sexual function is rarely considered during the provision of medical care.[61] This results in underestimation of quality-of-life impairment and insufficient counseling regarding psychologic and sexual function. This omission represents a serious disservice to our patients.

References

1. Chevalier T. *The Virgin Blue*. New York: Penguin, 1997: 34–5.
2. Chen SC, Bayoumi AM, Soon SL et al. A catalogue of dermatology utilities: a measure of the burden of skin diseases. *J Investig Dermatol Symp Proc* 2004; 9: 160–8.
3. Chren M-M, Weinstock MA. Conceptual issues in measuring the burden of skin diseases. *J Investig Dermatol Symp Proc* 2004; 9: 97–100.
4. Halioua B, Beumont MG, Lunel F. Quality of life in dermatology. *Int J Dermatol* 2000; 39: 801–6.
5. Chren M-M, Lasek RJ, Quinn EN et al. Skindex, a quality-of-life measure for patients with skin disease: reliability, validity, and responsiveness. *J Invest Dermatol* 1996; 107: 707–13.
6. Qureshi AA, Freedberg I, Goldsmith L et al. Report on "burden of skin disease" workshop NIAMS, September 2002. *J Investig Dermatol Symp Proc* 2004; 9: 111–19.
7. Murray CJ, Lopez AD. Mortality by cause for eight regions of the world. Global burden of disease study. *Lancet* 1997; 349: 1269–76.
8. Wolkenstein P, Grob J-J, Bastuji-Garin S et al. French people and skin disease. Results of a survey using a representative sample. *Arch Dermatol* 2003; 139: 1614–19.
9. Ware JE Jr, Sherbourne CD. The MOS 36-item short-form health survey (SF-36). I. Conceptual framework and item selection. *Med Care* 1992; 30: 473–83.
10. Wallenhammer L-M, Nyfall M, Lindberg M et al. Health-related quality of life and hand eczema –a comparison of two instruments, including factor analysis. *J Invest Dermatol* 2004; 122: 1381–9.
11. Lewis V, Finlay AY. 10 years experience of the Dermatology Life Quality Index (DLQI). *J Investig Dermatol Symp Proc* 2004; 9: 169–80.
12. Chren M-M, Lasek RJ, Flocke SA et al. Improved discriminative and evaluative capability of a refined version of Skindex, a quality-of-life instrument for patients with skin diseases. *Arch Dermatol* 1997; 133: 1433–40.
13. Chren M-M, Lasek RJ, Sahay AP et al. Measurement properties of Skindex-16: a brief quality-of-life measure for patients with skin diseases. *J Cutan Med Surg* 2001; 5: 105–10.
14. Anderson RT, Rajagopalan R. Development and validation of a quality of life instrument for cutaneous diseases. *J Am Acad Dermatol* 1997; 37: 41–50.
15. Morgan M, McCreedy R, Simpson J et al. Dermatology quality of life scales – a measure of the impact of skin diseases. *Br J Dermatol* 1997; 136: 202–6.

16. Johnson M-LT. Defining the burden of skin disease in the United States – a historical perspective. *J Investig Dermatol Symp Proc* 2004; 9: 108–10.

17. Dalgard F, Svensson A, Holm JO. Self-reported skin morbidity among adults: associations with quality of life and general health in a Norwegian Survey. *J Investig Dermatol Symp Proc* 2004; 9: 120–5.

18. Wolkenstein P, Grob J-J, Bastuji-Garin S. French people and skin diseases. *Arch Dermatol* 2003; 139: 1614–19.

19. Niemeier V, Gieier U. Skin disease and sexuality. In JYM Koo, CS Lee, eds. *Psychocutaneous Medicine*. New York: Marcel Decker, 2003: 375–82.

20. Harlow D, Poyner T, Finlay AY et al. Impaired quality of life of adults with skin disease in primary care. *Br J Dermatol* 2000; 143: 979–82.

21. Jowett S, Ryan T. Skin disease and handicap: an analysis of the impact of skin conditions. *Soc Sci Med* 1985; 20: 425–9.

22. Krowchuk DP, Stancin T, Keskin R et al. The psychological effects of acne on adolescents. *Pediatr Dermatol* 1991; 8: 332–8.

23. Smithard A, Glazebrook C, Williams HC. Acne prevalence, knowledge about acne and psychological morbidity in mid-adolescence: a community-based study. *Br J Dermatol* 2001; 145: 274–9.

24. Lasek RJ, Chren M-M. Acne vulgaris and the quality of life of adult dermatology patients. *Arch Dermatol* 1998; 134: 454–8.

25. Mallon E, Newton JN, Klassen A et al. The quality of life in acne: a comparison with general medical conditions using generic questionnaires. *Br J Dermatol* 1999; 140: 672–6.

26. Yazici K, Baz K, Yazici AE et al. Disease-specific quality of life is associated with anxiety and depression in patients with acne. *J Eur Acad Dermatol Venereol* 2004; 18: 435–9.

27. Cash TF, Price VH, Savin RS. Psychological effects of androgenetic alopecia on women: comparisons with balding men with female control subjects. *J Am Acad Dermatol* 1993; 29: 568–75.

28. van der Donk J, Passchier J, Knegt-Junk C et al. Psychological characteristics of women with androgenetic alopecia: a controlled study. *Br J Dermatol* 1991; 125: 248–52.

29. Williamson D, Gonzalez M, Finlay AY. The effect of hair loss on quality of life. *J Eur Acad Dermatol Venereol* 2000; 15: 137–9.

30. Schmidt S, Fischer TW, Chren M-M et al. Strategies of coping and quality of life in women with alopecia. *Br J Dermatol* 2001; 144: 1038–43.

31. Dolte KS, Girman CJ, Hartmaier S et al. Development of a health-related quality of life questionnaire for women with androgenetic alopecia. *Clin Exp Dermatol* 2000; 25: 737–42.

32. Eckert J. Diffuse hair loss in women: the psychopathology of those who complain. *Acta Psychiatr Scand* 1976; 53: 321–7.

33. Porter JR, Beuf AH, Lerner A et al. Psychosocial effect of vitiligo: a comparison of vitiligo patients with "normal" control subjects, with psoriasis patients, and with patients with other pigmentary disorders. *J Am Acad Dermatol* 1986; 15: 220–4.

34. Finlay AY, Khan GK. Dermatology Life Quality Index (DLQI): a simple, practical measure for routine clinical use. *Clin Exp Dermatol* 1994; 19: 210–16.

35. Kent G, Al'Abadie M. Psychologic effects of vitiligo: a critical incident analysis. *J Am Acad Dermatol* 1996; 35: 895–8.

36. Parsad D, Pandhi R, Dogra S et al. Dermatology Life Quality Index score in vitiligo and its impact on the treatment outcome. *Br J Dermatol* 2003; 148: 373–4.

37. Rumpf HJ, Lontz W, Uessler S. A self-administered version of a brief measure of suffering: first aspects of validity. *Psychother Psychosom* 2004; 73: 53–6.

38. Porter JR, Beuf AH, Lerner AB et al. The effect of vitiligo on sexual relationships. *J Am Acad Dermatol* 1990; 22: 221–2.

39. von der Werth JM, Jemec GBE. Morbidity in patients with hidradenitis suppurativa. *Br J Dermatol* 2001; 144: 809–13.

40. Jemec GBE, Heidenheim M, Nielsen NH. Hidradenitis suppurativa – characteristics and consequences. *Clin Exp Dermatol* 1996; 21: 419–23.

41. Updike J. *Self-Consciousness*. New York: Fawcett Crest, 1989: 42–80.

42. de Korte J, Sprangers MAG, Mombers FMC et al. Quality of life in patients with psoriasis: a systematic literature review. *J Investig Dermatol Symp Proc* 2004; 9: 140–7.

43. Lin PS, Koo JYM. Health-related quality-of-life instruments for psoriasis. In Koo JYM, CS Lee, eds. *Psychocutaneous Medicine*. New York: Marcel Dekker, 2003: 305–20.

44. Rapp SR, Feldman SR, Exum ML et al. Psoriasis causes as much disability as other major medical diseases. *J Am Acad Dermatol* 1999; 41: 401–7.

45. Gupta MA, Gupta AK. Age and gender differences in the impact of psoriasis on quality of life. *Inter J Dermatol* 1995; 34: 700–3.

46. Ramsay B, O'Reagan M. A survey of the social and psychological effects of psoriasis. *Br J Dermatol* 1988; 118: 195–201.

47. Ginsburg IH, Link BG. Feelings of stigmatization in patients with psoriasis. *J Am Acad Dermatol* 1989; 20: 53–63.

48. Finlay AY, Coles EC. The effect of severe psoriasis on the quality of life of 369 patients. *Br J Dermatol* 1995; 132: 236–44.

49. Gupta MA, Gupta AK. Psoriasis and sex: a study of moderately to severely affected patients. *Int J Dermatol* 1997; 36: 259–62.

50. Krueger G, Koo J, Lebwohl M et al. The impact of psoriasis on quality of life. Results of a 1998 National Psoriasis Foundation patient-membership survey. *Arch Dermatol* 2001; 137: 280–4.

51. Koo J. Population-based epidemiologic study of psoriasis with emphasis on quality of life assessment. *Dermatol Clin* 1996; 14: 485–96.

52. Badia X, Mascaro JM, Lozano R et al. Measuring health-related quality of life in patients with mild to moderate eczema and psoriasis: clinical validity, reliability and sensitivity to change of the DLQI. *Br J Dermatol* 1999; 141: 698–702.

53. Herd RM, Tidman MJ, Ruta DA et al. Measurement of quality of life in atopic dermatitis: correlation and validation of two different methods. *Br J Dermatol* 1997; 136: 502–7.

54. Kiebert G, Sorenson SV, Revicki D et al. Atopic dermatitis is associated with a decrement in health-related quality of life. *Int J Dermatol* 2002; 41: 151–8.

55. Lundberg L, Johanesson M, Silverdahl M et al. Quality of life, health-state utilities and willingness to pay in patients with psoriasis and atopic eczema. *Br J Dermatol* 1999; 141: 1067–75.

56. Shum KW, Lawton S, Williams HC et al. The British Association of Dermatologists audit of atopic eczema management in secondary

care. Phase 3: audit of service outcome. *Br J Dermatol* 2000; 142: 721–7.

57. Kurwa HA, Finlay AY. Dermatology in-patient management greatly improves life quality. *Br J Dermatol* 1995; 133: 575–8.

58. Linnet J, Jemec GB. An assessment of anxiety and dermatology life quality in patients with atopic dermatitis. *Br J Dermatol* 1999; 140: 268–72.

59. Drake L, Prendergast M, Maher R et al. The impact of tacrolimus ointment on health-related quality of life of adult and pediatric patients with atopic dermatitis. *J Am Acad Dermatol* 2001; 44: S65–72.

60. van Dorssen IE, Boom BW, Hengeveld MW. Experience of sexuality in patients with psoriasis and constitutional eczema. *Ned Tijdschr Geneeskd* 1992; 136: 2175–8.

61. Niemeier V, Winckelsesser T, Gieler U. Skin disease and sexuality. An empirical study of sex behavior on patients with psoriasis vulgaris and neurodermatitis in comparison with skin-healthy probands. *Hautarzt* 1997; 48: 629–33.

16.4 Cancer, sexuality and sexual expression

Michael L Krychman, Alison Amsterdam, Jeanne Carter

Introduction

Sexual concerns are common for patients during the diagnostic, treatment, and recovery phases of their cancer. As patients move away from the acute phase of illness, healthy sexual function is an important step toward re-establishing their sense of normalcy and well-being.[1] Approximately one-half of women who survive a breast or gynecologic malignancy report severe and long-lasting sexual problems.[2] Andersen[3] noted that sexual function morbidity occurs in up to 90% of women who have been diagnosed with cancer. Others have reported post-treatment sexual dysfunction incidences of 30–100%.[2,4] Most commonly, these patients report hypoactive desire disorder and/or dyspareunia (see Chapters 11.1–11.3 and 12.1–12.6 of this book).

Several physiologic and psychologic factors that are specific to oncology patients, such as radical surgical procedures, pelvic radiation, menopausal symptoms, premorbid sexual dysfunction, and negative self-concept, can increase sexual morbidity[5,6] (see Chapters 7.1–7.4). In addition, body-image concerns present a psychologic barrier to intimacy and sexual desire (see Chapter 6.1). Partner conflicts and relationship miscommunications can be severe and debilitating[7] (see Chapters 3.1–3.4).

Technological advances have changed clinicians' views of cancer; it is now often seen as chronic illness. The medical community continues to improve therapeutic modalities by focusing on techniques that not only improve cancer survival rates but also decrease long-lasting side effects. In many cases, cancer has come to resemble a chronic, rather than terminal, illness. Survivorship initiatives are now a critical focus of many cancer institutions and governmental organizations. Post-treatment resources as well as sexual health programs are integral parts of these survivorship initiatives.

Sexual function is identified by cancer survivors as a critical component of quality of life.[8,9] Typically, sexual problems have an acute onset, appearing shortly after treatment ends or when sexual intercourse is resumed. Studies investigating the interaction between a woman's sexual self-concept and her sexual function show that women with a negative sexual self-concept are more likely to have greater sexual morbidity.[8] Many patients report that sadness and grief emerge during sexual experiences, leaving them vulnerable to sexual dysfunction and a sense of sexual inadequacy.[1] Sexual dysfunction may threaten the integrity of relationships, limiting this source of social support at a time when it is most needed.[1,7,10] With a healthy sexual life, interpersonal relationships can be more intimate, romance can be more meaningful, and life can be approached with greater enthusiasm.[11]

Breast cancer

Treatment of breast cancer and sexual concerns

Introduction

Breast cancer is the most common malignancy in women (see Chapter 7.4).[12] In 2004, there were an estimated 215 990 new cases of female breast cancer, and approximately 40 110 women died from this disease.[13] Twenty-five percent of new cases present before menopause, and 15% present before the age of 45.[14–16] Women who receive a diagnosis of breast cancer often receive combination therapy with surgical excision, followed by chemotherapy,[17,18] radiation therapy, and/or hormonal manipulation. The duration, dosage, and type of therapy, along with the patient's age, are strong determinants of whether or not the patient will undergo premature ovarian failure and enter menopause.[19,20] The constellation of menopausal symptoms (hot flashes, sleep disturbances, vaginal atrophy, and mood alterations) can affect the sexual response cycle and have a major impact on patients' sexual function.

Surgery

Operative procedures can change structural anatomy and compromise the neurovascular integrity of organ systems critical to sexual responsiveness. The surgical removal of organs or tissues can also affect self-image and self-esteem. Several scientific reviews examined the impact of breast surgery on sexual function and concluded that conservative operative procedures and/or reconstruction played only minor roles in sexual function.[21,22] Patients who have undergone breast conservation surgery may be more likely to engage in breast caressing than women who have undergone mastectomy. However, the two groups do not differ with respect to coital frequency, ease of orgasm, or overall sexual satisfaction. Women who have undergone total mastectomy often have issues relating to altered body image and may develop a negative sexual self-schema. Some women complain of decreased breast stroking, while others may enjoy heightened erotic sensations when having their surgical incision caressed. Those who suffer from lymphedema, which can be painful and discomforting, complain of arm pain, paresthesia, skin sensitivity, swelling, and stiffness. These symptoms can limit mobility and affect sexual positioning. Compression garments, which are often used as standard therapy, may influence activities of daily living, such as sporting activity choices or wardrobe selection.

The BRCA1 and BRCA2 genes belong to a class of genes known as tumor suppressor genes. Like many other tumor suppressor genes, BRCA1 and BRCA2 regulate the cycle of cell division by keeping cells from growing. In particular, BRCA1 and BRCA2 inhibit the growth of cells that line the milk ducts in the breast. Up to 10% of women with breast cancer may have a genetic predisposition. The majority of these (55–70%) are caused by mutations in either BRCA1 or BRCA2 and are associated with an increased risk of ovarian cancer.[23] Some women may choose to undergo a risk-reducing bilateral salpingo-oophorectomy if they are found to be at increased risk of developing ovarian cancer. In a recent study by van Oostrom et al.,[24] women who underwent a risk-reducing bilateral salpingo-oophorectomy were negatively affected with respect to sexuality and body image. In addition to surgically induced menopausal symptoms, they may also develop the other symptoms mentioned previously.

As well as risk-reducing bilateral salpingo-oophorectomy, many women may choose to undergo prophylactic mastectomy on the breast unaffected by breast cancer. Fear of bilaterality or another primary breast cancer may influence women to proceed with this surgical intervention. Some women opt for reconstruction while others do not. The issues surrounding reconstruction, satisfaction with cosmetic result, and the impact on sexual function should not be underestimated.

Radiation

Radiation therapy often causes skin damage and changes, fatigue, alopecia, diarrhea, nausea, and vomiting. Many radiation-induced symptoms contribute to general malaise and may affect the sexual response cycle, most commonly libido. In addition, patients and/or their partners sometimes believe the myth of being "radioactive". Skin thickening and discoloration of the irradiated breast can affect self-esteem and sexual

function. Moreover, scars and fibrosis of the skin of the breast and axillary region can limit range of motion and contribute to lymphedema.

Chemotherapy

Many chemotherapeutic agents cause nausea, diarrhea, mucous membrane irritation, hot flashes, and vaginal atrophy. Hair loss on the head, eyebrows, eyelashes, and genitals is also common and may lead to changes in self-esteem and sexual attractiveness.

Premature ovarian failure can result from treatment with radiation and chemotherapy. The probability that a woman will enter menopause as a result of chemotherapy increases dramatically at the age of 35. More than 40% of women receiving chemotherapy at the age of 40 may become amenorrheic from treatment.[25] This may lead to menopausal symptoms, such as dyspareunia, vaginal atrophy, and hot flashes. This syndrome has been attributed to alterations in estrogen and/or androgen hormone levels. The vaginal lining may become thin and lose its pliability and elasticity, leading to pain with coital penetration. Patients may also complain of hypoactive desire disorder when their levels of sexual interest had been adequate prior to the entering of menopause. Hot flashes can affect mood and can lead to sleep disturbances and irritability, and ultimately affect the sexual response cycle.

Since breast cancer is often hormonally sensitive and tumor cells possess estrogen and progesterone receptors, treatment of menopausal sequelae with systemic hormone therapy is contraindicated. The use of alternative medications, including selective serotonin reuptake inhibitors, antihypertensive medications, and environmental modifications (rhythmic breathing, acupuncture, avoiding spicy foods and alcohol, and dressing in layers) is becoming more widely accepted to help decrease the intensity and severity of menopausal symptoms.

The potential for ovarian failure and cessation of menses can lead to a constellation of psychologic stressors surrounding the potential loss of reproductive capacity. One should not underestimate the impact that loss of reproductive capacity can have on a woman; the anxiety, stress, and mood changes can be severe when the survivor recognizes that she will no longer be able to bear children.

Hormonal therapy

Selective estrogen receptor modulators and aromatase inhibitors can exacerbate menopausal symptoms (see Chapters 5.5 and 6.1–6.3). Tamoxifen is a selective estrogen receptor modulator prescribed to block estrogen receptors in the breast, but it also acts as a weak estrogen agonist on the uterine lining. It has been linked to reports of vaginal dryness, excessive vaginal discharge, vaginal soreness, delayed orgasm, and changes in libido.[26] Studies that have looked at the impact of tamoxifen on sexual function have proven inconclusive.[22,27,28] According to the Breast Cancer Prevention Trial, only minor differences in sexual function were seen in women taking tamoxifen versus those not on the drug. In contrast, Mortimer et al.[29] noted no alteration in desire, arousal, or orgasm in patients on tamoxifen. However, more than 50% complained of vaginal discomfort and dyspareunia in spite of continued vaginal lubricant use. This was supported by Day et al.,[30] who reported that women on tamoxifen had increased vaginal discharge with associated genital pruritus.

Aromatase inhibitors are also used in women with various stages of breast cancer. In the pathway of steroidogenesis, the aromatase inhibitors halt the conversion of testosterone to estrogen, thus lowering levels of circulating estrogens. Although this is often a desired oncologic result, it may exacerbate menopausal sequelae and bone loss. There are limited data available that specifically address the impact of this class of drugs on sexuality and other parameters of quality of life.

Psychologic concerns

The psychologic adjustment of female survivors of breast cancer has been extensively studied (see Chapters 3.1–3.4). The literature shows that many women adapt well after they learn of their diagnosis. However, a subset of women report continued anxiety, depressive symptoms, distress concerning body image, fear of recurrence, post-traumatic stress disorder, and sexual problems even after they are treated and deemed free of disease.[25]

Sometimes, prior negative sexual experiences may be inappropriately linked to cancer and/or its recurrence. Past sexual behavior (involving promiscuity, extramarital affairs, and sexually transmitted diseases) may be erroneously attributed to the cancer diagnosis. Depression, changes in body image, and stress can contribute to female sexual difficulty.

Weight gain with chemotherapy and hormonal manipulation may also be an important determinant, and it has been linked to women's feelings of attractiveness.[31] Goodwin et al.[32] noted a mean overall weight gain of 1.6 kg, with an average gain of 2.5 kg, in newly diagnosed breast cancer patients receiving chemotherapy, and a 1.3-kg gain in those taking tamoxifen. This increase in weight was not explained by increased caloric intake or decreased physical activity.

The dynamics of relationships can be strained and changed with a cancer diagnosis and therapy. Women may have to take time off from their roles as caregivers and/or wage earners. This affects their partners, who often have to assume more or different responsibilities. This modification of roles can create marital and financial tension for the couple. Worries regarding partner abandonment and sexual rejection can affect dating and hinder the development of intimate relationships. Single women who are breast cancer survivors may also face unique stressors, such as negotiating new relationships while deciding when to disclose sensitive medical information regarding medical illnesses, fertilities issues, and longevity. Other forms of distress include fear of recurrence, early death, and disfigurement, as well as financial, employment and insurance concerns.

Gynecologic cancer and sexuality

Gynecologic cancer accounts for 13.4% of all cancers affecting women[33] (see Chapters 7.1–7.4). Tumors of the female reproductive tract include cancers of the vulva, vagina, cervix, uterus, fallopian tubes, and ovaries. Ten percent of cancer deaths in women can be attributed to gynecologic malignancy, with the largest proportion attributable to ovarian cancer. The side effects of treatment for gynecologic cancer may include hormonal disruption, reproductive failure, sexual morbidity, and bowel and bladder changes, in addition to the potential emotional and relationship alterations.[1,34–36]

The reproductive organs, the vagina, and the vulvar areas are obviously pivotal to female identity. Problems with these tissues and their function can adversely affect sexual interest and response. A woman's sense of her own reproductive status, regardless of her actual childbearing history, is central to her identity as well. Ovarian failure secondary to treatment signifies both reproductive loss and the advent of menopause, a state with its own profound significance, including a host of symptoms.[37]

A woman receiving treatment for gynecologic cancer may undergo multiple treatment modalities, often delivered sequentially.[1] Bowel resections and anterior/posterior exenterations for advanced gynecologic malignancy can result in stomas, colostomies, and ileoconduits for the patient. All these can affect self-image, and all have the potential of negative impact on the sexual response cycle. Many cancer institutes often have designated ostomy nurses who can help educate patients who have stomas or other medical appliances on proper hygiene and can provide useful techniques so that these devices do not hinder sexual activity.

Cancer treatment can negatively affect female fertility in several ways – by surgical removal of all or part of the reproductive organs; through chemotherapy with alkylating drugs, which can be toxic to the ovary; and/or by radiation therapy, which can cause sterility (permanent ovarian failure) by high doses to the ovaries.[34]

The trend over the past decade has been to provide adequate cancer treatment while also attempting to reduce long-term negative consequences.[38] One technique that has gained recognition in the field of gynecologic oncology is the fertility-preserving treatment of radical vaginal trachelectomy, with laparoscopic pelvic lymphadenectomy for treatment of early-stage cervical cancers.[39–44] The overall recurrence rate for women who have undergone laparoscopic vaginal radical trachelectomy is estimated to be 3%, which is not significantly different from radical hysterectomy.

With the prospect of radical surgery, a discussion regarding sexuality is often considered a low priority. However, sexual dysfunction is more than likely to occur, and adequate preparation may facilitate adjustment.[45] After radical surgery, women experience changes in body image, self-esteem, and feminine identity.[46–50] Significant loss in sexuality after pelvic exenteration has been reported in several studies.[45,49–52] Many women report no sexual interest or ability to achieve sexual satisfaction due to the loss of sexually responsive tissue.[47,51–53]

The correlation between radiation therapy and sexual dysfunction is documented in the literature.[54–56] Women experience problems with vaginal stenosis, loss of lubrication, and pain due to scarring after pelvic and vaginal radiation treatment.[56] Direct intense vaginal radiation can cause severe fibrosis, loss of elasticity, and decreased pliability of vaginal tissues and vaginal inflammation. It is not uncommon for women to be apprehensive about sexual activity for fear of bleeding and pain, symptoms that may be associated with initial diagnosis and may elicit concerns about recurrence.[57]

Chemotherapy can also negatively affect sexual function. As with breast cancer patients, pre- and perimenopausal women receiving chemotherapy may abruptly experience menopausal symptoms resulting from estrogen deficiency. These symptoms can contribute to sexual difficulties and quality-of-life impairments.[58]

Sexual rehabilitation and treatment

Sexual assessment and/or counseling are seldom provided in the oncology setting. There are a number of different reasons for this – time constraints and the need to prioritize critical and complex treatment issues, practitioner discomfort in initiating a conversation regarding sexual function, and patient discomfort or embarrassment with this subject.[9] However, a study exploring sexual function after gynecologic cancer treatment found that 78% of the women wanted to have a discussion about sexual matters but did not ask questions due to fear of rejection or inappropriate setting.[59] Questions that are important to keep in mind when assessing sexual difficulties include information about a woman's precancer sexual function, as well as her current sexual function. This will help to determine the degree of dysfunction experienced by the cancer patient. It is also very important to pay attention to a patient's relationship with her partner.[60]

The assessment of the cancer patient includes a detailed history, physical examination, psychologic examination, and, when appropriate, laboratory or radiologic evaluation. Sexual status, orientation, and past sexual experience are also assessed. Patients are encouraged to see both the gynecologist and psychologist for initial evaluations and follow-up surveillance. The Memorial Sloan-Kettering Cancer Center has established a comprehensive multidisciplinary program to help female cancer patients cope with sexual difficulties that may be experienced during or after cancer diagnosis and treatment. The model focuses on both the psychosexual and physical aspects of sexuality by providing an evaluation that includes both a medical examination by a gynecologist and a psychosexual evaluation by a psychologist.

Once the comprehensive evaluation is completed, a therapeutic management scheme is formulated. Several of the following issues should be addressed.

Treatment of systemic illness(es)

Cancer patients often have other underlying medical issues that can affect sexual health. A detailed history and physical examination can identify medical concerns that may been neglected in the midst of cancer therapy. Evaluation and treatment of chronic illnesses, such as undiagnosed anemia, uncontrolled hypertension, hypercholesterolemia, and/or underlying thyroid dysfunction, can identify a factor that may affect sexual function. Treatment of chronic illnesses can also improve general well-being, thus facilitating improved sexuality.

Identification of medications

Often cancer patients are on multiple medications. Some of them may directly affect the sexual response cycle and cause sexual dysfunction. Antidepressants and antihypertensive medications can alter sexual desire, arousal, and orgasm. Physicians and nurses should check pharmacologic guides to identify potential offending agents. If possible, specific antidotes to sexual side effects of these treatments, such as oral selective phosphodiesterase type 5 inhibitors,[61] can be prescribed alongside antidepressants and antihypertensives.

Behavioral modification

Patients with a cancer history are encouraged to make lifestyle modifications that improve quality of life. Well-balanced nutrition, active exercise regimes, discontinuing tobacco use, and minimizing alcohol consumption should be encouraged. Similarly, patients with sexual dysfunction are often given specific structured sexual tasks to help with specific sexual complaints. Examples include sensate focusing, guided imagery, relaxation techniques, and the exploration of sexual fantasies (see Chapters 11.1–11.5). Radiation-induced fatigue can be problematic for many patients, and many are encouraged to take frequent naps and plan sexual intimacy when well rested and fatigue is minimal. Alternate forms of sexual expression, such as erotic fantasy, mutual massage, intimate fondling and caressing, or manual, digital, or oral stimulation may be introduced. Patients and their partners may be encouraged to engage in alternative sexual positions. The missionary position may be the most uncomfortable sexual position for those with foreshortened vaginas. The side-to-side or female superior position may help limit deep pelvic thrusting to minimize vaginal discomfort during penetration.

Pain management

Chronic pain can influence a woman's sexual response and limit her interest in sexual activity (see Chapters 12.1–12.6). When pain and fatigue are minimal, sexual expression should be encouraged. Techniques, such as warm soaks and physical therapy, to help loosen and strengthen tense muscles should be encouraged. Guided imagery, meditation, deep-muscle relaxation, and avoidance of lethargy are options that can also be explored. Pain-management specialists should be consulted to adjust or reduce opioid regimens, add adjunctive analgesics, and modify dosing schedules to decrease fatigue and lethargy while maintaining adequate pain relief.

Education

Patients should be educated about their genital anatomy and on how a cancer diagnosis and therapeutic procedures can affect their sexual function. The debunking of many long-standing sexual myths and instruction by trained professionals are also an important part of the educational process (see Chapters 18.1 and 18.2). Take-home items, such as pamphlets, books, digital videodisks, videos, and other visual aids, can provide reinforcement and future reference. The American Cancer Society's booklet entitled *Cancer and Sexuality* is an excellent patient reference guide.

Psychotherapy

Certified sexual therapists are trained to deal with patients with cancer and with their associated body-image issues and changes in intimacy, sexuality, self-esteem, and mood. Sexual health patients are offered marital, individual, couples, and group therapy by trained therapists who deal with both oncologic and sexually based issues.

In general, most patients can benefit from brief psycho-sexual interventions, including education, counseling/support, and symptom management. Robinson[2] conducted an intervention to increase compliance with vaginal dilation recommendations – a recognized method of maintaining vaginal health and good sexual function after radiation therapy. The intervention consisted of a psychoeducational group providing information and support regarding effective use of dilators and lubricants. The women attending the intervention were significantly more likely to follow recommendations for vaginal dilation than the control group.[2] Local and national organizations relating to cancer support, sexual education, and fertility may also be useful references.

Pharmacologic intervention

Concerns regarding hormonal manipulation are common in breast and gynecologic cancer patients. Lifestyle changes (avoidance of spicy food, decreasing intake of caffeine and alcohol, and lowering the thermostat) and nonhormonal medications (selective serotonin reuptake inhibitors, clonidine patch, and megestrol acetate) can be used to help reduce systemic hot flashes when systemic estrogen is contraindicated or declined by patients. Patients with estrogen-sensitive tumors rarely agree to hormone therapy, probably due to the perception of an increased cancer risk associated with hormone therapy and/or

the side-effect profiles. On the other hand, some patients may choose the systemic hormones estrogen and progesterone; these can be prescribed for menopausal symptom managements for short durations (see Chapters 13.1–13.3).

Local use of nonmedicated, nonhormonal vaginal moisturizers, or vitamin E suppositories, can provide alternative relief for the symptoms of vaginal atrophy. It is recommended that these agents be used two or three times weekly. Nonmedicated, nonhormonal vaginal moisturizers and estrogen were compared in a randomized, control trial that demonstrated that nonmedicated, nonhormonal vaginal moisturizers improved vaginal cytology.[62] Patients are instructed to wear a light pad when using vitamin E suppositories, because it may stain undergarments. The use of water-based vaginal lubricants with intercourse is also encouraged. However, lubricants and moisturizers that contain microbicides, perfumes, coloration, and flavors should be discouraged because these additives may irritate the vaginal mucosa. Patients and oncologists more often use local estrogen for the treatment of vaginal atrophy. Many clinicians have chosen to use a 17-β-estradiol tablet, which is minimally absorbed into the systemic circulation.[63] Patients report that the tablets are also easy to use, less messy than cream preparations, and technically easier to insert than estrogen rings.[64] Studies are currently under way at several institutions to further investigate the safety of this agent in the breast cancer population. Other topical preparations include vaginal creams, rings, gels, and lotions.

The safety of androgen therapy in the breast cancer population has not been adequately studied. There is concern that the testosterone can be aromatized to estrogen, which may reactivate or promote further tumor growth. Many breast cancer cells have androgen receptors. The experimental testosterone transdermal matrix patch has proven to be effective for libido issues; however, further randomized, controlled trials and safety data are warranted before consideration in this patient population.

Sexual devices

For patients who have undergone pelvic surgery or radiation therapy, vaginal shortening, vaginal narrowing, and scar tissue can often impede penetration, causing dyspareunia. Vaginal dilators with water- or hormone-based lubricants can help lengthen and widen the vagina and loosen the scar tissue that contributes to the pain and discomfort associated with vaginal intercourse. Supportive behavioral therapy is instrumental for continued compliance. The prescribed regimen for dilator use is often individualized; some benefit from short (5 min) daily use, while others use dilators three times a week for 15 min per usage. Dilators should be cleansed with gentle soap and water, rinsed completely, and stored in a cool location between uses. Devices, such as the EROS clitoral stimulator, can be prescribed for patients who have had cervical cancer or other pelvic cancers, such as rectal and vaginal cancers. Preliminary data presented by Schroder et al.[65] at the 2003 annual conference of the International Society for the Study of Women's Sexual Health show promise that this device may be helpful in combating arousal difficulty after cervical cancer therapy.

Sexually active survivors should always be informed about sexually transmitted disease prevention, and condom use should always be encouraged.

Alternative and complementary medicine

Many nonmedical pharmacologic therapies have worrying and potentially detrimental side effects without scientific evidence of their benefit in alleviating sexual dysfunction. Although patients try agents such as chocolate, ginseng, oysters, and black cohosh to enhance sexuality, randomized, controlled clinical trials are needed to ensure patient safety and efficacy, and to demonstrate a low side-effect profile.

Consultation

Referral for an evaluation by a subspecialist may be appropriate for certain clinical conditions. Such consultants may include oncologists, social services providers, nutritionists, exercise therapists, and psychiatrists. A list of clinicians and ancillary staff who are sensitive to sexual issues should be readily available for patients who take part in sexual health programs.

In addition, pain and palliative care providers need to reassure patients and their partners that even at the end of life, when intercourse may not be feasible, intimacy and emotional closeness should be encouraged.

Conclusions

Quality-of-life concerns in survivorship are at the forefront of importance for both clinicians and patients. Sexual concerns and dysfunctions, during or after cancer therapy, are often overlooked. The diagnosis and treatment of malignancy are very complicated and stressful. Physical changes and psychologic issues are complex in a cancer patient suffering from sexual complaints. The goal of a comprehensive sexual health evaluation and the resulting therapy is to promote sexual health by fostering open communication, providing anticipatory guidance, and validating normalcy with respect to sexual thoughts and feelings. Individual treatment plans are created and implemented by the sexual health-care professional team to educate patients and survivors so they can enjoy fulfilling and pleasurable sexual repertoires with their partners during and after cancer therapy.

References

1. Schover LR. *Sexuality and Fertility After Cancer*. New York: Wiley, 1997.
2. Robinson JW. Sexuality and cancer. Breaking the silence. *Aust Fam Physician* 1998; 27(1–2): 45–7.
3. Andersen BL. How cancer affects sexual functioning. *Oncology (Huntingt)* 1990; 4: 81–8; discussion, 92–4.
4. Andersen BL, Woods XA, Copeland LJ. Sexual self-schema and sexual morbidity among gynecologic cancer survivors. *J Consult Clin Psychol* 1997; 65: 221–9.
5. Devita VT, Rosenberg SA, Hellman S, eds. *Cancer: Principles and Practices of Oncology*, 6th edn. Philadelphia: Lippincott Williams & Wilkins, 2000: 3032–49.
6. Andersen BL. Surviving cancer: the importance of sexual self-concept. *Med Pediatr Oncol* 1999; 33: 15–23.
7. Van de Wiel HB, Weijmer MC, Wouda EJ et al. Sexual functioning of partners of gynecologic oncology patients. *Sex Marital Ther* 1990; 1: 479–94.
8. Andersen BL, Cyranowski JM. Women's sexuality: behaviors, responses, and individual differences. *J Consult Clin Psychol* 1995; 63: 891–906.
9. Schover LR. Counseling cancer patients about changes in sexual function. *Oncol (Huntingt)* 1999; 13: 1585–92, 95–6.
10. Auchincloss SS. Sexual dysfunction in cancer patients: issues in evaluation and treatment. In JC Holland, JH Rowland, eds. *Handbook of Psycho-Oncology, Psychological Care of the Patient with Cancer*. New York: Oxford University Press, 1990: 383–413.
11. Laumann EO, Paik A, Rosen RC. Sexual dysfunction in the United States: prevalence and predictors. *JAMA* 1999; 281: 537–44.
12. National Cancer Institute. PDQ treatment summary for health professionals. Cervical cancer. Bethesda: National Institutes of Health, 2002. Available at http://cancernet.nci.gov/cgi-bin/srchcgi.exe?DBID=pdq&TYPE=search&SFMT=pdq_statement/1/0/0&Z208+208_00103H.
13. Jemal A, Tiwari RC, Murray T et al. Cancer statistics, 2004. *CA Cancer J Clin* 2004; 54: 8–29.
14. Hankey BF, Miller B, Curtis R et al. Trends in breast cancer in younger women in contrast to older women. *J Natl Cancer Inst Monogr* 1994; 16: 7–14.
15. Higgins S, Haffty BG. Pregnancy and lactation after breast conservation therapy for early breast cancer. *Cancer* 1994; 73: 2175–80.
16. Bines J, Oleske DM, Cobleigh MA. Ovarian function in premenopausal women treated with adjunctive chemotherapy for breast cancer. *J Clin Oncol* 1996; 14: 1718–29.
17. Hortobagyi GN. Progress in systemic chemotherapy of primary breast cancer: an overview. *J Natl Cancer Inst Monogr* 2001; 30: 72–9.
18. National Institute of Health Consensus Development Panel. National Institutes of Health Consensus Development Conference Statement. Adjuvant therapy for breast cancer. 1–3 November 2000. *J Natl Cancer Inst Monogr* 2001; 30: 5–15.
19. Meirow D, Epstein M, Lewis H et al. Administration of cyclophosphamide at different stages of follicular maturation in mice; effects on reproductive performance and fetal malformations. *Hum Reprod* 2001; 16: 632–7.

20. Goodwin PJ, Ennis M, Pritchard KI et al. Risk of menopause during the first year after breast cancer diagnosis. *J Clin Oncol* 1999; 17: 2365–70.

21. Schover LR. Sexuality and body image in younger women with breast cancer. *J Natl Cancer Inst Monogr* 1994; 16: 177–82.

22. Schover LR, Yetman RJ, Tuason LJ et al. Partial mastectomy and breast reconstruction. A comparison of their effects on psychosocial adjustment, body image, and sexuality. *Cancer* 1995; 75: 54–64.

23. Offit K. *Clinical Cancer Genetics*. New York: Wiley-Liss, 1998.

24. van Oostrom I, Meijers-Heijboer H, Lodder LN et al. Long-term psychological impact of carrying a BRCA1/2 mutation and prophylactic surgery: a 5-year follow-up study. *J Clin Oncol* 2003; 21: 3867–74.

25. Kornblith AB, Ligibel J. Psychosocial and sexual functioning of survivors of breast cancer. *Semin Oncol* 2003; 30: 799–813.

26. Kaplan HS. A neglected issue: the sexual side effects of current treatments for breast cancer. *J Sex Marital Ther* 1992; 18: 3–19.

27. Ganz PA, Rowland JH, Desmond K et al. Life after breast cancer: understanding women's health related quality of life and sexual functioning. *J Clin Oncol* 1998; 16: 501–14.

28. Meyerowitz BE, Desmond KA, Rowland JH et al. Sexuality following breast cancer. *J Sex Marital Ther* 1999; 25: 237–50.

29. Mortimer JE, Boucher L, Baty J et al. Effect of tamoxifen on sexual function in patients with breast cancer. *J Clin Oncol* 1999; 17: 1488–92.

30. Day R, Ganz PA, Costantino JP et al. Health-related quality of life and tamoxifen on breast cancer prevention. A report from the National Surgical Adjuvant Breast and Bowel Project P-1. *J Clin Oncol* 1999; 17: 2659–69.

31. Demark-Wahnefried W, Rimer BK, Winer EP. Weight gain in women diagnosed with breast cancer. *J Am Diet Assoc* 1997; 97: 519–26, 29.

32. Goodwin PJ, Ennis M, Pritchard KI et al. Adjuvant treatment and onset of menopause predict weight gain after breast cancer diagnosis. *J Clin Oncol* 1999; 17: 120–9.

33. Fields AL, Jones JG, Thomas GM et al. Gynecologic cancer. In RE Lenhard, RT Osteen, T Gansler, eds. *American Cancer Society's Clinical Oncology*. Altanta: The Society, 2001: 455–96.

34. American Cancer Society. *Cancer Facts and Figures*. Atlanta. Available at www.cancer.org.

35. Auchincloss S, McCartney C. Gynecologic cancer. In J Holland, ed. *Psych-Oncology*. New York: Oxford University Press, 1998: 359–70.

36. Byrne J. Infertility and premature menopause in childhood cancer survivors. *Med Pediatr Oncol* 1999; 33: 24–8.

37. Lagana L, McGarvey EL, Classen C et al. Psychosexual dysfunction among gynecologic cancer survivors. *J Clin Psych Med Setting* 2001; 8: 73–83.

38. Plante M, Roy M. Radical trachelectomy. *Oper Tech Gynecol Surg* 1997; 2: 187–99.

39. Dargent D, Brun JL, Roy M et al. Pregnancies following radical trachelectomy for invasive cervical cancer. *Gynecol Oncol* 1994; 52: 105.

40. Dargent D, Martin X, Sacchetoni A et al. Laparoscopic vaginal radical trachelectomy: a treatment to preserve the fertility of cervical carcinoma patients. *Cancer* 2000; 88: 1877–82.

41. Dargent D. Using radical trachelectomy to preserve fertility in early invasive cervical cancer. *Contemp Ob Gyn* 2000; 5: 23–49.

42. Roy M, Plante M. Pregnancies after radical vaginal trachelectomy for early-stage cervical cancer. *Am J Obstet Gynecol* 1998; 179: 1491–6.

43. Covens A, Shaw P, Murphy J et al. Is radical trachelectomy a safe alternative to a radical hysterectomy for patients with stage IA-B carcinoma of the cervix? *Cancer* 1999; 86: 2273–9.

44. Shepard JH, Mould T, Oram DH. Radical trachelectomy in early stage carcinoma of the cervix: outcome as judged by recurrence and fertility rates. *Br J Obstet Gynaecol* 2001; 100. 882–5.

45. Gleeson N, Baile W, Roberts WS et al. Surgical and psychosexual outcome following vaginal reconstruction with pelvic exenteration. *Eur J Gynaecol Oncol* 1994; 2: 89–95.

46. Andersen BL. Sexual functioning complications in women with gynecologic cancer. *Cancer* 1987; 60: 2123–8.

47. Andersen BL, Hacker NF. Psychosexual adjustment following pelvic exenteration. *Obstet Gynecol* 1983; 61: 331–8.

48. Corney RH, Crowther ME, Everett H et al. Psychosexual dysfunction in women with gynecologic cancer following radical pelvic surgery. *Br J Obstet Gynaecol* 1993; 100: 73–8.

49. Fisher SG. Psychosexual adjustment following total pelvic exenteration. *Cancer Nurs* 1979; 2: 219–25.

50. Sewell HH, Edwards DW. Pelvic genital cancer: body image and sexuality. *Front Radiat Ther Oncol* 1980; 14: 35–41.

51. Dempsey GM, Buchsbaum HJ, Morrison J. Psychosocial adjustment to pelvic exenteration. *Gynecol Oncol* 1975; 3: 325–34.

52. Vera MI. Quality of life following pelvic exenteration. *Gynecol Oncol* 1981; 12: 355–66.

53. Brown RS, Haddox V, Posada A et al. Social and psychological adjustment following pelvic exenteration. *Am J Obstet Gynecol* 1972; 114: 162–71.

54. Andersen BL, Andersen B, deProsse C. Controlled prospective longitudinal study of women with cancer: sexual functioning outcomes. *J Consult Clin Psychol* 1989; 57: 683–91.

55. Schover LR, Fife M, Gershenson DM. Sexual dysfunction and treatment for early stage cervical cancer. *Cancer* 1989; 63: 204–12.

56. Bruner DW, Lanciano R, Keegan M et al. Vaginal stenosis and sexual dysfunction following intracavitary radiation for the treatment of cervical and endometrial carcinoma. *Int J Radiat Oncol Biol Phys* 1993; 27: 825–30.

57. Gamel C, Hengeveld M, Davis B. Informational needs about the effects of gynecologic cancer on sexuality: a review of the literature. *J Clin Nurs* 2000; 9: 678–88.

58. Ganz PA, Coscarelli A, Fred C et al. Breast cancer survivors: psychosocial concerns and quality of life. *Breast Cancer Res Treat* 1996; 38: 183–99.

59. Lancaster J. Women's experiences of gynecologic cancer treated with radiation. *Curationis* 1993; 16: 37–42.

60. Schultz WC, Van de Wiel HB. Sexuality, intimacy, and gynecologic cancer. *J Sex Marital Ther* 2003; 29(Suppl 1): 121–8.

61. Shen WW, Urosevich Z, Clayton DO. Sildenafil in the treatment of female sexual dysfunction induced by selective serotonin reuptake inhibitors. *J Reprod Med* 1999; 44: 535–42.

62. Nachtigall LE. Comparative study: Replens versus local estrogen in menopausal women. *Fertil Steril* 1994; 61: 178–80.

63. *Vagifem* [package insert]. Denmark: Novo Nordisk A/S, 2003.

64. Rioux JE, Devlin MC, Gelfand MM et al. 17 beta estradiol vaginal tablet versus conjugated equine estrogen vaginal cream to relieve menopausal atrophic vaginitis. *Menopause* 2000; 7: 156–61.

65. Schroder M, Mell LK, Waggoner S et al. A clinical trial of EROS therapy for treatment of sexual dysfunction in irradiated cervical cancer patients. In International Society for the Study of Women's Sexual Health, 16–19 October 2003, The Netherlands. Abstract (Poster no. 15).

16.5 Spinal cord injury

Marca L Sipski, Craig J Alexander

Our understanding of the impact of spinal cord injury on female sexual response and sexuality is probably greater than that of any other physical problem (see Chapter 16.6 of this book). Despite this fact, our understanding of and ability to document the presence of sexual dysfunction in women with spinal cord injury remain in their infancy. Moreover, our ability to treat sexual dysfunction in this population remains unproven. The goal of this chapter is to review our knowledge of the natural history of spinal cord injury in relation to female sexual response and sexuality, to discuss the diagnosis of sexual dysfunction in the population of women with spinal cord injury, and to discuss potential treatment methods currently being evaluated.

The impact of spinal cord injury on female sexuality

A number of questionnaire studies have addressed the impact of injury on women's sexuality.[1-4] As this population is heterogeneous in their neurologic injuries, these data are mainly useful in issues such as frequency of, patterns of, and satisfaction with sexual activities. The frequency of sexual activity has been shown to decrease in women after spinal cord injury.[2] Additionally, sexual satisfaction has been shown to decrease in women after spinal cord injury.[1,4] Women have not demonstrated a significant change in their sexual activities after spinal cord injury;[1] however, more recent unpublished data reveal that a surprisingly low percentage of women with spinal cord injuries masturbate. This information should be considered when coming up with a plan for treatment of sexual concerns in women with spinal cord injury.

What is a spinal cord injury?

Before any discussion of the impact of spinal cord injury on female sexual response, one must understand the effects of spinal cord injury (see Chapters 4.1–4.4). Spinal cord injury can occur at any level of the spinal cord and can produce varying degrees of neurologic dysfunction.[5] Depending on where the injury occurs, the person will sustain either tetraplegia, which implies some loss of neurologic function in both the arms and legs, or paraplegia, which implies only loss of neurologic function in the legs and potentially torso. Spinal cord injuries are classified according to the International Standards for Spinal Cord Injury (Figure 16.5.1).[6] These standards allow us to describe a specific level of neurologic injury, the degree of motor and sensory dysfunction, and the pattern of neurologic dysfunction as determined by physical examination.

Performance of the spinal cord injury examination

A detailed neurologic assessment, using the international standards,[6] is of paramount importance in accurately assessing the impact of spinal cord injury on a woman's sexual response. Specifically, one should document whether the injury is complete or not by determining whether the person has voluntary rectal contraction and/or sensation. Those with incomplete injuries would have one or both of these functions present, while those with complete injuries should have neither. Additionally, one should document whether the ability to perceive pinprick and light touch sensation in the T11–L2 dermatomes has been preserved, and quantify how much function is preserved, utilizing the international standards.[6] The score for the remaining sensation in the area is a 2-point score completed for both light touch and pinprick sensation with 0 being no sensation preserved; 1, partial sensation; and 2, normal sensation. Scores are tested on both sides of the body, so that a person could have a score of 0-32 for the combined scores in both dermatomes.

The impact of the spinal cord injury on reflex function in the sacral region is also an important consequence of the injury. Spinal cord injury can result in upper motor neuron (damage to the first neuron coming down from the brain to the cord) or lower motor neuron dysfunction (damage of the second neuron going directly to the muscle) in this area. The type of injury that affects the sacral segments is determined by testing the bulbocavernosus reflex; that is, by inserting the finger into the rectum and then pulling on the pubic hairs or stimulating the clitoris.

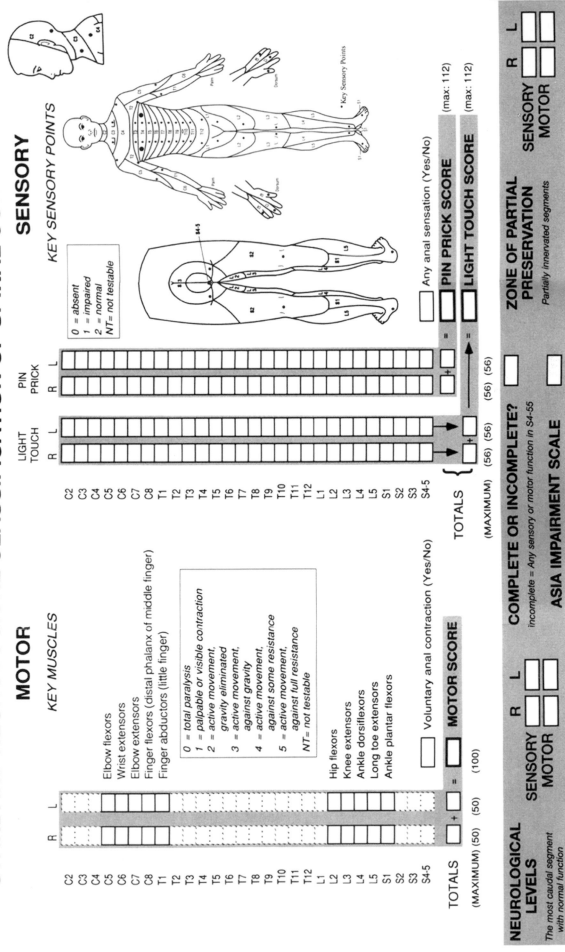

Figure 16.5.1

Table 16.5.1. Female spinal sexual function classification

Function	Response	Criteria
A: Sexual dysfunction	Present	Desire disorders
		Arousal disorders
		Orgasm disorders
		Pain disorders
	Absent	
B: Psychogenic genital arousal	Intact/normal	SS = 32
		T11–L2
	Likely	SS = 16–31
		T11–L2
	Unlikely	SS = 1–15
		T11–L2
	Not possible	SS = 0
		T11–L2
C: Reflex genital arousal	Intact	Normal or hyperactive BC and anal wink reflexes
	Possible	Hypoactive or partially intact BC and/or anal wink reflexes
	Not possible	Absent BC and anal wink reflexes
D: Orgasm	Not possible	No S2–S5 sensation; absent BC and anal wink reflexes
	Possible	All other neurologic lesions

Reprinted with permission from Sipski and Alexander.[22] (BC = Bulbocavernosus reflex; SS = sensation score)

Women with upper motor neuron injury demonstrate a quick contraction about the finger, women without neurologic injuries also demonstrate a contraction, and women with lower motor neuron complete injuries do not have any reflex contraction around the examiner's finger. Persons with incomplete injuries should have some voluntary rectal contraction preserved regardless of whether the injury is upper motor neuron or lower motor neuron in nature.

It is important to note that the standards do not contain a description of the effects of the spinal cord injury on autonomic function. Consequently, although persons may have "complete" injuries – defined by the absence of sensory and motor function going to the anal area – they may still perceive internal, autonomically driven sensory experiences, such as menstrual cramps, neurogenic pain, and sometimes vague sensation of the need to move their bowels. In addition to damage to external neurologic function, there are various effects on other organ systems as a result of spinal cord injury. For instance, patients with spinal cord injury may suffer from neurogenic bowel and bladder dysfunction, both with characteristics of upper motor neuron or lower motor neuron injuries.

Effect of spinal cord injury on female sexual response

The effect of spinal cord injury on female sexual response has been evaluated in numerous laboratory-based studies.[7–10] The neurologic control of sexual response relies on two separate pathways to control genital sexual arousal: a psychogenic pathway and a reflex pathway. Thus, the impact of spinal cord injury on sexual response depends on which of these pathways is affected. In order to understand most clearly and thereby treat the dysfunction, one should consider the individual and the specific pattern of injury.

In women with all levels of spinal cord injury, the control of psychogenic arousal has been studied in a laboratory with vaginal pulse amplitude[11] as a means to record genital vasocongestion. In women with all levels of injury, the ability to achieve psychogenic genital arousal has been shown to be related to the preservation of the ability to perceive pinprick and light touch sensation in the T11–L2 dermatomes.[6] Those women with combined scores of 24–32 in these dermatomes were significantly more likely to demonstrate psychogenic genital vasocongestion than women with scores of 9–23. Moreover, women with scores of 9–23 were significantly more likely to achieve psychogenic vasocongestion than those with scores of 0–8. Practically speaking, these dermatomes include the area between the umbilicus and the middle of the thigh, so that women with spinal cord injury that have better sensation in these areas have a greater likelihood of achieving genital arousal through psychogenic stimulation, such as watching sensual movies, kissing, or hearing or reading erotic passages.

The control of reflex arousal has also been studied in the laboratory. Women with spinal cord injury who were first subjected to psychogenic stimulation and then to manual stimulation were shown to have further increases in their level of genital arousal by manual stimulation regardless of whether they had concomitant increases in their level of subjective arousal.[3,5] This is thought to be evidence of the maintenance of reflex genital arousal in women with upper motor neuron injuries affecting their sacral spinal segments. Further research also compared the effect of the addition of manual stimulation to psychogenic stimulation in women with upper motor neuron versus lower motor neuron injuries affecting their sacral segments.[10]

Results revealed greater increases in vaginal pulse amplitude (see Chapter 10.1) and thus genital vasocongestion in the group with upper motor neuron injuries; however, these findings were not statistically significant. Despite the lack of significance in these results, the overall psychophysiologic data tend to validate the hypothesis that reflex lubrication should be preserved in women with upper motor neuron injuries affecting their sacral segments, and that women with lower motor neuron incomplete injuries should still have partial preservation of reflex lubrication. The only subset of women who should not have the potential for reflex lubrication would be women with complete lower motor neuron injuries.

The ability to achieve orgasm in women with spinal cord injury has also been assessed via questionnaire studies and in the laboratory.[12,13] In the largest laboratory-based series to date,[6] the ability to achieve orgasm was found to be significantly diminished in women with complete lower motor neuron injuries affecting their sacral spinal cord (see Chapter 6.4). Women with all other levels and degrees of spinal cord injury were significantly less likely than able-bodied control subjects to achieve orgasm. Fifty-five percent of women with spinal cord injury reported the ability to achieve orgasm as opposed to 100% of able-bodied control subjects, and 44% of spinal cord injury subjects were orgasmic in the laboratory as opposed to 100% of able-bodied controls. These results were taken as evidence that the occurrence of orgasm depends on the presence of an intact sacral arc.

The authors also noted that when two of the investigators were masked to the subjects' descriptions of orgasms they were unable to distinguish whether the women had complete or incomplete spinal cord injury, or were able-bodied control subjects. This finding, in addition to the above, led to the hypothesis that orgasm is a reflex response of the autonomic nervous system that can be either facilitated or inhibited by cerebral input.

Other recent research also points to the fact that orgasm may be associated with a pattern generator in the spinal cord. The suggestion has been made that an ejaculation generator is present in the spinal cord[14] of male rats. These researchers also documented activation of a subset of lumbar spinothalamic neurons after copulatory behavior in male, but not in female, rats.[15] This finding in male rats is similar to that of the urogenital reflex that is found in spinalized, anesthetized animals above T9. It comprises rhythmic firing of the hypogastric, pelvic, and pudendal motor nerves;[16,17] and appears to be similar to the finding of orgasm in women with spinal cord injury. The peripheral activity displayed during the urogenital reflex strongly resembles that seen during human orgasm.[18] Vaginal, uterine, and anal sphincter rhythmic contractions are present in both the urogenital reflex and orgasm, and both are relatively insensitive to gonadal hormones.

The characteristics of orgasm in able-bodied versus spinal cord injury subjects were also analyzed. Despite previous reports that nongenital stimulation is often used as a means to achieve orgasm, only one woman in this study[10] chose nongenital stimulation in combination with genital stimulation. The average latency to orgasm was significantly greater in spinal cord injury than able-bodied subjects (26 vs 16 min). The heart rate, systolic blood pressure, and respiratory rate at orgasm compared to baseline were significantly greater for both spinal cord injury and able-bodied subjects; however, there were no significant differences between groups at any time period. Diastolic blood pressure was similar in both groups of subjects at orgasm and baseline; moreover, there was no significant increase in diastolic blood pressure at orgasm versus baseline.

The authors hypothesized that if the neurologic potential to achieve orgasm exists in approximately 50% of women with all levels of spinal cord injuries, then those women who did not achieve orgasm must have some intervening variable precluding them from achieving orgasm. Lack of education and interfering psychologic issues were mentioned as possible problems, in addition to the overall negative viewpoint in the medical literature that has previously existed.[19,20] Therefore, the authors concluded that women with spinal cord injury should be instructed that a longer and more intense degree of genital stimulation may be necessary to achieve orgasm, and that the development of treatment methods to remediate orgasmic dysfunction is warranted.

Documentation of sexual dysfunction in women with spinal cord injury

The above documentation of the impact of spinal cord injury on sexual response provides a framework for understanding how the injury affects sexual response (see Chapters 10.5 and 10.6). But it does not give us any information about whether a woman with a spinal cord injury has sexual dysfunction. According to the International Consensus Development Conference on Female Sexual Dysfunction,[21] in order for patients to have sexual dysfunction they must complain of personal distress. Therefore, a woman with spinal cord injury could have alterations in her sexual response related to her injury but still not complain of distress and therefore not have sexual dysfunction. In addition, a woman with spinal cord injury could have no injury-related alterations in her sexual response but still complain of sexual distress and thus suffer from sexual dysfunction. In order to remedy this lack of a means of documentation, the "female spinal sexual function classification" was proposed.[22] This classification system relies on previous research to define four categories of sexual function after spinal cord injury, and document their presence, the associated characteristics, and which aspects of the neurologic examination should be used to determine the likely response (Table 16.5.1). From the neurologic examination and detailed history, one should be able to document the expected effects of the injury on specific components of sexual response and also document whether the subject reports any sexual dysfunction. This latter issue becomes especially important when the issue of clinical trials for remediation of sexual dysfunction after spinal cord injury is addressed. The female spinal sexual function classification is currently being utilized in a study of women with spinal cord injuries and multiple sclerosis in order to assess its utility for documentation of the remaining sexual function and presence or absence of sexual dysfunction in women with spinal cord injury.

Improving sexual responsiveness

The PLISSIT model[23] offers specific suggestions for initiating and maintaining discussions for sexual counseling. The PLISSIT model describes the process of permission, limited information, specific suggestions, and intensive therapy/ counseling. This is a useful model for describing how to address the issue of talking about sexuality with women with spinal cord injury, and it underscores the importance of education about changes in sexual response and sexuality that occur after spinal cord injury. Education about the impact of injury on sexual response is the first and probably most important thing that needs to be done to improve the sexual responsiveness of women with spinal cord injury. In light of this need, a consumer-friendly video about the impact of spinal cord injury on female sexual response was recently made available.[24]

Education alone will probably help a number of women with spinal cord injury to improve their sexual response. However, some women will need more intensive therapy.

A number of studies have begun to develop therapies to improve sexual responsiveness in women with spinal cord injury. The majority of these studies have been based on treatments previously used in able-bodied women, although one drug study was based upon testing the efficacy of medications utilized in men.[25]

The first series of therapies can be described as psychologic in nature. False-positive feedback was used in a laboratory-based study[26] to increase the level of sexual arousal in a sample of women with spinal cord injury. It is unknown whether these women complained of sexual dysfunction or not. In this study, false-positive feedback was shown to increase psychogenic arousal in both complete and incomplete spinal cord injury. However, genital arousal was increased only in women with incomplete injuries who had preservation of sensory function in the T11–L2 dermatomes. This study concluded that psychologically based treatments may help to improve function in this subset of women with spinal cord injury.

In another study, the same authors investigated the impact of an anxiety-provoking video on sexual arousal.[27] Subjects viewed two erotic videos, one of which was preceded by exposure to a neutral video, while the other was preceded by exposure to an anxiety-provoking video. In subjects with impaired genital responsiveness to psychogenic erotic stimulation (T11–L2

combined American Spinal Injury Association scores less than 23), anxiety pre-exposure resulted in a small increase in genital responsiveness to erotic stimulation as compared to neutral pre-exposure. For those subjects who had mostly intact genital responsiveness (spinal cord injury subjects with T11–L2 combined American Spinal Injury Association scores greater than 23) and able-bodied subjects, anxiety pre-exposure resulted in decreased genital responsiveness as compared to neutral pre-exposure. The authors concluded that these results document the potential usefulness of manipulation of the sympathetic nervous system in subjects with impaired, but not absent, ability to achieve psychogenic genital vasocongestion. In addition, the authors noted that these data are further evidence of the regulatory role of the sympathetic nervous system in psychogenic arousal.

Only one published study has looked at the effects of medications on sexual responsiveness after spinal cord injury in females. In a laboratory-based, double-blind, crossover-design study,[17] the effects of sildenafil 50 mg versus placebo were compared on vaginal pulse amplitude, subjective arousal, and autonomic function. Subjects underwent a 78-min protocol in which audiovisual erotic stimulation and audiovisual erotic combined with self-applied manual stimulation were experienced. A statistically significant increase in subjective arousal was noted with the use of the medication in addition to the sexual stimulation conditions. A borderline significant effect of drug administration was noted on vaginal pulse amplitude. Modest increases in heart rate (±5 beats/min) and blood pressure (±4 mmHg) were also documented.

Although the above studies begin to outline some possible methods of treatment for sexual arousal dysfunction in women with spinal cord injury, data are still preliminary and have yet to be translated into clinical utility. Other studies currently in progress will examine the effect of medical sympathetic stimulation on sexual responsiveness. As new medications, such as the testosterone patch, become available, it will be warranted to assess their effects on sexual desire and arousal dysfunction after spinal cord injury.

With regard to orgasmic dysfunction after spinal cord injury, we are unaware of any previous clinical trials designed to treat this problem. If the orgasm is a reflex response of the autonomic nervous system and if a spinal pattern generator exists, it may be possible to train the pattern generator. This concept is similar to work that is being done on ambulation training[28,29] and is the foundation for a study to test the efficacy of EROS therapy[30] versus vibratory stimulation that is currently underway. Both of these therapies that are designed to stimulate a reflex response should be useful to treat sexual dysfunction in women with spinal cord injury. Until the results of this research are available, either method could be considered potentially useful as a supplement to targeted sexual education in women with spinal cord injury and sexual dysfunction.

As compared to other neurologic injuries, our knowledge of the impact of spinal cord injury on female sexual response is relatively advanced. We have recently begun a study of predominantly women with spinal multiple sclerosis to see whether the impact on sexual response in women with spinal lesions as a result of multiple sclerosis is similar to that of spinal cord injury. It is hoped that our knowledge about the impact of spinal cord injury on female sexual response can serve as a model to study not only multiple sclerosis but also other neurologic disabilities.

Acknowledgment

This work was supported in part by funds from the US National Institutes of Health, R01 HD 30149.

References

1. Sipski ML, Alexander CJ. Sexual activities, response and satisfaction in women pre- and post-spinal cord injury. *Arch Phys Med Rehabil* 1993; 74: 1025–9.
2. Charlifue SW, Gerhart KA, Menter RR et al. Sexual issues of women with spinal cord injuries. *Paraplegia* 1992; 30: 192–9.
3. Jackson AB, Wadley V. A multicenter study of women's self-reported reproductive health after spinal cord injury. *Arch Phys Med Rehabil* 1999; 80: 1420–8.
4. Fisher TL, Laud PW, Byfield MG et al. Sexual health after spinal cord injury: a longitudinal study. *Arch Phys Med Rehabil* 2002; 83: 1043–51.
5. Staas WE, Formal CS, Freedman MK et al. *Spinal Cord Injury and Spinal Cord Injury Medicine in Rehabilitation Medicine: Priniciples and Practice*, 3rd edn. Philadelphia: DeLisa & Gans, 1993: 1259–91.
6. American Spinal Injury Association. *International Standards for Neurological and Functional Classification of Spinal Cord Injury*, revised. Chicago: American Spinal Injury Association, 1992.
7. Sipski ML, Alexander CJ, Rosen RC. Physiologic parameters associated with psychogenic sexual arousal in women with complete spinal cord injuries. *Arch Phys Med Rehabil* 1995; 76: 811–18.
8. Sipski ML, Alexander CJ, Rosen RC. Physiologic parameters associated with the performance of a distracting task and genital self-stimulation in women with complete spinal cord injuries. *Arch Phys Med Rehabil* 1996; 77: 419–24.
9. Sipski ML, Alexander CJ, Rosen RC. Physiologic parameters associated with psychogenic sexual arousal in women with incomplete spinal cord injuries. *Arch Phys Med Rehabil* 1997; 78: 305–13.
10. Sipski ML, Alexander CJ, Rosen RC. The neurologic basis of sexual arousal and orgasm in women: effects of spinal cord injury. *Ann Neurol* 2001; 49: 35–44.
11. Lann E, Everaerd W. Physiological measures of vaginal vasocongestion. *Int J Impot Res* 1998; 10: 107–10.
12. Sipski ML, Alexander CJ, Rosen RC. Orgasm in women with spinal cord injuries: a laboratory-based assessment. *Arch Phys Med Rehabil* 1995; 76: 1097–1102.
13. Whipple B, Gerdes CA, Komisaruk BR. Sexual response to self-stimulation in women with complete spinal cord injury. *J Sex Res* 1996; 33: 231–40.
14. Truitt WA, Coolen LM. Identification of a potential ejaculation generator in the spinal cord. *Science* 2002; 297(5586): 1566–9.
15. Truitt WA, Shipley MT, Veening JG et al. Activation of a subset of lumbar spinothalamic neurons after copulator behavior in male but not female rats. *J Neurosci* 2003; 23: 325–31.
16. Chung SK, McVary KT, McKenna KE. Sexual reflexes in male and female rats. *Neurosci Lett* 1988; 94: 343–8.
17. McKenna KE, Chung SK, McVary KT. A model for the study of sexual function in anesthetized male and female rats. *Am J Physiol* 1991; 30: R1276–85.
18. Bohlen JG, Held JP, Sanderson MO et al. The female orgasm: pelvic contractions. *Arch Sex Behav* 1982; 11: 367–86.
19. Money J. Phantom orgasm in the dreams of paraplegic men and women. *Arch Gen Psychiatry* 1960; 3: 373–82.
20. Fitting M, Salisbury S, Davies N et al. Self-concept and sexuality of spinal injured women. *Arch Sex Behav* 1978; 7: 143–56.
21. Basson R, Berman J, Burnett A et al. Report of the international consensus development conference on female sexual dysfunction: definitions and classification. *J Urol* 2000; 163: 888–93.
22. Sipski, ML, Alexander CJ. Documentation of the impact of spinal cord injury on female sexual function: the female spinal sexual function classification. *Top Spinal Cord Inj Rehabil* 2002; 8: 63–73.
23. Annon J. *The Behavioral Treatment of Sexual Problems: Brief Therapy*. New York: Harper & Row, 1976.
24. Sipski ML. *Women's Sexuality After SCI: Understanding the Changes and Finding Ways to Respond*. Video, 2003.
25. Sipski ML, Rosen RC, Alexander CJ et al. Sildenafil effects on sexual and cardiovascular responses in women with spinal cord injury. *Urology* 2000; 55: 812–15.
26. Sipski ML, Rosen R, Alexander CJ et al. A controlled trial of positive feedback to increase sexual arousal in women with spinal cord injuries. *NeuroRehabilitation* 2000; 15: 145–53.
27. Sipski ML, Rosen RC, Alexander CJ et al. Sexual responsiveness in women with spinal cord injuries: differential effects of anxiety-eliciting stimulation. *Arch Sex Behav* 2004; 33: 295–302.
28. Wernig A, Muller S, Nanassy A et al. Laufband therapy based on "rules of spinal locomotion" is effective in spinal cord injured persons. *Eur J Neurosci* 1995; 7: 823–9.
29. Wernig A, Nanassy A, Muller S. Maintenance of locomotor abilities following Laufband (treadmill) therapy in para- and tetraplegic persons: follow-up studies. *Spinal Cord* 1998; 36: 744–9.
30. Billups KL, Berman L, Berman J et al. A new non-pharmacological vacuum therapy for female sexual dysfunction. *J Sex Marital Ther* 2001; 27: 1435–41.

16.6 Neurologic disorders: female neurosexology

P O Lundberg

Introduction

The mechanisms behind sexual dysfunction in women with neurologic disorders are of three different types. Firstly, the dysfunction may result from specific lesions to those parts of the nervous system that are directly involved in sexual physiology (see Chapters 4.1–4.4 of this book). Secondly, the dysfunction may result from lesions in the nervous system that impair cognition, movements, and communication (see Chapter 5.3). Thirdly, the dysfunction may refer to psychologic, social, and cultural issues (see Chapters 3.1–3.4). As we will see from the following, these mechanisms may work entirely differently in many well-known neurologic disorders.

Neurologic disorders may be congenital, leading to defect development of sexual anatomy and physiology. In such a case as well as in disorders starting before puberty, pubertal development may be retarded or missing. Defect anatomic development and hormone insufficiency may also lead to lack of organization of those parts of the nervous system involved in sexual physiology.

In evaluating a patient with a disease or a handicap, issues such as attraction and partner relationship have to be considered. The sexual prognosis is often highly dependent upon "sex before", that is, how well the patient functioned sexually and how sexually experienced the patient was before the start of the disease or time of physical trauma.

Central and peripheral nervous system

From a neurologic point of view, female sexual physiology is largely dependent upon which sensory (afferent) mechanisms (Table 16.6.1) are actually stimulated in the women and what kinds of effects (efferent mechanisms) (Table 16.6.2) the sexual stimulation has in the body.[1] This model is of essential importance for clinical understanding of the many different types of sexual symptoms summarized in the concept of female sexual dysfunction.

Our knowledge about what we could call "peripheral" sexual physiology is rather good. However, we know much less about what is actually going on in the brain, and where, during sexual arousal and activity. Here we have to rely on data from a limited number of patients with more or less precisely localized lesions of the brain. Now we also have a few studies with modern imaging techniques, such as positron-emission tomography (PET) and functional magnetic resonance imaging (fMRI) of the brain.[2]

Hypothalamo–pituitary disorders and malformations

In women with hypothalamo-pituitary disorders and malformations, amenorrhea and infertility are usually the problems that

Table 16.6.1. Stimulation of sexual arousal in women

Visual stimulation – through the eyes and optic nerves to the brain

Olfactory stimulation (pheromones) – through the nose and the olfactory nerves to the rhinencephalon of the brain

Breast stimulation – sensory impulses via segmental peripheral nerves and the thoracic part of the spinal cord to the brain

Clitoral stimulation – sensory impulses through the pudendal nerve via the cauda and the spinal cord to the brain

Vaginal stimulation – sensory impulses through the pelvic nerves via the spinal cord to the brain and possibly also through the vagus nerve to the brainstem

Table 16.6.2. Sexual efferent mechanisms in women

A. From the brainstem via the spinal cord
1. Through the sympathetic nervous system to the hypogastric nerves and pelvic plexus to the vaginal vessels, resulting in lubrication
2. Through the sacral parasympathetic nerves to the pelvic plexus and the cavernosal nerves, giving erection of the clitoris and increased blood flow in the spongious tissue
3. Through the sacral parasympathetic nerves to the pelvic plexus and peripheral nerves to glandular tissue (the paraurethral and Bartholin's glands), resulting in secretion
4. Through the spinal nerves S3–4 to the pelvic floor muscles, resulting in contractions during orgasm

B. From the hypothalamus
1. To the posterior pituitary, resulting in oxytocin release and giving uterine contractions
2. To the anterior pituitary, giving a number of hormonal effects

take the patient to the doctor (see Chapters 6.1 and 7.3). In women aged 20–60 years with morphologically verified hypothalamo-pituitary disorders,[3] two-thirds noticed absence of, or a considerable and troublesome decrease in, sexual desire. This problem was much more common among women with hyperprolactinemia than among those with normal serum prolactin.[4] Most of these women also had amenorrhea as well as problems with lubrication and/or orgasms.

Besides pituitary adenomas (Figs 16.6.1 and 16.6.2), hormone-producing or nonfunctional, there is a large group of other types of tumors and pathologic processes in the hypothalamo-pituitary region also causing decrease in sexual desire, decreased lubrication, and anorgasmia. Among the tumors, craniopharyngiomas and meningiomas are the most important in women.

Congenital malformations of the pituitary, visualized as dystopia of the posterior pituitary and/or dysplasia of the sella turcica, the olfactogenital dysplasia with anosmia and the septo-optic dysplasia also with malformations of the optic nerves, all with hypogonadotropic hypogonadism, are easily diagnosed with modern computed tomography or magnetic resonance imaging.

There are a number of acquired hypothalamo-pituitary disorders, such as spontaneous pituitary apoplexy, pituitary bleeding during labor (Sheehan's syndrome), sequela after traumatic hypothalamic bleeding, ruptured arterial aneurysm, and acute asphyxia. Spontaneously arrested infantile hydrocephalus, delayed radiation necrosis, meningo-encephalitis, sarcoidosis, and lymphocytic hypophysitis are further examples of hypogonadotropic hypogonadism with sexual dysfunction.[5]

Cerebellar disorders

In a number of families with cerebellar atrophy and ataxia, hypogonadism of the hypogonadotropic form, thus indicating hypothalamo-pituitary insufficiency, has been found.[6–8] There is evidence of a hypothalamic gonadotropin-releasing hormone deficiency. This is in contrast to the hypergonadotropic hypogonadism indicating primary ovarian failure in, for example, mitochondrial disorders or sex-chromosome abnormalities. The women present with primary amenorrhea, lack of secondary sexual characteristics, and absence of sexual desire. The mechanism behind these syndromes is unknown.

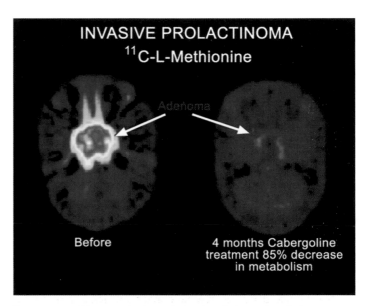

Figure 16.6.1. A huge, prolactin-producing, invasively growing pituitary adenoma visualized by positron-emission tomography (PET) with ^{11}C-L-methionine. "Before" indicates before treatment. The image to the right shows the result of 4-month treatment with the dopamine agonist carbergoline. Now only traces of the tumor remain. After further treatment, the tumor entirely disappeared.

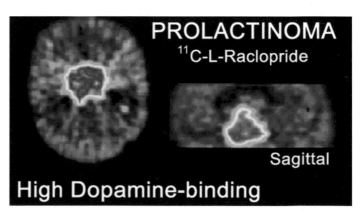

Figure 16.6.2. High dopamine binding of the same tumor as in Fig. 16.6.1, visualized by PET with the dopamine agonist ^{11}C-L-raclopride, indicating that the tumor should be treated with dopamine agonists. Left horizontal, right sagittal image of the brain with tumor.

Traumatic brain injuries and encephalopathies

Disability and cognitive impairment occur rather often after traumatic brain injury. Sexual impairment is not rare, as a consequence of either the cerebral lesions or psychologic factors.[9] Both decreased and increased sexual desire have been reported in women. Lesions of the frontal, temporal, and limbic cortex are the most important. Little is known about female sexual arousal after such injuries. However, in women, endocrine abnormalities are the most sensitive predictors of sexual dysfunction.[10]

Stroke

Because of the vascular anatomy, infarcts or bleedings in stroke patients are usually not localized to those parts of the brain directly involved in sexual physiology (see Chapter 7.3). Thus, the high frequency of sexual dysfunction and difficulty in desire, orgasm, and sexual activity in women who were sexually active before stroke can usually be explained in terms of coping.[11,12] Orgasmic dysfunction is seen in three-quarters of the females.[13] Decreased desire, sexual arousal, and satisfaction are related particularly to the presence of hemisensory symptoms.[14]

Sexual activity can provoke vascular catastrophes, such as subarachnoidal hemorrhage,[15] or transitory ischemic attacks, such as transient global amnesia.[16]

Epilepsy

Epilepsy and sexuality have many interconnections. Sexual activity can provoke an epileptic fit. For example, hyperventilation during sexual encounters may in itself provoke an attack. Reflex mechanisms from the cortical area corresponding to the genitalia could also trigger a partial epileptic attack. Sexual fantasies as well as genital stimuli (masturbation or orgasm)[17] are typical examples of triggering phenomena.

Sexual phenomena may be a part of an epileptic attack. Partial seizures generated from the genital sensory cortical area mentioned may result in sensations in the genital organs.[18] Such sensations may be described as clitoral warmth, hot feelings in the vagina, and pleasant sensations of anal or vaginal constriction or of penetration, but also as attacks of actual genital pain. Most of the described cases have been associated with a parasagittal tumor involving the primary sensory cortex. Epileptic sensations of sexual excitement and orgasm also occur in patients with temporal lobe epilepsy.[19]

The sexual life of the epileptic patient may also be changed between attacks. Many female epilepsy patients[20,21] report decreased sexual arousability, vaginismis, and dyspareunia. A diminution in genital vasocongestion in response to sexually arousing stimuli not accompanied by a decrease in self-perceived sexual arousal was observed in some women with temporal lobe epilepsy.[22] In another study, epileptic female patients had a lower marriage rate than the general population. Married epileptic females have fewer children.[23] Social and psychologic factors play an important role. Epileptic patients describe poorer psychologic health than healthy subjects. Paranoid delusions of being violated, abused, or seduced are another problem in epileptic women.

Antiepileptic drugs, especially phenytoin, phenobarbital, primidone, carbamazepine, and valproic acid, may cause hormonal changes,[24] as well as decreased sexual desire and performance in women. Epileptic attacks are particularly common during the menstrual phase.[25] Precocious puberty has been observed in a number of epileptic girls treated with carbamazepine, clonazepam, or valproic acid. Some antiepileptic drugs (gabapentin, clonazepam, and valproic acid) may influence orgasmic capacity.

Narcolepsy-cataplexy syndrome

The narcolepsy-cataplexy syndrome is a distinct neurologic disorder, usually without a recognized neuropathology. The main components are irresistible but short episodes of sleep during daytime and short-lived attacks of loss of muscular tone often provoked by emotions. The patients often also have sleep paralysis, which means being awake without being able to move, and hyponagogic hallucinations. Anorgasmia is also a component of the syndrome, and sexual activity can sometimes provoke an attack of cataplexy.[26] Drugs used to treat the sleep attack may interfere with sexual function.

Kleine–Levin syndrome

Kleine–Levin syndrome is a rare but very typical syndrome of unknown etiology with onset in adolescence. Periods of somnolence, hyperphagia, and hypersexuality with a time correlation to menstruation are the cardinal features.[27] The sexual phenomenology is characterized by aggressiveness, sadomasochistic behavior, and delusions.

Parkinson's disease and other movement disorders

Bladder, bowel, and sexual dysfunction is prominent in patients with Parkinson's disease compared to controls of the same ages.[28] The rate of sexual dysfunction was not increased with increasing handicap stage. About 80% of female Parkinson's disease patients had less frequent sexual activity than before the disease.[29] There was a decrease in both sexual interest and sexual drive in 71% and 62%, respectively, of these women. Vaginal dryness was noted in 38% and anorgasm also in 38%. Another study[30] showed similar figures. When Parkinson's disease women were compared with controls matched for age and marital status, the Parkinson's disease women were less satisfied with their sexual relationships and partners, and they were also more depressed.[31] In a further study,[32] the partners of the Parkinson's disease women were also questioned. Among these partners, a high level of sexual dysfunction was found. These observations show that, in Parkinson's disease women, all the three different mechanisms behind sexual dysfunction (see above) have to be taken into account, and a multimodal therapeutic approach is needed. Treatment with dopaminergic drugs has resulted in increase of sexual desire in a number of women.

Multiple sclerosis

Changes in sexual function become very common during the evolution of the disease. In a recent study of 47 women with advanced multiple sclerosis, 60% reported decreased sexual desire; 36%, decreased lubrication; and 40%, diminished orgasmic capacity during the course of the disease. Sensory dysfunction in the genital area was experienced by 62% of the women, and 77% had weakness of the pelvic muscles.[33] In a review of other studies, reduced interest was reported by 29–86% of female multiple sclerosis patients, reduced sensation by 43–62%, reduced orgasmic capacity by 24–58%, vaginal dryness by 12–40%, and dyspareunia by 6–40%.[34]

However, sexual dysfunction may also occur in early and mild cases of multiple sclerosis. Half of the women in one study of 25 females with multiple sclerosis aged 20–42 and with a low handicap score reported sexual problems. None of them had had sexual problems before the start of the disease.[35] In this study, 25 women with migraine matched for age and parity served as controls. Here sexual problems were few and mild.

Sensory dysfunction seems to be the most important reason for sexual problems in multiple sclerosis women. Because of severe external dysesthesia, some patients reported that during a certain period they could not bear direct genital or nongenital contact with their partner. The dysesthesia was of maximum intensity from the beginning of an episode of neurologic symptoms, but resolved fairly rapidly, as is usual in multiple sclerosis.

Most multiple sclerosis patients report diminished sexual desire during the course of the disease. Some patients may experience a temporary decrease during an episode; in others, the problem continues. In certain cases, increased sexual desire has also been described. When this phenomenon is transitory and concurrent with an episode of new symptoms, there is reason to believe that the hypersexuality is the result of a distinct cerebral multiple sclerosis lesion, the localization of

which is unknown. Another important symptom of sexual dysfunction in women with multiple sclerosis is deterioration of orgasmic capacity, intensity, and quality. In most cases, the orgasmic sensations are reduced, becoming shorter lasting, less intense, and/or less agreeable. These changes may be temporary. However, better orgasms have also been noticed. The orgasms may be more easily triggered, longer lasting, stronger, and more pleasant. Paroxysmal attacks of different types are common in multiple sclerosis. Attacks of pelvic pain are one type of such attacks.[36]

Sexual dysfunction correlates with bladder and bowel dysfunction (see Chapter 17.4),[33–35,37,38] but it correlates more mildly with motor and sensory dysfunction in the legs.[33] The correlation is poor with disability scale, clinical course, and disease duration. Sexual dysfunction also correlates with lesions in the pons as detected by magnetic resonance imaging.[39] Brainstem lesions seen on magnetic resonance imaging seem to be of particular importance for anorgasmia.[40]

Symptoms related to multiple sclerosis, such as fatigue, muscle contractures in the lower limbs, urinary disturbances and the use of aids to manage incontinence, and paroxysmal motor and sensory disturbances triggered by sexual intercourse, can indirectly exert a negative effect on sex life as well as social and physical changes. Depression and cognitive impairment play an important role.[40,41]

Neurophysiologic data, such as cortical evoked potentials of the dorsal nerve of the clitoris or pudendal nerve,[39,42,43] as well as measurements of vibratory thresholds in the clitoris,[44] imply that pudendal somatosensory innervation is necessary for one type of female sexual stimulation, that of the clitoris. To compensate for such a loss, more direct stimulation of the anterior vaginal wall (G-spot) is recommended (Table 16.6.1).

Amyotrophic lateral sclerosis

Amyotrophic lateral sclerosis is a rapidly progressive motor disease leading to almost total paralysis of the whole body, including respiratory muscles. However, the patients do not have sensory or autonomic symptoms. Thus, the patients can usually control bladder and bowel functions, and sexual functions are possible. Patients with amyotrophic lateral sclerosis only late, or do not at all, lose their sexual desire. A recent study[45] found sexuality to be an important issue for a high proportion of these patients, despite the fact that they were ventilated.

Diabetes mellitus

Studies of sexual function in women with diabetes mellitus have given conflicting results (see Chapters 7.3 and 17.1). In one early study, 35% of the diabetic women were reported to have had orgasmic dysfunction in the preceding year, as compared to

6% of the controls.[46] In another study, the frequency of sexual dysfunction was around 25% both in insulin-treated diabetic women and in age-matched controls.[47] A more recent, structured-interview study of 42 women with insulin-dependent diabetes, compared both with matched controls and results from the Sweden 1986 national sex survey study,[48] found that 26% of the insulin-dependent diabetes mellitus women had decreased sexual desire, 22% had decreased vaginal lubrication, and 10% had decreased capacity to acquire orgasm. Several of the women reported more than one dysfunction. Overall, the figure for sexual dysfunction was 40%. Among the age-matched controls without diabetes or neurologic disease, only 7% reported some kind of sexual dysfunction.

When compared, type I diabetes was found to have little or no effect on women, while type II diabetes had a pervasively negative impact on sexual desire, lubrication, orgasmic capacity, sexual satisfaction, and sexual activity, and on the relationship with the sexual partner.[49]

Inadequate lubrication is described as the most important sexual problem in many studies.[50] Diabetic women also often have dyspareunia from *Candida* infection. Loss of desire as a major problem has been reported in some other studies.[51,52]

Subjective sexual arousal as measured by vaginal lubrication was often found to be inadequate or to require prolonged stimulation in insulin-dependent diabetes mellitus women compared to controls.[53] Two psychophysiologic studies in women with diabetes mellitus have been published. One of them found no difference from controls,[54] but in the other, diabetic women experienced significantly less physiologic arousal to erotic stimuli than controls.[55]

Impaired subjective vulvar sensibility was noticed more often in women with insulin-dependent diabetes mellitus than in controls.[48] The diabetic patients also had significantly higher vibration perception thresholds in the hands and clitoris than controls. Reduced foot perspiration, increased gustatory perspiration, constipation, and incontinence were also correlated with sexual dysfunction. This indicates that autonomic polyneuropathy is an important mechanism behind sexual dysfunction in diabetic women.

Tissue samples taken postmortem in 17 diabetic women showed evidence of both clitoral nerve degeneration and changes in blood vessels in the clitoris.[56] A nondiabetic control group did not show any signs of neuropathy or vascular damage. However, so far, this study does not seem to have been replicated.

However, sexual problems in patients with diabetes mellitus may have many pathophysiologic mechanisms besides polyneuropathy. The metabolic process in itself, with variations in blood sugar, acidosis, and high-molecular-weight sugars, certainly plays a role. Vascular damage to small vessels as well as larger arteries may result in decreased blood flow to the clitoris and other cavernous tissues. However, other types of endocrine insufficiency, such as hypogonadism, are not considered to play an important role in either sexual desire or sexual arousal. Women with more diabetic complications have more sexual

dysfunction.[57] However, female sexual dysfunction may also precede other symptoms of insulin-dependent diabetes mellitus, and good glycemic control may restore normal sexual function at least in early cases.[58]

Peripheral poly- and mononeuropathies

Peripheral mononeuropathies of the pudendal nerve or branches of that nerve in particular are not uncommon in women. Solitary neurofibromas are one type.[59] The pudendal nerve may also be involved in patients with hereditary motor and sensory neuropathies.[60] Also in the polyneuropathy of primary systemic amyloidosis, changes of the pudendal as well as the autonomic pelvic nerves can lead to sexual dysfunction combined with bladder and bowel dysfunction.[61] Autonomic polyneuropathy may also be a problem in malignant disorders, such as plasma cell dyscrasia.[62] The nerve lesions often result in so much pain and dyspareunia that coitus becomes impossible or at least unpleasant.

Myopathies and encephalomyopathies

In some types of progressive muscular dystrophy, such as myotonic dystrophy,[63,64] Becker's myopathy, and ocular myopathy of the autosomal progressive external ophthalmoplegia type,[65,66] and in Marinesco–Sjögren syndrome,[67,68] secondary amenorrhea, in combination with disturbances of desire and sexual function, has been described. This is also the case in mitochondrial encephalomyopathies, such as myoclonus epilepsy with ragged red fibers and mitochondrial encephalomyopathy with lactic acidosis and stroke syndromes.[69] The hypogonadism in these cases is of a hypergonadotropic type, indicating primary ovarian failure, in contrast to the situation in hypothalamo-pituitary insufficiency (see above).

Headache

Women may have sudden severe headaches precipitated by sexual activity, occurring at the moment of orgasm or shortly after. Many of these attacks have a migraine-like appearance. The attacks are usually recurrent, and all symptoms disappear. This type of attack is called benign orgasmic headache in contrast to the malignant attacks resulting from subarachnoidal hemorrhage, as mentioned above.[15] However, the attacks may be associated with a segmental reversible cerebral artery vasospasm.[70] Beta-receptor blockers taken before sexual activity can prevent the attacks.

Sexual adverse reactions to psychopharmacologic drugs

Antidepressant drugs

Sexual dysfunction, decrease in libido in particular, is very often seen in women with depression. Many reports indicate that sexual desire may decrease during antidepressive treatment instead of being normalized, as would be expected in parallel to otherwise good therapeutic results. However, it is often difficult to decide what is caused by the disease itself and what by its pharmacologic treatment.

In contrast, anorgasmia is not a symptom of depression but instead a very typical adverse drug reaction to the antidepressant selective serotonin reuptake inhibitors. It is particularly common with fluoxetine, paroxetine, sertraline, and citalopram but less common with fluvoxamine. There are much fewer reports of anorgasmia in patients with the nonselective monoamine reuptake inhibitors, with the exception of clomipramine. Pharmacologically, this drug is rather close to the selective serotonin reuptake inhibitors. Among the other types of antidepressant drugs, mianserine, mirtazapine, and nefazodone have very few reports of anorgasmia, but venlafaxine has rather many.[71,72]

Neuroleptic drugs

Neuroleptic drugs often cause sexual endocrine effects, such as amenorrhea, galactorrhea, and hyperprolactinemia. Decrease in sexual desire has been observed, but the number of reports of dysfunction of female sexual arousal and anorgasmia is rather low. However, one should remember that many patients treated with neuroleptic drugs have severe psychiatric disorders, making this group of patients difficult to evaluate.

Therapy and rehabilitation

For treatment of female sexual dysfunction in patients with neurologic disorders, the reader is referred to other chapters of this book and to European Federation of Neurologic Sciences' Official Guidelines for Neurologists.[73] Here more details about female neurosexology are to be found. The procedure of sexual rehabilitation in neurologic patients is described in the textbook on sexual rehabilitation.[74]

References

1. Lundberg PO. The peripheral innervation of the genital organs of women. Scand J Sexol 2001; 4: 213–25.
2. Whipple B. Where in the brain is a woman's sexual response? Laboratory studies including brain imaging (fMRI and PET) during orgasm. Sex Relatsh Ther 2004; 19(Suppl 1): S57–8.
3. Hulter B, Lundberg PO. Sexual function in women with hypothalamo-pituitary disorders. Arch Sex Behav 1994; 23: 171–83.
4. Lundberg PO, Muhr C, Hulter B et al. Sexual libido in patients with hypothalamo-pituitary disorders. In Proceedings of the 7th World Congress of Sexology. Bombay: Indian Association of Sex Educators, 1986: 126–8.
5. Lundberg PO. Neurological disorders in andrology. In J Bain, ESE Hafez, eds. Diagnosis in Andrology. The Hague: Martinus Nijhoff, 1980: 195–213.
6. Neuhäuser G, Opitz JM. Autosomal recessive syndrome of cerebellar ataxia and hypogonadotropic hypogonadism. Clin Genet 1975; 7: 426–34.
7. Berciano J, Amado JA, Freijanes J et al. Familial cerebellar ataxia and hypogonadotropic hypogonadism: evidence for hypothalamic LHRH deficiency. J Neurol Neurosurg Psychiatry 1982; 45: 747–51.
8. Seminara SB, Acierno JS, Abdulwahid NA et al. Hypogonadotropic hypogonadism and cerebellar ataxia: detailed phenotypic characterization of a large, extended kindred. J Clin Endocr Metab 2002; 87: 1607–12.
9. Aloni R, Katz S. Sexual Difficulties After Traumatic Brain Injury and Ways to Deal with It. Springfield, IL: Thomas, 2003.
10. Hibbard MR, Gordon WA, Flanagan S et al. Sexual dysfunction after traumatic brain injury. NeuroRehabilitation 2000; 15: 107–20.
11. Boldrini P, Basaglia N, Calanca MC. Sexual changes in hemiparetic patients. Arch Phys Med Rehabil 1991; 72: 202–7.
12. Sjögren K. Sexuality after stroke II, with special regard to partnership adjustment and to fulfillment. Scand J Rehab Med 1983; 15: 63–9.
13. Sjögren K, Damber J-E, Lilieqvist B. Sexuality after stroke I. Aspects of sexual function. Scand J Rehabil Med 1983; 15: 55–61.
14. Korpelainen JT, Kaulhanen M-L, Kemola H et al. Sexual dysfunction in stroke patients. Acta Neurol Scand 1998; 98: 400–5.
15. Lundberg PO, Osterman PO. The benign and malignant forms of orgasmic cephalgia. Headache 1974; 14: 164–5.
16. Monzani V, Rovellini A, Schinco G et al. Transient global amnesia or subarachnoidal haemorrhage? Eur J Emerg Med 2000; 7: 291–3.
17. Hoenig J, Hamilton CM. Epilepsy and sexual orgasm. Acta Psychiatr Neurol Scand 1960; 35: 448–56.
18. Calleja J, Carpizo R, Berciano J. Orgasmic epilepsy. Epilepsia 1988; 29: 635–9.
19. Rémillard GM, Andermann F, Testa GF et al. Sexual ictal manifestations predominate in women with temporal lobe epilepsy: a finding suggesting sexual dimorphism in the human brain. Neurology 1983; 33: 323–30.
20. Demerdash A, Shalaan M, Midani A et al. Sexual behavior of a sample of females with epilepsy. Epilepsia 1991; 32: 82–5.
21. Morrell MJ, Guldner GT. Self-reported sexual function and sexual arousability in women with epilepsy. Epilepsia 1996; 37: 1204–10.
22. Morrell MJ, Sperling MR, Stecker M et al. Sexual dysfunction in partial epilepsy: a deficit in physiological arousal. Neurology 1994; 44: 243–7.
23. Dansky LV, Andermann E, Andermann F. Marriage and fertility in epileptic patients. Epilepsia 1980; 21: 261–71.

24. Isojärvi JIT. Serum steroid hormones and pituitary function in female epileptic patients during carbamazepine therapy. *Epilepsy* 1990; 31: 438–45.

25. Lundberg PO. Catamenial epilepsy: a review. *Cephalalgia* 1997; 17(Suppl 20): 42–5.

26. Roy A. Anorgasmia and cataplexy. *Arch Sex Behav* 1977; 6: 437–9.

27. Billiard M, Guilleminault C, Dement WC. A menstruation-linked periodic hypersomnia. *Neurology* 1975; 25: 436–43.

28. Sakakibara R, Shinotoh H, Uchiyama T et al. Questionnaire-based assessment of pelvic organ dysfunction in Parkinson's disease. *Auton Neurosci* 2001; 17: 76–85.

29. Koller WC, Vetere-Overfield B, Williamson A et al. Sexual dysfunction in Parkinson's disease. *Clin Neuropharmacol* 1990; 13: 461–3.

30. Wermuth L, Stenager E. Sexual problems in young patients with Parkinson's disease. *Acta Neurol Scand* 1995; 91: 453–5.

31. Welsh M, Hung L, Waters CH. Sexuality in women with Parkinson's disease. *Movement Disord* 1997; 12: 923–7.

32. Brown RG, Jahanshahi M, Quinn N et al. Sexual function in patients with Parkinson's disease and their partners. *J Neurol Neurosurg Psychiatry* 1990; 53: 480–6.

33. Hulter B, Lundberg PO. Sexual function in women with advanced multiple sclerosis. *J Neurol Neurosurg Psychiatry* 1995; 59: 83–6.

34. Ghezzi A. Sexuality and multiple sclerosis. *Scand J Sexol* 1999; 2: 125–40.

35. Lundberg PO. Sexual dysfunction in female patients with multiple sclerosis. *Int Rehab Med* 1981; 3: 32–4.

36. Miró J, García-Moncó C, Leno C et al. Pelvic pain: an undescribed paroxysmal manifestation of multiple sclerosis. *Pain* 1988; 32: 73–5.

37. Beck KP, Warren KG, Whitman P. Urodynamic studies in female patients with multiple sclerosis. *Am J Obstet Gynecol* 1981; 139: 273–6.

38. Hennessey A, Robertson NP, Swinger R et al. Urinary, faecal and sexual dysfunction in patients with multiple sclerosis. *J Neurol* 1999; 246: 1027–32.

39. Zivadinov R, Zorzon M, Locatelli L et al. Sexual function in multiple sclerosis: a MRI, neurophysiological and urodynamic study. *J Neurol Sci* 2003; 210: 73–6.

40. Barak Y, Achiron A, Elizur A et al. Sexual dysfunction in relapsing-remitting multiple sclerosis: magnetic resonance imaging, clinical, and psychological correlates. *J Psychiatr Neurosci* 1996; 21: 255–8.

41. Foley FW, Sanders A. Sexuality, multiple sclerosis and women. International MS Support Foundation. www.imssf.org/sex3.shtml.

42. Yang CC, Bowen JR, Kraft GH et al. Cortical evoked potentials of the dorsal nerve of the clitoris and female sexual dysfunction in multiple sclerosis. *J Urol* 2000; 164: 2010–13.

43. DasGupta R, Kanabar G, Fowler C. Pudendal somatosensory evoked potentials in women with female sexual dysfunction and multiple sclerosis. *Int J Impot Res* 2002; 14(Suppl 3): S83.

44. Hulter B, Lundberg PO. Genital vibratory perception threshold (VPT) measurements in women with sexual dysfunction and/or sexual pain disorders. International Academy of Sex Research (IASR) 31st Annual Meeting: Ottawa, July 2005. Book of abstracts, 44.

45. Kaub-Wittemer D, von Steinbüchel N, Wasner M et al. Quality of life and psychosocial issues in ventilated patients with amyotrophic lateral sclerosis and their caregivers. *J Pain Symptom Manage* 2003; 26: 890–6.

46. Kolodny RC. Sexual dysfunction in diabetic females. *Diabetes* 1971; 20: 557–9.

47. Buus Jensen S. Diabetic sexual dysfunction: a comparative study of 160 insulin treated diabetic men and women and an age-matched control group. *Arch Sex Behav* 1981; 10: 493–504.

48. Hulter B, Berne C, Lundberg PO. Sexual function in women with insulin dependent diabetes mellitus. I. Correlation with neurological symptoms and signs. *Scand J Sex* 1998; 1: 43–50.

49. Schreiner-Engel P, Schiavi RC, Victorisz D et al. The differential impact of diabetes type on female sexuality. *J Psychosom Res* 1987; 31: 23–33.

50. Enzlin P, Mathieu C, Vanderschueren D et al. Diabetes mellitus and female sexuality: a review of 25 years' research. *Diabet Med* 1998; 15: 809–15.

51. Campbell LV, Redelman MJ, Borkman M et al. Factors in sexual dysfunction in diabetic female volunteer subjects. *Med J Aust* 1989; 151: 550–2.

52. Newman AS, Bertelson AD. Sexual dysfunction in diabetic women. *J Behav Med* 1986; 9: 261–70.

53. Tyrer G, Steel JM, Ewing DJ et al. Sexual responsiveness in diabetic women. *Diabetologia* 1983; 24: 166–71.

54. Slob AK, Koster J, Radder JK et al. Sexuality and psychophysiological functioning in women with diabetes mellitus. *J Sex Marital Ther* 1990; 16: 59–69.

55. Wincze JP, Albert A, Bansal S. Sexual arousal in diabetic females: physiological and self-report measures. *Arch Sex Behav* 1993; 22: 587–601.

56. Zrustová M, Vísek V. Sexuální porchy u zen úplavicí cukrovou. *Cesc Gynekol* 1978; 43: 277–80.

57. Enzlin P, Mathieu C, Van Den Bruel A et al. Sexual dysfunction in women with type 1 diabetes: a controlled study. *Diabetes Care* 2002; 25: 672–7.

58. Bultrini A, Carosa E, Colpi EM et al. Possible correlation between type 1 diabetes mellitus and female sexual dysfunction. *J Sex Med* 2004; 1: 337–40.

59. Tognetti F, Poppi M, Gaist G et al. Pudendal neuralgia due to solitary neurofibroma. *J Neurosurg* 1982; 56: 732–3.

60. Vodusek DB, Zidar J. Pudendal nerve involvement in patients with hereditary motor and sensory neuropathy. *Acta Neurol Scand* 1987; 76: 457–60.

61. Kelly JJ, Kyle R, O'Brian PC et al. The natural history of peripheral neuropathy in primary systemic amyloidosis. *Ann Neurol* 1979; 6: 1–7.

62. Takatsuki K, Sanada I. Plasma cell dyscrasia with polyneuropathy and endocrine disorder: clinical and laboratory features of 109 reported cases. *Jpn J Clin Oncol* 1983; 13: 543–55.

63. Marinkovic Z, Prelevic G, Würzburger M et al. Gonadal dysfunction in patients with myotonic dystrophy. *Exp Clin Endocrinol* 1990; 96: 37–44.

64. Olsson T, Olofsson B-O, Hägg E et al. Adrenocortical and gonadal abnormalities in dystrophia myotonica – a common enzyme defect? *Eur J Intern Med* 1996; 7: 29–33.

65. Lundberg PO. Observations on endocrine function in ocular myopathy. *Acta Neurol Scand* 1966; 42: 39–61.

66. Melberg A, Arnell H, Dahl N et al. Anticipation of autosomal progressive external ophthalmoplegia with hypogonadism. *Muscle Nerve* 1996; 19: 751–7.

67. Lundberg PO. Hereditary myopathy, oligophrenia, cataract, skeletal abnormalities and hypergonadotropic hypogonadism. *Eur Neurol* 1973; 10: 261–80.

68. Skre H, Bassöe HH, Berg K et al. Cerebellar ataxia and hypergonadotropic hypogonadism in two kindreds. *Clin Genet* 1976; 9: 661–7.

69. Chen CM, Huang CC. Gonadal dysfunction in mitochondrial encephalomyopathies. *Eur Neurol* 1995; 35: 281–6.

70. Valenca MM, Valenca LP, Bordini CA et al. Cerebral vasospasm and headache during sexual intercourse and masturbatory orgasms. *Headache* 2004; 44: 244–8.

71. Lundberg PO, Biriell C. Sexual dysfunction as a suspect adverse reaction to antidepressant drugs. *Scand J Sexol* 1998; 1: 97–105.

72. https://vigisearch.who-umc.org.

73. Lundberg PO, Ertekin C, Ghezzi A et al. Neurosexology. Guidelines for neurologists. *Eur J Neurol* 2001; 8(Suppl 3): 1–24.

74. Fugl-Meyer A, Fugl-Meyer K, Lundberg PO. Sexual rehabilitation. In P Frommelt, H Grötzbach, eds. *NeuroRehabilitation*. Berlin: Blackwell, 1999: 370–88.

16.7 Hysterectomy and alternative therapies

Andrea Bradford, Cindy M Meston

Despite a recent series of well-controlled investigations into the effects of hysterectomy, the potential impact of the surgery on sexual function remains difficult to ascertain. It has become clear that, for many women, hysterectomy relieves symptoms that stand in the way of enjoyable sexual activity. However, past research has consistently revealed a significant minority of women who report that some aspect of their sexuality suffers as a result of hysterectomy. Understanding the mechanisms by which hysterectomy may influence sexual function, for better or worse, is important for assisting women in informed treatment decisions. With advances in nonsurgical alternatives to the treatment of uterine fibroids and other common indications for hysterectomy, appreciating the costs and benefits of this surgery has become particularly relevant. The majority of hysterectomies are not performed to treat life-threatening illness but rather are elective surgeries performed for benign conditions ("simple" hysterectomy); these procedures will be the primary focus of this chapter.

Historical perspectives

The symbolic importance of the uterus

The view of the uterus as a vital organ was embraced by many ancient physicians and philosophers in Western civilization. Interestingly, sexual gratification, defined in terms of orgasm, was for centuries considered a remedy for the "hysteria" caused by the diseased and displaced uterus.[1] More recent theoretic perspectives, particularly psychoanalytic interpretations, modernized the idea of an intrinsic association of the uterus with mental health.[2] However, the directionality of this relationship shifted, as typified by the explanation of many women's complaints as, "a psychic conflict sailing under a gynaecological flag".[3] Thus, by the twentieth century, the view of hysteria had shifted to a psychically based, rather than organically based, phenomenon.

Politics and practice

Public concern has been raised about the appropriateness of hysterectomy for the treatment of benign conditions such as uterine fibroids and menorrhagia. The invasiveness, risks, and irreversibility of hysterectomy are prominent when compared to less invasive surgical and medical alternatives. An expert review panel recently determined that a substantial number of hysterectomies are performed in the absence of evidence-based indications,[4] echoing earlier concerns about the possible misuse of the procedure.[5]

Citing deficiencies in patient education, decision-making autonomy, and informed consent among candidates for hysterectomy, some researchers and women's health advocates have sharply questioned the manner in which hysterectomies are recommended to women. Anecdotal reports of uninformed and even coercive treatment decisions abound.[6-8] Previous studies suggest that concerns about sexuality are common among women who plan to undergo hysterectomy, although they might go undisclosed.[9-11] Inconsistent findings for negative sexual outcomes, in addition to the broad range of subjective experiences that may follow hysterectomy, create a difficult scenario for the clinician who wishes to provide patients with comprehensive but accurate information about hysterectomy.

Research on hysterectomy and sexual function

The effects of hysterectomy on sexual function are potentially numerous and difficult to measure reliably (see Chapters 7.1–7.3, 13.1–13.3, and 17.4 of this book). The majority of studies that have attempted to assess sexual outcomes have been based on retrospective self-reports, although prospective studies have become more common in recent years. Recent studies of hysterectomy have generally been more careful to examine potentially relevant moderators, such as hormonal status and surgical technique. However, relatively little research to date has used valid and reliable self-report measures, diagnostic interviews, or physiologic indices of sexual function to assess outcomes. Several important design issues for future research are described below.

Timeline of the research

Prospective studies are generally preferable to retrospective studies because they allow changes in sexual function to be assessed pre- to posthysterectomy. It is possible, however, that assessment of sexual function just prior to hysterectomy does not provide a valid baseline.[12] Alterations of sexual function prior to surgery could inflate estimates of improvement in sexual function, although the magnitude of such an effect is debatable. Generally speaking, it is preferable to collect baseline data as far in advance of hysterectomy as possible, and at multiple time points if feasible.

Assessment instruments

The choice of appropriate assessment instruments is essential. Simple yes/no questions or vague, overly general questions (e.g., how is your sex life?) are inappropriate for studies that are designed to measure sexual outcomes. Measuring the frequency of sexual activity as an outcome variable is unreliable at best, since it does not reflect specific aspects of sexual function. Ideally, the researcher should use an instrument that has good internal consistency and test–retest reliability. The instrument should also be internally valid and able to discriminate between sexually functional and dysfunctional populations (for a review of validated instruments for measuring sexual function, see Meston and Derogatis[13]). To date, the self-report measures used in hysterectomy research have rarely met these criteria. Several valid methods of psychophysiologic assessment are also available to the researcher when physiologic sexual response is an outcome of interest (for review, see Janssen[14]).

Control for moderating variables

Hysterectomy is not a single, uniform procedure, and therefore it is preferable to control both for variables within the individual (such as menopausal status and psychologic symptoms) and variables pertaining to the surgery itself (such as surgical approach and ovarian status). Control for these variables may be accomplished by the design of the research or the data-analysis strategy, although the latter option may entail a substantial cost of statistical power. A discussion of putative outcome moderators appears later in this chapter.

Control or comparison groups

Within-group designs are appropriate for many research questions addressing hysterectomy and sexual function. However, two studies have noted that sexual outcomes after hysterectomy are similar to those of other, nongynecologic surgical operations.[15,16]

None of the larger prospective studies on sexual outcomes have attempted to replicate these findings. Moreover, no research to date has prospectively compared the incidence of sexual complaints among women undergoing hysterectomy with that of the general population. Thus, it is unclear from many studies of hysterectomy and sexual function whether sexual outcomes reflect women's experiences of hysterectomy, surgery in general, poor health, or other causes. Including both no-surgery and nongynecologic surgery control groups in large-scale prospective research may help clarify effects that are specific to hysterectomy.

It is difficult to design and execute an outcome study that will yield meaningful results. Practical limitations too often force the exclusion of a desirable study procedure or study group. On the other hand, an overly controlled protocol may hold a number of variables constant at the expense of external validity. Thus, one of the researcher's most important tasks is to clearly define research objectives in a manner that will facilitate the delicate balancing of methodological rigor with methodological economy. Although there is great room for improvement in the body of research on hysterectomy and sexual function to date, the findings from these studies should not be wholly discredited. The remainder of this chapter will review key findings from past research.

Mechanisms by which hysterectomy may affect sexual function

Estimates of the prevalence of sexual problems after hysterectomy vary widely due to methodological inconsistencies among studies. Retrospectively, 17–27% of women report worse sexual adjustment after hysterectomy, whereas 22–71% report improved sexual function.[17–20] However, retrospective comparisons are difficult to interpret due to a multitude of factors that may or may not be directly associated with hysterectomy.[18] Only a handful of published studies have reported the number of new sexual complaints that have surfaced postoperatively. Rates of new sexual problems are 2–7% for dyspareunia, 9–21% for vaginal lubrication difficulty, 5–11% for low sexual desire, and 2–11% for orgasmic difficulty.[20–24] Although these estimates are relatively low, they nevertheless represent a large number of women, given the high utilization of hysterectomy. At present, it is unclear which factors play a role in sexual outcomes after hysterectomy, although both psychologic and physiologic factors are likely to be influential.

Psychologic consequences

Anxiety prior to hysterectomy is common, and many women express specific worries about the impact of surgery on their sexuality (see Chapters 3.1–3.4). Dennerstein et al.[17] found that women who endorsed anxiety about sexual issues prior to hysterectomy also tended to experience poorer sexual outcomes after hysterectomy, although no prospective studies have investigated this possibility.

Qualitative research suggests that concerns about sexual function after hysterectomy are seldom addressed effectively by health-care providers;[11] this may signify an opportunity to improve outcomes with proactive, sexuality-focused education prior to surgery.

The incidence of depression after hysterectomy has been studied closely over the past several decades (see Chapter 16.2). Depression has been associated with sexual problems[25] and may complicate sexual adjustment after hysterectomy.[22] Earlier studies suggested that depression was alarmingly prevalent after hysterectomy, although most of these studies were poorly designed and did not account for psychiatric symptoms prior to hysterectomy (for review, see Khastgir et al.[26]). More recent studies have failed to support a posthysterectomy depressive syndrome; in fact, they have revealed significant improvements in psychologic adjustment after surgery.[27-29] Whether women who present with more severe psychosocial impairments are more likely to be recommended for hysterectomy is an interesting but unresolved question.

A source of confusion about the incidence of depression after hysterectomy is the fact that psychiatric morbidity may be elevated among women with gynecologic problems.[27-29] It is reasonable to assume that stress due to pain and other symptoms of gynecologic conditions may contribute to psychologic maladjustment. Indeed, Ferroni and Deeble[30] noted that women with unresolved gynecologic illness reported more severe depressive symptoms than an age-matched group of women who had undergone hysterectomy for similar conditions. There is strong evidence that psychologic improvements after hysterectomy are attributable to symptom relief and improved health.[21,24,31,32] Improved psychologic adjustment may also largely account for improvements on sexuality measures.[33] Not surprisingly, sexual function scores may be most improved among women who experienced the greatest health-related impairment prior to hysterectomy.[34,35]

Psychologic adjustment to hysterectomy and its impact on sexual function may be affected by concerns about femininity, loss of fertility, and sexual attractiveness. Some women may view themselves as defeminized by hysterectomy surgery,[11,30,32] and similar concerns may affect male partners of hysterectomized women.[36] Culture-specific beliefs may be influential in the perception of sexual changes and should be addressed sensitively.[8,10,36] The scar left by abdominal hysterectomy may also raise body-image concerns, although vaginal and laparoscopic surgical approaches are viable alternatives in many cases. Hormonal changes after hysterectomy can also affect body image and health-related quality of life,[11,37] and should be addressed comprehensively prior to surgery.

Physiologic consequences

The role of the uterus in the sexual response is unclear. Early studies by Kinsey et al.[38] suggested that uterine contractions accompany sexual arousal, but Masters and Johnson[39] later claimed that contractions occurred only at orgasm (see Chapter 6.4). Objective measurements of uterine tone during sexual stimulation are scarce,[39,40] and the extent to which uterine activity influences subjective sexual experiences is speculative.

Far more concern has been expressed regarding the impact of hysterectomy on the autonomic nervous pathways that are essential to the sexual response (see Chapters 4.1–4.4). The inferior hypogastric plexus is the immediate supplier of autonomic nerve fibers to the genital organs. This structure and its extensions may be at risk of damage by conventional hysterectomy techniques.[41] It has been hypothesized that hysterectomy may disrupt pelvic autonomic pathways through the excision of the cervix and separation of the uterus from its supportive ligaments.[42-45] Evidence of urinary, bowel, and sexual dysfunction after hysterectomy is scarce in most of the recent literature,[20,21,46-48] although a few studies do suggest long-term adverse effects.[15,49,50]

Using vaginal laser Doppler flowmetry, Richman and Sarrel[51] observed no differences in resting vaginal blood flow pre- to posthysterectomy, suggesting no evidence of overt vascular damage to the vaginal tissues. However, disturbance of autonomic pathways could hypothetically interfere with the vaginal vasocongestive response during sexual arousal. Three studies have examined this possibility by measuring physiologic responses to sexual stimulation by vaginal photoplethysmography. Comparing women who had and had not undergone hysterectomy, with or without oophorectomy, Bellerose and Binik[37] found no significant differences in the magnitude of vaginal pulse amplitude or vaginal blood-volume responses to sexual film clips (see Chapter 10.1). In contrast, using a comparison group of women with uterine fibroids, Meston[52] found that vaginal pulse amplitude responses to a sexual film were significantly lower among women who had undergone hysterectomy to treat fibroids. Maas et al.[53] compared vaginal pulse amplitude responses to sexual stimulation among women who had undergone both radical and simple hysterectomy, along with age-matched control women. The authors found that vaginal pulse amplitude responses to sexual stimulation were significantly less robust in the radical hysterectomy group than in controls. The authors noted a trend suggesting that the average magnitude of vaginal pulse amplitude responses among the simple hysterectomy group was between those of the radical and control groups; however, this trend was statistically nonsignificant. These three studies are limited by the fact that they involve retrospective, between-subject comparisons of vaginal pulse amplitude responses. To minimize the inherent variability in psychophysiologic data due to individual differences, the impact of hysterectomy on sexual arousal should ideally be investigated by within-subject, prospective designs.

Moderators of sexual outcomes after hysterectomy

Previous work has concentrated on several key factors that may influence sexual function after hysterectomy. Given conflicting findings, as well as the quality and scope of past studies, it is premature to declare a consensus about any of these potential moderators. However, these factors should be closely examined in practice and future research.

Radicality of hysterectomy

Radical hysterectomy for gynecologic cancer has received considerable attention due to higher levels of postoperative urinary, bowel, and sexual dysfunction than are typically reported with simple hysterectomy (see discussion[54–58]). Because radical hysterectomy entails a higher degree of tissue removal and tissue damage than simple hysterectomy, the two procedures should be examined separately in terms of outcomes. Comparing sexual outcomes of the radical and simple procedures is also confounded by psychologic factors, namely, that the former is performed to treat lethal illness, whereas the latter is an elective treatment for benign conditions. Among the few studies that have directly compared sexual outcomes of both surgeries, Maas et al.[53] found that vaginal pulse amplitude responses to sexual stimuli were lower among women who had undergone radical hysterectomy compared to simple hysterectomy. The authors hypothesized that radical hysterectomy may cause greater neurologic impairment than simple hysterectomy, thereby attenuating the vasocongestive response. This hypothesis is supported by anatomic studies of the uterus and its supportive ligaments. Butler-Manuel et al.[42,59] found that the cardinal and uterosacral ligaments contain significant amounts of autonomic (particularly sympathetic) nerves and ganglia that are associated with the inferior hypogastric plexus. The authors noted that transection of these ligaments at their origin (as in radical hysterectomy) was associated with more extensive nerve damage than transection at the insertion point at the uterus (as in simple hysterectomy). Radical hysterectomy techniques designed to minimize nerve damage show promise (for review, see Maas et al.[60]), but as yet have not been compared rigorously to traditional techniques.

Surgical approach

Most hysterectomies are performed either vaginally or via abdominal incision, with laparoscopically assisted procedures comprising a third, less utilized approach. Although one retrospective study concluded that the abdominal route has a more negative impact on sexual function than other approaches,[61] the majority of studies that have specifically examined this question have found no differences in sexual outcomes among the surgical approaches.[21–23,34,62]

Removal of the cervix

In modern practice, the uterine cervix is often removed during hysterectomy. However, concern has been raised regarding the potential role of the cervix in the sexual response. The cervix is innervated with autonomic and sensory nervous tissue, and stimulation of the cervix may contribute to sexual arousal and orgasm (for discussion, see Hasson[43]). To the extent that the cervix can appreciably influence sexual responses, its removal may result in less satisfactory sexual outcomes. This hypothesis was supported by Kilkku et al.,[63,64] who reported that subtotal (supracervical) hysterectomy was associated with better outcomes in terms of dyspareunia and orgasm. More recently, several well-controlled, prospective trials of total and subtotal hysterectomy have reported no significant differences in sexual outcomes between the total and subtotal procedures.[23,65,66] These findings suggest that the role of the cervix in sexual response, if any, is not likely to be uniform across women.

Ovarian conversion or removal

Although concerns about the long-term safety of hormone therapy may give pause to many clinicians, it is common for women to undergo oophorectomy (surgical removal of ovaries) at the same time as hysterectomy (see Chapters 5.5 and 7.2). In premenopausal women, this procedure brings about immediate "surgical menopause", characterized by significant reduction in levels of estrogen, testosterone, and other sex steroids.[67] The loss of these hormones could affect sexual function broadly. In particular, estrogen loss may be accompanied by insufficient vaginal lubrication, whereas reduced testosterone may affect sexual desire and subjective sexual arousal.[68,69] Retrospective studies have found that women who have preserved their ovaries tend to experience more positive sexual outcomes than women who have undergone oophorectomy, even when hormone therapy is considered.[19,37,70,71] However, findings are inconsistent across studies,[22] and the specific aspects of sexual function that are affected by oophorectomy are not well established.

Psychiatric morbidity prior to hysterectomy

Prospective studies have largely invalidated the view that hysterectomy is a risk factor for mental illness, while at the same time suggesting that preoperative mental health may affect psychologic and sexual outcomes. Rhodes et al.[22] reported that preoperative depression negatively influenced outcomes of sexual desire, lubrication, orgasm, and pain, although Helstrom et al.[35] failed to find any effect of psychiatric history on sexual function. This discrepancy may be attributable to different definitions of psychiatric complaints (e.g., limited to depression in the Rhodes et al. study), and it calls for the inclusion of psychiatric variables in future outcome studies (see Chapters 17.2 and 17.3).

Sexual function prior to hysterectomy

Among studies to date, one of the most consistent predictors of sexual difficulties after hysterectomy has been poor sexual function prior to surgery.[18,22,34,66,72] A notable exception to this trend is the presence of dyspareunia prior to hysterectomy, which is often relieved after the removal of diseased uterine tissue.[20–22,48,66]

Relationship with partner

Several studies have reported a significant influence of the sexual partner's emotional support and quality of relationship on sexual outcomes after hysterectomy (see Chapters 8.1 and 8.2).[18,22,66,72] The sexual partner's attitudes and beliefs regarding hysterectomy have the potential to dramatically influence a woman's posthysterectomy sexual life, although drastic shifts in the partner's behavior appear to be more prevalent in myth than in reality. Lalos and Lalos[73] reported numerous misconceptions about female anatomy and fears about hysterectomy among a sample of male partners of women scheduled to undergo hysterectomy. The extent to which this may affect sexual feelings for the partner undergoing surgery is unclear. However, women themselves may feel apprehensive about their partners' (particularly men's) ignorance of hysterectomy and sexuality.[36]

Alternatives to hysterectomy

A number of treatment alternatives are available for benign gynecologic conditions.[74] To date, few studies have directly compared the sexual outcomes of hysterectomy and alternative treatments. However, a few recent clinical trials suggest that alternatives to hysterectomy do not necessarily result in better sexual outcomes.

Endometrial ablation and resection

A randomized trial of endometrial ablation versus vaginal hysterectomy failed to show any differences between the two patient groups on a measure of sexual function.[75] Similarly, a retrospective comparison of abdominal hysterectomy and roller-ball endometrial ablation revealed no significant differences in sexual outcomes.[76]

Medical management

Hurskainen et al.[77] reported 5-year follow-up comparisons of treatment with a levonorgestrel-releasing intrauterine device or hysterectomy for menorrhagia. Five-year change scores on measures of sexual satisfaction, sexual problems, and partner satisfaction were minimal and not significantly different between the two groups. Kupperman et al.[78] studied a group of women who were dissatisfied with their current medical treatment regimens for abnormal uterine bleeding and were randomized to receive either hysterectomy or expanded medical treatment. This study allowed for flexibility in medical management as well as crossover to hysterectomy when additional medical treatments were unsuccessful. The results indicated that women who underwent hysterectomy showed greater improvement in sexual desire at the 6-month and 2-year follow-up periods, and less interference of pelvic problems during sexual activity at the 6-month follow-up.

Because sexual function was not assessed comprehensively in these studies, these results should be interpreted cautiously. The lack of data from validated sexual function measures, the limitations of the study samples (e.g., willingness to be randomized), and the absence of controlled studies of other hysterectomy alternatives (such as myomectomy and uterine fibroid embolization) suggest a strong need for additional research on alternative treatments before drawing conclusions about their sexual outcomes relative to hysterectomy.

Conclusions and recommendations

Less invasive alternatives to hysterectomy are not effective or appropriate for all patients, and a number of women will ultimately face the choice of whether to undergo hysterectomy. Although many studies have suggested that sexual function is unchanged or improved after hysterectomy, there is compelling evidence that a significant proportion of women undergoing hysterectomy experience undesirable sexual outcomes. Preliminary evidence suggests that negative sexual outcomes may have a physiologic basis, although psychologic reactions may also contribute. Assessing the risk of negative sexual outcomes for any given individual is a daunting task. Collaborative and deliberative treatment planning is recommended to help women fully understand, and ultimately accept or reject, the risks of surgery. The patient's consent to hysterectomy should be prefaced by substantial instruction and an opportunity to discuss any viable alternatives.

It should be recognized that the potential for negative sexual outcomes may be substantially outweighed by the need to relieve symptoms of illness. Optimally, health-care providers should be proactive and sensitive in addressing the sexual concerns of patients considering hysterectomy. A discussion of sexual function prior to surgery may reveal important considerations for treatment and recovery. A woman with severe dyspareunia secondary to uterine fibroids, for example, may face a dramatically different posthysterectomy experience than a woman whose otherwise enjoyable sexual activity has been disrupted by unpredictable uterine bleeding. Given the complexity of individual cases, caution should be exercised in the interpretation of frequently publicized claims that hysterectomy "improves" sexual function for "most" women.

Finally, considering the patient's psychologic well-being prior to surgery may be an important but overlooked aspect of clinical management. Pre-existing psychologic problems may hinder adjustment to hysterectomy and should be carefully monitored. Psychosocial support may play a vital role in adjustment after surgery. Although the role of the patient's sexual partner in outcomes is understudied, it seems reasonable to assume that the partner should usually be considered in the discussion of hysterectomy. Reactions from partners, friends, family, community, and other social supports are potentially critical factors in the woman's psychologic and sexual outcomes after hysterectomy.

References

1. Maines RP. The *Technology of Orgasm*. Baltimore: Johns Hopkins University Press, 1999.

2. Drellich MG, Bieber I. The psychologic importance of the uterus and its functions. *J Nerv Ment Dis* 1958; 126: 322–36.

3. Rogers FS. Emotional factors in gynecology. *Am J Obstet Gynecol* 1950; 77: 806–23.

4. Broder MS, Kanouse DE, Mittman BS et al. The appropriateness of recommendations for hysterectomy. *Obstet Gynecol* 2000; 95: 199–205.

5. Miller NF. Hysterectomy: therapeutic necessity or surgical racket? *Am J Obstet Gynecol* 1946; 51: 804–10.

6. Cloutier-Steele L. *Misinformed Consent: Women's Stories About Unnecessary Hysterectomy*. Chester: Next Decade, 2003.

7. Uskul AK, Ahmad F, Leyland NA et al. Women's hysterectomy experiences and decision-making. *Women Health* 2003; 38: 53–67.

8. Williams RD, Clark AJ. A qualitative study of women's hysterectomy experience. *J Womens Health Gend Based Med* 2000; 9(Suppl 2): S15–25.

9. Dragisic KG, Milad MP. Sexual functioning and patient expectations of sexual functioning after hysterectomy. *Am J Obstet Gynecol* 2004; 190: 1416–18.

10. Groff JY, Mullen PD, Byrd T et al. Decision making, beliefs, and attitudes toward hysterectomy: a focus group study with medically underserved women in Texas. *J Womens Health Gend Based Med* 2000; 9(Suppl 2): S39–S50.

11. Wade J, Pletsch PK, Morgan SW et al. Hysterectomy: what do women need and want to know? *J Obstet Gynecol Neonatal Nurs* 2000; 29: 33–42.

12. Cutler WB, Zacher MG, McCoy NL et al. The impact of hysterectomy on sexual life of women. *Obstet Gynecol* 2001; 97(4 Suppl): 23S.

13. Meston CM, Derogatis LR. Validated instruments for assessing female sexual function. *J Sex Marital Ther* 2002; 28(Suppl): 155–64.

14. Janssen E. Psychophysiological measurement of sexual arousal. In MW Wiederman, BE Whitley, eds. *Handbook for Conducting Research on Human Sexuality*. Mahwah: Lawrence Erlbaum Associates, Inc., 2001: 139–71.

15. Cosson M, Rajabally R, Querleu D et al. Long term complications of vaginal hysterectomy: a case control study. *Eur J Obstet Gynecol Reprod Biol* 2001; 94: 239–44.

16. Galyer KT, Conaglen HM, Hare A et al. The effect of gynecological surgery on sexual desire. *J Sex Marital Ther* 1999; 5: 81–8.

17. Dennerstein L, Wood C, Burrows GD. Sexual response following hysterectomy and oophorecomy. *Obstet Gynecol* 1977; 49: 92–6.

18. Helstrom L. Sexuality after hysterectomy: a model based on quantitative and qualitative analysis of 104 women before and after subtotal hysterectomy. *J Psychosom Obstet Gynaecol* 1994; 15: 219–29.

19. Nathorst-Boos J, von Schoultz B. Psychological reactions and sexual life after hysterectomy with and without oophorectomy. *Gynecol Obstet Invest* 1992; 34: 97–101.

20. Weber AM, Walters MD, Schover LR et al. Functional outcomes and satisfaction after abdominal hysterectomy. *Am J Obstet Gynecol* 1999; 181: 530–5.

21. Carlson KJ, Miller BA, Fowler FJ Jr. The Maine Women's Health Study. I. Outcomes of hysterectomy. *Obstet Gynecol* 1994; 83: 556–65.

22. Rhodes JC, Kjerulff KH, Langenberg PW et al. Hysterectomy and sexual functioning. *JAMA* 1999; 282: 1934–41.

23. Roovers J-PWR, van der Born JG, van der Vaart CH et al. Hysterectomy and sexual well-being: prospective observational study of vaginal hysterectomy, subtotal abdominal hysterectomy, and total abdominal hysterectomy. *Br Med J* 2003; 327: 774–8.

24. Schofield MJ, Bennett A, Redman S et al. Self-reported long-term outcomes of hysterectomy. *Br J Obstet Gynaecol* 1991; 98: 1129–36.

25. Cyranowski JM, Frank E, Cherry C et al. Prospective assessment of sexual function in women treated for recurrent major depression. *J Psychiatr Res* 2004; 38: 267–73.

26. Khastgir G, Studd JW, Catalan J. The psychological outcome of hysterectomy. *Gynecol Endocrinol* 2000; 14: 132–41.

27. Donoghue AP, Jackson HJ, Pagano R. Understanding pre- and post-hysterectomy levels of negative affect: a stress moderation model approach. *J Psychosom Obstet Gynaecol* 2003; 24: 99–109.

28. Gath D, Rose N, Bond A et al. Hysterectomy and psychiatric disorder: are the levels of psychiatric morbidity falling? *Psychol Med* 1995; 25: 277–83.

29. Ryan MM, Dennerstein L, Pepperell R. Psychological aspects of hysterectomy. A prospective study. *Br J Psychiatry* 1989; 154: 516–22.

30. Ferroni P, Deeble J. Women's subjective experience of hysterectomy. *Aust Health Rev* 1996; 19: 40–55.

31. Lambden MP, Bellamy G, Ogburn-Russell L et al. Women's sense of well-being before and after hysterectomy. *J Obstet Gynecol Neonatal Nurs* 1997; 26: 540–8.

32. Rannestad T, Eikeland OJ, Helland H et al. Are the physiologically and psychosocially based symptoms in women suffering from gynecological disorders alleviated by means of hysterectomy? *J Womens Health Gend Based Med* 2001; 10: 579–87.

33. Bernhard LA. Consequences of hysterectomy in the lives of women. *Health Care Women Int* 1992; 13: 281–91.

34. Gutl P, Greimel ER, Roth R et al. Women's sexual behavior, body image and satisfaction with surgical outcomes after hysterectomy: a comparison of vaginal and abdominal surgery. *J Psychosom Obstet Gynaecol* 2002; 23: 51–9.

35. Helstrom L, Weiner E, Sorbom D et al. Predictive value of psychiatric history, genital pain and menstrual symptoms for sexuality after hysterectomy. *Acta Obstet Gynecol Scand* 1994; 73: 575–80.

36. Richter DL, McKeown RE, Corwin SJ et al. The role of male partners in women's decision making regarding hysterectomy. *J Womens Health Gend Based Med* 2000; 9(Suppl 2): S51–61.

37. Bellerose SB, Binik YM. Body image and sexuality in oophorectomized women. *Arch Sex Behav* 1993; 22: 435–59.

38. Kinsey AC, Pomeroy WB, Martin CE et al. *Sexual Behavior in the Human Female*. Philadelphia: WB Saunders, 1953.

39. Masters WH, Johnson V. *Human Sexual Response*. Boston: Little, Brown, 1966.

40. Fox CA, Wolff HS, Baker JA. Measurement of intra-vaginal and intra-uterine pressures during human coitus by radiotelemetry. *J Reprod Fertil* 1970; 22: 243–51.

41. Maas CP, DeRuiter MC, Kenter GG et al. The inferior hypogastric plexus in gynecologic surgery. *J Gynecol Tech* 1999; 5: 55–62.

42. Butler-Manuel SA, Buttery LD, A'Hern RP et al. Pelvic nerve plexus trauma at radical and simple hysterectomy: a quantitative study of nerve types in the uterine supporting ligaments. *J Soc Gynecol Investig* 2002; 9: 47–56.

43. Hasson HM. Cervical removal at hysterectomy for benign disease: risks and benefits. *J Reprod Med* 1993; 38: 781–90.

44. Munro MG. Supracervical hysterectomy: a time for reappraisal. *Obstet Gynecol* 1997; 89: 133–9.

45. Thakar R, Manyonda I, Stanton SL et al. Bladder, bowel and sexual function after hysterectomy for benign conditions. *Br J Obstet Gynaecol* 1997; 104: 983–7.

46. Clarke A, Black N, Rowe P et al. Indications for and outcome of total abdominal hysterectomy for benign disease: a prospective cohort study. *Br J Obstet Gynaecol* 1995; 102: 611–20.

47. Gimbel H, Zobbe V, Anderson BM et al. Randomised controlled trial of total compared with subtotal hysterectomy with one-year follow up results. *Br J Obstet Gynaecol* 2003; 110: 1088–98.

48. Virtanen H, Makinen J, Tenho T et al. Effects of abdominal hysterectomy on urinary and sexual symptoms. *Br J Urol* 1993; 72: 868–72.

49. Altman D, Zetterstrom J, Lopez A et al. Effect of hysterectomy on bowel function. *Dis Colon Rectum* 2004; 47: 502–8.

50. Prior A, Stanley K, Smith ARB et al. Effect of hysterectomy on anorectal and urethrovesical physiology. *Gut* 1992; 33: 264–7.

51. Richman SM, Sarrel PM. Vaginal laser Doppler flowmetry pre- and posthysterectomy. *J Sex Marital Ther* 2004; 30: 43–7.

52. Meston CM. The effects of hysterectomy on sexual arousal in women with a history of benign uterine fibroids. *Arch Sex Behav* 2004; 33: 31–42.

53. Maas CP, ter Kuile MM, Laan E et al. Objective assessment of sexual arousal in women with a history of hysterectomy. *Br J Obstet Gynaecol* 2004; 111: 456–62.

54. Bergmark K, Avall-Lundqvist E, Dickman PW et al. Patient-rating of distressful symptoms after treatment for early cervical cancer. *Acta Obstet Gynecol Scand* 2002; 81: 443–50.

55. Bergmark K, Avall-Lundqvist E, Dickman PW et al. Vaginal changes and sexuality in women with a history of cervical cancer. *N Engl J Med* 1999; 340: 1383–9.

56. Corney RH, Crowther ME, Everett H et al. Psychosexual dysfunction in women with gynaecological cancer following radical pelvic surgery. *Br J Obstet Gynaecol* 1993; 100: 73–8.

57. Jensen PT, Groenvold M, Klee MC et al. Early-stage cervical carcinoma, radical hysterectomy, and sexual function. *Cancer* 2004; 100: 97–106.

58. Weijmar Schultz WCM, Van de Wiel HBM, Hahn DEE. Sexuality and cancer in women: an integrative model of sexual function in women after treatment for cancer. *Annu Rev Sex Res* 1992; 3: 151–200.

59. Butler-Manuel SA, Buttery LD, A'Hern RP et al. Pelvic nerve plexus trauma at radical hysterectomy and simple hysterectomy: the nerve content of the uterine supporting ligaments. *Cancer* 2000; 89: 834–41.

60. Maas CP, Trimbos JB, DeRuiter MC et al. Nerve sparing radical hysterectomy: latest developments and historical perspective. *Crit Rev Oncol Hematol* 2003; 48: 271–9.

61. Ayoubi JM, Fanchin R, Monrozies X et al. Respective consequences of abdominal, vaginal, and laparoscopic hysterectomies on women's sexuality. *Eur J Obstet Gynecol Reprod Biol* 2003; 111: 179–82.

62. Ellstrom MA, Astrom M, Moller A et al. A randomized trial comparing changes in psychological well-being and sexuality after laparoscopic and abdominal hysterectomy. *Acta Obstet Gynecol Scand* 2003; 82: 871–5.

63. Kilkku P. Supravaginal uterine amputation vs. hysterectomy. Effects on coital frequency and dyspareunia. *Acta Obstet Gynecol Scand* 1983; 62: 141–5.

64. Kilkku P, Gronroos M, Hirvonen T et al. Supravaginal uterine amputation vs. hysterectomy. Effects on libido and orgasm. *Acta Obstet Gynecol Scand* 1983; 62: 147–52.

65. Thakar R, Ayers S, Clarkson P et al. Outcomes after total versus subtotal abdominal hysterectomy. *N Engl J Med* 2002; 347: 1318–25.

66. Zobbe V, Gimbel H, Anderson BM et al. Sexuality after total vs. subtotal hysterectomy. *Acta Obstet Gynecol Scand* 2004; 83: 191–6.

67. Beksac MS, Kisnisci HA, Cakar AN et al. The endocrinological evaluation of bilateral and unilateral oophorectomy in premenopausal women. *Int J Fertil* 1983; 28: 219–24.

68. Sarrel P, Dobay B, Wiita B. Estrogen and estrogen-androgen replacement in postmenopausal women dissatisfied with estrogen-only therapy: sexual behavior and neuroendocrine responses. *J Reprod Med* 1998; 43: 847–56.

69. Sherwin BB, Gelfand MM. The role of androgens in the maintenance of sexual functionining on oophorectomized women. *Psychosom Med* 1987; 49: 397–409.

70. Farquhar CM, Sadler L, Harvey S et al. A prospective study of the short-term outcomes of hysterectomy with and without oophorectomy. *Aust N Z J Obstet Gynaecol* 2002; 42: 197–204.

71. Nathorst-Boos J, von Schoultz B, Carlstrom K. Elective ovarian removal and estrogen replacement therapy – effects on sexual life, psychological well-being and androgen status. *J Psychosom Obstet Gynaecol* 1993; 14: 283–93.

72. Helstrom L, Lundberg PO, Sorbom D et al. Sexuality after hysterectomy: a factor analysis of women's sexual lives before and after subtotal hysterectomy. *Obstet Gynecol* 1993; 81: 357–62.

73. Lalos A, Lalos O. The partner's view about hysterectomy. *J Psychosom Obstet Gynaecol* 1996; 17: 119–24.

74. American College of Obstetricians and Gynecologists. Surgical alternatives to hysterectomy in the management of leiomyomas. *Int J Gynecol Obstet* 2001; 73: 285–94.

75. Crosignani PG, Vercellini P, Apolone G et al. Endometrial resection versus vaginal hysterectomy for menorrhagia: long-term clinical and quality-of-life outcomes. *Am J Obstet Gynecol* 1997; 177: 95–101.

76. Mousa HA, El Senoun GMSA, Mahmood TA. Medium-term clinical outcome of women with menorrhagia treated by rollerball endometrial ablation versus abdominal hysterectomy with conservation of at least one ovary. *Acta Obstet Gynecol Scand* 2001; 80: 442–6.

77. Hurskainen R, Teperi J, Rissanen P et al. Clinical outcomes and costs with the levonorgestrel-releasing intrauterine system or hysterectomy for treatment of menorrhagia. JAMA 2004; 291: 1456–63.

78. Kupperman M, Varner RE, Summitt RL Jr et al. Effect of hysterectomy vs. medical treatment on health-related quality of life and sexual functioning. JAMA 2004; 291: 1447–55.

16.8 Sexuality and genital cutting

Jean L Fourcroy

Almighty God created sexual desire in ten parts; then he gave nine parts to women and one to men.

—Attributed to Ali ihn Abu Taleb, husband of Muhammed's daughter[1]

Does female genital cutting or female genital circumcision/female genital mutilation affect female sexuality? To understand the impact of a cultural custom on a woman's sexuality, one must first understand the origin, perpetuation, and prevalence of the custom as well as understand the procedure itself.

The question of a woman's sexuality must also be understood within the culture where female genital cutting/female genital mutilation is practiced. Cultural and social mores play an important role in the acceptance and achievement of normal sexual function for both men and women. These mores limit a woman's freedom during her entire life, including menses, marriage, pregnancy, and postpartum. Cultural mores also identify specific customs that should or must be followed. Thus, tradition, law, education, and the status of women are important indicators of sexual health.

Sexual health is an assumed right for every individual.[2] Sexual health is a state of physical, emotional, mental, and social well-being related to sexuality; it is not merely the absence of disease, dysfunction, or infirmity.[3] Sexual health requires a positive and respectful approach to sexuality and sexual relationships, as well as the possibility of having pleasurable and safe sexual experiences. A sexual experience must be free of coercion, discrimination, and violence. For many women, discrimination and violence are part of their lives. For sexual health to be attained and maintained, the sexual rights of all persons must be respected, protected, and fulfilled.[2] Sexual rights embrace human rights that are already recognized in international human rights documents, national laws, and other consensus documents. Education of women may be the most important socioeconomic piece of the puzzle of how to preserve the sexual health of women.[4–6]

Sexual health assumes that each individual:

- receive the highest attainable standard of health in relation to sexuality, including access to sexual and reproductive health-care services
- be able to seek, receive, and impart information in relation to sexuality
- have sexuality education
- have respect for bodily integrity
- have a choice of partner
- be able to decide whether to be sexually active or not
- be able to have consensual sexual relations and/or marriage
- be able to decide whether or not, and when, to have children
- be able to pursue a satisfying, safe, and pleasurable sexual life.

The responsible exercise of human rights requires that all persons respect the rights of others.[7]

History and prevalence of female genital cutting/female genital mutilation

The current preferred term for our subject is female genital cutting (FGC), but female genital mutilation (FGM) and cutting (FGC) are used interchangeably.

The origin of female cutting rituals cannot be traced but appears to have been practiced as early as the time of the Pharaohs. Even though female genital cutting/female genital mutilation is practiced mostly in Islamic countries, it is *not* an Islamic practice, and there does not appear to be a religious connection. The "circumcision" of girls, in any form, predated Islam by many centuries. It was practiced in some parts of Arabia at the time of the Prophet Muhammad and was evidently a custom of the time that may have been a practice of some, but not all, of the local tribes. Female genital cutting/female genital mutilation is practiced by Muslims and non-Muslims alike residing in sub-Saharan African in countries that include, but are not limited to, Egypt, Sudan, Somalia, Ethiopia, Kenya, and Chad (Fig. 16.8.1). A minor form of the procedure is also performed in some parts of the Middle East and south Asia.[8] In Africa and the Middle East, it is performed by Muslims, Coptic Christians, members of various indigenous groups, Protestants, and Catholics. The procedure is also found among some ethnic groups in Oman, the United Arab Emirates, and Yemen, as well as in parts of India, Indonesia, and Malaysia. It is important to remember that, within a country, tribes or cultures may vary in the practice or the type of cutting employed.[9] Country-specific "Demographic and Health Surveys", listing the prevalence rates of female genital cutting/female genital mutilation, are maintained by the US State Department.[10]

Patterns of immigration have spread this practice worldwide. Estimates of the prevalence of female genital cutting/female genital mutilation in the USA are based on the numbers of such immigrant families throughout the country. In 1990, it was estimated that nearly 168 000 immigrant women and girls in the USA had either undergone female genital cutting/female genital mutilation or were at risk of it.[12,13]

The Qur'an refers to the sexual relationship in marriage as one of mutual satisfaction that is considered a mercy from

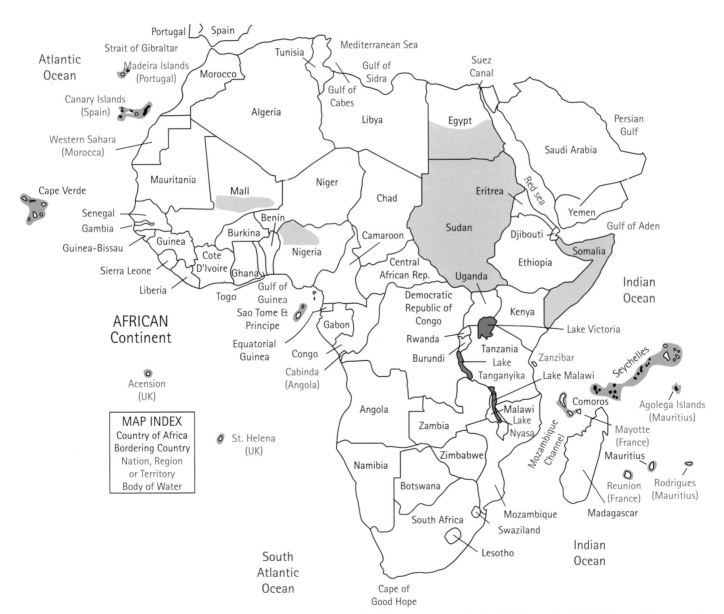

Figure 16.8.1. Map of African continent. Main areas where female genital cutting (FGC)/female genital mutilation (FGM) is practiced.[11] Sub-Saharan African countries practicing some form of FGC include Egypt, Sudan, Somalia, Ethiopia, Kenya, and Chad.

Allah. "It is lawful for you to go in unto your wives during the night preceding the [day's] fast; they are as a garment for you and you are as a garment for them (2:187) … and he has put love and mercy between you" (30:21).[8]

Female genital cutting/female genital mutilation is thought to preserve a family's honor and prevent promiscuity and immorality. The virginity of the girl-child is economically important, and the value placed upon this virginity probably dates back to the days of nomadic existence. However, it is claimed that the custom of genital mutilation is perpetuated because a circumcised woman provides more sexual pleasure for her husband. In a community when the majority of women have been circumcised, those who are not are considered abnormal by themselves or their families. It is a mark of cultural identity. Within a culture, female genital cutting/female genital mutilation is a powerful marker of belonging and affirms a woman's identity. To be circumcised is to be normal. Belonging to the culture has tremendous significance in terms of the desirability of a young woman as a wife; a daughter's marriageability is a major means for her family to achieve economic advancement and independence. Thus, a woman's being unsuitable for marriage affects the ability of her family to prosper. The procedure is believed to ensure cleanliness and chastity and to minimize the sexual appetite of women, thus reducing the likelihood that they will bring shame on themselves or their families through sexual indiscretion. These guarantees of a young woman's purity further enhance her attractiveness to potential suitors.[8,14-16]

In summary, the proponents of female genital cutting/ female genital mutilation believe that:

- The practice reinforces a woman's place in her society.
- It establishes eligibility for marriage.
- It initiates a girl into womanhood.
- Female genitals are unhygienic and in need of cleaning.
- Female genitals are ugly and will grow unwieldy if not cut back.
- The practice safeguards virginity.
- It prevents maternal and infant mortality.
- It improves fertility.
- It enhances a husband's sexual pleasure.

Cultural issues and social mores play an important role in the acceptance and achievement of normal sexual function for both men and women. Tradition, law, education, and the status of women are important indicators of the reproductive function of and freedom of women.[17-19] Cultural mores limit women's freedom during her entire life.

Female genital cutting has been considered one of the "three feminine sorrows": that is, the sorrow on the day of the mutilation, that of the wedding night, and that of childbirth, reflecting the pain associated with these crucial points of a woman's life.[20]

The cutting is usually done in infancy or just before puberty, but practice varies from tribe to tribe. It is a rite of passage, but also the physical sign of a woman's marriageability, the assurance of virginity, and the formation of a chastity belt of her own tissue. The perpetuation of this custom is difficult to understand, since the risks to the health of women are so great, but harm is not the intention.

The term "female circumcision" is clearly inaccurate, as "circumcision" denotes the removal of part of the male prepuce. The World Health Organization has defined female genital cutting/female genital mutilation as all procedures that involve the partial or total removal of the female external genitalia and/or injury to the female genital organs for cultural or any other nontherapeutic reasons.[2] Although the term "female genital mutilation" was previously used to describe this practice, it is now more widely known as "female genital cutting" to avoid the stigma previously associated with female genital mutilation.

Female genital cutting/female genital mutilation refers to a spectrum of surgical excisions from partial to complete clitoridectomy, including the removal of the labia minora and/or majora, scarifying the remnants, and even inserting a matchstick to maintain a sufficient opening for urination. The procedure can be classified according to the extent of the excision. Type I, often referred to as "sunna circumcision", involves the removal of the clitoral prepuce (also called the clitoral hood), but it can also include either partial or total removal of the clitoris (clitoridectomy). Removal of the hood is similar to male circumcision but would be very difficult in a small, prepubertal girl. Types II, III, and IV are more traditional surgical excisions, and are all more damaging to the female urogenital system. Extensive genital excisions may require that the girl remain with her legs bound together from hip to ankle for 1 month or longer to ensure the adequate formation of scar tissue around the raw edges of the labia[3,15,16,20-29,32,33] (Table 16.8.1 and Fig. 16.8.2a–c).

Associated complications can be either immediate or delayed. At the time of the procedure, hemorrhage, shock, infection, and even septicemia and death are possible; severe pain because of the lack of anesthesia can contribute to shock and death. Urinary retention is often the immediate result of the procedure.

Table 16.8.1. Female genital cutting/female genital mutilation classifications

Type I	Also known as "sunna" and involves the excision of the prepuce and/or partial or total clitoridectomy
Type II	Procedure involves removal of the clitoris and partial or total excision of the labia minora
Type III	This is also known as "Pharaonic" and involves clitoridectomy, and excision of the labia minora and majora; infibulation is the reapproximation of the cut ends
Type IV	Refers to any other form of genital manipulation, e.g., burning, pricking, or piercing

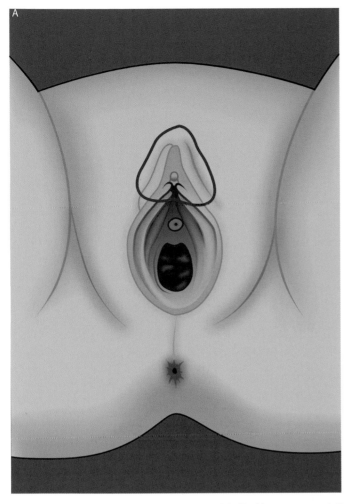
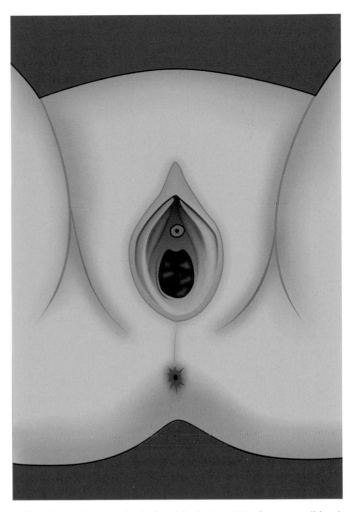

Figure 16.8.2a. Type I – excision of prepuce, partial clitoridectomy, or total clitoridectomy. Type 1 is also known as "sunna", an Islamic term that refers to a traditional practice, or a customary procedure or action. The image on the left has red highlighting the area cut, and the healed area on the right.

Although the age of circumcision ranges from newborn to adult years, it is primarily a prepubertal custom done while the child is held down by a family member. When one considers the anatomy of the underdeveloped prepubertal female external genitalia, one can begin to understand the associated adverse events. It is a procedure done *without* anesthesia, sterile instruments, or visual accuracy. Miscalculations are disastrous. The clitoris, like the penis, is rich in vascular, lymphatic, and neural supply; and extensive bleeding is common.

Delayed gynecologic complications include hematocolpos, menstrual disorders, vaginal stenosis, and future infertility or sterility (see Chapters 9.2–9.5 of this book). An uncommon occurrence can be hematocolpos secondary to imperforate hymen unrelated to female genital cutting. When a young a girl presents with an enlarging abdominal mass and apparent amenorrhea, she may be killed for the honor of the family if they assume that she is pregnant and fail to realize that her menstrual flow is obstructed. The urologic complications relate to the extent of the adnexal damage from infection, bleeding, or the wideness of the excision of the clitoris and adnexal labia. Either

incontinence, because of loss of sphincter function, or urethral stenosis and inability to void appropriately can result. The latter is associated with increased urinary infections because of the relative or complete obstruction. Obstetric complications include prolonged labor and fistula formation between the vagina and the bladder or urethra because of the prolonged labor secondary to the altered birth canal[4,30,33–35] (see Chapter 7.5).

Late-appearing scars include dermoid inclusions, neuromas, vulvar cysts and abscesses, and keloid formation.[36,37] All of these are especially troublesome and painful when nerve endings become entrapped. Sexual "scars" also include the pain and fear that may accompany intercourse and lead to marital problems. Depression and other psychiatric complications may be secondary to a system built on distrust. The person holding the child at the time of the procedure is usually a trusted family member such as the mother; this breach of trust has long-term effects on child and parent.

Each of these complications can obviously affect a woman's sexuality. However, there has been little research on the effects

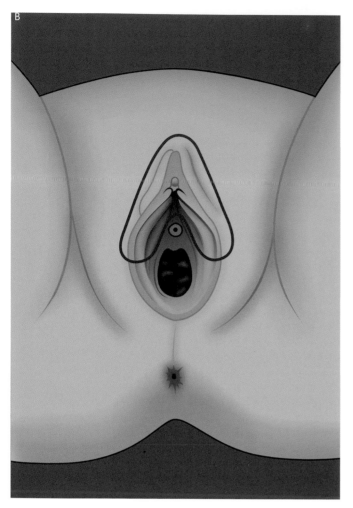 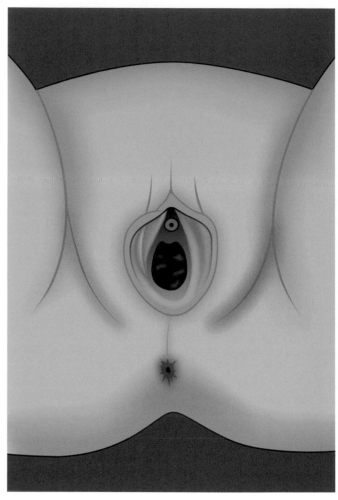

Figure 16.8.2b. Type II involves the removal of the clitoris accompanied by partial or total excision of the labia minora. It is thought that this is the most common form of circumcision practiced throughout central and western Africa. No stitching takes place, but deep cutting of the labia minora may result in raw surfaces that fuse together during healing, creating a false infibulation or pseudo-infibulation. The image on the left has red highlighting the area cut, and the healed area on the right.

of these procedures on women's sexuality. Women with extensive female genital cutting/female genital mutilation may find vaginal intercourse impossible or impeded, although they may be fertile. Childbirth in such women also requires appropriate care, including anesthesia and a midlongitudinal cut, to avoid extensive tearing and obstetric delay.[29,38] Nour notes that the two main causes of infertility are anatomic and psychologic barriers. Women with type III have infertility rates as high as 25–30%. Dyspareunia and the inability to achieve penetration can create stress and frustration in a couple's sexual life (see Chapters 12.1–12.6).

The sexual complications of female genital cutting/female genital mutilation have not been well researched, and there are conflicting reports. The removal of a woman's external sexual organs (such as the clitoris) and infibulation may leave the woman with little sexually sensitive genital tissue. Although female genital cutting/female genital mutilation does not affect the hormones that contribute to sexual arousal, the missing

structures and tissue can have a negative effect on sexual desire, arousal, pleasure, and satisfaction. Other sexually sensitive parts of the body, such as the breasts, nipples, lips, neck, and earlobes, may become increasingly sensitive in women who have undergone female genital cutting to make up for the lack of clitoral stimulation.[31] The type and depth of the genital cut also affect sexual responsiveness. Each of these factors plays an important role in the sexual life of women with female genital cutting/female genital mutilation.[21] Although type I may be practiced in one culture, the cutter may have missed his aim with a screaming child. It has been reported that women with type I were unaffected, while those with type III were significantly affected.[39] A report and curriculum developed by Dr Morris at San Diego State University confirmed some of the problems.[14,46] One woman reported to the investigators: "When I make love with my husband, I can't handle it. I don't want to see him because I have a lot of pain."

Lightfoot-Klein[24–26] reported that "close to 90% of Sudanese

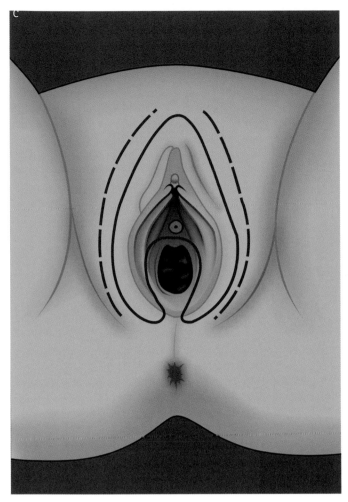
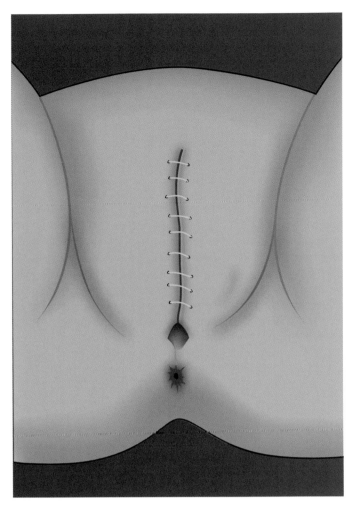

Figure 16.8.2c. Type III involves the most extensive alteration and constitutes approximately 15% of all procedures. This is referred to as "Pharaonic" circumcision or infibulation. It involves the removal of the clitoris, labia minora, and labia majora with reapproximation of the raw surfaces. A small opening is preserved to ensure passage for urine and menstrual blood. The image on the left has red highlighting the area cut, and the healed area is shown on the right.

women interviewed claimed to achieve, or had at some time in their lives achieved, orgasm". It should be observed that orgasmic responses may vary according to the amount of tissue removed, and there is variation in erogenous stimulation as well as cultural expectations.

Gruenbaum[23] concluded that "the effect of female circumcision on sexuality is not uniform or sufficiently well understood. It would appear that the various forms of female circumcisions are not equally devastating to female sexuality. There can be no doubt that many of the circumcision practices can alter physical well-being, including sexual responsiveness. Psychologic aspects of sexuality must also impact on sexual responses. The trauma of circumcision may always influence a woman's sex life."

Measures of female sexual function often use coital frequency as a surrogate marker of normal sexual function. Unfortunately, there is no way to identify in these studies who initiated the sex act. In a study evaluating Nigerian women attending family planning and antenatal clinics, a structured questionnaire was used which asked about the frequency of orgasm achieved during sexual intercourse and symptoms of reproductive tract infections.[4] Forty-five percent of the women were circumcised, including 71% with type I and 24% with type II. The researchers found no significant differences between cut and uncut women in the frequency of reports of sexual intercourse, the frequency of reports of early arousal during intercourse, and the proportions reporting experience of orgasm during intercourse. Uncut women were significantly more likely to report that the clitoris is the most sexually sensitive part of their body, while cut women were more likely to report that their breasts are their most sexually sensitive body parts. Cut women were significantly more likely than uncut women to report having lower abdominal pain and vaginal discharge. Female genital cutting in this group of women did not attenuate sexual feelings. However, female genital cutting may predispose women to adverse sexuality outcomes, including early pregnancy and reproductive tract infections.

Depression and other psychologic disorders may be important sequelae of female genital cutting/female genital mutilation and would also be important markers of the perception of women's sexuality. No research has been done to determine the effect of depression or possible anxiety on sexuality in these women.

Do male expectations determine the prevalence of female genital cutting/female genital mutilation and the sexual response of women? "If men say they don't want the external genitalia, then women won't want to have it."[23] An important aspect of assumed male sexual pleasure is the culturally defined anatomic appearance. Male preference is for smoothness of the vulva in cultures practicing female circumcision; a husband may find a woman's body distasteful if the vulva is not smooth. Female sexual desires may reflect the cultural norm set by men. In many of these cultures, the fidelity of the partners will be an important aspect of a woman's sexuality. Does the presence of the husband's multiple partners outside the home affect a woman's sexual response? Partner reduction and fidelity have been important concepts in the reduction of human immuno-deficiency virus.[41] There are few jobs in rural areas, and most men in rural areas must travel far for migrant work. The acceptance and availability of prostitutes in a particular country will also be important determinants in the spread of disease.

In many of the cultures practicing female genital cutting/female genital mutilation, a dry vagina is also deemed important. The role of agents thought to dry and tighten a woman's vagina and serve as love potions to attract sexual partners and ensure their faithfulness is unclear. It is presumed that these agents draw out moisture, but such astringent agents may be important to reduce secretions from the high prevalence of vaginal infections.[42–45]

Does female genital cutting/female genital mutilation allow women to have a normal and fulfilling sexual relationship? The ability to engage in a mutually fulfilling sexual relationship is an important element in reproductive health. The role of female genital cutting/female genital mutilation in the normal cycle of sexuality is unclear. It is also difficult to understand if we look through Western eyes. Although female genital cutting/female genital mutilation is supposed to control sexuality before marriage, these same women are expected to be sexually responsive to their husbands in marriage. Coital difficulty or inability to have vaginal intercourse at all because of stenosis of the vagina may affect up to 35% of "Pharaonically" circumcised women, and dyspareunia may be common. It is probable that sexual pain disorders may play a role and have an indirect effect on desire, arousal, and orgasmic sexual responses. Sexual dysfunction is highly associated with negative experiences in sexual relationships and reduction of overall well-being. Sexual complications include the pain and fear that may accompany sexual intercourse and can lead to marital problems.

Cultural sensitivity in addressing these problems with a circumcised woman is critical. Most immigrant women do not feel comfortable discussing intimate problems with health-care workers they view as strangers. Toubia[31] cautions health workers to assume that satisfactory sexual and emotional relationships exist in couples regardless of the degree of the women's genital cutting. In interviews with genitally cut women, it was found they had experienced orgasm at some time. Their statements were "qualified by the fact that they were not always sexually satisfied, and it was the nature of the relationship and the sensitivity of the partner that made the difference". Many couples can have a fulfilling relationship because of the deep emotional bond, camaraderie, and social compatibility even if the sexual aspect is missing.

Although both US and Canadian law, as well as many state laws and international laws,[44,45] prohibit the circumcision of any woman under the age of 18 years, there are still many women in the USA who have undergone this procedure. Changes in reproductive rights and information must challenge the culture of silence that has been associated with sex education and contraceptive understanding. Education for women and their daughters will be key to improving their sexuality.

References

1. Brooks G. *Nine Parts of Desire: The Hidden World of Islamic Women.* New York: Doubleday, 1977.

2. Constitution of the World Health Organization, 22 July 1946. www.WHO.int/ (last accessed 25 January 2005).

3. Cook RJ. *Women's Health and Human Rights. The Promotion and Protection of Women's Health Through International Human Rights Law.* Geneva: World Health Organization, 1994.

4. Okonofu F, Larsen U, Oronsaye F et al. The association between female genital cutting and correlates of sexual and gynaecological morbidity in Edo State, Nigeria. *Br J Obstet Gynaecol* 2002; 109: 1089–96.

5. Research, Action and Information Network for the Bodily Integrity of women: RainBo. www.rainbo.org/ (last accessed 15 June 2004).

6. www.un.org (last accessed 1 June 2004).

7. www.who.int/reproductive-health/gender/sexual_health.html#4).

8. www.mwlusa.org (last accessed 25 January 2005).

9. www.fgmnetwork.org/ (last accessed 25 January 2005).

10. www.state.gov (last accessed 25 January 2005).

11. www.fgmnetwork.org/intro/africa_types_maps_type3.htm (last accessed 25 January 2005).

12. Jones W, Smith J, Kieke B et al. Female genital mutilation, female circumcision. Who is at risk in the U.S.? *Public Health Rep* 1997; 112: 368–77.

13. www.path.org/files/FGM-The-Facts.htm (last accessed 1 June 2004).

14. Morris RJ, Gulino C, eds. *Reproductive Health Promotion in Special Populations Curriculum.* San Diego: San Diego State University, 2001.

15. Fourcroy JL. L'éternel couteau: review of female circumcision. *Urology* 1983; 22: 458–61.

16. Wasunna A. Towards redirecting the female circumcision debate: legal, ethical and cultural considerations. *McGill J Med* 2000; 5: 104–10.

17. Osaku GI, Martin-Hilber A. Women's sexuality and fertility;

Nigeria breaking the culture of silence. In *Negotiating Reproductive Rights: Women's Perspectives Across Countries and Cultures*. New York: Zed Books, 1998: 180–216.

18. Petchesky R, Judd K. *Negotiating Reproductive Rights*. London: Zed Division of St Martin's Press, 2001.

19. Wolff B, Blanc A. Who decides? Women's status and negotiation of sex in Uganda. *Cult Health Sex* 2000; 2: 303–22.

20. Fourcroy JL. The three feminine sorrows. *Hosp Pract* 1998; 33: 15–21.

21. Elchalai U, Ben-ami B, Brzezinski A. Female circumcision: the peril remains. *BJU Int* 1999; 83(Suppl 1): 103–8.

22. el Saadawi RE. *The Hidden Face of Eve. Women in the Arab World*. Boston: Beacon Press, 1980.

23. Gruenbaum E. *The Female Circumcision Controversy. An Anthropological Perspective*. Philadelphia: University of Pennsylvania Press, 2001: 154.

24. Lightfoot-Klein H. The sexual experience and marital adjustment of genitally circumcised and infibulated females in the Sudan. *J Sex Res* 1989; 26: 375–92.

25. Lightfoot-Klein H. *Prisoners of Ritual – an Odyssey into Female Genital Circumcision in Africa*. Binghamton: Haworth Press, 1989.

26. Lightfoot-Klein H. *A Woman's Odyssey into Africa*. New York: Haworth Press, 1992.

27. Morris R. The culture of female circumcision. *Adv Nurs Sci* 1996; 19: 43–53.

28. Morris R. Female genital mutilation: perspectives, risks, and complications. *Urol Nurs* 1999; 19: 13–19.

29. Nour NM. Female genital cutting: a need for reform. *Obstet Gynecol* 2003; 101: 1051–2.

30. Nour N. Female genital cutting: clinical and cultural guidelines. *Obstet Gynecol Surv* 2004; 59: 272–9.

31. Toubia N. *Caring for Women with Circumcision – A Technical Manual for Health Care Providers*. New York: Research, Action and Information Network for the Bodily Integrity of Women: RainBo, 1999.

32. Toubia N. Female circumcision as a public health issue. *N Engl J Med* 1994; 331: 712–16.

33. Okonofua F, Larsen U, Oronsaye F et al. The association between female genital cutting and correlates of sexual and gynaecological morbidity in Edo State, Nigeria. *Br J Obstet Gynaecol* 2002; 109: 1089–96.

34. Okonofua F. Female circumcision and obstetric complications. *Int J Gynaecol Obstet* 2002; 77: 255–65.

35. Rushwan H. Female genital mutilation (FGM) management during pregnancy, childbirth and the postpartum period. *Int J Gynaecol Obstet* 2000; 70: 99–104.

36. Slanger T, Snow R, Okonofua F. The impact of female genital cutting on first delivery in southwest Nigeria. *Stud Fam Plann* 2002; 33: 173–84.

37. Fernandez-Aguilar S, Noel J-C. Neuroma of the clitoris after female genital cutting. *Obstet Gynecol* 2003; 101: 1053–4.

38. Young W, Shakya R, Sanders B et al. Clitoral inclusion cyst: a complication of type I female genital mutilation. *J Obstet Gynaecol* 2004; 24: 98–9.

39. Chen G, Dharia S, Steinkampf MP et al. Infertility from female circumcision. *Fertil Steril* 2004; 81: 1692–4.

40. Morris R. Attitudes of Somali men in San Diego toward Female Genital Mutilation. Final Report to the Department of Health Services San Diego County. San Diego: San Diego State University, June 1996.

41. Epstein H. The fidelity fix. *New York Times Sunday Magazine*, 13 June 2004.

42. Brown J, Ayowa O, Brown R. Dry and tight: sexual practices and potential AIDs risk in Zaire. *Soc Sci Med* 1993; 37: 989–94.

43. Brown RC, Brown J, Ayowa O. The use and physical effects of intravaginal substances in Zairian women. *Sex Transm Dis* 1993; 20: 96–9.

44. Dallabetta GA. Traditional vaginal agents: use and association with HIV infection in Malawian women. *AIDS* 1995; 9: 293–7.

45. Wagner G, Bondil P, Dabees K et al. Ethical, socio-cultural and educational aspects of sexual medicine. In T Lue, R Basson, R Rosen et al., eds. *Sexual Medicine: Sexual Dysfunctions in Men and Women. 2nd International Consultation on Sexual Dysfunctions*. Paris: Distributor Editions 21, Health Publications, 2004: 117–38.

46. *Laws of the World on Female Genital Mutilation*. http://annualreview.law.harvard.edu/population/fgm/fgm.htm (last accessed 24 January 2005).

16.9 Persistent sexual arousal syndrome and clitoral priapism

Irwin Goldstein, Elise JB De, Julie A Johnson

Introduction

Many organs and tissues are involved in the physiologic regulation of sexual arousal and orgasm in women. Physiologic sexual activity requires the integration of activity from key brain regions, the central and peripheral nervous systems, and sex steroid hormones. A healthy and intact circulatory system to and from genital tissues is necessary to support the hemodynamic changes associated with sexual arousal. Finally, sexual arousal is dependent upon functionally intact genital tissues, including the various tissue types (smooth muscle, connective tissue, endothelial cells, epithelial cells, neurologic tissue) within the clitoris, corpora spongiosa, vestibular glands, urethral meatus, periurethral glans, vagina, cervix, G-spot, and pelvic floor muscles.[1]

The exact physiologic mechanisms and pathways involved in the complex regulation of peripheral genital arousal and orgasm are not yet known. What is known is that during sexual excitement, genital tissue vascular and nonvascular smooth muscle undergoes loss of baseline contraction, and this relaxation leads to genital tissue engorgement. Following sexual excitement and/or orgasm, the physiologic genital changes eventually return to the baseline condition with restoration of the vasoconstrictive state.[1]

This chapter will address two unusual women's sexual health conditions, persistent sexual arousal syndrome[2,3] and clitoral priapism.[4-9] Both conditions are extremely rare and both are usually associated with significant personal distress. These conditions are defined by physiologic peripheral genital arousal that persists for hours or days despite the absence of sexual desire or sexual stimulation. Specifically in patients with "persistent sexual arousal syndrome", orgasm may temporarily resolve the persistent arousal for a short time, but without sexual thoughts or stimulation, or after what may appear to be a seemingly nonsexual stimulus (vibrations of a moving car), the arousal state returns. The purpose of this chapter is to describe what is currently known concerning these rarely reported conditions. There are limited evidence-based data on the epidemiology, pathophysiology, diagnosis, and treatment of both of these syndromes.

Relation to priapism conditions

Women's sexual dysfunctions are common, complicated, and multidimensional. In the case of medical and biologic sexual dysfunctions, pathophysiologic factors may include abnormalities in the central and peripheral nervous system, hormonal milieu, and/or vascular system. Other pathophysiologic factors include the use of medications, such as antidepressants, that have an adverse effect on sexual function.[10] Persistent sexual arousal syndrome and clitoral priapism are not among the more common sexual complaints, such as lack of interest, inability to achieve orgasm, lack of sexual pleasure, difficulty with lubrication, and sexual pain.[11] A key question, then, is how persistent sexual arousal syndrome and clitoral priapism are distinct from these more often interrelated problems.

The extent to which persistent sexual arousal syndrome and clitoral priapism are similar to male priapism is unclear. In men, priapism is defined as a pathologic condition of peripheral genital arousal that persists beyond or is unrelated to sexual stimulation. There are three recognized forms of priapism: ischemic, low-flow priapism; arterial, high-flow priapism; and a stuttering or recurrent form of priapism.[12] Clitoral priapism best fits the general conceptual definition of ischemic, low-flow priapism, whereas persistent sexual arousal syndrome more closely resembles arterial, high-flow and/or stuttering or recurrent priapism.

Clitoral priapism

The clitoris consists of two paired corpora cavernosa that form a midline shaft with attachment to the pubic bone by the suspensory ligament and two paired crura that attach to the ischiopubic ramus. The most distal aspect, the pars descendens, extrudes only a short distance from the suspensory ligament. Each corporal body is surrounded by a fibrous sheath, the tunica albuginea, that encases cavernosal tissue consisting of sinusoids and surrounding smooth muscle. The glans clitoris appears to emanate from the paired corpora spongiosa (Fig. 16.9.1).

There has been little research on the basic physiology of clitoral engorgement/erection. At present, most researchers believe that nitric oxide is released from the autonomic nerves and from the corpora cavernosal endothelial cells after pelvic nerve stimulation. In one animal study, the mean baseline clitoral intracavernosal pressure was 6 mmHg and the mean internal pudendal arterial blood flow was 5 ml/min. Cavernous nerve stimulation resulted in an increase in the mean clitoral intracavernosal pressure to 10 mmHg and an increase in mean internal pudendal arterial blood flow to 13 ml/min. Pudendal nerve stimulation increased the mean clitoral intracavernosal pressure to 24 mmHg without associated increase in arterial blood flow. It is presumed that the pressure increase in the clitoral corpora cavernosa provides deep anatomic support for extrusion of the sensory nerve-rich glans clitoris[13] (Fig. 16.9.2).

During clitoral engorgement and erection, the ability to induce complete corporal venous outflow resistance or corporal veno-occlusive function is limited. The clitoral intracavernosal pressure at any time during sexual arousal is the result of the equilibrium between the cavernosal artery perfusion pressure and the resistance to blood outflow through the compressed subtunical venules. In the clitoris, during cavernous nerve stimulation, mean clitoral intracavernosal pressure increases approximately twofold from flaccid state measurements. In addition, mean clitoral intracavernosal pressure values decay quickly to baseline pressure values seconds after termination of cavernous stimulation. This would imply that, in the absence of overt clitoral cavernosal arterial disorder, there is limited veno-occlusive function in the clitoral corpora cavernosa. This is quite consistent with overall clitoral function; that is, tumescence/engorgement, pars descendens extrusion, support, and enhanced glans clitoris exposure.[13]

If the draining subtunical venules within the clitoral corpora cavernosa became obstructed, the result would be consistent with ischemic, low-flow priapism. Although this form of priapism is the most common form of priapism in men, this may not be the case in women. Ischemic, low-flow priapism in either gender is related to inability to drain blood from within the corporal bodies. This may occur in an extravascular sense, secondary to drug-induced, *persistent*, corporal smooth muscle

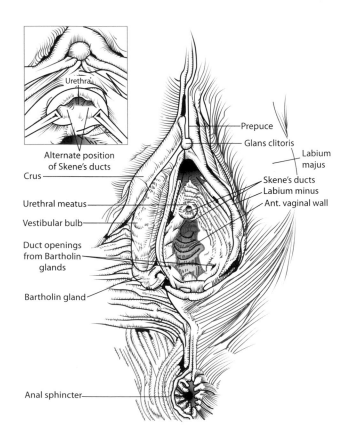

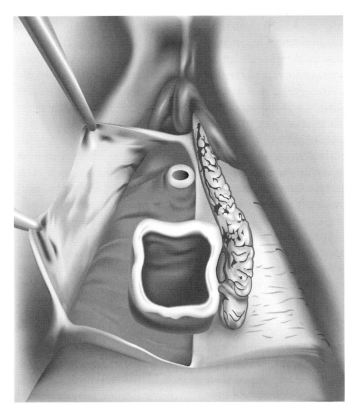

Figure 16.9.1. Clitoral anatomy. The clitoris consists of two paired corpora cavernosa that form a midline shaft with attachment to the pubic bone by the suspensory ligament and two paired crura that attach to the ischiopubic ramus. The glans clitoris appears to emanate from the paired corpora spongiosa.

Baseline state   Aroused state

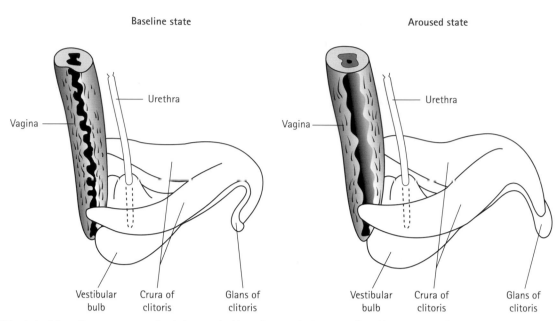

Figure 16.9.2. Clitoral physiology. Cavernous nerve stimulation resulted in an increase in the mean clitoral intracavernosal pressure and an increase in mean internal pudendal arterial blood flow. It is presumed that the pressure increase in the clitoral corpora cavernosa provides deep anatomic support for extrusion of the sensory nerve-rich glans clitoris.

relaxation. Priapism of the clitoris can occur after the use of oral psychotropic agents such as trazodone,[5,9] citalopram,[8] nefazodone,[7] and olanzapine.[6]

Unusual clitoral erectile activity has been observed after the use of several oral pharmacologic agents. Bromocryptine has been noted to induce recurrent clitoral tumescent episodes of only several minutes in duration and occurring only in the upright position.[14] Fluoxetine, a bicyclic propylamine antidepressant with potent inhibition of serotonin reuptake, has been observed to induce recurrent, short-duration, painless clitoral engorgement in association with yawning and multiple, spontaneously occurring orgasms.[15,16]

Ischemic, low-flow priapism may also occur by an intravascular mechanism such as mechanical obstruction within draining subtunical venules. Clinical conditions associated with intravascular mechanisms include metastatic invasive carcinomas.[17]

Ischemic, low-flow priapism of the clitoris presents as acute clitoral pain and is a genuine medical emergency, since it is a closed compartment syndrome with potentially irreversible genital tissue damage.

Persistent sexual arousal syndrome

Persistent sexual arousal syndrome is *not* an acute state of clitoral priapism with acute pain in the clitoris. Persistent sexual arousal syndrome is, on the other hand, chronic and recurrent, and is not likely to be curable given our limited understanding of its pathophysiology. In most women, the persistent arousal state is not sought and interferes greatly with their quality of life. In our experience, women affected with the condition are

frequently suicidal, socially ostracized, isolated, frustrated, miserable, embarrassed, and extremely humiliated. Persistent sexual arousal syndrome therefore is more consistent with the two other recognized forms of priapism. One is high-flow, arterial priapism, which is considered to be the inability to regulate physiologic arterial inflow to the corporal cavernosal bodies. Clinical conditions associated with persistent arterial inflow that bypasses sympathetic arteriolar regulation include arterial-lacunar fistulas from blunt or penetrating perineal trauma and pelvic arterial-venous malformations. In high-flow priapism, the state of abnormally increased arousal is persistent, not associated with pain, not wanted, felt to be intrusive, and not associated with sexual desire.[12]

The other form of priapism is stuttering or recurrent priapism. This condition is characterized by repeated episodes of unwanted genital arousal that may or may not proceed to classic ischemic, low-flow priapism. Stuttering priapism in men is reported in sickle cell disease and in those with so-called recurrent idiopathic prolonged erection. Preliminary data suggest that hypoxia might downregulate phosphodiesterase type 5A promoters, implying an involvement of phosphodiesterase type 5 in recurrent or stuttering priapism.[18] Such patients cannot efficiently metabolize the second messenger cyclic guanosine monophosphate, resulting in a tendency to unrelenting genital smooth muscle relaxation. Ischemic, low-flow priapism associated with genital tissue damage from hypoxia, hypercapnia, and severe acidosis most commonly results in permanent erectile dysfunction. In unusual cases, however, ischemic, low-flow priapism has been reported to result in stuttering or recurrent priapism. One hypothesis to explain this unusual sequela of tissue ischemia is that the damage interfered with the biochemistry of contraction, resulting in a tendency to recurrent genital arousal. Unfortunately, there is little research on the topic.[12]

In both arterial, high-flow and stuttering or recurrent forms of priapism, the abnormal arousal condition is chronic and persistent, unsolicited, and not associated with sexual interest, and it adversely affects patients' lives. There appear to be many parallels between these two forms of priapism and persistent sexual arousal syndrome in women.

Classification

The definition and classification of women's sexual dysfunctions, especially disorders of arousal and orgasm, have been recently reconsidered. Persistent sexual arousal syndrome, but not clitoral priapism, has also been addressed in recent attempts at nomenclature and classification.[19] The authors propose the following conditions for future consideration.

Clitoral priapism is a pathologic condition of clitoral engorgement/erection that is usually painful and persists beyond or is unrelated to sexual stimulation. Clitoral priapism is an important medical condition that requires evaluation and may require emergency management. Potential consequences are irreversible corporal fibrosis and permanent sexual dysfunction.

Persistent sexual arousal syndrome is a persistent, recurrent, or continuous unwanted state of sexual excitement, causing personal distress. It may be expressed as excessive subjective excitement or excessive genital (lubrication, swelling, engorgement) or other somatic responses. If the woman with persistent sexual arousal syndrome experiences repeated orgasm, another pathologic condition may exist, persistent orgasmic disorder. Persistent orgasmic disorder would be considered the persistent, recurrent, or continuous attainment of or need to attain orgasm after minimal or absent sexual stimulation and arousal, causing personal distress.

Epidemiology

Clitoral priapism has been reported rarely.[4–9,14–17] Persistent sexual arousal syndrome has been reported in a few publications. At our outpatient sexual medicine clinic, we are managing approximately 20 women with persistent sexual arousal syndrome and are in communication with over 20 others. An Internet survey of women afflicted with persistent sexual arousal has been established.[20] Women around the world have registered with this group and appear to have symptoms consistent with persistent sexual arousal syndrome. It is possible that the condition is more common than previously thought.

Case examples

The following are case examples of patients from our out-patient sexual medicine clinic who have been diagnosed with clitoral pri-apism and persistent sexual arousal syndrome. As in other portions of this textbook relating to difficult case management, all efforts have been made to protect the privacy of patients and to maintain the management strategies utilized in the case for teaching purposes.

Clitoral priapism

A 34-year-old woman reported a past history of alcohol and drug abuse and a positive family history for depression. She was diagnosed with adjustment disorder with anxious mood and major depression. The patient was prescribed fluoxetine 40 mg daily with a resultant effective clinical response for a period of 10 months. Due to drug-associated insomnia, trazodone hydrochloride was initiated at 25 mg a night for the first two nights, and then increased to 50 mg nightly, while fluoxetine was concomitantly decreased to 20 mg daily. Five days after initiating trazodone, the patient experienced a new onset irritation and itch-like discomfort in the region of the clitoris. Four days later, upon awakening from sleep, the patient observed a marked change in the quality of the introital discomfort, describing it as an intense pain, unlike anything she had previously encountered. The patient denied any history of trauma to the introitus. She denied any history of blood dyscrasia or previous malignancies. Physical examination by a gynecologist the same day confirmed introital changes consistent with clitoral priapism, including an erect, reddened, distended, tender, firm, and painful clitoris. The treatment strategy, which involved discontinuation of all psychotropic medications (fluoxetine and trazodone) and administration of phenylpropanolamine twice daily, successfully resolved the priapism, and no long-term sexual sequelae were reported.[9]

Persistent sexual arousal syndrome

Case 1

A 68-year-old woman with numerous medical problems presented with complaints of unrelenting orgasms. She had never had a problem reaching orgasm with masturbation and oral sex. Shortly after she had brain surgery for an arteriovenous malformation, she began to experience throbbing and fluttering sensations in the area of her clitoris and vagina, followed by multiple orgasms. The ability to have 100–200 orgasms per day without masturbation persisted. Sitting became unbearable, sometimes causing pressure to orgasm, and traveling by car became torture. Her only relief was standing, with orgasmic activity increasing throughout the course of the day. The sensations were in the clitoris, the right wall of the outer labia, and the G-spot. Physical examination revealed a distended glans clitoris in the absence of sexual stimulation (Fig. 16.9.3). Merely touching the vaginal opening would cause her to reach orgasm. Her husband remains sympathetic to her plight and relieves her pressure whenever asked. Her physician tried to help by prescribing paroxetine, which had no effect. While

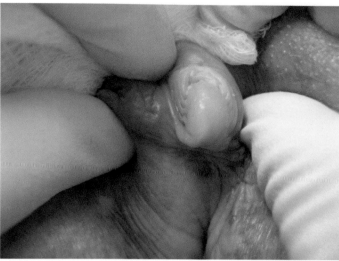

A

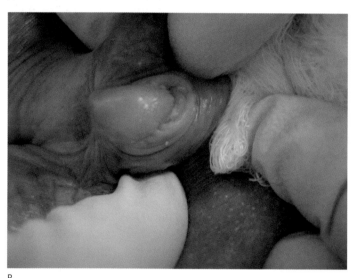

B

Figure 16.9.3. Physical examination revealed a distended glans clitoris in the absence of sexual stimulation.

having an active sex life at 68 would be rewarding, this patient is miserable living with this condition.

Case 2

A 43-year-old woman, who had experienced neck problems for a year, began having anxiety and panic attacks and was prescribed sertraline. Her neck pain worsened. Treatment included acupressure, physical therapy, soma, and hydrocodone. Within 2 months, she noticed an increase in libido and a need to reach orgasm once or twice a day rather than once a week as usual. She and her husband rarely had sexual activity due to her chronic neck pain and intense headaches. After surgery, she regained mobility in her neck and relief from the chronic pain and debilitating headaches, but the feelings of pulsation in her clitoris and need to reach orgasm became constant. Her release from orgasm lasted only

2–5 min at a time. Her gynecologist found her hormone values within normal limits and joked that she was every man's dream. Her psychiatrist tried several medications including divalproex, citalopram, imipramine, and fluoxetine. While none of these decreased her libido, they did decrease her ability to reach orgasm, her only source of relief. Consequently, she discontinued these medications.

She calls her life sheer hell, resulting in depression, reclusiveness, weight gain, and inability to participate in normal activities. The vibration from the activities she used to enjoy causes so much stimulation as to be unacceptable. She continues to search for answers, and believes that there may be some relation between her problems and persistent sexual arousal syndrome.

Case 3

Another patient experienced similar symptoms, but with the additional complication of having survived sexual abuse. The patient was unable to sleep through the discomfort. She felt her level of arousal was increasing, and that orgasm was progressively less effective in relieving these feelings, sometimes taking hours over several days to reach orgasm with little relief afterward. The patient was diagnosed with a prolapsed urethra resulting in a hyperactive urethral-clitoral neurologic reflex (Fig. 16.9.4). After using topical estradiol cream twice daily, eliminating treatment with methylphenidate, and having the prolapse surgically repaired, she now goes for days and even weeks symptom-free, but is afraid to have sexual relations with her husband for fear of the persistent sexual arousal returning. Indeed, even after treatment, the patient's feelings of sexual arousal continued to persist into the day after intercourse. However, this condition has improved over time, with sexual arousal eventually subsiding about 1 h after intercourse.

Case 4

"I was constantly feeling overwhelming sensations of sexual arousal, which were purely physical and not accompanied by romantic or sexual fantasies." This patient needed to have repeated orgasms, but experienced little relief from them. She felt insatiable, and the constant sensation was "dreadful" in her words. Disabled from Lyme disease, the patient considered suicide rather than spending day after day masturbating continually. Treatment with oral contraceptives lessened the persistent sexual arousal, but gave her a cluster migraine. Treatment with nafarelin acetate nasal spray diminished the persistent sexual arousal syndrome somewhat but also lessened her ability to achieve orgasm. After years of using trazodone for insomnia, the patient eliminated the medication from her regimen, and her persistent sexual arousal syndrome symptoms decreased by 80%.

Case 5

Persistent sexual arousal syndrome severely impairs everyday life and relationships, often leading to feelings of depression and thoughts of suicide. One patient explained, "it continues to rule my life and I schedule my work and personal life around my

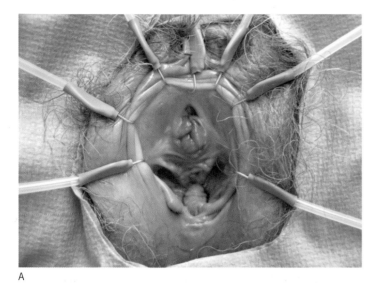

A

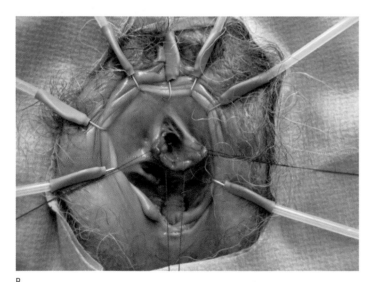

B

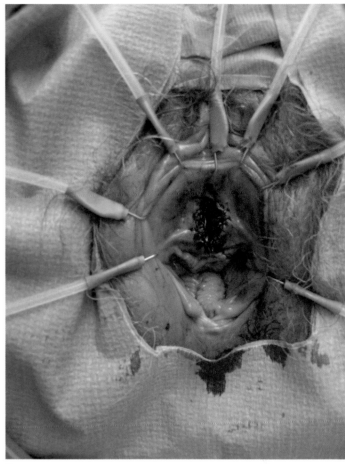

C

Figure 16.9.4. The patient was diagnosed with prolapsed urethra. Surgical repair involved excision of the redundant urethral mucosa.

physical pain and discomfort. It is still difficult to concentrate, focus, or achieve what I would like to both at work and at home. It has led to a renewed problem of depression and angry outbursts that are affecting my personal relationships. I have begun to contemplate suicide because I cannot imagine living like this for the rest of my life." At the age of 12, this patient had perineal trauma, causing bleeding for 2 weeks. During her teen years, she experienced sensations of extreme pressure in her groin area. The heavy pressure and engorgement in the clitoris started in her late teens around the time she became sexually active, although it was not as intense as in later years. This was always managed by reaching orgasm every 2–3 days. However, after hysterectomy, it became more difficult for her to reach orgasm. The patient also began experiencing occasional acute pain in the groin that lasted for up to 10 min. This was not associated with any activity, but would force her to lie down.

Pressure on her bowels and bladder during sexual stimulation interrupted activity for toileting, causing further distress and lessening enjoyment of sexual activity. Reaching orgasm continued to be difficult, and normal function and normal relationships became increasingly disrupted. Although her clitoris was painfully engorged, she had no interest in sex. While the symptoms were lessened somewhat by eliminating hormone therapy and using ice packs, gradually her symptoms worsened and she contemplated suicide more often. She was ultimately diagnosed as having a pelvic, arteriovenous malformation (Fig. 16.9.5). After multiple embolizations, her condition has improved greatly.

Case 6

A 47 year old health-care professional, married for 24 years, with a lifelong history of depression, has been treated with a

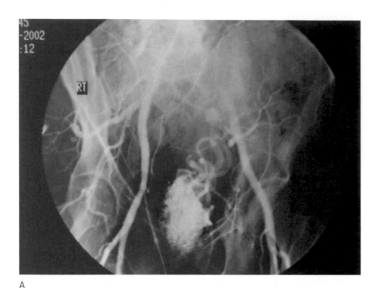

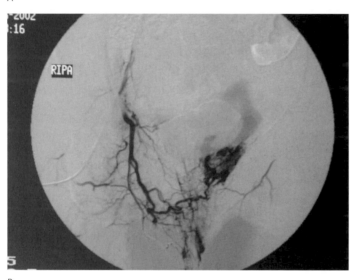

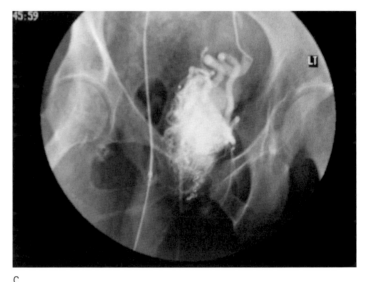

Figure 16.9.5. Aortography revealed a left internal iliac arteriovenous malformation. Selective internal pudendal arteriography revealed clitoral arteries communicating with the left arteriovenous malformation.

multitude of antidepressant medications. Despite the use of antidepressants, she had a healthy sex life and was multi-orgasmic all her life. After being put on lamotrigone (lamictal) 2 years ago for treatment of depression, she developed symptoms of persistent sexual arousal. The symptoms of constant, unre-lenting clitoral and genital engorgement remained 24 h a day, 7 days a week, with virtually no relief. In addition, despite the continual feeling of engorgement, she could not easily achieve orgasm for 2 years. "I never knew such a horrible, hideous thing could happen to someone."

She was an avid antique coin dealer, and this hobby went downhill. She lived in an old farmhouse, and projects that used to get completed with passion just sat untouched. She felt the need to spend a large amount of time alone in her bedroom just trying to get some kind of relief, but that was not often possible.

She is a professional, and she had to go to work with very little sleep literally for days on end.

She was referred to both a multidisciplinary sexual medi-cine clinic and to a psychoneurologist. She was started on val-proic acid (depakote) 125 mg/day for 1 week, and this was then increased each week by 125 mg until 1000 mg/day was adminis-tered. Although she had initial nausea, she tolerated the medication well. She felt some relief shortly after starting the medication, and every dose increase improved the persistent sexual arousal symptoms. While the valproic acid kept the per-sistent engorgement to a tolerable level, the medication did not fully resolve the symptoms.

She was also found to have very low androgen levels with low free testosterone, low total testosterone, low dehydro-epiandrosterone sulfate, low androstenedione, and modestly elevated sex hormone-binding globulin. She also had modest clitoral and labial atrophy, partial clitoral phimosis, and mild dyspareunia. She was also started on oral dehydroepiandros-terone, testosterone gel, vestibular estradiol, and intravaginal estradiol. She was temporarily happy. Life was better. She was orgasmic more easily. She stated that persistent sexual arousal without orgasm was infinitely worse than persistent sexual arousal with orgasmic release.

After 6 months of the valproic acid, she felt immobilized on the medication and gained over 45 pounds. Due to persistent depression, feelings of despair and suicide, and the persistent sexual arousal, she was offered electroconvulsive therapy as an extreme treatment for an extreme problem. Ultimately, after 3 years of persistent sexual arousal, she agreed.

Three months after undergoing 19 electroconvulsive therapy sessions, the persistent sexual arousal symptoms were completely gone. She stated she never thought she would be normal again. She felt reborn, so no more than six treatments were necessary at the time. She has no residual persistent sexual arousal symptoms and takes no antidepressant medication at present. She continues on the four sexual medications. She is sexually active, and says her sexual function, including desire, arousal, and orgasm, is back to normal, a statement she never thought she would get to make again.

Pathophysiology

The pathophysiology of clitoral priapism appears to be relatively straightforward. There are cases of drug-induced, persistent, smooth muscle relaxation and cases of infiltrative malignancy.[4–9,14–17] The remainder of this chapter will focus on the biologic pathophysiologies of persistent sexual arousal syndrome, using the arbitrary classifications of neurologic, vascular, pharmacologic, idiopathic, and hormonal etiologies.

Neurologic – central and/or peripheral genital

Little is known of the central nervous system pathways controlling sexual function in women. The central anatomic structures or networks involved in the mediation of women's genital arousal probably include the prefrontal cortex, hippocampus, amygdala, hypothalamus, midbrain, pons, and medulla. Supraspinal sites that project directly to the spinal cord center for women's genital arousal probably include the paraventricular nucleus, locus cereulus, nucleus paragigantocellularis, parapyramidal reticular formation, raphe magnus, raphe pallidus, A5-adrenergic cell group, and Barrington's nucleus. The suprasinal anatomic organization of centers and pathways involved in women's genital arousal can be theorized to function in terms of parallel processing.[20]

A generator system is theorized to exist within the spinal cord. This system can be activated by the pudendal, pelvic, and possibly the hypogastric nerve afferents. The spinal generator system is under inhibitory and excitatory descending modulatory control. Ascending pathways via the spinothalamic and spinoreticular pathways to the brainstem, hypothalamus, and forebrain modulate activity or level setting of the suprasinal sites. The ascending and descending pathways ultimately modulate the spinal generator system at the level of the spinal interneurons found in the intermediolateral column and dorsal interneurons.[21]

In the end, neurologic control of genital arousal consists of numerous spinal level reflexes, most activated by pudendal afferents. Theoretically, central or peripheral nervous system disorder may lead to persistent neurologic stimulation or facilitation of the motor autonomic nerves regulating smooth muscle control of the clitoris, labia, and/or vagina. The result would be persistent smooth muscle relaxation of the arterioles and corporal bodies of the clitoris and corpora spongiosa, leading to clitoral and labial engorgement. In addition, there would be increased blood flow in the vaginal lamina propria and relaxation of the vaginal muscularis, leading to vaginal engorgement. The end result would be consistent with persistent sexual arousal syndrome.

In our outpatient sexual medicine clinic, we have observed four women we considered to have persistent sexual arousal syndrome secondary to central neurologic pathophysiology. One woman developed persistent sexual arousal syndrome after neurosurgical intervention for arteriovenous malformation. Two noted persistent arousal after developing symptoms of cerebrovascular accident, in one case after discontinuing estrogens and in the other case after discontinuing a cholesterol-lowering agent. The fourth developed persistent arousal after neurosurgical intervention for severe neck pain. In one woman, persistent sexual arousal syndrome was observed that may have been secondary to neurologic peripheral pathophysiology. This woman developed persistent arousal after surgery for urethral prolapse. It was hypothesized that the inflammation around the urethra activated local urethroclitoral and/or urethrolabial nerves, activating the spinal reflex leading to persistent arousal. Re-establishing estrogen treatment, performing steroid-lidocaine nerve blocks around the urethral meatus, and surgically correcting the urethral prolapse led to a marked improvement in her condition.

Vascular

The main arterial supply to the peripheral genitals is from the iliohypogastric-pudendal arterial bed. The internal pudendal artery is the last anterior branch off the internal iliac artery. Distally, the internal pudendal artery traverses Alcock's canal, and lies on the inner side in apposition to the ischiopubic ramus. The internal pudendal artery terminates as it supplies the inferior rectal and perineal artery, which supplies the labia. The common clitoral artery continues to the clitoris. This artery bifurcates into a dorsal clitoral artery and a cavernosal clitoral artery.[20]

The arterial supply to the vagina is derived from an extensive network of branching vessels surrounding it on all sides. The anterior branch of the internal iliac artery continually bifurcates as it descends through the pelvis with a series of the newly generated vessels, each supplying the vagina to some degree. After giving off an obturator artery branch, the umbilical, and the midrectal arteries diverge to supply a superior and inferior vesicle artery, respectively. Between the umbilical and the midrectal branches, there is a generation of a uterine artery, which further bifurcates to give the vaginal artery. The internal pudendal and accessory pudendal artery also sends a branch. Finally, the common clitoral artery sends a branch to the vaginal muscularis.[20]

Arterial blood flow through the iliohypogastric-pudendal-cavernosal bed or through the ilio-obturator-uterine-vaginal bed is regulated by the arteriolar resistance tone, as determined by the sympathetic nervous system. A pelvic arteriovenous malformation may bypass arteriolar regulation and lead to unregulated arterial inflow to the clitoris, labia, and/or vagina, resulting in persistent engorgement of the corporal bodies of the clitoris and corpora spongiosa. In addition, there would be increased blood flow in the vaginal lamina propria leading to vaginal engorgement. The end result would be consistent with persistent sexual arousal syndrome.

In our outpatient sexual medicine clinic, a woman, presenting with lifelong persistent sexual arousal syndrome, was found on clitoral ultrasound to have high baseline arterial blood flow. She subsequently underwent a selective internal pudendal arteriogram and was discovered to have a pelvic arteriovenous malformation with multiple branches feeding the clitoral corporal bodies (Fig. 16.9.5). After a series of embolizations, the patient's condition improved.

Pharmacologic

Physiologic and pharmacologic investigations of the arousal phase of the female sexual response involve, in part, an understanding of the various local regulatory mechanisms that modulate smooth muscle tone in the clitoral and corpora spongiosal erectile tissue and the vaginal muscularis. Immunohistochemical studies in human vaginal tissues have shown the presence of nerve fibers containing neuropeptide Y, vasoactive intestinal polypeptide, nitric oxide synthase, calcitonin gene-related peptide, and substance P.[1,20] The effects of sex steroid hormones on genital smooth muscle contractility are presently being studied. The state of tone of the genital smooth muscles in the clitoris, labia, and vagina determines the state of genital arousal. When the smooth muscles are relaxed, engorgement results. Pharmacologically induced inhibition of contraction or enhanced relaxation of the clitoral, labial, and/or vaginal smooth muscle results in persistent engorgement of the corporal bodies of the clitoris and corpora spongiosa, and increased blood flow in the vaginal lamina propria. This causes symptoms consistent with persistent sexual arousal syndrome.

Trazodone administration in men is associated with the development of prolonged penile erections, especially nocturnal erections.[21] The mechanism is unknown but thought to be related in part to alpha-blocking activity and serotonergic

blocking activity.[21] The effect on erectile tissue is inability to induce smooth muscle contraction, with persistence of smooth muscle relaxation. While we and others have reported that trazodone induces clitoral priapism,[5,9] we have also documented that chronic trazodone use is associated with persistent sexual arousal.[22] In our outpatient sexual medicine clinic, two women presenting with persistent sexual arousal syndrome were found on history-taking to be long-term users of trazodone. In both cases, discontinuation of trazodone led to improvement of the condition.

We have one patient who believes her symptoms of persistent sexual arousal began after administration of lamotrigone. Her symptoms remained despite discontinuing the medication.

Idiopathic

Patients who do *not* have a distinct history of a central or peripheral nervous system pathophysiology, evidence of a vascular arteriovenous malformation, or use a medication such as an antipsychotic or trazodone have an idiopathic form of persistent sexual arousal syndrome. It would appear that most patients should be classified into this category because, for the most part, clearly recognized causes for the syndrome are limited.

Clues to the pathophysiology of the idiopathic form of persistent sexual arousal come from listening to what our patients claim to be responsible for initiating an attack. Precipitating factors have been categorized into arbitrary subheadings. Enhanced sensory input states, for example, are reported, such as pressure against the genitals, riding a bicycle or horse, or vibrations transmitted to the genital area, especially from riding in a car. Sexual stimulation states such as sexual intercourse, sexual foreplay, and/or masturbation can activate the persistent arousal response. Changed hormone states, such as pregnancy, premenstrual syndrome, high dietary intake of soy, menopause, and initiating or discontinuing hormone therapy, may also precipitate symptoms. These precipitating factors have in common the potential inclination to initiate genital smooth relaxation and/or inhibit genital smooth muscle contraction.

Other hints and signs of the pathophysiology of the idiopathic form of persistent sexual arousal come from paying attention to what *terminates* an attack. In virtually all patients with persistent sexual arousal syndrome, orgasmic relief by masturbation may for varying periods of time conclude an event of persistent arousal. Other patients assert that pain and the distraction from pain, as well as distraction via physical exercise and the application of cold to the genitals, can temporarily stop an event of persistent arousal. Orgasm, pain, and cold temperature all activate the sympathetic nervous system. These factors that induce loss of persistent arousal have in common the potential inclination to initiate genital smooth contraction and/or negate genital smooth muscle relaxation.

What is the unifying characteristic of idiopathic persistent sexual arousal syndrome? We hypothesize that these patients are vulnerable to persistent sexual arousal syndrome on the basis of unusual genital tissue biochemistry. Theoretically, patients with idiopathic persistent sexual arousal syndrome lack the ability to induce genital smooth muscle contraction once genital smooth muscle relaxation has been initiated. More specifically, as discussed earlier, persistent sexual arousal syndrome has much in common with stuttering or recurrent priapism. If the smooth muscles cannot be contracted once relaxed, the state of arousal will persist.[23]

What are the recognized biochemical regulatory controls over genital smooth muscle contraction once genital tissue is relaxed? Vascular and nonvascular smooth muscle contraction is under the control of several mechanisms. The one best studied is the contribution by alpha-adrenergic receptor activation from norepinephrine released by the sympathetic nervous system. Adrenergic activation involves alpha receptors, dissociation of G-protein receptor subunits, activation of phospholipase C, synthesis of inositol triphosphate and diacylglycerol, and activation of protein kinase C. The end result is an increase in intracellular calcium that promotes phosphorylation of myosin light chain and a contractile response of actin and myosin.[23]

Another contributory mechanism to induce vascular and nonvascular smooth muscle is endothelin-1 secreted by genital tissue endothelial cells. Endothelin-1 binds to endothelin-A receptors, leading to increased levels of intracellular calcium. The importance of endothelin in inducing genital tissue contractility remains to be determined.[23]

An additional fundamental means of inducing vascular and nonvascular smooth muscle contraction is by the RhoA and Rho-kinase system. The contractile effects of RhoA/Rho-kinase appear to be the result of Rho-kinase-mediated inhibition of myosin light-chain phosphatase through phosphorylation of the myosin-binding subunit. The end result is maintenance of phosphorylated myosin light chain, promoting the binding of actin and myosin and smooth muscle contractile force generation.[23]

Another contributory mechanism promoting termination of genital smooth muscle relaxation after sexual stimulation is activation of the enzyme phosphodiesterase 5. The action of phosphodiesterase type 5 is to hydrolyze the second messenger cyclic guanosine monophosphate. Since high intracellular cyclic guanosine monophosphate concentrations decrease intracellular calcium by increasing the flux of calcium out of the cell and by increasing calcium binding to the sarcoplasmic reticulum, decreasing cyclic guanosine monophosphate by phosphodiesterase type 5 hydrolysis would promote and encourage increased intracellular calcium and genital smooth muscle contraction.[23]

In theory, alterations, modifications, or changes to any or all of the four mechanisms promoting increase in intracellular calcium and genital smooth muscle contraction may place an individual at risk of persistent sexual arousal syndrome. In such cases, once genital smooth muscle is relaxed, these theorized biochemical alterations would make it difficult to induce smooth muscle contraction and thereby inhibit further arousal.

Another theory is that in some patients with persistent sexual arousal, there are the equivalent of "mini-seizures", with unregulated, excitatory central neurons firing constantly and activating peripheral genital arousal. Antiseizure medications may have some inhibitory effect on these individuals with uninhibited activated neurons. At least in one case, the dramatic effects of the electroconvulsive therapy suggest that once the "mini-seizure-like" activity was discontinued, the persistent sexual arousal symptoms were terminated.

The role of psychologic factors in the pathophysiology of the syndrome remains unclear. Precipitating psychologic factors reported to initiate persistent arousal include nervousness, concern, fretfulness, worry, strain, and tension. It is not understood how psychologic factors associated with stress and anxiety precipitate genital smooth muscle relaxation, and it is possible there is simply no obvious relation of psychologic factors to induction of persistent genital arousal. Once genital smooth muscle relaxation has been initiated and the persistent arousal response occurs, patients often become angry, mortified, and preoccupied. No matter how upset they become, afflicted patients continue to experience this condition and generally are unable to terminate the symptoms. This observation is consistent with an underlying biochemical contribution. The role of psychology in persistent sexual arousal syndrome perhaps is less in pathophysiology and more in treatment. Psychotherapy is an imperative and central additional treatment for women with persistent sexual arousal syndrome to assist in the management of the devastating psychologic sequelae, especially the helplessness associated with the condition.

Hormonal

The pathophysiology of persistent sexual arousal syndrome should be discussed in terms of a possible hormonal pathophysiology, such as a hyperandrogenic or a hyperestrogenic state. Theoretically, this can result in a persistent sexual arousal state, although this has not been observed in our sexual medicine clinic to date. The measurement of sex steroid hormone blood tests in all patients who were evaluated at our outpatient clinic has not revealed abnormally high levels of sex steroids. Most patients either had a normal or a hypoandrogen and/or hypoestrogen state. Luteinizing hormone-releasing hormone agonists, such as leuprolide acetate, were provided to several women with persistent sexual arousal syndrome, but no benefit was observed. While no patient has yet been encountered with persistent sexual arousal syndrome with an abnormal hormonal pathophysiology, blood test values are constantly being checked in light of this possibility.

Management paradigm

The management strategy for clitoral priapism is based on an underlying pharmacologic etiology. Under such pathophysiology, all potential offending medications (psychotropic, alpha-blocking agents) need to be discontinued. In addition, alpha-agonists need to be administered orally. If such treatment fails, clitoral intracavernosal administration of alpha-agonists (phenylephrine, 100 μg) should be considered.[4–9]

It is somewhat premature to discuss treatment of persistent sexual arousal syndrome, since the pathophysiologies are not fully elucidated. The following represent various biologic treatments, under the proposed classification system, that we have employed with varying success in the patients we have managed with persistent sexual arousal syndrome.

Neurologic – central

1. The medical treatment of irritating central nervous system lesion is as follows: neurosurgical excision of irritating space-occupying lesion; physical therapy, especially if there is a cervical disk lesion; acupressure; pain medications; and muscle relaxants.
2. Use medications that stabilize nerve transmission, theoretically decreasing excitation of the genital arousal reflex: divalproex, citalopram, gabapentin, clonazepam, imipramine, fluoxetine, paroxetine, olanzapine, and lorazepam.
3. Use local topical anesthetic agents, ice.
4. Normalize sex steroid hormonal milieu to improved orgasmic function, as orgasmic release consistently offers patients temporary relief.

Neurologic – peripheral genital

1. Medical treatment of irritating lesion, especially genital estrogen, may diminish the local inflammation of the sensory nerves.
2. Use local topical anesthetic agents, ice.
3. Use steroid nerve blocks (repeated).
4. Normalize sex steroid hormonal milieu to improved orgasmic function, as orgasmic release consistently offers patients temporary relief.
5. Surgical excision of the irritating lesion is another treatment.

Pharmacologic

Discontinue offending medication.

Arterial

1. Embolization of arteriovenous malformation.
2. Surgical excision of arteriovenous malformation.

Idiopathic

1. Use medications that stabilize nerve transmission, theoretically decreasing excitation of the genital arousal reflex: divalproex, citalopram, gabapentin, clonazepam, imipramine, fluoxetine, paroxetine, olanzapine, and lorazepam.
2. Local topical anesthetic agents, ice.

3. Normalize sex steroid hormonal milieu to improved orgasmic function, as orgasmic release consistently offers patients temporary relief.

For all patients who cannot be relieved of their symptoms, psychotherapy should be considered to manage the chronic adverse effects of the syndrome. In our experience, the reaction to persistent sexual arousal syndrome is unique for each individual. The initial distress, including confusion, shame, and isolation, is frequently compounded by a lack of access to health care. The overwhelming majority of women we evaluated at our clinic complain of depression. Work, family, and relationship roles are severely altered by the condition. Loss of employment due to poor concentration or time spent managing symptoms is common. Children are often aware that something has changed. In one case, a mother had to lock herself in her bedroom for entire afternoons to manage her persistent arousal.

The woman's relationship with her partner frequently is adversely affected. Partners experience helplessness and confusion, uncertainty in providing relief, inadequacy, frustration, and isolation. A decline in the quality of life often occurs for not only the woman, but also her family, as she becomes less available emotionally.

For some of the patients, persistent sexual arousal syndrome was long-standing and manageable, but became unmanageable when new-onset orgasmic difficulty occurred, often due to aging or a medical change such as androgen insufficiency. Couples who had been managing the symptoms through frequent sexual activity suddenly were met with unsatisfactory sexual encounters, and extreme discomfort and frustration on the part of the woman. Both members of the couple have communicated a sense of relief at finding professional help and hope about treatment options. The awareness of other individuals regarding the diagnosis has decreased the sense of isolation that the overwhelming majority of individuals describe.

Consultation with a sex therapist should be standard practice. This can occur either in the physician's office setting or by referral to a nearby practice with an understanding of the diagnosis. It should be made clear that the consultation is a standard adjunct of treatment while a diagnosis is being sought or treatment undertaken, and not because the physician considers the diagnosis to be psychogenic.

References

1. Giraldi A, Marson L, Nappi R et al. Physiology of female sexual function: animal models. *J Sex Med* 2004; 1: 237–53.
2. Leiblum S, Nathan S. Persistent sexual arousal syndrome: a newly discovered pattern of female sexuality. *J Sex Marital Ther* 2001; 27: 365–80.
3. Leiblum S, Nathan S. Persistent sexual arousal syndrome in women: a not uncommon but little recognized complaint. *J Sex Relatsh Ther* 2002; 17: 191–8.

4. Xiao H, Liu J, Wang S et al. One case report of clitoral priapism and literature review. *Zhonghua Nan Ke Xue* 2004; 10: 524–5.

5. Medina CA. Clitoral priapism: a rare condition presenting as a cause of vulvar pain. *J Clin Psychopharmacol* 2004; 24: 572–3.

6. Bucur M, Mahmood T. Olanzapine-induced clitoral priapism. *Obstet Gynecol* 2002; 100: 1089–91.

7. Brodie-Meijer CC, Diemont WL, Buijs PJ. Nefazodone-induced clitoral priapism. *Int Clin Psychopharmacol* 1999; 14: 257–8.

8. Berk M, Acton M. Citalopram-associated clitoral priapism: a case series. *Int Clin Psychopharmacol* 1997; 12: 121–2.

9. Pescatori ES, Engelman JC, Davis G et al. Priapism of the clitoris: a case report following trazodone use. *J Urol* 1993; 149: 1557–9.

10. Nappi R, Salonia A, Traish AM et al. Clinical biologic pathophysiologies of women's sexual dysfunction. *J Sex Med* 2005; 2: 4–25.

11. Laumann E, Paik A, Rosen R. Sexual dysfunction in the United States: prevalence and predictors. *JAMA* 1999; 281: 537–44.

12. Pryor J, Akkus E, Alter G et al. Priapism. *J Sex Med* 2004; 1: 116–20.

13. Diederichs W, Lue T, Tanagho EA. Clitoral response to cavernous nerve stimulation in dogs. *Int J Impot Res* 1991; 3: 7.

14. Blin O, Schwertschlag US, Serratrice G. Painful clitoral tumescence during bromocriptine therapy. *Lancet* 1991; 337: 1231–2.

15. Modell JG. Repeated observations of yawning, clitoral engorgement and orgasm associated with fluoxetine administration. *J Clin Psychopharmacol* 1989; 9: 63–5.

16. Ciraulo DA, Shader RI. Fluoxetine drug–drug interactions. I. Antidepressants and antipsychotics. *J Clin Psychopharmacol* 1990; 10: 48–50.

17. DiGiorgi S, Schnatz PF, Mandavilli S et al. Transitional cell carcinoma presenting as clitoral priapism. *Gynecol Oncol* 2004; 93: 540–2.

18. Lin C-S. Tissue expression, distribution and regulation of PDE_5. *Int J Impot Res* 2004; 16: S8–S10.

19. Basson R, Leiblum S, Brotto L et al. Revised definitions of women's sexual dysfunction. *J Sex Med* 2004; 1: 40–8.

20. Hartman S, Herman RA, Nolan CL et al. Men and women differ in amygdala responses to visual sexual stimuli. *Nature Neurosci* 2004; 7: 411–16.

21. Saenz de Tejada I, Ware JC, Blanco R et al. Pathophysiology of prolonged penile erection associated with trazodone use. *J Urol* 1991; 145: 60–4.

22. Webb RC. State of the art: ying yang of corporal smooth muscle control. *J Sex Med* 2004; 1: S1–2.

23. Levine FJ, Saenz de Tejada I et al. Recurrent prolonged erections and priapism as a sequela of priapism: pathophysiology and management. *J Urol* 1991; 145: 764–7.

STRATEGIES BY HEALTH-CARE CLINICIANS FOR MANAGEMENT OF FEMALE SEXUAL DYSFUNCTION

17.1 Role of the primary care and internal medicine clinician

Sharon J Parish

Introduction

Sexuality involves the integration of an individual's intellectual and emotional aspects, personal development, social mores, and biologic function.[1] It influences happiness, self-esteem, and interpersonal relationships (see Chapter 17.6 of this book). It may involve intimacy with a partner, masturbation, integration of religious or cultural views, and the definition of one's sexual identity and orientation.[2,3] Sexual expression requires the acquisition of skills that involve the complex integration of emotional and physical behaviors. The human sexual response is multifaceted and therefore is vulnerable to dysfunction (see Chapters 3.1–3.4 and 5.1–5.6). Primary care clinicians are accustomed and ideally situated to deal with such complex issues, and patients hope that their physicians will be able to help.

This chapter will discuss the role of the primary care practitioner in the detection, evaluation, and management of female sexual problems. Internal medicine and family medicine office-based outpatient care of female sexual disorders is explicitly considered. In actual practice, internal medicine subspecialists, gynecologists, urologists, pediatricians, and psychiatrists often manage these problems; and the principles can be applied to these practice settings. We will describe the rationale for screening and a primary care approach to sexual disorders that includes the sexual history, the biopsychosocial model, physical examination, laboratory and diagnostic testing, classification, treatment, and referral.[4]

Epidemiology in community and clinic populations

Surveys of community samples suggest that sexual problems in women are common (see Chapters 2.1–2.4). In the early 1990s,

Spector and Carey concluded that the prevalence of sexual dysfunction was 20–63% in sexually active women of all ages.[5] A 1999 analysis by Lauman et al. of a survey of adult sexual behavior at ages 18–59 revealed that 43% of women experience sexual problems that negatively affect their quality of life.[6] A comprehensive review of the literature in 2001 by Simons and Carey reported a community prevalence of 7–10% for female orgasmic disorder, and that the current stable prevalence of other female sexual dysfunctions was difficult to estimate because of wide methodological variation of the study designs.[7]

Moreover, most studies Simons and Carey reviewed did not distinguish between the presence of sexual dysfunction and a meaningful sexual disorder. An example they cited was a large Swedish community study in which the prevalence of the presence of a dysfunction was compared to the prevalence of those who perceived the dysfunction as a problem. For example, only 45% of women with orgasmic disorder saw it as a problem causing psychosocial distress; the 1-year prevalence of anorgasmia was 22%, but the prevalence of orgasmic disorder causing distress was 10%.[8]

In a review in 2004, Lewis et al. stated that 40–45% of adult women have at least one sexual dysfunction and that low sexual desire increased from 10% before age 50 to 47% at age 74.[9] Arousal and lubrication disorders were estimated to be 8–28% and dyspareunia 2–20%. Orgasm dysfunction was present in at least 25% of women of all ages, and vaginismus was reported in 6% of women worldwide.

Simons and Carey's review reported that prevalence rates in primary care and sexuality clinics were generally higher.[7] However, the data had methodological problems and did not apply uniform criteria. Only some studies utilized all of the criteria for sexual disorders used in the Diagnostic and Statistical Manual of Mental Disorders, fourth edition (DSM-IV): interpersonal or intrapersonal distress; and the absence of another Axis I disorder, medical condition, or the physiologic effects of a substance.[10] The DSM-IV system was designed to classify and label psychiatric disorders and has limited applicability in medical settings. In 2000, Basson et al. composed an International Consensus Statement that proposed a new uniform scheme to define female sexual disorders.[11] This classification system applied to both organic and psychogenic causes of female sexual dysfunction and included the personal distress criterion as an integral component of the definition of a disorder. Although the consensus statement called for research trials to define "clearer specification of clinical endpoints and outcomes", few subsequent studies, including those reviewed by Lewis et al., have applied this new classification to determine accurate current prevalence rates in clinical populations.[9] Moreover, well-validated questionnaires, such as the Female Sexual Function Index, and standard physiologic measures, such as vaginal photoplethysmography, have not been used uniformly in existing studies.[12]

Although the accuracy of clinical data has limitations, numerous studies have demonstrated that the prevalence of female sexual problems increases with certain medical illnesses and psychosocial factors. Medical and psychologic risk factors and comorbidities include general health status, diabetes mellitus, cardiovascular disease, genitourinary disease, breast and gynecologic cancer, chronic diseases, and psychiatric conditions.[11] Sociodemographic factors include low educational attainment, minority status, deterioration in social/economic status, and sexual trauma.[6]

Screening and detection

Although sexual disorders are common, only 10–20% of affected women spontaneously report these concerns to medical practitioners.[6] Since clinicians rarely screen for sexual problems, detection rates are low. In an analysis of the detection of sexual dysfunction in an English general practice population, the majority (70%) of the 177 patients surveyed considered sexual issues to be appropriate for the general practitioner to discuss.[13] However, physicians recorded sexual problems in only 2% of their notes, despite a survey prevalence of female sexual dysfunction of 42%. Improving screening procedures does improve recognition. In one study in which clinic physicians were trained to take a screening sexual history, 53% of the patients reported a sexual problem.[14] Most (91%) of the patients said they considered questions about sexuality to be an appropriate part of the interview. These data demonstrate the high prevalence of sexual problems, improved detection with focused training in history-taking skills, and patients' acceptance of such discussions.[3,4]

Although 50% of patients may report sexual problems when asked, not everyone wants treatment. Generally, less than half of women experience personal distress regarding their sexual dysfunction such that it would meet established criteria for a sexual disorder and require clinical intervention.[9] The challenge in primary care is to identify existing sexual issues and discern which problems require further assessment and which

patients would benefit from addressing problems that would not otherwise be addressed (see Chapter 9.4).

Barriers to addressing sexual problems

Practitioners may be reluctant to discuss sexual issues because of lack of knowledge or skills, discomfort with sexual language, concern over the effect of such a discussion, and fear of opening "Pandora's box".[15] Both adolescents and adults perceive that physicians are often uncomfortable in discussing sexual issues and lack adequate communication skills to do so effectively.[16] An Israeli study examined the attitudes and sexual dysfunction management of 179 primary care physicians who attended a family practice and general practice conference.[17] While 79% of the respondents thought that the primary care physician should address most sexual problems, 50% or fewer actually treated patients for sexual dysfunction. They perceived that only 12% of their sexual dysfunction patients were female; and the main barriers to treating sexual problems were lack of time (62%) and knowledge (47%).

Physicians may have difficulty in remaining objective and separating their personal beliefs and values from those of their patients.[18] They may have limited sexual experience, unresolved issues regarding their own sexuality, or concern about developing sexual feelings toward patients.

Patients fear their doctor will dismiss their sexual concerns or that the topic might embarrass their physician. Consequently, they are often grateful when their practitioner initiates discussions. Patients may be unaware of potential treatments or may be concerned about side effects or adverse outcomes. Gott and Hincliff studied the barriers to older female patients seeking treatment in an English general practice setting.[19] The women, of ages 50–92, reported that the most significant barriers were the general practitioner's attitudes toward later-life sexuality, the attribution of sexual problems to "normal aging", shame/embarrassment and fear, perceiving sexual problems as "not serious", and lack of knowledge about available resources.

While physicians and patients should not go beyond their comfort in discussing sexual issues, barriers can be addressed through patient and physician education. While physicians typically do not receive adequate training in sexual medicine and sexual history taking, primary care physicians believe that they should address sexual problems and that they need more training to overcome knowledge deficits.[17] Physicians can gain increased comfort and experience in managing sexual problems by incorporating routine sexual health questions into their practice, by sharing cases with colleagues, and by exploring their own attitudes toward sexuality.[18]

Sexual function and sexual concerns

Patients frequently present questions to their doctors about whether or not their sexual behavior is consistent with sexual dysfunction. Sexuality is subjective, and sexual behavior varies widely. The World Health Organization has proposed definitions of biologic, psychologic, and social components of sexual activity.[20] Biologic dimensions include the usual sequence of sexual development and the ability to experience the physical events of the sexual response cycle. Psychologic aspects involve psychosexual maturation and the capacity for intimacy. Social elements relate to societal norms of sexual behavior as they compare with an individual's sexual expression.[4,20]

The sexual response cycle (desire, arousal, orgasm, and resolution as a linear model) has been the standard framework for understanding physiologic sexual function (see Chapter 9.1). This approach has been challenged by Tiefer, Basson, and others, who assert that this model assumes that the sexual experiences of men and women are equivalent, when in fact the female sexual response does not always proceed according to the prescribed sequence.[4] For example, many women experience desire only after sexual stimulation has led to arousal.[21] Moreover, the sexual response cycle model may be too "genitally focused" and limited, defining heterosexual intercourse as the normative sexual experience, when in fact many women experience sexual satisfaction and pleasure through other behaviors.[22] Furthermore, women may not see sexuality as a necessary component of satisfying intimate relationships. The sexual response cycle model may not adequately account for the wide spectrum of sexual expression and does not attend to communication and intimacy, both central to female sexual satisfaction. To enhance the quality of sexual discussions with female patients, physicians can learn about and integrate these alternative views of physiologic female sexuality.

Although the classic sexual disorders are prevalent, more commonly seen in primary care are sexual concerns. Women may have questions about their sexual behavior with regard to frequency, techniques to reach orgasm, masturbation, and fantasy. Women may have concerns about communication, disparate attitudes or value systems, sexual orientation, and the role of sexuality in their overall relationship. They may have inadequate knowledge about sexual function regarding developmental issues in adolescence; sexual changes with aging, medical illness, disability, or pharmacologic treatment; and changes with pregnancy, breastfeeding, or infertility.

The generalist can play a key role in sexuality by explaining the medical perspective, providing education, giving permission, and offering reassurance. According to Bullard and Caplan, the most common issues needing clarification are the following.[18]

Masturbation

From the medical perspective, masturbation is a commonly performed and universal behavior. It is physically safe and can offer individuals practice and sexual self-esteem. It may be problematic if it is associated with excessive guilt or used compulsively to avoid intimacy.

Frequency

There is a wide range of sexual frequency, from monthly to several times daily. Partner disparities in desired frequency may result in interpersonal conflict.

Fantasy

Sexual fantasies are normal as long as they are not associated with disturbing or intrusive thoughts that may indicate deeper psychologic issues.

Clitoral stimulation

Most women need direct stimulation to reach orgasm manually or orally. Approximately one-third of women reach orgasm only through clitoral stimulation, whereas other women require vaginal penetration; and some respond to both forms of stimulation.

Homosexuality

While some women may need support during the "coming out process" (the formation and evolution of sexual identity into a homosexual lifestyle), most lesbian women do not wish to have their sexual orientation questioned or changed. They have similar rates of sexual problems and have comparable sexual concerns. Up to one-fifth of adults, who may not identify themselves as homosexual, have had at least one same-sex encounter.[6]

Sexual changes with aging

As women age, they may note decreased vaginal muscle tension and expansion, delay in clitoral reaction time, and lack of breast size increase during stimulation. Consequently, they may require more direct genital stimulation and more time for arousal. Estrogen levels decline with menopause, which may be associated with atrophic changes and dyspareunia. Appropriate treatment of this condition often restores sexual function. Although orgasmic capacity is retained with age, there is a decrease in the number and intensity of vaginal contractions. The most important factors for postmenopausal women in maintaining sexual activity are partner availability and the partner's physical health.[23] Many women over age 70 continue to enjoy sexuality; and in response to changes in their sexual physiology, they may become less focused on intercourse and engage in alternate forms of sexual and physical intimacy. The physician can offer information and advice about how to accommodate to these physiologic changes.

Sexual difficulties versus disorders

(see Chapter 2.4)

Sexual concerns may evolve into sexual difficulties or dysfunctions if they result in intrapsychic distress or conflict between partners. In community and primary care samples, sexual difficulties are more common than classic sexual disorders. Frank et al.'s survey (1978) of couples with a high degree of marital satisfaction reported that 63% of the women reported arousal or orgasmic dysfunction and an even higher percentage (77%) reported sexual "difficulties".[24] Survey respondents in an English general practice population reported sexual dysfunction (43%) less frequently than "general sexual dissatisfaction": 68% of the women reported at least one problem with avoidance, infrequency, and noncommunication.[13] The generalist may identify and intervene with sexual difficulties before they amplify into complex disorders.

Organizing a generalist approach to sexual dysfunction

The primary care practitioner can best understand sexual problems by using a model that combines the affected phase(s) of the sexual response cycle; the biologic, psychologic, and social causes; and the predisposing, precipitating, and maintaining factors.[25] The three-dimensional model depicted in Fig. 17.1.1 provides a framework for this analysis. The following general considerations may be helpful:

- Psychologic problems can produce sexual dysfunction in the absence of physical disorder.
- Almost all organic problems evoke psychologic reactions, such as performance anxiety and "spectatoring" (obsessive self-observation during sex), which inevitably exacerbate the disorder.
- Sexual function and dysfunction can be a learned phenomenon, subject to behavioral conditioning and learned inhibition.

While specific characteristics may help differentiate organic from psychogenic etiologies, most sexual problems managed by the generalist are multifactorial, especially in older patients with complex medical illness. The best approach is to identify and focus on those causes and factors that are amenable to intervention.

Clinical assessment of female sexual disorders

Detailed discussions of the causes and factors discussed above, sexual history and classification, medical history, physical examination, and physiologic testing are provided in Chapters 9.2–9.5 and 10.1–10.7. Selected highlights of specific recommendations for a practical approach to female sexual disorders in a primary care setting will be presented.

Sexual history taking

The goals of sexual history taking in primary care are listed in Table 17.1.1. While the sexual history can address numerous

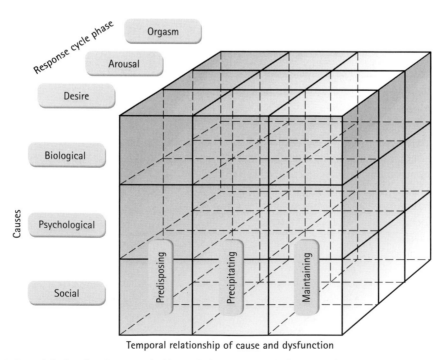

Figure 17.1.1. Integrated model of sexual dysfunction. Reproduced with permission from Parish S, Salazar W. Sexual Problems. In FV DeGruy, WP Dickinson, EW Staton, eds. *Twenty Common Problems in Behavioral Health.* New York: McGraw Hill, 2002:143–172.[3]

Table 17.1.1. Goals of sexual history taking in primary care

Identify any questions or concerns related to sexuality

Identify sexual dysfunction and assess possible organic or psychogenic etiologies

Assess effects of illness, disability, surgery, medication, or substances on sexual function

Assess effects of psychiatric disorders and sociocultural issues on sexual function

Identify and assess the impact of psychologic reactions on sexual function

Identify sexual problems that may be clues to psychosocial problems or organic illness

Identify high-risk sexual behavior requiring education or counseling

Identify sexually transmitted diseases and sexual pain

Assess reproductive concerns, including contraception, infertility, pregnancy, and abortion

Identify and explore the impact of sexual trauma, including molestation, rape, and incest

issues relevant to the female patient, sexual problems are an important and frequently overlooked agenda. A screening sexual problem history aims to detect sexual disorders that cause the patient distress. The sexual history can be incorporated into the medical interview where the clinician finds it appropriate and when the questions arise naturally. Opportunities appear during the urogenital or gynecologic review of systems or the social history, or when discussing a relationship. The clinician can initiate the discussion by asking permission and universalizing the process: "May I ask you some questions that I ask all my patients?" The interviewer can determine whether a patient is in a sexual relationship and ask about the nature of that relationship: "Are you having a meaningful relationship at this time?"; "How is it?"; "Are you sexually involved in this relationship?" Then sexual problem-screening questions might include: "Are you satisfied with your sexual function?" or "How has your illness affected your sexual function?" The clinician can also assess psychologic reactions to medical illnesses that do not have a direct effect on sexual function but do have symbolic implications. For example, after mastectomy, as a result of the perceived disfigurement, women may experience shame or fear of rejection.

In the sexual problem history, the interviewer can lead a patient through a typical sexual experience, using the sexual response cycle as a guide. Because a dysfunction in one phase can actually result from a dysfunction in another phase (e.g., decreased lubrication may cause pain and lead to decreased sexual desire), a problem should be characterized from its onset as it evolves over time. The interviewer should determine whether the problem occurs in specific situations or is generalized, as well as explore the nonsexual aspects of the relationship, the biopsychosocial context, the influence of cultural or religious mores, and the partner's sexual function.

Contrary to what is recommended for the general medical interview, it may be useful to model the level of explicitness by starting with a close-ended question instead of open-ended questions. Examples include: "Do you experience any difficulty with lubrication?" or "Have you ever reached orgasm with your partner?" Then one can follow up with an open-ended question such as, "Could you tell me more about that?"

The interviewer should avoid making assumptions about the patient's sexuality and that the first relationship mentioned is the only one that the patient is having. A patient may be having an affair, and an apparently happily married woman may be having homosexual contacts. The interviewer may include "safety net" questions such as, "Do you have any other questions or concerns about sex?" or "Are there other sexual relationships that I should know about?"[4]

The interviewer should use language that is clear, explicit, and mutually understood. The physician should avoid language that is excessively technical or informal, and instead use language that the patient understands and that is comfortable for the interviewer.[26]

Discussions about sexuality may bring up sensitive issues. The interviewer may uncover issues the patient has never discussed with anyone and which may require specific interventions. For example, a woman may disclose a history of sexual trauma in a very emotional manner, so the clinician needs to be prepared to refer to a qualified resource person who could provide timely and appropriate therapeutic follow-up.[3]

Clinical evaluation

In analyzing a sexual problem in the primary care setting, the medical history, physical examination, laboratory testing, and physiologic testing will be guided by an understanding of the probable biologic causes and the physiology of the female sexual response. The Female Sexual Function Index is a multidimensional, self-report instrument that has been used to identify and classify the severity of female sexual dysfunctions in research trials (see Chapter 11.2). While validated questionnaires such as the Female Sexual Function Index provide detailed information, they have limited applicability in the clinical setting as routine screening and assessment tools.[12] A detailed medical history and general physical examination is recommended for all sexual dysfunctions, with particular attention to the common medical comorbidities, depression, substance use, and side effects of frequently prescribed medications (e.g., selective serotonin reuptake inhibitors, antihypertensive drugs). The genital examination should be targeted to the assessment of specific physical complaints, such as vulvar pain. It can be diagnostic and educational, as, for example, in women with lifelong dyspareunia and difficulty with penetration. A detailed neuro-genital and vascular examination may be helpful in women with arousal complaints and suggestive medical or traumatic histories. There are no recommended routine laboratory tests for sexual dysfunctions, especially with those with apparent psychogenic problems. Blood and radiologic testing should be dictated by the clinical suspicion of medical disease, such as lipids or serum glucose, and by gynecologic concerns, such as cervical cultures or pelvic ultrasound. Accurate assays of total testosterone and sex hormone-binding globulin are required with investigational testosterone therapy.[27] Physiologic testing (e.g., vaginal photoplethysmography) has been used primarily in research trials and is not used routinely in the primary care evaluation of a sexual problem.

Therapy recommendations

The generalist can effectively diagnose and treat an array of sexual problems. The primary care setting is often the only place where patients can receive treatment, especially in urban or underserved areas. Access to sexual medicine specialists or sex therapists may be limited by geography, cost, language barriers, or managed care restrictions.

Empathic sexual history taking and delineation of problems can be therapeutic. Patients can be coached in enhanced communication. The clinician may suggest that the patient involve her partner. The P-LI-SS-IT model, a widely recognized stepwise approach to sex therapy, provides behavioral and psychologic techniques easily integrated in general practice, as detailed in the following:[28]

- (P) Permission: patients are given permission to discuss their problems and emotions and to explore new solutions.
- (LI) Limited information: the practitioner may instruct the patient about sexual physiology or suggest educational resources such as literature, videos, and erotica.
- (SS) Specific suggestions might include more tailored approaches designed to improve sexual and emotional communication, such as the sensate focus exercises, which emphasize replacing traditional intercourse with gradual, nondemanding pleasuring techniques; masturbation; Kegel exercises, technical advice regarding sexual positions; and the use of lubricants or dilators.
- (IT) Intensive therapy may involve referral for individual therapy to deal with intrapsychic issues, or couples therapy to improve communication or address conflict.

Treatment and referral for specific sexual disorders

The sexual disorders are categorized by the revised definitions of Basson et al. in Table 17.1.2.[27] The recommended primary care intervention and indications for referral are outlined. Referral

Table 17.1.2. Sexual dysfunction treatment and referral

Sexual disorder*	Primary care intervention	Indications for referral to specialist treatment
Sexual desire/interest disorder; Subjective and combined (subjective and genital) Sexual arousal disorder**	Systemic estrogen/progesterone therapy with attention to risks/benefits; Investigational androgen therapy with attention to potential side effects; Listening exercises to enhance communication: temporary intercourse ban, sensate focus, genital caressing; Kegel exercises; Relaxation techniques; Suggested readings, erotica, and other techniques to enhance sensuality	Psychiatry referral: Psychogenic lifelong disorder, Complex interpersonal conflict, Psychiatric disorders refractory to primary care treatment (depression, panic disorder), History of sexual trauma
Genital sexual arousal disorder	Local estrogen therapy; Investigational use of PDE5 inhibitors; Consider clitoral vacuum device; Lubricants (Astroglide, K-Y, Albolene); Zestra (massage oil)	Gynecology or urology referral: Refractory to estrogen therapy
Orgasmic disorder (psychogenic)	Lifelong generalized orgasmic disorder: directed masturbation, relaxation techniques if anxiety present; Situational (orgasmic with masturbation, not with partner): focus on trust and safety in relationship, use of vibrators with intercourse, "women on top" position	Sex therapy referral: Refractory to basic behavioral counseling techniques
Orgasmic disorder (organic or drug induced)	SSRI-induced anorgasmia: Buproprion, investigational use of PDE5 inhibitor, drug holiday, dose reduction	Sexual medicine specialist or urology referral: Neurologic condition (multiple sclerosis, spinal cord injury, late diabetes)
Dyspareunia** Vaginismus**	Treatment of vaginal/cervical infections; Vulvar vestibulitis syndrome (VVS): irritant avoidance, tricyclic antidepressants, anti-convulsants; Adequate stimulation and female control of thrusting with intercourse; Progressive vaginal inserts (finger or dilator)	Gynecology referral: Complex VVS; Sex and/or pelvic floor physical therapy referral: Lifelong vaginismus refractory to dilator therapy

*Based on the revised classification of female sexual disorders.[27]
**Disorders which often present together and have similar treatment considerations.
PDE5: phosphodiesterase type 5; SSRI: selective serotinin reuptake inhibitors.

may involve specialists in urology, gynecology, psychiatry, sex therapy, and pelvic floor physiotherapy.

There are currently no US Food and Drug Administration-approved pharmacotherapies for female sexual dysfunction. However, the generalist may consider investigational uses of prescription medications, such as selective phosphodiesterase type 5 inhibitors and testosterone, or over-the-counter supplements,[29] with attention to the considerations regarding these therapies discussed above. The generalist can treat gynecologic conditions, such as atrophic vaginitis, with topical estrogen and address drug side effects, such as with serotonin reuptake inhibitor-induced anorgasmia.

Conclusion

Female sexual concerns and disorders are common, inadequately recognized, and under-treated. Although these disorders may be challenging, a set of clinical skills within the grasp of primary care clinicians can enhance detection and permit successful treatment for many woman. Generalists that naturally and commonly apply a holistic, comprehensive, biopsychosocial approach can make a world of difference by learning how to manage female sexual disorders effectively.

References

1. Klingman EW. Office evaluation of sexual function and complaints. *Clin Geriatr Med* 1991; 7: 15–36.
2. Parish S, McGinn T. Sexual dysfunction in men and women. In LM Rucker, ed. *Essentials of Adult Ambulatory Care*. Baltimore: Williams and Wilkins, 1997: 432–41.
3. Parish S, Salazar W. Sexual problems. In FV DeGruy, WP Dickinson, EW Staton, eds. *Twenty Common Problems in Behavioral Health*. New York: McGraw Hill, 2002: 143–172.
4. Parish S, Salazar W. Sexuality. In J Ryden, PD Blumenthal, eds. *Practical Gynecology: A Guide for the Primary Care Physician*. Philadelphia: American College of Physicians, 2002: 26–51.
5. Spector IP, Carey MP. Incidence and prevalence of the sexual dysfunctions: a critical review of the empirical literature. *Arch Sex Behav* 1990; 19: 389–407.
6. Laumann E, Paik A, Rosen RC. Sexual dysfunction in the United States: prevalence and predictors. *JAMA* 1999; 281: 537–44.
7. Simons JS, Carey MP. Prevalence of sexual dysfunctions: results from a decade of research. *Arch Sex Behav* 2001; 30: 177–219.
8. Fugi-Meyer AR, Sjogren Fugi-Meyer K. Sexual disabilities, problems, and satisfaction in 18–74 year old Swedes. *Scand J Sexol* 1999; 3: 79–105.
9. Lewis RW, Fugi-Meyer KS, Bosch R et al. Epidemiology/risk factors of sexual dysfunction. *J Sex Med* 2004; 1: 35–9.
10. *Diagnostic and Statistical Manual of Mental Disorders*, 4th edn (DSM-IV). Washington, DC: American Psychiatric Association, 1994.
11. Basson R, Berman J, Burnett A et al. Report of the international consensus development conference on female sexual dysfunction: definitions and classification. *J Urol* 2000; 163: 888–93.
12. Rosen RC, Brown C, Heiman J et al. The Female Sexual Function Index (FSFI); a multidimensional self-report instrument for the assessment of female sexual function. *J Sex Marital Ther* 2000; 26: 191–208.
13. Read S, King M, Watson J. Sexual dysfunction in primary medical care: prevalence, characteristics and detection by the general practitioner. *J Public Health Med* 1997; 19: 387–91.
14. Ende J, Rockwell S, Galsgow M. The sexual history in general medical practice. *Arch Int Med* 1984; 144: 558–61.
15. Risen CD. A guide to taking a sexual history. *Psychiatr Clin North Am* 1995; 18: 39–53.
16. Croft CA, Asmussen L. A developmental approach to sexuality education: implications for medical practice. *J Adolesc Health* 1993; 14: 109–14.
17. Press Y, Menahem S, Shvartzman P. [Sexual dysfunction – what is the primary physician's role?] *Harefuah* 2003; 142: 662–5, 719.
18. Bullard DG, Caplan H. Sexual problems. In MD Feldman, JF Christensen, eds. *Behavioral Medicine in Primary Care: A Practical Guide*, 2nd edn. Stamford: Lange Medical Books/McGraw-Hill, 2002: 274–92.
19. Gott M, Hincliff S. Barriers to seeking treatment for sexual problems in primary care: a qualitative study with older people. *Fam Pract* 2003; 20: 690–5.
20. Schover LR, Jensen SB. *Sexuality and Chronic Illness. A Comprehensive Approach*. New York: Guilford Press, 1998.
21. Basson R. The female sexual response revisited. *J Soc Obstet Gynecol Can* 2000; 22: 383–7.
22. Tiefer L. *Sex Is Not a Natural Act and Other Essays*. Boulder: Westview Press, 1995.
23. Greendale GA, Hogan P, Shumaker S. Sexual functioning in postmenopausal women: the postmenopausal estrogen/progestin interventions (PEPI) trial. *J Womens Health* 1996; 5: 445–58.
24. Frank E, Anderson C, Rubenstein D. Frequency of sexual dysfunction in "normal" couples. *N Engl J Med* 1978; 299: 111–15.
25. Wincze JP, Carey MP. *Sexual Dysfunction. A Guide for Assessment and Treatment*. New York: Guildford, 1991.
26. Williams S. The sexual history. In A Lipkin, S Putnam, A Lazare, eds. *The Medical Interview: Clinical Care, Education, and Research*. New York: Springer-Verlag, 1995: 235–50.
27. Basson R, Altholf S, Davis S et al. Summary of the recommendations on sexual dysfunctions in Women. *J Sex Med* 2004; 1: 24–34.
28. Annon JS. *Behavioral Treatment of Sexual Problems: Brief Therapy*. Hagerstown: Harper & Row, 1976.
29. Ferguson DM, Steidle CP, Singh GS et al. Randomized placebo-controlled, double-blind, crossover trial of the efficacy and safety of Zestra for women in women with and without female sexual arousal disorder. *J Sex Marital Ther* 2003; 29(Suppl 1): 33–44.

17.2 The role of the psychologist

Aline P Zoldbrod

Introduction

Sexuality is a biopsychosocial phenomenon. Sexual feelings and expression are infinitely malleable. Thus, each individual woman's sexuality is different from every other woman's, a result of all of the various forces and experiences that have affected her over her lifetime. Our patients come to us for help, yet there is no single goal in treating sexual problems in women, and no one formula for healthy sexuality or perfect functioning. Each woman's "sexual recipe" for success and pleasure is unique and complex.

This chapter focuses on the responsibility of the psychologist, a nonphysician, to understand, assess, and explain the impact of intrapsychic, familial, historic, relational, and cultural forces on each woman's sexuality; to understand her special vulnerabilities, strengths, and goals; and to interpret and explain all this information to the patient and to the medical team. The psychologist helps the patient assimilate medical and psychologic findings and remain hopeful. Finally, the psychologist applies her professional knowledge, skills, empathy, creativity, and resources to enhance each patient's sexual pleasure and comfort.

This is an exciting and promising time to be working in the field of female sexual dysfunction (see Chapter 1.1 of this book). Medical information is expanding and changing; understanding of female anatomy is improving; old diagnoses are being challenged; and new medications, treatments, and devices are being quantified and tested scientifically[1,2] (see Chapters 4.1–4.4). New treatments show promise for specific groups of women, including the use of selective phosphodiesterase type 5 inhibitors in treating antidepressant-associated sexual dysfunction,[3] and the use of the EROS pump, selective phosphodiesterase type 5 inhibitors, and/or topical vasodilators in certain cases of female sexual arousal disorder (see Chapters 13.1–13.3, 14.1, and 14.2). Our understanding of vulvar pain has been enhanced by new conceptualizations of the disorder[4] (see Chapters 12.1–12.6). In addition, new advances in understanding of and success in treating the sexual sequelae of emotional, physical, and sexual trauma are an important innovation in sex therapy for women (see Chapters 11.1–11.5).[5,6]

It is not a simple time to work in the field of sex therapy, however. Women demand the latest medical treatments, hoping for a rapid solution, as selective phosphodiesterase type 5 inhibitors have been for men. However, given the complexity and highly contextual nature of women's sexual experience, medical advances, in and of themselves, will not be able to solve most women's sexual problems.[7] The history of psychologic treatments has been reviewed in Chapter 11.1. For many diagnoses, there is no standard, reliable psychologic protocol of treatment at this time.[8] Before beginning any treatment approach, the psychologist must be prepared to deal with patients' and partners' high expectations, impatience, and disappointment at the lack of a quick fix.

Women's feelings about sexuality are embedded in nonphysiologic factors

Most women's sexual problems have a mixed etiology, part psychologic, part relational, part cultural, part biologic; all areas must be evaluated. Meston[9] cautioned that medications that promote physiologic arousal in men may not be effective in the opposite sex, because, for women, "Evidence suggests that external stimulus information (e.g., relationship issues, sexual scenarios) may play a more important role in assessing feelings of sexual arousal than do internal physiological cues."

Studies have found that relationship satisfaction is the most important contributor to sexual satisfaction.[10,11] Beck found that anger reduces sexual desire in women, but not in men.[12] Thus, evaluating the woman's current and past satisfaction with her partner is a critical piece of the diagnostic puzzle.

Women juggle multiple roles and many have difficulty allowing themselves to take the time to focus on eroticism, even when desired. This may create a "vicious cycle" in which a lack of satisfying erotic encounters diminishes positive sexual imagery and memories, reducing future sexual desire and per-petuating the problem. Further, cultural demands on women to look young and sexy are relentless and, in some women, con-tribute to body dissatisfaction. Women with poorer body images reported less sexual satisfaction, lower rates of orgasm, and more sexually dysfunctional experiences in general.[13,14]

The woman with the sexual problem: the psychology of being "the patient"

Patients who come into treatment for sexual problems feel vulnerable. Many of them feel defective, unable to have or to enjoy normal sexual relations. They may feel hopeless or frightened. The clinician's questions about sexual function and history can themselves seem intimidating, awkward, meddling, humiliating, and even inappropriate. The health-care provider can enhance her empathy with the patient by considering whether or when she has ever discussed these topics with anyone.[15]

Some women come to treatment under duress to try to save a troubled relationship. Others have never experienced sexual pleasure and believe that women's sexual pleasure is a myth. Some women, who have embraced and valued their own sexuality, come highly motivated to resolve a secondary sexual dysfunction that has taken away one of life's great pleasures.

It is common for patients to hope for an easy cure. Unfortunately, some must confront the fact that their sexuality was damaged by the abuse or neglect they suffered in their family of origin. It is painful to identify oneself as a victim, and the standard set of physical examinations and procedures can be especially stressful for women with a history of sexual abuse. Westerlund's[16] research on sexual abuse survivors found that survivors may experience uncomfortable feelings in any situa-tion that appears to be sexual, such as a vaginal ultrasound or sensory testing. Thus, the psychologist must screen for sexual or physical abuse. When an abusive history is present, the psycho-logist should alert the other members of the medical team, with the patient's permission. In turn, physicians and other staff members who will come in contact with an abuse survivor should be asked to take care to modify treatment protocols to help her maintain a sense of control during evaluation and treatment. Changes to medical protocols might include giving the patient written descriptions of all possible procedures in advance, taking care to explain orally what will occur in the office each step of the way, helping the patient determine whether she will need any help in feeling safe during each described process, and making sure that no unnecessary personnel are present during procedures.

The pros and cons of diagnosis

Many patients come to treatment in search of a diagnosis, hoping that a correct identification of the problem equals a cure. Sometimes receiving the accurate diagnosis feels like a triumph, but at other times it can feel like a death knell.

The physician and the psychologist's language and imagery with patients can have a far-reaching influence on sexuality, sexual self-image, and self-esteem.[17] For example, terms such as "senile vaginitis" can be shocking and demoralizing. Test results can be devastating,[18] and negative results should be described to the patient in a way that will minimize negative psychologic impact. For example, if Doppler ultrasound shows severe nerve damage in the pelvis, the patient should be advised of the results gently and told that the psychologist on the team can help her learn other physical and mental ways to raise her sexual arousal.

Evaluating intrapsychic, historic, cultural, and relational factors

Creating a safe environment in the therapist–patient relationship

To learn about the genesis and history of the woman's problem, the psychologist must create a safe environment in the patient–therapist relationship. The patient must feel curious about her sexual history and feel secure in sharing private and potentially upsetting information. In the interests of time, the sexual questions posed to the patient by the medical team may be framed in an objective manner. The psychologist's stance during the initial interview needs to be less goal-driven and more relaxed, with attention to the woman's communicated sense of discomfort, hesitancy, embarrassment, or shame. Once rapport has been formed, the psychologist can use standardized tests, questionnaires, and interview sessions to gather data, generate hypotheses, and plan treatment.

Assessing family-of-origin factors: issues with touch, trust, empathy, gender, and power (Fig. 17.2.1)

Part of the psychologist's role is to find the hidden, unconscious factors that cause sexual inhibition and discomfort. Many patients have never recognized deep-seated problems with sexuality and intimacy,[19] based on their early childhood experi-ences with milestones of sexual development[20] such as touch, empathy, trust, and power. Touch is the "ground zero" of sexuality. Good associations with touch allow caresses by a loved partner to create a cascade of pleasurable associations, leading to feelings of safety and sexual arousal. Without positive experiences with touch as an infant and a girl, the woman will not grow up to be able to enjoy embodied feelings of pleasure, including appropriate familiarity with the sights, touches, tastes, and smells of bodily intimacy, even with a beloved partner. Adult body image also is affected by whether or not the girl was touched lovingly by her parents. The psychologist must evaluate and treat early devel-opmental blocks to experiencing physical pleasure.

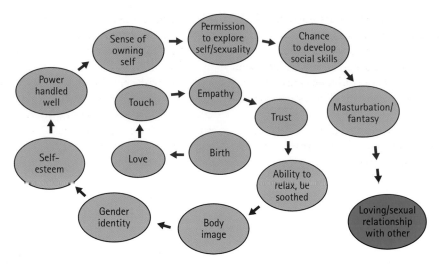

Figure 17.2.1. Milestones in Sexual Development (with permission[20]).

Childhood experiences with trust and empathy are basic determinants of whether a woman will be motivated to be in a psychologically and physically intimate relationship.[21] If she learned that it was safe to trust her parents to address her emotional and physical needs as a child, now she will allow herself to share deep sentiments with her partner. If her parents had empathy and could tolerate her strong feelings, as an adult she can feel safe with intense, visceral feelings and can choose to lose control and experience deep sexual pleasure in her body.[22]

Sexual and nonsexual traumatic events in past family life cause sexual dysfunction

The startling prevalence of sexual abuse among women is reviewed elsewhere in this book. However, many kinds of families inflict "sexual trauma" in a more diffuse way, affecting the platform upon which healthy sexuality must be built. Male violence against women, including wife abuse, is an international epidemic, affecting from one in five to four out of five families, depending on the nation involved.[23] Women who witnessed their mothers being physically and emotionally abused but who were not battered themselves may present with varied sexual dysfunctions, according to their changed associations with touch, trust, feelings about their own gender, and concerns about male/female power.

Alcoholism,[24] drug abuse, child abuse, and mental illness are problems in families around the globe. For women who grew up in families with parents who were alcoholics, emotionally or physically abusive, neglectful, or mentally ill, sexual trauma and inhibition occur because of negative assumptions about human relationships, which can interfere with the woman's wish for sexual vulnerability and closeness as an adult.[20]

Guilt, inhibition, and socialization

The double standard exists worldwide, and women's socialization to be pure, non-sexual beings is an obstacle to achieving sexual fulfillment. Cultural influences have been reviewed by Amaro et al.[25] One part of the psychologist's role with the patient is to give her permission to explore her sexuality through masturbation, touch, sexual fantasy, erotica, books, movies,[26] and the internet.[27] However, research has shown that experiencing negative familial and cultural attitudes toward sex does not, by itself, create adults who have problematic sexual functioning.[28] The psychologist "giving permission to be sexual" may be a minor part of treatment for many women. If early associations to touch, trust, empathy and power were negative, giving patients permission to be sexual and assigning standard sexual homework is premature and will not lead to clinical success. Similarly, if a patient has any kind of trauma, appropriately staged work on safety must be the first therapeutic step.

Women come late for help, often in crisis

Oftentimes, even when the medical team identifies an important, even crucial, aspect of the difficulty, simply remediating the problem medically is not enough. Patients frequently address sexual problems with us only after suffering for a long time, fruitlessly. Some tried resolution by themselves. Others ignored sexual issues for years, even decades. Sex therapists see quarreling, angry couples with serious, longstanding sexual dysfunctions who spent years in conjoint therapy which avoided the sexual issues completely. Their therapists believe that sexual harmony will miraculously be restored when the couple's other tribulations abate. Instead, conflicts and hurts escalate. When such a woman reaches us, the situation is much more complicated psychologically, relationally, and biologically than it would have been had she sought treatment earlier. Her sexual self-esteem, self-image, sexual imagery, and memories are damaged. Patients commonly report feeling "unlike other women" or "broken".

If she has a partner, the patient's relationship may be in distress from the lack of sexual intimacy. Her partner may feel "revolting" or lacking because sexual advances have been spurned repeatedly, or sexual interludes have been obligatory, wooden, and joyless. Tension and blame creates years of hurtful interaction. Impairment may even have occurred in her sexual organs, from lack of proper medical attention. Patience and skill are required to treat such cases and promote forgiveness and trust between partners (Table 17.2.1).

Future directions

Women's sexuality will forever be a complicated, multidimensional phenomenon. Each patient, no matter what her past history or medical status, can maximize her sexual function and work to find her unique recipe for sexual pleasure. The psychologist can be of great assistance in this exploration. There are few situations in which a motivated patient or couple cannot be helped by psychotherapy, resources, and education. However, outreach is essential to ensure that this information is available. Educating colleagues in mental health and medicine to refer patients and couples with sexual issues to certified sex therapists for specialized treatment can prevent prolonged suffering and treat the sexual problems more efficiently.

The Internet provides support for women around the globe. Problems with sexuality are private, and patients are helped if they do not feel isolated in their struggles. Confidential, anonymous chatrooms and groups are available for women with many different sexual issues, including low sexual desire, effects of prior abuse, vulvodynia, sexual fears and inhibitions, or sexual side effects as a result of illness. Clinicians should be familiar with these resources.

Patience and skill is required to treat cases of sexual dysfunction. Clinical work with highly distressed couples is often intense, particularly in the beginning of treatment. Couples may need to be seen more than once a week in order to learn how to manage their anger and increase positive interactions. Couples in crisis may need referral to a therapist who has the time and the setting best to meet their needs. If so, the psychologist will make the referral, communicate with the other therapist, and coordinate the couple's sexual and marital treatment.

Psychologists must stay abreast of the latest safe and effective advances in sexual medicine that can help patients. As women live longer, rates of illness and disability increase. Advancement in sexual medicine has the potential to help women regain lost sexual function or even to transform their sexuality in their forties, fifties, sixties, and beyond. While some women choose to phase out the sexual part of their lives as they age, another group will embrace their sexuality into old age. At its best, sexual pleasure is as life-affirming an activity as has ever existed.

Table 17.2.1. The psychologist's clinical stance in providing sex therapy

Good communication skills. Patients perceive that most health-care providers are uncomfortable when discussing sexuality and often lack adequate communication skills.[29] The psychologist speaks comfortably and competently about sexual matters, combining sensitivity and frankness.

Expertise. The psychologist is a credentialed expert, with the responsibility of providing accurate information on sexuality. The psychologist assesses the patient's need for appropriately staged and executed treatment. If a patient needs more intense care than can be provided in the current setting, she will refer that patient only to another suitable specialist.

Empathy. The psychologist treats the patient's conversations as privileged, not routine, communication and is aware of her vulnerability when divulging and discussing sexual material.

Patience. The psychologist understands that it takes time to repair the emotional and physical aspects of sexual problems and models a treatment stance for the woman and her partner that is simultaneously active and patient.

Permission. The psychologist is the antidote to cultural and familial forces that declare that the patient should not take pleasure in her sexuality.

Resources. Health psychology research documents the psychologic and physical benefits of social support during stressful events.[30] Because patients with sexual problems tend to stay isolated, the psychologist encourages patients to reach out. She stays up to date on relevant community and confidential Internet support groups.

Providing hope. The psychologist has a broad, nonlinear definition of sexual contentment, knowledge of alternative paths to pleasure,[31] and a creative approach to solving sexual problems. Even when a patient is confronted with a discouraging diagnosis or prognosis, the psychologist explores avenues for enhanced sexual pleasure.

Team member. The psychologist works with medical and allied professionals to share information and ideas and provide comprehensive care for the patient.

Privacy. The psychologist respects the patient's privacy in all written and verbal communications with others.

References

1. Berman L, Berman J. Viagra and beyond: where sex educators and therapists fit in from a multidisciplinary perspective. *J Sex Educ Ther* 2000; 25: 17–24.

2. Goldstein I, Berman JR.Vasculogenic female sexual dysfunction: vaginal engorement and clitoral erectile insufficiency syndrome. *Int J Impot Res* 1998; 10: S84–90.

3. Nurnberg HG, Hensley PL, Lauriello J et al. Sildenafil for women patients with antidepressant-induced sexual dysfunction. *Psychiatry Serv* 1999; 50: 1076–8.

4. Pukall C, Reissing E, Binik Y et al. New clinical and research perspectives on the sexual pain disorders. *J Sex Educ Ther* 2000; 25: 36–44.

5. Shapiro F. *Eye Movement Desensitization and Reprocessing: Basic Principles, Protocols, and Procedures.* New York: Guilford, 1995.

6. Schore A. *Affect Regulation and the Repair of the Self.* New York: Norton, 2003.

7. Kaschuk E, Tiefer L, eds. *A New View of Women's Sexual Problems.* Binghamton: Haworth Press, 2000.

8. Williams S, Lieblum SL. Sexual dysfunction. In GM Wingood, R DiClemente, eds. *Handbook of Women's Sexual and Reproductive Health.* New York: Plenum, 2002: 303–28.

9. Meston C. The psychophysiologial assessment of female sexual function. *J Sex Educ Ther* 2000; 25: 6–16.

10. Lawrance K, Byers ES. Sexual satisfaction in long term heterosexual relationships: the interpersonal exchange model of sexual satisfaction. *Pers Relatsh* 1995; 2: 267–85.

11. MacNeil S, Byers ES. The relationships between sexual problems, communication and sexual satisfaction. *Can J Hum Sex* 1997; 6: 277–83.

12. Beck JG. Hypoactive sexual desire disorder: an overview. *J Consult Clin Psychol* 1995; 63: 919–27.

13. Cash TF. Women's body images. In GM Wingood, R DiClemente, eds. *Handbook of Women's Sexual and Reproductive Health.* New York: Plenum, 2002: 175–94.

14. Rieves LC, Cash TF. Social developmental factors and women's body-image attitudes. *J Soc Behav Pers* 1996; 11: 63–78.

15. Zoldbrod AP. Sexuality and infertility: special considerations for practice. *Clin Consult Obstet Gynecol* 1994; 6: 109–15.

16. Westerlund E. *Women's Sexuality After Childhood Incest.* New York: Norton, 1992.

17. Zoldbrod A. *Men, Women and Infertility: Intervention and Treatment Strategies.* New York: Macmillan, 1993.

18. Keye WR. Psychosexual responses to infertility. *Clin Obstet Gynecol* 1984; 27: 760–6.

19. Scharff D. *The Sexual Relationship: An Object Relations View of the Family.* Boston: Routledge and Kegan Paul, 1982.

20. Zoldbrod A. *SexSmart: How Your Childhood Shaped Your Sexual Life and What to Do About It.* Oakland: New Harbinger, 1998.

21. Levine SB. Intrapsychic and individual aspects of sexual desire. In S Lieblum, R Rosen, eds. *Sexual Desire Disorders.* New York: Guilford, 1988.

22. Zoldbrod A. Assessing intrapsychic blocks to sexual pleasure using the milestones of sexual development model. *Contemp Sex* 2003; 37: 7–14.

23. Seager J. *The State of Women in the World Atlas.* New York: Penguin, 1997: 26–7.

24. Helzer J, Canino G. *Alcoholism in North America, Europe and Asia.* London: Oxford University Press, 1992: 14.

25. Amaro H, Navarro A, Conron KJ et al. Cultural influences on women's sexual health. In GM Wingood, R DiClemente, eds. *Handbook of Women's Sexual and Reproductive Health.* New York: Plenum, 2002: 71–92.

26. Heiman J, LoPiccolo J. *Becoming Orgasmic.* New York: Fireside, 1987.

27. Foley S, Kope S, Sugrue D. *Sex Matters for Women: A Complete Guide to Taking Care of Your Sexual Self.* New York: Guilford, 2002.

28. Heiman J, Gladue B, Roberts C et al. Historical and current factors discriminating sexually functional from sexually dysfunctional married couples. *J Marital Fam Ther* 1986; 12: 163–74.

29. Croft CA, Asmussen L. A developmental approach to sexuality education: implications for medical practice. *J Adolesc Health* 1993; 14: 109–14.

30. Taylor SE. Health psychology: the science and the field. *Am Psychol* 1990; 45: 40–50.

31. Whipple B, Komisaruk BR. Beyond the G spot: recent research of female sexuality. *Psychiatr Ann* 1999; 29: 34–7.

17.3 Role of the psychiatrist

Robert Taylor Segraves

The differential diagnosis and treatment of sexual disorders in women is complicated because of their diverse and often interactive biologic, psychologic, and interpersonal etiologies. Few physicians are qualified to be the sole providers of sexual medicine services to female patients with sexual dysfunction, as the requisite knowledge base extends across medical specialty boundaries (see Chapter 17.6 of this book). The ideal solution is a multidisciplinary team approach to diagnosis and treatment, although anomalies in insurance coverage may make this approach difficult to implement in many settings. The treatment team needs to involve a clinician skilled in assessing psychologic aspects of sexual behavior, as the full impact of psychologic and interpersonal forces on female sexuality may not always be fully appreciated by physicians from many specialties. This chapter will focus specifically on how most psychiatrists would approach the diagnosis and treatment of sexual disorders to illustrate what a psychiatric referral or consult might provide. It is important to emphasize that not all psychiatrists are interested in treating or knowledgeable about human sexuality. It is important to select someone with expertise in this area. As well as providing an understanding of the psychologic factors influencing human behavior, the psychiatrist also has expertise in the effects of various psychiatric disorders and their treatment on sexual dysfunction.

The specific contribution of the psychiatric clinician is to broaden the diagnostic and treatment options to include psychiatric and psychosocial etiologies and interventions. In particular, the psychiatrist should be able to recognize and treat female sexual dysfunction secondary to other psychiatric syndromes or secondary to psychopharmacologic interventions, as well as problems related to couple dynamics and individual psychopathology. Similarly, the psychiatrist should be able to target interventions based on the etiologic factors identified. Treatment may include changing medication, treating underlying syndromes, couple psychotherapy, individual psychotherapy, or targeted behavioral therapy (see Chapters 11.1–11.5 and 16.2). In this chapter, the psychiatric approach to diagnosis and treatment of female sexual disorders will be summarized.

Diagnostic assessment

The major instrument in psychiatric assessment is the psychiatric interview. The psychiatric interview is central to all psychiatric care and is of the same importance to the psychiatrist as the physical examination to physicians in many other specialties.[1] In sexual disorders, a multidimensional assessment is important.[2] Each dimension will offer a different perspective from which to view the problem and plan possible interventions. Realizing that many sexual problems have multiple interactive etiologies, the clinician will attempt to identify the most easily correctable factor.[3]

The primary component will be the differential diagnosis, which will be based on a detailed understanding of the primary complaint, its onset and course, and its relationship to other medical events and to environmental factors. The primary complaint will be classified as global or situational, lifelong, or acquired. These subtypes will help to provide tentative hypotheses as to whether the complaint has a predominantly biologic or psychogenic etiology, and whether it is related to a major psychiatric syndrome or is drug induced. If the problem appears related to a major psychiatric syndrome, it is usually treated first to see whether the sexual complaint will resolve as well.

The next dimension of assessment, particularly if the etiology is hypothesized to be psychogenic, is to examine couple dynamics. As well as overt discord, one may observe that one partner subtly prevents his or her partner from recovering. This diagnosis may be based on a careful assessment of antecedents and consequences of sexual behavior. In these cases, conjoint behavioral psychotherapy with a particular focus on couple dynamics might be the intervention of choice. For example, the author treated a recently married woman with a complaint of low sexual desire in conjoint behavioral psychotherapy. As the woman became increasingly more comfortable in experiencing her own sexual feelings, her husband became increasingly emotionally distant. His withdrawal dampened his wife's sexual interest. Once the therapist was able to help the husband be comfortable with his wife's experience of her own sexuality, she was then able to experience a heightened awareness of her own libido.

A third factor in assessment is individual personality traits. If the patient has difficulty with trust and control in interpersonal interactions, it is likely that these issues will also affect her experience of sexual activities, as many behaviors appear to be consistent across different interpersonal settings. These issues may require targeted individual educative psychotherapy as well as behavioral interventions. In this regard, it is of note that the major effect of childhood sexual abuse on women in midlife appears to be on the quality of relationships with the partner rather than on sexual function *per se*.[4] The effects of incest on sexual behavior are reviewed in more detail in Chapter 3.4.

A fourth perspective is the individual's sexual life story.[5] The patient will reveal a sexual narrative in which the inner symbolic meaning and cultural significance of sexual behavior to her are revealed. This information may be utilized in individual psychotherapy or kept in mind as one proceeds with targeted behavioral therapy.

Disorders commonly treated by psychiatrists are difficulties with sexual desire and sexual arousal, orgasm problems, and vaginismus uncomplicated by pelvic pain. Most psychiatrists would collaborate closely with a gynecologist for complaints of sexual pain[6] (see Chapters 12.1–12.6). The psychiatrist may help in the multidisciplinary evaluation of sexual pain disorders primarily by excluding psychiatric etiologies of the complaint, thereby reinforcing the need to find somatic solutions to the problem. Referral or collaboration with an endocrinologist or gynecologist would be common in issues concerning hormone therapy or androgen augmentation.[7]

Subsequent sections will review psychiatric syndromes associated with female sexual dysfunction, psychiatric drugs causing sexual dysfunction, a differential diagnostic approach, and psychotherapeutic approaches.

Psychiatric disorders and comorbid female sexual dysfunction

Studies of sexual function in psychiatric patients indicate that female sexual dysfunction is more common in women with a variety of psychiatric disorders.[8] High rates of hypoactive sexual desire disorder have also been found in women with anxiety disorders such as panic disorder, obsessive compulsive disorder,[9] and post-traumatic stress disorder,[10] as well as in anorexia nervosa[11] and in schizophrenia.[12] In many cases, treatment of the underlying psychiatric disorder may resolve the sexual problem. Thus, it is important that a differential psychiatric assessment be part of the evaluation of female sexual dysfunction. For example, low desire resulting from panic attacks during sexual activity might be misdiagnosed as hypoactive sexual desire disorder. Depression may also present as low libido as part of generalized anhedonia.

Population surveys have found a high concordance of female sexual dysfunction with relationship discord and symptoms of depression and anxiety.[13] For decades, clinicians have recognized that decreased libido is part of the symptomatic presentation of depressive disorders.[14] Kennedy et al.[15] investigated the prevalence of sexual disorders in 79 untreated female patients with major depressive disorder. Fifty percent reported a marked decrease in libido as well as arousal. Another 15% reported difficulty in achieving orgasm. Kivela and Pahkala[16] studied depressive symptoms in elderly citizens in Ahtari, Finland. In women aged 60–70, loss of libido was significantly more common in women diagnosed with depression. After the age of 70, loss of libido was common in the entire population and no longer more common in depressed women than in nondepressed cohorts. Psychiatric disorders that have a high comorbidity with sexual disorders are listed in Table 17.3.1.

Table 17.3.1. Psychiatric disorders highly comorbid with hypoactive sexual desire disorder

Major depressive disorder
Dysthymic disorder
Anorexia nervosa
Panic disorder
Obsessive compulsive disorder
Post-traumatic stress disorder
Schizophrenia

Effects of psychiatric drugs on female sexual dysfunction

Psychiatric drugs have a high propensity to cause sexual side effects. The most common side effects are orgasmic dysfunction and decreased libido, although there have been some reports of decreased arousal on psychiatric drugs.[17] Case reports and even double-blind studies in the 1980s indicated that antidepressants (see Chapter 16.2), benzodiazepines, and antipsychotic drugs cause sexual dysfunction.[18] However, the sexual side effects of commonly prescribed psychiatric drugs were not generally appreciated until these drugs had been in general use for a number of years. The reason for the delayed recognition by physicians has been attributed to the fact that most patients do not volunteer this information unless directly asked by their physicians.[19]

Considerable evidence establishes that most antidepressants cause sexual dysfunction, especially orgasmic delay. Double-blind studies have demonstrated that phenelzine, imipramine,[20] clomipramine,[21] and most selective serotonin reuptake inhibitors cause orgasmic delay.[22]

Controlled studies indicate that nefazodone and bupropion have extremely low incidence of sexual side effects.[23,24] The sexual side-effect profiles of mirtazapine and venlafaxine are unclear but are probably close to that of the selective serotonin reuptake inhibitors.[25,26] Newer antidepressants and the incidence of sexual side effects are listed in Table 17.3.2. It should be emphasized that one needs to know the spectrum of action of antidepressants prior to substituting drugs. For example, selective serotonin reuptake inhibitors may be prescribed for a depressed patient with comorbid obsessive compulsive symptoms, and bupropion is not effective against obsessive compulsive symptoms. In addition to switching drugs, antidotes can be employed. To date, double-blind studies support the efficacy of 60 mg buspirone[27] or 150 mg bupropion[28] as antidotes. Case reports suggest that sildenafil may reverse selective serotonin reuptake inhibitor-induced anorgasmia in women, but this has never been demonstrated in a double-blind study.[29]

Case reports and clinical studies indicate that antipsychotic drugs can cause sexual difficulty, particularly orgasmic delay and decreased libido. This is important as these drugs are increasingly being utilized to augment treatment of affective disorders including major depressive disorder. These difficulties appear to be more pronounced in older antipsychotic drugs (e.g., haloperidol, thioridazine) as well as the new antipsychotic risperidone, all of which are associated with prolactin elevation.[30–32] Large case studies suggest that quetiapine and olanzapine have the lowest incidence of sexual side effects in both sexes.[33] Switching from an antipsychotic that causes prolactin elevation to a prolactin-sparing antipsychotic has been reported to resolve sexual dysfunction. Dopamine agonists, such as bromocriptine and cabergoline, have also been reported to reverse antipsychotic-induced sexual dysfunction.[34,35] The effects of antipsychotic drugs on sexual function are listed in Table 17.3.3.

Other drugs utilized in psychiatric practice, such as lithium carbonate,[36] valproate,[37] gabapentin,[38] and carbamazepine,[39] have been reported to cause sexual dysfunction. One controlled study found that diazepam may cause orgasmic delay in adult women.[40] There is minimal evidence concerning the prevalence of sexual dysfunction due to these agents.

Table 17.3.2. Sexual side effects and antidepressant therapy

High incidence
 Fluoxetine (Prozac)
 Sertraline (Zoloft)
 Paroxetine (Paxil)
 Citalopram (Celexa)
 S-Citalopram (Lexapro)

Intermediate incidence
 Fluvoxamine (Luvox)
 Venlafaxine (Effexor)
 Mirtazapine (Remeron)

Low incidence
 Bupropion (Wellbutrin)
 Nefazodone (Serzone)

Table 17.3.3. Antipsychotic drugs and sexual dysfunction

High incidence
 Thioridazine (Mellaril)
 Risperidone (Risperdal)
 Haloperidol (Haldol)

Possibly intermediate incidence
 Olanzapine (Zyprexa)

Low incidence
 Quetiapine (Seroquel)

Unknown incidence
 Ziprasidone (Geodon)
 Aripiprazole (Abilify)

General issues in the evaluation and treatment of female sexual disorder

The treatment of female sexual disorders will be partly determined by the presenting symptoms and partly by the patient's life story. The life story may reveal difficulties with trust, control, or past sexual trauma which may direct treatment as much as the formal diagnosis. Although there is considerable overlap between different sexual disorders, assignment to a primary diagnostic group while noting associated disorders will usually guide treatment decisions. A careful subtyping by duration and pervasiveness of the disorder may give clues as to etiology. For example, disorders present from the first sexual experience are thought to be related to sexual attitudes learned in the family of origin, whereas acquired disorders may be organic or psychogenic in etiology. Perhaps the most useful subtyping is whether the disorder is generalized to all sexual situations (global) or specific to one situation alone (situational). In general, situational disorders are more likely to be psychogenic in etiology.

If a psychogenic etiology is diagnosed, treatment is usually symptom-oriented and derived from behavioral models with deviations from this approach when necessary. Situations in which treatment might be altered from a symptom-oriented approach present when significant relationship discord exists or when the resolution of a sexual symptom is blocked by the personal meaning of the symptom.

Lifelong low sexual desire

The psychologic treatment of global, lifelong low sexual desire usually consists of various attempts to achieve attitude change if the problem appears to reside in restrictive attitudes about sexual pleasure. A typical patient may be a young female with minimal sexual experience from a home in which there were strong prohibitions against the experience of sexual pleasure. An exploration of the origins of the patient's sexual attitudes and reflection on whether her family's attitudes are applicable in independent adult life can help the patient experience less guilt about experiencing sexual pleasure. In individuals who are highly religious, referral to a well-chosen pastoral or rabbinical counselor may help tremendously. In symptom-oriented treatment, the therapist may give the patient homework assignments of reading romantic/erotic material, bodily self-exploration, or visiting erotic art in a local museum or bookstore. The therapist may also assist the patient to develop sexual fantasies. An example would be to give the patient the assignment of first noticing which male in her office she finds most attractive and then to imagine kissing him. These interventions are usually accompanied by sexual homework assignments. Most therapists share the belief that the patient is more likely to have a positive response to therapy if the patient herself desires change rather than desiring to change in order to please her partner.[41] A few case reports suggest organic causes for lifelong low libido, but these have not been confirmed in large studies.[42,43] One encounters a subset of women with lifelong histories of low sexual desire whose difficulties are not clearly related to psychologic, psychiatric, or interpersonal matters. One often suspects a normal variation in sexual drive of biologic origin. In these cases, experimental approaches such as androgen supplementation, the use of dopaminergic agonists, or the use of bupropion may be considered.[44]

An alternative viewpoint is that age-related declines in women in long-term relationships is normative. Situational lifelong low libido may reflect an atypical arousal pattern.[45] An example would be a woman in a heterosexual relationship who complains of low libido but masturbates by herself on a frequent basis. Underlying factors may be uncovered by examining the patient's usual masturbatory fantasies. If the patient desires greater sexual pleasure with the partner, she may be asked to change gradually her masturbatory fantasies to include the partner and to change her sexual activity with the partner to resemble the masturbatory fantasy. An examination of the masturbatory fantasies might sometimes reveal that the woman's primary sexual attraction is to same sex. In such cases, a frank discussion of this with the patient and consideration of the social and financial consequences of living an openly homosexual life can help the patient resolve life choices, although obviously this will not alter the patient's sexual attraction pattern. Rarely, one encounters a female patient with an alternative sexual arousal pattern (e.g., involving sadomasochistic activities). It is important to remember that paraphilic behavior is not always constant and may wax and wane with external stress and relationship discord. Depending on the particular paraphilia, it may be possible to have a conjoint session with both partners to see whether some of their sexual activity can be adapted to include the specific paraphilic behavior which is arousing to the patient.[46] In female patients with a history of repeated sexual abuse, decreased libido may be characterized by extreme ambivalence toward any sexual activity that might be interpreted as aggressive. In such cases, psychotherapy may be useful in ameliorating the aversion to sexual activity.[47]

Acquired hypoactive sexual desire disorder

Acquired hypoactive sexual desire disorder is an extremely common complaint in most medical practices (see Chapter 11.3).[48] One first needs to ascertain whether the problem is situational (occurring in one context) or global (occurring in all situations). A clear example of a situational loss of libido would be a woman who has lost interest in sexual activity with her partner but continues to have sexual fantasies about a past lover. Alternatively, the patient could report absence of sexual interest but daily masturbation. In these cases, it is highly likely that the problem is related to interpersonal issues with the partner.[49] Conjoint marital therapy is the treatment of choice.

Acquired global loss of desire can be due to a variety of factors. One first tries to rule out causes that can be treated by well-established therapies. Psychiatric disorders to rule out include major depressive disorder, social anxiety, panic disorder, obsessive compulsive disorder, and post-traumatic stress disorder. For these disorders, one would attempt to treat the underlying psychiatric disorder in the hope that it would resolve the problem with libido.[50]

As mentioned in another section, a number of psychiatric drugs have been reported to be associated with decreased libido. The influence of nonpsychiatric drugs on female libido has been minimally studied. Hypertensive disease and its treatment may be associated with decreased libido.[51,52] It appears that angiotensin-converting enzyme inhibitors are less likely to cause libido problems than other antihypertensive agents. There is some evidence that hypothyroidism and hyperprolactinemia are also treatable causes of decreased libido.[53] Evidence from numerous studies suggests that oral contraceptives may decrease libido in many women. There is no definitive evidence of which agents are worse.[54] Clinically, it seems logical to assume that any agent might cause sexual dysfunction, and always to consider whether the onset of a sexual problem coincided with the introduction of a new agent or with a dose change. It is also reasonable to do a trial of suspected agents to see whether libido returns.

In postmenopausal women, especially post-oophorectomy, decreased libido is common and has been attributed to decreased androgen production,[55] although the evidence for beneficial effects of androgen therapy at physiologic levels is unclear.[48] In cases involving hormonal therapy, most psychiatrists would collaborate with a gynecologist or endocrinologist.

Female arousal problems

A important differential in diagnostic evaluation is whether the problem is with subjective arousal, physiologic arousal (vaginal lubrication), or both (see Chapter 11.3). A lack of physiologic arousal in the presence of subjective arousal has a high probability of organic etiology. In premenopausal women, arousal problems are frequently associated with diminished libido as well. Although numerous pharmacologic agents have been reported to cause erectile dysfunction, the effects of these agents on female arousal have been little studied.[17] A reasonable approach is to assess whether the onset of the arousal difficulty appears to coincide with drug initiation and to do a trial of suspected drugs. Psychiatrists should also inquire about the sexual relationship and whether sufficient foreplay occurs. Many women require continuous stimulation to maintain adequate lubrication. If a woman becomes aware of diminished lubrication, she may become apprehensive about what is happening and begin self-observation, distancing herself from perception of further stimulation. In many cases, the clinician can help the woman become aware of this cycle and gradually retrain her to stop excessive self-observation.

In postmenopausal women, arousal problems are often associated with atrophic vaginitis due to decreased estrogen. The psychiatrist might begin estrogen therapy, although in most cases he or she would seek gynecologic consultation. For women who choose to avoid any form of hormone therapy, various artificial lubricants may be suggested.[56]

Female orgasmic disorder

Lifelong anorgasmia is relatively common and usually easily treated (see Chapter 11.4). Most often, it reflects relative inexperience combined with some anxiety about experiencing sexual pleasure, although the scenario may be more complex in women with a history of sexual abuse. Most psychiatrists would treat such problems with symptom-oriented therapy, including masturbatory training and systematic desensitization to sexual pleasure. Most women can learn to be orgasmic with masturbation. Occasionally, the use of a vibrator is needed. Once the woman can reliably experience orgasm during masturbation, the therapist usually attempts to integrate masturbatory activities gradually into partner-related activities. Controlled outcome studies indicate that the woman can usually be taught to reach orgasm by self-stimulation. The transfer of that skill to partner related-activities is more problematic.[57] Recent research indicates that bupropion enhances orgasmic capacity in women with a diagnosis of global, acquired hypoactive sexual desire disorder.[44] It is unclear whether bupropion would be similarly successful in women with a primary orgasmic disorder. A double-blind, placebo-controlled study of bupropion in premenopausal women found that doses of 300–450 mg per day of bupropion had a statistically and clinically significant positive effect on orgasm completion in a sample of women with global, acquired hypoactive sexual desire disorder.

General psychotherapeutic considerations

Evidence-based approaches form the basis of most sexual psychotherapy. These approaches usually involve a series of "homework assignments" of exercises designed to increase sexual intimacy over a period of weeks, with an absolute prohibition against coitus. These behavioral interventions are often referred to as "sensate focus" and provide a way for each partner to focus on sensual pleasure in the absence of performance pressure. As previously mentioned, orgasmic dysfunction usually also involves masturbation training. In the case of vaginismus, dilators of progressive size may be utilized. An alternative approach is to have the patient insert one and then two fingers into her vagina until the muscle spasm subsides. Subsequently, the patient guides her partners' fingers for insertion and subsequently allows the partner to insert his fingers without assistance. This method can serve to desensitize the patient gradually to the feeling of loss of control.

These targeted behavioral interventions are usually accompanied by individual and/or couple psychotherapy. Couple psychotherapy usually focuses on communication training. Couples are taught how to express, and coached in expressing, their wishes and feelings clearly in the first person without attributing blame. The other partner is taught active listening skills and may be instructed to repeat what he thinks his partner just said. Individual cognitive-behavioral therapy may be utilized to challenge negative attitudes about sexuality and intimate interpersonal relationships.[49] Evidence-based psychologic approaches to the female sexual disorders are covered in more detail in earlier chapters.

Conclusion

Because female sexual dysfunction frequently involves psychiatric issues, it is important to include a psychiatric assessment in the evaluation. A multidimensional approach to diagnosis and intervention can offer an orderly and systemic way to assess psychiatric and psychologic factors involved in the etiology and maintenance of sexual problems. Given the complexity of female sexual dysfunction and the limitations of our current knowledge base, multidisciplinary assessment is critical for effective interventions. The psychiatrist offers a distinct biopsychosocial approach to diagnosis and treatment. In addition, the psychiatrist has special expertise in the comorbidity of sexual dysfunction with other psychiatric disorders and their treatment.

References

1. Andreasen NC, Black DW. *Introductory Textbook of Psychiatry*, 2nd edn. Washington: American Psychiatric Press, 1995.
2. Pagan P. *Sexual Disorders: Perspectives on Diagnosis and Treatment.* Baltimore: Johns Hopkins University Press, 2004.
3. Segraves RT, Segraves KB. Female sexual disorders. In N Stotland, D Stewart, eds. *Psychological Aspects of Women's Health Care.* Washington: American Psychiatric Press, 2001: 379–400.
4. Dennerstein L, Guthrie J, Alford S. Childhood abuse and its association with mid-aged women's sexual functioning. *J Sex Marital Ther* 2004; 30: 225–34.

5. Risen C. Listening to sexual stories. In S Levine, C Risen, S Althof, eds. *Handbook of Clinical Sexuality for Mental Health Professionals*. New York: Brunner-Routledge, 2003: 3–19.

6. Bergeron S, Meana M, Binik Y et al. Painful genital sexual activity. In S Levine, C Risen, S Althof, eds. *Handbook of Clinical Sexuality for Mental Health Professionals*. New York: Brunner-Routledge, 2003: 131–52.

7. Dennerstein LL. The sexual impact of menopause. In S Levine, C Risen, S Althof, eds. *Handbook of Clinical Sexuality for Mental Health Professionals*. New York: Brunner-Routledge, 2003: 187–98.

8. Segraves RT. Female sexual disorders: psychiatric aspects. *Can J Psychiatry* 2002; 47: 419–24.

9. Minnen AV, Kampman M. The interaction between anxiety and sexual functioning: a controlled study of sexual functioning in women with anxiety disorders. *Sex Relatsh Ther* 2000; 15: 47–57.

10. Van Berlo W, Ensink B. Problems with sexuality after sexual assault. *Annu Rev Sex Res* 2000; 11: 235–57.

11. Morgan JF, Lacey JH, Reid F. Anorexia nervosa: changes in sexuality with weight restoration. *Psychosom Med* 1999; 61: 541–5.

12. Lyketos GC, Sakka P, Mailis A. The sexual adjustment of chronic schizophrenics: a preliminary study. *Br J Psychiatry* 1983; 143: 376–82.

13. Dunn KM, Croft PR, Hackett GI. Satisfaction in the sex life of a general population sample. *J Sex Marital Ther* 2000; 26: 141–51.

14. Mathew R, Weinman M. Sexual dysfunctions in depression. *Arch Sex Behav* 1982; 11: 323–8.

15. Kennedy SH, Dickens SE, Eisfeld BS et al. Sexual dysfunction before antidepressant therapy in major depression. *J Affect Disord* 1999; 56: 201–8.

16. Kivela SL, Pahkala S. Symptoms of depression in aged Finns. *Int J Soc Psychiatry* 1988; 34: 274–84.

17. Segraves RT, Balon R. *Sexual Pharmacology: Fast Facts*. Philadelphia: WW Norton, 2003.

18. Segraves RT. Psychiatric drugs and orgasm in the human female. *J Psychosom Obstet Gynec* 1985; 4: 125–8.

19. Nkanginieme I, Segraves RT. Neuropsychiatric aspects of sexual disorders. In R Schiffer, S Rao, B Fogel, eds. *Neuropsychiatry*. Baltimore: Williams and Wilkins, 2003: 338–57.

20. Harrison W, Rabkin J, Erhardt A et al. Effect of antidepressant medication on sexual function: a controlled study. *J Clin Psychopharmacol* 1986; 6: 144–9.

21. Monteiro W, Noshirvani H, Marks I et al. Anorgasmia from clomipramine in obsessive compulsive disorder: a controlled study. *Br J Psychiatry* 1987; 151: 107–12.

22. Waldinger M, Hengeveld M, Zwinderman AH et al. Effect of SSRI antidepressants on ejaculation: a double-blind, randomized, placebo-controlled study with fluoxetine, fluvoxamine, paroxetine, and sertraline. *J Clin Psychopharmacol* 1998; 18: 274–81.

23. Ferguson J, Shrivastava R, Stahl S et al. Reemergence of sexual dysfunction in patients with major depressive disorder: double-blind comparison of nefazodone and sertraline. *J Clin Psychiatry* 2001; 62: 24–9.

24. Croft H, Settle E Jr, Houser T et al. A placebo-controlled comparison of the antidepressant and effects on sexual functioning of sustained-release bupropion and sertraline. *Clin Ther* 1999; 21: 643–58.

25. Clayton A, Pradko J, Croft H et al. Prevalence of sexual dysfunction among newer antidepressants. *J Clin Psychiatry* 2002; 63: 357–66.

26. Montejo A, Llorca G, Izquiedo J et al. SSRI induced sexual dysfunction. Fluoxetine, paroxetine, sertraline and fluvoxamine in a prospective multicenter and descriptive study. *J Sex Marital Ther* 1997; 23: 176–94.

27. Landen M, Eriksson E, Agren H et al. Effect of buspirone on sexual dysfunction in depressed patients treated with selective serotonin reuptake inhibitors. *J Clin Psychopharmacol* 1999; 19: 268–71.

28. Clayton AH, Warnock JK, Kornstein SG et al. A placebo-controlled trial of bupropion SR as an antidote for selective serotonin reuptake inhibitor-induced sexual dysfunction. *J Clin Psychiatry* 2004; 65: 62–7.

29. Numberg G, Lauriello J, Hensley et al. Sildenafil for iatrogenic serotonergic antidepressant medication-induced sexual dysfunction in four patients. *J Clin Psychiatry* 1999; 60: 33–5.

30. Baldwin D. Schizophrenia, antipsychotic drugs and sexual function. *Prim Care Psychiatry* 1999; 60: 33–5.

31. Dickson R, Seeman M, Corenblum B. Hormonal side effects in women: typical versus atypical antipsychotic treatment. *J Clin Psychiatry* 2000; 61: 10–15.

32. Ghadirian A, Choviard G. Sexual dysfunction and plasma prolactin levels in treated schizophrenic patients. *J Nerv Ment Dis* 1982; 10: 463–73.

33. Bobes J, Garcia-Portilla MP, Rejas J et al. Frequency of sexual dysfunction and other reproductive side effects in patients with schizophrenia treated with risperidone, olanzapine, quetiapine A or haloperidol; results of the EIRE study. *J Sex Marital Ther* 2003; 29: 125–47.

34. Gazzola L, Opier L. Return of menstruation after switching from risperidone to olanzapine. *J Clin Psychopharmacol* 1998; 18: 486–7.

35. Tollin S. Use of the dopamine agonists bromocriptine and cabergoline in the management of risperidone induced hyperprolactinemia in patients with psychotic disorders. *J Endocrinol Invest* 2000; 23: 765–70.

36. Kristensen E, Jorgensen P. Sexual function in lithium-treated manic-depressive patients. *Pharmacopsychiatry* 1987; 20: 165–7.

37. Schneck CD, Thomas MR, Gundersen D. Sexual side effects associated with valproate. *J Clin Psychopharmacol* 2002; 22: 532–4.

38. Montes JM, Ferrando L. Gabapentin-induced anorgasmia as a cause of noncompliance in a bipolar patient. *Bipolar Disord* 2001; 3: 52.

39. Morrell MJ. Sexual dysfunction in epilepsy. *Epilepsia* 1991; 32: 38–45.

40. Riley A, Riley E. The effect of single dose diazepam on sexual response induced by masturbation. *J Sex Marital Ther* 1986; 1: 49–53.

41. Rosen R, Leiblum S. Hypoactive sexual desire. *Psychiatr Clin North Am* 1995; 18: 107–21.

42. Riley AJ. Lifelong absence of sexual drive in a woman associated with 5-dihydrotestosterone deficiency. *J Sex Marital Ther* 1999; 25: 73–8.

43. Riley A, Riley E. Controlled studies on women presenting with

sexual desire disorder: endocrine status. *J Sex Marital Ther* 2000; 26: 269–83.

44. Segraves RT, Clayton A, Croft H et al. Bupropion sustained release for the treatment of hypoactive sexual desire disorder in premenopausal women. *J Clin Psychopharmacol* 2004; 24: 339–42.

45. Friedman R, Downey J. Male and female homosexuality in heterosexual life. In S Levine, C Risen, S Althof, eds. *Handbook of Clinical Sexuality for Mental Health Professionals*. New York: Brunner-Routledge, 2003: 277–90.

46. Federoff J. The paraphilic world. In S Levine, C Risen, S Althof, eds. *Handbook of Clinical Sexuality for Mental Health Professionals*. New York: Brunner-Routledge, 2003: 333–56.

47. McCarthy B. Sexual trauma. In S Levine, C Risen, S Althof, eds. *Handbook of Clinical Sexuality for Mental Health Professionals*. New York: Brunner-Routledge, 2003: 425–42.

48. Basson R. Women's difficulties with low sexual desire and sexual avoidance. In S Levine, C Risen, S Althof, eds. *Handbook of Clinical Sexuality for Mental Health Professionals*. New York: Bmnner-Routledge, 2003: 111–30.

49. Wincze JP, Carey MP. *Sexual Dysfunction. A Guide for Assessment and Treatment*, 2nd edn. New York: Guilford, 2003.

50. Segraves RT, Rahman MI. Sexual disorders. In L Goldman, T Wise, D Brody, eds. *Psychiatry for Primary Care Physicians*. Chicago: American Medical Association, 1998: 197–216.

51. Duncan L, Lewis C, Jenkins P et al. Does hypertension and its pharmacotherapy affect the quality of sexual function in women. *Am J Hypertens* 2000; 13: 640–7.

52. Gandhi S, Kong S. Quality of life measures in the evaluation of antihypertensive drug therapy: reliability, validity and quality of life domains. *Clin Ther* 1996; 18: 1276–95.

53. Lombardo F, Gandini L, Santuli M et al. Endocrinological diagnosis in sexology. *J Endocrinol Invest* 2003; 20: 112–14.

54. Sanders SA, Graham CA, Bass JL et al. A prospective study of the effects of oral contraceptives on sexuality and well-being and their relationship to discontinuation. *Contraception* 2001; 64: 51–8.

55. Palacios S, Tobar A, Menendez C. Sexuality in the climacteric years. *Maturitas* 2002; 43: 69–77.

56. Ellison CR. Facilitating orgasmic responsiveness. In S Levine, C Risen, S Althof, eds. *Handbook of Clinical Sexuality for Mental Health Professionals*. New York: Brunner-Routledge, 2003: 167–86.

57. Segraves RT, Althof S. Psychotherapy and pharmacotherapy of sexual dysfunction. In P Nathan, J German, eds. *A Guide to Treatments That Work*. New York: Oxford University Press, 1998: 447–71.

17.4 Role of the female urologist/ urogynecologist

Susan Kellogg-Spadt, Kristene E Whitmore

Today, more than ever in the specialties of urology and urogynecology, comprehensive sexual health care is available for women. Sexual medicine centers devoted to the diagnosis and treatment of sexual disorders are opening across the USA, many of which are comprised of multidisciplinary teams (see Chapter 17.6 of this book). Women in these centers are typically seen by a team of specialty clinicians, advanced practice nurses, sexologists, psychologists, and physical therapists, under the direction of a female urologist or urogynecologist.

Historical perspective

Historically, recognition and treatment of female sexual health issues mirrored the recognition and treatment of female urologic disorders. Both were poorly understood, and therefore, under-diagnosed and undertreated. This was due, in part, to the absence of accurate definitions and controlled research. Topics including female pelvic anatomy (see Chapters 4.1–4.3) and muscular support (see Chapter 4.4) were given little attention in traditional urologic texts. Women's anatomy was simply considered to be a duplication of the male pelvic anatomy. Then, in the 1980s, several key urologists, including Raz, McGuire, and Kursh, began studying the effects of female sex hormones on urinary tract smooth muscle as well as delineating the function of the female pelvic floor and its surgical management.[1-3] In 1983, the first edition of the textbook *Female Urology* was published.[4]

In a similar fashion, the field of urology dealt with sexual concerns as they related to men only. Textbooks contained chapters on "sexual dysfunction" which pertained exclusively to erectile and ejaculatory dysfunction related to vascular and/or sensory insufficiency. In 1998, investigators examined the physiology of female engorgement during arousal and identified vasculogenic sexual dysfunction in females[5] (see Chapters 5.4–5.6). These researchers were also members of the American Foundation for Urologic Diseases international consensus conference convened in 1999 to define and formally classify female sexual dysfunction (see Chapter 9.1). Internationally recognized diagnostic criteria for female desire, arousal, orgasm, and pain disorders, as well as for hypersensitivity disorders and pelvic floor dysfunction, all prime causes of sexual dysfunction in women, were established at this conference. These assist a more scientific approach to therapeutics and research in female sexual dysfunction.[6]

Unlike urologists of the past, today's resident and attending urogynecologists understand the specialized anatomy and physiology of the female pelvic floor, in terms of muscular support, physiology, restoration of function, affects of pharmacology, and relationship to sexual function.[7-10] In the last 20 years, there has been a redefinition of urogynecology as a specialty that excels in the diagnosis and treatment of women with disorders that affect any aspect of the female pelvic floor. Those disorders may involve the "front" compartment, e.g., bladder dysfunction; the "middle" compartment, e.g., genital/sexual dysfunction; or the "rear" compartment, e.g., bowel dysfunction.

Pelvic floor dysfunction

Normal function of the pelvic floor musculature is essential in maintaining appropriate function of the pelvic organs, as well as appropriate sexual function. Abnormal function of this musculature is seen in an estimated 70% of women with genitourinary, bowel, and sexual disorders.[9-11] Pelvic floor dysfunction refers to conditions in which the pelvic floor muscular support system is functioning suboptimally. Disorders of abnormal pelvic floor laxity, termed "low-tone pelvic floor dysfunction", or disorders that cause spasticity and tightness of the pelvic floor, termed "high-tone pelvic floor muscle dysfunction", may be closely associated with sexual dysfunction.[10–12]

Hypotonus of the pelvic floor is a familiar disorder in urologic literature because of the relationship of the pelvic floor muscles to incontinence and pelvic organ prolapse. Low-tone pelvic floor dysfunction can result from childbirth, trauma, and/or senescence, and it can contribute to pelvic organ prolapse, transurethral urinary incontinence during orgasm, vaginal laxity, thrusting dyspareunia, and fecal incontinence related to or not related to sexual intercourse.[11,12]

"Hypertonus or spasm of the pelvic floor" is a newer term, although the concept has been used extensively in the colorectal literature by Thiele and others, referred to as "tension myalgia of the pelvic floor" and "levator ani syndrome".[13,14] High-tone pelvic floor dysfunction can result from childbirth, postural stressors, microtrauma, infection, adhesions, and surgical trauma, and can contribute to symptoms of frequency, urgency, dysuria, urinary retention, fecal retention, penetrative dyspareunia, and/or vaginismus.[8–12]

Assessment of tone in the pelvic floor is performed to determine a woman's ability to isolate, contract, and relax the pelvic floor muscles. When the clinician conducts a digital examination exerting light pressure on the inferior lateral walls of the vagina, the woman is asked to squeeze the examining finger and to "lift" the pelvic floor, without simultaneously tightening the abdominal, gluteal, or adductor muscle groups. If the patient is unable to produce sufficient muscle strength to "squeeze" the finger or to sustain that squeeze for a period of 5 s, she may be exhibiting the low-tone pelvic floor dysfunction pattern. If, conversely, the woman experiences muscle tenderness or pain when pressure is applied to the lateral vaginal wall or during an attempted squeeze against resistance, she may be exhibiting the spastic or high-tone pelvic floor dysfunction pattern. Results of the simple digital examination can be verified by the placement of a measurement tool, such as a perineometer or an electromyography probe, designed to measure muscle activity.[11–12,14]

Conservative therapy for pelvic floor dysfunction is aimed at muscle reeducation. A physical therapist who specializes in the pelvic floor can be a valuable asset to the female sexual dysfunction team in designing a pelvic floor rehabilitation program aimed at facilitating sexual comfort and pleasure for patients. Such a program might involve directed sling massage of the pelvic floor to elongate shortened muscles and decrease high-tone spasm for a woman with involuntary spasm of the pelvic floor muscles or vaginismus.[11–13] Thiele reported a case series of 31 patients with pelvic floor related pain, in which 19 (61.3%) were "cured" and 17 (35.5%) were "improved" after a series of directed transrectal massage of the pelvic floor muscles.[14] Pelvic floor massage can precede and facilitate the gradual introduction of dilators and movement toward sexual penetration for vaginismus patients.[12,13]

For a woman with low-tone pelvic floor dysfunction, which can manifest as incontinence with sex, decreased sensation, or poor orgasm amplitude, the physical therapist may design a program focusing on pelvic floor muscle strengthening with Kegel exercises, augmented with biofeedback and/or electrical stimulation of the pelvic floor.[10–12,15]

The concepts of pelvic floor dysfunction and muscle reeducation will appear throughout the remainder of this chapter as specific disorders and therapeutic regimens are discussed.

Hypersensitivity disorders associated with high-tone pelvic floor dysfunction

Hypersensitivity or sensory disorders of the lower urinary tract represent a spectrum of symptoms and conditions that includes chronic bacterial cystitis, urgency and frequency syndrome, sensory urgency, urethral syndrome, and interstitial cystitis. These entities, as well as vulvar pain, vaginal pain, and perineal and pelvic pain, are associated with spasm or hypertonus of the pelvic floor musculature.[16,17] They are classified by the International Continence Society as "genitourinary pain syndromes" and account for a large percentage of the concerns of female patients who present to urogynecologic and sexual medicine practices.[8]

During assessment of any genitourinary complaints in women, the undeniable link between the hormonal status, sexual activity, and development or exacerbation of urinary symptoms becomes apparent.

Sexual activity can cause direct pressure on vulvovaginal structures as well as a displacement of the bladder neck, creating an uncomfortable coital experience for some women, and potentially resulting in urinary trauma. Frequent and painful voiding, as well as anticipation of genital pain during sex play, can result in pelvic floor muscle guarding, which, over time, can become a spastic or high-tone pelvic floor.

The situation can be further complicated by any relative estrogen deficiency. Up to 40% of women experience atrophic urogenital symptoms at some time during the life cycle, whether during the peri- and postmenopausal years, during lactation, or while using low- or non-estrogen contraceptive alternatives. Discomfort during sex play, due to trauma or increased fragility of the urogenital tissues, can alter arousal and lubrication. In an evaluation of 90 peri- and postmenopausal women, Sarrell noted marked dyspareunia, burning, penetrative pain, and decreased sexual satisfaction in women whose serum estradiol levels were less than 50 pg/ml when compared with women whose serum estradiol levels were greater than 50 pg/ml.[15] Estrogen-deficiency symptoms include dryness, itching, burning, penetrative pain, irritative leukorrhea, urethral pressure, urinary urgency, and fissures associated with loss of tissue elasticity. In addition, poor estrogen binding in genitourinary tissues leads to ischemia, a decreased urethral mucosal cushion, and increased susceptibility of the bladder to bacterial adherence. The result is potential exposure of the neurovascular elements of the bladder wall to urinary toxins and infectious agents, the ramifications of which may be the development of recurrent urinary tract infection and/or a lower urinary tract hypersensitivity syndrome.[8,17] Of the 8.5 million women with urinary incontinence, up to 40% have detrusor instability and/or sensory urgency. Symptoms include urinary frequency (greater than eight episodes per 24 h) and uncomfortable urgency with or without leakage. Women with sensory urgency often name sexual intercourse as an inciting event for their symptoms, and report hypoactive sexual desire as a result of this association.[17,18] An estimated 5 million women are diagnosed with urinary tract infections each year. Among the 15% of these women who are classified as recurrent urinary tract infection sufferers (more than two episodes in 6 months or three in 1 year), coitus is cited as a major contributing factor for their symptoms[17] (see Chapter 7.7).

Interstitial cystitis

Interstitial cystitis is one of the most severe and challenging hypersensitivity disorders. Symptoms of interstitial cystitis can be greatly exacerbated by sexual activity, and the disorder can severely disrupt a couple's satisfying sexual relations over time.

Interstitial cystitis is a chronic bladder condition characterized by urgency, frequency and pain; it affects as many as 1 million Americans, the majority of whom are women.[19,20] Although the term "interstitial cystitis" was first suggested in 1887 by Skene, the exact etiology of the disorder remains unclear.[21] In 1915, Hunner reported the presence of ulcers on congested bladder mucosa associated with a contracted fibrotic bladder that hemorrhaged after bladder hydrodistention.[22] In 1987, the US National Institutes of Health established the following diagnostic criteria for interstitial cystitis: urinary frequency (more than eight times while awake; more than two times at night) and/or pain associated with the bladder, as well as diffuse glomerulations in three quadrants of the bladder and/or a classic Hunner ulcer on cystoscopy.[23]

Although the exact etiology of interstitial cystitis is currently unknown, most authors believe that it is multifactorial. Proposed causes include infectious agents; quantitative glycosaminoglycan layer deficiency; and ultrastructural abnormality of the lamina propria, interstitium, and/or mast cells of the bladder with neurogenic inflammation.[24]

Interstitial cystitis, like all hypersensitivity disorders of the lower urinary tract, is a diagnosis of exclusion. Infections such as vaginitis, urethritis, ureaplasm, or herpes cannot be present. In addition, carcinoma, diverticulum or stricture of the urethra, radiation exposure, allergic reactions, and tuberculosis must be excluded. Physical examination yields many typical signs of interstitial cystitis. During a bimanual examination, a woman with interstitial cystitis will often have tenderness just under the posterior bladder wall and/or behind and above the pubic bone. This feature will markedly differ from the condition of a woman who expresses only mild pressure during palpation of her urethra and bladder. The typical experience of a woman with interstitial cystitis is pain rather than light pressure. In addition,

a rigid or spastic state of the pelvic floor muscles is often present. Conclusive diagnosis of interstitial cystitis is made in conjunction with other diagnostic procedures.[11,17,25]

Several office and/or operating room procedures can suggest a diagnosis of interstitial cystitis. Findings on a 24-h voiding diary quantify voiding as over eight times per day and/or over two times per night. Urodynamic testing can verify low volume at first sensation of bladder filling, first and strong desires to void at low volume, increased bladder sensation, presence of detrusor overactivity, and reproduction of the patient's symptoms during filling. Cystoscopy with hydrodistention can verify the presence of Hunner's ulcers, linear scarring, hypervascularity, bloody effluent, and glomerulations after hydrodistention. Potassium sensitivity testing can verify increased epithelial permeability when the instillation of a mild potassium chloride solution exacerbates a woman's symptoms of urgency and pain.[26-30]

Although no treatment is considered curative for interstitial cystitis, multimodal management includes behavioral, pharmacologic, and surgical therapies. Behavioral therapies include dietary modification, bladder training, and pelvic floor physical therapy. Pharmacologic therapy begins with pentsosan polysulfate. Antihistamines, tricyclic antidepressants, anticholinergics, antiepileptics, muscle relaxants, anti-inflammatory agents, and narcotics are employed for symptom relief. Intravesical instillations are used for symptom flare. Surgical therapy includes hydrodistention and sacral nerve stimulation. Rarely, augmentation cystoplasty or urinary diversion, with or without cystectomy, is performed[11,20,23,25,28-30] (see Chapter 14.2).

Vulvar vestibulitis

Frequently, the discomfort experienced by women with hypersensitivity disorders of the bladder is compounded by vulvar vestibulitis syndrome. Vulvar vestibulitis syndrome, also referred to as vulvar adenitis, focal vulvitis, vestibulodynia, or vulvodynia, affects up to 15% of women in the general population and up to 40% of women with interstitial cystitis.[18,31] Vulvar vestibulitis syndrome is characterized by focal erythema and hypersensitivity of the vulvar vestibule, dyspareunia, and dysesthesia[31-33] (see Chapters 12.1–12.6).

Definitive causes of vulvar vestibulitis syndrome have not been identified; research suggests that neurogenic inflammation of the vulvar vestibule can occur in response to a variety of noxious environmental stimuli, including mechanical or chemical trauma, infections, viral exposure, and localized allergic responses.[31-34]

A key factor in managing vulvar vestibulitis syndrome is competent and early diagnosis. In the "touch test", vulvar structures such as the labia, interlabial sulci, and periclitoral and perirectal areas are touched firmly with a saline-moistened cotton swab, and the patient is asked to respond if she feels discomfort. As the openings of the Skene's and vestibular glands are tested, women with vulvar vestibulitis syndrome will respond that these touches are painful. If the diagnosis is in doubt, the procedure can be repeated after application of 5%

lidocaine to the glandular ostia. If the touch test becomes negative after this application, a diagnosis of vulvar vestibulitis syndrome is likely. Touch testing should be performed in conjunction with a thorough pelvic and vaginal examination, including cultures for bacteria and fungi. Vulvar colposcopy often reveals inflammatory vascular ectasia in gland areas, and can be a useful adjunct to diagnosis.[34,35]

At present, no treatment for vulvar vestibulitis syndrome is considered "curative". Traditional management includes anti-irritant hygiene regimens, low oxalate diets, tricyclic antidepressant therapy, topical cortico- or hormone steroids, antifungal therapy, intradermal interferon, pelvic muscle biofeedback, and/or vestibulectomy. Newer investigational approaches include use of topical creams containing capsaicin, cromolyn, atropine, or nitroglycerin; pelvic floor physical therapy; and acupuncture.[33-41]

Irritable bowel syndrome

Hypersensitivity disorders of the bladder and genitals are often accompanied by bowel symptoms. Irritable bowel syndrome affects more than 5 million people and is characterized as a hypersensitivity syndrome. Symptoms include abdominal bloating and cramping, painful diarrhea and/or constipation, mucoid stools, and sensations of incomplete emptying. Symptoms can be incited by ingestion of large meals, certain foods (milk products; fatty foods; or alcoholic, caffeinated, or carbonated beverages), gaseous overdistention, hormonal fluctuations, exercise, and sexual activity. Treatments include dietary modifications, stress management, antispasmotics, and antidepressants.[42]

Strategies for managing sexuality with hypersensitivity disorders

Sexuality is adversely affected in up to 80% of women with hypersensitivity disorders of the bladder, bowel, and vulva and accompanying high-tone pelvic floor dysfunction. Those that are able to tolerate coitus often suffer a flare of their symptoms for days as a result of sexual activity, which then becomes a negative reinforcement for future sexual activity, and research has documented "avoidance of intimacy most of the time".[25,35,45] Avoidance can result in negative outcomes for both the woman and her partner. As the result of a Western cultural "script" that equates penile-vaginal sex with adequate sexual function, women who avoid contact may feel "abnormal" and inadequate from a cultural standpoint. Lack of physical intimacy can also result in generalized loss of interest in sex, decreased ability to respond sexually, and feelings of depression.[16,25,44]

An important intervention when working with women who have hypersensitivity-related sexual dysfunction is to introduce the concept of sexual "rescripting". Encourage the woman and her partner to develop a unique definition of adequate pleasuring (which may or may not involve genital contact) and to make a commitment to pleasure each other with agreed-upon regularity. A way to reframe pleasuring for a couple is by introducing the concept of "his and hers intimacy". Explain that intimacy, for one partner, might involve a quiet dinner out or going to a movie, while, for the other partner, intimacy might be defined as oral or genital sex play that leads to orgasm. With this technique, intimacy needs are met through activities that are appropriate to physical limitations. Encourage couples to follow their own sexual script, not one that the culture has written for them.[43-46]

Consistent with the concept of rescripting is the premise of noncoital pleasuring. Since many women with hypersensitivity are unable to engage in pain-free penile-vaginal sex, they may turn to their health-care provider to suggest alternate strategies. For some, oral and manual pleasuring of the clitoris and/or penis (without penetration) are viable options, but others may be unwilling or unable to consider these. Many women find the option of "outercourse" appealing and pain free. In this technique, a man mounts a woman in a traditional intercourse fashion, but instead of thrusting his penis inside of her vagina, he thrusts on the "outside". Rubbing against her lubricated lower abdomen and pubic bone area, or between a woman's inner thighs, often creates friction sufficient to result in both male and female orgasm.[43,45]

For other women with hypersensitivity, sexual intercourse can be accomplished on a limited basis. Comfort measures (Table 17.4.1) that facilitate intimate expression may include applying 2–5% lidocaine jelly to the vaginal introitus 20 min before stimulation to decrease the hypersensitivity of the urethra and vestibular gland areas; applying liberal amounts of a water-soluble lubricant or small amounts of estrogen-based vaginal cream to aid penetration; premedicating with a sublingual smooth muscle relaxer and/or an anticholinergic to decrease sensory urinary or fecal urgency; premedicating with a skeletal muscle relaxant 1 h before sex play to decrease pelvic floor spasm; or inserting a belladonna rectal suppository 1 h before sex play to calm both the bladder and pelvic floor. In addition, many women find that precoital pelvic floor massage, pre- and postcoital voiding, and postcoital application of an ice pack to the genital/suprapubic area enhance comfort.[11,25,43,45] Choosing coital positions that are least likely to affect the pelvic floor include having the woman lying on her side or inferior with raised hips. Thrusting in a circular movement and limiting thrusting time to 5–10 min helps to minimize discomfort.[45]

A couples' sexual therapist or psychologist can often help the woman and her partner deal with the "long-term prospect" of altered comfort with sexual intercourse and may suggest alternative pleasuring strategies.

Laxity disorders associated with low-tone pelvic floor dysfunction

A second major class of disorders encountered in the urogynecologic setting is disorders associated with weakness and laxity

Table 17.4.1. Medications that facilitate comfortable sexual relations

Drug class	Examples	Action	Indication
Topical anesthetic	Lidocaine gel Prilocaine gel	Blocks pain and hypersensitivity of vulvar tissues	Apply to introitus and/or urethra 5–20 min before lovemaking
Anticholinergic/ antispasmodic/ antimuscarinic	Hyoscyamine Tolterodine Oxybutynin Trospium	Decreases sensory urgency; smooth muscle relaxer	Dosed 10–60 min before sex play, decreases urinary and/or fecal urgency, urethral spasms, and/or urge incontinence that can interfere with sexual expression
Central skeletal muscle relaxant/alpha adrenergic agonist	Soma Metaxalone Tizanidine Cyclobenzaprine	Decreases involuntary pelvic floor muscle guarding and spasm	Dosed 60 min before sex play, inhibits painful muscle spasms that can interfere with penetration and thrusting
Topical estrogen	Estradiol cream	Enhances elasticity and moisture in vulvar tissues	Applied nightly and/or just before sex play, enhances comfort with penetration, and decreases introital microfissures

of the pelvic floor muscles. Predominant symptoms among this group of patients are pelvic organ prolapse with or without urinary or fecal incontinence.

An incidence of involuntary loss of urine is experienced by an estimated 95% of women during their lifetime, with an estimated one in four women leaking before the age of 59. Approximately 50% of female residents in nursing homes are incontinent.[47] Urinary incontinence can be broadly classified as urge incontinence, related to sensory urgency (see previous section on hypersensitivity disorders); stress incontinence, which occurs with increased intra-abdominal pressure and maneuvers such as sneezing, coughing, and straining; or mixed incontinence. Abnormalities in urethral closure and poor pelvic muscle support are the primary mechanisms underlying stress incontinence.[17,23]

Factors predisposing a woman to stress incontinence include age; heredity; vaginal birth trauma; previous pelvic/vaginal surgery; history of radiation therapy; menopausal status; lifestyle factors, such as strenuous lifting; and chronic medical conditions, including obstructive pulmonary disease, obesity, and constipation. Assessment strategies for incontinence include evaluation of voiding diaries, urinalysis, cytology, and urodynamic testing.[47]

Incontinence can be improved in 8 of 10 women by treatment options that include nonsurgical and surgical strategies. Nonsurgical strategies include behavioral bladder retraining, pelvic floor strengthening (Kegel exercises), pessary placement, urethral plugs, and implants. Surgical procedures, including sling and tension-free vaginal tape placement, provide cure rates as high as 95% when performed in appropriate candidates.[8,47]

Fecal incontinence

Fecal incontinence, or involuntary leakage of solid, liquid, or gaseous stool from the rectum, affects as many as 5.5 million Americans. It is more common in women and in the elderly.[47,48]

Muscle damage is involved in most cases of fecal incontinence. In women, this damage commonly occurs during childbirth, especially after a difficult vaginal delivery that involves forceps and/or episiotomy. Studies suggest that 3–25% of woman experience some degree of fecal incontinence after childbirth.[47] Damage to the nerves that control the anal muscle or that are responsible for rectal sensation is also a common cause of fecal incontinence. Nerve injury can occur during childbirth, with severe and prolonged straining for stool, or in association with chronic medical conditions such as diabetes, spinal cord tumors, and multiple sclerosis. Muscle damage can also occur during rectal surgery, as well as in people with inflammatory bowel disease or a history of abscess in the perirectal area.

Fecal incontinence is often associated with reduction in the elasticity of the rectum, which shortens the time between the sensation of the stool and the urge for a bowel movement. Surgery, radiation injury, and history of inflammatory bowel disease are associated with poor elasticity of the rectum. Medical evaluation may include physical examination, ultrasonography, defacography, and anorectal manometry, which tests anal pressures, rectal elasticity, and rectal sensation.[48]

The treatment of fecal incontinence varies, depending upon its etiology. Behavioral strategies include dietary modifications that eliminate irritants and add fiber, bowel-retraining strategies to prevent diarrhea and enhance formation of a regular bowel movement pattern, Kegel exercises, and anorectal biofeedback. Pelvic floor reconstructive surgery can be an effective treatment for structural defects.[47]

Strategies for managing sexuality with incontinence

Data from several recent studies suggest that women with mild to moderate incontinence self-report commensurate levels of sexual activity, comfort, and enjoyment with sex as women without incontinence. Mild to moderate prolapse did not usually interfere with sex, as the herniated tissues tended to be pushed into the vagina with penile penetration and thrusting. Prolapse pressure was considered less bothersome during intercourse because of being in a recumbent position. Studies indicate that when incontinence and prolapse are severe, symptoms are a source of anxiety and interfere with the overall sense of sexual satisfaction. Interestingly, studies suggest that women under age 65 report being incontinent during intercourse at a higher rate than women over age 65. The reasons for the findings are unclear and may be related to more frequent and/or more vigorous sex play among the younger age group. The younger women may have had greater urge incontinence, which is harder to control during sex play than stress incontinence, a more common finding among older women.[49-52]

Women who experience incontinence during intercourse express concern about feeling unclean, undesirable, and "unsexy". They fear embarrassment, rejection, and possible infection of themselves or their partner. Encouraging a woman to be open and communicative with her partner about incontinence will often decrease anxiety by bringing the issue into the forefront rather than being veiled in secrecy. Instructing the woman with urinary leakage that urine is sterile and poses no health threats will often decrease the fear associated with unavoidable leakage.[47,49] Other strategies for women who experience any type of incontinence during sexual activity include daily performance of 30–60 Kegel exercises (taught by a healthcare provider with a return demonstration in the office), emptying the bladder or colon before sexual activity, avoiding ingestion of food or fluids for 1 h before lovemaking, and coital positioning to decrease leakage (e.g., female in superior or side-lying position). Use of a water-soluable lubricant or vaginal estrogen before penetration will decrease urethral trauma and facilitate comfortable entry.[47-51,53]

Conclusion

When managing female sexual dysfunction patients, it is important that the urogynecology team be confident in their diagnostic and therapeutic capabilities, or be able to triage the patient for optimal care. The adage, "if the treatment isn't working, reconsider the diagnosis", should always be kept in mind.

Showing empathy for the patient with sexual concerns is paramount, because of the quality-of-life threats that this problem poses. Advising the patient that if sexual dysfunction has begun to make her feel aversive to intimacy, she should abstain for several weeks (while medical testing and treatment are conducted) may provide a much needed "break" from the stress and discomfort and a chance to re-establish healthy sexual feelings between partners.

A woman's sense of well-being is closely tied to the quality of her relationships, including her intimate physical relationships. By taking the time to assess and address patients' sexual concerns, health-care providers can assist women with chronic genitourinary disorders reclaim a sense of themselves as competent women capable of intimacy, rather than "sexually dysfunctional".

References

1. Raz S. *Female Urology*. Philadelphia: WB Saunders, 1996: 30–55.
2. Sant G. *Interstitial Cystitis*. Philadelphia: Raven-Lippincott, 1997.
3. Kursh ED, McGuire EJ. *Female Urology*. Philadelphia: JB Lippincott, 1994.
4. Raz S. *Female Urology*. Philadelphia: WB Saunders, 1983.
5. Goldstein I, Berman J. Vasculogenic female sexual dysfunction: vaginal engorgement and clitoral erectile insufficiency syndrome. *Int J Impot Res* 1998; 10: S84–8.
6. Basson R, Berman J, Burnett A et al. Report of the international consensus of development conference on female sexual dysfunction: definitions and classifications. *J Urol* 2000; 163: 888–94.
7. Bump RC, Mattisson A, Bo K et al. The standardization of terminology of female pelvic organ prolapse and pelvic floor dysfunction. *Am J Obstet Gynecol* 1996; 175: 10–17.
8. Abrams P, Cardozo L, Fall M et al. The standardization of terminology in lower urinary tract function. Report from the standardization subcommittee of the International Continence Society, 2002.
9. Moldwin RM, Mendelowitz F. Pelvic floor dysfunction and interstitial cystitis. *J Urol* 1994; 151: 285–7.
10. Travell J, Simons DG. *Myofascial Pain and Dysfunction: The Triggerpoint Manual*. Baltimore: Williams and Wilkins, 2002.
11. Lukban JC, Whitmore KE. Pelvic floor muscle re-education: treatment of the overactive bladder and painful bladder syndrome. *Clin Obstet Gynecol* 2000; 45: 273–80.
12. Whitmore K, Kellogg-Spadt S, Fletcher E. Comprehensive assessment of the pelvic floor. *Issues Incontinence* 1998; Fall: 1–10.
13. Fitzgerald MP, Kotarinos R. Rehabilitation of the short pelvic floor. *Int Urogynecol J* 2003; 14: 269–75.
14. Thiele GH. Coccygodynia: cause and treatment. *Dis Colon Rectum* 1963; 6: 422–4.
15. Sarrell PM. Sexuality and menopause. *Obstet Gynecol* 1990; 7: 26–32.
16. Steege JF, Metzger DA, Levy BA. *Chronic Pelvic Pain*. Philadelphia: WB Saunders, 1998.
17. Goldwasser B. Urodynamics. In Wein AJ, Barrett DM, eds. *Voiding Function and Dysfunction: A Logical and Practical Approach*. Chicago: Year Book Medical Publishers, 1988.
18. Erickson DR, Morgan KC, Ordille S et al. Nonbladder related symptoms in patients with interstitial cystitis. *J Urol* 2001, 166: 557–60.
19. Curhan GC, Speitzer FE Hunter DJ et al. Epidemiology of interstitial cystitis: a population based study. *J Urol* 1999; 161: 549–54.
20. Alagiri M, Chottiner S, Ratner V et al. Interstitial cystitis: unexplained associations with other chronic disease and pain syndromes. *Urology* 1997; 49S (5A): 52–7.
21. Skene AJC. *Diseases of the Bladder and Urethra in Women*. New York: William Wood, 1887: 167.

22. Hunner GL. A rare type of bladder ulcer in women: report of cases. *Trans South Surg Gynecol Assoc* 1915; 27: 247–92.

23. Gillenwater JY, Wein AJ. Summary of the National Institutes of Arthritis, Diabetes, Digestive and Kidney Diseases Workshop on Interstitial Cystitis, National Institutes of Health, Bethesda. *J Urol* 1988; 140: 203–6.

24. Christmas TJ. Historical aspects of interstitial cystitis. In Sant GR, ed. *Interstitial Cystitis*. Philadelphia: Raven-Lippincott, 1997.

25. Whitmore K. Self-care regimens for patients with interstitial cystitis. *Urol Clin North Am* 1994; 21: 121–4.

26. Kirkemo A, Peabody M, Diokno AC et al. Association among urodynamics findings and symptoms in women enrolled in the interstitial cystitis data base (ICDB) study. *Urology* 1997; 49S(5A): 76–7.

27. Parsons CL, Greenberger M, Gabal L. The role of urinary potassium in the pathogeneses and diagnoses of interstitial cystitis. *J Urol* 1998; 159: 1862–6.

28. Bade JJ, Peters JM, Mensink HJ. Is the diet of patients with interstitial cystitis related to their disease? *Eur Urol* 1997; 2: 179–81.

29. Brookoff D. The causes and treatment of pain in interstitial cystitis. In Sant GR, ed. *Interstitial Cystitis*. Philadelphia: Raven-Lippincott, 1997.

30. Comiter CV. Sacral neuromodulation for the symptomatic treatment of refractory interstitial cystitis: a prospective study. *J Urol* 2003; 261: 1369–72.

31. Goetsch MF. Vulvar vestibulitis: prevalence and historic features in a general gynecologic practice population. *Am J Obstet Gynecol* 1991; 164: 1609–13.

32. Bohm-Starke N, Hilligres M, Falconer C et al. Increased intraepithelial innervation in women with vulvar vestibulitis syndrome. *Gynecol Obstet Invest* 1998; 46: 256–8.

33. Metts J. Vulvodynia and vulvar vestibulitis: challenges in diagnosis and management. *Am Fam Physician* 1999; 15: 1547–50.

34. McKay M. Vulvitis and vulvovaginitis: cutaneous considerations. *Am J Obstet Gynecol* 1991; 165: 1176–9.

35. Paavonem J. Diagnosis and treatment of vulvodynia. *Am Med* 1995; 27: 175–8.

36. Nyirjesy P, Sobel JD, Weitz MV et al. Cromolyn cream for idiopathic vulvar vestibulitis: results of a placebo controlled study. *Sex Transm Infect* 2001; 77: 53–8.

37. Miles M, Niezen P, Berman L et al. Relief of vaginal and labial pain and burning with 0.2% nitroglycerin cream in women with vulvodynia. Proceedings from the Female Sexual Function Forum. Boston: 2001.

38. Ekgren JS. Vulvovaginitis treated with anticholinergics. *Gastroenterol Int* 2000; 13: 72.

39. Zyczynski HM, Culbertson S, Gross J et al. Topical capsaicin in the treatment of vulvar vestibulitis. *Gynecol Invest* 1997; 4: 107a.

40. Daniellson I, Sjoberg I, Ostrum C. Acupuncture for the treatment of vulvar vestibulitis: a pilot study. *Acta Obstet Gynecol Scand* 2001; 80: 437.

41. Glazer HI, Rodk G. *The Vulvodynia Survival Guide*. Oakland: New Harbinger Publications, 2002.

42. Steinhart MJ. Irritable bowel syndrome: how to relieve symptoms enough to improve daily function. *Postgrad Med* 1992; 91: 315–21.

43. Webster D, Brennan T. Use and effectiveness of sexual self-care strategies for interstitial cystitis. *Urol Nurs* 1995; 15: 14–18.

44. Herman S. Interstitial cystitis: impact on female sexual function. Paper presented at the Society for the Scientific Study of Sex, Toronto, Canada, 2000.

45. Kellogg-Spadt S. *Listening to the Voices of Women Diagnosed with Vulvodynia*. Ann Arbor: Proquest Press, 2002.

46. Leiblum S. Libido and lubrication: tips for sexual counseling. *Menopause Manage* 1993; March: 16–19.

47. Parker WH, Rosenman AE, Parker R. *The Incontinence Solution*. New York: Simon and Schuster, 2002: 940–1010.

48. NIH Publication. *Fecal Incontinence*. March 2004.

49. Berglund A, Eisemann M, Lalos A et al. Social adjustment and sexual relationships among women with stress incontinence before and after surgical treatment. *Soc Sci Med* 1996; 42: 1537–42.

50. Berglund A, Fugl-Meyer K. Some sexological characteristics of stress incontinent women. *Scand J Urol Nephrol* 1996; 30: 207–301.

51. Roe B, May C. Incontinence and sexuality: findings from a quality prospective. *J Adv Nurs* 1999; 30: 573–7.

52. Weber A, Walters M, Peidmonte M. Sexual function and vaginal anatomy in women before and after surgery for pelvic organ prolapse and incontinence. *Am J Obstet Gynecol* 2000; 182: 1610–15.

53. Glazener CMA, Herbison GP, Wilson PD et al. Conservative management of persistent postnatal urinary and fecal incontinence. *Br Med J* 2001; 323: 593–9.

17.5 Role of the nonphysician health-care clinician

Amy L Gamez

Introduction

It is an exciting and dynamic time, as the specialty of female sexual health is developing into an independent field that can improve the quality of life of our patients. Nonphysician health-care clinicians play an integral part in an interdisciplinary team in the management of female sexual dysfunction. They can be instrumental in helping patients with female sexual dysfunction confront their sexual health issues, as well as in the planning and carrying out of a successful treatment strategy.

Nonphysician health-care clinicians, including nurse practitioners and physician assistants, can provide a critical part of comprehensive care to the patient with female sexual dysfunction. Among other things, the nurse practitioner and physician assistant are trained to educate patients on sexual health issues, perform health assessments, conduct patient interviews, and take a thorough medical history that incorporates a sexual health history. Evaluation of sexual dysfunction should become a part of the routine history and physical examination. Nonphysician health-care clinicians have the opportunity to address sexual health proactively with female patients, mostly because they are the first clinicians encountered by the patient in a primary care setting. Health-care professionals in endocrinology, urology, gynecology, and family practice settings are in key roles to identify females experiencing sexual dysfunction[1] (see Chapters 17.1–17.4 and 17.6).

This chapter will explore how the nonphysician health-care clinician can assist in the integration of awareness, diagnosis, and treatment of female sexual health issues in the primary care setting. A brief historical perspective will provide the developmental background of sexual health treatment. The next section supplies suggestions on how to create an office environment that is "sexual health friendly", and guidance to the clinician on how to promote a permissive atmosphere in which patients can effectively communicate their sexual problems. The chapter will then delve into the intricacies of the interaction with the patient, such as taking a sexual health history and breaking the barriers that currently exist, as well as discussing the physical examination and appropriate laboratory testing. Then, suggestions will be provided on how to integrate the evaluation techniques to be utilized. Lastly, this chapter will provide suggestions on how to incorporate treatment-management strategies to help patients in their everyday lives.

Historical perspective

From the start of the twentieth century until the late 1960s, sexual dysfunction had been treated within a psychoanalytic framework.[2] Sex therapy, as it is known today, was essentially founded by Masters and Johnson in 1970, whose published report on a "new" approach to sexual problems revolutionized what health professionals saw as the appropriate treatment for such difficulties[2] (see Chapters 1.1 and 11.1). This linear model of the sexual response cycle, in contrast to the psychoanalytic practices, focused primarily on the vascular and neurologic changes, which included four stages: (1) excitement; (2) plateau; (3) orgasm; and (4) resolution.[3] Subsequently, a biopsychosocial model was presented that combined biologic, psychologic, and sociocultural influences, and interpersonal relationships, and suggested that emotional intimacy, commitment, sharing, and tenderness to another person are often required for a woman to respond to sexual stimuli.[3] Based on those models, the criteria of the *Diagnostic and Statistical Manual of Mental Disorders*, fourth edition (DSM-IV), provide guidance in the diagnosis of female sexual dysfunction; these criteria include the four main categories of sexual desire disorder, sexual arousal disorder, orgasm disorder, and sexual pain disorder.[4] The

1999 Consensus Classification System further expanded the DSM-IV criteria to include physical as well as psychologic causes of female sexual dysfunction. Several changes were made in the specific definitions and criteria for each diagnosis, including use of a personal distress criterion for most diagnostic categories[5] (see Chapter 9.1).

Recently, with the advent of oral therapies in the treatment of male erectile dysfunction, sexual health issues have become an easier topic to discuss for both men and women (see Chapters 13.1–13.3, 14.1, and 14.2). An increasing number of patients are discussing sexual problems with their health-care providers, requiring the nonphysician health-care clinician to keep abreast of the latest treatment options as well as knowing the available resources. As the field of female sexual dysfunction continues to progress, nonphysician health-care clinicians will have the responsibility of furthering the development of their role in the management of female sexual dysfunction.

Creating an environment that promotes sexual health

Identifying patients with sexual issues

The first step in identifying female patients with sexual health issues is to recognize that this is a common problem. Sexual dysfunction in women is age-related, progressive, and highly prevalent, affecting 30–50% of American women[6] (see Chapters 2.1–2.4). Potentially, every other female patient to enter the office could be experiencing some type of sexual dysfunction.

Even after recognition, many patients are reluctant to disclose their sexual problems to their primary care physician and/or endocrinologist, urologist, or gynecologist despite good patient rapport. Usually, patients do not present with female sexual dysfunction symptoms in the primary care setting as they do with other disorders; therefore, it is important to ask appropriate questions to elicit their concerns (see Chapter 17.1).

So, how are we to identify female patients with sexual health issues? Generally, nonphysician health-care clinicians have more time to spend with their patients, enabling them to establish better rapport. In turn, the time spent encourages patients to feel more comfortable in disclosing sensitive issues, particularly those that have to do with sexuality. By our increasing the comfort level through a good patient–clinician relationship, the patient will feel more at ease when asked questions of a sexual nature. However, if the patient is unwilling to bring up the subject on her own, it is essential for the clinician to introduce the subject in a sensitive manner. But what is the right way to "ask the question"? What question will make the patient comfortable? We have certainly learned from approaching men with erectile dysfunction that there is no one correct question for everyone. Questions to consider when introducing sexual health are as follows:

- Are you sexually active?
- Are you experiencing any difficulties with your sex life?
- Are you having any difficulties sexually, such as problems with desire, sexual arousal, or reaching orgasm? (This is more direct and will probably elicit a clarifying question from the patient if she is interested.)

One final suggestion about approaching the subject is to ask questions concerning sexual health on the history intake form. This will let the patient know that her health-care clinician is receptive to sexual health issues as well as to her overall well-being.

Creating the environment

A goal of the clinician is to create and promote an environment that is "sex-discussion friendly". There are several ways to achieve this goal. One way is to encourage the clinician to be aware of exhibiting negative nonverbal cues.

Conducting interviews while standing or making minimal eye contact are prime examples of negative nonverbal cues. Conversely, by sitting down, actively listening, and making good eye contact, the clinician will promote a more comfortable environment for the patient.

Secondly, the office can convey its interest in patients' sexual health by the availability of patient education materials such as brochures and patient questionnaires. As mentioned earlier, history intake forms provide another vehicle to display the commitment of the office to sexual health care. The inclusion of sexual health concerns on the intake form shows the patient that the clinical staff are interested in all of her medical issues, including those about sex. By implementing these suggestions, an office will go a long way toward creating a more conducive and "friendly" environment for sexual health discussions (see Chapter 11.2).

Establishing the roles in the office

Due to lack of specific academic education, few urologists and gynecologists are skillful in sexual medicine. For this reason, it is crucial for the physician with a surgical background to convey the message that the nonphysician health-care clinician is a valuable resource in the office in regard to sexual health issues. Although the physician has the final responsibility for the patient's treatment, the nonphysician health-care clinician can assist in providing patient information, diagnosis, treatment, and integration of care so as to provide a comprehensive evaluation of the patient's sexual health concerns.

Additionally, there must be clear guidelines as to the relationship between the physician and nonphysician health-care clinician regarding care of sexual health patients. Items to clarify include the following: who should conduct the initial interview? When should the sexual health questions be posed, and by whom, the nonphysician health-care clinician, the physician, or both? What treatment protocols are to be used?

Furthermore, while it is important to create a conducive environment, it is worth ensuring that the office staff are instructed on their respective roles. For nurses, medical assistants, and ancillary staff, it might be as simple as teaching each person to be sensitive to the patients who are being given sexual health brochures or medication samples.

Interaction with the patient

Addressing sexual health history

Once a comfortable environment has been established, it is necessary to incorporate a detailed and thorough sexual health evaluation in addition to the routine history and physical examination. The nonphysician health-care clinician must be open, empathetic, and nonjudgmental during the interview to allow the patient to feel comfortable in disclosing sensitive and private matters. Moreover, the clinician should make a concerted effort to avoid making moral or religious judgments regarding the patient's behaviors; instead, the clinician should relate the information from a point of view that includes emotional and psychologic health.[7]

For appropriate evaluation and management, it is important to establish the patient's sexual orientation early in the interview process. Since gender identity conflicts are often a cause of sexual dysfunction, the mode and type of the questions posed by clinicians should ease patients into openly expressing their concerns.[8] Ideally, these patients should be referred to a sex therapist/psychologist for further evaluation.

Regardless of sexual orientation, the patient should be asked questions about sexual activity such as whether or not she is currently sexually active. If so, one should ascertain frequency of intercourse, the number of partners over the past year, and any associated symptoms with sexual activity (e.g., pain, burning, bleeding).

Next, the clinician should evaluate the patient's scope of sexual dysfunction. For instance, the patient's concern over sexual desire and how that relates to her partner relationship should be discussed. The assessment should include the patient's past as well as current information regarding sexual arousal, her ability to achieve orgasm, and any associated pain during sexual intercourse.

Additionally, discussions may involve overall sexual satisfaction. The clinician should determine whether the dysfunction is a lifelong or acquired problem, and whether the dysfunction is generalized or situational.

The variations of questions will differ from practitioner to practitioner, depending on comfort level and experience. Table 17.5.1 lists sample questions.

Sometimes the patient's own testimonials provide the best insight.[8] For example, the patient may disclose relationship problems or possible embarrassments about urinary incontinence during intercourse. Obtaining this information early in the interview may expedite diagnosis, treatment initiation, and/or proper referral to another health-care clinician.

Table 17.5.1. Sample questions to elicit sexual health concerns

- Do you have any sexual concerns that you would like to discuss today?
- Are you experiencing any difficulties with your sex life?
- Do you have any difficulty becoming lubricated with sexual intercourse?
- Do you have difficulty achieving orgasm?
- Do you experience pain with intercourse?
- Do you currently suffer from a sexually transmitted disease?

Alternatively, questionnaires may be used prior to the office visit to save time. There are a variety of validated scales, such as the Female Sexual Function Index, that assess the domains of desire, arousal, orgasm, and pain. Another useful instrument is the Female Sexual Distress Scale, which helps to quantify the patient's level of bother and distress.[9,10]

Consequently, a sexual history may help to explain the patient's current health problems, or aid in identifying new health problems such as depression/anxiety, diabetes, or hypertension.

Barriers to discussing sexual health issues

It is important to recognize some of the barriers to discussing sexual health issues by clinicians to illustrate the importance of sexual health evaluation in women. Female sexual dysfunction is a common problem. Although the available literature demonstrates the importance of sexuality to patients, physicians often do not introduce the subject during clinical encounters.[11] Patients report that physician discomfort and anticipated nonempathetic response to sexual problems are the primary barriers to discussing sexual health.[7] The intent is to treat the whole person. The ability to understand and overcome the barriers will allow clinicians to better identify sexual dysfunction among their female patients.

Many clinicians, due to feelings of embarrassment or unfamiliarity, feel uncomfortable discussing sexual issues with their patients. Clinicians may also worry that their patients will find the questioning offensive. In one study, only 35% of primary care physicians reported that they often or always took a sexual history.[7] However, research conducted on healthy women has indicated that they would seek advice from their family physicians if the physicians raised the issue of sexual function rather than the women themselves having to volunteer the information.[12]

Furthermore, the clinician should practice sexual health interviews on a regular basis in order to become more comfortable in discussing sexual issues with patients. As the level of comfort exhibited by the clinician increases, the expression of patient concerns will be enhanced.

Appropriate timing in discussing sensitive sexual health issues is another element the clinician must consider. The patient may feel uneasy discussing sexual issues while being physically examined and become hesitant in disclosing information. For better results, the comfort level should be established during the interview process.

Another barrier is the perceived lack of time by clinicians during a patient visit. Clinicians worry that asking patients about their sexual issues will take too much time for evaluation and treatment. In actuality, asking about sexual issues may save time, as underlying issues are uncovered. Clinicians can decide to what level they want to delve with each patient and at what point a referral to another health-care clinician is necessary.

An additional obstacle is the reluctance to address sexual function due to the clinician's lack of expertise. Generally, clinicians do not feel comfortable discussing issues on which they do not have a great deal of knowledge. More often than not, primary care practitioners have received little training on how to assess female sexual function.[13] Clinicians can inform themselves about female sexual dysfunction through continuing education programs, attending educational conferences on female sexual health, and reading journal articles, other current research, and other published material. The DSM-IV criteria provide the current diagnostic and classification system for female sexual dysfunction; however, they do not provide a background for understanding the patients' sexual problems. Clinicians need to address possible contributing factors such as relationship difficulties, and biologic or psychosocial issues. By taking a thorough history, nonphysician health-care clinicians can perform the initial assessment for biologic, psychosocial, interpersonal, and emotional factors that will enable them to recommend the appropriate referral.

Lastly, the clinician may harbor the misconception that female sexual dysfunction requires a more complicated treatment plan. Male sexual dysfunction is perceived to be an uncomplicated diagnosis compared to female sexual dysfunction and easier to treat. Hence, many clinicians avoid the issue of female sexual dysfunction altogether.

Medical history and physical examination

The medical history (see Chapter 9.2) should include focused questions on the patient's overall health condition. The nonphysician health-care clinician can be instrumental in helping patients to understand how the medical history indicates the etiology of female sexual dysfunction. It is an opportunity for patients to understand that female sexual dysfunction can potentially be a normal consequence of their health issues.

In addition to a thorough sexual health history (see Chapter 9.4) to identify sexual problems, the nonphysician health-care clinician can perform a focused physical examination and laboratory blood tests (see Chapter 9.5). Sexual dysfunction may be symptomatic of organic or psychiatric disorders or a combination of both. Some of the possible risk factors associated with female sexual dysfunction are listed in Table 17.5.2.

The patient's current medications should be reviewed, including prescription, over-the-counter drugs, and street drugs, as some may contribute to the etiology of a patient's sexual

Table 17.5.2. Risk factors for female sexual dysfunction

- Cancer
- Cardiovascular disease
- Depression/anxiety
- Endocrine disease
- Fatigue
- Genital surgery
- Genital atrophy
- Hormonal abnormality
- Interpersonal relationships
- Medications
- Neurologic disease
- Psychosocial factors
- Sexual or physical abuse
- Urogenital disorders

dysfunction (Table 17.5.3). Additionally, the patient's current medical therapy can be turned into an opportunity for the nonphysician health-care clinician to educate the patient, and to clarify how some of these medicinal interventions may contribute to sexual health issues.

Moreover, the clinician should review the patient's surgical history, including pelvic surgery, back surgery, and cardiovascular surgery. For example, a hysterectomy may reduce blood flow to the vagina and decrease lubrication. A thorough physical examination should be performed, including a gynecologic examination to assess physiologic etiologies, pain, and trauma. The goal of the examination is detection of disease; however, the examination also provides an opportunity to educate the patient about normal anatomy and sexual function, and to reproduce and localize pain encountered during sexual activity.[8] After a comfortable rapport has been established, the clinician can teach the patient during the examination and when appropriate, make use of readily available mirrors, illustrations, and pictures to make the patient feel more comfortable with her own anatomy.

The nonphysician health-care clinician should coordinate with the physician to establish a protocol of laboratory tests to be ordered at the initial evaluation. This initial blood testing may identify an underlying disease such as diabetes or hypercholesterolemia. Treating these organic disorders may improve or reverse the patient's sexual dysfunction.

Table 17.5.3. Medications associated with female sexual dysfunction

- Antihistamines
- Antihypertensives
- Anticonvulsants
- Benzodiazepines
- Diuretics
- Narcotics
- Antiandrogens
- Oral contraceptives
- Antidepressants
- Antiestrogens

Incorporating an integrated treatment strategy

Integration and multidisciplinary treatment coordination

In coordinating the sexual health evaluation and interdisciplinary treatment plan, the nonphysician health-care clinician is likely to enhance treatment outcomes through follow-up. Another added benefit is that the nonphysician health-care clinician can collaborate with the clinical staff in determining which treatment options are most appropriate for this list. The responsibilities include maintaining continual communication and synchronizing the interventions proposed by the interdisciplinary team members, such as the endocrinologist, urologist, or gynecologist, as well as a sex therapist, psychologist, or psychiatrist, depending on the resources of the community. One way to implement team communication is through scheduled teleconferences or meetings to discuss patient progress. Integrating each team member's assessment allows better understanding of the patient's problem for an optimal treatment plan. The coordination of the services of these specialists is paramount if the goal is to keep patients knowledgeable and interested in addressing their original sexual health issues. The nonphysician health-care clinician can assist in devising a comprehensive treatment plan and determining which treatments the physician deems appropriate to utilize in the armamentarium of the practice.

The nonphysician health-care clinician's own sexual health education

As previously mentioned, nonphysician health-care clinicians must continue to educate themselves to increase the knowledge base regarding female sexual dysfunction, as this is a rapidly growing field. By making a commitment to self-education, the nonphysician health-care clinician can help to educate other staff members in the office through periodic in-service programs.

Education can be furthered by reading textbooks and journal articles, and attending conferences, such as the annual meeting of the International Society for the Study of Women's Sexual Health. There is a growing list of national, regional and community-sponsored continuing medical education talks and teleconferences with emphasis on the field of sexual health.

The nonphysician health-care clinician certainly is in a strategic position to educate the patient and office staff about the clinical trials underway on female sexual dysfunction. In order to integrate this additional service into the office, the nonphysician health-care clinician needs to be aware of the research protocols that are available in the office as well as any research opportunities that are available in the community.

How the nonphysician health-care clinician can incorporate patient education into female sexual dysfunction treatment and management

For clinicians to be successful in the treatment of sexual dysfunction, the most crucial aspects of medical care are coordination and implementation. The nonphysician health-care clinician can be instrumental in assisting patients with female sexual dysfunction to confront sexual health issues, and can assist in planning and carrying out a successful treatment strategy. Educating the patient and partner about normal female physiologic response and female pelvic and genital anatomy is often necessary. Additionally, physiologic changes associated with aging, pregnancy, menopause, and vascular dysfunction should be explained. The clear correlation between the patient's general health and sexual function must be emphasized.[14] The nonphysician health-care clinician can play a significant role in informing the female patient about the definition of female sexual dysfunction through handouts and brochures.

Patients may need education on how to modify harmful lifestyle behaviors (i.e., alcoholism, recreational drug use, smoking, sedentary lifestyle, and promiscuity) that could be a factor in their sexual dysfunction. Sexually transmitted disease prevention through education and awareness may be prudent, depending on the patient's risk factors.

Educating patients on their prescribed sexual health medications and sexual health interventions is very important. Patients often need reinforcement on how and when to take their medications as well as discussion of possible side effects that they may experience that could lead to discontinuation of treatment. Partner education and sexual evaluation are a critical component in the management of female sexual dysfunction.

The nonphysician health-care clinician should be aware of the current literature on female sexual dysfunction to be able to provide patients with information on available treatments.

Expanding the "sexual health friendly" environment beyond the office setting

Once the nonphysician health-care clinician is comfortable with the field, it may be time to expand the area of academic influence. The first step is promoting intraoffice appreciation of the field of sexual medicine. Essentially, this involves teaching the staff to "spread the word" that the health-care team is interested in being attuned to the sexual health needs of female patients. The next step is to consider out-of-the-office medical education. This enables other clinicians and their office staff as well as the general community to become aware of the practice's special expertise in female sexual dysfunction. With continued knowledge, the nonphysician health-care clinician may eventually consider delivering local talks to other nonphysician health-care clinicians. It is an opportunity to teach and excite them about the field of sexual medicine in the expectation that some may eventually see patients in their own offices.

Conclusion

It is an exciting time in the field of female sexual dysfunction as it ventures to become an independently recognized field in the practice of medicine. The treatment of female sexual dysfunction is progressively evolving, as new approaches and treatment options are discovered through basic and clinical research.

A collaborative approach is ideal in the management of female sexual dysfunction, including both medical and psychosocial evaluation. The nonphysician health-care clinician, as part of the necessarily multidisciplinary team, can play a significant role in the management of the complexity of the female patient with sexual dysfunction. While the physician is ultimately responsible for the patient's overall management, the nonphysician health-care clinician can assist by performing the initial evaluation, providing patient education, and assisting in the protocol development for the practice/office staff, thus playing an integral role in the management of patients with female sexual dysfunction.

References

1. Keller M. Female sexual dysfunction: definitions, causes, and treatment. *Urol Nurs* 2002; 22: 237–44, 284.
2. Weiderman MW. The state of theory in sex therapy (the use of theory in research and scholarship on sexuality). *J Sex Res* 1998; 35: 88–99.
3. Walton B, Thorton T. Female sexual dysfunction. *Curr Womens Health Rep* 2003; 3: 319–26.
4. Anastasiadis AG, Davis AR, Ghafar MA et al. The epidemiology and definition of female sexual disorders. *World J Urol* 2002; 20: 74–8.
5. Basson R, Berman J, Burnett A et al. Report of the international consensus development conference on female sexual dysfunction: definitions and classifications. *J Urol* 2000; 163: 888–93.
6. Berman JR, Bassuk J. Physiology and pathophysiology of female sexual function and dysfunction. *World J Urol* 2002; 20: 111–18.
7. Nusbaum MR, Hamilton C, Lenahan P. Chronic illness and sexual functioning. *Am Fam Physician* 2003; 67: 347–54, 357.
8. Nusbaum MR, Hamilton CD. The proactive sexual health history. *Am Fam Physician* 2002; 66: 1705–12.
9. Rosen R, Brown C, Heiman J et al. The female sexual function index (FSFI): a multidimensional self-report instrument for the assessment of female sexual function. *J Sex Marital Ther* 2000; 26: 191–208.
10. Derogatis LR, Rosen R, Leiblum S et al. The female sexual distress scale (FSDS): initial validation of a standardized scale for assessment of sexually related personal distress in women. *J Sex Marital Ther* 2002; 28: 317–30.
11. Phillips NA. Female sexual dysfunction: evaluation and treatment. *Am Fam Physician* 2000; 62: 127–36, 141–2.
12. Sarkadi A, Rosenqvist U. Contradictions in the medical encounter: female sexual dysfunction in primary care contacts. *Fam Pract* 2001; 18: 161–6.
13. Coons HL. Women's health in primary care: interdisciplinary interventions. *Fam Syst Health* 2002; 20: 237–51.
14. Lightner DJ. Female sexual dysfunction. *Mayo Clin Proc* 2002; 77: 698–702.

17.6 Integration of medical and psychologic diagnosis and treatment

Dongwoo Kang, Stanley H Ducharme

In recent years, female sexual dysfunction has gained considerable attention in the medical literature. Both biologic and psychosocial scientists have gained basic understanding of the etiology and clinical treatment of the various female sexual dysfunctions. Scientific studies[1-4] have demonstrated that the prevalence of female sexual dysfunction is much higher than previously believed. They have also shown that both the prevalence of female sexual dysfunctions and the overlap or comorbidity of female sexual dysfunction is higher than those of sexual dysfunction in men. Nevertheless, there are few data on the biologic and psychologic efficacy of the various treatment modalities. Even well-controlled clinical trials have failed to provide a clear picture of the most effective treatment protocols. As a result, health-care clinicians who treat female sexual dysfunction face a variety of obstacles in determining the most effective treatment approach. To further complicate this clinical picture, there have been very few treatment protocols thus far approved by the US Food and Drug Administration. Thus, clinicians have been forced to develop treatment modalities that remain off-label.

A wide range of treatment modalities for female sexual dysfunction have been independently developed and implemented in a variety of clinical settings. Specialists in departments of psychiatry, urology, gynecology, endocrinology, and psychology have found various management paradigms to be effective under particular conditions. In our clinical experience, the most effective treatment for female sexual dysfunction has been a multidisciplinary integration of biologic and psychologic perspectives. Unfortunately, however, there is still a lack of understanding of how these biologic and psychologic treatment modalities can be integrated into the clinical setting.

In this chapter, various models of integrating biologic and psychologic assessment and treatment will be discussed. Furthermore, this chapter will also consider various methods of systemically integrating these biologic and psychologic issues in the clinical setting to achieve optimal patient satisfaction.

Diagnosis

Female sexual dysfunction is a multicausal and multidimensional disorder combining biologic, psychologic, and interpersonal determinants.[5] We emphasize that although the primary diagnosis may be based on either a biologic or psychologic etiology, the clinician must always maintain a holistic perspective, keeping in mind both ends of this spectrum. The possibility of other diagnoses should be repeatedly considered from the initial interview until the end of treatment.

Clinical practice has demonstrated that, despite the presence or absence of organic disease, mood and psychologic issues significantly affect sexual response and can strongly correlate with female sexual dysfunction.[6,7] In a similar manner, organic problems with or without psychologic issues can also affect a woman's sexual response directly or indirectly. In cases where the care provider believes there is a predominantly biologic etiology, psychologic and relational factors can often play a role in maintaining the dysfunction, making the condition difficult to treat. In addition, psychologic issues may emerge as a consequence of the biologic condition. For this reason, considering a diagnosis as strictly biologic or psychologic can be inaccurate and a disservice to the woman and her partner.

Many specialists tend to regard problems beyond their own field as an indication for "further" evaluation and treatment, but both biologic and psychosocial evaluations should be considered as basic and essential procedures. This comprehensive assessment is highly recommended for all sexual dysfunctions and is especially critical in the initial conceptualization and treatment planning. Without early attention to emotional and relational issues, women may find it difficult to address these concerns later in the treatment process. Once treatment has been initiated, many women and their partners may be reluctant to seek referrals to mental health professionals and to address the less tangible psychologic aspects of the sexual dysfunction.

With this in mind, one effective and ideal model for the treatment of female sexual dysfunction has been to integrate the mental health professional or sex therapist into the medical setting. In this way, both mental health professional and treating physician can participate in the diagnosis collaboratively. Psychosocial issues can be identified at the time of the initial office visit, and relevant psychologic factors can be communicated to the treating physician prior to the full medical evaluation. Ultimately, not only can a comprehensive assessment be made, but the therapeutic strategies can be individually designed to address the biologic components as well as the emotional and relational issues. In this clinical setting, therapeutic strategies can be promptly shared and modified as changes occur during the treatment process.

Psychosocial evaluation

It is strongly recommended that the psychodynamic or psychosocial evaluation be made under the responsibility of a mental health professional. In taking the psychologic history, the following factors should be included in the assessment: developmental history, cultural and religious influences, sexual history, family background, early trauma or abuse, life stresses, past psychiatric treatments, alcohol and substance abuse, and relational factors. In addition, it is extremely important to have a broad understanding of the partner's reaction to the sexual dysfunction and the impact of the dysfunction on the quality of the relationship. This information often provides important insight into the motivation for treatment and the relationship demands being placed on the patient.

In many clinical settings, the presence of a mental health professional may be difficult or impractical. In such cases, the treating physician should always take a detailed history that includes the emotional and relationship components. Although patients may initially be reluctant to discuss such issues, there is often a sense of relief in communicating such factors after many years of distress. For the clinician, it is imperative to be open, supportive, and nonjudgmental throughout the interview and diagnostic process. The use of standard, objective psychologic instruments and questionnaires can also be an adjunct to the treating physician. The Female Sexual Function Inventory,[8] the

Brief Index of Sexual Functioning for Women,[9] the Derogatis Interview for Sexual Functioning,[10] and numerous other instruments can be beneficial in understanding the subjective status of the sexual functions. Moreover, standardized psychologic instruments such as the Minnesota Multiphasic Personality Inventory, the Beck Depression Inventory, the Perceived Stress Scale, and others can be used to evaluate psychologic factors that are indirectly related to sexual functions. In spite of their widespread usage, the psychosocial information gathered from these instruments carries the risk of being fragmentary and is often difficult to use by biologically minded physicians who are not familiar with the interpretation of validated questionnaires. Naturally, the use of psychologic questionnaires should never replace the clinical interview itself. Questionnaires are best used when they can supplement and add additional information to the clinical interview. Questionnaires can also provide personal insight into issues of which the patient may not be aware.

In medical settings where the mental health profession is not integrated into the treatment team, referrals should be made to knowledgeable mental health clinicians in the community. In such cases, it is important to identify clinicians who have previously worked in the field of sexual medicine and are knowledgeable, skilled, and comfortable working with sexual material. Having an available mental health clinician as a resource can often be beneficial to the woman and her partner at some point during the treatment process. For many couples, counseling may be beneficial at any time in the treatment process, as new issues often emerge as the treatment proceeds.

Traditionally, marital and relational issues have been neglected not only by biologically minded physicians, but also in the psychologic field. It is not unusual for clinicians to focus on the sexual function of the individual while neglecting the environmental and relational factors. The presence of the partner during the early diagnostic process provides another source of objective and trustworthy information. This can improve the long-term prognosis of the patient. Since the presence of female sexual dysfunction may itself induce conflicts in the relationship, it is critically important to explore and address this aspect of the presenting problem. Health clinicians working in the field of female sexual dysfunction should routinely meet with the partner at the beginning of treatment and periodically throughout the treatment process.

In general, a comprehensive psychosocial evaluation is required either prior to the biologic evaluation or simultaneously.

Biologic evaluation

The major predisposing factors of the biologic etiologies are vascular, urogynecologic, hormonal, neurologic, and medication (see Chapters 6.1–6.5 and 7.1–7.7 of this book). Evaluation of these factors is the core of a good biologic assessment. The danger in evaluating female sexual dysfunction is that physicians may neglect psychologic issues while, at the same time, mental health clinicians or sex therapists may neglect the underlying biologic aspects of the dysfunction. In cases where there are clear psychologic concerns and an apparent psychologic etiology, there may also be biologic issues that contribute to the underlying dysfunction. Mental health professionals should be especially careful not to neglect the basic biologic evaluation. This is particularly true if the clinician works in the community rather than an academic institution where the full team may be available. In all cases, good clinical practice demands that a medical evaluation be performed prior to beginning a course of sex therapy. It is not uncommon for various physical problems, underlying medical illness, and medications to be contributing factors.

The specific evaluation procedure could include focused history and physical examination, laboratory tests,[11] and laboratory evaluation[12] (see Chapters 9.2–9.5). At times, the results of various physiologic tests can be inconsistent with the patient's clinical presentation. As Bancroft[13] has indicated, women are more prone to sexual inhibition than men. Furthermore, the laboratory or office setting can be an unnatural and inhibiting environment for many women. Aberrations in the clinical evaluation can be a function of the office setting rather than a true picture of the underlying dysfunction. Subsequently, before the physiologic data are interpreted, individual differences, such as sexual inhibition (e.g., lack of privacy, performance anxiety, fear) and exhibition factors[14,15] (e.g., sexual stimuli, intimacy), should be considered. For example, when evaluating pain or arousal, it may be difficult to determine whether the clinical presentation is a function of the office setting or whether it occurs in the home environment as well. As a result, a comprehensive sexual history is important to gather before the physician begins to interpret the data from any physiologic testing. In cases where the patient is reluctant to provide a complete sexual history, some psychologic testing or consultation with a psychologic specialist may prove beneficial in better understanding the patient.

The importance of a good physical evaluation is twofold. Not only is it critical in uncovering the basic physiology, but also it is helpful for the patient to understand cognitively the physical aspects of the disorder. This benefit of physical examination can be compared to the initial psychologic evaluation, since both assessments must focus on the development of a therapeutic alliance in the clinician–patient relationship (see Chapters 9.5, 12.1, and 12.4).

In all cases, the physician should be aware of the doctor–patient relationship and of the psychologic impact of the examination on the patient. Even the interview and sexual history taking can raise anxiety because of their obvious sexual content and personal nature. When discussing sensitive sexual material, it is not uncommon for patients to develop erotic feelings toward the clinician. This is referred to as an erotic transference. This phenomenon can develop when the patient begins to convey intimate sexual details to the physician. Erotic feelings can often be mistaken as genuine feelings of love and

longing for the physician. They can often be accompanied by sexual fantasies. Such feelings may be a function of the patient's current psychologic condition or may represent some unresolved concerns from the patient's childhood. For many patients, a focused genital examination can be extremely sensitive and can act as the source of erotic transference toward the doctor. The presence of such erotic feelings can cause discomfort for the physician and can interfere with providing an effective treatment plan. Ultimately, such erotic feelings from the patient need to be addressed so that they do not intensify. In some cases, it may be important for the physician to remind the patient of the professional relationship. Such discussions are often described as ones that help establish boundaries and set limits.

Erotic feelings toward the treating physician are especially common for women with a psychiatric diagnosis such as histrionic or borderline personality disorder.[16] These patients typically have high attention needs and a tendency to somatization. In addition, patients who are experiencing a manic episode of bipolar mood disorder may easily demonstrate serious erotic transference because of hypersexuality, as these patients often have increased sexual thoughts and urges. In more unstable patients, erotic or paranoid delusion may indicate an underlying psychotic disorder such as schizophrenia. These cases demand that the treating physician work concurrently with a psychiatrist to ensure the patient's emotional stability and safety.

The psychiatrist has advantages over other mental health professionals such as psychologists, family/couple therapists, and sex therapists. Because of their medical training, psychiatrists not only understand the emotional context of the sexual dysfunction, but also have the biologic knowledge relating to neurotransmitters, neuropeptides, and other key functions of the brain. Psychiatrists are also trained in the secondary sexual dysfunctions associated with psychiatric illness (e.g., hyper/hyposexual symptoms of mood disorder) or psychiatric medications. Therefore, psychiatric consultation can be an important component in the overall treatment of female sexual dysfunction, especially in patients with psychiatric disorders or medications.

Multidiagnosis and descriptors

Considering the multidimensional characteristics of female sexual dysfunction with its high comorbidity and multicausality, Basson et al.[17,18] have recommended that the clinician be aware of the need to consider multiple diagnoses for an individual patient (e.g., sexual desire disorder and combined arousal disorder). In addition, as descriptors are integral components of diagnosis(es), it is strongly recommended that the contextual factors be considered. Often, the contextual factors of an individual case are based on the main etiologic considerations of each diagnosis. As Maurice[19] has previously noted in his discussion of contextual factors, this proposed classification system differs little from the multiaxial diagnostic system of the *Diagnostic and Statistical Manual of Mental Disorders*, fourth edition, text revised (DSM-IV-TR).[20] Utilizing a multidiagnostic classification that includes the contextual descriptors for each diagnosis (e.g., hypoactive sexual desire disorder with androgen deficiency and marital conflict, or Axis I: hypoactive sexual desire disorder/Axis III: androgen deficiency/Axis IV: marital conflicts in the DSM-IV-TR[20]) can reflect the specific diversity of female sexual dysfunction. One advantage of utilizing this diagnostic classification is that it specifies both the underlying medical diagnosis and the psychologic and relationship factors. When these issues are clearly presented in the diagnostic formulation, communication is enhanced among providers, and treatment goals are more clearly articulated. Ultimately, this comprehensive diagnostic formulation improves the overall integration of the biologic/psychologic diagnosis and treatment.

Treatment

The initial diagnosis and development of an individualized management plan are the starting point of the treatment for female sexual dysfunction. Good clinical practice demands that the treatment approach be a shared decision-making process,[21,22] defined as the process by which clinicians and patients agree on a specific course of action based on a common understanding of the treatment goals and pros and cons of the chosen course compared with any available alternatives. In this process, the health-care provider is the expert in diagnosis, treatment alternatives, and prognosis. In contrast, the patient is good at her own history, preferences, and goals. In addition, the patient, treating physician, and other providers can work collaboratively in addressing the biologic, emotional, and relationship components of the dysfunction. The ultimate focus of the treatment is to improve the female sexual function itself, but if the associated problems are not checked or corrected, clinicians may find themselves facing resistance to treatment. In our experience, women will more often follow through with recommendations if they are part of the decision-making process. Successful treatment is also more likely if the partner is involved early in the treatment process. In cases where both partners are involved, marital therapy to improve communication or various sensate focus techniques may help the couple to resume sexual activity as biologic treatment progresses.

In many cases, biologic treatment alone is insufficient. Although psychologic treatment can be the mainstay of management of female sexual dysfunction, it is not reasonable to make partial edits of the traditional sex therapy with sensate focus and to apply it alone to all kinds of female sexual dysfunction as "one size fits all". Therefore, psychologic and biologic management is often combined. However, specialists should also be cautious of excessive blending. It may result in too much pressure on the patient, low cost-effectiveness, and low efficacy. Specialists should always attempt to balance combined therapy with facilitation. To avoid this difficulty, multidisciplinary

discussion about individualized management, primary treatments, other treatment alternatives, and the patient's decision should be pursued.

As the treatment progresses, biologic etiologies tend to have linear results and be comparatively predictable due to their distinct relation between cause and effect. On the other hand, psychologic issues can spread like wildfire in all directions or can newly develop at any time. Therefore, continuous re-evaluation is more frequently required throughout the treatment. Commonly, if the problem persists for a long period or if there is no response despite continuous main treatment, there must be a referral in mind in case different causes or other diseases are suspected.

Sexual desire/interest disorder

As the relationship between the patient and her partner must be considered in all cases of female sexual dysfunction, the presence of a male sexual dysfunction should also be evaluated and considered (see Chapter 8.2). Male erectile dysfunction or premature ejaculation may be contributing, causal, or maintaining factors in the woman's lack of sexual interest or orgasmic disorder. In these cases, female sexual dysfunction usually cannot be restored unless the partner's sexual dysfunction is also addressed. In addition, environmental hygiene care (i.e., privacy, etc.) and sex education should be prepared as occasion demands.

Androgen therapy, which is often the treatment in the desire disorder related to androgen insufficiency, has various biologic adverse effects[23,24] (see Chapters 13.1–13.3). In addition to those, however, the psychologically potential adverse risk should also be considered. Testosterone has sometimes been associated with feelings of anger, rage attacks, and aggressive behavior.[25,26] In view of a number of studies[27,28] outlining the antidepressant effects of testosterone, mood fluctuations and related psychologic change are not uncommon and can be expected during androgen therapy.

Especially for women with bipolar disorder, the use of antidepressants and the mood-altering effects of testosterone overlap. In these cases, there is a danger that the combination of the antidepressant and testosterone may trigger manic symptoms of bipolar disorder.[29,30] Therefore, drug holidays, switching, dosage adjustment, or discontinuation of the medications should be determined by considering the triangular relationships among antidepressant, testosterone, and mood. Again, psychiatric consultation should be considered given the severity of the underlying psychiatric disorder. Bupropion can also be used in the treatment of low sexual desire or orgasmic disorder.[31–33] A careful decision about existing antidepressants and secondary mood-related psychologic changes should take place beforehand.

There are more complicated cases of hypoactive sexual desire that require constant consultation and communication between the treating physician and the psychologic specialist. If hypoactive sexual desire is associated with ovarian cancer, oophorectomy, and hormone therapy, it is imperative that the clinician work closely with the endocrinologist. In cases of hypoactive sexual desire associated with major depression, bipolar disorder, schizophrenia, and sexual trauma, the treating physician must work in conjunction with the psychiatrist or other mental professional. This strategy can be applicable not only to hypoactive sexual desire, but also to arousal, orgasmic, and pain disorders of female sexual dysfunction (see Chapter 17.3).

Although testosterone level, general mood, and subjective sexual desire may be restored by various treatments, the patient may continue to report that sexual activity and desire are problematic. In these cases, it is recommended that the clinician re-evaluate sexual desire discrepancy with her partner. Referral to a couples therapy specialist or a structured sensate focus exercise by a mental health professional is strongly recommended.

Arousal disorders

It is helpful to distinguish between subjective and genital arousal. In the clinical presentation, it may be difficult to distinguish clearly between these two conditions (see Chapter 11.3). In cases where the lack of arousal may be due to subjective causes, sex therapy and especially sensate focus are suggested. This form of sex therapy is commonly utilized for an extended period of time during the treatment process. In some cases, the addition of vasoactive agents[34] or a clitoral vacuum device[35] can help to reduce the length of treatment while increasing arousal response. In other cases, local estrogen therapy may be recommended for sexual symptoms that result from estrogen-deficient vulvovaginal atrophy.[36] Again, the re-evaluation of secondary psychologic change after these biologic approaches is needed.

Biologically minded treating physicians should keep in mind that sensate focus exercises may help to improve the patient's comfort level and reduce anxiety. The typical approach to these issues often involves the partner as well as the woman. The couples are instructed in nondemanding sensual exercises in which they explore techniques and areas of stimulation that increase arousal. They are further instructed to maintain journals, to communicate with each other regarding their erogenous zones, and perhaps to share their sexual fantasies with each other. In some cases, sex therapy may be supplemented with individual psychotherapy to uncover conflicts regarding childhood experiences, sexual traumas, and familial relationships.

Orgasmic disorder

For women with lifelong generalized orgasmic disorder, directed masturbation with the bridge maneuver is often recommended.[37,38] Couples therapy, individual psychotherapy, or cognitive-behavioral therapy can also be very beneficial (see Chapter 11.4). The success of treatment relies on maximizing stimulation while simultaneously minimizing feelings of inhibition.[38] Sex therapy in these cases can often be very effective, but it can progress slowly and systematically. For therapy to be successful, the patient and her partner must be motivated to complete homework assignments and to follow the instructions of the therapist. If feelings of resentment or rejection are present in the relationship, these may need to be dealt with before the couple can engage in sex therapy exercise and assignments.

As in men's orgasmic mechanism, investigation with anti-serotonergic agents and central nervous system stimulants should be utilized with caution. Even today, there is a lack of scientific data on the possible adverse effects of these medications. In addition, Kegel exercise or electromyography biofeedback, which are designed to improve pelvic floor musculature, are often helpful in treating orgasmic disorder, arousal, or sexual pain disorders. However, there is some controversy regarding the effectiveness of these treatments.[39,40] The use of these modalities needs to be determined on a case-by-case basis, depending on the needs of the patient.

Dyspareunia and vaginismus

For women with dyspareunia and vaginismus, a general multi-dimensional and multidisciplinary approach with specific attention to the following six major areas is recommended (see Chapters 12.1–12.6): mucous membrane, pelvic floor, pain, sexual partner relationship, emotional profile, and genital mutilation/sexual abuse.[41] For these patients, a program in pain management is often critical.

Tricyclic antidepressants, serotonin norepinephrine reuptake inhibitors (e.g., venlafaxine, duloxetine), and anticonvulsants (e.g., gabapentin, carbamazepine) can also be beneficial for pain relief. Classical triyclic antidepressants should be started with a low dosage of 10 mg daily and then gradually increased to 40–60 mg daily. If a far higher dosage is needed, re-evaluation of the initial diagnosis and treatment is recommended. Cognitive-behavioral therapy, electromyography biofeedback, pelvic floor physical therapy, vestibulectomy, or a combination can also be attempted after exploring the severity of the problem, cost-effectiveness, and the concerns of the patient.

In the treatment of women with painful intercourse, the patient's phobic anxiety regarding penetration is an additional factor that must be addressed. Anxiety is often present regardless of the psychologic or biologic etiology of the presenting problem. In these cases, general anxiety or the development of a phobia regarding penetration can intensify the woman's experience of pain. She will subsequently avoid sexual contact or will attempt to have intercourse in spite of the pain she is experiencing. It is not unusual to hear of women who are tearful throughout intercourse as a result of pain, anxiety, guilt, and/or fear. The treatment of this psychologic reaction often requires more than emotional support and reassurance by the physician. Severe phobic reactions or generalized anxiety regarding penetration require psychotherapy or a specific cognitive-behavioral intervention by a trained mental health professional.

Of all the female sexual dysfunction diagnoses, vaginismus is especially well suited for a comprehensive psychologic approach. In the treatment, the patient is encouraged to explore her genital area and to develop an increased level of comfort with her sexual organs and her sexuality in general. While the central focus of the treatment is graduated vaginal penetration, it does not mean vaginal penetration is the final goal of treatment. At the same time, attention needs to be focused, as required, on underlying or newly developed issues in the relationship of the couple if intercourse is possible.

Re-evaluation during the treatment

In view of the comprehensive assessment and continuing changes in the patient, the treating physician should always keep in mind the possibility of additional diagnoses and the need for changes in the treatment plan. It is not uncommon for circumstances, symptoms, or sexual responses to change during the course of treatment. Obviously, any significant change will require a re-evaluation of the treatment approach. For example, if the patient is being treated primarily for psychologic problems, additional biologic factors may emerge and change

the patient's medical condition. These include newly developed medical illness, pregnancy and delivery, or menopause. In such cases, a biologic re-evaluation will be needed as soon as possible. On the other hand, if the woman is receiving primarily biologic treatment, psychologic issues may develop that have great impact on the patient. Such changes include a newly developed psychiatric and medical illness and major life stresses (e.g., divorce, death of an important family member, remarriage, childbirth, sexual abuse, infidelity of partner). In a similar manner, psychologic re-evaluation will be needed. It is also important to remember that as a specific sexual dysfunction is treated and sexual activities are more frequently attempted, new sexual problems with the patient or her partner may emerge.

Conclusion

In summary, it has been our experience that the integration of both biologic and psychologic aspects is essential in the treatment of a woman with female sexual dysfunction. A concise outline of this integrated approach is shown in Fig. 17.6.1. The figure provides a schematic overview of an integrated approach in which both the biologic assessment and psychologic evaluation are used in determining the initial diagnosis of the patient. The figure also demonstrates how the treatment approach can

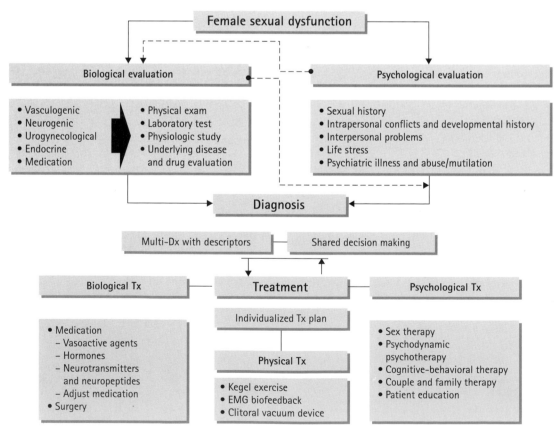

Figure 17.6.1. Integrated algorithm of psychologic/biologic diagnosis and treatment for female sexual dysfunction. Dx: diagnosis; Tx: treatment.

comprise biologic, physical, and psychologic components. Most importantly, this model focuses on the development of an individualized treatment program based on the input from an interdisciplinary team.

For women who have difficult and complicated forms of female sexual dysfunction, it is important to have specialists who have an understanding of both the biologic and psychologic factors. However, in our current situation, there are many places to reach beyond each clinician's individual capacity. An immediate way to overcome such a barrier is to understand the importance of the tightly knit referral system and to establish a method to address all aspects of the presenting problem.

References

1. Laumann EL, Paik A, Rosen RC. Sexual dysfunction in the United States: prevalence and predictors. JAMA 1999; 10: 537–45.
2. Bancroft J, Loftus J, Long JS. Distress about sex: a national survey of women in heterosexual relationships. Arch Sex Behav 2003; 32: 193–208.
3. Segraves KB, Segraves RT. Hypoactive sexual desire disorder: prevalence and comorbidity in 906 subjects. J Sex Marital Ther 1991; 17: 55–8.
4. Rosen RC, Taylor JF, Leiblum SR et al. Prevalence of sexual dysfunction in women: results of a survey study of 329 women in an outpatient gynecological clinic. J Sex Marital Ther 1993; 19: 171–88.
5. Basson R, Berman J, Burnett A et al. Report of the international consensus development conference on female sexual dysfunction: definitions and classifications. J Sex Marital Ther 2001; 27: 83–94.
6. Barber M, Visco AG, Wyman JF et al. Sexual function in women with urinary incontinence in pelvic organ prolapse. Obstet Gynecol 2002; 99: 281–9.
7. Enzlin P, Mathieu C, van DenBruel A et al. Sexual dysfunction in women with type 1 diabetes. Diabetes Care 2002; 25: 672–7.
8. Rosen R, Brown C, Heiman J et al. The Female Sexual Function Index (FSFI): a multidimensional self-report instrument for the assessment of female sexual function. J Sex Marital Ther 2000; 26: 191–208.
9. Taylor JF, Rosen RC, Leiblum SR. Self-report assessment of female sexual function: psychometric evaluation of the Brief Index of Sexual Functioning for Women. Arch Sex Behav 1994; 23: 627–43.
10. Derogatis LR. The Derogatis Interview for Sexual Functioning (DISF/DISF-R): an introductory report. J Sex Marital Ther 1997; 23: 291–304.
11. Davis S, Guay A, Shifren J et al. Endocrine aspects of female sexual dysfunction. J Sex Med 2004; 1: 82–6.
12. Berman J, Berman L, Goldstein I. Female sexual dysfunction: incidence, pathophysiology, evaluation, and treatment options. Urology 1999; 54: 385–91.
13. Bancroft J. The medicalization of female sexual dysfunction: the need for caution. Arch Sex Behav 2002; 31: 451–5.
14. Bancroft J, Janssen E. The dual control model of male sexual

response: a theoretical approach to centrally mediated erectile dysfunction. Neurosci Biobehav Rev 2000; 24: 571–9.
15. Graham CA, Sanders SA, Milhausen R et al. Turning on and turning off: a focus group study of the factors that affect women's sexual arousal. Arch Sex Behav 2004; 33: 527–38.
16. Pope KS, Bouhoutsos JC. Sexual Intimacy Between Therapists and Patients. New York: Praeger, 1986.
17. Basson R, Berman J, Bernett A et al. Report of the international consensus development conference on female sexual dysfunction: definitions and classification. J Urol 2000; 163: 888–93.
18. Basson R, Leiblum S, Brotto L et al. Definitions of women's sexual dysfunction reconsidered: advocating expansion and revision. J Psychosom Obstet Gynaecol 2003; 24: 221–9.
19. Maurice WL. Understanding female sexual dysfunction and the consensus conference: this is progress? J Sex Marital Ther 2001; 27: 171–4.
20. American Psychiatric Association. Diagnostic and Statistical Manual for Mental Disorders, 4th edn (DSM-IV-TR). Washington: American Psychiatric Press, 2000.
21. Hatzichristou DG, Bertero E, Goldstein I. Decision making in the evaluation of impotence: the patient profile-oriented algorithm. Sex Dis 1994; 12: 81–95.
22. Kaplan SH, Greenfield S, Gandek B et al. Characteristics of physicians with participatory decision-making styles. Ann Intern Med 1996; 124: 497–504.
23. Slayden SM. Risks of menopausal androgen supplementation. Semin Reprod Endocrinol 1998; 16: 145–52.
24. Simon JA. Safety of estrogen/androgen regimens. J Reprod Med 2001; 46(Suppl 3): 281–90.
25. Pope HG Jr, Kouri EM, Hudson JI. Effects of supraphysiologic doses of testosterone on mood and aggression in normal men: a randomized controlled trial. Arch Gen Psychiatry 2000; 57: 133–40; discussion 155–6.
26. George DT, Umhau JC, Phillips MJ et al. Serotonin, testosterone and alcohol in the etiology of domestic violence. Psychiatry Res 2001; 104: 27–37.
27. Seidman SN, Spatz E, Rizzo C et al. Testosterone replacement therapy for hypogonadal men with major depressive disorder: a randomized, placebo-controlled trial. J Clin Psychiatry 2001; 62: 406–12.
28. Pope HG Jr, Cohane GH, Kanayama G et al. Testosterone gel supplementation for men with refractory depression: a randomized, placebo-controlled trial. Am J Psychiatry 2003; 160: 105–11.
29. Barbenel DM, Yusufi B, O'Shea D et al. Mania in a patient receiving testosterone replacement postorchidectomy taking St John's wort and sertraline. J Psychopharmacol 2000; 14: 84–6.
30. Weiss EL, Bowers MB Jr, Mazure CM. Testosterone-patch-induced psychotic mania. Am J Psychiatry 1999; 156: 969.
31. Segraves RT, Croft H, Kavoussi R et al. Bupropion sustained release (SR) for the treatment of hypoactive sexual desire disorder (HSDD) in nondepressed women. J Sex Marital Ther 2001; 27: 303–16.
32. Modell JG, May RS, Katholi R. Effect of bupropion-SR on orgasmic dysfunction in nondepressed subjects: a pilot study. J Sex Marital Ther 2000; 26: 231–40.

33. Gitlin MJ, Suri R, Altshuler L et al. Bupropion-sustained release as a treatment for SSRI-induced sexual side effects. *J Sex Marital Ther* 2002; 28: 131–8.

34. Berman J, Berman L, Lin H et al. Effect of sildenafil on subjective and physiologic parameters of the female sexual response in women with sexual arousal disorder. *J Sex Marital Ther* 2001; 27: 411–20.

35. Billups KL, Berman L, Berman J et al. A new non-pharmacological vacuum therapy for female sexual dysfunction. *J Sex Marital Ther* 2001; 27: 435–41.

36. Crandall C. Vaginal estrogen preparations: a review of safety and efficacy for vaginal atrophy. *J Womens Health* 2002; 11: 857–77.

37. Heiman J, Meston M. Empirically validated treatment for sexual dysfunction. *Annu Rev Sex Res* 1997; 8: 148–94.

38. Kaplan HS. *The Illustrated Manual of Sex Therapy*, 2nd edn. New York: Brunner Mazel, 1987: 72–98.

39. Chambless DL, Stern T, Sultan FE et al. The pubococcygeus and female orgasm: a correlation study with normal subjects. *Arch Sex Behav* 1982; 11: 479–90.

40. Hoon PW. Physiologic assessment of sexual response in women: the unfulfilled promise. *Clin Obstet Gynecol* 1984; 27: 767–80.

41. Basson R, Weijmar Shultz WCM, Binik YM et al. Women's sexual desire and arousal disorders and sexual pain. In TF Lue, R Basson, R Rosen et al., eds. *Second International Consultation on Sexual Medicine: Sexual Dysfunctions in Men and Women*. Paris: Health Publications, 2004: 851–974.

Section 4

OUTREACH

EDUCATION

18.1 Medical student curricula/sexual medical education

Anita H Clayton, Sharon J Parish

Given the broad range of areas that need to be addressed in medical school and residency training, even fundamental subject matter may not be allotted the appropriate amount of curriculum time. Sexual health education is an example of an often neglected, but very important topic. Sexuality and associated issues play an incredibly important role in the lives almost all patients, yet this weight is not adequately reflected in most undergraduate and graduate medical education programs. Recently, educators are paying more attention to this gap, assessing it and piloting new curricula. The current interest in this topic will hopefully, in the next decade, generate medical school curricula that focus proper attention on this critical subject.

The current state of sexual health

A recent US poll indicates that 94% of adults feel that sexual pleasure adds to quality of life.[1] Another national study published in 1999 showed that 43% of women and 31% men have sexual complaints.[2] These statistics signify that sex is a vital part of many people's lives, and problems can undercut the enjoyment it provides. Sexual dysfunction may occur at any point in the sexual response cycle (desire, arousal, or orgasm) and can be a primary problem or a secondary issue related to another disease process or medications (see Chapters 3.1–3.4 and 6.1–6.5 of this book). The consequences of untreated sexual dysfunction may include, for example, depression, conflicts within interpersonal relationships, or noncompliance with prescribed medication regimens.[3,4,5] Researchers have made significant strides in understanding the mechanisms powering the male and female sexual response. This knowledge has enabled the development of new drugs capable of treating some forms of sexual dysfunction (see Chapters 13.1–13.3, 14.1, and 14.2). The next milestone will be the widespread distribution of this once considered taboo information to the patient population at large.

Doctor–patient barriers

Despite the recognition of sexual dysfunction and the availability of treatment options, physicians and their patients still hesitate to discuss these issues (see Chapters 17.1–17.6). One study reports that 47% of patients have never been asked by their primary care physician if they are engaged in a sexual relationship.[6] (see Chapters 17.1 and 17.5). Only 25% of primary care physicians actually take a patient's sexual history, citing lack of training as the most common reason for not doing so.[7,8,9] Physicians report other barriers such as insufficient knowledge of sexual function and dysfunction, lack of information about treatment options, time constraints during the patient encounter, personal biases about sexual issues, apprehension that their inquiries may offend the patient, and their own feelings of embarrassment about the subject.[1,10,11,12]

Patients are reluctant to bring up sexual issues with their doctors. A survey indicated that 75% of patients believe that their doctors would dismiss their sexual health concerns if their patients confronted them with that information. A substantial number (68%) feel that they would embarrass their doctors if they were to broach the topic.[1] Ninety-one percent of patients, however, do believe that it is a physician's role to address sexual health concerns; but only 10% of patients request assistance with these concerns if not prompted by their doctor.[13]

The data show that a chasm exists between doctor and patient. Physician education targeted at increasing knowledge and encouraging the recognition of personal biases is the key to minimizing obstacles that interfere with doctors addressing and optimizing sexual health.

The importance of sexual health in medical education

Sex is certainly a topic given much coverage in today's popular society. However, medical school education and, consequently, accurate patient education on this subject have fallen far behind. Given the amount of misinformation that is available, it is critical that physicians disseminate correct information to their patients. Medical school and postgraduate training are the primary forums in which doctors need to acquire the necessary knowledge and skills.

In 1974, the World Health Organization assumed the task of clarifying the term "sexual health".[14] Their definition, revised in 2000, states that sexual health is:

> the experience of the ongoing process of physical, psychologic and socio-cultural well-being related to sexuality. Sexual health is evidenced by the free and responsible expression of sexual capabilities that foster harmonious personal and social wellness, enriching individual and social life. It is not merely the absence of disease, dysfunction or infirmity.[15]

Following this definition, 11 sexual rights were enumerated, including the right to sexual information based on scientific inquiry, the right to comprehensive sexuality education, and the right to sexual health care.[16]

Medical schools are charged with the responsibility of ensuring that these needs are met. Crucial areas to cover in medical school include conducting a comprehensive sexual health interview, awareness of causes and treatments of sexual dysfunction, recognizing and responding to signs of sexual violence, prevention and treatment of sexually transmitted infections, and understanding issues related to gay and lesbian sexual health. As well, medical schools should teach about the relationship between sexual dysfunction and other, more life-threatening health problems. They also need to teach students to recognize and handle their personal biases about sex. While it is important for students not to compromise their own values, it is equally imperative that these principles not interfere with patient care.[17] The combination of increasing knowledge and confronting biases about sexual health in the forum of undergraduate medical education is an excellent start to dismantling the communication barriers that exist between doctor and patient concerning the issue of sexual health.

The current state of sexual education in medical school

Despite the statistics indicating that sexual dysfunction is prominent, affecting men and women of all age groups, races, and socioeconomic levels, sexual health education in the medical profession has only recently become a subject of interest. The slow dissolution of the taboo associated with this topic is associated with a concomitant rise in society's willingness to discuss the subject. It should follow that physicians are adequately prepared to accommodate this paradigm shift, and the training to do so should begin in medical school.

A study in 2003 assessed the state of sexual health education in medical schools: a questionnaire was issued to 125 medical schools in the USA and 16 in Canada asking several questions about their education techniques.[18] This survey was the first of its kind since the 1970s, when Harold Lief and his colleagues, fueled by the reform brought about by the sexual revolution, attempted a similar undertaking.[19]

In this recent study, the investigators received 101 valid responses. Two schools that did not complete the survey admitted that their curriculum dedicated no hours to sexual health education, and five other schools that did submit the survey stated that they were embarrassed at how little time their school devoted to the topic. At many schools, no one particular person was in charge of the sexual health curriculum. Most schools (83.1%) reported that they used a lecture format, and 81.2% of schools made attendance mandatory. Two-thirds of the schools used a multidisciplinary approach to teach sexual health. Members of the Department of Psychiatry were the most frequently utilized teachers and were incorporated into the curriculum at 75.3% of schools. About half of the schools offered 3–10 hours of training, whereas one-third spent 11 hours or more on the subject. The most common topics discussed were sexual dysfunction and its treatment, sexual identity/orientation, and issues of sexuality in disabled or medically ill patients. Approximately half the schools allowed students to interact with patients receiving treatment for or education on sexual issues during their clinical experience.[18]

Postgraduate education in sexual health is understudied and unaddressed, lagging behind even the rudimentary efforts made in medical school. Much work is needed to create adequate curriculum and skills training in sexual health assessment and treatment in residency programs and beyond.

Research on sexual health education

Clearly, a wide range of effort is dedicated to sexual health education in medical schools. This disparity was also recognized by the pharmaceutical company, Pfizer, Inc., with the recent offer of seven grants to medical schools to evaluate and enhance their sexual health curricula. To apply, schools presented an outline of course work spanning the four years of undergraduate medical education covering the medical, psychologic, social, and ethical issues of sexual health care, and proposed assessments of and enhancements to the curriculum. Among the schools selected, the University of Virginia School of Medicine, Case Western Reserve University School of Medicine, and the University of Massachusetts Medical School have published data. Internationally, there have been also been efforts to evaluate the state of sexual health education.

In 2003, the University of Virginia School of Medicine released a study comparing knowledge of, comfort with, and attitudes toward the importance of sexual health among first-, second-, and third-year medical students.[20] The University of Virginia uses a multidisciplinary approach to teaching sexual health, providing pertinent information within the following courses: Anatomy, Embryology, Histology, Physiology, Human Behavior, Pathology, Introduction to Psychiatry, and Practice of Medicine. The Practice of Medicine training included lectures on obtaining a sexual health history and screening for domestic violence, sexual history taking while role-playing and interacting with standardized patients, and gynecologic and genitourinary examinations performed on female and male standardized patients. First- and second-year students were given questionnaires on the first day of their autumn term before any curriculum improvements had been implemented, and third-year students participated via an email survey.

First-year students felt that they knew the least about obtaining a sexual history and the most about medications for treating sexual dysfunction.[20] Interestingly, these students have not yet had a course in pharmacology, so their responses may reflect the prevalence of this information in the media. Both second- and third-year students claimed to be the most knowledgeable about taking a sexual history. Second-year students believed that they knew the least about sexual side effects of medications, while third-year students indicated that they knew the least about medications for treating sexual dysfunction.[20] This difference in the perception of second- and third-year students about their knowledge and skills from first-year students may indicate that this information is not frequently addressed during the clinical years.

All three groups of students felt the least comfortable discussing sexually related health problems and the most comfortable discussing sexual side effects of medications.[20] These responses may reflect students' overall discomfort with discussing sensitive psychosocial issues. Of note, female students reported significantly less comfort in discussing these topics than male students.[20]

All three groups also agreed that discussing sexual health during a routine checkup was more important than during a problem-focused appointment. Second-year students thought that it was more important to discuss sex during office visits than either first- or third-year students. This decrease in perceived importance in the third year, which is the first clinical year the student experiences, may reflect the attending physician's negative attitude toward a thorough sexual history in the inpatient setting, or the attending physician's embarrassment in discussing sexual health with patients.[20]

In 2003, an Australian study reported the status of lesbian health care in medical education. Lesbians often delay seeking care despite specific risk factors associated with the population.[21] This hesitance is understandable given that 23% of lesbian, gay, bisexual, and transgendered patients felt that they experienced discrimination in these situations.[22] In 1994, half (52%) of the members of a US-based gay and lesbian medical association

stated that they had observed colleagues providing less than adequate care to patients according to sexual orientation, and 88% have overheard fellow physicians make disparaging remarks about their patients' sexual orientation.[23] Finally, in a US survey, eight of the 82 medical schools that responded stated that they offered no teaching on gay and lesbian issues.[24] This is clearly a gap in sexual health education that needs to be addressed.

An Australian study published in 1996 compared students' personal sexual experiences with their confidence and ability to perform female pelvic examinations.[25] Both male and female students who had sexual experience (153 of 286 students) felt more comfortable performing the examination, explaining their actions to their patients, and being able to detect disorder. The male students who had no sexual experience felt an overall lack of confidence and were more likely to want to perform gynecologic examinations with the patient under anesthesia.[25]

These data provide some insight into the current status of sexual health education in medical schools. Perhaps these data will motivate schools to conduct investigations into their own training programs, assess student knowledge and biases, and ascertain the most appropriate way to correct the problems that they discover.

New developments in medical sexual education

Some schools have already begun to reform their sexual health education programs. Case Western Reserve University School of Medicine is "in the process of implementing a comprehensive, cross-disciplinary and innovative curriculum that is based on three primary objectives for teaching sexual health: attitude change, behavior change, and knowledge acquisition".[26] The first goal, attitude change, is being accomplished by encouraging the students to achieve a sense of self-awareness. The new curriculum emphasizes normal variations of sexuality and provides exposure to them, dispels myths, and teaches boundary setting, as well as appropriate ways to handle situations in which those boundaries are challenged. The second objective, behavior change, is being approached by enhancing communications skills among both faculty and students. Patients often will not initiate a discussion with their physicians if they appear uncomfortable or unwilling to discuss sexual health. The third goal, knowledge acquisition, involves a multidisciplinary approach to ensuring that all facets of sexual health are taught.

The school outlines several arenas in which these changes will take place, including "faculty development, additional didactics, case-based learning, testing and assessment, and electronic (computer/web-based) enhancements".[26] This innovative, multidisciplinary sexual health education initiative appears to be an excellent model for other schools.

The University of Massachusetts Medical School is also

enhancing its current sexual health education curriculum. In the 1999–2000 academic year, several topics were added to the third-year curriculum, including teenage sexuality, health care for gay youth, lesbian health care, reproduction counseling in relation to HIV risk, and sexual dysfunction caused by medications.[27] In autumn 2001, the University of Massachusetts Medical School surveyed first- and second-year medical students to find the gaps in sexual health education. The problems identified included the idea that sex is private, students' lack of knowledge, patient and student discomfort with the subject, and cultural differences. Specific topics that were considered to be particularly difficult were extramarital affairs, multiple partners, sexual violence, gathering sexual information from older patients, and patients who continue with high-risk sexual behavior despite education.[27]

Based on this survey data, the curriculum was further modified throughout the four years of medical education. During the first year, Anatomy students participated in a reflection session to discuss the thoughts and feelings they might have concerning the dissection of the female pelvis. Half of those who participated (with a 25% class participation rate) felt that the session reduced their apprehension about the dissection, and 95% wanted to have more sessions of a similar nature in the future.[27] A one-hour session on the medical risks of the gay, lesbian, bisexual, and transgendered community was instituted during an interclerkship day in the students' third year. About half of the class participated; and of those that did, 95% evaluated it as effective.[27] The third modification was the addition of a one-week women's health course available as an elective for fourth-year students. In this program, a multidisciplinary group of faculty utilized a variety of teaching methods. After attending this course, the students felt that their comfort level in discussing these subjects with their patients improved.[27]

In 1998, at the Stanford University School of Medicine, the medical students took the initiative to provide their own sexual health education. Second-year students organized a nine-session, weekly, lunchtime, elective lecture series entitled "Current Issues in Reproductive Health".[28] Students were given credit for simply attending the course. By 2001, attendance had grown to one-sixth of the preclinical medical student body. At this time, a "reproductive health fair" was added as part of the course, and opened to the university community with great success.[28] Students who attended were surveyed in 2000 and 2001. They reported that the two most frequently acquired skills were the ability to discuss an unwanted pregnancy and the ability to communicate with patients of varying gender, sexual orientation, and culture. The survey also identified what the students considered the most useful learning methods, including having discussions with fellow students, engaging in interactive presentations with faculty, listening to traditional lectures, and teaching their peers.[28] Stanford's program offers a number of novel strategies that extend beyond the traditional methods, and that certainly could be implemented by other institutions.

Developments in international sexual medicine education

The recognition of and effort to correct the lack of sexual health education is not limited to the USA. Medical schools in the UK have also been reviewing and revising their curricula. The University of Cambridge initiated role-playing as a means of exploring sexual health issues.[29] One of 14 scenarios was given to students, who alternate playing the physician and the patient. Two examples include a young homosexual man who has just "come out" but doesn't know how to use a condom, and a woman interested in having an intrauterine device fitted. The goal of these mock clinic scenarios is to allow students to react to such situations, empathize with the patient, and discover and test beneficial behaviors.[29] The University of Cambridge also has, for the last 20 years, conducted a session for its medical students dedicated to increasing awareness of homosexuality in the patient population.[30] There are two main goals of the course. The first is to allow students "to explore internalized prejudice"; this is accomplished by having students brainstorm all the slang terms they know relating to homosexuality and then reflect silently on them for a few minutes. The second goal is "to look at the effects of prejudice"; students are asked to imagine that they are gay and decide how those terms would make them feel and what their subsequent behavior would be.[30]

Another medical school in the UK, Leicester-Warwick Medical School, recognized the importance of how medical students' attitudes and values may influence their interactions with patients. This school initiated a course designed to help students to recognize their feelings; this involved the techniques of desensitization, problem solving, and reflection with the ultimate goal of self-development.[31] Human sexuality is covered as part of a 12-week module on human diversity in the second year. A combination of teaching techniques is used, and the course moves from relatively unthreatening topics to those that may challenge students more. Sessions often contain attempts to desensitize the students to embarrassment by the discussion of sexual topics, including becoming familiar with slang and medical terms.[31] The intent of these sessions is to provide students with a safe environment in which they can rehearse their reactions and responses to difficult topics related to sexual health. Most students (78%) felt that the course offered some benefit, and a similar number believed that it made them more sensitive to the needs of patients and the duties of doctors.[31] This program is another thoughtful and innovative approach to the correction of the deficiency of sexual health education.

Conclusion

Society has become more willing to recognize and discuss sexual health, and physicians should be at the forefront of this campaign; yet, according to the data, that is not currently the case. To correct this deficiency, the process must begin with appropriate training in medical schools. The first step involves the analysis of the current state of sexual health education in medical schools. When the various needs are ascertained, new curricula can be developed that will give medical students the tools to provide good patient care to those with sexual health concerns. Such changes are being undertaken in both the USA and abroad. Hopefully, these schools will establish a trend that will inspire all medical schools to modernize their curriculum in sexual health education. Graduate medical education in sexual health is in its infancy, with much work remaining in order to enhance the practitioner's ability to meet patient needs.

References

1. Marwick C. Survey says patients expect little physician help on sex. *JAMA* 1999; 281: 2173–4.
2. Laumann EO, Paik A, Rosen RC. Sexual dysfunction in the United States: prevalence and predictors. *JAMA* 1999; 281: 537–44.
3. Prisant LM, Carr AA, Bottini PB et al. Sexual dysfunction with antihypertensive drugs. *Arch Intern Med* 1994; 154: 730–6.
4. Salazar WH. Management of depression in the outpatient office. *Med Clin North Am* 1996; 80: 431–55.
5. Ernst JL, Hahnstadt WA, Piskule AM et al. The self-identified long-term care needs of persons with spinal cord injury. *SCI Psychosoc Process* 1998; 10: 127–32.
6. Matthews WC, Linn LS. AIDS prevention in primary care clinics: testing the market. *J Gen Intern Med* 1989; 4: 34–38.
7. McCance KL, Moser Jr R, Smith KR. A survey of physicians' knowledge and application of AIDS prevention capabilities. *Am J Prev Med* 1991; 7: 141–5.
8. Association of American Medical Colleges Medical School Graduation Questionnaire. Final School Report: University of Massachusetts Medical School, 1999–2001.
9. Jonassen JA, Ferrara E, O'Dell K. An intensive, multidisciplinary mini-selective course improves senior students' knowledge and self-confidence about women's healthcare and women's health research. Presented at the 113th Annual Meeting of the Association of Medical Colleges, San Francisco, 11 November 2002.
10. Maheux B, Haley N, Rivard M et al. Do physicians assess lifestyle health risks during general medical examinations? A survey of general practitioners and obstetrician-gynecologists in Quebec. *Can Med Assoc J* 1999; 160: 1830–43.
11. Epstein R, Frankel RM, Frarey L et al. Awkward moments in patient–physician communication about HIV risk. *Ann Intern Med* 1998; 128: 435–42.
12. Piazza LA et al. Sexual dysfunction and antidepressant therapy. Presented at the 148th Annual Meeting of the American Psychiatric Association, Miami, 20–25 May 2002.
13. Ende J, Kazis L, Ash A et al. Measuring patients' desire for autonomy: decision-making and information-seeking preferences among medical patients. *J Gen Intern Med* 1989; 4: 23–30.
14. World Health Organization Meeting. Education and treatment in human sexuality: the training of health professionals. Extracts from WHO technical report no. 572, 1975: 5–16.
15. World Health Organization. Education and treatment in human sexuality: the training of health professionals. *Report of a WHO Meeting*, Albany, NY 12210, 2000.
16. Ng EMI, Borras-Valls JJ, Perez-Conchillo M et al. *Sexuality in a New Millennium*. Bologna: Editrice, 2000.
17. Wagner G, Bondil P, Dabees K et al. Ethical aspects of sexual medicine. *J Sex Med* 2005; 2: 163–8.
18. Solursh DS, Ernst JL, Lewis RW et al. The human sexuality education of physicians in North American medical schools. *Int J Impot Res* 2003; 15(Suppl 5): S41–5.
19. Lief HI. Sex education in medical schools. *Med Educ* 1971; 46: 684.
20. McGarvey E, Peterson C, Pinkerton R et al. Medical students' perceptions of sexual health issues prior to a curriculum enhancement. *Int J Impot Res* 2003; 15(Suppl 5): S58–66.
21. McNair R. Outing lesbian health in medical education. *Women Health* 2003; 37: 89–103.
22. Victorian Gay and Lesbian Rights Lobby. *Enough Is Enough. A Report on Discrimination and Abuse Experienced by Lesbians, Gay Men, Bisexuals and Transgender People in Victoria*. 2002.
23. Schatz B, O'Hanlan K. *Anti-Gay Discrimination in Medicine: Results of a National Survey of Lesbian, Gay and Bisexual Physicians*. San Francisco: American Association of Physicians for Human Rights, 1994.
24. Wallick MM, Cambre KM, Townsend MH. How the topic of homosexuality is taught at US medical schools. *Acad Med* 1992; 67: 601–3.
25. Abraham S. The effect of sexual experience on the attitudes of medical students to learning gynecological examinations. *J Psychosom Obstet Gynecol* 1996; 17: 15–20.
26. Kingsberg SA, Malemud CJ, Novak T et al. A comprehensive approach to enhancing sexual health education in the Case Western Reserve University School of Medicine. *Int J Impot Res* 2003; 15(Suppl 5): S51–7.
27. Ferrara E, Pugnaire MP, Jonassen JA et al. Sexual health innovations in undergraduate medical education. *Int J Impot Res* 2003; 15(Suppl 5): S46–50.
28. Meites E, Wagner JL, Choy MKW et al. A student-initiated interactive course as a model for teaching reproductive health. *Am J Obstet Gynecol* 2002; 187(3, Pt 2): S30–3.
29. Henderson P, Johnson MH. Assisting medical students to conduct empathic conversations with patients from a sexual medicine clinic. *Sex Transm Infect* 2002; 78: 246–9.
30. Johnson MH, Henderson P. Acquiring and demonstrating attitudes in medical education: attitudes to homosexuality as a case study. *Med Teach* 2000; 22: 585–91.
31. Dixon-Woods M, Regan J, Robertson N et al. Teaching and learning about human sexuality in undergraduate medical education. *Med Educ* 2002; 36: 432–40.

18.2 Patient outreach and education

Lillian Arleque

Introduction

Until recently, when women complained of sexual health problems to their physicians, their only treatment option was referral to a mental health professional (see Chapters 17.2 and 17.3 of this book). As a result of this historical reliance on a psychologic model for treatment, many women suffering from sexual health problems are unaware that their symptoms may actually be caused by a physical problem (see Chapters 13.1–13.3, 14.1, and 14.2). Recent findings have demonstrated that in many cases of female sexual dysfunction, there is both a psychologic cause and an underlying physiologic cause, and that with proper medical and psychologic intervention a significant number of women have been able to regain their sexual function completely. Therefore, it is incumbent upon health-care professionals to reach out to women to make them aware that their sexual health is an integral component of their physical health and well-being, and to educate them about symptoms and possible medical and psychologic treatments for female sexual dysfunction (see Chapters 17.4, 17.5, and 18.1).

The purpose of this chapter is to provide health-care professionals with suggestions and information on how to effectively inform and educate women and their partners about the symptoms as well as the possible cures for female sexual dysfunction. A number of possible models and educational strategies are presented so that the reader may replicate and/or enhance or expand upon each suggestion. Many of these strategies and ideas utilize technology that makes patient outreach and education a dynamic and interactive process.

Key factors necessary for outreach and education

When designing and planning for patient outreach and education, it is important to be cognizant of key components that will contribute to their effectiveness and success. It is also important to be aware that many women are hesitant to broach the subject of sexual health with their health-care professionals out of embarrassment or as a result of experiences when their concerns were patronizingly minimized and/or they received inadequate treatment (i.e., exclusively psychologic management that was not successful). Accordingly, it is critical for health-care professionals to feel comfortable in asking their patients questions regarding sexual health thus giving patients the opening to discuss any issues and concerns they may have. Moreover, by posing questions on sexual health, health-care professionals can better care for their patient's physical health and well-being and/or refer them to other resources for treatment.

Educational environment

All education should take place in a safe and secure environment. Whether a woman is sitting in a health-care professional's office in a one-on-one situation or attending an off-site seminar on female sexual dysfunction, it is crucial that she feel comfortable and safe in discussing the details of her sexual function or hearing a lecture on the physiologic intricacies of a women's body and sexual response.

Provide ample time for questions and concerns

The subject of sexual health and dysfunction is extremely difficult for many women to discuss; in fact, many women are so sensitive about the issue that they may not have discussed their problems even with their partners. For this reason, all outreach and education programs need to provide patients or participants with ample time to express their feelings and articulate their questions and concerns. Women need to believe that they are listened to, acknowledged, and respected, especially when they are talking about the most intimate details of their lives.

Provide resources for active involvement and self-directed learning

Since the Internet has many sites focused on health, women who are suffering from sexual health problems may have already become actively involved in educating themselves through online searches. The purpose of their research is often to locate information and resources to assist them in understanding and articulating their sexual health concerns as well as finding health-care professionals to treat their problems. Therefore, all outreach and educational programs on female sexual dysfunction should include information on additional resources available to women, so they may continue to be actively involved in seeking information and solutions. These may include bibliographies, websites, newsletters, outreach programs, etc. Furthermore, as self-directed learners, they will need the opportunity to seek feedback and to interact with their health-care professionals to determine and clarify their understanding of their issues and concerns. This can be accomplished through patient visits, telephone conversations, e-mail, and on-site and off-site educational seminars.

Outreach and education strategies

Newsletters

Printed

A quarterly newsletter is an excellent tool that provides useful and up-to-date information to patients as well as other interested individuals and health-care professionals who are seeking education and knowledge about women's sexual health. Investing significant time, discussion, and preparation prior to its initial publication in order to determine intended outcomes and a target readership are critical to the newsletter's long-range success and effectiveness. Having a stated purpose and specific outcomes will assist the editors of the newsletter in decision making regarding future content. In addition, determining a target readership will enable the editors and writers to maintain focus on the needs and level of understanding of the readers. For example, if the primary audience is lay people, the articles need to be informative and "translated" into appropriate language. If it is necessary to include complex vocabulary in order to present a concept, it is helpful to provide definitions within the context of the article and/or to provide a glossary of terms within the newsletter. The ultimate value of the newsletter, as an educational tool, is contingent upon its ability to meet the informational needs and knowledge level of the reader.

The content of the newsletter may vary, but a standard format is more effective, as it creates consistency and a sense of predictability for the reader. For example, a newsletter could start with a message from the physician. A message about sexual medicine education from the health-care professional responsible for education could also be included as well as summaries from recent sexual medicine information sessions. Other possibilities are announcements of upcoming events devoted to sexual medicine issues, and highlights of recent sexual medicine meetings. Along with the standard format, "special features" may be included that enhance the educational value of a newsletter. Summaries of research, book reviews, patient stories, articles by experts in the field, in-depth articles focusing on specific sexual health problems, interviews, a listing of resources such as a bibliography, recent publications, and related websites are all ways to educate and reach out to interested individuals through the newsletter.

Before the Internet, a newsletter was typically a printed document that was mailed through the postal service. The cost of doing a printed newsletter four times a year may be substantial, especially if the printing and mailing are done by an outside company. However, given the sophisticated, yet user-friendly and relatively inexpensive software that is available, printing and publishing a newsletter can be a viable educational tool for even the smallest health-care practice. In-house printing can be easily accomplished by software with a newsletter template allowing two- or three-column design. In addition, a number of paper companies offer high-quality and colorfully designed papers for two- or four-sided newsletters that ensure a professional appearance yet utilize inexpensive black-and-white printing.

The most efficient and timely way to send a printed newsletter is by first-class mail, which is also the most expensive. On the other hand, using bulk mail through the US postal service can minimize mailing costs. However, this approach can add significant amounts of time to the process, as the items to be mailed need to be sorted and grouped by zip code. Delivery time is not guaranteed, and it may actually take 2–3 weeks for some people to receive their newsletter. Consequently, if the choice is bulk mail rather than first class, and there are announcements in the newsletter pertaining to upcoming events, it is important that ample time be given for the mailing process.

Electronic

Another way to minimize the expense of publishing a newsletter is to use e-mail as a delivery mechanism. In addition to the environmental benefit of saving paper, an e-newsletter enables one to reach a significant number of individuals in a more cost-effective manner. People interested in receiving the newsletter via e-mail can register through the practice website. Furthermore, current patients and interested individuals who have participated in on-site informational sessions or off-site seminars can also be invited to register for the newsletter via e-mail. Utilizing the Internet to "distribute" the newsletter, however, does not necessarily eliminate the need for a printed version, as there are still people who do not have access to or chose not to use e-mail. Accordingly, when offering a newsletter as a resource tool, it is important to provide people with the choice of receiving it through e-mail or traditional mail.

Information sessions and seminars

Effective communication

All effective communication is tailored to and delivered with the "receiver" in mind. Based on that premise, it is clearly the responsibility of the "speaker" to design and present concepts in a manner that will ensure that individuals understand as well as remember the information presented to them. Consequently, when health-care professionals are planning to educate and/or reach out to women regarding female sexual dysfunction, it is important to consider and utilize strategies for effective communication.

Since most adults rely on visual forms of communication rather than oral communication as their primary source for learning new concepts and remembering information, it is critical to incorporate written documentation as well as visual representations of data and information to support verbal instruction and explanation. In most situations, patient education is presented orally, whether it is in a one-on-one setting with the health-care professional or in a group program. This oral information can be supported with graphic representations such as pictures, diagrams, graphs, and flowcharts to illustrate concepts. Written information can also be enhanced by similar types of graphic representations, thus aiding the comprehension and retention of the data. Furthermore, since the terminology describing sexual health issues and diagnosis may be unfamiliar to patients and other lay people, a glossary of specific vocabulary used by health-care professionals would enable individuals to feel competent and comfortable enough to engage in discussion and articulate their concerns, as well as read, with comprehension, additional literature on the topic of female sexual dysfunction.

Information sessions

Information sessions typically attract small to middle-sized groups and are usually held in a clinical setting such as a hospital conference room, auditorium, or practice waiting room. Since the meetings are usually no longer than 2 h, it is more effective to plan a series of sessions, thus providing participants with the opportunity to attend several sessions and experience a more in-depth discussion of a focused topic at each session. Current patients and their partners often attend these sessions, and this venue can be utilized to enhance and clarify the education that was presented during their office visit. Advertising for on-site informational sessions entails little or no expense and can be accomplished through the practice website, within the office, through hospital newsletters, in local newspapers and any other available publication resource.

Successful model – information sessions

The instructional design of an information session may consist of the following: a lecture by a health-care professional who is an expert in the session topic, the opportunity to hear a patient speak of her experience, and a question-and-answer period. This format provides education, clarity, and concept reinforcement for patients and their partners. It gives them an opportunity to ask questions and meet other patients in a nonthreatening and safe environment. It also gives nonpatients the opportunity to learn about female sexual dysfunction and to meet health-care professionals who treat sexual medicine issues.

Off-site educational seminars

The off-site educational seminar is a comprehensive educational program designed to attract a large group of people. The seminar is held in a nonclinical setting, usually a hotel or a conference center that is centrally located to major roads with ample parking. With a concerted advertising effort, off-site seminars will often attract current patients and their partners, individuals who are seeking more information about female sexual dysfunction, and health-care professionals who desire to learn about treatment options for their patients.

Because the intent of this seminar is to reach a larger and wider population beyond the practice and into the community at large, planning for an off-site seminar is significantly more time-consuming than an informational session. Moreover, because the printed material informing the public about the seminar is a reflection of the practice, it is strongly recommended that all promotional materials be professional yet eye-catching. Preparation for the seminar should also include a marketing plan that incorporates both free and paid advertising. Brochures and flyers announcing the seminar can also be distributed to local and regional physician practices by utilizing a professional mailing list. A well-designed brochure to promote the seminar can include educational information on female sexual dysfunction that will heighten the awareness of anyone who has the opportunity to read it and thus be of value as an outreach tool well past the program date. Needless to say, promotional materials, advertising, and mailing can be costly, but educational grants and other creative financial approaches can be used to defray expenses.

Successful model – off-site seminar

An example of a successful model is as follows. The seminar program begins with a 1–2 h lecture by a physician who specializes in sexual medicine. The purpose of this educational lecture is to explain the background science, the symptoms, up-to-date supporting research, and current treatments for female sexual dysfunction. The physician establishes a strong science foundation for the participants, and, of equal importance, the lectures are designed to use slides and language that are appropriate for the layperson.

After the lecture, a panel with five to six volunteer patients provides participants in the seminar with the opportunity to hear individual women describe their stories of dealing with their personal sexual dysfunction. The effective selection of women for the panel includes patients of varying ages with a wide range of problems and solutions, thus enabling participants to hear real-life experiences to which they can relate. One very powerful strategy for the patient panel is to have each patient sit with her sexual medicine physician in front of the participants.

In addition to facilitating the discussion and helping the patient to feel at ease, the physician can provide a brief history of the patient's story, ask clarifying questions, and contribute specificity to patient remarks during the interview. If the volunteer patient feels comfortable, a brief question-and-answer session after each interview gives participants the opportunity to gain additional insight and knowledge from the prior discussion.

After the patient panel and a break, participants return to a room set up for focus groups. An effective strategy for the focus groups is to assign a specific topic to each group and to include a health-care professional as well as the patient from the panel who spoke on that topic to act as facilitators. Participants of the seminar are then invited to select the group that is the most relevant to them. Utilizing focus groups as a seminar strategy allows for more specific discussion and interaction on a particular issue and provides participants with a comfortable and secure setting to ask additional questions as well as a feeling of security that encourages the sharing of information and personal experiences.

The last segment of the seminar is the expert panel. Members of the panel may include health-care professionals who specialize in sexual medicine or who treat women with female sexual dysfunction, such as physicians, psychologists, physical therapists, nurses, or any other specialist who could contribute knowledge and information that would enhance and extend the understanding of the participants.

Patient-to-patient support

E-mail can also be used as a strategy for physician-to-patient and patient-to-patient education and outreach. Many health-care professionals are now asking patients for e-mail addresses; as a result, they can now communicate directly with their patients for education and clarity and to provide patients with e-mail addresses, with permission, of other women with similar experiences. For example, although the physician provides education and direction about the therapy, a patient concerned about using a particular therapy can communicate through e-mail with another willing patient to ease her concerns and anxiety. This strategy provides the level of anonymity that a patient desires yet enables her to gain from the knowledge and personal experiences of another woman.

Brochures and pamphlets

Publishing software makes it possible to create brochures and pamphlets for distribution within the office. These bi-fold or tri-fold documents can be utilized to provide current patients with information to enhance and extend their understanding of female sexual dysfunction. For example, a pamphlet or brochure describing the symptoms and risk factors of female sexual dysfunction would contribute to the patient's knowledge base and could be easily taken home by the patient for reference. Because they are printed in the office, they can be easily updated with current information and resources.

Websites

Any individual or group seeking to provide education and outreach programs on the topic of female sexual dysfunction must have a website. The Internet has become the first step in the research/education process for both lay people and health-care professionals. A typical practice website includes contact information for making an appointment and directions to the location. It may also include the mission statement and goals so that future patients will know that the approach of the health-care professionals in the practice is in alignment with their personal philosophies. It may provide the background information and credentials as well as the achievements and affiliations of the health-care professionals in the practice. These components enable women to feel confident that their health-care needs would be met and that any information on the site is credible and reliable.

On the other hand, a more comprehensive website designed to educate patients, health-care professionals, and researchers looking for information and resources on female sexual dysfunction can be an excellent and versatile tool for education and outreach. Visitors to the website can read summaries of state-of-the-art research as well as information about upcoming programs and seminars. A section of frequently asked questions might give more specific information about various aspects of female sexual dysfunction. For example, an individual may learn the symptoms of female sexual dysfunction or what tests are used to diagnose it. The website can also lead Web researchers to other sites and resources, enabling individuals to learn about organizations such as the International Society for the Study of Women's Sexual Health (ISSWSH) and upcoming professional conferences. It is critical to be continually cognizant of the level of understanding of the visitors to the website. While many health-care professionals may use the site as a tool, there may also be many lay people visiting the site for information. Consequently, providing a glossary of terms will enable all visitors to comprehend and understand the content on the site.

Patient support groups

The website can also provide for patient-to-patient support groups through a chat room. Health-care professionals can also arrange for focus/support groups within the practice. In this venue, a health-care professional facilitates and guides the discussion between patients with similar issues and concerns. This opportunity enables individuals to ask questions both of the health-care professional and other patients, providing both clarity and support.

Media

Utilizing various media outlets as a tool for education is another inexpensive yet extremely effective strategy that can reach out to a large number of women. When a health-care professional is considered an expert in a specialty, print and media journalists often contact him or her for interviews for magazine and newspaper articles as well as television and radio interviews. Health-care professionals can also write articles for large and small print publications and websites that target women readers.

Summary

Because of the past treatment focus totally on a psychologic model, women need to be educated that new findings have demonstrated that female sexual dysfunction is often caused by a physiologic problem that is treatable. The first step that health-care professionals can take to alleviate the emotional suffering and physical distress that many women are experiencing is to develop outreach and education programs that heighten women's awareness and understanding of sexual health problems as well as informing them of possible treatments.

FUTURE DIRECTIONS

19 Future directions

Irwin Goldstein, Cindy M Meston, Abdulmaged M Traish, Susan R Davis

The chapters in this book provide comprehensive reviews of what is known about the epidemiology (Chapters 2.1–2.4), psychology (Chapters 3.1–3.4, 11.1–11.5, 17.2, and 17.3), biology (Chapters 6.1–6.5, 13.1–13.3, 14.1, and 14.2), and complex pathophysiologies (Chapters 7.1–7.7 and 16.1–16.9) of female sexual function. However, a recurrent theme is that our understanding of these dimensions of female sexual health remains limited.

It is only in recent years that acceptance of the high prevalence of female sexual dysfunction has broadened. A contributing factor was the publication of *The Social Organization of Sexuality* by Laumann et al. in 1994,[1] which presented the results of the National Health and Social Life Survey of 1410 men and 1749 women aged 18–59 years. Results from comprehensive interviews on sexuality brought to public attention that 43% of women aged 18–59 in the USA experience sexual concerns.[2] This report was criticized for labeling what was defined as sexual problems in the survey interviews as sexual dysfunctions in the results, the concern being that the high prevalence statistic would contribute to the over-medicalization of women's sexuality and consequent over-prescribing of drugs to treat psychologic problems.[3,4] Notwithstanding these valid concerns for women who are not clinically sexually dysfunctional, the National Health and Social Life Survey proved beneficial in spreading the word about women's sexual concerns for the significant number of women who meet the clinical diagnosis for sexual dysfunction. Starkly lacking, however, is comparable detailed information for women 60 years and older, since, clearly, sexual health is not limited to women of younger years.

The increased discourse and awareness of the extent of women's sexual dysfunctions has subsequently helped many women with sexual problems feel more comfortable in talking about their sexual concerns and justified in seeking help. Clinicians in the field of sexuality are now, more than ever, faced with the challenge of effectively diagnosing the many women who present with sexual dysfunction and offering them the best available treatment options.

In addition, the National Health and Social Life Survey brought to our attention the need for further exploration of a number of psychologically relevant variables affecting sexuality. Substantial differences in gender, age, marital status, race, and, less often, education were noted for a number of sexuality variables.[1] It is now incumbent upon future researchers to explore why these differences exist and the degree to which factors such as learning, sexual schemas and scripts, choices and opportunities, and network ties moderate these group differences.

Other events that have significantly influenced the assessment and management of female sexual dysfunction and research directions are the conferences devoted to the definition and classification of female sexual dysfunction. One of the first of these was a gathering of clinicians, researchers, government regulating agency representatives and pharmaceutical company representatives in Cape Cod in 1997[5] (see Chapter 1.2). This was followed by the first international consensus development conference of thought leaders in Boston in October 1988;[6] and, more recently, by a second series of multidisciplinary international consensus meetings in 2002 and 2003.[7] These were held during a time in which there has been increased advocacy from diverse groups for women's sexual rights internationally. The outcome has been the realization that the definitions of female sexual dysfunction listed by the American Psychiatric Association's *Diagnostic and Statistical Manual of Mental Disorders*, fourth edition, text revised (DSM-IV-TR), and the *International Statistical Classification of Diseases and Related Health Problems* (ICD) are unsatisfactory. As noted in the second conference publication,[6] this stems in part from the problematic conceptualization of women's sexual response cycle underlying those definitions. That is, the traditional models of women's sexual response[8,9] are based on a model more characteristic of men than of women, with the assumed linearity and sequential stages of desire, arousal, and orgasm. The most recent panel challenged six fundamental assumptions underlying the definitions of women's sexual dysfunctions listed by the DSM-IV-TR and ICD, and provided a revised classification system[7] (see Chapter 9.1). The most notable changes include a division of sexual arousal disorder into genital and subjective subtypes and the recognition of persistent sexual arousal. The panel also recommended that all diagnoses be accompanied by descriptors relating to associated contextual factors and degree of distress. These revised definitions and descriptors, although a significant improvement, still do not adequately take into account the global sociocultural diversity in female sexual health. Future research needs to include the influences of culture and age on female sexual dysfunction as well as provide a more in-depth examination of individual differences in order to provide better insight into a number of key psychologic contributors to women's sexual health.

It is important to acknowledge that our understanding of women's sexual function from the physiologic and biochemical point of view is far from complete.

The physiology of genital arousal is highly dependent on the structural and functional integrity of the tissue, involving complex neurovascular processes modulated by numerous local neurotransmitters, vasoactive agents, sex steroid hormones, and growth factors. The vascular nature of genital tissue lends itself to many parallel comparisons from the already established field of cardiovascular biology. However, it is also well known that different vascular beds can yield diverse responses to the same disease state. Thus, there are probably mechanisms unique to the genital tissues and their vasculature. For example, delta-5-androstenediol, a steroid hormone possessing both androgenic and estrogenic activity, binds to a unique nuclear receptor that may be preferentially expressed in the vagina (see Chapter 5.5). In addition, the alpha-adrenergic, nitric oxide and purinergic signaling systems, the neurotransmitter vasoactive intestinal polypeptide, and the enzyme arginase have all been shown to regulate the genital arousal response in animal models (see Chapters 5.3–5.6). Whether any of these mediate genital arousal dysfunction remains to be seen. Additional understanding of the cellular and molecular mechanisms of normal physiology, as well as of pathogenesis, will help to identify potential points of intervention for the treatment of female genital arousal dysfunction. Much of this work will be facilitated by recently established tissue culture and female animal models.

The physiology of sex steroid hormones, the consequences of the depletion of these hormones, and their potential use in the management of female sexual dysfunction are yet to be established. With respect to the last, studies involving large numbers of women of adequate duration, and providing extensive safety data, are required before any therapy can be recommended for use. Furthermore, it is critical to understand the impact of imbalances in sex steroid hormone levels on the synthesis and function of growth factors and neurotransmitters, which play a key role in regulating genital tissue structure and the genital arousal response. These studies must first delineate the effects of sex steroid hormones on the expression of steroid receptors.

The basic premise of biologic management of women with sexual health concerns is that physiologic processes can be altered by pathologic states. Biologic pathophysiologies that adversely affect genital tissue structure and function now include genital tissue infections, genital tissue inflammatory conditions, mechanical compartment syndromes of the prepuce and labia, blunt or penetrating traumatic injuries to the perineum or vulva, pelvic support tissue weakness states with genitourinary organ prolapse, genital tissue alterations in immunologic defense capabilities, systemic alterations in hormonal milieu, peripheral and central nervous alterations, alterations in iliopudenal arterial blood inflow integrity, genital and nongenital tissue tumors and/or malignancies, and the adverse effects of cardiovascular, hormonal, and/or chemotherapeutic pharmacologic agents. The recorded number of biologic pathophysiologies keeps increasing as researchers expand biologic investigations.

The problem of how specific medical conditions modulate female sexual health urgently requires consideration and investigation. For example, the effects of diabetes on the physiology of sexual function in women have been poorly investigated, and the available information is limited and inconsistent. Similarly, all the other medical conditions that affect vascular function and endothelial integrity, and that are common in women, such as cardiovascular disease, rheumatoid arthritis, and systemic lupus, need to be included in female sexual dysfunction research (see Chapter 7.3).

From the perspective of the biologically focused clinician, the essential principle guiding medical decision making is identification of the underlying pathophysiology of the sexual dysfunction. If the biologic basis of the dysfunction can be diagnosed, management outcome may be successfully directed to the source pathophysiology.

Despite the research done so far, the paucity of proven medical interventions to help women with various forms of female sexual dysfunction is of concern. In the contemporary clinical armamentarium to treat female sexual dysfunction, the following medications and treatments are available with at least some level of evidence supporting safety and efficacy (see Chapters 14.1 and 14.2). Oral fluconazole is used to treat genital tissues (vagina, clitoris, and labia) infected with *Candida*. Oral acyclovir can treat genital tissues (vagina, clitoris, and labia) infected with genital herpes. Imiquimod, cryotherapy, electrotherapy, and silver nitrate are used to treat genital tissues (vagina, clitoris, and labia) affected by genital warts. Topical clobetasol can be used to treat genital tissues (vagina, clitoris, and labia) involved with lichen sclerosus or lichen planus. Topical lidocaine on the vestibule can lower genital sexual pain. Amitriptyline and gabapentin can lower genital sexual pain. Systemic testosterone may help manage low libido and sexual function. The therapeutic effects of dehydroepiandrosterone are yet to be determined in quality randomized, placebo-control trials. Systemic and local estrogen can improve diminished arousal, decreased lubrication, symptoms of atrophic vaginitis, and sexual function. Systemic progesterone can lower the opportunity for uterine epithelial hypertrophy in a woman with an intact uterus receiving systemic estrogen therapy. Systemic agents that are dopamine agonists, such as bupropion, can improve low libido, orgasmic function, and sexual function.

Oral phosphodiesterase inhibitors may improve arousal, genital sensation, orgasm, and sexual function in some women with sexual dysfunction, primarily those with normal hormonal profiles. However, two findings that emerged from the many clinical trials of the phosphodiesterase inhibitors for women warrant mention. First is the finding of a substantial placebo effect of up to about 40% in women with sexual concerns, and second is the finding that often these drugs increased physiologic sexual arousal (e.g., vaginal pulse amplitude) in women without showing a congruent increase in subjective or mental sexual arousal.[10] The first finding points to the powerful influence of nonspecific drug effects on women's sexuality. That is, factors such as expectancies of improvement, simply enrolling in a study about sexuality, talking to a professional about one's sexual difficulties, and/or monitoring one's sexual responses may alone have enhanced women's sexual experience. Research is now needed to analyze the potential contribution of each of these factors to improved sexual well-being, and explore how best these beneficial elements might be applied in therapeutic settings.

The lack of a clinically meaningful drug influence on mental sexual arousal in women, despite evidence of an increase in genital engorgement, also highlights the limitations of applying a male template to study women's sexual concerns. That is, there may be substantial gender differences in the degree to which individuals focus on genital cues to estimate their degree of sexual arousal. As best described by Basson[11] in her model of the female sexual response, there are myriad factors that contribute to women's sexual desire and psychologic arousal, only one of which may be genital vasocongestion. Clinicians and theorists have noted endless contextual factors, past negative experiences, self-image, mood, and intimacy and relationship issues (e.g., commitment, sharing, tenderness, communication) that affect women's desire and ability to become sexually aroused and/or satisfied. The field could now benefit from an empirical examination of how and to what degree these factors affect a woman's sexual functioning, and how this may change across the life span. Research is also needed to clarify the relation between mental and physiologic sexual arousal in women. The degree to which these responses change in synchrony with sexual stimuli does not seem to be predicted by a woman's sexual functioning status.[12] Knowledge of what does affect the synchrony between responses would help to inform us of what subgroup of women might benefit from drugs that act primarily on physiologic mechanisms.

As a consequence of limited clinical and basic science research, the requisite knowledge underlying contemporary clinical decision making is quite rudimentary. This will change in the future as basic science investigations probe the physiologic principles of women's sexual activity. We also expect evidence-based management to be derived from double-blind, placebo-controlled, multi-institutional, and multicultural clinical trials (see Chapter 16.1).

Finally, effective care of women with female sexual dysfunction will depend on the education of health professionals and the community (see Chapters 18.1 and 18.2). Health professional education should not be limited to those with a special interest in this field, but rather, all health professionals must be cognizant of the importance, high prevalence, and potential consequences of women's sexual health problems and how they may adversely affect quality of life every day.

At present, in 2005, women's sexual health is hardly on the radar screen of afflicted patients or health-care professionals. Most women who have a sexual health concern do not even know they can seek help for their problem. Most do not know that any medical therapies are available to improve their function. There has not been universal acceptance of the biologic component of women's sexual disorders as a valid medical condition. Government granting agencies have not encouraged basic science research in this area. Government regulatory agencies have not yet approved pharmaceutic therapies to treat women's sexual health concerns safely and effectively. Sexual medicine practitioners in medical schools are not given the academic respect or teaching time enjoyed by other medical specialties. This situation must change.

As in any other area of medicine, primary care physicians, general psychologists, allied health-care professionals, physical therapists, and others should ask their female patients basic sexual health questions upon evaluation of any physical and/or mental health concern. Such primary care health-care professionals need to be knowledgeable regarding the broad management paradigms in women's sexual health. When health-care providers are uncomfortable with the subject, they are unable to manage effectively the sexual health problem; and when the issues exceed the realm of knowledge of the health-care clinician, patients must be referred to appropriate psychologic and biologic specialists in sexual medicine or women's sexual health.

The lack of academic representation of male and female sexual medicine in the core curricula of medical schools needs to be globally addressed. This will be substantially aided by the establishment of departments, divisions, or sections of sexual medicine in medical schools and teaching hospitals. To achieve these aims, we need a process by which sexual medicine specialists with expertise in the study, diagnosis, and treatment of sexual dysfunction can be "certified", such that this discipline achieves equal status with other specialties. Ideally, this will involve the development of a residency program to allow medical graduates the opportunity to choose a career in sexual medicine.

In summary, the contemporary ideal clinical management of women with sexual health concerns and sexual dysfunction is by multidisciplinary teams whose essential members include both psychologically focused and biologically focused health-care professionals.

We look forward to the future when the biologically focused health-care clinician has more pharmaceutical agents available with high levels of robust evidence supporting their safe and effective use in women with sexual health problems.

References

1. Laumann EO, Gagnon JH, Michael RT et al. *The Social Organization of Sexuality: Sexual Practices in the United States.* Chicago: University of Chicago Press, 1994.

2. Laumann EO, Paik A, Rosen RC. Sexual dysfunction in the United States: prevalence and predictors. *JAMA* 1999; 281: 537–44.

3. Bancroft J. The medicalization of female sexual dysfunction: the need for caution. *Arch Sex Behav* 2002; 31: 451–5.

4. Tiefer L. The medicalization of sexuality: conceptual, normative, and professional issues. *Annu Rev Sex Res* 1996; 7: 252–82.

5. Special supplement. The Cape Cod conference: sexual function assessment in clinical trials, 30–31 May 1997, Hyannis, Massachusetts, USA. *Int J Impot Res* 1998; 10(Suppl 2): S1–142.

6. Basson R, Berman J, Burnett A et al. Report of the international consensus development conference on female sexual dysfunction: definitions and classifications. *J Urol* 2000; 163: 888–93.

7. Basson R, Leiblum S, Brotto L et al. Definitions of women's sexual dysfunction reconsidered: advocating expansion and revision. *J Psychosom Obstet Gynec* 2003; 24: 221–9.

8. Kaplan HS. *Disorders of Sexual Desire*. New York: Brunner/Mazel, 1979.

9. Masters WH, Johnson VE. *Human Sexual Response*. Boston: Little, Brown, 1970.

10. Laan E, van Lunsen RHW, Everaerd W et al. The effects of sildenafil on women's genital and subjective sexual response. Paper presented at the 26th Annual Meeting of the International Academy of Sex Research, Paris, France, 21–24 June 2000.

11. Basson R. The female sexual response: a different model. *J Sex Marital Ther* 2000; 25: 51–65.

12. Meston CM. Determinants of women's subjective sexual arousal. Presentation to the Annual Meeting of the International Society for the Study of Women's Sexual Health (ISSWSH), Amsterdam, The Netherlands, October 2003.

Index

Page numbers in *italics* refer to tables and figures.